DATE DUE

The American Pharmaceutical Association
Practical Guide to Natural Medicines

THE AMERICAN PHARMACEUTICAL ASSOCIATION

Practical Guide to Natural Medicines

ANDREA PEIRCE

Foreword by John A. Gans, Pharm.D.

Introduction by Andrew T. Weil, M.D.

A Stonesong Press Book

WILLIAM MORROW AND COMPANY, INC. • **New York**

For Fred

Copyright © 1999 by The Stonesong Press, Inc.

It is the policy of William Morrow and Company, Inc., and its imprints and affiliates, recognizing the importance of preserving what has been written, to print the books we publish on acid-free paper, and we exert our best efforts to that end.

Library of Congress Cataloging-in-Publication Data

Peirce, Andrea.
The American Pharmaceutical Association practical guide to natural
medicines/Andrea Peirce.
p.   cm.
Includes bibliographical references.
ISBN 0-688-16151-0
1. Herbs—Therapeutic use. 2. Naturopathy. 3. Dietary
supplements. I. American Pharmaceutical Association. II. Title.
RM666.H33.P45 1999
615' .321—dc21   98-26810
                    CIP

Printed in the United States of America

First Edition

     2 3 4 5 6 7 8 9 10

A STONESONG PRESS BOOK
BOOK DESIGN BY HELENE BERINSKY

www.williammorrow.com

Acknowledgments

Of the many organizations to which the author is indebted for help in researching this book, none stands out more than the New York Botanical Garden in the Bronx. The remarkable collection of books in the library there, not to mention the kind and consistently helpful library staff, provided me with an invaluable concentration of resources and encouragement. Also extremely helpful was the staff at the American Botanical Council in Austin, Texas, who fielded multiple queries regarding the Commission E Monographs in particular (they were in the process of being translated into English as I worked on this book). The National Library of Medicine's source on biomedical literature, MEDLINE, facilitated my research in innumerable ways, as did the comprehensive medicinal plants database, Natural Products Alert (NAPRALERT), at the University of Illinois at Chicago. The same can be said for the prodigious resources of the Herb Research Foundation in Boulder, Colorado.

Thanks also to the dedicated editors and production people at William Morrow, including Toni Sciarra, Joan Amico, Bruce Giffords, Lisa Healy, Ronny Johnson, and Nora Reichard, who did so much to make this enormous undertaking into a book.

My deepest thanks to Paul Fargis and Ellen Scordato at The Stonesong Press for seeing to it that these words actually made it into print. And for all the friends and family who tolerated my extended absences, you know how much I appreciate your steady support and understanding.

Contents

ACKNOWLEDGMENTS   vii

FOREWORD by John A. Gans, Pharm.D.   xi

INTRODUCTION by Andrew T. Weil, M.D.   xiii

AUTHOR'S NOTE: WHY USE NATURAL REMEDIES?   xv

Definitions, Standards, and Other Fundamentals   1

  WHAT YOU GET IN A NATURAL MEDICINE   1

    Is It an Herb? A Food? A Drug?   1

    Herbal Medicine and Homeopathy: Critical Distinctions   2

  REGULATIONS AND STANDARDS: STAYING IN TUNE WITH THE TIMES   2

    How the United States Regulates Herbal Medicines   2

    How Other Countries Regulate Herbal Medicines:
The German Example   3

    Applying Western Standards to Other Healing Traditions   4

Do's and Don'ts for Wise Consumers   5

How to Use This Book   8

  SETTING YOUR OWN STANDARDS   8

    Assessing Efficacy   8

    Assessing Safety   10

    The Rating System   12

  WHAT YOU WILL FIND IN EACH LISTING   13

Natural Medicines and Their Common Uses: A Guide   17

INDEX OF SYMPTOMS 699

INDEX OF REMEDIES 711

APPENDIX A: SOURCES USED FOR COMPILING THE DOSAGE INFORMATION 725

APPENDIX B: SOURCES FREQUENTLY CONSULTED 727

Foreword

From the American Pharmaceutical Association, the National Professional Society of Pharmacists

John A. Gans, Pharm.D., Executive Vice President

The mission of the American Pharmaceutical Association (APhA), the national professional society of pharmacists, is to help pharmacists help you, the patient, use your medicines safely and effectively. Herbal products and other natural remedies are categorized as "dietary supplements" (see Definitions, Standards, and Other Fundamentals, page 1), which is different from prescription and nonprescription medicines. Yet, because American consumers increasingly are using herbs and other natural remedies for medicinal purposes, your doctor and pharmacist need to know what you are taking.

Afraid of criticism, only about half of patients using vitamins, dietary supplements, and herbal and homeopathic products will admit it to their doctors, according to the Institute for Safe Medication Practices. We strongly encourage you to inform both your doctor and your pharmacist which of these alternative products you are taking, particularly if you have a medical condition. This is good communication, in general, but also there may be interactions with your conventional medicines that need to be considered. And we urge you to report to your doctor and pharmacist any adverse effects you may experience. "Natural" products can cause side effects just as conventional ones can.

The list of the Do's and Don'ts for Wise Consumers on pages 5–7 provides important practical suggestions to help you make informed decisions about the array of natural remedies available. So, here, let me make a few overriding recommendations that will help you get the most out of your conventional medications and alternative products alike.

Choose a Pharmacist

- with whom you feel comfortable discussing health-related matters;
- who maintains complete records on the medicines and alternative products you and your family members take;
- who will answer all your questions, counsel you, and monitor your response to the products; and
- who will help you understand dosage instructions, potential side effects, and food and drug interactions.

When you find such a pharmacist, keep going back to that person to build a relationship, much as you would with a physician. Use only one pharmacy, so that all your medication records are at one location.

We all want to take charge of our own health care, and this book by Andrea Peirce will help you do so when you are considering natural remedies. But no book replaces the direct interaction you can have with a health professional. Don't hesitate to ask your pharmacist how to make the best use of your medications and dietary supplements.

Introduction

Andrew T. Weil, M.D.

This book is a rich compilation of natural products in use as remedies, especially derivatives of plants. I did not learn about most of these substances in medical school, nor have many health professionals learned their benefits and risks in the course of their professional education.

My involvement in natural product medicine dates back to my undergraduate days as a botany major at Harvard College in the early 1960s. I developed a strong interest in economic botany, the study of plants of economic importance other than ornamentals. Economic botany concerns plant sources of foods, spices, fibers, medicines, intoxicants, dyes, and so forth. I also set out to study ethnobotany, the use of plants by indigenous peoples and subcultures throughout the world, and ethnopharmacology, the traditional use of natural drugs.

In the early 1960s, none of these subjects was in fashion. In the previous decade, isolation of reserpine, an antihypertensive drug from Indian snakeroot (*Rauwolfia serpentina*), and anticancer alkaloids from the Madagascar periwinkle (*Vinca minor*) led to a flurry of interest in natural product medicine on the part of pharmaceutical companies. Grant money was then available for botanical and ethnobotanical investigations and field work. Unfortunately, most of these efforts did not pay off with further marketable discoveries, and pharmaceutical industry interest in natural products entered a phase of decline that persisted through the 1970s and midway into the 1980s, the period when I was most active in ethnopharmacological research.

My work in that field gave me the knowledge base and motivation to begin using natural remedies in my medical practice. Since 1982, when I began seeing patients in Tucson, Arizona, I have treated many hundreds of patients with herbs, vitamins, and other natural products, in addition to recommending changes in diet, exercise, and other aspects of lifestyle. I first called myself a practitioner of natural and preventive medicine, but I now prefer the term Integrative Medicine, because it emphasizes the need to incorporate this "alternative" approach into conventional medicine.

In my practice, I write prescriptions for pharmaceutical drugs when they are indicated, but, much more frequently, I recommend natural remedies, especially botanicals. I have never seen even one significant adverse reaction to these recommendations. That is not to say that "natural" is synonymous with "nontoxic." Certainly, poisonous plants exist, but the great advantage of using herbal remedies is that the active principles are present in low concentrations, making the risk of toxicity much less than that of purified, concentrated derivatives of plants.

The relative safety of natural products is a major reason for their popularity with the general public. Another reason is enthusiasm for environmental protection, especially rain forest preservation, and the preservation of knowledge of indigenous peoples. Ethnobotany, once an obscure academic field, is suddenly fashionable. And the rapidly expanding market for natural remedies has once again excited the interest of industry. The very fact of publication of this book is testimony to the current importance of natural product medicine, both scientific and economic.

The explosion of sales of herbs, vitamins, and the rest also raises important concerns. First is the growing gap between consumer demand and professional response. At this writing, most physicians and pharmacists remain uninformed about the benefits and risks of most of the products described in these pages. That situation must and will change. The pioneering Program in Integrative Medicine that I direct at the University of Arizona College of Medicine is a first effort in that direction. We are developing new models of medical education that include adequate instruction in the use of botanicals, vitamins, and other natural products, and we are working with pharmacists, nurses, and other health professionals in order to keep them informed about what people are using to maintain and improve health.

We are also encouraging the development of new generations of natural medicines that conform to the standards of safety and efficacy that physicians expect. A great problem is that many products in the marketplace do not now meet those standards. For example, feverfew (*Tanacetum parthenium*) has been shown in good studies done in England to be an effective treatment for migraine, but it is not clear that any of the feverfew products on the American market have the efficacy of English feverfew, whether or not they are standardized for content of parthenolide, which may not be the active component. If Integrative Medicine is going to become mainstream, practitioners and patients must have access to remedies that are reliable.

Our program is also committed to public education. One of the most common complaints I hear from people today is that the experience of walking into a health food store is completely bewildering. How do you select from the confusing array of products and evaluate the claims of manufacturers and distributors? It seems that new miracle supplements captivate the attention of the public with great regularity. In very few cases is there scientific research to back up the claims made for these products.

This guide to natural remedies is an excellent addition to the information available on the subject. It is comprehensive, clear, well researched, and useful. I expect that it will be helpful not only to consumers but to health professionals as well.

Natural remedies are not a fad. Interest in them is part of a worldwide socio-cultural trend that is beginning to transform health care and medicine. I welcome the publication of this book and congratulate the American Pharmaceutical Association for recognizing the importance of the renewal of interest in an old form of medicine.

Author's Note:
Why Use Natural Remedies?

Frustration, nostalgia, a desire for control—these constitute the impulses driving Americans to look back in time and to other regions of the world for the types of natural healing remedies so familiar to our ancestors and to other cultures.

Frustration that the much-marveled engine of American medicine, fueled by the prosperity of the post–World War II economy, has failed to live up to the promise of a balm for every itch, a cure for every ill, and a transplant for every faltering organ. Instead, certain old diseases remain prevalent or uncured, new diseases threaten to emerge, and troublesome side effects still plague the consumer of modern medicines.

Nostalgia, perhaps unfounded but seductive nonetheless, for a time when the remedy for a cough or congestion, an ache or wart, involved a simple visit to the village meadow to pick an herb, or a stroll into a majestic stand of virgin forest to scrape some bark off a tree—a time when we lived closer to and better understood the earth and its prodigious healing fruits.

And of course, the yearning for control in a medical system that seems to be sliding into unknown territory where the doctor barely knows you, the remedy often annoys you, the bill intimidates you, and the explanations confuse you.

When the Federal Drug Administration (FDA) attempted to tighten its regulation of herbs and various supplements in the early 1990s, consumers across the country showered Capitol Hill with some beyond-the-beltway news: Do not take away our right to decide what we will put into (or onto) our own bodies. Ironically, the legislation that Congress subsequently passed—the Dietary Supplement Health and Education Act of 1994—not only resulted in a looser set of regulations than America has seen in decades, but also sent consumers on a ride into the frontiers of misinformation.

Signs of the surge in natural remedies are not hard to spot: sales of herbs and plant medicines totaled $2.5 billion in 1996 and are estimated to increase by 25 percent every year.[1] According to a 1993 survey, one in three Americans, if asked by their doctor if they take any herbal medicine, would answer yes.[2] Some insurance companies have started to accept alternative medicines.

Stroll through a typical downtown or suburban mall, and one storefront or another will beckon you with the latest herbal remedy or cure for obesity, memory loss, impotence. And who lacks an impassioned friend ready to extol the wonders of echinacea, goldenseal, or melatonin?

This book offers you some signposts through the thickets. It contains information on substances that we have loosely identified as natural remedies—primarily herbs and plant medicines, as well as a few vitamins and minerals, amino acids, pollens, microorganisms, and homeopathic remedies. It neither advocates the use of these substances nor denies their value. It attempts, instead, to extend a helping hand to the determined consumer looking for an unbiased answer to the questions: What is known about this substance? Has it helped others? Has it hurt any? Weighing benefit and risk in the current frenzy of misinformation, mistrust, and drug companies' bottom lines can be challenging indeed.

This book recognizes that you are the one who will judge the standards to which you want to hold the substances you put into your mouth, smooth onto your skin, gargle in your throat, or inhale into your lungs.

Whatever your standard—perhaps the one you hope to develop through the help of this book—we hope that the information you find here provides you with the raw data to make intelligent, independent decisions.

TEXT CITATIONS:

1. C. Grauds, "Botanicals: Strong Medicine for Health and Profit." *Association of Natural Medicine Pharmacists*, 3 (1) (1997). A. Vann, "The Herbal Medicine Boom: Understanding What Patients Are Taking," *Cleveland Clinic Journal of Medicine*, 65(3) (1998): 129–34.
2. Vann, op. cit.

The American Pharmaceutical Association
Practical Guide to Natural Medicines

DEFINITIONS, STANDARDS, AND OTHER FUNDAMENTALS

What You Get in a Natural Medicine

IS IT AN HERB? A FOOD? A DRUG?

Our earliest ancestors probably made little distinction between the foods they ate to sustain themselves and the healing properties these foods provided. A bowl of flaxseed gruel not only nourished them, it helped them soothe a sore throat and form a healthy stool. Caraway seeds enhanced the flavor of meats and breads, but also eased their digestion. Through observation of people and animals, test and trial, a pharmacopeia was developed and handed down through the ages.

Though many of us live amid concrete and steel, some of these foods, like flaxseed and caraway, still constitute part of our diet. When we use them specifically to prevent or treat an ailment—when we take them in therapeutic doses as our forebears sometimes did—they effectively become drugs. Today we refer to drugs of this type as *natural medicines or remedies*, largely because the medical establishment has not yet accepted them as proven agents that merit being patented, stamped into tablets, subjected to quality-control standards, and sold as regulated substances. Nevertheless, they can in many cases act upon our bodies, to heal or harm, in much the same ways that conventional drugs do.

Natural does not, however, necessarily mean safe. Consider some of the most poisonous substances known to humankind: strychnine, ricin, aconite; all are found in plants. Humans have survived by recognizing and respecting that the environment offers harmful as well as healing substances.

Despite appearances, conventional Western medicine has never strayed far from natural remedies. Many of the substances in this book were actually pharmaceutical standards of another era, materials which a traveler back in time would find crammed into the frayed leather bag of every family doctor from Philadelphia to rural Oklahoma to frontier towns of the Pacific. Arnica, sarsaparilla, and senna were included in such official publications as the *United States Pharmacopeia* (*USP*; the official listing of U.S. drugs) and the *National Formulary* (the pharmacist's handbook), which had legal standards for identifying and assuring the quality of the substances. Even today, approximately 25 percent of prescription drugs in the United States are derived from natural sources. Consider the contribution of foxglove to treating heart disease (digitalis), or willow bark to alleviating pain (aspirin), or the Pacific yew to cancer (taxol).

As the twenty-first century is upon us, as much as 80 percent of the world's population still relies on herbal medicines. Although most of this book is devoted to herbs, you will also find information on other natural substances popularly used in healing, such as foods (nuts, seeds, fruits), minerals, microorganisms, and amino acids. We consider them all natural remedies. Nearly all are sold in America as **dietary supplements** rather than as drugs.

HERBAL MEDICINE AND HOMEOPATHY: CRITICAL DISTINCTIONS

Do not confuse herbal medicine with homeopathy, a common mistake that even professionals make. The practice of homeopathy was imported from Europe in the early 1800s and taught in a number of medical colleges. After decades of popularity—in 1900 as many as one out of every six health-care practitioners was a homeopath—it slipped into obscurity until the 1970s, when a virtual renaissance occurred.[1]

Homeopathy relies on herbs, but it uses them in a completely different way than herbalism does. The practice of homeopathy is founded on the Law of Similars, or "like heals like." According to this theory, a disease is treated with a substance that produces the same symptoms as those of the disease itself. Thus, a cough, for example, should be treated with a substance believed to cause or promote the cough, not suppress it. Homeopaths believe that this "stimulates the body to recover itself."

In addition, homeopathy rejects the conventional proposition that a larger quantity of active substance is likely to produce a greater response. Instead, it ascribes to the Law of Infinitesimals, which holds that the *lower* the dose of the active substance, the greater its effectiveness. Homeopathic medicines are made by placing an herb or other active substance in a diluting agent such as water, milk sugar, or alcohol, and then diluting it further, usually six to thirty times, to a point where very little (if any) of the original material remains. Believers say some "memory" of the drug lingers.

Homeopathy has attracted its share of critics. Many ascribe apparent benefits to the role of the placebo effect: in up to a third of cases, people will experience the desired therapeutic effect if they *think* they are being treated. No reliable scientific or clinical evidence can be found to confirm the validity of homeopathy.

Regulations and Standards: Staying in Tune with the Times

HOW THE UNITED STATES REGULATES HERBAL MEDICINES

In response to rampant fraud and outrageous claims among drug and food producers in the early part of the twentieth century—not to mention a few public health disasters—the government started to tighten its regulation of herbal medicines. As of 1962, all substances marketed as drugs had to be proven effective and safe in the classic randomized, double-blind, placebo-controlled clinical trial. Few herbs met these standards. (The only exceptions were for substances marketed before 1938, which were grandfathered.) From the early 1960s until 1994, many classic herbs lingered in a netherworld between foods and drugs, with the FDA forbidding marketers from listing any medical benefits.

The Dietary Supplement Health and Education Act of 1994 shifted the rules once again, leaving Americans with a curiously ironic mix of choices. The nation's prescription and nonprescription drug supply certainly qualifies as one of the safest and most carefully regulated in the world, but the same is not true of natural remedies sold as dietary supplements. In fact, American consumers have less assurance of safety and efficacy when they take one of these formulations than many other consumers around the globe have.

The FDA does not establish or regularly enforce any quality standards for dietary supplements. When a substance is sold as such, the FDA has not been presented with sufficient data to declare it safe and/or effective; it may be both or neither. Given that most natural remedies cannot be patented, the odds of a drug company's investing the time and resources—hundreds of millions of dollars in most cases—in conducting the necessary testing are low indeed. The onus is also on the FDA to prove that the supplement is unsafe before it can demand that it be taken off the market. To critics, this provision effectively turns the public into a set of laboratory guinea pigs. To others, it returns the right to make free choices to the individual.

Manufacturers are not allowed to make health claims for dietary supplements on the label. They are, however, allowed to describe the product's role in affecting the "structure or function in humans" and in accompanying publications to present a "balanced view of available scientific information." Many skirt the issue by giving the product a very suggestive name, such as "EnergyBoost" for a supplement containing stimulants. More guidance may be on the way, however. According to requirements that go into effect in 1999, products labeled as dietary supplements will carry a Supplement Facts panel similar to the Nutritional Facts panels found on foods.[2] An appropriate serving size will also be noted, and the manufacturer will be required to place the words *high potency* on a product that contains a nutrient in concentrations higher than 100 percent of the Reference Daily Intake for that vitamin or mineral.

HOW OTHER COUNTRIES REGULATE HERBAL MEDICINES: THE GERMAN EXAMPLE

The regulatory situation in the United States contrasts dramatically with that in many other countries, including Germany, where hundreds of herbs and other natural remedies are tested and regulated by the government and sold in standardized form by the manufacturer. As a result, consumers have much more assurance of exactly what they are purchasing. There, becoming a doctor involves studying herbs and plant medicines, as well as standard Western medicine, and passing an exam on the subject. In 1978, the German Federal Health Agency created an independent organization, Commission E, to develop monographs on herbs and plant medicines based on a review of clinical trial results, field studies, case reports, medical association opinions, scientific literature, and a host of other sources. Much like the FDA controls prescription medicines in the United States, this commission requires manufacturers of natural remedies to prove that their products are effective and safe. The Commission's monographs, which are published in official German publications, declare an herb "Approved" or "Unapproved." More than three hundred of these monographs have been translated into English in *The Complete German Commission E Monographs* edited by M. Blumenthal, J. Gruenwald, T. Hall, and R. S. Rister (Boston: Integrative Medicine Communications, 1998).

Many references made to "German health authorities" in this book refer to the Commission E findings. Keep in mind that the Commission bases much of its approval (or disapproval) of particular herbal formulations on the use of tightly regulated substances. Standardized amounts of the herb and its active ingredients are often ensured in the products sold there. United States consumers, on the other hand, can often find only crude or powdered forms of an herb, in which case similar benefits or even risks cannot be expected.

APPLYING WESTERN STANDARDS TO OTHER HEALING TRADITIONS

Based on Western scientific standards, a natural remedy merits acceptance only if a specific ingredient can be proved to cause a specific action. Adequate amounts of tannins in an herb, for example, explain its astringent effect on wounds. Some herbalists argue that science cannot penetrate the mystery of a healing substance or explain how and why the human body responds in a particular way. A herb may represent a complex mixture of healing elements dependent on one another, which makes judging its value by isolated derivatives unfair. Heated debate on this subject continues within the herbal community, with detractors arguing that shielding herbs with a "magical umbrella" ignores the enormous contribution that modern science has made to human health.

Ancient healing traditions in India, China, and other parts of the world have unique and complex ways of interpreting health and disease. It would be not only unwise, but also arrogant to try to encapsulate these traditions in a few sentences. Traditional Chinese medicine aims in a very general sense to achieve a sense of balance and harmony in the body by using plant medicines, acupuncture, and a variety of other means. Plant medicines are judged through this lens. As a rule, Chinese herbal remedies also consist of multiple herbs and other substances and are expected to produce subtle effects that science may not readily explain. To honor and respect these traditions, we mention them but do not go into great detail on natural remedies common to these traditions unless they are very popular and well known in the United States, such as ginseng.

TEXT CITATIONS:

1. R. M. Henig, *Civilization*, April–May 1997.
2. *Journal of the American Medical Association*, 278 (17) (1997) 1394.

DO'S AND DON'TS FOR WISE CONSUMERS

Some basic do's and don'ts apply to the use of all herbs and natural remedies. As you read through these, you will likely notice that they reflect simple common sense. When considering taking any new substance, for example, it is always important to question the source of your information, be it a salesperson, magazine ad, book, article in the popular press, or promotional speaker. Is the source trying to make a profit? Or seeking to promote your health for altruistic reasons? A healthy blend of openness and skepticism in these and other matters should not only protect you from unnecessary harm (both to your health and to your pocketbook), but enable you to take advantage of the many herbs and other natural remedies that our forebears relied on and about which we continue to learn so much.

Do's:

DO QUESTION YOUR INFORMATION SOURCE.
- What motivates your source? Altruism? Profit? A personal crusade? The spread of knowledge?
- Where do they get their information? Do they draw broad conclusions from personal anecdote, animal studies, or unconfirmed, or even unpublished, human studies?
- Are they qualified to advise you? What are their credentials?
- Do they show telltale signs of a hard sell or of quackery? Do they claim they have:
  —Discovered a cure-all, an effortless weight-loss strategy, or a single-step cure for a complex disease such as cancer?
  —Access to the one and only source for reliable information, and are on a crusade (sometimes at great personal sacrifice) to help save you and other honest, unsuspecting citizens?
  —Found a conspiracy on the part of the medical establishment to keep information from the public or banish herbal and other types of natural remedies?
  —Evidence that natural remedies can only cure, and never harm?
  —Convincing data that Americans are poorly nourished, and require vita-

min or mineral supplementation to make up for what cannot be absorbed or properly processed because of stress, exercise, disease, and other factors? (Other than a few notable exceptions, this argument has never been well justified.)

DO SELECT HIGH-QUALITY PRODUCTS.

• Buy only dried herbs that appear to be fresh, clean, and free of infestation. Store these in a tightly closed container, preferably glass, in a cool, dry place away from direct sunlight.

• Buy only commercial products from reliable sources. The label should include the scientific name of the herb, list the ingredients in detail, note a batch or lot number, and cite the date of manufacture and expiration. It should also include the name and address of the manufacturer and provide a number to call with questions.

• Buy standardized extracts whenever possible. This provides you with some assurance that the active ingredient is present. Be suspicious of any products that do not inform you of the quantity of herbs they contain.

• Make sure you know how to identify a plant properly if you are picking it yourself. This book does not contain information about the collection of wild plants or the home preparation of fresh herbs, however, and should not be used as a reference for these purposes.

DO REPORT ADVERSE REACTIONS.

• If you suffer an adverse reaction to a dietary supplement (herbal or other natural medicine) product, see your doctor and help yourself and the community by calling the Centers for Disease Control (CDC) at 404-639-3311 or the Food and Drug Administration (FDA) at 800-332-1088.

Don'ts:

DON'T TAKE UNNECESSARY RISKS.

• Pregnant or nursing women and young children (especially infants) should not take most herbal or other natural remedies, including most herbal teas. Children under two years of age have immature livers incapable of detoxifying many substances. With such little data available on the potential for harm, the risks clearly outweigh the potential benefits in such cases. Elderly individuals with impaired liver function, cardiovascular problems, or other serious conditions should also avoid most natural remedies.

DON'T ASSUME THAT MORE IS BETTER.

• When turning to a natural remedy, avoid the temptation to flood your system with more than the typically recommended amounts. The notion that more is better is based on foggy thinking, is almost always bad medicine, and could produce a toxic reaction. Avoid taking a natural remedy every day or for weeks, as some pose health risks by accumulating in your system.

DON'T SELF-TREAT A SERIOUS DISEASE OR SYMPTOM.

- A simple cold, headache, or itch may well respond to a natural remedy. But serious illnesses such as diabetes, high blood pressure, cancer, AIDS, and heart disease demand professional care. It would be foolish to self-medicate for these illnesses. The same is true for symptoms that may signal the presence of a condition that requires vigorous treatment, such as burning or pain during urination or swelling due to fluid retention. Talk to your doctor about your desire to integrate natural remedies into your regimen.

DON'T MAKE DRUG SUBSTITUTIONS ON YOUR OWN.

- Some natural remedies contain potent chemicals that can interfere with the absorption or metabolism of other medicines you might be taking. The same is true of certain types of food. For example, regularly taking an herb that has demonstrated monoamine-oxidase (MAO) inhibitor actions and then consuming tyramine-containing red wine or cheese could be dangerous. Talk to your doctor before adding a natural remedy to your regimen.

DON'T IGNORE ADVERSE REACTIONS TO A SUBSTANCE.

- Stop taking a natural remedy if it causes any adverse reactions, from stomach upset to a skin rash or headache. See your doctor.

HOW TO USE THIS BOOK

Setting Your Own Standards

Within these pages you will find a wealth of information on more than three hundred natural remedies. We have consulted numerous sources—medical and botanical databases, primary research studies, government analyses, sound secondary sources—to amass as much reliable data as we can. In a few notable cases, abundant research provides the information needed to make a confident decision about whether or not to take a natural remedy. But most of the time, the substance has not been extensively studied, and only scant or confusing information is available. Sometimes there is none at all.

To help you make a judgment about whether or not to use a natural remedy, for each entry in the guide we let you know what research has been done (or, by implication, has not), and provide a rating that reflects *our* overall impression of the substance's potential to help and harm. Our hope is that this will enable you to make a decision for yourself with confidence.

ASSESSING EFFICACY

Not surprisingly, our standards for efficacy are as different we are. For some people, simply knowing that folk healers around the world have been treating an ailment with a certain herb for centuries will be good enough, or that a friend or colleague has reaped some apparent benefit. For others, only the twentieth-century medical gold standard will do: the randomized, double-blind, placebo-controlled clinical trial. Still others may simply want to confirm that what they are taking is unlikely to harm them.

Sometimes science offers fascinating and satisfying explanations for why an herb or other natural remedy has earned its reputation. Other times it points out health hazards to watch for. At still other times it offers us nothing because no researcher has ever taken an interest in the substance or found information on the subject that they (or a medical journal) deemed worthy of print.

When considering the significance of research, you need to be aware of the difference among the various types of studies that are reported and decide how exacting you want your evidence to be. Will you accept only the findings of well-designed clinical trials? Or will suggestive animal testing suffice? Or personal anecdote?

The following hierarchy represents a rough ranking of the types of studies in which results would be deemed significant and reliable by many scientists and clinicians. For each entry in the guide, we let you know what type of studies we found and what results they produced.

1. At the top of the hierarchy for nearly any scientist shimmers the clinical gold standard of modern medicine: the *large, randomized, placebo-controlled, double-blind, human trial.* For many government agencies, including the FDA, only this standard will do. Such studies involve a large enough number of subjects that clinical differences can be detected statistically. Subjects who have qualified are randomly selected to receive either the drug being tested or a placebo (an inert but identical-appearing substance— a "dummy drug"). A *placebo-controlled study* involves roughly equal numbers of subjects who are given the drug and the placebo. If enough of the treated subjects have a different outcome than the placebo subjects, then the investigators can ascribe some efficacy to the treatment. In a *double-blind study,* neither the subjects nor the investigators know which subject has been assigned the drug, further protecting the results from bias. In a *crossover* study, the subjects switch regimens (taking either an active substance or a placebo), but are not told which regimen they have been switched from and to. This type of study, in most cases, reduces bias. The best studies involve subjects with similar physical and mental health.

There are many other variations on this classic type of study, and students of medicine spend many hours analyzing why some are well designed and others are not. Not many natural remedies have been put through the sophisticated and often costly process of conducting a top-notch study.

2. Second in the hierarchy stands the *large-scale, clinical human trial* conducted without a placebo, albeit with trained observers and objective measurements of effectiveness and adverse reactions.

3. Third in the hierarchy is the *large, placebo-controlled animal experiment.* Although many consumers are concerned about animal testing and do not wish to use products tested on animals, it remains true that computer simulation is as yet inadequate for testing pharmaceuticals. In general terms, the more evolved the animal, the more meaningful the results. One classic type of study, which involves testing the anti-inflammatory potency of a substance by treating a rat paw that has been artificially made to swell, is cited many times in these pages. Many herbs have been tested only on rodents. Of course, consumers are free to choose to purchase natural remedies from companies that do not do animal testing themselves and whose formulations contain no animal products.

4. Fourth in the hierarchy is the *in-vitro* (Latin for "in glass") study, which for the sake of brevity and clarity we refer to as "test-tube studies." By definition, an in-vitro study is carried out in an artificial environment such as a test tube or culture medium. It contrasts with *in vivo,* meaning within a living body.

5. Fifth in the hierarchy is *decades-long* or *centuries-long use* of a particular substance for a particular condition by cultures unknown to one another. For example, Mediterranean and Chinese cultures independently turned to basil to soothe stomach spasms.

6. Sixth in the hierarchy is a *relatively large collection of cases* for which one can cite apparent benefit from a treatment with a substance as judged by an independent professional.

7. At the bottom of the hierarchy is the most common type of "study" that the consumer is exposed to: the *personal anecdote*. On purely scientific grounds, this type of evidence is considered very weak because we differ so much as humans in the way we metabolize medicines, the way we perceive an illness, and how we judge "improvement." Often, the body simply heals itself regardless of what we do. A third of the time, the placebo effect plays an important role.

When it comes to efficacy, there are also less obvious variables at play. Does the product contain what it claims to? Does it contain another substance altogether? Does it contain substances that could even harm you?

No U.S. government agency checks the quality of dietary supplements. Studies have found highly variable amounts of active ingredients in products randomly tested. A 1995 *Consumer Reports* investigation reported finding "huge variations" in ginseng concentration of the ten different brands they tested.[1] In short, you must rely completely on the seller's reputation for assurance of quality. A 1998 independent test commissioned by the *Los Angeles Times* found that four of ten brands of St. John's wort contained less than 90 percent of the listed potency, and that three of the ten had no more than half the listed potency.[2]

ASSESSING SAFETY

Now that the onus of proving that a substance is potentially harmful rests with the government, you as a consumer must decide which safety standards are comfortable for you. Most medicinal herbs handed down through the generations have withstood an important safety test: time. Although there are important exceptions to this rule, such as comfrey (for anything other than external use), one can presume that people would have stopped using an herb if it caused intolerable or dangerous reactions. Many people are satisfied knowing that serious adverse reactions have not been reported.

For many natural remedies, all that scientific research reveals is that they contain no known toxic ingredients. Sometimes animal testing indicates a potential risk; these findings should be taken seriously. Most alarming are indications from human trials or case studies that a substance can cause serious adverse reactions, such as liver damage. Few natural remedies have been subjected to human trials that specifically test for toxic reactions.

There are also less obvious safety variables to consider, all of which highlight the importance of buying high-quality products:

- *Cleanliness.* Was the substance processed in a sanitary environment, largely free of vermin and other contaminants? The FDA does not check for this.

- *Identification.* If the plant was picked in the wild, is there any way of knowing if the pickers correctly identified the plant each time they plucked it from the ground? Are they collecting the substance you think they are, one that is widely recognized by its Latin name?

- *Purity.* Does the product contain only the substances listed? Or could there be others, some of which you might be allergic to, for example?

When judging safety, never forget that numerous herbs and other natural remedies are potentially potent drugs which can be dangerous, particularly if improperly used. Consider, for example, ephedra. For years, the drug industry extracted the key ingredient—ephedrine—for use in decongestants, bronchodilators, and other upper respiratory tract remedies. Traditional Chinese healers have used the plant this way for millennia. More recently, supplement manufacturers started to mix ephedrine with caffeine to create a potent but potentially harmful nonprescription "upper." They claim the substance is safe as long as it is used in recommended amounts by healthy individuals. However, as a central nervous stimulant, ephedra can increase heart rate and blood pressure to the point of shock and death, particularly when misused by being taken in large doses or mixed with other stimulants, such as caffeine. The FDA has blamed these "uppers" for dozens of deaths, most of them linked to this type of abuse.

Moreover, almost any substance can cause an allergic reaction. For the sake of space, we note this within the entry only if there have been cases documented in the literature, or if the plant belongs to a plant family known for its tendency to cause allergic reactions, such as the Asteraceae (formerly called Compositae) family, which includes daisies, ragweed, and asters.

The risks a natural remedy poses to pregnant or nursing women, or to young children (especially infants), are often unknown. With little data on safety risks, the potential benefits of a natural remedy rarely outweigh the risks. The same holds true for elderly individuals with impaired liver function, cardiovascular problems, or other serious conditions. Warnings are included in the "Will It Harm You?" section if the risks are particularly notable, but consider these precautions a part of every entry.

The safety of using natural remedies has a lot to do with common sense:

- If you are *pregnant,* or think you may be, see your doctor. During pregnancy, consult your doctor before taking any prescription, nonprescription, or herbal or natural medication or remedy.

- Be sensible in treating *wounds.* Always clean a wound properly before applying any substance.

- If a *cough* lasts for more than three days, see a doctor.

- If *diarrhea* persists, see a doctor.

- If you suffer from acute *stomach inflammation, ulcers,* or *hyperacidity,* avoid herbs known to stimulate gastric juices, such as bitters.

- Beware of diuretics touted as *"slimming agents"* or *"weight-reduction aids"*; any weight loss represents only a transitory loss of fluids.

- If you suffer from serious illness that could compromise your body's ability to process a drug, such as *liver* or *kidney impairment,* talk to your doctor before using a natural remedy for any condition.

THE RATING SYSTEM

Based on our interpretation of the data, we rate each natural remedy from 1 to 5. While these ratings will give you a general sense of what to expect in terms of effectiveness and safety, you should always read the rest of the entry for perspective and for specific safety warnings. Also take the time to read the complete rating in each instance, as there may be important distinctions.

1 = Years of use and extensive, high-quality studies indicate that this substance is very effective and safe when used in commonly reported dosages for the indication(s) noted in the "Will It Work for You?" section.

Few substances receive this rating, which is not to say that there are not many effective and safe natural remedies; the remedy being rated may not have been put through the rigorous testing that definitely proves, by Western medical standards, that you can expect it to work and not to cause any unexpected reactions. There is a simple reason why so few substances earn a "1": these studies are expensive, and no one has offered to foot the bill. Drug companies stand to earn no profit from substances they cannot patent.

2 = According to a number of well-designed studies and common use, this substance appears to be relatively effective and safe when used in commonly reported dosages for the indication(s) noted in the "Will It Work for You?" section.

Many more "2s" than "1s" were handed out because the standard set is far less strict. Common use also comes into play here, a critical factor for substances relied on for generations.

3 = Studies on the effectiveness and safety of this substance are conflicting, or there are not enough studies to draw a conclusion.

Not surprisingly, the majority of natural remedies fall into this category. They may well be effective and safe or they may not; there is simply too little information to judge.

4 = Research indicates that this substance will not fulfill the claims made for it, but that it is also unlikely to cause any harm.

A rating of "4" implies that scientists have uncovered enough information based on the ingredients or evidence from animal or test-tube studies to conclude that the substance is unlikely to help prevent or cure any ill. On the other hand, they have also learned enough to be able to declare that it is probably safe.

5 = Studies indicate that there is a definite health hazard in using this substance, even in recommended amounts.

This rating indicates that even if there is evidence that a substance has active and potentially beneficial ingredients—and it often will—the risks involved in taking it are relatively high.

What You Will Find in Each Listing

Each listing contains the following sections:

—Primary Name
—Scientific Name
—Common Names
—Rating
—What Is It?
—What It Is Used For
—Forms Available Include
—Dosage Commonly Reported
—Will It Work for You? What the Studies Say
—Will It Harm You? What the Studies Say
—General Sources
—Text Citations

N/A indicates that no other names are available.

PRIMARY NAME: The name by which the herb or other substance is commonly known in herbal guides, the media, sales catalogs, and other sources.

SCIENTIFIC NAME: The full botanical name, including the Latin name in italics (genus and species), is followed by the standard abbreviation for the individual who named it. For example, "L." stands for Carolus Linnaeus, an eighteenth-century Swedish scientist who set out to categorize everything in the plant, animal, and mineral kingdom. The original classifier is noted in parentheses if, for any reason, the botanical name is later changed. The line ends with the name of the plant family to which the herb belongs. Family names that appear in parentheses after the first are older names being phased out of use.

COMMON NAMES: Other names by which the herb or natural remedy may be identified in herbal guides, the media, sales catalogs, and other sources.

RATING: Our rating of the effectiveness and safety of each natural remedy, based on the available data.

WHAT IS IT?

- A simple physical description of the herb or other substance.
- Usually a notation as to whether or not it is grown in North America.
- Indication of which parts of the plant are used medicinally and whether they are used in dried or fresh form.

WHAT IT IS USED FOR:

- Traditional uses by Western and Eastern healers through the ages.
- Common uses proposed by contemporary herbalists, supplement makers, or other sources.

FORMS AVAILABLE INCLUDE:

- The forms typically available to you as a U.S. consumer.
- If the substance is commonly used both internally and externally, the forms available are distinguished. Several forms appear quite commonly:

  -A *capsule* containing a powder is typically the most concentrated form of an herb, as making it involves evaporating all of the solvent used to remove the active constituents.

  -A *decoction* is made by boiling a plant part, usually a tougher part such as the root, in hot water, and then straining the liquid. The longer it boils, the stronger the decoction will be.

  -An *infusion* is made by pouring boiling water over the herb and allowing it to steep; as with a decoction, the amount of time it is allowed to steep will roughly determine its strength. Some substances do not have very water-soluble components and may need to be exposed to the hot water for longer periods to render them effective medicines.

  -A *tea* typically refers to an infusion, although some sources may in fact be referring to a decoction in such cases. When the distinction is not clear, the preparation is described more generally in this text as a tea.

  -A *tincture* is an alcohol-based solution of a substance that is then diluted in water.

  -An *extract* is made by percolating or macerating (softening in a liquid) a plant part in a solvent such as alcohol, glycerin, or water. It is generally more concentrated than a tincture.

DOSAGE COMMONLY REPORTED:

- What you find here is exactly what the heading suggests: dosage commonly reported. These are not dosages that we have tested or necessarily endorse; they simply represent a rough guide to the dosages that can be found in commonly used books and reference sources. See the Appendix for a listing of the sources that were used to compile this information.

WILL IT WORK FOR YOU? WHAT THE STUDIES SAY:

- An explanation of the data we found on the substance, from clinical trials to test-tube studies.

- Traditional or proposed uses noted in the "What It Is Used For" section are not repeated here if there are no scientific data available on them. There are often multiple uses for herbs and other natural remedies and many do not make it into this section.

WILL IT HARM YOU? WHAT THE STUDIES SAY:

- Here you will find information, if available, on the potential toxicity of the substance, including results of animal studies and common side effects noted in humans. Sometimes no studies at all have been conducted, and only years of use indicate it is relatively safe to take. With a few very important exceptions, generations of use attest to the relative safety of a natural remedy.

- The FDA maintains a list of about 250 substances "Generally Recognized as Safe" (the GRAS list) based on their use as food additives (e.g., foods and drinks). Often, the list does not make clear whether the approval applies to the substance as a therapeutic agent (and generally in higher medicinal doses), but in most cases it can be assumed that it does not. While we often make mention of an herb's inclusion on this list, bear in mind that the list was never intended to be comprehensive, so the fact that a substance did not get listed means relatively little. At one time the FDA also kept lists of "Herbs of Undefined Safety" and "Unsafe Herbs," and while we frequently mention these, but keep in mind that both lists were eliminated in 1986 because of major flaws and inappropriate conclusions.[3]

GENERAL SOURCES:

- This section lists sources that have been used to create the entry. The fact that a source is listed here does not mean that it contains accurate or reliable information, although many do. Often, the source has simply offered insight into what modern herbalists are recommending.

TEXT CITATIONS:

- Text citations refer to the specific source, usually a scientific journal or one of the general sources that offers a unique idea or point. The citations are also intended to help you track down a particular study if it interests you.

---

1. *Consumer Reports*, November 1995, pp. 698–705.
2. Los Angeles AP, *CNN Interactive*, August 31, 1998.
3. V. F. Tyler, *Herbs of Choice: The Therapeutic Use of Phytomedicinals* (Binghamton, NY: Haworth Press/Pharmaceutical Products Press, 1994).

NATURAL MEDICINES AND THEIR COMMON USES: A GUIDE

PRIMARY NAME:
ACIDOPHILUS

SCIENTIFIC NAME:
Lactobacillus acidophilus

COMMON NAME:
N/A

RATING:
3 = Studies on the effectiveness
and safety of this substance are
conflicting, or there are not
enough studies to draw a
conclusion.

What Is Acidophilus?

Acidophilus is a beneficial, live bacterial organism that is naturally present in the human body. Many sources use "acidophilus" as a generic term for other types of naturally occurring, beneficial live bacteria, such as *Lactobacillus bulgaris*.

What It Is Used For:

Acidophilus normally lives in the healthy gastrointestinal tract and vagina. It is considered "friendly" bacteria. Some sources suggest taking acidophilus supplements to ensure plentiful supplies of the bacteria, both to keep the digestive tract healthy and to help prevent disease in the area. Many recommend taking acidophilus supplements if you are on antibiotics or sulfonamides, or are undergoing irradiation, as these treatments can kill the "good" bacteria and disrupt the delicate balance of flora. Some sources claim that acidophilus supplements can protect against traveler's diarrhea, aid digestion, lower the risk of colon cancer, reduce cholesterol levels, control cold sores, improve lactose intolerance, and "detoxify" harmful substances. A commercial preparation combining dried *Lactobacillus acidophilus* and *Lactobacillus bulgaris* is marketed for simple diarrhea.

Forms Available Include:

Capsule, granule, liquid, powder, tablet. Acidophilus is often combined with other "friendly" bacteria or added to milk, yogurt (see **Yogurt**), and nondairy products.

Dosage Commonly Reported:

A common daily dosage is 8 ounces of yogurt containing live acidophilus cultures, one enteric-coated capsule containing two to three billion viable organisms, or ½ to 1 teaspoon of the powder or liquid. To use commercial acidophilus formulations, follow the package instructions. Avoid taking live bacteria products within two hours of taking antibiotics.

Will It Work for You? What the Studies Say:

Scientific evidence to justify acidophilus supplements for certain purposes—to promote a healthy digestive tract and aid digestion, and to restore the intestinal or vaginal flora after antibiotic therapy—is accumulating, albeit slowly. Skeptics, however, question the efficacy of taking the bacteria as an oral supplement because it may not survive the acidic environment of the stomach.[1]

Antibiotics can disrupt the natural flora of the gastrointestinal tract, sometimes causing diarrhea, dehydration, and other complications. The notion that diarrhea can be prevented by destroying bacteria with a commercial supplement —acidophilus in particular—has been examined by investigators with mixed results. A review of numerous studies on the subject found that acidophilus supplements may well have a role to play in preventing antibiotic-associated diarrhea.[2] But study results have not been consistent. According to a 1979 study in fifty adults, prophylactic (preventive) ingestion of *lactobacilli* for one week does not reduce the incidence or duration of traveler's diarrhea either during that week or over the following three weeks.[3] Similarly, a 1981 study found that the supplements did not prevent or alter the course of diarrhea caused by the common bacterial culprit, *Escherichia coli*.[4] Acidophilus failed to consistently prevent diarrhea in children treated with amoxicillin in a 1990 trial.[5]

The value of acidophilus supplements for treating stomach pain caused by acid-peptic disease is similarly unclear. In the test tube at least, acidophilus-containing products have suppressed the growth of organisms considered responsible for this disorder (*Helicobacter pylori*, for example).[6] But more research is needed to determine whether supplementation will help prevent or treat the symptoms of the disorder.

Lactobacilli such as acidophilus have long been considered protective organisms in the vagina. According to several small but relatively well designed studies, acidophilus may help prevent vaginal yeast infections caused by overgrowth of the fungus *Candida albicans*.[7] Women who consume adequate amounts of yogurt with live acidophilus cultures (at least 1 cup—8 ounces—daily, for example) may reduce the risk of new infections of this type and the associated itching, a cheesy-thick discharge, and general discomfort in the vaginal area. In one six-month trial, this regimen notably reduced the rate of new infections.[8] Viable live and active *Lactobacillus acidophilus* bacteria must be present for this strategy to work, however, and unfortunately not all products such as yogurts accurately document their presence.[9] Capsules containing this bacteria may work as well, although more research is needed.[10] Researchers have also found that acidophilus inhibits the growth of other types of organisms in the vagina, such as *Escherichia coli*, and *Gardnerella vaginalis*,[11] which can cause urinary tract infections.

People who are lactose-intolerant, meaning that they have problems digesting lactose in dairy products, may find relief with milk products that have had acid-tolerant strains of acidophilus added.[12] This should make it easier for them to digest the lactose in the milk.

Scientists had hopes that certain *Lactobacillus* compounds might show the same cholesterol-assimilating properties in humans that they do in the laboratory.[13] But study results have not been promising. A major 1989 study found no significant, positive cholesterol changes associated with taking acidophilus in the form of Lactinex, a commercial product that combines *Lactobacillus acidophilus* with *Lactobacillus bulgaricus*. In the double-blind study, 354 individuals with high cholesterol took the tablets four times a day for six weeks and then switched to a placebo for six weeks after a three-week period in which they took neither.[14]

There are no good data to support the use of acidophilus for cold sores[15] or to protect against cancer.

Will It Harm You? What the Studies Say:

The medical literature contains no reports of toxic reactions to acidophilus-containing products. If you are on antibiotics, take the acidophilus at least two hours before or after taking the drug.

GENERAL SOURCES:

American Pharmaceutical Association. *Handbook of Nonprescription Drugs.* 11th ed. Washington, D.C.: American Pharmaceutical Association, 1996.

Balch, J.F., and P.A. Balch. *Prescription for Nutritional Healing: A Practical A to Z Reference to Drug-Free Remedies Using Vitamins, Minerals, Herbs & Food Supplements,* 2nd ed. Garden City Park, NY: Avery Publishing Group, 1997.

Barrett, S., and V. Herbert. *The Vitamin Pushers: How the "Health Food" Industry Is Selling America a Bill of Goods.* Amherst, NY: Prometheus Books, 1994.

Lawrence Review of Natural Products. St. Louis: Facts and Comparisons, November 1991.

Mayell, M. *Off-the-Shelf Natural Health: How to Use Herbs and Nutrients to Stay Well.* New York: Bantam Books, 1995.

Tyler, V.E. *Herbs of Choice: The Therapeutic Use of Phytomedicinals.* Binghamton, NY: Haworth Press/Pharmaceutical Products Press, 1994.

TEXT CITATIONS:

1. S. Barrett and V. Herbert, *The Vitamin Pushers: How the "Health Food" Industry Is Selling America a Bill of Goods* (Amherst, NY: Prometheus Books, 1994).
2. G.W. Elmer et al., *Journal of the American Medical Association,* 11 (1996): 870–76.
3. J. de Dios Pozo Olano, *Gastroenterology,* 74(5 Pt 1) (1978): 829–30.
4. M.L. Clements et al., *Antimicrobial Agents & Chemotherapy,* 20(1) (1981): 104–8.
5. R.M. Tankanow et al., *DICP,* 24(4) (1990): 382–84.
6. S.J. Bhatia et al., *Journal of Clinical Microbiology,* 27 (1989): 2328. M.R. Gismondo et al., *Clin Ter,* 134(l) (1990): 41. *Lawrence Review of Natural Products* (St. Louis: Facts and Comparisons, November 1991).
7. Elmer et al., op. cit.
8. E. Hilton et al., *Annals of Internal Medicine,* 116 (1992): 353–57.
9. V.E. Tyler, *Herbs of Choice: The Therapeutic Use of Phytomedicinals* (Binghamton, NY: Haworth Press/Pharmaceutical Products Press, 1994).
10. Ibid.
11. V.L. Hughes and S.L. Hillier, *Obstetrics & Gynecology,* 75(2) (1990): 244.
12. Barrett and Herbert, op. cit.
13. *Lawrence Review of Natural Products,* op. cit.
14. S.Y. Lin et al., *Journal of Dairy Science,* 72(11) (1989): 2885–99.
15. American Pharmaceutical Association, *Handbook of Nonprescription Drugs,* 11th ed. (Washington, D.C.: American Pharmaceutical Association, 1996). R.L. Gertenrich and R.W. Hart, *Oral Surgery, Oral Medicine, Oral Pathology,* (1970): 196–200.

PRIMARY NAME:

ACTIVATED CHARCOAL

SCIENTIFIC NAME:

N/A

COMMON NAMES:

Activated organic charcoal, animal charcoal,

What Is Activated Charcoal?

Made from charred wood, peat moss, or other vegetable matter, this fine black powder is specially processed to enhance its absorption capacity.

What It Is Used For:

Activated charcoal has been used to treat poisonings for nearly a century. Its tiny particles have an enormous surface area capable of absorbing large amounts of complex toxic substances and transporting them through the bowels and out of the body, thereby preventing their absorption into the bloodstream. For poisonings, however, *use activated charcoal ONLY under the*

A

ACTIVATED CHARCOAL
(Continued)

charcoal, gas black, lampblack

RATING:
- *For flatulence and cholesterol control:* 3 = Studies on the effectiveness and safety of this substance are conflicting, or there are not enough studies to draw a conclusion.
- *For other proposed uses:* 4 = Research indicates that this substance will not fulfill the claims made for it, but that it is also unlikely to cause any harm.

guidance of a doctor or Poison Control Center agent, as there are certain circumstances in which it should never be used. This is very important, for charcoal's use in poisonings is *not fully discussed here.*

Other proposed uses include reducing flatulence (stomach or intestinal gas and associated pains), relieving bloating and other symptoms of digestive system upset, lowering cholesterol levels, "detoxifying" the body, and combating hangovers, infections, and hiccups.

Forms Available Include:

Capsule, liquid, powder, tablet. Capsules are the form typically used to treat conditions other than poisonings. Activated charcoal often appears in multi-ingredient formulations.

Dosage Commonly Reported:

A common dosage for digestive problems is 500 milligrams at the onset of symptoms and another 500 to 1,000 milligrams every two hours as needed. Doses in excess of 20 grams may interfere with nutrient absorption. Avoid taking activated charcoal within one hour of taking nutritional supplements. For poisonings, the charcoal should be taken *under the guidance of a doctor or Poison Control Center agent only,* as a mixture made with 60 to 100 grams of activated charcoal (15 to 30 grams for children) per 8 ounces of water as soon as possible after ingestion of the toxin; the dose is repeated as necessary.

Will It Work for You? What the Studies Say:

Although not all studies have come to the same conclusion,[1] at least one well-designed though small human trial indicates that activated charcoal, when taken at certain dosages and appropriate times (about thirty minutes before a meal, for example), may reduce flatulence.[2] In the study, the nine subjects taking charcoal experienced significantly less gas (as measured by breath analysis) and abdominal bloating or discomfort than when they took a placebo or a conventional over-the-counter antiflatulent drug (simethicone) after eating a cup of baked beans.[3] Activated charcoal's antigas mechanism remains something of a mystery. Still, claims that it will somehow "detoxify" the intestines by adsorbing gases, as some promoters assert, appear to be unfounded; not only have test-tube studies indicated that this theory is false,[4] but intestinal "toxins" are effectively removed through the body's normal elimination process anyway.

Much remains to be learned about the capacity of activated charcoal to lower cholesterol levels, from the consistency of the effect to the appropriate dosage and risk for side effects.[5] In a small but frequently cited 1986 study, total cholesterol and levels of "bad" low-density lipoprotein (LDL) cholesterol dropped by 25 percent and 41 percent, respectively, in seven individuals with high cholesterol levels. The reduction was seen after four weeks in which they took 8 grams activated charcoal three times a day.[6] Levels of the "good" cholesterol—high-density lipoprotein (HDL) cholesterol—increased. Similar cholesterol shifts have occurred in individuals taking activated charcoal for other reasons, as well as in diabetic laboratory rats.[7]

Will It Harm You? What the Studies Say:

Decades of experience in poisoning emergencies attest to the relative safety of activated charcoal. If taken regularly over time, however, the charcoal may start to interfere with the absorption of important nutrients or even pose the risk of gastrointestinal obstruction.[8] The safety of megadoses has also not been determined. Take any vitamins or oral medications at least two hours after or one hour before the activated charcoal because they too may be adsorbed, allowing them no chance to enter your bloodstream. At high doses, activated charcoal may cause stomach upset, diarrhea, constipation, or vomiting.

GENERAL SOURCES:

American Pharmaceutical Association. *Handbook of Nonprescription Drugs*. 11th ed. Washington, D.C.: American Pharmaceutical Association, 1996.

Barrett, S., and V. Herbert. *The Vitamin Pushers: How the "Health Food" Industry Is Selling America a Bill of Goods*. Amherst, NY: Prometheus Books, 1994.

Lawrence Review of Natural Products. St. Louis: Facts and Comparisons, April 1996.

Mayell, M. *Off-the-Shelf Natural Health: How to Use Herbs and Nutrients to Stay Well*. New York: Bantam Books, 1995.

TEXT CITATIONS

1. T. Potter et al., *Gastroenterology*, 1985; 88: 620–4. R.G. Hall et al., *American Journal of Gastroenterology*, 75 (1981): 192–96.
2. N.K. Jain et al., *Annals of Internal Medicine*, 105(1) (1986): 61–62.
3. Ibid.
4. Potter et al., op. cit.
5. *Lawrence Review of Natural Products* (St. Louis: Facts and Comparisons, April 1996).
6. P. Kuusisto et al., *Lancet*, 2(8503) (1986): 366–67.
7. E.A. Friedman et al., *Clinical Nephrology*, 11(2) (1979): 79–80. T. Manis et al., *Transactions—American Society for Artificial Internal Organs*, 25 (1979): 19–23.
8. *Lawrence Review of Natural Products*, op. cit.

PRIMARY NAME:
AGRIMONY

SCIENTIFIC NAME:
Agrimonia eupatoria L. Family: Rosaceae

COMMON NAMES:
Church steeples, cocklebur, liverwort, stickwort, xian he cao

RATING:
- *For external use:* 2 = According to a number of well-designed studies and common use, this herb

What Is Agrimony?

Agrimonia eupatoria is an aromatic perennial found throughout the northern hemisphere, the yellow flowering tops of which are used medicinally. The star-shaped flowers bloom along an erect stem, forming tall spikes. Although not as commonly, the small hooked fruits, leaves, and roots have been used medicinally as well.

What It Is Used For:

Scores of contemporary herbalists consider this ancient healing herb a valuable astringent and tonic. European herbalists in particular recommend it for soothing inflamed mucous membranes such as occur with a sore throat, gastroenteritis, and congested nasal passages. It is widely hailed as a diarrhea remedy. Poultices and other external formulations, reportedly common on the battle fields of yore, are still used as healing astringents on bleeding and inflamed hemorrhoids, oozing wounds, sores, ulcers, blemishes, varicose veins, rashes, appears to be relatively effective and safe when used in recommended amounts for the indication(s) noted in the "Will It Work for You?" section.

- *For diarrhea:* 2 = According to a number of well-designed studies and common use, this herb appears to be relatively effective and safe when used in recommended amounts for the indication(s) noted in the "Will It Work for You?" section.
- *For other internal uses:* 4 = Research indicates that this herb will not fulfill the claims made for it, but that it is also unlikely to cause any harm.

and the like. In Europe today, gallbladder, stomach, bowel, liver, and urinary tract "teas" and other remedies containing agrimony can be purchased in many shops. Other folk uses, from fighting kidney stones to controlling diabetes, have also been reported in India, Argentina, and Iraq. Traditional Chinese healers have long relied on a related *Agrimonia* variety—*Agrimonia pilosa*—for healing. The herb has also served as a dye and flavoring.

Forms Available Include:

- *For external use:* Bath formulation, compress, eye wash, gargle, poultice, tincture.
- *For internal use:* Decoction, infusion, tincture.

Dosage Commonly Reported:

A common daily dose is 3 to 6 grams. A decoction or infusion is made from 1 teaspoon of herb per cup of boiling water. The decoction is used to make a poultice, which is applied several times a day.

Will It Work for You? What the Studies Say:

Agrimony contains substantial amounts of tannins (4 percent to 10 percent) and other ingredients, which explains its enduring use as an astringent. Astringents constrict (tighten) tissue, encouraging healing by reducing bleeding and oozing of secretions. German health authorities approve of sipping agrimony tea for simple diarrhea (when it is due to something other than an underlying disease), gargling the tea to soothe a sore throat or other oral mucous membrane inflammation, and applying poultices to mild and superficial skin inflammations.[1] The tea is quite flavorful.

Although much remains to be confirmed about its action in humans, test-tube studies indicate that alcoholic extracts and parts of the dried herb are mildly antiseptic, capable of fighting certain disease-causing viruses, bacteria, and fungi, including the fungus *Candida albicans* responsible for many cases of oral thrush and vaginal yeast infections.[2] Extracts have shown promise as antidiabetic agents in laboratory mice.[3]

Overall, evidence for agrimony's effectiveness for internal ailments is much weaker.[4] No scientific evidence can be found to support its use as a remedy for gallbladder disorders, for example.[5] Taiwanese researchers found an agrimony extract active against chemically induced hyperglycemia (high blood sugar) in rats, but further examination is needed to determine if it has this effect in humans.[6] Considerably more research has been done on the Chinese variety of the plant, *Agrimonia pilosa*. While much of this research is intriguing, most demands fuller substantiation.

Will It Harm You? What the Studies Say:

Agrimony appears to be relatively safe to use in moderation based on the limited animal studies done so far, not to mention its many centuries of common use in Europe and other regions of the world. No human trials to confirm its safety have been done, however. German health authorities cite no conditions in which it should be avoided, or notable interactions with other medicines.[7] They also cite no significant known side effects, although sun sensitivity reactions have been reported after taking the herb.[8] Given the herb's astringency, you may want to avoid infusions and other internal formulations if you suffer from constipation. No high-tannin herb, such as black tea, should be taken internally for long periods of time (more than several months).

GENERAL SOURCES:

Balch, J.F., and P.A. Balch. *Prescription for Nutritional Healing: A Practical A to Z Reference to Drug-Free Remedies Using Vitamins, Minerals, Herbs & Food Supplements.* 2nd ed. Garden City Park, NY: Avery Publishing Group, 1997.

Bisset, N.G., ed. *Herbal Drugs and Phytopharmaceuticals.* Stuttgart: medpharm GmbH Scientific Publishers, 1994.

Blumenthal, M., J. Gruenwald, T. Hall, and R.S. Rister, eds. *The Complete German Commission E Monographs: Therapeutic Guide to Herbal Medicine.* Boston: Integrative Medicine Communications, 1998.

Duke, J.A. *CRC Handbook of Medicinal Herbs.* Boca Raton, FL: CRC Press, 1985.

Hylton, W.H., ed. *The Rodale Herb Book: How to Use, Grow, and Buy Nature's Miracle Plants.* Emmaus, PA: Rodale Press, Inc., 1974.

Lawrence Review of Natural Products. St. Louis: Facts and Comparisons, August 1995.

Ody, P. *The Herb Society's Complete Medicinal Herbal.* London: Dorling Kindersley Limited, 1993.

Stary, F. *The Natural Guide to Medicinal Herbs and Plants.* New York: Barnes & Noble, Inc.; Prague: Aventinum Publishers, 1996.

Tierra, M. *The Way of Herbs.* New York: Pocket Books, 1990.

Weiss, R.F. *Herbal Medicine,* trans. A.R. Meuss, from the 6th German edition. Beaconsfield, England: Beaconsfield Publishers, Ltd., 1988.

TEXT CITATIONS:

1. M. Blumenthal, J. Gruenwald, T. Hall, and R.S. Rister, eds., *The Complete German Commission E Monographs: Therapeutic Guide to Herbal Medicine* (Boston: Integrative Medicine Communications, 1998).
2. S.C. Chon et al., *Medicina et Pharmacologia Experimentalis,* 16 (1987): 407. H.M. Peter, *Pharmazie,* 24 (1969): 632–35. G. May and G. Willuhn, *Arzneimittel-Forschung,* 28(1) (1978): 1–7.
3. S.K. Swanston-Flatt et al., *Diabetologia,* 33(8) (1990): 462–64.
4. *Lawrence Review of Natural Products* (St. Louis: Facts and Comparisons, August 1995).
5. N.G. Bisset, ed., *Herbal Drugs and Phytopharmaceuticals* (Stuttgart: medpharm GmbH Scientific Publishers, 1994).
6. F.L. Hsu and J.T. Cheng, *Phytotherapy Research,* 62 (1992): 108–11.
7. Blumenthal et al., op. cit.
8. J.A. Duke, *CRC Handbook of Medicinal Herbs* (Boca Raton, FL: CRC Press, 1985).

PRIMARY NAME:
ALFALFA

SCIENTIFIC NAME:
Medicago sativa L. Family:
Leguminosae

COMMON NAMES:
Buffalo grass, Chilean clover,
lucerne

RATING:
4 = Research indicates that this
herb will not fulfill the claims
made for it, but that it is also
unlikely to cause any harm
under most circumstances. See
"Will It Harm You?" section for
more details.

What Is Alfalfa?

This bushy perennial forage plant is cultivated worldwide. Its three-leaflet clusters and pale blue, purple, or yellow flowers are used medicinally.

What It Is Used For:

In addition to its age-old reputation as a nutritious food and forage for livestock, alfalfa has been used by traditional healers from Europe to China as a diuretic ("water pill") and treatment for arthritis, diabetes, asthma, digestive system upset, weight loss, ulcers, high cholesterol, kidney and bladder problems, prostate disorders, asthma and hay fever, and other disorders. Many herbalists hail it as a vitalizing tonic. Alfalfa is a major source of chlorophyll. (See **Chlorophyll**.)

Forms Available Include:

Capsule, infusion, powder, sprouts (to eat raw), tablet, tincture. Most formulations contain dried alfalfa leaves, although contamination with other substances has been reported.[1]

Dosage Commonly Reported:

An infusion is made using 1 to 2 teaspoons dried leaves per cup of water and is drunk up to three times per day. To use commercial alfalfa formulations, follow the package instructions.

Will It Work for You? What the Studies Say:

Alfalfa's long list of ingredients includes nutritious proteins, trace minerals (iron, calcium, phosphorous), beta carotene, minerals, vitamins (including vitamins K, C, A, D, and E), and fiber. The presence of saponin glycosides (2 to 3 percent) may help explain why in certain studies, laboratory monkeys and other animals fed alfalfa leaves (and sprouts to a lesser degree) experience a drop in cholesterol levels and some protection against the formation of plaque deposits on artery walls, both conditions widely viewed as risk factors for heart disease and stroke.[2] Much remains to be learned about how and why these reactions occur, however, and whether the same will hold true for humans. Unfortunately, test-tube studies indicate that these same substances also interfere with the body's use of vitamin E and break up important red blood cells.[3]

No scientific research and none of the ingredients identified in alfalfa so far indicate that eating the leaves or taking them in any other form will increase urine output as a diuretic should, or significantly benefit diabetics, aid bladder disorders, reduce inflammation, allay rheumatic illnesses such as arthritis, counter ulcers, improve asthma or hay fever, stimulate the appetite, promote menstruation, or function as a vitalizing tonic.[4]

Will It Harm You? What the Studies Say:

Alfalfa tablets and other formulations are probably safe for most people to take in moderation, although there are important exceptions. If you suffer from the autoimmune disease systemic lupus erythematosus, avoid alfalfa; not only have monkeys fed the seeds or sprouts developed new cases of the disease, but latent disease has been reactivated in people taking alfalfa tablets.[5] Experts hold the amino acid L-canavanine responsible for this reaction; it appears in all parts of the plant, but especially the seeds. Consuming large amounts of alfalfa seeds can also lead to a buildup of this amino acid and result in a serious, although reversible, blood clotting disorder called pancytopenia.[6]

Treating asthma or hay fever with alfalfa tablets is probably unwise; no scientific evidence indicates that it works, and there have been allergic reactions to alfalfa tablets contaminated with other substances.[7] In a 1971 study, investigators observed worrisome cell changes in rats fed alfalfa, but the implications for an increased susceptibility to colon cancer in the rats—or humans who consume alfalfa—remain unclear.[8] Rats fed sprouts rather than the whole plant showed fewer of these cellular changes.[9]

GENERAL SOURCES:

Balch, J.F., and P.A. Balch. *Prescription for Nutritional Healing: A Practical A to Z Reference to Drug-Free Remedies Using Vitamins, Minerals, Herbs & Food Supplements.* 2nd ed. Garden City Park, NY: Avery Publishing Group, 1997.

Castleman, M. *The Healing Herbs: The Ultimate Guide to the Curative Power of Nature's Medicines.* New York: Bantam Books, 1995.

Der Marderosian, A., and L. Liberti. *Natural Product Medicine: A Scientific Guide to Foods, Drugs, Cosmetics.* Philadelphia: George F. Stickley, 1988.

Lawrence Review of Natural Products. St. Louis: Facts and Comparisons, March 1991.

Leung, A.Y. *Chinese Healing Foods and Herbs.* Glen Rock, NJ: AYSL Corp., 1984.

Leung, A.Y., and S. Foster. *Encyclopedia of Common Natural Ingredients Used in Food, Drugs, and Cosmetics.* 2nd ed. New York: John Wiley & Sons, 1996.

Mindell, E. *Earl Mindell's Herb Bible.* New York: Simon & Schuster/Fireside, 1992.

Tierra, M. *The Way of Herbs.* New York: Pocket Books, 1990.

Tyler, V.E. *The Honest Herbal.* Binghamton, NY: Haworth Press/Pharmaceutical Products Press, 1993.

Tyler, V.E., L.R. Brady, and J.E. Robbers, eds. *Pharmacognosy.* Philadelphia: Lea & Febiger, 1988.

TEXT CITATIONS:

1. A.Y. Leung, *Chinese Healing Foods and Herbs* (Glen Rock, NJ: AYSL Corp, 1984).
2. M.R. Malinow et al., *American Journal of Clinical Nutrition,* 30 (1977): 2061. M.R. Malinow et al., *Journal of Clinical Investigations,* 67 (1981): 156. M.R. Wilcox and L.S. Galloway, *American Journal of Clinical Nutrition.,* 9 (1961): 236. M.R. Malinow et al., *Science,* 216 (1982): 415.
3. A.Y Leung and S. Foster, *Encyclopedia of Common Natural Ingredients Used in Food, Drugs, and Cosmetics,* 2nd ed. (New York: John Wiley & Sons, 1996). E. Small et al., *Economic Botany,* 44 (1990): 226.
4. Leung and Foster, op. cit. V.E. Tyler, L.R. Brady, and J.E. Robbers, eds., *Pharmacognosy* (Philadelphia: Lea & Febiger, 1988). *Lawrence Review of Natural Products* (St. Louis: Facts and Comparisons, March 1991). I.J. Polk, *Journal of the American Medical Association,* 247 (1982): 1493.
5. M.R. Malinow et al., *Science,* 216 (1982): 415. J.L. Roberts and J.A. Hayashi, *New England Journal of Medicine,* 308 (1983): 1361.
6. M.R. Malinow et al., *Lancet,* 1 (1981): 615.
7. Polk, op. cit.
8. H. Sprinz, *Cancer,* 28 (1971): 71.

9. *Lawrence Review of Natural Products*, op. cit. J.A. Story et al., *American Journal of Clinical Nutrition*, 39 (1984): 917.

PRIMARY NAME:
ALLSPICE

SCIENTIFIC NAME:
Pimenta dioica (L.) Merr. Sometimes referred to as *Pimenta officinalis* Lindl. or *Eugenia pimenta* DC. Family: Myrtaceae

COMMON NAMES:
Clove pepper, Jamaica pepper, pimenta, pimento

RATING:
2 = According to a number of well-designed studies and common use, this substance appears to be relatively effective and safe when used in recommended amounts for the indication(s) noted in the "Will It Work for You?" section.

What Is Allspice?

The green fruits ("berries") known as allspice develop on the *Pimenta*, a tall tropical South and Central American tree. They are picked and dried while mature but unripe. The allspice powder on food store shelves is made from these. The berries and the plant's leathery, oblong leaves are used medicinally, as is an oil derived from both. The *Pimenta* tree is not cultivated in the United States.

What It Is Used For:

Allspice, readily recognized by North Americans as a spice and fragrance, has been used as a folk remedy in many Central and South American countries and the West Indies, where the aromatic *Pimenta* tree is widely cultivated. A whiff brings to mind a mélange of nutmeg, cloves, cinnamon, juniper, and pepper. Allspice has traditionally been used to encourage good digestion, relieve stomach or intestinal gas and soothe stomachaches, control diarrhea, stimulate the appetite, allay rheumatic aches, relieve pain (including toothaches, menstrual cramps, and nerve pain), reduce vomiting, lessen corns, control diabetes (in a specially prepared decoction), and stimulate the body in the form of a tonic. The oil is used externally.

Contemporary herbalists recommend a number of these practices. Controlling toothache pain with a few drops of allspice oil is particularly popular, as is applying a poultice to muscle aches and pains, and sipping an infusion of allspice powder to soothe indigestion.

Forms Available Include:

Berry (whole, powdered), drops, infusion, oil, poultice. Except for the oil, formulations are typically made with powdered berries.

Dosage Commonly Reported:

An infusion is made using 1 to 2 teaspoons powder per cup of water and is drunk up to three times per day. For toothache pain the drops are applied one at a time using a cotton swab. The oil is used as an aromatic carminative (gas-relieving digestive aid) at a dose of 0.05 to 0.2 milliliters.

Will It Work for You? What the Studies Say:

Allspice's volatile oil (about 4 percent) likely contributes to its long-standing use as relief for gas and griping (sharp abdominal pains), a property that the pharmaceutical industry has taken advantage of at times.[1] Of the dozens of chemical constituents identified in the herb, a substance called eugenol in the berry's volatile oil (60 to 80 percent) and leaves (up to 96 percent) ranks as the most important in terms of healing powers. The presence of this active substance, which also appears in clove, myrrh, and other herbs, may help explain its long-standing use as a local antiseptic and anesthetic. Numerous test-tube studies have shown that it vigorously fights certain viruses, fungi, parasites, larvae, and bacteria, including strains of *Staphylococcus aureus* and *Pseudomonas bacteria*, both organisms that can cause skin infections, as well as the fungus *Candida albicans*, a common cause of vaginal yeast infections.[2] Eugenol functions as a local anesthetic by depressing the sensory receptors critical to perceiving pain. This property helps explain allspice's enduring reputation for reducing muscle aches and pains. Rubbed on sore gums, allspice oil should offer several hours of pain relief. Dentists use eugenol as a local antiseptic and anesthetic for teeth and gums.

The berries, their oil, and the eugenol extract promote the activity of the digestive enzyme trypsin, which may help explain why allspice has traditionally been used as a digestive aid.[3] The volatile oil probably contributes as well. Investigators have uncovered a number of other interesting properties that may one day prove useful, although they require more research and the implications for human health are still unclear. For example, researchers have identified anticonvulsant, antispasmodic, and other properties in eugenol, and studies in humans indicate that it depresses (slows down) the central nervous system.[4] Primarily on the basis of its eugenol content, some experts consider allspice a potential new source of natural antioxidants.[5] Antioxidants help prevent the formation of dangerous chemicals capable of becoming toxic (free radicals), possibly inducing the formation of cancer cells. Much remains to be learned about this subject, however.

Will It Harm You? What the Studies Say:

This ancient spice and folk remedy appears to be safe to use in moderation. Never ingest the concentrated oil (after applying it to a throbbing tooth, spit it out), as even 1 teaspoon has been shown to cause nausea, vomiting, and in serious cases a slowing down of the central nervous system and convulsions.[6] Applied externally, the oil can cause irritation and inflammation in individuals with sensitive skin.

GENERAL SOURCES:
Castleman, M. *The Healing Herbs: The Ultimate Guide to the Curative Power of Nature's Medicines.* New York: Bantam Books, 1995.
Chevallier, A. *The Encyclopedia of Medicinal Plants: A Practical Reference Guide to More Than 550 Key Medicinal Plants & Their Uses.* New York: Dorling Kindersley Publications, 1996.
Duke, J.A. *CRC Handbook of Medicinal Herbs.* Boca Raton, FL: CRC Press, 1985.
Lawrence Review of Natural Products. St. Louis: Facts and Comparisons, December 1993.
Leung, A.Y., and S. Foster. *Encyclopedia of Common Natural Ingredients Used in Food, Drugs, and Cosmetics.* 2nd ed. New York: John Wiley & Sons, 1996.

TEXT CITATIONS:
1. A.Y. Leung and S. Foster, *Encyclopedia of Common Natural Ingredients Used in Food, Drugs, and Cosmetics,* 2nd ed. (New York: John Wiley & Sons, 1996).
2. D.E. Conner and L.R. Beuchat, *Applied and Environmental Microbiology,* 47 (1984): 229–33. H. Hitokoto et al., *Applied and Environmental Microbiology,* 39 (1980):818–22. M.A. El-Naghy et al., *Zentralblatt für Mikrobiologie,* 147(3–4) (1992): 214–20. W.J. Zhang, *China Journal of Chinese Materia Medica,* 19(9) (1994): 532–74. J. Briozzo et al., *Journal of Applied Bacteriology,* 66(1) (1989): 69–75.
3. K. Oishi et al., *Nippon Suisan Gakkaishi,* 40 (1974): 1241. Leung and Foster, op. cit.

4. Leung and Foster, op. cit.
5. Ibid.
6. *Lawrence Review of Natural Products* (St. Louis: Facts and Comparisons, December 1993).

PRIMARY NAME:
ALMOND, SWEET

SCIENTIFIC NAME:
Prunus amygdalus (Mill.) D.A. Webb. Family: Rosaceae

COMMON NAME:
Ba dan xing ren

RATING:
• *For external use:* 1 = Years of use and extensive, high-quality studies indicate that this substance is very effective and safe when used in recommended amounts for the indication(s) noted in the "Will It Work for You?" section.
• *For internal use:* 3 = Studies on the effectiveness and safety of this substance are conflicting, or there are not enough studies to draw a conclusion.

What Is Sweet Almond?

The small, flowering tree *Prunus amygdalus* bears fleshless fruits (drupes) containing stony pits, inside of which are nutlike edible seeds known as sweet almonds. The tree is a deciduous member of the rose family native to western Asia, although it is now widely cultivated in California, Italy, Spain, and East Asia. In China, "almond" refers not only to the sweet almond seeds taken from this tree, but also to bitter almond or apricot pits found on other kinds of trees (see **Apricot Pit** for more information on bitter almond).

What It Is Used For:

Westerners have been eating sweet almonds for thousands of years. The Bible refers to them frequently. A fixed oil pressed from the nut, known as sweet almond oil or simply almond oil, is widely used as a flavoring and its skin-soothing and softening properties are frequently put to work in lotions and ointments. It often serves as a base for massage oil and as a lubricant and emulsifier in cosmetics and other products. The oil purportedly has laxative properties, and both the oil and the seed have been used to treat breast, mouth, bladder, and other cancers.[1] Recent research suggests that when taken internally, the oil may help reduce cholesterol levels, which has implications for preventing heart disease. Almond meal often appears in face soaps and scrubs.

Forms Available Include:

Meal (from the kernel), oil, and seed.

Dosage Commonly Reported:

Sweet almond is used as a laxative in doses up to 30 milliliters. A handful of meal is used as a face scrub, and is rubbed onto dry skin.

Will It Work for You? What the Studies Say:

Almonds qualify as a good source of protein, fats, iron, potassium, calcium, phosphorous, and trace minerals. Research indicates that the oil has emollient and demulcent properties, which means it can soften, soothe, and protect skin and mucous membranes and is likely to be effective as a laxative in commercial products. It also fights certain bacteria, though not vigorously, so do not count on it as an antiseptic.[2]

Data on substituting almond oil for other dietary oils to lower cholesterol levels (and possibly help prevent heart disease) are promising but still preliminary. A 1992 study reported rapid and sustained reductions in total cholesterol and low-density lipoprotein cholesterol (LDL), the so-called "bad" cholesterol, during periods in which twenty-six subjects supplemented their diets with raw almonds, which are high in monounsaturated fat. The subjects had already shifted their overall diet to make it low in saturated fat, low in cholesterol, and high in fiber. The only oil allowed for food preparation was almond oil. Levels of the "good" high-density lipoprotein (HDL) cholesterol did not change.[3] A 1990 study of forty-five individuals reported a serum cholesterol reduction of about 11 percent among those whose dietary oil was confined to almond oil, a greater reduction than that observed in those whose diets were confined to olive oil. All the subjects in the three-week California study followed a fixed diet.[4] No other studies have apparently been done to confirm this cholesterol-lowering action.

Will It Harm You? What the Studies Say:

Experts consider both almond oil and almond meal safe to use, and neither appears to irritate or sensitize human skin.[5] Almonds themselves have been enjoyed by millions. As with any food, an allergic reaction is always a risk.

GENERAL SOURCES:

Leung, A.Y. *Chinese Healing Foods and Herbs.* Glen Rock, NJ: AYSL Corp, 1984.

Leung, A.Y., and S. Foster. *Encyclopedia of Common Natural Ingredients Used in Food, Drugs, and Cosmetics.* 2nd ed. New York: John Wiley & Sons, 1996.

Mindell, E. *Earl Mindell's Herb Bible.* New York: Simon & Schuster/Fireside, 1992.

Weiss, R.F. *Herbal Medicine*, trans. A. R. Meuss, from the 6th German edition. Beaconsfield, England: Beaconsfield Publishers, Ltd., 1988.

TEXT CITATIONS:

1. A.Y. Leung and S. Foster, *Encyclopedia of Common Natural Ingredients Used in Food, Drugs, and Cosmetics*, 2nd ed. (New York: John Wiley & Sons, 1996).
2. Ibid.
3. G.A. Spiller et al., *Journal of the American College of Nutrition*, 11(2) (1992):126–30.
4. *INSIGHT*, 1990.
5. Leung and Foster, op. cit. K.T. Fisher, *Journal of the American College of Toxicology*, 2 (1983): 85.

PRIMARY NAME:
ALOE VERA

SCIENTIFIC NAME:

Aloe vera (L.) N.L. Burm., sometimes referred to as *Aloe barbadensis* Mill., is the most commonly recognized and widely used of the hundreds of *Aloe* species for medicinal purposes. Family: Liliaceae

What Is Aloe Vera?

Aloe vera is a hardy perennial succulent with yellow flowers and stiff, spearlike leaves that grow in rosettes. The leaves yield two very different substances that should never be confused with one another. Aloe vera gel is a thin, clear, colorless, and jellylike substance obtained from the inner part of the leaf. Aloe juice or latex, on the other hand, refers to a bitter yellow liquid extracted from specialized cells of the inner leaf skin. It is most commonly sold in dried powder form. Aloe gel and aloe juice are used in different ways.

What It Is Used For:

Many traditional systems of medicine have used aloe gel and juice for millennia. Ancient Egyptians and Greeks valued the gel as a topical healer and beauty

ALOE VERA (Continued)

COMMON NAMES:
Barbados, Cape, Curacao, Natal, Socotrine, Uganda, and Zanzibar aloes

RATING:

- *For external use* (fresh gel for healing wounds and burns): 2 = According to a number of well-designed studies and common use, this substance appears to be relatively effective and safe when used in recommended amounts.

- *For internal use* (juice as a laxative): 2 = According to a number of well-designed studies and common use, this substance appears to be relatively effective and safe when used in recommended amounts. Certain groups of people should avoid it, however; see the safety warnings in the "Will It Harm You?" section.

aid; Cleopatra reportedly kept her skin supple and glowing with it. Traditional Chinese healers began focusing on the topical uses of aloe relatively recently, after centuries of focus on the juice as a remedy for ailments such as constipation, fungal infections, and internal worms.[1]

Today, aloe vera gel probably qualifies as the most widely used herbal folk remedy in America.[2] Many people keep a plant at home for promoting scar-free healing of cuts and for soothing burns (especially sunburns), wounds, and minor skin irritations. The gel is commonly billed as one of nature's finest moisturizers. Dozens of other external and internal applications for the gel have been proposed, from treating hemorrhoids, to insect bites, premenstrual syndrome (PMS), ringworm, radiation burns, peptic ulcers, diabetes, boils, asthma, and cough.

Aloe juice's fame as a purgative (a very potent laxative) is older than the gel's renown for skin treatments. A few contemporary herbalists recommend the juice internally for constipation, for liver problems, and to promote "internal healing."[3]

Forms Available Include:

- *Gel:* Fresh from the plant (readily found in North American plant shops). Many commercial products, from sunburn lotions to moisturizers, first aid creams, and shampoos, feature aloe vera gel as a key ingredient. Products labeled "Aloe vera gel extract" contain pulverized whole plant leaves.[4]
- *Juice (latex):* Typically sold in dried form in capsules and pills, frequently in multi-ingredient formulas.

Dosage Commonly Reported:

The gel is applied directly to the skin. As a laxative, the powder or dry extract is often taken in doses of 0.05 to 0.2 grams, for short periods of time only. The juice or gel is taken in doses of 1 tablespoon up to three times per day. Many commercial aloe preparations contain very little aloe. Check the list of ingredients.

Will It Work for You? What the Studies Say:

Although research findings are not consistent, most studies indicate that aloe vera gel helps speed healing in minor wounds and burns. Animal studies have demonstrated the gel's capacity to inhibit further skin tissue damage in burns and frostbite,[5] and human studies have shown that it can speed healing of partial thickness burns faster than a placebo,[6] help heal various types of skin ulceration, promote skin healing following dermabrasion and electrical trauma,[7] and encourage blood circulation, thus reducing tissue loss following frostbite injuries (using an aloe vera cream).[8] Overall, the gel's value in treating minor burns is less certain than its ability to accelerate wound healing.[9]

Despite intensive study, scientists still have a somewhat foggy picture of how aloe vera gel works. They know it consists largely of polysaccharides (complex carbohydrate molecules) and that one of these may well contribute to the gel's skin-softening properties. They have also identified a pain reliever and anti-

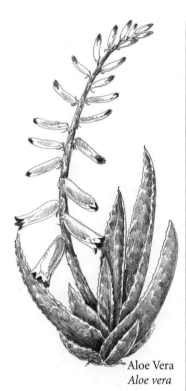

Aloe Vera
Aloe vera

swelling agent (bradykininase), an anti-inflammatory substance (an antiprostaglandin), an anti-itch component (magnesium lactate, a histamine-blocker),[10] as well as antibacterial and antifungal constituents. The gel appears to encourage healing by increasing the blood supply to injured tissue.[11]

Always check the label of commercial products to determine whether pure aloe is listed as one of the first ingredients; quality products typically contain a very high percentage (more than 95 percent) of pure aloe. Controversy persists over whether the skin-healing properties of fresh aloe remain after storage and in commercialized form, including those billed as stabilized (preserved) or even pure, naturalized, or purified.[12] At least one test-tube study using cultured human cells gave a stabilized commercial form a failing grade; there was even evidence of cell damage.[13] Although the FDA remains skeptical about the effectiveness of aloe gel for any condition, evidence to support the use of fresh gel and even some standardized commercial gels is accumulating.[14]

Solid evidence cannot be found to confirm the value of many of the other proposed uses for aloe vera gel. Despite antifungal action, for example, no sound evidence exists to support the use of aloe for treating vaginal yeast infections. A study indicating that seventeen of eighteen patients were cured of their peptic ulcers was poorly designed and the results have not been duplicated.[15]

Aloe juice (as opposed to the gel) contains such powerful laxative chemicals (anthraquinones) that most herbalists discourage its use. These substances work by irritating the large intestine, and thus they are also capable of causing severe intestinal cramping and diarrhea. Europeans use small doses, often mixed with other agents, to treat chronic constipation. German health authorities approve of concentrated dried aloe leaf juice as a stool softener to make defecation easier for people suffering from such conditions as persistent constipation and hemorrhoids.[16]

An extract (aloe-emodin) showed potential in fighting leukemia in one test-tube study, but for various reasons, National Cancer Institute experts deemed it unworthy of further testing.[17] The implications are unclear. A limited 1989 Chinese study found that an aloe extract administered by injection could protect the liver in individuals with chronic hepatitis.[18] The same is true of a 1985 study reporting success using oral aloe vera extracts to treat adults with bronchial asthma.[19]

A patent granted in 1994 to a Texas company for an aloe vera derivative, acemannan, states that this substance directly stimulates the immune system and may therefore prove valuable in treating such conditions as cancer and viral infections, including HIV and the virus that causes measles.[20] Results of animal studies that involved injecting acemannan into sarcomas and spontaneous tumors were promising.[21]

Although the implications for treating HIV infection and AIDS in humans remain far from clear, it is important to note that acemannan has been studied for this purpose. Injections of the substance have extended survival times and improved health in cats with confirmed feline leukemia.[22] This is considered intriguing in part because feline leukemia, like AIDS, is caused by a retrovirus. Some proponents claim that studies in HIV-infected individuals and AIDS patients given injections or oral formulations of acemannan have been likewise promising, especially when it is administered in the early stages of infection.[23] Test-tube studies suggest that acemannan may prove most beneficial in enhancing the actions of other AIDS medications, such as AZT, possibly reducing the need for them.[24] Much more confirmatory evidence—and sound clinical trials reported in established, peer-reviewed journals—is needed to verify these claims. Many of these studies were reported in one journal, *Molecular Biotherapy*, which was published for only a few years in the late 1980s and early 1990s.

Will It Harm You? What the Studies Say:

Aloe vera gel is considered safe for skin care, although in rare cases it can cause an allergic reaction. Do not use it on anything other than a minor surface wound and always clean the wound before applying any substance. The gel may actually delay healing of complex or deeper wounds. In a study that involved applying the gel or a placebo (in addition to standard wound therapy) to twenty-one women with complicated wounds related to a laparotomy or cesarean delivery, the wounds treated with aloe vera gel healed in a mean of eighty-three days, compared with a mean of only fifty-three days without the gel.[25] The gel may cause severe stomach cramping if taken internally; few herbalists recommend ingesting it and U.S. regulatory agencies do not approve of it as an internal medication.[26]

If you decide to use aloe juice as a laxative, take care not to exceed the recommended dose and stop using it if you develop stomach cramps or other worrisome reactions. Excessive doses may cause kidney inflammation.[27] Also, long-term abuse of this kind of anthranoid-containing laxative has been linked to an increased risk of colorectal cancer.[28] Pregnant women should never take aloe internally in any form because it may stimulate uterine contractions. It is probably best to avoid during the menstrual period as well. Children, the elderly, nursing women, and people with gastrointestinal inflammation or disorders should never take it internally.

GENERAL SOURCES:

American Pharmaceutical Association. *Handbook of Nonprescription Drugs*. 11th ed. Washington, D.C.: American Pharmaceutical Association, 1996.

Blumenthal, M., J. Gruenwald, T. Hall, and R.S. Rister, eds. *The Complete German Commission E. Monographs: Therapeutic Guide to Herbal Medicine*. Boston: Integrative Medicine Communications, 1998.

Bradley, P.C., ed. *British Herbal Compendium: A Handbook of Scientific Information on Widely Used Plant Drugs.*, vol. 1. Bournemouth, England: British Herbal Medicine Association, 1992.

Castleman, M. *The Healing Herbs: The Ultimate Guide to the Curative Power of Nature's Medicines*. New York: Bantam Books, 1995.

Duke, J.A. *CRC Handbook of Medicinal Herbs*. Boca Raton, FL: CRC Press, 1985.

Lampe, K.E., and M.A. McCann. *AMA Handbook of Poisonous and Injurious Plants*. Chicago: American Medical Association, 1985.

Lawrence Review of Natural Products. St. Louis: Facts and Comparisons, April 1992.

Leung, A.Y. *Chinese Healing Foods and Herbs*. Glen Rock, NJ: AYSL Corp, 1984.

Leung, A.Y., and S. Foster. *Encyclopedia of Common Natural Ingredients Used in Food, Drugs, and Cosmetics*. 2nd ed. New York: John Wiley & Sons, 1996.

Mindell, E. *Earl Mindell's Herb Bible.* New York: Simon & Schuster/Fireside, 1992.

Murray, M.T. *The Healing Power of Herbs: The Enlightened Person's Guide to the Wonders of Medicinal Plants.* rev. ed. Rocklin, CA: Prima Publishing, 1995.

Tierra, M. *The Way of Herbs.* New York: Pocket Books, 1990.

Tyler, V.E. *Herbs of Choice: The Therapeutic Use of Phytomedicinals.* Binghamton, NY: Haworth Press/Pharmaceutical Products Press, 1994.

———. *The Honest Herbal.* Binghamton, NY: Haworth Press/Pharmaceutical Products Press, 1993.

Tyler, V.E., J.R. Brady, and J.E. Robbers, eds. *Pharmacognosy.* Philadelphia: Lea & Febiger, 1988.

Weiner, M.A., and J.A. Weiner. *Herbs That Heal: Prescription for Herbal Healing.* Mill Valley, CA: Quantum Books, 1994.

Weiss, R.F. *Herbal Medicine,* trans. A. R. Meuss, from the 6th German edition. Beaconsfield, England: Beaconsfield Publishers, Ltd., 1988.

TEXT CITATIONS:

1. A.Y. Leung, *Chinese Healing Foods and Herbs* (Glen Rock, NJ: AYSL Corp, 1984).

2. A.Y. Leung and S. Foster, *Encyclopedia of Common Natural Ingredients Used in Food, Drugs, and Cosmetics,* 2nd ed. (New York: John Wiley & Sons, 1996).

3. M. Tierra, *The Way of Herbs* (New York: Pocket Books, 1990).

4. *Lawrence Review of Natural Products* (St. Louis: Facts and Comparisons, April 1992).

5. A.D. Klein and N.S. Penneys, *Journal of the American Academy of Dermatology,* 18 (1988): 714–20. M. Rodriguez-Bigas et al., *Plastic and Reconstructive Surgery,* 81(3) (1988): 386–89.

6. V. Visuthikosol et al., *Journal of the Medical Association of Thailand,* 78(8) (1995): 403–9.

7. American Pharmaceutical Association, *Handbook of Nonprescription Drugs,* 11th ed. (Washington, D.C.: American Pharmaceutical Association, 1996).

8. R.L. McCauley et al., *Postgraduate Medicine,* 88(8) (1990): 67–68, 73–77.

9. *Lawrence Review of Natural Products,* op. cit.

10. Ibid.

11. J.P. Heggers et al., *Phytotherapy Research,* 7 (1993): S48–S52.

12. Leung, op. cit.

13. W.D. Winters et al., *Economic Botany.,* 35 (1981): 89–95.

14. *Lawrence Review of Natural Products,* op. cit.

15. J.J. Blitz et al., *Journal of the American Osteopath Association,* 62 (1963): 731.

16. M. Blumenthal, J. Gruenwald, T. Hall, and R.S. Rister, eds., *The Complete German Commission E Monographs: Therapeutic Guide to Herbal Medicine* (Boston: Integrative Medicine Communications, 1998).

17. K. Kupchan, *Journal of Natural Products,* 39 (1976): 223.

18. Y.J. Fan et al., *Chung Kuo Chung Yao Tsa Chih,* 14(12) (1989): 746.

19. T. Shida et al., *Planta Medica,* 51 (1985): 273–75.

20. Patent assigned to Carrington Laboratories, Inc., Irving TX. U.S. Patent #5,308,838. Issued May 3, 1994.

21. C. Harris et al., *Molecular Biotherapy,* 3 (1991): 207–13.

22. M.A. Sheets et al., *Molecular Biotherapy,* 3 (1991): 41–45.

23. M.T. Murray, *The Healing Power of Herbs: The Enlightened Person's Guide to the Wonders of Medicinal Plants,* rev. ed. (Rocklin, CA: Prima Publishing, 1995).

24. J.B. Kahlon et al., *Molecular Biotherapy,* 3 (1991): 214–23.

25. J.M. Schmidt and J.S. Greenspoon, *Obstetrics and Gynecology,* 78(1) (1991): 115–17.

26. *Lawrence Review of Natural Products,* op. cit.

27. K.E. Lampe and M.A. McCann, *AMA Handbook of Poisonous and Injurious Plants* (Chicago: American Medical Association, 1985).

28. C.P. Siegers et al., *Gut,* 38(8) (1993): 1099–101.

ANGELICA

SCIENTIFIC NAME:
Angelica archangelica L., sometimes referred to as *Archangelica officinalis* (Moench) Hoffm. Other *Angelica* species, including the North American *Angelica atropurpurea*, are sometimes used medicinally as well. Family: Umbelliferae (Apiaceae)

COMMON NAMES:
American angelica, bai zhi, European angelica, garden angelica, masterwort, wild angelica, wild celery

RATING:
5 = Studies indicate that there is a definite health hazard to using this substance, even in recommended amounts.

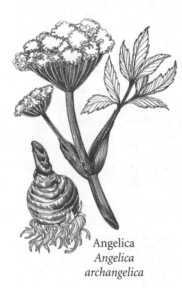
Angelica
*Angelica
archangelica*

What Is Angelica?

Angelica is a tall and striking, hardy aromatic plant with large leaves and greenish-white flowers. It belongs to the parsley family and bears a resemblance to celery. The roots, large leaves, and fruits ("seeds") are used medicinally. Other *Angelica* species are used as well, including ten or more different varieties in Chinese medicine. Refer to **Dong Quai** for information on the most common Chinese variety, *Angelica sinensis*, as none of the following information applies to that herb.

Angelica roots must be thoroughly dried before using because they are poisonous while fresh. Do not collect angelica on your own; it closely resembles the extremely poisonous water hemlock (*Cicuta maculata* L.).

What It Is Used For:

According to legend, angelica is named after an angel who appeared before a monk in plague-ridden Europe centuries ago and revealed the herb to him as a cure. Magical qualities and a good measure of witchcraft have been attributed to the herb, long a popular folk remedy for colds and other respiratory ailments such as cough and bronchitis, arthritis and other rheumatic complaints, stomach cancer, painful or irregular menstrual cycles, and ailments requiring a diuretic ("water pill") or diaphoretic (sweat-inducer). Native Americans were reportedly treating respiratory ailments with angelica when Europeans arrived. As a bitter-tasting herb, angelica has a long-standing reputation for stimulating the appetite, relieving gas, and soothing other digestive problems.

External preparations have been used as counterirritants for rheumatic pains and to treat skin disorders and lice. In America today, angelica's primary use is as a flavoring for alcoholic beverages, most notably gin and Benedictine, and as a scent. Candied leaves and stalks appear in sweets.

Forms Available Include:

Capsule, concentrated drops, decoction (typically of powdered root), extract, infusion (typically of powdered seeds or leaves), tincture. Because the fresh root is poisonous, only dried roots are used.

Dosage Commonly Reported:

A common dosage for infusions is 1 teaspoon of powdered seeds or leaves per cup of boiling water, steeped for ten to twenty minutes. Decoctions are made with 1 teaspoon of the powdered roots per cup of water, simmered for two minutes and drunk in quantities of up to 2 cups a day.

Will It Work for You? What the Studies Say:

Evidence that angelica will successfully fulfill any of the claims made for it is not only slim but somewhat academic, given significant health risks associated with it. Scientists have learned much more about Asian *Angelica* varieties. The fragrant volatile oil (about 1 percent in fresh roots and fruits and 0.5 percent when dried) accounts for the plant's use as a flavoring agent and probably as a folk cure. Angelica does not fight bacteria, and it probably offered little more than psychological help in battling plague. In test-tube studies the oil has been shown to inhibit fungal growth, but whether this translates into useful antifungal activity in humans remains unclear.[1]

German health authorities consider preparations of angelica root (but not herb or seed) effective in stimulating the appetite and relieving gas, stomach cramps, bloating, and similar digestive system upsets. Herbal bitters such as angelica are believed to work by stimulating taste receptors on the tongue, promoting salivation and the production and flow of digestive juices.

Preliminary results from studies in mouse bone marrow cells indicate that the herb may help prevent potentially cancerous mutations.[2] What this means for a future role in preventing or reversing cancerous changes in humans is unknown.

Will It Harm You? What the Studies Say:

Scientists have found reason to consider angelica quite hazardous under certain circumstances, unlike most herbs that people have relied on steadily over the centuries. It contains substances called psoralens (furocoumarins) that can incite a severe sunburn, a rash, or other signs of a sensitivity reaction in a person using it internally or externally who is then exposed to the sun or another source of ultraviolet rays. According to animal studies, furocoumarins can also cause cancer and instigate dangerous cell changes without exposure to light.[3]

GENERAL SOURCES:

Balch, J.F., and P.A. Balch. *Prescription for Nutritional Healing: A Practical A to Z Reference to Drug-Free Remedies Using Vitamins, Minerals, Herbs & Food Supplements.* 2nd ed. Garden City Park, NY: Avery Publishing Group, 1997.

Castleman, M. *The Healing Herbs: The Ultimate Guide to the Curative Power of Nature's Medicines.* New York: Bantam Books, 1995.

Duke, J.A. *CRC Handbook of Medicinal Herbs.* Boca Raton, FL: CRC Press, 1985.

Lawrence Review of Natural Products. St. Louis: Facts and Comparisons, November 1995.

Mindell, E. *Earl Mindell's Herb Bible.* New York: Simon & Schuster/Fireside, 1992.

Murray, M.T. *The Healing Power of Herbs: The Enlightened Person's Guide to the Wonders of Medicinal Plants.* Revised and expanded 2nd ed. Rocklin, CA: Prima Publishing, 1995.

Tierra, M. *The Way of Herbs.* New York: Pocket Books, 1990.

Tyler, V.E. *The Honest Herbal.* Binghamton, NY: Haworth Press/Pharmaceutical Products Press, 1993.

Tyler, V.E., L.R. Brady, and J.E. Robbers, eds. *Pharmacognosy.* Philadelphia: Lea & Febiger, 1988.

TEXT CITATIONS:

1. N. Saksena and H.H.S. Tripathi, *Fitoterapia,* 564 (1985): 243.
2. R.A. Salikhova and G.G. Poroshenko, *Vestnik Rossiiskoi Akademii Meditsinskikh Nauk (Moskva),* (1) (1995): 58–61.
3. G.W. Ivie et al., *Science,* 213 (1981): 909–10.

PRIMARY NAME:
ANISE
(and STAR ANISE)

SCIENTIFIC NAME:
Pimpinella anisum L., sometimes referred to as *Anisum vulgare* Gaertn. or *Anisum officinarum* Moench. Family: Umbelliferae (Apiaceae). Star anise: *Illicium verum* Hook. filius. Family: Magnoliaceae

COMMON NAMES:
Anise: aniseseed, sweet cumin; star anise: Chinese anise, Chinese star anise, illicium

RATING:
2 = According to a number of well-designed studies and common use, this substance appears to be relatively effective and safe when used in recommended amounts for the indication(s) noted in the "Will It Work for You?" section.

What Is Anise?

Anise and star anise are two separate plants. Anise, *Pimpinella anisum*, a highly aromatic annual indigenous to Greece and Egypt and now cultivated world-wide, produces feathery leaves; small white and yellow flowers; and ribbed, gray-green fruits ("seeds"). The seeds have been used medicinally. The considerably larger, star-shaped seeds of an evergreen known as star anise (*Illicium verum*), indigenous to southeastern Asia, are often used in similar ways. China is a major producer. Steam distillation of the dried seeds of both anise and star anise produces essential oils similar in their licoricelike aroma and flavor; they are used interchangeably in American commerce.[1] Neither plant should be confused with the highly poisonous Japanese anise (*Illicium lanceolata* or *Illicium anisatum*).

What It Is Used For:

Since ancient times, both Western and Asian healing traditions have treasured their respective anise variety as a spice and fragrance. Modern herbalists carry on the torch, continuing to recommend anise and star anise as remedies for clearing respiratory tract congestion and cough, encouraging good digestion, and treating indigestion, gas, stomach cramps, infant colic, bad breath, nausea (including morning sickness), and numerous other ailments. Many still consider anise valuable as a female hormonal agent, using it to stimulate a mother's milk production, facilitate birth, and increase libido.[2] The seeds and oil are used in similar ways. Anise oil has reportedly been used externally for lice and scabies and as an inhalant for congestion. The oil is also widely used to mask the unpleasant smell and taste of other medicines. It serves as the licorice flavor in many American candies and appears in numerous liqueurs.

Forms Available Include:

Infusion (typically made with crushed or powdered seeds), oil, seed, tincture. In China, star anise almost always appears in herbal blends.

Dosage Commonly Reported:

As an expectorant and gastrointestinal spasmolytic, anise is often taken in doses of 3 grams. *Do not take the essential oil internally except under professional supervision*—it is usually used as an inhalant. A tea is made using 1 teaspoon crushed seeds per cup of water and is drunk up to three times per day. The tincture is taken in doses of ¹/₂ to 1 teaspoon up to three times per day.

Will It Work for You? What the Studies Say:

Chemists investigating anise and star anise have found that both have a volatile oil with high concentrations (up to 90 percent) of a substance called *trans*-anethol. Many plant experts consider this substance to be an effective expectorant for loosening bronchial secretions in coughs and congestion, thereby making the secretions easier to cough up, and a carminative for helping to prevent and reduce stomach and intestinal gas and griping (sharp abdominal pains). Neither property appears to have been tested in humans with anise preparations per se. But on the basis of the presence of anethol and common experience with it, German health authorities have officially approved the seed and essential oil of both anise varieties for clearing upper respiratory tract congestion and for calming spasm-related indigestion problems, such as colic and flatulence.[3] Anise appears in numerous German cough-, congestion-, gas-, and stomach-soothing remedies.[4] Many of the gas and stomach remedies are considered appropriate for infants and small children.

Some herbalists point to the presence of scientifically accepted active estrogenic compounds (polymers of anethole)[5] to help explain the traditional use of anise as a milk stimulant for nursing mothers, as a sexual arousant, and for its other properties. The estrogenic action is considered mild, however, and has never been formally tested in women. Anise has displayed antibacterial and insecticidal properties,[6] which may explain why so many people through the years have used it topically to treat lice and scabies.

Anise tea may have a role to play in preventing or treating such conditions as iron-deficiency anemia in children and adults, according to the authors of a 1990 study who found that it (and certain other herbs) notably increased intestinal iron absorption in laboratory rats.[7]

Will It Harm You? What the Studies Say:

Generations have used the seeds from these two plants without suffering major adverse reactions. The FDA considers them a safe herb for food use. But exercise caution when taking medicinal concentrations. Do not swallow the essential oil directly. There are government standards determining safe concentrations for humans. At certain doses—possibly even a few teaspoons—the oil can cause vomiting, seizures, and pulmonary edema.[8] Concerns have also been raised by the finding that rats fed 1 percent anethole for fifteen weeks developed microscopic changes in liver cells.[9] However, those fed less over a longer time (0.25 percent for one year) showed no adverse reactions at all. Researchers are still exploring whether anise oil contains a potential cancer-causing agent called safrole.[10]

People sensitive to anethole may develop redness, scaling, blistering, or other signs of an allergic or adverse reaction with topical formulations. Respiratory and gastrointestinal tract reactions to anise have also occurred; avoid the herb if you have ever had an allergic response to it or to anethole.[11] German health authorities recommend limiting the use of anise oil to inhalation solutions for respiratory tract congestion.[12] Given the potential estrogenlike effect of anethole, some herbalists advise pregnant women not to exceed culinary amounts of the herb; no human or animal studies have ever proved it is hazardous, however.

GENERAL SOURCES:

Balch, J.F., and P.A. Balch. *Prescription for Nutritional Healing: A Practical A to Z Reference to Drug-Free Remedies Using Vitamins, Minerals, Herbs & Food Supplements*. 2nd ed. Garden City Park, NY: Avery Publishing Group, 1997.

Bisset, N.G., ed. *Herbal Drugs and Phytopharmaceuticals*. Stuttgart: medpharm GmbH Scientific Publishers, 1994.

Blumenthal, M., J. Gruenwald, T. Hall, and R.S. Rister, eds. *The Complete German Commission E. Monographs: Therapeutic Guide to Herbal Medicine. Boston: Integrative Medicine Communications, 1998.

Castleman, M. The Healing Herbs: The Ultimate Guide to the Curative Power of Nature's Medicines. New York: Bantam Books, 1995.

Chevallier, A. The Encyclopedia of Medicinal Plants: A Practical Reference Guide to More Than 550 Key Medicinal Plants & Their Uses. 1st American ed. New York: Dorling Kindersley Publications, 1996.

Duke, J.A. CRC Handbook of Medicinal Herbs. Boca Raton, FL: CRC Press, 1985.

Lawrence Review of Natural Products. St. Louis: Facts and Comparisons, October 1990.

Leung, A.Y. Chinese Healing Foods and Herbs. Glen Rock, NJ: AYSL Corp, 1984.

Leung, A.Y., and S. Foster. Encyclopedia of Common Natural Ingredients Used in Food, Drugs, and Cosmetics. 2nd ed. New York: John Wiley & Sons, 1996.

Mindell, E. Earl Mindell's Herb Bible. New York: Simon & Schuster/Fireside, 1992.

Stary, F. The Natural Guide to Medicinal Herbs and Plants. Prague: Barnes & Noble, Inc., in arrangement with Aventinum Publishers, 1996.

Tyler, V.E. Herbs of Choice: The Therapeutic Use of Phytomedicinals. Binghamton, NY: Haworth Press/Pharmaceutical Products Press, 1994.

TEXT CITATIONS:

1. A.Y. Leung and S. Foster, Encyclopedia of Common Natural Ingredients Used in Food, Drugs, and Cosmetics, 2nd ed. (New York: John Wiley & Sons, 1996).
2. M. Albert-Puleo, Journal of Ethnopharmacology, 2(4) (1980): 337–44.
3. M. Blumenthal, J. Gruenwald, T. Hall, and R.S. Rister, eds. The Complete German Commission E Monographs: Therapeutic Guide to Herbal Medicine (Boston: Integrative Medicine Communications, 1998).
4. N.G. Bisset, ed., Herbal Drugs and Phytopharmaceuticals (Stuttgart: medpharm GmbH Scientific Publishers, 1994).
5. Albert-Puleo, op. cit. Leung and Foster, op. cit.
6. Leung and Foster, op. cit. Blumenthal et al., op. cit.
7. F.A. el-Shobaki et al., Zeitschrift für Ernahrungswissenschaft. 29(4) (1990): 264–69.
8. D.G. Spoerke, Herbal Medications (Santa Barbara: Woodbridge Press, 1980).
9. R.L. Buchanan, Journal of Food Safety, 1 (1978): 275.
10. Lawrence Review of Natural Products (St. Louis: Facts and Comparisons, October 1990).
11. Blumenthal et al., op. cit.
12. Bisset, op. cit.

PRIMARY NAME:
APPLE

SCIENTIFIC NAME:
Malus pumila or sylvestris (L.) Mill. Family: Rosaceae

COMMON NAMES:
Common apple, wild apple

What Is Apple?

Apple is the fleshy, seeded, edible fruit of trees of the Malus genus. The graceful, flowering apple tree grows across North America and other temperate climates. The Malus genus includes one of more than one thousand cultivated varieties. Its seeded fruits come in various sizes, tastes (sweet, tart), colors (red, yellow, green), and textures (mealy, snappy).

What It Is Used For:

Generations have celebrated not only the taste but the healing properties of apples. Folk healers in prehistoric times, in ancient Egypt and India, and finally in modern China and America have extolled their value in encouraging good digestion; preventing and resolving constipation; controlling diarrhea (includ-

RATING:
2 = According to a number of well-designed studies and common use, this substance appears to be relatively effective and safe when used in recommended amounts for the indication(s) noted in the "Will It Work for You?" section.

ing infectious diarrhea); cleaning the teeth; and relieving fever, infant intestinal disorders, heart disease, rheumatic joint stiffness and pain, high cholesterol, warts, cancer, and other ills. Traditional Chinese doctors have long used apple bark to treat diabetes.

Forms Available Include:

Bark, fruit (whole, peeled, sliced, grated), juice.

Dosage Commonly Reported:

Enjoy as many apples—whole, peeled, grated, juiced—as satisfy your appetite. No dosage information is available for the bark.

Will It Work for You? What the Studies Say:

Apples have a well-deserved reputation for regulating the consistency of the stool and in this way controlling diarrhea and relieving constipation. Scientists attribute these properties to the pulp's considerable levels (17 percent) of a high-fiber substance called pectin and to pectic acids. As pectin travels through the stomach and intestines, it absorbs water and expands into a gelatinous clump, thus moisturizing dry, hard stools and making them easier to pass. The sheer bulk provided by the fiber also stimulates bowel contractions and ultimately a bowel movement. Loose stools are likewise endowed with form and substance. Pectin appears in many commercial antidiarrheal preparations.[1]

Researchers are continuing to examine pectin's potential to steady blood sugar levels (valuable in diabetes), reduce cholesterol levels, help prevent certain kinds of cancer, and perform a range of other functions.[2] While this is promising, no definitive findings have been made, and the blanket claim that apples will help reduce cholesterol, for example, is premature given negative findings in some human trials.[3] A substance in various parts of the apple tree called phloretin fights—albeit weakly—certain disease-causing bacteria in the test tube, but whether this translates into anything meaningful for fighting human infections is still unclear.[4]

Will It Harm You? What the Studies Say:

While the fruit of the apple is harmless by all accounts, the seeds are not. They contain cyanide, a deadly poison. Swallowing just a few is unlikely to lead to any symptoms, especially in an adult, but more than that may cause stomach upset, diarrhea, and constipation, and large doses can induce even more serious and potentially fatal reactions. Symptoms of poisoning may appear several hours later because cyanide takes a while to be absorbed into the body.[5]

If you are interested in eating apples to help manage such potentially serious illnesses as high cholesterol or diabetes, talk to your doctor; apples are best viewed as a supplement, not a substitute for treatment.

GENERAL SOURCES:
Castleman, M. *The Healing Herbs: The Ultimate Guide to the Curative Power of Nature's Medicines.* New York: Bantam Books, 1995.

Duke, J.A. *CRC Handbook of Medicinal Herbs*. Boca Raton, FL: CRC Press, 1985.

Lawrence Review of Natural Products. St. Louis: Facts and Comparisons, January 1995.

Leung, A.Y., and S. Foster. *Encyclopedia of Common Natural Ingredients Used in Food, Drugs, and Cosmetics*. 2nd ed. New York: John Wiley & Sons, 1996.

Mindell, E. *Earl Mindell's Herb Bible*. New York: Simon & Schuster/Fireside, 1992.

TEXT CITATIONS:

1. A.Y. Leung and S. Foster, *Encyclopedia of Common Natural Ingredients Used in Food, Drugs, and Cosmetics*, 2nd ed. (New York: John Wiley & Sons, 1996).
2. Ibid.
3. F. Delbarre et al., *American Journal of Clinical Nutrition*, 30 (1977): 463.
4. W.H. Lewis and M.P.F. Elvin-Lewis, *Medical Botany: Plants Affecting Man's Health* (New York: John Wiley & Sons, 1977). *Lawrence Review of Natural Products* (St. Louis: Facts and Comparisons, January 1995).
5. K.E. Lampe and M.A. McCann, *AMA Handbook of Poisonous and Injurious Plants* (Chicago: American Medical Association, 1985).

PRIMARY NAME:

APRICOT PIT

SCIENTIFIC NAME:

Prunus armeniaca L. Family: Rosaceae

COMMON NAMES:

Apricot kernels, apricot seed, bitter almond, xing ren

RATING:

5 = Studies indicate that there is a definite health hazard to using this substance, even in recommended amounts. *It is potentially fatal.*

What Is Apricot Pit?

Apricot pit is the kernel of the edible golden fruit plucked from the apricot tree. Used in Chinese medicine, it contains an extract called laetrile, which promoters claim can prevent and cure cancer. Almond, peach, apple, and cherry pits also contain laetrile, as do certain other fruits, but apricot pit is the most commonly marketed source in the United States. Laetrile spelled with a capital *L* connotes a synthetic substance patented in 1961 but never sold in the United States, although it can be found in Mexico and is distributed covertly.[1] Laetrile spelled with a small *l* is, for lay purposes, synonymous with "amygdalin." The American inventor Ernst T. Krebs, M.D., also marketed laetrile as "vitamin B-17," although it is not actually a vitamin. In China, "almond" refers to two substances: almond pit and **Almond, Sweet**.[2] An oil is pressed from the apricot pits.

What It Is Used For:

In traditional Chinese medicine, small amounts of carefully prepared apricot kernel have been used for centuries to treat cough, congestion, asthma, tumors, constipation, and other disorders. Topical formulations made with mashed kernels are applied to skin sores, snake and dog bites, and toothaches, and more recently to the vulvar area to reduce itching.[3] Since the 1970s, enthusiasts in the United States have promoted apricot pit as a source of laetrile, which they claim can effectively prevent and cure cancer. This cancer treatment is highly controversial. Although the FDA banned laetrile from interstate commerce in 1971, many states eventually legalized its use. It still proves hard to get, however, so many people decide to treat themselves with the apricot pits directly. A single call to a major dietary supplement wholesaler in 1997 proved successful in locating a pound of pits.

Forms Available Include:

Oil, raw kernel.

Dosage Commonly Reported:

Apricot pit should not be used medicinally.

Will It Work for You? What the Studies Say:

Laetrile consists of 6 percent cyanide (prussic or hydrocyanic acid), a highly poisonous substance that can kill by depriving the brain of oxygen. Advocates contend that small amounts of laetrile taken over an extended period will selectively starve cancerous tissue of oxygen, thus destroying it. The theory holds that healthy cells and tissue are spared, partly because cancer tissue is less capable of detoxifying cyanide. No scientific studies in animals or humans have ever proved the validity of this theory or demonstrated that laetrile exerts any anticancer action. An extensive National Cancer Institute study involving terminal cancer patients at four major medical centers found that laetrile from apricot pits or other natural sources did not make cancer regress, extend the lifespan of the patients, improve their symptoms, or help them gain weight or become more physically active.[4]

Several clinical trials in China were reportedly successful in treating chronic bronchitis as well as vulvar itching and vaginal trichomoniasis (a type of infection) with apricot kernels that had been mashed or made into an oil paste.[5]

Will It Harm You? What the Studies Say:

Ingesting apricot pits poses a significant risk of potentially fatal cyanide poisoning. The literature contains many reports of apricot pit poisoning among children particularly.[6] The amygdalin in the pits can cause cyanide toxicity, according to animal studies, although they are primarily known for containing an emulsion that releases the toxic cyanide. Heating the pits does not always inactivate this emulsion, as some sources claim. Fatal cyanide poisoning has occurred in people taking laetrile directly. Symptoms of such poisoning include dizziness, severe headache, convulsions, irregular breathing, and collapse. In terms of effectiveness and toxicity, it is important to keep in mind that the laetrile content of apricot pits varies considerably, from as much as 8 percent in some apricot varieties to twenty times that amount in wild varieties.[7]

In China, where apricot pits are relatively common in herbal medicine shops, their toxicity is well recognized and respected.

GENERAL SOURCES:
Barrett, S., and V. Herbert. *The Vitamin Pushers: How the "Health Food" Industry Is Selling America a Bill of Goods.* Amherst, NY: Prometheus Books, 1994.
Jukes, T.H. *Journal of the American Medical Association.* 242 (1979): 719–20.
Leung, A.Y. *Chinese Healing Foods and Herbs.* Glen Rock, NJ: AYSL Corp, 1984.
Leung, A.Y., and S. Foster. *Encyclopedia of Common Natural Ingredients Used in Food, Drugs, and Cosmetics.* 2nd ed. New York: John Wiley & Sons, 1996.
Tierra, M. *The Way of Herbs.* New York: Pocket Books, 1990.
Tyler, V.E. *The Honest Herbal.* Binghamton, NY: Haworth Press/Pharmaceutical Products Press, 1993.

————. *Herbs of Choice: The Therapeutic Use of Phytomedicinals.* Binghamton, NY: Haworth Press/Pharmaceutical Products Press, 1994.

Tyler, V.E., L.R. Brady, and J.E. Robbers, eds. *Pharmacognosy.* Philadelphia: Lea & Febiger, 1988.

Weiss, R.F. *Herbal Medicine*, trans. A. R. Meuss, from the 6th German edition. Beaconsfield, England: Beaconsfield Publishers, Ltd., 1988.

TEXT CITATIONS:
1. V.E. Tyler, *The Honest Herbal* (Binghamton, NY: Haworth Press/Pharmaceutical Products Press, 1993).
2. A.Y. Leung, *Chinese Healing Foods and Herbs* (Glen Rock, NJ: AYSL Corp, 1984).
3. Ibid.
4. T.H. Jukes, *Journal of the American Medical Association*, 242 (1979): 719–20.
5. Leung, op. cit.
6. J.W. Sayre and S. Kaymakcalan, *New England Journal of Medicine*, 270 (1964): 1113–15.
7. Tyler, op. cit.

PRIMARY NAME:
ARNICA

SCIENTIFIC NAME:
Arnica montana L. and related species. In the United States, species used include *Arnica fulgens* Pursh., *Arnica sororia* Green., *Arnica latifolia* Bong, and *Arnica cordifolia* Hook. Family: Asteraceae (Compositae)

COMMON NAMES:
Leopard's bane, mountain snuff, mountain tobacco, wolfsbane

What Is Arnica?

Arnica consists of the dried flower heads of *Arnica montana* or other *Arnica* species, perennials that boast bright-yellow flowers reminiscent of daisies. The rhizomes (underground stems) are sometimes used as well.

What It Is Used For:

For centuries, arnica equaled royalty among medicinal herbs of the West. Oral formulations were used to suppress coughs, invigorate the heart, and stimulate the central nervous system. American settlers took arnica to break a fever and enhance blood circulation, often at the recommendation of their doctors. In recent years, however, health concerns have seriously eroded its reputation as an internal healer.

External formulations do not pose the same hazards, however, and continue to be heavily used among Europeans, particularly as general counterirritants, anti-inflammatories, and pain relievers. Arnica formulations have been rubbed into countless swollen ankles, dislocated shoulders, muscle aches, arthritic joints, bruises, abrasions, insect bites, boils, inflamed gums, and acne eruptions. Some herbalists recommend gargling with an arnica infusion to soothe a sore throat. It can be used on a moist compress to cool inflamed hemorrhoids. Many herbal psoriasis and seborrheic eczema preparations contain arnica extracts. Homeopaths prescribe minute amounts for various ailments. (See page 2 for a discussion of homeopathy.)

Forms Available Include:

- *For external use:* Gel, infusion (used for gargles, compresses, and poultices), ointment, tincture. Arnica-containing creams are popular in Europe.
- *For internal use:* Arnica should not be used internally.

RATING:
- *For external use:* 1 = Years of use and extensive, high-quality studies indicate that this substance is very effective and safe when used in recommended amounts for the indication(s) noted in the "Will It Work for You?" section below.
- *For internal use:* 5 = Studies indicate that there is a definite health hazard to using this substance, even in recommended amounts.

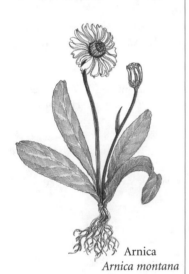

Arnica
Arnica montana

Dosage Commonly Reported:

A compress is made using 1 tablespoon tincture per ¹/2 liter water. An infusion is made using 2 grams arnica per 100 milliliters water. For use in poultices, the tincture is diluted three to ten times with water. The ointment is used in maximum concentrations of 15 percent arnica oil or 20 to 25 percent tincture. Do not use arnica internally or on broken skin.

Will It Work for You? What the Studies Say:

In the early 1980s, German investigators made a breakthrough when they identified two critical substances in arnica—the sesquiterpene lactones helanalin and dihydrohelanalin, and their derivatives—both of which help reduce inflammation, alleviate pain, and fight bacteria, albeit mildly.[1] Many of the traditional uses for the herb make sense in the light of this discovery, especially given previous knowledge about counterirritant chemicals in arnica. Just as millions of Europeans suspected, arnica may indeed help soothe scrapes and aches. German health authorities approve of using arnica externally as an antiseptic, an anti-inflammatory, and a numbing agent for pain.[2]

Although most experts now consider it too risky to take internally, arnica was probably used to exert various effects. Animal studies indicate that extracts mildly boost the resistance to infection (probably by stimulating the immune system)[3] and can increase bile output, promote excess fluid loss (as a diuretic, or "water pill"), and improve blood flow.[4] Most of these properties appear to be relatively weak, however. For example, in a mid-1980s study, individuals having their impacted wisdom teeth removed suffered more postoperative pain and inflammation if they were given arnica than if they took an antibiotic (metronidazole) *or* a placebo.[5]

Will It Harm You? What the Studies Say:

Experts around the world strongly discourage taking internal forms of arnica, as they can irritate mucous membranes and cause burning pains in the stomach, vomiting, diarrhea, and drowsiness. As little as 1 ounce of the tincture may generate shortness of breath, elevated blood pressure, and heart damage, according to studies with small animals.[6] An overdose can be fatal. The FDA classifies arnica as an unsafe herb.

In contrast, most people tolerate external formulations well. They appear to pose no risk of a toxic systemic reaction. Allergic reactions with contact dermatitis are relatively common, however,[7] so if you are sensitive to other members of the daisy family, or you have ever had an allergic reaction to arnica, avoid the plant altogether.

Stick to recommended amounts. Swelling, redness, eczema, pain, itching, and small blisters may develop if you apply arnica very frequently or for prolonged periods.[8] The risk is particularly high if you place it on broken skin such as an abrasion. Some herbalists warn against making external preparations at home because they could irritate the skin if they turn out too strong.

Because arnica is classified as a protected species in many countries, it is sometimes hard to come by and other plants are surreptitiously used instead. Buy it from a reputable source.

GENERAL SOURCES:

Bisset, N.E., ed. *Herbal Drugs and Phytopharmaceuticals.* Stuttgart: medpharm GmbH Scientific Publishers, 1994.

Blumenthal, M., J. Gruenwald, T. Hall, and R.S. Rister, eds. *The Complete German Commission E. Monographs: Therapeutic Guide to Herbal Medicine.* Boston: Integrative Medicine Communications, 1998.

Duke, J.A. *CRC Handbook of Medicinal Herbs.* Boca Raton, FL: CRC Press, 1985.

Lawrence Review of Natural Products. St. Louis: Facts and Comparisons, February 1991.

Leung, A.Y., *Encyclopedia of Common Natural Ingredients Used in Food, Drugs, and Cosmetics.* New York: John Wiley & Sons, 1980.

Tyler, V.E. *Herbs of Choice: The Therapeutic Use of Phytomedicinals.* Binghamton, NY: Haworth Press/Pharmaceutical Products Press, 1994.

Wagner, H., et al. *Arzneimittel-Forschung,* 35(7) (1985): 1069–75.

Weiss, R. F. *Herbal Medicine.* Trans. A. R. Meuss, from the 6th German edition. Beaconsfield, England: Beaconsfield Publishers, Ltd., 1988.

TEXT CITATIONS:

1. V.E. Tyler, *The Honest Herbal* (Binghamton, NY: Haworth Press/Pharmaceutical Products Press, 1992). N.E. Bisset, ed., *Herbal Drugs and Phytopharmaceuticals* (Stuttgart: medpharm GmbH Scientific Publishers, 1994). S.D. Sokolova et al., *Uch Zap Pyatigorskii Farmatsevt. Inst.* 5 (1961): 309–16.

2. M. Blumenthal, J. Gruenwald, T. Hall, and R.S. Rister, eds., *The Complete German Commission E Monographs: Therapeutic Guide to Herbal Medicine* (Boston: Integrative Medicine Communications, 1998).

3. H. Buschmann, *Fortschritte Vetrinarmedizin,* 20 (1974): 98.

4. A.W. Forst, *Naunyn-Schmeid,* 201 (1943): 242. N.O. Skakun and V.A. Zhulkevich, *Farmakologiai I Toksikologia,* 18, No. 2 (1955): 45–46. Bisset, op. cit. H. Schroder et al., *Thrombosis Research,* 57 (1990): 839.

5. G.S. Kaziro, *British Journal of Oral Maxillofacial Surgery,* 22 (1984): 42.

6. A.Y. Leung, *Encyclopedia of Common Natural Ingredients Used in Food, Drugs, and Cosmetics* (New York: John Wiley & Sons, 1980).

7. J.C. Mitchell, *Recent Advances in Phytochemistry,* vol. 9, V.C. Runeckles, ed. (New York: Plenum, 1975).

8. Bisset, op. cit.

PRIMARY NAME:
ARTICHOKE

SCIENTIFIC NAME:
Cynara scolymus L. Family: Asteraceae (Compositae)

COMMON NAME:
Globe artichoke

What Is Artichoke?

This widely cultivated, thistlelike perennial has large lobed leaves and violet flower heads. Primarily the leaves are used medicinally.

What It Is Used For:

For centuries, Europeans have not only relished artichokes as a delicacy but relied on them to treat a broad spectrum of ailments: liver disease, jaundice, indigestion, atherosclerosis, anemia, and snakebite are just a few. Their reputation as a diuretic, or "water pill," is long-standing. A recently identified ingredient—cynarin—in the leaves is believed to stimulate bile production. It is now commonly extracted and added to indigestion remedies as well as cholesterol-lowering drugs. Some sources cite cynarin as a liver protectant.

ARTICHOKE (Continued)

RATING:

- *For the extract cynarin:* 2 = According to a number of well-designed studies and common use, this substance appears to be relatively effective and safe when used in recommended amounts for the indication(s) noted in the "Will It Work for You?" section.
- *For the rest of the plant:* 3 = Studies on the effectiveness and safety of this substance are conflicting, or there are not enough studies to draw a conclusion.

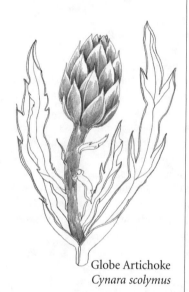

Globe Artichoke
Cynara scolymus

Contemporary herbalists encourage a number of the traditional and newer uses for the artichoke. Some even suggest it can enhance sexual desire. Cynarin and other artichoke extracts serve as sweeteners and as flavors in alcoholic drinks, including aperitif liqueurs that also rely on the plant's bitter attributes to encourage good digestion.

Forms Available Include:

Capsule, tablet, tincture. The whole plant can be purchased in grocery stores, and the leaves cooked and eaten as a vegetable. Artichoke and certain extracts (e.g., cynarin) appear in multi-ingredient formulations, particularly in Europe. Products with standardized amounts of caffeoylquinic acids—cynarin is one of them—are available in the United States.

Dosage Commonly Reported:

A daily dosage of two to three 100-milligram capsules standardized with 15 milligrams of caffeoylquinic acids is a common recommendation. Otherwise there are no uniform standards for artichoke.

Will It Work for You? What the Studies Say:

The aromatic bitter attributes in the leaves, stem, and root of this plant not only account for its distinctive bitter taste but explain why people have instinctively turned to it to encourage gastric juice secretion and good digestion. Cynarin is widely accepted among experts as a choleretic, meaning that it stimulates bile output and can thus be expected to help settle dyspeptic symptoms such as nausea, pain, vomiting, and bloating. This property is particularly valuable for individuals suffering from digestive disorders characterized by poor fat assimilation due to inadequate bile secretion, according to a well-designed randomized and placebo-controlled 1994 trial.[1] Artichoke extract significantly increased bile production in the trial's twenty male subjects. German health authorities endorse the use of artichoke juice (from the fresh plant) and other preparations made from the leaves for dyspeptic problems.[2]

Investigators have uncovered a number of other interesting properties in artichoke and its extracts that may one day prove useful, although they all require more research. For example, intriguing but still weakly substantiated evidence indicates that artichoke possesses liver-protectant properties. In a study of rats, liquid extracts of the roots and leaves of the fresh plant demonstrated this property by encouraging regeneration of the liver.[3] Another study found that artichoke compounds had a protective effect on rat liver cells examined in the test tube.[4] In a study of traditional anti-snake-venom remedies, investigators discovered that the plant has anti-inflammatory and even antitumor actions in test mice.[5] Cynarin has been used to treat human nephritis (kidney inflammation).[6] And several sources have reported that the plant has mild diuretic properties, meaning that it can be expected to increase urine output, and that it can lower blood sugar levels, a property valued in managing diabetes.[7]

Results of studies examining cynarin's capacity to lower cholesterol levels have been mixed, with some investigators reporting that it reduces blood cholesterol and triglyceride levels in humans[8] and serum and hepatic cholesterol levels in rats,[9] and others finding no benefits at all. One team reported that cynarin failed to significantly improve cholesterol and triglyceride concentrations in seventeen individuals with familial Type II hyperlipoproteinaemia who took daily supplements of the extract for three months.[10] Some German physicians view the possible ability to reduce cholesterol levels as a sign that artichoke extracts may help prevent gallstone formation.[11]

Will It Harm You? What the Studies Say:

Most people tolerate artichoke and its extracts well. Obviously, if you are allergic to the plant, you should avoid it and also avoid formulations that contain cynarin or other extracts. Allergic contact dermatitis has occurred when sensitized individuals touch the fresh plant. German health authorities cite no side effects but do advise anyone with gallstones or a bile duct obstruction to take cynarin only under a doctor's advice.[12] The FDA classifies the leaves as safe for use as a food ingredient.

GENERAL SOURCES:

Balch, J.F., and P.A. Balch. *Prescription for Nutritional Healing: A Practical A to Z Reference to Drug-Free Remedies Using Vitamins, Minerals, Herbs & Food Supplements*. 2nd ed. Garden City Park, NY: Avery Publishing Group, 1997.

Blumenthal, M., J. Gruenwald, T. Hall, and R.S. Rister, eds. *The Complete German Commission E. Monographs: Therapeutic Guide to Herbal Medicine*. Boston: Integrative Medicine Communications, 1998.

Lawrence Review of Natural Products. St. Louis: Facts and Comparisons, November 1992.

Leung, A.Y., and S. Foster. *Encyclopedia of Common Natural Ingredients Used in Food, Drugs, and Cosmetics*. 2nd ed. New York: John Wiley & Sons, 1996.

Mindell, E. *Earl Mindell's Herb Bible*. New York: Simon & Schuster/Fireside, 1992.

Stary, F. *The Natural Guide to Medicinal Herbs and Plants*. Prague: Barnes & Noble, Inc., in arrangement with Aventinum Publishers, 1996.

Weiss, R.F. *Herbal Medicine*, trans. A. R. Meuss, from the 6th German edition. Beaconsfield, England: Beaconsfield Publishers, Ltd., 1988.

TEXT CITATIONS:

1. R. Kirchhoff et al., *Phytomedicine*, vol. 1 (1994): 107–15.
2. M. Blumenthal, J. Gruenwald, T. Hall, and R.S. Rister, eds., *The Complete German Commission E Monographs: Therapeutic Guide to Herbal Medicine* (Boston: Integrative Medicine Communications, 1998).
3. T. Maros et al., *Arzneimittel-Forschung*, 16(2) (1966): 127–29.
4. T. Adzet et al., *Journal of Natural Products*, 50(4) (1987): 612–17.
5. B.M. Ruppelt et al., *Memorias do Instituto Oswaldo Cruz* (86 Suppl 2) (1991): 203–5. K. Yasukawa et al., *Oncology*, 53(4) (1996): 341–44.
6. K. Cieslinska and J. Wojcicki, *World Health Organization Technical Report Series*, 27(5) (1974): 457–62.
7. *Lawrence Review of Natural Products* (St. Louis: Facts and Comparisons, November 1992).
8. P.E. Altman, Jr., and I.L. Honigberg, *Journal of Pharmaceutical Sciences*, 61 (1972): 610.
9. J. Wojcicki, *Drug & Alcohol Dependence*, 3(2) (1978): 143–45.
10. H. Heckers et al., *Atherosclerosis*, 26(2) (1977): 249–53.

11. R.F. Weiss, *Herbal Medicine*, trans. A.R. Meuss, from the 6th German edition. (Beaconsfield, England: Beaconsfield Publishers, Ltd., 1988).

12. Blumenthal et al., op. cit.

PRIMARY NAME:

ASHWAGANDHA

SCIENTIFIC NAME:
Withania somnifera Dunal;
Withania coagulans Dunal.
Family: Solanaceae

COMMON NAMES:
Aswagandha, Indian ginseng, winter cherry, withania

RATING:
3 = Studies on the effectiveness and safety of this substance are conflicting, or there are not enough studies to draw a conclusion.

What Is Ashwagandha?

This small evergreen undershrub can be found in drier parts of India, the Mediterranean, and the Middle East. It bears showy greenish or yellow flowers. Primarily the dried roots, fruits ("berries"), and oval leaves are used medicinally.

What It Is Used For:

For more than two thousand years, traditional Eastern systems of healing, especially India's Ayurvedic system, have celebrated ashwagandha as a rejuvenating tonic instrumental in boosting strength, stamina, vigor, and sexual energy. It is considered helpful in "balancing life forces." Ashwagandha has also been recommended for more specific ailments such as nausea, bronchitis, tuberculosis, arthritis and other inflammatory conditions, tumors, anemia, and fluid retention (as a diuretic, or "water pill"). Skin ulcerations and swelling are treated with topical formulations.

Numerous Western herbalists refer to ashwagandha as "Ayurvedic ginseng" and highlight its presumed value as an adaptogen, antistress proponent, and agent for promoting drowsiness-free relaxation and sedation.

Forms Available Include:

Capsule, decoction (of root bark), powder (of leaves or root).

Dosage Commonly Reported:

Many capsules are standardized for 2 to 5 milligrams withanolides, with a commonly recommended daily dosage of 150 to 300 milligrams. Recommendations of 2 to 3 grams of the root powder taken three times a day are common in India.

Will It Work for You? What the Studies Say:

Intensive research over decades, much of it done in India, has yielded a formidable body of information about the chemical constituents of this complex, ancient herb. Test-tube and small-animal studies indicate that the plant has anti-inflammatory, sedative, and antistress properties, although results are not always consistent. Firm conclusions about the significance of these findings for humans are difficult to draw, particularly given that few if any human trials have apparently been done. (Examinations in humans with herbal blends containing ashwagandha are not considered because the herb's specific contribution is difficult to discern).

Ashwagandha contains, among other substances, an essential oil (ipuranol), a crystalline alkaloid (withania), and a number of steroidal lactones commonly designated withanolides. The plant's cancer-fighting potential has been a subject of intense research. Carefully selected doses of withaferin A have inhibited tumor growth and increased survival in laboratory mice.[1] Concentrations of the antitumor constituents appear to vary widely, however.[2] Rodent studies indicate that ashwagandha extracts can counter inflammation similarly or more vigorously than other anti-inflammatory herbs[3] and in some cases just as well as an established anti-inflammatory medicine, hydrocortisone.[4] Whether this is meaningful for people suffering from inflammatory diseases remains unexplored. In terms of ashwagandha's value as a relaxant and sedative, some investigators found that mice and dogs fed certain types of the plant's extracts experience a mild depression (slowing down) of the central nervous system and attendant sedation, but others found no such reaction at all.[5]

In asserting that ashwagandha qualifies as an "adaptogen" capable of bolstering the body's ability to withstand stress, many herbalists cite a constellation of studies that found that root extracts significantly improved the performance of rodents in classic stress tests such as swimming endurance.[6] No human trials have been done to verify this, however. Further research is also needed to elaborate on intriguing but limited rodent studies indicating that certain ashwagandha extracts may protect against liver toxicity,[7] counter arthritis,[8] and reverse cognitive deficits (in rats chemically induced with a type of Alzheimer's disease).[9] Experiments to test its antibacterial and antifungal activity have yielded mixed results.

Will It Harm You? What the Studies Say:

Centuries of use and extensive animal testing suggest that ashwagandha is relatively safe to use. Moderation may be justified, however. A study of seventy Sri Lankan medicinal plants identified ashwagandha as one of two that produced marked renal (kidney) lesions in test rats.[10] Male rats repeatedly injected with alcoholic extracts died at certain doses, with the weight of various critical organs declining significantly as well.[11] If you decide to use ashwagandha, keep in mind the plant's potential to cause sedation and other central nervous system effects.[12]

GENERAL SOURCES:

Balch, J.F., and P.A. Balch. *Prescription for Nutritional Healing: A Practical A to Z Reference to Drug-Free Remedies Using Vitamins, Minerals, Herbs & Food Supplements.* 2nd ed. Garden City Park, NY: Avery Publishing Group, 1997.

Chevallier, A. *The Encyclopedia of Medicinal Plants: A Practical Reference Guide to More Than 550 Key Medicinal Plants & Their Uses.* 1st American ed. New York: Dorling Kindersley Publications, 1996.

Duke, J.A. *CRC Handbook of Medicinal Herbs.* Boca Raton, FL: CRC Press, 1985.

Lawrence Review of Natural Products. St. Louis: Facts and Comparisons, July 1988.

Mayell, M. *Off-the-Shelf Natural Health: How to Use Herbs and Nutrients to Stay Well.* New York: Bantam Books, 1995.

Tyler, V.E. *Herbs of Choice: The Therapeutic Use of Phytomedicinals.* Binghamton, NY: Haworth Press/Pharmaceutical Products Press, 1994.

TEXT CITATIONS:

1. A.C. Sharad et al., *Acta Oncologica*, 35(1) (1996): 95–100. P.U. Devi et al., *Cancer Letters*, 95(1–2) (1995): 189–93. P.V. Devi et al., *Indian Journal of Experimental Biology*, 30(3) (1992): 169–72.
2. S.K. Chakraborti et al., *Experientia*, 30(8) (1974): 852–53.
3. M.K. al-Hindawi et al., *Journal of Ethnopharmacology*, 26(2) (1989): 163–68.
4. M.K. al-Hindawi, *Journal of Ethnopharmacology*, 1992;37(2):13–16.
5. R. Fontaine and A. Erdoes, *Planta Medica*, 30 (1976): 242.
6. S.K. Bhattacharya, *Phytotherapy Research*, 1(1) (1987): 32–37. H. Wagner et al., *Zeitschrift für Phytotherapie*, 13 (1992): 42–54.
7. S. Sudhir et al., *Planta Medica*, 1 (1986): 61–63.
8. J. Sadique et al., *Acta Pharmacologica Toxicol Suppl*, 59(7) (1986): 406–9.
9. S.K. Bhattacharya et al., *Phytotherapy Research*, 9(2) (1995): 110–13.
10. S.N. Arseculeratne et al., *Journal of Ethnopharmacology*, 13(3) (1985): 323–35.
11. A.C. Sharada et al., *International Journal of Pharmacognosy*, 31(3) (1993): 205–12.
12. *Lawrence Review of Natural Products* (St. Louis: Facts and Comparisons, July 1988).

PRIMARY NAME:
ASPARAGUS

SCIENTIFIC NAME:
Asparagus officinalis L. Family: Liliaceae

COMMON NAME:
Garden asparagus

RATING:
- *Root preparation as a mild diuretic:* 2 = According to a number of well-designed studies and common use, this substance appears to be relatively effective and safe when used in recommended amounts and by people free from certain complications (see "Will It Harm You?" section).
- *For all other purposes:* 3 = Studies on the effectiveness and safety of this substance are conflicting, or there are not enough studies to draw a conclusion.

What Is Asparagus?

This perennial herb is cultivated worldwide for its tall, slender, edible stalks (spears or shoots), which are customarily cooked as a vegetable. It has scalelike leaves, bright-red berries, and yellow-green flowers. The stalks, roots, and occasionally the seeds have been used medicinally.

What It Is Used For:

Asparagus spears are a widely recognized and enjoyed vegetable. Over the centuries, many traditional healing cultures, including those in China and India, have come to consider the vegetable a part of their healing repertoire and treated ailments ranging from toothaches to cancer, parasitic disease, rheumatism, and constipation with it. In China, the seeds are used to treat parasitic diseases and the roots treasured as a fatigue-fighting (*yin*) tonic. Root preparations appear in diuretic ("water pill") preparations in Germany and other parts of the world, as well as in formulas for urinary tract inflammation and infection and kidney stone prevention. External formulations of the spears and extracts have been used in folk medicine for cleaning the face and drying up sores and pimples. Seed and root extracts can be found in alcoholic beverages.

A number of contemporary herbalists recommend asparagus spear preparations for reducing rheumatic joint pain and swelling, and for treating bladder infections, female reproductive system problems including hormonal imbalances, dryness in the lungs and throat, and AIDS. Some contend that the herb can reduce fluid retention as well as help prevent anemia due to folic acid deficiency. The powdered seeds have been recommended for calming stomach upset.

Forms Available Include:

Decoction (of the root), powder (of seeds), root, seeds, spears.

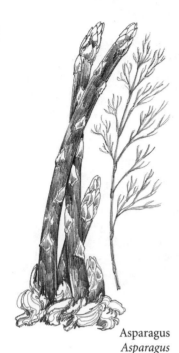

Asparagus
*Asparagus
officinalis*

Dosage Commonly Reported:

The young stalks are eaten as part of the diet. The seed is taken in powder form at a dose of 1 teaspoon in juice.

Will It Work for You? What the Studies Say:

Evidence to confirm the value of most traditional uses for asparagus is sketchy at best. Perhaps the most substantiated effect is a diuretic one; studies have shown that root preparations increase urine production. Asparagus herb preparations do as well, but the action is apparently much weaker.[1] Both the reliability and the potency of asparagus in any form remain quite unclear. After examining the evidence, German health authorities decided to approve preparations of asparagus root—but not asparagus herb—as diuretics for helping to prevent kidney stones and treat inflammatory diseases of the urinary tract.[2]

Although the implications for humans are still far from clear, there is evidence that asparagus has promise as a cancer-preventing agent; in test-tube studies it inhibited dangerous cell mutations that could lead to cancer.[3] In 1996, a team of investigators reported that substances called saponins in asparagus spears effectively inhibited the growth of human leukemia HL-60 cells in the laboratory dish.[4]

Scientists have identified steroidal glycosides in asparagus roots, but the claim that the plant is therefore an aphrodisiac, a hormone regulator, or a powerful anti-inflammatory agent for such ailments as rheumatism-related joint pain still requires confirmation in human testing. Other intriguing findings that likewise demand further examination are the plant's use as an antibacterial agent,[5] an antiviral agent (related species have tested positive for this in the test tube),[6] and blood-pressure reducer.[7]

Will It Harm You? What the Studies Say:

Centuries of use attest to the relative safety of asparagus and its extracts for healing. The distinctive, pungent odor that it produces in the urine of some individuals (about 40 percent, according to a study of eight hundred volunteers) after eating the spears is also harmless.[8] In fact, the ability to detect the odor may represent a specific genetic trait, as only certain individuals can smell it.[9]

If you use the root as a diuretic, be sure to drink plenty of water. German health authorities warn that neither individuals with fluid retention (edema) from functional heart or kidney disease nor those suffering from an inflammatory kidney disease should use medicinal-strength asparagus root preparations.[10]

GENERAL SOURCES:

Blumenthal, M., J. Gruenwald, T. Hall, and R.S. Rister, eds. *The Complete German Commission E. Monographs: Therapeutic Guide to Herbal Medicine.* Boston: Integrative Medicine Communications, 1998.

Lawrence Review of Natural Products. St. Louis: Facts and Comparisons, July 1995.

Leung, A.Y., and S. Foster. *Encyclopedia of Common Natural Ingredients Used in Food, Drugs, and Cosmetics.* 2nd ed. New York: John Wiley & Sons, 1996.

Mindell, E. *Earl Mindell's Herb Bible.* New York: Simon & Schuster/Fireside, 1992.

Tierra, M. *The Way of Herbs.* New York: Pocket Books, 1990.

TEXT CITATIONS:

1. M. Blumenthal, J. Gruenwald, T. Hall, and R.S. Rister, eds., *The Complete German Commission E Monographs: Therapeutic Guide to Herbal Medicine* (Boston: Integrative Medicine Communications, 1998). A.Y. Leung and S. Foster, *Encyclopedia of Common Natural Ingredients Used in Food, Drugs, and Cosmetics*, 2nd ed. (New York: John Wiley & Sons, 1996).
2. Blumenthal et al., op. cit.
3. Leung and Foster, op. cit. R. Edenharder et al., *Zeitschrift für Die Gesamte Hygiene und Ihre Grenzgebiete (Berlin)*, 36(3) (1990): 144.
4. Y. Shao et al., *Cancer Letters*, 104(1) (1996): 31–36.
5. D. Bensky and A. Gamble, eds., *Chinese Herbal Medicine: Materia Medica* (Seattle: Eastland Press, Inc., 1986).
6. R. Aquino et al., *Journal of Chemotherapy*, 3(4) (1991): 305.
7. Leung and Foster, op. cit.
8. S.C. Mitchell et al., *Experientia*, 43(4) (1987): 382.
9. M. Lison, *The British Medical Journal*, 281 (6256) (1980): 1676.
10. Blumenthal et al., op cit.

PRIMARY NAME:

ASTRAGALUS

SCIENTIFIC NAME:
Astragalus membranaceous (Fisch.) Bge., *Astragalus mongholicus* Bge., and various other *Astragalus* species. Family: Leguminosae

COMMON NAMES:
Hunag bai, milk vetch, Mongolian milk vetch, yellow leader

RATING:
3 = Studies on the effectiveness and safety of this substance are conflicting, or there are not enough studies to draw a conclusion.

What Is Astragalus?

There are several species of *Astragalus*, hairy-stemmed perennials native to northern China and neighboring regions. The best known and most extensively studied are *Astragalus membranaceous* and *Astragalus mongholicus*. The dried root is used medicinally, sometimes in cured (honey-treated) form. A yellow core is at the center of the sweet-tasting black roots.

What It Is Used For:

While only recently introduced in the West, astragalus root has been valued in China as a tonic and medicine for more than two thousand years. Healers there consider it one of their tradition's premier immune-system tonics for nourishing and fortifying the constitution, especially in chronic immune deficiency states such as cancer. It is believed to function as a warming tonic for increased resistance to cold. Many contend it can replenish vital energy (*qi*), aiding the body in overcoming fatigue and weakness, regenerating tissue growth and promoting muscle growth, and boosting stamina and endurance in young people especially.[1] The Chinese attribute most of the energizing elements to cured forms of the root. Astragalus also has a reputation for promoting urine output (as a diuretic, or "water pill"), reducing swelling, resolving diarrhea due to spleen deficiency, correcting rectal prolapse, and stopping uterine bleeding.[2]

In recent years particularly, traditional healers in many other parts of the world have recommended astragalus to prevent and treat the common cold, boost the body's immune system to fight AIDS[3] and endure the rigors of chemotherapy and radiation for cancer, control diabetes, soothe stomach ulcers,[4] prevent viral heart damage (from Coxsackie B virus), reduce blood pressure, and help heal burns and abscesses.[5]

Forms Available Include:

Capsule, concentrated drop, decoction, extract, root (fresh, dried, cured slices), tea, tincture.

Dosage Commonly Reported:

One dropperful of tincture is taken two to three times per day. The dried root is taken in dosages of 1 to 4 grams three times per day.

Will It Work for You? What the Studies Say:

Chinese researchers in particular have carefully investigated this complex herb, conducting dozens of studies in the past decade alone. Most appear to have been done in the test tube or on rodents or other small animals, and collectively they indicate that this ancient remedy holds promise as an immune system stimulant (especially for chronic rather than acute problems), anticancer agent, and heart tonic, among other things. Few studies have involved humans, however, and of these the majority involved herbal blends, making the specific contribution of astragalus difficult to discern. Some sources have made extravagant claims for what are revealed on closer inspection to be relatively insignificant findings. Many factors must be taken into account in evaluating the research on this herb, from the standards of Chinese researchers (sometimes different from those of Western researchers) to the limitations of Western bias in the interpretation of Eastern herbs. The polysaccharides (carbohydrates) and saponins (glucoside molecules) the herb contains probably contribute enormously to the numerous actions that have been demonstrated.[6]

Several studies suggest that astragalus can stimulate the immune system, supporting its long-term reputation as a "vital energy" tonic and system strengthener.[7] Mice subjected to standard Chinese tests for stamina and resistance to stress such as swimming long distances and being exposed to temperature extremes perform better when fed astragalus extracts (saponins).[8] A component of the herb has been examined as an immune system stimulant for AIDS patients, with one study reporting intriguing findings that may merit further investigation.[9] The same investigation revealed that the herb could inhibit immune system suppression by a chemotherapy drug.

In a frequently cited and often misinterpreted study done at the University of Texas Medical Center in Houston, researchers found that in blood taken from cancer patients, astragalus extracts restored function in immune system cells damaged by chemotherapy. The condition of the patients themselves was not examined, only their blood was. This is an intriguing finding but a far cry from the claim that the herb can actually boost the immune systems of AIDS or cancer patients. More studies are needed.

According to various studies, astragalus may have beneficial effects on the damaged heart in particular. In one investigation, heart attack victims treated with the herb suffered less angina pectoris (chest pain) and experienced more improvement in EKG readings and other measurements than subjects given such standard heart medicines as nifedipine.[10] One team of Chinese researchers reported that the herb had tonic effects on the heart (left ventricular function in particular) of patients hospitalized with heart attacks over a four-week period, compared with patients not given the herb.[11] They hypothesized that the herb's beneficial impact on free radicals (that is, its antioxidant effects) may have made the difference. Other beneficial actions on the cardiovascular system have also been reported.[12]

Several test-tube and rodent studies have shown that the herb fights the Coxsackie B virus, which can cause scarring, inflammation, and other heart damage.[13] Authors of a 1995 study who examined the herb's impact on immune system cells in blood from individuals with viral myocarditis suggested that the improved cell immunity they observed was a good argument for considering the herb as part of treatment for such patients in the future.[14]

Studies have also shown that the herb in various formulations can fight inflammation, improve learning and memory, protect against hepatitis-related liver damage, improve stamina, inhibit aberrations in blood sugar levels, impair the growth of certain kinds of cancers, and increase urine output as a diuretic.[15]

Will It Harm You? What the Studies Say:

The toxicity of astragalus appears to be very low, according to centuries of continued use as a healing food in parts of Asia, the ingredients identified, and results of rodent studies.[16] Its safety has yet to be properly examined in clinical trials, however, and information on common side effects—if any—is hard to obtain.

GENERAL SOURCES:

Balch, J.F., and P.A. Balch. *Prescription for Nutritional Healing: A Practical A to Z Reference to Drug-Free Remedies Using Vitamins, Minerals, Herbs & Food Supplements.* 2nd ed. Garden City Park, NY: Avery Publishing Group, 1997.

Chevallier, A. *The Encyclopedia of Medicinal Plants: A Practical Reference Guide to More Than 550 Key Medicinal Plants & Their Uses.* 1st American ed. New York: Dorling Kindersley Publications, 1996.

Leung, A.Y., and S. Foster. *Encyclopedia of Common Natural Ingredients Used in Food, Drugs, and Cosmetics.* 2nd ed. New York: John Wiley & Sons, 1996.

Mayell, M. *Off-the-Shelf Natural Health: How to Use Herbs and Nutrients to Stay Well.* New York: Bantam Books, 1995.

Mindell, E. *Earl Mindell's Herb Bible.* New York: Simon & Schuster/Fireside, 1992.

TEXT CITATIONS:

1. A. Chevallier, *The Encyclopedia of Medicinal Plants: A Practical Reference Guide to More Than 550 Key Medicinal Plants & Their Uses,* 1st American ed. (New York: Dorling Kindersley Publications, 1996).
2. A.Y. Leung and S. Foster, *Encyclopedia of Common Natural Ingredients Used in Food, Drugs, and Cosmetics,* 2nd ed. (New York: John Wiley & Sons, 1996).
3. S.M. Bao, *Zhongguo Zhongyao Zazhi,* 14(5) (1989): 59.
4. J. Grujic-Vasic et al., *Planta Medica,* 55 (1989): 649.
5. Leung and Foster, op. cit.
6. Ibid.
7. B.H.S. Lau et al., *Phytotherapy Research,* 3(4) (1989): 148. D.T. Chu et al., *Journal of Clinical and Laboratory Immunology,* 25 (1988): 125. D.C. Wang et al., *Chinese Journal of Oncology,* 25 (1989):119. Leung and Foster, op. cit.
8. Y. Zhang et al., *Nanjing Yizueyuan Xuebao,* 12(3) (1992): 244–48.

9. D.T. Chu et al., *Chinese Journal of Oncology*, 16(3) (1994): 167–71.

10. S.Q. Li et al., *Chung-Kuo Chung Hsi I Chieh Ho Tsa Chih*, 15(2) (1995): 77–80.

11. L.X. Chen et al., *Chung-Kuo Chung Hsi I Chieh Ho Tsa Chih*, 15(3) (1995): 141–43.

12. Z.Y. Lei, *Chung-Kuo Chung Hsi I Chieh Ho Tsa Chih*, 13(7) (1993): 443–46.

13. Q. Guo et al., *Chung-Kuo Chung Hsi I Chieh Ho Tsa Chih*, 15(8) (1995): 483–85. T. Peng et al., *Chinese Medical Sciences Journal*, 10(3) (1995): 146–50.

14. Z.Q. Huang et al., *Chung-Kuo Chung Hsi I Chieh Ho Tsa Chih*, 15(6) (1995): 328–30.

15. Leung and Foster, op. cit. G.X. Hong et al., *Chung-Kuo Chung Yao Tsa Chih (China Journal of Chinese Materia Medica)*, 19(11) (1994): 687–88, 704. K.W. Zhao and H.Y. Kong, *Chung-Kuo Chung Hsi I Chieh Ho Tsa Chi*, 13(5) (1993): 259, 263–65.

16. Leung and Foster, op. cit.

PRIMARY NAME:
BALM

SCIENTIFIC NAME:
Melissa officinalis L. Family: Labiatae (Lamiaceae)

COMMON NAMES:
Bee balm, common balm, cure-all, lemon balm, melissa, oswego tea, sweet balm

RATING:
1 = Years of use and extensive, high-quality studies indicate that this substance is very effective and safe when used in recommended amounts for the indication(s) noted in the "Will It Work for You?" section.

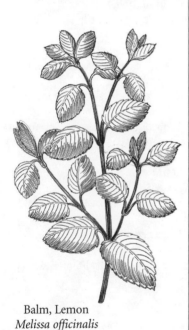

Balm, Lemon
Melissa officinalis

What Is Balm?

The lemon-scented leaves of this perennial member of the mint family are used medicinally, as are its small white or yellow flowers on occasion. Steam distillation of the leaves produces an essential oil. Do not confuse this herb with the common garden plant *Monarda didyma*, also called bee balm.

What It Is Used For:

Many of balm's calmative, antispasmodic, carminative (gas-relieving), and antiseptic properties were recognized by the ancient Greeks and Arabs. By the Middle Ages, folk healers considered balm something of a cure-all. Herbalists today enthusiastically carry on the tradition, recommending balm for relieving nervousness and anxiety, dissipating tension-related sleep problems, easing indigestion and nervousness-related stomach upset, stimulating the appetite, alleviating tension headaches, reducing nervous heart palpitations, and resolving menstrual cramps. Topical formulations are considered soothing healers for cuts, stings, wounds, and herpes-related cold sores and genital lesions.

Forms Available Include:

- *For internal use:* Concentrated drops, extracts, infusion, leaf (fresh and dried), oil, tincture.
- *For external use:* Compress, ointment, poultice.

A number of commercial preparations available abroad cannot be found in the United States.

Dosage Commonly Reported:

An infusion is made using 1 to 3 teaspoons crushed leaves per cup of water. The tincture is taken in dosages of ½ to 1½ teaspoons up to three times per day.

Will It Work for You? What the Studies Say:

Studies have substantiated the wisdom of several traditional uses for this herb. German researchers have shown that the volatile oil in the leaves—0.1 to 0.2 percent—calms the central nervous system (specifically, the limbic system) of laboratory animals.[1] The resulting tranquilizing, sedative, and antispasmodic actions (including relaxation of the smooth muscles of the digestive tract) are considered valuable for treating nervousness-related insomnia, stomach upset, and gas. German health authorities approve of balm for these conditions, and some physicians there extend the recommendations to conditions such as anxiety-related palpitations.[2] Balm also contains a bitter principle that may help control digestive upset and gas.

Based on human testing, even more evidence has been found for the capacity of specially prepared balm ointments and solutions to speed healing and reduce the recurrence of cold sores and genital lesions caused by the herpes simplex virus (types 1 or 2, respectively). An ointment for this purpose has been sold in Germany for a while and can now be found in some American outlets.[3] In one randomized double-blind trial involving 116 individuals, both those treated with the ointment and the physicians caring for them reported the cream more effective than the placebo it was tested against.[4] The ointment was most effective when treatment began at the first signs of infection. A cotton compress soaked in a strong infusion may have a similar effect.[5] A tannin and some polyphenols are believed to be responsible for the herb's antiviral actions.[6]

Research shows that balm fights certain other infection-causing viruses and bacteria as well, possibly helping to explain its enduring popularity as a first-aid treatment for cuts, stings, and other minor wounds.[7] Its astringent tannins may also contribute to healing and reducing oozing. Clinical trials to confirm its effectiveness in humans do not appear to have been done, however.

Will It Harm You? What the Studies Say:

No reports of significant adverse reactions to balm can be found after centuries of use. However, people with thyroid problems such as Graves' disease should probably avoid the herb (or get a doctor's approval) because research indicates that it inhibits certain thyroid hormones.[8] The FDA places balm on its list of herbs regarded as safe for food use.

GENERAL SOURCES:

American Pharmaceutical Association. *Handbook of Nonprescription Drugs.* 11th ed. Washington, D.C.: American Pharmaceutical Association, 1996.

Bisset, N.E., ed. *Herbal Drugs and Phytopharmaceuticals.* Stuttgart: medpharm GmbH Scientific Publishers, 1994.

Blumenthal, M., J. Gruenwald, T. Hall, and R.S. Rister, eds. *The Complete German Commission E Monographs: Therapeutic Guide to Herbal Medicine.* Boston: Integrative Medicine Communications, 1998.

Castleman, M. *The Healing Herbs: The Ultimate Guide to the Curative Power of Nature's Medicines.* New York: Bantam Books, 1995.

Chevallier, A. *The Encyclopedia of Medicinal Plants: A Practical Reference Guide to More Than 550 Key Medicinal Plants & Their Uses.* 1st American ed. New York: Dorling Kindersley Publications, 1996.

Leung, A.Y., and S. Foster. *Encyclopedia of Common Natural Ingredients Used in Food, Drugs, and Cosmetics.* 2nd ed. New York: John Wiley & Sons, 1996.

Mayell, M. *Off-the-Shelf Natural Health: How to Use Herbs and Nutrients to Stay Well.* New York: Bantam Books, 1995.

Tyler, V.E. *Herbs of Choice: The Therapeutic Use of Phytomedicinals.* Binghamton, NY: Haworth Press/Pharmaceutical Products Press, 1994.

Weiss, R.F. *Herbal Medicine,* trans. A. R. Meuss, from the 6th German edition. Beaconsfield, England: Beaconsfield Publishers, Ltd., 1988.

TEXT CITATIONS:

1. R.F. Weiss, *Herbal Medicine,* trans. A. R. Meuss, from the 6th German edition. (Beaconsfield, England: Beaconsfield Publishers, Ltd., 1988).
2. M. Blumenthal, J. Gruenwald, T. Hall, and R.S. Rister, eds., *The Complete German Commission E Monographs: Therapeutic Guide to Herbal Medicine* (Boston: Integrative Medicine Communications, 1998).
3. American Pharmaceutical Association, *Handbook of Nonprescription Drugs,* 11th ed. (Washington, D.C.: American Pharmaceutical Association, 1996).
4. R.H. Wobilng and K. Leonhardt, *Phytomedicine,* 1 (1994): 25–31.
5. V.E. Tyler, *Herbs of Choice: The Therapeutic Use of Phytomedicinals* (Binghamton, NY: Haworth Press/Pharmaceutical Products Press, 1994).
6. A.Y. Leung and S. Foster, *Encyclopedia of Common Natural Ingredients Used in Food,*

Drugs, and Cosmetics, 2nd ed. (New York: John Wiley & Sons, 1996). L.S. Kucera and E.C. Herrmann, Jr., *Proceedings of the Society for Experimental Biology and Medicine*, 124 (1967): 865, 869.

7. Leung and Foster, op. cit.
8. H. Sourgens et al., *Planta Medica*, 45(2) (1982): 78–86. M. Auf'mkolk et al., *Endocrinology*, 116(5) (1985): 1687–93. M. Auf'mkolk et al., *Hormone and Metabolic Research*, 16(4) (1984): 188–92.

PRIMARY NAME:
BARBERRY

SCIENTIFIC NAME:
Berberis vulgaris L. Family: Berberidaceae

COMMON NAMES:
Berberis, common barberry, European barberry, pepperidge bush, sour-spine, sowberry, woodsour

RATING:
3 = Studies on the effectiveness and safety of this substance are conflicting, or there are not enough studies to draw a conclusion.

What Is Barberry?

Berberis vulgaris is a native European shrub now found in eastern North America. Primarily the dried stem and root bark of this deciduous perennial are used medicinally. Bright yellow flowers bloom in clusters and eventually turn into edible red berries. For information on the closely related (indigenous) American variant, *Berberis aquifolium*, see **Wild Oregon Grape**.

What It Is Used For:

Although this herb is far less popular today, folk healers from Russia to India for centuries turned to it to remedy stomach upset and ulcers, diarrhea, heartburn, high blood pressure, cough-related congestion, mouth ulcers and sore throat, fever, infections, and abnormal uterine bleeding. The ancient Egyptians reportedly took barberry to prevent plague. Large doses have a powerful laxative effect. Traditional healers in medieval Europe, believing that the appearance of a plant holds clues to its healing powers, treated symptoms of liver disease with it; the yellow flowers and root brought to mind the yellowing skin and eyes produced by jaundice.[1]

Interestingly, independent of the rest of the world, Native Americans turned to the indigenous American version of barberry (wild oregon grape) as a healing agent too, as did Chinese healers using their native variants. Barberry appeared in controversial cancer therapies of the early 1900s. Homeopaths recommend minute amounts for ailments ranging from arthritis to intestinal disorders, sciatica, and herpes. (See page 000 for more information on homeopathy.) The edible, vitamin-C-rich berries appear in jams and jellies and the roots were once popular as a source of yellow dye.

Forms Available Include:

- *For internal use:* Bark, capsule, decoction, root (powdered), tincture. Herbalists recommend masking the bark's bitter taste by adding honey or mixing it into an herbal blend.
- *For external use:* Eye compress (made with infusion), eyedrops, eyewash. The drops may not be available in the United States.

Dosage Commonly Reported:

A decoction is made using ½ teaspoon of powdered root bark per cup of water and is drunk once per day. The decoction is also used in a compress. The tincture is taken in dosages of 1½ to 3 teaspoons three times per day. The recommendation depends in part on whether the formula contains a high concentration of alcohol; the dropperful may be a more appropriate dosage if the alcohol content is high, for example.

Will It Work for You? What the Studies Say:

Researchers have identified several active ingredients in barberry, shedding light on numerous traditional uses. Similar active properties can be expected from closely related *Berberis* species; see **Wild Oregon Grape** and **Goldenseal**. All contain high concentrations of active alkaloid salts—berberine in particular—that fight bacteria, fungi, and parasites responsible for certain wound and urinary tract infections, vaginal yeast infections, cholera, and diarrhea. In one experiment, berberine's bacteria-killing powers proved more powerful than those of a widely accepted antibiotic, chloramphenicol.[2]

Another alkaloid—berbamine—appears to help fight infection by stimulating the white blood cells (macrophages) critical to the body's defense force, as was observed in a mouse study.[3] One study found that individuals suffering from cholera-induced diarrhea experienced significant relief from acute watery diarrhea (and reduced excretion of the virus) after twenty-four hours when they took berberine (100 milligrams four times a day; in some cases combined with tetracycline), at least in comparison with sufferers taking a placebo.[4] Barberry's ability to fight diarrhea caused by other organisms is less clear. Experts do not consider the herb's astringent tannins, substances normally linked with an antidiarrheal effect, responsible for this.[5] Scientists have also identified sedative, anticonvulsant, antifibrillatory (preventing disorganized electrical activity in the heart), and uterine stimulant properties in berberine, and other alkaloids and substances have shown notable blood-pressure-lowering, antispasmodic, and amebicide properties.[6]

The herb's practical use in today's world is unclear, however, and, citing a lack of proven effectiveness in humans, German health authorities have declined to officially approve of the herb for any ailment.[7] Although very uncommon in the United States today, berberine salts isolated from the plant were once frequently used in the form of eyedrops to soothe inflamed lids, control allergic conjunctivitis (pinkeye), and revive sore, sensitive, and bloodshot eyes. The antiseptic, astringent, and anti-inflammatory properties of the herb were considered responsible for this effect. Physicians in some other countries including Germany still recommend this, claiming good tolerance and rapid results.

Will It Harm You? What the Studies Say:

Berberine and berberine-containing plants are generally considered nontoxic at commonly reported doses. Take note, however, that although poisonings from the herb itself have not been documented, berberine doses greater than 0.5 gram have been associated with skin and eye irritation, nosebleeds, shortness of breath, lethargy, nausea, vomiting, and diarrhea.[8] Kidney irritation and inflammation have occurred, and there have been cases of fatal poisonings in humans.[9] Normal metabolism of vitamin B may be altered with high doses. Pregnant women should probably avoid the herb, given still unconfirmed reports that it can stimulate the uterine muscles.

GENERAL SOURCES:

Blumenthal, M., J. Gruenwald, T. Hall, and R.S. Rister, eds. *The Complete German Commission E Monographs: Therapeutic Guide to Herbal Medicine.* Boston: Integrative Medicine Communications, 1998.

Castleman, M. *The Healing Herbs: The Ultimate Guide to the Curative Power of Nature's Medicines.* New York: Bantam Books, 1995.

Lawrence Review of Natural Products. St. Louis: Facts and Comparisons, July 1991.

Leung, A.Y., and S. Foster. *Encyclopedia of Common Natural Ingredients Used in Food, Drugs, and Cosmetics.* 2nd ed. New York: John Wiley & Sons, 1996.

Murray, M.T. *The Healing Power of Herbs: The Enlightened Person's Guide to the Wonders of Medicinal Plants.* Revised and expanded 2nd ed. Rocklin, CA: Prima Publishing, 1995.

Tyler, V.E. *The Honest Herbal.* Binghamton, NY: Haworth Press/Pharmaceutical Products Press, 1993.

Weiss, R.F. *Herbal Medicine*, trans. A. R. Meuss, from the 6th German edition. Beaconsfield, England: Beaconsfield Publishers, Ltd., 1988.

TEXT CITATIONS:

1. M. Castleman, *The Healing Herbs: The Ultimate Guide to the Curative Power of Nature's Medicines* (New York: Bantam Books, 1995).

2. A.Y. Leung and S. Foster, *Encyclopedia of Common Natural Ingredients Used in Food, Drugs, and Cosmetics*, 2nd ed. (New York: John Wiley & Sons, 1996).

3. L. Lin and W.Z. Sui, *Zhongguo Yaoli Xuebao*, 7 (1986): 475.

4. K.U. Maung et al., *British Medical Journal*, 291 (1985): 1601. M.H. Akheter et al., *Indian Journal of Medical Research*, 70 (1979): 233. *Lawrence Review of Natural Products* (St. Louis: Facts and Comparisons, July 1991).

5. *Lawrence Review*, op. cit. Akhtar, *International Journal of Pharmacology*, 30 (1992): 97.

6. Leung and Foster, op. cit.

7. M. Blumenthal, J. Gruenwald, T. Hall, and R.S. Rister, eds., *The Complete German Commission E Monographs: Therapeutic Guide to Herbal Medicine* (Boston: Integrative Medicine Communications, 1998). V.E. Tyler, *The Honest Herbal* (Binghamton, NY: Haworth Press/Pharmaceutical Products Press, 1993).

8. Blumenthal et al., op. cit.

9. Ibid.

PRIMARY NAME:

BARLEY (and BARLEY GRASS)

SCIENTIFIC NAME:
Hordeum vulgare L. Family: Gramineae

COMMON NAME:
Hordeum

What Is Barley?

Barley is a cereal grass. The name refers to the seeds or grain of that grass as well. It has been cultivated in virtually all parts of the inhabited earth. The grass is an annual with straight, hollow stems that mature to a golden brown and taper off into characteristic long bristles, atop which spikelets bear rows of husk-covered seeds—the grain. There are many varieties of barley.

What It Is Used For:

Humans have been cultivating barley since ancient times as a nourishing food and healing agent. Gladiators ate barley to strengthen themselves before a fight. As late as the 1500s, it served as the primary bread grain in Europe. Today barley appears in cereals, soups, countless other foods, and animal feed, and plays an important role in brewing beer. Many herbalists carry on a tradition begun by the ancient Greeks of soothing a sore or inflamed throat or bowel (some-

BARLEY (and BARLEY GRASS) (Continued)

RATING:

- *Barley:* 2 = According to a number of well-designed studies and common use, this substance appears to be relatively effective and safe when used in recommended amounts for the indications noted in the "Will It Work for You?" section.
- *Barley grass:* 4 = Research indicates that this substance will not fulfill the claims made for it, but that it is also unlikely to cause any harm.

times involving diarrhea) with barley porridge or water. Many a convalescent of yore was reportedly coaxed back to health with such a regimen. Traditional Chinese healers recommend barley to strengthen digestion and stimulate the appetite. Contemporary Western herbalists also consider barley a good cholesterol-lowering source of fiber. It is occasionally drunk as a tea or coffee. Teas and poultices are applied topically to treat sores, swellings, and blemishes, and many herbal facial masks contain the grain.

Supplement manufacturers sell a "green food" supplement made of barley grass (harvested before the grain develops). They bill it as an immune system booster, an antioxidant, a chlorophyll source, and a preventive agent and cure for cancer, diabetes, arthritis, heart disease, and many other ailments.

Forms Available Include:

- *Barley grain:* Dry-roasted, malted, pearled. Also available in numerous commercial products, including flour, tea, and barley water.
- *Barley grass:* Capsule, powder (for liquid mixtures). Often included in herbal blends.

Dosage Commonly Reported:

Barley is most commonly consumed as a food. For commercial dietary supplements of barley grass, follow package instructions.

Will It Work for You? What the Studies Say:

The grain's vitamin- and amino-acid–rich hull is polished to produce "pearl" barley, the form in which most people consume it. The high-fiber material remains. According to preliminary but promising studies, high-fiber foods such as barley may encourage lower cholesterol levels, help control high blood sugar, and even help prevent certain kinds of cancer. Research indicates that a fiber in barley—beta-glucan (also found in oat bran)—can reduce cholesterol levels.[1] In a well-designed 1994 study involving seventy-nine individuals with high cholesterol, the addition of barley bran flour or barley oil significantly enhanced the cholesterol-lowering effect of the diet they undertook. Importantly, while total serum cholesterol levels and damaging low-density lipoprotein (LDL) cholesterol significantly decreased in the barley-consuming subjects, they did not decrease in those taking a placebo.[2]

Another important study, this one with potential implications for diabetes sufferers, recorded lower sugar and insulin levels in healthy subjects consuming barley-based breads than in subjects using white or pumpernickel bread.[3] Cancer-related findings have also been intriguing. Spent barley grain has been shown to protect against the risk of colon cancer in rats, and in a related finding, barley bran flour significantly accelerated the time it took for food to pass through the stomach and intestines of subjects in a medium-sized (forty-four-subject) placebo-controlled trial.[4] Germinated barley seeds also contain the alkaloids hordenine and gramine, both of which have shown interesting pharmacological properties.[5]

Barley "green" products offer the consumer relatively insignificant amounts of usable nutrients, and none that cannot be obtained in a balanced diet.[6] The grass does contain chlorophyll, the pigment responsible for making green plants green, but researchers have yet to demonstrate any beneficial therapeutic activity of chlorophyll taken as a dietary supplement. The FDA has ordered manufacturers of the "green food" product called "Barley Grass" to stop making unsubstantiated and often inconsistent claims regarding its ability to help prevent or cure a wide variety of serious ailments, including cancer and heart disease.[7]

Will It Harm You? What the Studies Say:

Countless millions have consumed barley over the centuries with no apparent ill effect. However, people who have difficulty digesting gluten, such as those with celiac disease, should avoid the grain because it does contain low levels of this substance.[8]

GENERAL SOURCES:

Barrett, S., and V. Herbert. *The Vitamin Pushers: How the "Health Food" Industry Is Selling America a Bill of Goods.* Amherst, NY: Prometheus Books, 1994.

Bremness, L. *Herbs.* 1st American ed. Eyewitness Handbooks. New York: Dorling Kindersley Publications, 1994.

Chevallier, A. *The Encyclopedia of Medicinal Plants: A Practical Reference Guide to More Than 550 Key Medicinal Plants & Their Uses.* 1st American ed. New York: Dorling Kindersley Publications, 1996.

Lawrence Review of Natural Products. St. Louis: Facts and Comparisons, November 1994.

Mayell, M. *Off-the-Shelf Natural Health: How to Use Herbs and Nutrients to Stay Well.* New York: Bantam Books, 1995.

Tierra, M. *The Way of Herbs.* New York: Pocket Books, 1990.

Weiss, R.F. *Herbal Medicine,* trans. A. R. Meuss, from the 6th German edition. Beaconsfield, England: Beaconsfield Publisher, Ltd., 1988.

TEXT CITATIONS:

1. *Lawrence Review of Natural Products* (St. Louis: Facts and Comparisons, November 1994).
2. J.R. Lupton et al., *Journal of the American Dietetic Association,* 94(1) (1994): 65–70.
3. Y. Granfeldt et al., *American Journal of Clinical Nutrition,* Beaconsfield, England: Beaxonsfield Publishers, Ltd., 1988. 59 (1994): 1057.
4. *Lawrence Review of Natural Products,* op. cit. J.R. Lupton et al., *Journal of the American Dietetic Association,* 93 (1993): 881–85.
5. H.J. Hapke and W. Strathmann, *Deutsche Tierarztliche Wochenschrift,* 102(6) (1995): 228–32.
6. S. Barrett and V. Herbert, *The Vitamin Pushers: How the "Health Food" Industry Is Selling America a Bill of Goods* (Amherst, NY: Prometheus Books, 1994).
7. Ibid.
8. P.G. Ciclitira et al., *Panminerva Medica,* 33 (1991): 75.

PRIMARY NAME:

BASIL

What Is Basil?

Basil is a beloved culinary herb, used particularly in Mediterranean cuisine. Many varieties of this fragrant annual grow wild and are cultivated in North America. Its flowering tops and dried leaves are used medicinally. Steam distillation produces an essential oil.

SCIENTIFIC NAME:

Ocimum basilicum L. Family: Labiatae (Lamiaceae)

COMMON NAMES:

Common basil, garden basil, St. Josephwort, sweet basil

RATING:

3 = Studies on the effectiveness and safety of this substance are conflicting, or there are not enough studies to draw a conclusion.

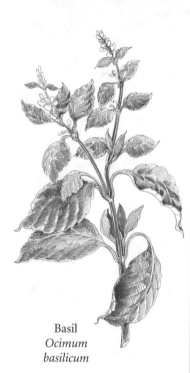

Basil
*Ocimum
basilicum*

What It Is Used For:

Generations have celebrated the distinctive, slightly peppery taste of this member of the mint family. As an herbal remedy, it has had a remarkably mixed reputation over the centuries: Some have hailed it as a healer, others as a poison. Today the former perspective prevails, and many people around the world sip basil tea for such broad-ranging ailments as intestinal parasites, congestive heart failure, alcoholism, and depression, as well as to promote urine flow (as a diuretic) and stimulate the body's defense system against chills, colds, and nervous exhaustion.

American herbalists carry on the age-old practice, still healthful in Mediterranean countries, of enlisting basil as an appetite stimulant; digestive aid; and soothing agent for stomach cramps, nausea, constipation, and excess gas. External preparations have been used to encourage wound healing, control itching and swelling from snakebites; fight ringworm and warts; and disinfect and calm throat inflammation. Inhaling the steam rising from basil leaves boiling in water is said to ease a head cold. Basil commands great respect in the repertoires of Asian traditional healers. The Chinese have used it for centuries to encourage good blood circulation after labor and treat kidney ailments and stomach spasms.

Forms Available Include:

- *For internal use:* Extracts, fresh or dried leaf, infusion, medicinal-strength oil, tincture.
- *For external use:* Extracts, gargle, infusion, medicinal-strength oil, ointment, tincture.

Dosage Commonly Reported:

A tea is made using 1 to 2 heaping teaspoons of chopped herb per cup of water and is drunk two to three times per day between meals. Plant experts advise caution, however, as all forms may contain safrole (see "Will It Harm You?" section for more information).

Will It Work for You? What the Studies Say:

Of the dozens of healing powers attributed to basil, only a handful have withstood the rigors of scientific examination and none appears to have been subjected to well-designed clinical trials in humans. Investigators have discovered that basil's essential oil fights intestinal parasites, which may help explain its long-standing reputation as a remedy for related stomach upset.[1] Germans and others commonly drink basil tea for bloating and excess gas, apparently on the theory that its essential oil can help alleviate such conditions. Researchers studying laboratory mice have reported finding antiulcer activity in leaf extracts.[2]

Basil displays bacteria-killing properties when applied to the skin, so it is no surprise to find extracts in wound ointments. One study indicated that the essential oil could successfully treat acne.[3] Relatively high concentrations of antioxidant vitamins (A and C) in basil may help scavenge toxic by-products that contribute to cancer cell formation. In a test-tube study of spices and vegetables, basil leaves performed well enough to be classified as "protective" against carcinogenesis (cancer formation).[4] Much more research is needed, however. Basil leaves have also shown potential in preventing dental plaque.[5]

Will It Harm You? What the Studies Say:

Medicinal concentrations of this herb have never caused anyone apparent harm. Even the essential oil appears to be nontoxic.[6] U.S. health authorities and plant experts apparently consider minimal the risk of tumor formation raised by reports in the mid-1970s; at that time it was reported that a chemical in basil called estragole could cause liver tumors in mice.[7] The mice were given the herb's essential oil, of which estragole is a major ingredient. Another constituent, safrole, is reportedly carcinogenic as well. The FDA continues to classify basil as a safe food. German health authorities, on the other hand, concerned about the potential carcinogenic effect of substances in basil oil, do not approve of its use in medicinal concentrations.[8] They also warn that infants, toddlers, and pregnant and nursing women should not take basil oil. Many cultures consider basil a menstruation promoter and labor inducer, although no evidence can be found in the literature to indicate that these reactions occur or that the herb in any way stimulates the uterus.

GENERAL SOURCES:

Bisset, N.E., ed. *Herbal Drugs and Phytopharmaceuticals.* Stuttgart: medpharm GmbH Scientific Publishers, 1994.

Blumenthal, M., J. Gruenwald, T. Hall, and R.S. Rister, eds. *The Complete German Commission E Monographs: Therapeutic Guide to Herbal Medicine.* Boston: Integrative Medicine Communications, 1998.

Castleman, M. *The Healing Herbs: The Ultimate Guide to the Curative Power of Nature's Medicines.* New York: Bantam Books, 1995.

Drinkwater, N.R., et al. *Journal of the National Cancer Institute,* 57 (1976): 1323.

Duke, J.A. *CRC Handbook of Medicinal Herbs.* Boca Raton, FL: CRC Press, 1985.

Godhwani, B., et al. *Journal of Ethnopharmacology,* 24 (1988): 193.

Leung, A.Y. *Encyclopedia of Common Natural Ingredients Used in Food, Drugs, and Cosmetics.* New York: John Wiley & Sons, 1980.

Miller, E.C., et al. *Cancer Research.* 43 (1983): 1124.

Mindell, E. *Earl Mindell's Herb Bible.* New York: Simon & Schuster/Fireside, 1992.

Ody P. *The Herb Society's Complete Medicinal Herbal.* London: Dorling Kindersley Limited, 1993.

Opdyke, D.L.J. *Food & Cosmetics Toxicology.* 11 (1973): 867.

Tyler, V.E. *Herbs of Choice: The Therapeutic Use of Phytomedicinals.* Binghamton, NY: Haworth Press/Pharmaceutical Products Press, 1994.

TEXT CITATIONS:

1. S.R. Jain and M.L. Jain, *Planta Medica,* 24(3) (1973): 286–89. M.L. Jain and S.R. Jain, *Planta Medica,* 22 (1972): 66–70.
2. M.S. Akhtar et al., *International Journal of Pharmacology,* 30 (1992): 97.
3. R. Balambal et al., *Journal of the Association of Physicians of India,* 33 (1985): 507–8.
4. K. Aruna and V.M. Sivaramakrishnan, *Indian Journal of Experimental Biology,* 28(11) (1990): 1008–11.
5. V.E. Tyler, *Herbs of Choice: The Therapeutic Use of Phytomedicinals* (Binghamton, NY: Haworth Press/Pharmaceutical Products Press, 1994).

6. E.C. Miller et al., *Cancer Research*, 43 (1983): 1124.
7. N.R. Drinkwater et al., *Journal of the National Cancer Institute*, 57 (1976): 1323.
8. M. Blumenthal, J. Gruenwald, T. Hall, and R.S. Rister, eds., *The Complete German Commission E Monographs: Therapeutic Guide to Herbal Medicine* (Boston: Integrative Medicine Communications, 1998).

PRIMARY NAME:
BAY, SWEET

SCIENTIFIC NAME:
Laurus nobilis L. Family:
Lauraceae

COMMON NAMES:
Bay, bay laurel, Grecian laurel, green bay, laurel, Mediterranean bay, true bay, true laurel

RATING:
4 = Research indicates that this substance will not fulfill the claims made for it, but that it is also unlikely to cause any harm.

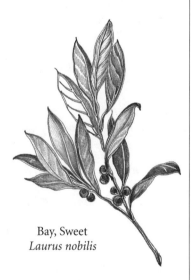

Bay, Sweet
Laurus nobilis

What Is Sweet Bay?

This small, aromatic flowering evergreen tree is widely cultivated but notoriously difficult to grow. The leathery dark green leaves and shiny black berries are dried and used medicinally. Steam distillation of the leaves and branches produces an essential oil.

What It Is Used For:

Aside from its rich symbolic and culinary history stretching back to biblical times, past cultures revered this now common household herb as a healer and protector. Various preparations of the dried or fresh leaves, the essential oil, and the berries have been used as relaxants, appetite stimulants, sweat-inducers (once valued for lowering fevers), indigestion and colic relievers, flatulence (gas) remedies, and menstruation promoters. Topical formulations have been applied to arthritic aches and pains, sprains, bruises, insect stings, sores, other skin irritations, and scalp conditions such as dandruff. Some contemporary herbalists continue to encourage a number of these uses.

Forms Available Include:

- *For internal use:* Infusion (typically made with crushed leaves), oil, tincture.
- *For external use:* Decoction, leaf (fresh and dried), oil, poultice.

Dosage Commonly Reported:

An infusion is made using 1 to 2 teaspoons crushed leaves per cup of water and is drunk up to three times per day. One or two drops of the oil are added to tea, brandy, or honey.

Will It Work for You? What the Studies Say:

Mice administered bay oil, which contains a substance called methyl eugenol (4 percent), have reportedly become sedated at low doses and showed signs of reversible narcosis at high doses.[1] The essential oil likewise mildly lowered blood pressure and slowed the heartbeat in laboratory animals in another study.[2] Whether the same changes occur in the human nervous system is impossible to say at this point, although this does not deter some herbalists who continue to recommend bay for making a relaxing infusion.[3]

As with many other herbs, the value of bay leaf infusion in settling the stomach, stimulating the appetite, and preventing gas may be explained by the presence of a volatile oil (up to 3 percent). The property has not been well described with bay, however. Test-tube studies indicate that bay extracts kill a number of disease-causing bacteria, fungi, and viruses, and some commercial German antiviral products contain bay extracts.[4] But just how effective or practical bay in homemade forms is for disinfecting minor cuts or other wounds remains unclear. No studies have ever shown that bay preparations can ease arthritis pain or reduce inflammation, nor can evidence be found to substantiate the millennia-old custom of using bay to promote menstruation. According to a 1981 study, bay contains cockroach-repelling compounds, including cineole (up to 50 percent in the volatile oil).[5]

Will It Harm You? What the Studies Say:

Bay infusions and other medicinal-strength preparations appear to be generally safe to use, although external formulations occasionally cause rashes and other skin reactions in people with sensitive skin. Avoid ingesting the essential oil. Pregnant women may want to avoid medicinal-strength preparations, given the very old—and still unproven—belief that the herb can stimulate the uterus.

GENERAL SOURCES:

Castleman, M. *The Healing Herbs: The Ultimate Guide to the Curative Power of Nature's Medicines.* New York: Bantam Books, 1995.

Chevallier, A. *The Encyclopedia of Medicinal Plants: A Practical Reference Guide to More Than 550 Key Medicinal Plants & Their Uses.* 1st American ed. New York: Dorling Kindersley Publications, 1996.

Duke, J.A. *CRC Handbook of Medicinal Herbs.* Boca Raton, FL: CRC Press, 1985.

Foster, S., and J.A. Duke. *The Peterson Field Guide Series: A Field Guide to Medicinal Plants. Eastern and Central North America.* Boston: Houghton Mifflin Company, 1990.

Hylton, W.H., ed. *The Rodale Herb Book: How to Use, Grow, and Buy Nature's Miracle Plants.* Emmaus, PA: Rodale Press, Inc., 1974.

Leung, A.Y., and S. Foster. *Encyclopedia of Common Natural Ingredients Used in Food, Drugs, and Cosmetics.* 2nd ed. New York: John Wiley & Sons, 1996.

Tierra, M. *The Way of Herbs.* New York: Pocket Books, 1990.

TEXT CITATIONS:

1. A.Y. Leung and S. Foster, *Encyclopedia of Common Natural Ingredients Used in Food, Drugs, and Cosmetics,* 2nd ed. (New York: John Wiley & Sons, 1996).
2. Ibid.
3. M. Castleman, *The Healing Herbs: The Ultimate Guide to the Curative Power of Nature's Medicines* (New York: Bantam Books, 1995).
4. S. Foster and J.A. Duke, *The Peterson Field Guide Series: A Field Guide to Medicinal Plants. Eastern and Central North America* (Boston: Houghton Mifflin Company, 1990).
5. M.M. Verma, *Dissertation Abstract International B,* 41(12, Pt.1) (1981): 4514.

PRIMARY NAME:
BAYBERRY

What Is Bayberry?

The native American bayberry shrub, an evergreen, populates southern and eastern regions of the country. It bears small bluish-white fruits ("berries") and yellow flowers. The dried root bark is used medicinally, although some folk traditions consider the waxy material on the berries healing as well.

BAYBERRY (Continued)

SCIENTIFIC NAME:
Myrica cerifera L. and *Myrica pennsylvanica* L. Family: Myricaceae

COMMON NAMES:
Candleberry, southern bayberry, southern wax myrtle, tallow shrub, waxberry, wax myrtle

RATING:
5 = Studies indicate that there is a definite health hazard to using this substance, even in recommended amounts.

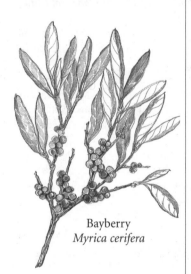

Bayberry
Myrica cerifera

What It Is Used For:

Only a handful of Native American tribes were reportedly using the bayberry for medicinal purposes when European settlers arrived. Some herbalists continue to recommend bayberry for the wide range of ailments proposed over the decades. Many consider it valuable as an internal stimulant, tonic, fever-reducer, astringent (for diarrhea and infectious diarrhea especially), headache remedy, and expectorant to clear congestion during colds and flu. A douche is recommended for excess vaginal discharge; a poultice for hard-to-heal ulcers, hemorrhoids, and varicose veins; a gargle for sore throats; and a mouthwash for sensitive gums. Large doses were once used to induce vomiting in poisonings. The root bark can be found in "Dr. Thompson's Composition" (possibly sold under an abbreviated name today), a treatment for colds, fever, and other ailments patented by nineteenth-century New England herbalist Samuel A. Thompson. The waxy berries have long been used to create scented candles.

Forms Available Include:

Capsule, decoction, extract, infusion, mouthwash, powder, tincture.

Dosage Commonly Reported:

Bayberry should not be used medicinally.

Will It Work for You? What the Studies Say:

Sound scientific evidence to support the use of bayberry internally for any ailment is lacking, and the potential hazard its high tannin content poses only reinforces the arguments against using it. (See "Will It Harm You?") Tannins are astringent, however, which probably explains why so many people once relied on it to control diarrhea (tannins are believed to reduce intestinal inflammation) and to treat ulcers, hemorrhoids, and sore throats topically.

Researchers have identified other notable ingredients in bayberry: three triterpenes, including one (myricadiol) with mineralocorticoid activity that can presumably influence the body's metabolism of sodium and potassium. Test-tube studies also indicate that a flavonoid glycoside (myricitrin) can stimulate bile flow, a property sometimes beneficial for liver and gallbladder ailments. Myricitrin apparently also kills sperm and certain kinds of bacteria and paramecia.[1] What these findings mean for treating disease is still unclear.

Will It Harm You? What the Studies Say:

Although some sources simply recommend avoiding excessive doses of this herb, a number of others consider the health risks of bayberry too great to justify its use, especially given the availability of safer and more proven herbal remedies.[2] Tannins in high concentrations can cause cancer in laboratory animals. In one study, a significant number of malignant tumors developed over a seventy-eight-week stretch of time in rats injected with tannins and phenols isolated from bayberry bark.[3] Much remains to be learned about the cancer risk posed by tannins and other possibly toxic ingredients in bayberry. Anecdotal evidence collected over decades suggests that the herb can cause stomach irritation, nausea, and vomiting, especially in large doses.

GENERAL SOURCES:

Castleman, M. *The Healing Herbs: The Ultimate Guide to the Curative Power of Nature's Medicines.* New York: Bantam Books, 1995.

Duke, J.A. *CRC Handbook of Medicinal Herbs.* Boca Raton, FL: CRC Press, 1985.

Lawrence Review of Natural Products. St. Louis: Facts and Comparisons, August 1991.

Leung, A.Y., and S. Foster. *Encyclopedia of Common Natural Ingredients Used in Food, Drugs, and Cosmetics.* 2nd ed. New York: John Wiley & Sons, 1996.

Mindell, E. *Earl Mindell's Herb Bible.* New York: Simon & Schuster/Fireside, 1992.

Tyler, V.E. *The Honest Herbal.* Binghamton, NY: Haworth Press/Pharmaceutical Products Press, 1993.

TEXT CITATIONS:

1. B.D. Paul et al., *Journal of Pharmaceutical Sciences*, 63 (1974): 958.

2. V.E. Tyler, *The Honest Herbal* (Binghamton, NY: Haworth Press/Pharmaceutical Products Press, 1993.). *Lawrence Review of Natural Products* (St. Louis: Facts and Comparisons, August 1991).

3. G.J. Kapadia et al., *Journal of the National Cancer Institute*, 57 (1976): 207.

PRIMARY NAME:

BEE POLLEN

SCIENTIFIC NAME:

N/A

COMMON NAMES:

Buckwheat pollen, maize pollen, pine pollen, pollen, puhuang, rape pollen, typha pollen[1]

RATING:

3 = Studies on the effectiveness and safety of this substance are conflicting, or there are not enough studies to draw a conclusion.

What Is Bee Pollen?

Bee pollen refers to the pollen collected by worker bees from the flowers of certain seed-bearing plants. True bee pollen also contains the insect's saliva and some plant nectar. Harvesters retrieve the pollen directly from the hive or from special wire-mesh, netlike traps that brush against the legs of worker bees as they enter the hive. Some products labeled as bee pollen may actually be harvested directly by humans, however. These are more accurately referred to as "bee-free pollen" or simply, "pollen."

What It Is Used For:

In some parts of the world, including China, people have been taking bee pollen for centuries as a nutrient and to remedy such wide-ranging ailments as eczema, mouth sores, hemorrhage, and menstrual irregularities. In the United States, pollen has long been used in carefully controlled medical environments (such as doctors' offices) to detect allergies and foster immunity against allergies, but has only recently been promoted as a general health tonic, a source of "natural vitality" to boost athletic stamina and ability, and a remedy for a host of debilitating conditions ranging from anemia to constipation, diarrhea, mental illness, premature aging, and obesity. (Interestingly, it has also been promoted for weight gain.) Many health food outlets bill bee pollen as a "perfect food," an energy-packed food supplement rich with protein and carbohydrates. Some tout it as an appetite stimulant. Bee pollen extracts appear in numerous skin-care products.

Forms Available Include:

Capsule, extracts (for internal and external use), granules, liquid (including syrup), tablet.

Dosage Commonly Reported:

Bee pollen is commonly sold in the form of 500- or 586-milligram tablets. A typical recommendation is to take three capsules three times a day.

Will It Work for You? What the Studies Say:

Individual testimonials extolling the benefits of bee pollen, particularly for athletic performance, are not hard to find. But the truth is that sound scientific evidence to support the use of bee pollen to enhance health or to treat any human disease is lacking. Not even its ingredients offer much promise.[2] The substance is clearly nutrient-rich; it consists of about 55 percent carbohydrates, 30 percent protein, 1 to 2 percent fat, 3 percent minerals, and trace vitamins (sometimes including high concentrations of vitamin C). Not only do these concentrations vary considerably, depending on the plant from which the bee collected the material, but similarly nutritious foods can be found at much lower prices.

Most studies describing enhanced athletic performance with bee pollen supplements have emanated from the former Soviet Union or Eastern Europe and were not very well monitored.[3] On the other hand, relatively rigorous Western studies on swimmers, weight lifters, and nonathletes indicate that these supplements endow the user with no greater strength, stamina, or superior performance than a placebo. For example, in a two-year double-blind study, the swim team members at Louisiana State University who were given bee pollen did not perform better, train better, or exhibit better metabolism than swimmers taking a placebo; to avoid bias, neither the athletes nor the testers knew who was receiving the bee pollen.[4]

Intriguing test-tube and animal studies of other properties in bee pollen demand further examination and repetition before any conclusions can be made about their value for human health.[5] The Chinese appear to have studied bee pollen most extensively. They and others report that the substance may help treat chronic prostatism,[6] inhibit prostate overgrowth (tested in aged dogs),[7] counter the effects of aging (tested in rats),[8] protect the liver from experimental injury (in laboratory animals),[9] boost the immune systems of medicated multiple sclerosis patients,[10] reduce symptoms of radiation sickness in people being treated for cancer,[11] and lower blood fat levels (in humans and laboratory animals).[12] German health authorities were satisfied enough with the scientific evidence presented to them to approve of raw pollen from various flowering plants (in the form of a tonic) for stimulating the appetite and treating feebleness.[13]

Will It Harm You? What the Studies Say:

Although infrequent, severe and even fatal allergic reactions to bee pollen are possible. Individuals with pollen-sensitive allergies are particularly at risk. Hay fever sufferers have experienced dramatic reactions, some after single doses of

1 tablespoon or less of the product.[14] There has been at least one case of life-threatening anaphylactic shock (a severe allergic reaction) to bee pollen in an individual with no history of such allergies.[15]

If you decide to take bee pollen products, stick to commercial sources. Some herbalists recommend starting out with small doses to test your reaction, but given the variability in pollen content among products, this approach poses some risk as well. One expert warns pregnant women to avoid bee pollen, given indications that certain pollens (puhuang) may stimulate the uterus.[16]

GENERAL SOURCES:

Balch, J.F., and P.A. Balch. *Prescription for Nutritional Healing: A Practical A to Z Reference to Drug-Free Remedies Using Vitamins, Minerals, Herbs & Food Supplements*. 2nd ed. Garden City Park, NY: Avery Publishing Group, 1997.

Barrett, S., and V. Herbert. *The Vitamin Pushers: How the "Health Food" Industry Is Selling America a Bill of Goods*. Amherst, NY: Prometheus Books, 1994.

Der Marderosian, A., and L. Liberti. *Natural Product Medicine: A Scientific Guide to Foods, Drugs, Cosmetics*. Philadelphia: George F. Stickley, 1988.

Duke, J.A. *CRC Handbook of Medicinal Herbs*. Boca Raton, FL: CRC Press, 1985.

Lawrence Review of Natural Products. St. Louis: Facts and Comparisons, November 1995.

Leung, A.Y., and S. Foster. *Encyclopedia of Common Natural Ingredients Used in Food, Drugs, and Cosmetics*. 2nd ed. New York: John Wiley & Sons, 1996.

Mayell, M. *Off-the-Shelf Natural Health: How to Use Herbs and Nutrients to Stay Well*. New York: Bantam Books, 1995.

Tyler, V.E. *The Honest Herbal*. Binghamton, NY: Haworth Press/Pharmaceutical Products Press, 1993.

Tyler, V.E., L.R. Brady, and J.E. Robbers, eds. *Pharmacognosy*. Philadelphia: Lea & Febiger, 1988.

TEXT CITATIONS:

1. A.Y. Leung and S. Foster, *Encyclopedia of Common Natural Ingredients Used in Food, Drugs, and Cosmetics*, 2nd ed. (New York: John Wiley & Sons, 1996).

2. V.E. Tyler, *The Honest Herbal* (Binghamton, NY: Haworth Press/Pharmaceutical Products Press, 1993).

3. M. Mayell, *Off-the-Shelf Natural Health: How to Use Herbs and Nutrients to Stay Well* (New York: Bantam Books, 1995).

4. *Lawrence Review of Natural Products* (St. Louis: Facts and Comparisons, November 1995). P.L. Montgomery, *The New York Times*, (February 6, 1977).

5. Tyler, op. cit.

6. Ibid.

7. Leung and Foster, op. cit.

8. X. Liu and L. Li, *Chung-Kuo Chung Yao Tsa Chih—China Journal of Chinese Materia Medica*, 15(9) (1990): 561.

9. Leung and Foster, op. cit.

10. A.A. Iarosh et al., *Vrach Delo*, (2) (199): 83.

11. Tyler, op. cit.

12. Leung and Foster, op. cit.

13. Ibid.

14. S.H. Cohen et al., *Journal of Allergy and Clinical Immunology*, 64(4) (1979): 270. F.L. Lin et al., *Journal of Allergy and Clinical Immunology*, 83(4) (1989): 793.

15. J.P. Geyman, *Journal of the American Board of Family Practice*, 7(3) (1994): 250.

16. Leung and Foster, op. cit.

PRIMARY NAME:
BETA-CAROTENE

SCIENTIFIC NAME:
N/A

COMMON NAME:
Carotenoid

RATING:
2 = According to a number of well-designed studies and common use, this substance appears to be relatively effective and safe when used in recommended amounts for the indication(s) noted in the "Will It Work for You?" section.

What Is Beta-Carotene?

Beta-carotene is a precursor of vitamin A, meaning the body converts it into this important vitamin. Since time immemorial, humans have been getting beta-carotene from the foods they eat. Carrots, broccoli, leafy green vegetables, squash, and cantaloupe are just a few of the particularly rich sources.

What It Is Used For:

Beta-carotene plays many important roles in the body, not the least of which is to serve as a precursor of vitamin A. Many sources claim that taking supplements of beta-carotene can help reduce the risk of certain types of cancer, boost the immune system, enhance the senses, and prolong life. They attribute these benefits to the fact that beta-carotene is a powerful antioxidant.

Forms Available Include:

Caplet, capsule (regular and soft-gel), liquid, tablet. Beta-carotene appears in many multivitamin and multimineral supplements. Many sources now sell beta-carotene as part of a larger carotenoid complex that also includes such carotenes as alpha-carotene, cryptoxanthin, and lutein.

Dosage Commonly Reported:

Dosage ranges from 6 to 30 milligrams (10,000 to 50,000 IU) per day. Average supplemental doses range from 15 milligrams to 30 milligrams (25,000 to 50,000 IU) a day.

Will It Work for You? What the Studies Say:

A mounting body of data, though still far from conclusive, indicates that beta-carotene is potentially beneficial to the body in several ways, primarily as an antioxidant. Whether antioxidants fulfill all the claims made for them is still a subject of debate, however. Antioxidants control the formation of dangerous substances in the body called free radicals. These substances can severely damage cells through oxidation and are believed to contribute to the risk of cancer-cell formation, cardiovascular disease, and inflammation. Some sources consider free radicals responsible for premature aging as well. Scientists are busy examining the true benefits of supplementing the diet with antioxidant vitamins such as beta-carotene, vitamin C, and vitamin E.

Data also indicate that antioxidants differ in their potency. Although much remains to be learned about whether beta-carotene is one of the most effective ones, preliminary findings indicate that it is. According to population studies, beta-carotene reduces the risk of certain cancers.[1] Several studies have shown that the risk of developing lung or colon cancer is increased if a person has low levels of beta-carotene in his or her bloodstream.[2]

Findings from controlled clinical trials have been mixed, however. In an often cited National Cancer Institute study reported in 1993, a placebo or a daily complex of antioxidants including beta-carotene, vitamin E, and selenium was given to 29,584 adults in China. By the end of the study, the incidence of stomach cancer was 16 percent lower in subjects taking the antioxidant complex than in those taking the placebo, and the risk of death from stomach cancer 21 percent lower.[3] But in a National Institutes of Health study reported just a few years later, high doses of beta-carotene not only failed to help but may actually have increased the risk of cancer among smokers. This long-term study involved 29,000 male Finnish smokers who took both beta-carotene and vitamin E for five to eight years. The incidence of lung cancer was 18 percent higher among those who took beta-carotene supplements (33,000 IU a day) than among those who took placebos.

Will It Harm You? What the Studies Say:

Although ingesting high levels of vitamin A is hazardous, this is not true for beta-carotene. The body converts only as much beta-carotene as needed to create vitamin A.[4] The more beta-carotene is ingested, the less efficient the intestines become in absorbing it. High levels of beta-carotene may cause the skin to acquire a harmless orange tint.

No Recommended Daily Allowance has been set for beta-carotene. It is generally considered safe to take in dosages up to 6 milligrams (10,000 IU) a day.[5] No specific dose has been reported to have caused a toxic reaction,[6] although some sources cite doses above 50,000 IU as toxic.[7]

GENERAL SOURCES:

Balch, J.F., and P.A. Balch. *Prescription for Nutritional Healing: A Practical A to Z Reference to Drug-Free Remedies Using Vitamins, Minerals, Herbs & Food Supplements.* 2nd ed. Garden City Park, NY: Avery Publishing Group, 1997.

Barber, D.A., and S.R. Harris. "Oxygen-Free Radicals and Antioxidants: A Review." *American Pharmacy.* NS34(9) (1994): 26–35.

Barrett, S., and V. Herbert. *The Vitamin Pushers: How the "Health Food" Industry Is Selling America a Bill of Goods.* Amherst, NY: Prometheus Books, 1994.

Mayell, M. *Off-the-Shelf Natural Health: How to Use Herbs and Nutrients to Stay Well.* New York: Bantam Books, 1995.

Pharmacy News. *American Pharmacy.* NS34(1) (1994): 7–9.

TEXT CITATIONS:

1. R.G. Ziegler, *Journal of Nutrition,* 119 (1989): 116–22.
2. F. Gey and G.B. Brubacher, *American Journal of Clinical Nutrition,* 45 (1987): 1368–77. H.B. Stahelin et al., *Journal of the National Cancer Institute,* 73 (1984): 1463–8.
3. *Journal of the National Cancer Institute,* 85 (1993): 1483–99.
4. Barber, P.A., and S.R. Harris. "Oxygen-Free Radicals and Antioxidants: A Review." *American Pharmacy,* NS34 (9) (1994): 26–35.
5. *American Pharmacy,* NS34(1) (1994): 7–9.
6. A. Bendich, *Nutrition and Cancer,* 11 (1988): 207–14.
7. *American Pharmacy,* op. cit.

BETEL NUT

SCIENTIFIC NAME:
Areca catechu L. Family:
Palmaceae

COMMON NAMES:
Areca nut, bing lang, pinang

RATING:
3 = Studies on the effectiveness of this substance are conflicting, or there are not enough studies to draw a conclusion. See the "Will It Harm You?" section for safety warnings.

What Is Betel Nut?

This hard nut grows on the betel palm, *Areca catechu*, cultivated in tropical parts of India, South China, Sri Lanka, the East Indies, and other tropical regions. The slender, tall, feathery palm bears whitish flowers and oval, orange-red fruits that contain small seeds. These seeds are referred to as betel nuts.

What It Is Used For:

Every day for centuries now, millions of Southeast Asians have chewed betel nut quids. These quids are typically composed of a mixture of betel nut in powdered or sliced form, tobacco, and slatted lime, all rolled in the leaf of the betel vine (*Piper betel*). Users not only enjoy the stimulant effects of this caffeine-containing concoction, but often rely on its powers to ease digestion, sweeten the breath, and strengthen the gums. Some claim that it relieves tension and actually offers a sedative action. It has long been considered an effective treatment for intestinal worms.

Forms Available Include:

Betel nuts may be found in some Asian grocery stores or health food outlets.

Dosage Commonly Reported:

In Southeast Asia, people commonly chew 4 to 15 betel nut quids per day.[1] Betel nuts are rarely used in Western medicine.

Will It Work for You? What the Studies Say:

Research has revealed the presence of a number of pharmacologically active components in betel nut, including high levels of astringent tannins (about 15 percent). But the alkaloids rank as the most important compounds by far.[2] One of the alkaloids, arecoline, accounts for the stimulant effect of betel nuts. The worm-killing properties of this oily liquid were recognized more than a century ago, and it is still used for this purpose in veterinary medicine.[3]

Human studies show that chewing betel nut increases salivation, which may well explain why it is considered good for treating digestive system upset.[4] Chewing betel nut quids turns the saliva red, an apparently harmless effect.

Will It Harm You? What the Studies Say:

There are definite health hazards to using betel nut, particularly over the long term. Mouse studies indicate that betel quids contain significant cancer-promoting substances, causing liver, lung, and gastrointestinal tract cancers in nearly 60 percent of the animals administered liquid extracts of the nut.[5] Precancerous lesions and certain types of oral cancer (squamous cell carcinoma) develop at unusually high rates in individuals with a betel-nut-chewing habit.[6] Whether these high cancer rates are due to certain substances in the quids, the alkaloids, or the high tannin concentrations remains to be determined,[7] but the danger of promoting cancer is definitely there.

Some asthma sufferers have experienced an exacerbation of their symptoms when chewing betel nuts.[8]

GENERAL SOURCES:

Dobelis, I.N., ed. *The Magic and Medicine of Plants: A Practical Guide to the Science, History, Folklore, and Everyday Uses of Medicinal Plants.* Pleasantville, NY: Reader's Digest Association, 1986.

Duke, J.A. *CRC Handbook of Medicinal Herbs.* Boca Raton, FL: CRC Press, 1985.

Lawrence Review of Natural Products. St. Louis: Facts and Comparisons, May 1992.

Weiner, M.A., and J.A. Weiner. *Herbs That Heal: Prescription for Herbal Healing.* Mill Valley, CA: Quantum Books, 1994.

TEXT CITATIONS:

1. *Lawrence Review of Natural Products* (St. Louis: Facts and Comparisons, May 1992).
2. J.A. Duke, *CRC Handbook of Medicinal Herbs* (Boca Raton, FL: CRC Press, 1985).
3. *Lawrence Review of Natural Products,* op. cit.
4. M.S. Reddy et al., *American Journal of Clinical Nutrition,* 33 (1980): 77.
5. S.V. Bhide et al., *British Journal of Cancer,* 40 (1979): 922.
6. C.A. McCallum, *Journal of the American Medical Association,* 247(19) (1982): 2715.
7. *Lawrence Review of Natural Products,* op. cit.
8. K.S. Kiyingi, *PNG Medical Journal,* 34(2) (1991): 117.

PRIMARY NAME:

BIFIDOBACTERIUM

SCIENTIFIC NAME:
Bifidobacterium bifidum

COMMON NAME:
Bifidophilus

RATING:
3 = Studies on the effectiveness and safety of this substance are conflicting, or there are not enough studies to draw a conclusion.

What Is Bifidobacterium?

Bifidobacterium is a "beneficial" live bacterium that, along with *Lactobacillus bulgaris*, *Lactobacillus acidophilus*, and other such bacteria, is naturally present in the human body.

What It Is Used For:

See **Acidophilus** for more information on what these type of bacteria can and cannot offer in dietary supplement form.

Forms Available Include:

Capsule, chewable tablet, liquid.

Dosage Commonly Reported:

A common dosage for maintaining a healthy gastrointestinal tract is one capsule containing 2 billion or 3 billion viable organisms per day, or 1/2 to 1 teaspoon powder or liquid. To replenish the intestinal flora while taking broad-spectrum antibiotics, up to 10 billion viable organisms are taken per day.

Will It Work for You? What the Studies Say:

See **Acidophilus**.

Will It Harm You? What the Studies Say:

See **Acidophilus**.

GENERAL SOURCES:

Balch, J.F., and P.A. Balch. *Prescription for Nutritional Healing: A Practical A to Z Reference to Drug-Free Remedies Using Vitamins, Minerals, Herbs & Food Supplements.* 2nd ed. Garden City Park, NY: Avery Publishing Group, 1997.

Mayell, M. *Off-the-Shelf Natural Health: How to Use Herbs and Nutrients to Stay Well.* New York: Bantam Books, 1995.

PRIMARY NAME:
BILBERRY

SCIENTIFIC NAME:
Vaccinium myrtillus L. Family: Ericaceae

COMMON NAMES:
Bog bilberry, dwarf bilberry, European blueberry, huckleberry, whortleberry

RATING:
For the dried berries: 1= Years of use and extensive, high-quality studies indicate that this substance is very effective and safe when used in recommended amounts for the indication(s) noted in the "Will It Work for You?" section.

What Is Bilberry?

This thickly branched, deciduous shrub belongs to the same plant family as cranberries and American blueberries. Its juicy, black, coarsely wrinkled berries (fruits) contain a purple meat and multiple brownish-red seeds. It is a flowering perennial and can be found in heaths, woods, and forest meadows across Europe and parts of North America. Both the dried berries and the oval leaves are used medicinally.

What It Is Used For:

Europeans in particular have long valued bilberry tea as a treatment for simple diarrhea. A mouthwash or gargle decocted from the boiled dried berries is used for gum disease, for sore throat, and to reduce other inflammation in the mucous membranes of the mouth and throat. Bilberry has also long been used for urinary tract infections. Studies following World War II supported the wisdom of British Royal Air Force pilots who had eaten bilberry preserves before heading out on night missions; many users believe bilberry can indeed improve visual activity, so it may have helped the pilots to adjust to darkness and light more quickly. Other eye complaints, including cataracts and glaucoma, have subsequently been treated with the herb in Europe. Some contemporary herbalists also recommend bilberry for diabetes, peptic ulcers, painful menstrual periods, and vascular disorders such as varicose veins.

Forms Available Include:

Formulations standardized for anthocyanidin content: Capsule, concentrated drops, extract, tablet. Also available: Berries (dried, sometimes powdered), decoction (made with dried berries), infusion (of leaves).

Dosage Commonly Reported:

Two 500-milligram capsules are taken two times a day. The dried berries are chewed in dosages of 1 to 2 teaspoonsful, along with some fluid. For an extract standardized for 25 percent anthocyanidin, follow the package instructions.

Will It Work for You? What the Studies Say:

Dried bilberries in the form of a concentrated decoction, or even chewed straight, will help control acute, simple diarrhea by virtue of the presence of astringent tannins (exactly how much they contain remains unclear) and pectin, an adsorbent. European authorities highly recommend the herb for diarrhea; Germans officially endorse the use of the fruits, but not the leaves.[1] Stick to bilberries that have been dried, as the drying process actually enhances tannin content, while fresh berries may actually encourage bowel movement and have even been used to treat constipation.[2] In Germany, infants suffering from infectious diarrhea or indigestion are occasionally given water or herb tea mixed (or boiled briefly) with bilberry powder for infectious diarrhea and indigestion; the stool should become firmer and bulkier under the influence of the fruit's astringent, antiseptic, and absorptive actions. One German physician reports that bilberries even help control vomiting.[3]

Astringent tannins and disinfectant properties also render the dried fruit (in decoction form) useful in mouthwashes and gargles to calm inflamed mucous membranes in the mouth and throat. German health authorities approve of the berries (but not the leaves) for this purpose.[4]

Bilberry has a rich reserve of valuable reddish-blue flavonoid pigments called anthocyanoides. Large clinical trials in humans are still needed to confirm promising findings from animal studies and small human trials indicating that concentrated anthocyanoside-containing berry extracts improve visual acuity, help correct day blindness or chronic eye fatigue, and protect against other eye disorders such as glaucoma and cataracts.[5] Experts hypothesize that anthocyanosides benefit these conditions primarily by boosting oxygen and blood supply to the eye. In one study, nearly all of the fifty individuals with senile cortical cataracts who supplemented their diets with vitamin E and bilberry extract experienced a halt in progression of their condition.[6]

Certain circulatory disorders such as varicose veins, venous insufficiency in the lower limbs, and atherosclerosis may benefit from treatment with bilberry fruit extracts, according to recent studies showing that these extracts can help prevent fragile capillaries (minute blood vessels) and decrease the permeability of blood vessels.[7] The fruits are reportedly used for such circulatory diseases in German, Italy, and other European countries.

More definitive research in humans is also needed to confirm intriguing preliminary findings from test-tube, animal, and a handful of small human trials indicating that the fruit anthocyanosides may help protect against or effectively treat edema, liver cell damage (as an antioxidant), inflammation, high blood sugar (important for diabetics), angina (chest pain), blood clots and atherosclerosis (by counteracting excessive platelet aggregation), and painful menstrual periods (by relaxing smooth muscles).[8] A 1996 test-tube study identified anticancer properties in certain bilberry compounds.[9] In a mouse study, bilberry extracts inactivated the virus that causes tick-borne encephalitis.[10] A 1988 investigation found antiulcer properties in anthocyanidin fed or injected into guinea pigs.[11] In one study, leaf extracts effectively lowered blood cholesterol levels.[12]

Will It Harm You? What the Studies Say:

Much remains to be learned about the risk of adverse reactions from bilberry. The evidence collected so far indicates that it is safe in typically recommended amounts. Rats fed high doses of bilberry anthocyanoside extracts do not appear to suffer any harm.[13] However, toxic reactions can develop with prolonged use or high doses of the leaves; in animal experiments, wasting, anemia, other complications, and some fatalities have occurred.[14] If you suffer from persistent diarrhea, see a doctor.

GENERAL SOURCES:

Bisset, N.E., ed. *Herbal Drugs and Phytopharmaceuticals.* Stuttgart: medpharm GmbH Scientific Publishers, 1994.

Blumenthal, M., J. Gruenwald, T. Hall, and R.S. Rister, eds. *The Complete German Commission E Monographs: Therapeutic Guide to Herbal Medicine.* Boston: Integrative Medicine Communications, 1998.

Lawrence Review of Natural Products. St. Louis: Facts and Comparisons, October 1995.

Leung, A.Y., and S. Foster. *Encyclopedia of Common Natural Ingredients Used in Food, Drugs, and Cosmetics.* 2nd ed. New York: John Wiley & Sons, 1996.

Mayell, M. *Off-the-Shelf Natural Health: How to Use Herbs and Nutrients to Stay Well.* New York: Bantam Books, 1995.

Mindell, E. *Earl Mindell's Herb Bible.* New York: Simon & Schuster/Fireside, 1992.

Murray, M.T. *The Healing Power of Herbs: The Enlightened Person's Guide to the Wonders of Medicinal Plants.* Revised and expanded 2nd ed. Rocklin, CA: Prima Publishing, 1995.

Ody, P. *The Herb Society's Complete Medicinal Herbal.* London: Dorling Kindersley Limited, 1993.

Tyler, V.E. *Herbs of Choice: The Therapeutic Use of Phytomedicinals.* Binghamton, NY: Haworth Press/Pharmaceutical Products Press, 1994.

Weiss, R.F. *Herbal Medicine,* trans. A. R. Meuss, from the 6th German edition. Beaconsfield, England: Beaconsfield Publishers, Ltd., 1988.

TEXT CITATIONS:

1. M. Blumenthal, J. Gruenwald, T. Hall, and R.S. Rister, eds., *The Complete German Commission E Monographs: Therapeutic Guide to Herbal Medicine* (Boston: Integrative Medicine Communications, 1998).

2. V.E. Tyler, *Herbs of Choice: The Therapeutic Use of Phytomedicinals* (Binghamton, NY: Haworth Press/Pharmaceutical Products Press, 1994).

3. R.F. Weiss, *Herbal Medicine,* trans. A. R. Meuss, from the 6th German edition (Beaconsfield, England: Beaconsfield Publishers, Ltd., 1988).

4. Blumenthal et al., op. cit.

5. A. Scharrer and M. Ober, *Klinische Monastblätter für Augenheilkunde,* 178 (1981): 386–9. D. Sala et al., *Minerva Oftalmologica,* 21 (1979): 283–85. E. Gloria and A. Peria, *Annali di Ottalmologia e Clinica Oculistica,* 92 (1966): 595–607.

6. G. Bravetti, *Annali di Ottalmologia e Clinica Oculistica,* 115 (1989): 109.

7. A.Y. Leung and S. Foster, *Encyclopedia of Common Natural Ingredients Used in Food, Drugs, and Cosmetics* (New York: John Wiley & Sons, 1996). A. Lietti et al., *Arzneimittel-Forschung,* 26(5) (1976): 829. M. Gabor, *Angiologica,* (9) (1972): 355–374. B. Havsteen, *Biochemical Pharmacology,* 32 (1983): 1141–48. G. Spinella, *Archivo di Medicina Interna,* 37 (1985): 21–29. J.M. Coget and J.F. Merlen, *I Mal Vasc,* 5 (1980): 43–46.

8. Leung and Foster, op. cit. *Lawrence Review of Natural Products* (St. Louis: Facts and Comparisons, October 1995). M. Marcollet et al., *Comptes Rendus de Seances de la Societe de Biologie et de Ses Filales,* 163 (1969): 8. P. Morazzoni and M.G. Magistretti,

Fitoterapia, 57 (1986): 11. J.C. Monboisse et al., *Agents Actions*, 15 (1984): 49–50. R.N. Zozulya et al., *Rastitel'nye Resursy*, 11 (1975): 87. F. Zaragoza et al., *Arch Pharmacol Toxicol*, 11 (1985): 183–88. D. Boftecchia et al., *Fitoterapia*, 48 (1987): 3–8. B. Bever and G. Zahnd, *Quarterly of Crude Drug Research*, 17 (1979): 139–96. M. Mitcheva et al., *Cellular Microbiology*, 39(4) (1993): 443. D. Colombo and R. Vescovini, *Giorno Italiano Obstetericali Ginecologia*, 7 (1985): 1033–38.

9. J. Bomser et al., *Planta Medica*, 62(3) (1996): 212–16.
10. G.I. Fokina et al., *Voprosy Virusologii*, 36(1) (1991): 18–21.
11. M.J. Magistretti et al., *Arzneimittel-Forschung*, 38(5) (1988): 686–90.
12. A. Cignarella et al., *Planta Medica*, 58S (1992): A581.
13. A. Detre et al., *Clinical Physiology and Biochemistry*, 4(2) (1986): 143.
14. Leung and Foster, op. cit.

BIRCH

SCIENTIFIC NAME:
Various *Betula* species, including *Betula lenta* L. and *Betula pendula* Roth. (also referred to as *Betula verrucose* Ehrh., *Betula alba* L., and *Betula pubescens* Ehrh.). Family: Betulaceae

COMMON NAMES:
There are many. Those discussed here include the following:
Black birch, cherry birch, sweet birch = *Betula lenta*.
Downy birch = *Betula pubescens*.
European white birch, silver birch = *Betula pendula, Betula alba, Betula pubescens*, and *Betula verrucosa*.

RATING:
2 = According to a number of well-designed studies and common use, this substance appears to be relatively effective and safe when used in recommended amounts for the indication(s) noted in the "Will It Work for You?" section.

What Is Birch?

There are some forty species of *Betula* (birch) around the world. The trees and shrubs of this genus all have a smooth outer grain and distinctive, close-grained wood. The leaves and bark have been used by various cultures over the years as a traditional remedy.

What It Is Used For:

Native Americans treated fevers, stomach upset, rheumatism, and other ailments with a tea made from the leaves and bark of sweet birch, and boiled the bark to make poultices for minor wounds. Early settlers reportedly made a mouthwash and (intestinal) worm treatment with parts of the tree. An oil made by distilling the bark of the sweet birch was traditionally used for bladder infections, rheumatism, gout, and nerve pain. Today the oil appears in medicinal ointments and other commercially prepared topical preparations as a counterirritant, painkiller, and antiseptic. Sweet birch extracts have a wintergreen (or root beer) flavor and scent widely used in foods (at commercially accepted concentrations) and fragrances.[1]

Traditional healers have long considered the leaves of the European white and silver birch effective in boosting urine output (a use particularly popular in Europe)[2] and remedying skin rashes, hair loss, rheumatic complaints, and conditions requiring that blood be "purified."[3] A birch tar oil formulated from European white birch is used to treat chronic eczema, psoriasis, and other skin diseases.[4]

Forms Available Include:

- *For internal use:* Infusion (made with leaves, sometimes available in tea bag form), juice (from fresh plant).
- *For external use:* European white birch tar oil, sweet birch oil, often sold as methyl salicylate in gels, liniments, lotions, ointments, and solutions.

Dosage Commonly Reported:

An infusion tea is made using 1 to 2 tablespoons chopped leaves per cup of water and is drunk several times per day. Sweet birch oil appears as an ingredient in

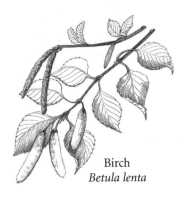

Birch
Betula lenta

many commercial liniments, gels, lotions, and ointments; carefully follow package instructions to avoid overexposure to the contained ingredient methyl salicylate.

Will It Work for You? What the Studies Say:

Of the many folk uses ascribed to this type of tree, scientific evidence can be found only for the use of European or silver birch as diuretics or eczema treatments, and sweet birch oil as a topical treatment for inflamed or irritated joints.

Silver or white birch tea may be a viable diuretic, according to research done over the years. Experts believe that flavonoids and possibly the volatile oil and other substances in the dried leaves are responsible for the increased urine output observed in laboratory rats.[5] Studies have not confirmed this diuretic property in humans, however.[6] Still, German health authorities approve of these birches for making teas to treat disorders such as inflammation and infections of the kidney and urinary tracts and to help prevent the formation of kidney stones.[7] When making a diuretic tea, avoid boiling the leaves because this could destroy the valuable volatile oil believed to contribute to the diuretic effect.[8]

In the case of birch tar oil, a doctor should oversee the treatment of chronic skin conditions, as increasing concentrations must be carefully monitored. Sweet birch oil contains high concentrations (98 percent) of a compound called methyl salicylate, which also appears in wintergreen oil and can be made synthetically.[9] Applied to the skin in the form of a gel, ointment, lotion, or topical solution, methyl salicylate is medically accepted as a mild counterirritant for inflamed or irritated joints. (Counterirritants cause superficial irritation to deflect deeper pain and discomfort.) Methyl salicylate is similar to aspirin and should also help reduce pain and inflammation.

Researchers are exploring the value of a substance called betulin, which is found in some birch species and bears important similarities to betulinic acid, to inhibit skin cancers called melanomas.[10]

Will It Harm You? What the Studies Say:

Infusions made of European or silver birch leaves are relatively safe to use, according to common usage in European countries, although anyone taking a diuretic should be sure to drink plenty of fluids.[11] German health authorities warn that individuals with swelling due to impaired heart or kidney function should not use this preparation, however. They report no adverse interactions with other medicines.[12] Most conditions requiring a diuretic are serious enough to merit a doctor's attention.

When using birch tar oil—or any wood tar, for that matter—remember that prolonged or extensive use (or over large parts of the body) merits regular testing of the urine for the presence of proteins and sediment, given the risk of kidney irritation.[13]

Whether derived from birch or wintergreen or synthesized in the laboratory, the oil from birch sold as methyl salicylate should be used very cautiously as a counterirritant. Follow package instructions and avoid applying it after vigorous exercise or in hot and humid weather because dangerous amounts could get absorbed into your system.[14] *Never swallow methyl salicylate;* it is much more toxic than most salicylates, such as acetylsalicylic acid found in aspirin, and fatal poisonings in children have been reported.[15]

GENERAL SOURCES:

Balch, J.F., and P.A. Balch. *Prescription for Nutritional Healing: A Practical A to Z Reference to Drug-Free Remedies Using Vitamins, Minerals, Herbs & Food Supplements.* 2nd ed. Garden City Park, NY: Avery Publishing Group, 1997.

Bisset, N.E., ed. *Herbal Drugs and Phytopharmaceuticals.* Stuttgart: medpharm GmbH Scientific Publishers, 1994.

Blumenthal, M., J. Gruenwald, T. Hall, and R.S. Rister, eds. *The Complete German Commission E Monographs: Therapeutic Guide to Herbal Medicine.* Boston: Integrative Medicine Communications, 1998.

Duke, J.A. *CRC Handbook of Medicinal Herbs.* Boca Raton, FL: CRC Press, 1985.

Leung, A.Y., and S. Foster. *Encyclopedia of Common Natural Ingredients Used in Food, Drugs, and Cosmetics.* 2nd ed. New York: John Wiley & Sons, 1996.

Tyler, V.E. *Herbs of Choice: The Therapeutic Use of Phytomedicinals.* Binghamton, NY: Haworth Press/Pharmaceutical Products Press, 1994.

Weiss, R.F. *Herbal Medicine,* trans. A. R. Meuss, from the 6th German edition. Beaconsfield, England: Beaconsfield Publishers, Ltd., 1988.

TEXT CITATIONS:

1. A.Y. Leung and S. Foster, *Encyclopedia of Common Natural Ingredients Used in Food, Drugs, and Cosmetics,* 2nd ed. (New York: John Wiley & Sons, 1996).
2. V.E. Tyler, *Herbs of Choice: The Therapeutic Use of Phytomedicinals* (Binghamton, NY: Haworth Press/Pharmaceutical Products Press, 1994).
3. N.E. Bisset, ed., *Herbal Drugs and Phytopharmaceuticals* (Stuttgart: medpharm GmbH Scientific Publishers, 1994).
4. Leung and Foster, op. cit.
5. Bisset, op. cit. H. Schilcher, *Deutscher Apotheker Zeitung,* 124 (1984): 2429.
6. R.F. Weiss, *Herbal Medicine,* trans. A. R. Meuss, from the 6th German edition (Beaconsfield, England: Beaconsfield Publishers, Ltd., 1988).
7. M. Blumenthal, J. Gruenwald, T. Hall, and R.S. Rister, eds., *The Complete German Commission E Monographs: Therapeutic Guide to Herbal Medicine* (Boston: Integrative Medicine Communications, 1998).
8. Weiss, op. cit.
9. Tyler. op. cit.
10. E. Pisha et al., *Nature Medicine,* 1(10) (1995): 1046–51.
11. Blumenthal et al., op. cit.
12. Ibid.
13. Tyler, op. cit.
14. Ibid.
15. Leung and Foster, op. cit.

PRIMARY NAME:
BITTER ORANGE

SCIENTIFIC NAME:
Citrus aurantium L. Family: Rutaceae

What Is Bitter Orange?

Citrus aurantium is an evergreen tree that bears scented flowers and very bitter, sour fruit. It is cultivated in many parts of the world including North America, but is native to China and India. The part most commonly used medicinally is the carefully dried, spicy, bitter-tasting fruit peel (devoid of the spongy inner white part). An oil known as bitter orange oil is pressed

COMMON NAMES:
Seville orange, sour orange

RATING:
2 = According to a number of well-designed studies and common use, this substance appears to be relatively effective and safe when used in recommended amounts for the indication(s) noted in the "Will It Work for You?" section.

from the fresh peel; the oil extracted from the blossoms is referred to as neroli oil or orange flower oil. The oil specially treated with distilled water is referred to as orange flower water. The plant's leaves have reportedly been used as well.

Do not confuse bitter orange with the commonly eaten sweet orange (*Citrus sinensis* [L.] Osb).

What It Is Used For:

Various folk healing traditions, including those in the United States, Europe, and China, have long used dried bitter orange peel to stimulate gastric juice secretions and encourage an appetite, promote digestion, relieve indigestion and gas, help clear cough-related phlegm and other congestion, and even fight cancers.[1] It appears in prepared tonics, gastrointestinal and digestive remedies, appetite stimulators, cholagogues (to promote bile flow), and laxatives. In some European and Central American countries (and possibly elsewhere), neroli oil is used as a mild sedative, particularly for individuals suffering from nervousness-related insomnia.[2] Traditional Chinese healers treat a wide range of illnesses with the peel, from diarrhea to bloody stools and prolapse of the uterus, anus, or rectum.[3] The *National Formulary* once officially listed bitter orange peel. Bitter orange oil finds use in many countries as a flavoring and fragrance.

Forms Available Include:

Dried peel, extract, flower water, infusion, oil, syrup, tincture.

Dosage Commonly Reported:

An infusion tea is made using 1 teaspoon pulverized peel per cup of water. The tincture is taken in dosages of 20 drops three times per day. Orange flower water is given by the tablespoon.

Will It Work for You? What the Studies Say:

As its name suggests, bitter orange ranks high on the bitter taste scale, largely owing to the presence of intensely bitter-tasting flavonoid glycosides such as naringin and neohesperidin. Bitters such as this are commonly used to stimulate gastric juices and jog the appetite. German health authorities endorse the use of bitter orange peel for appetite loss and dyspeptic complaints.[4] The peel also contains an essential oil (up to more than 2 percent), notable amounts of pectin, and other active ingredients. Experts consider the pectin responsible for high cholesterol-reducing actions seen in some studies in laboratory animals and humans treated with the fruit, although much remains unclear about its practical use for these purposes. (See **Apple** for a fuller discussion of pectin.)

The oil of the bitter orange proved very effective in fighting fungal skin infections in an uncontrolled 1996 clinical trial; 8 percent of the twenty patients treated with an emulsion of the oil three times a day were cured in one to two weeks, and 20 percent were cured in two to three weeks.[5] In comparison, those treated with a solution of the oil in alcohol or with pure bitter orange oil (once daily) took slightly longer to recover. Mild skin irritation was seen with the use of the pure form.

Although bitter orange is widely used as a sedative in some folk medicines, virtually no sound research on this subject appears to have been done so far. The oil from the blossoms (neroli oil) rather than the peel is often used for this purpose. A 1985 study of multiple plant oils found that bitter orange oil had certain muscle-relaxing properties; it relaxed the tracheal smooth muscle of the guinea pig.[6] Some German physicians suggest that the aroma or flavor in itself has a gentle sedative and calming effect.[7]

In various experiments over the years, most of them in the test tube and all with unclear implications for treating human disease, the peel and in some cases the unripe fruit have demonstrated antibacterial, anti-inflammatory, choleretic (bile-increasing), antitumor, blood-pressure-lowering (in rats), and even larvacidal properties.[8]

Will It Harm You? What the Studies Say:

Bitter orange peel and other formulations are generally considered safe to use in recommended amounts. No reports of serious adverse reactions appear in the medical literature. However, German health authorities warn that people with fair skin in particular may develop skin reactions to the sun (photosensitivity) after taking bitter orange peel preparations.[9] The presence of sun-sensitizing substances called furocoumarins no doubt accounts for this warning. If you have a stomach or intestinal ulcer, avoid the herb altogether. Severe adverse reactions including intestinal colic, convulsions, and fatalities have been reported in children who ate large amounts of the peel.[10]

Do not take the essential oil internally without professional supervision. The pure oil may mildly irritate your skin.

GENERAL SOURCES:

Bisset, N.E., ed. *Herbal Drugs and Phytopharmaceuticals.* Stuttgart: medpharm GmbH Scientific Publishers, 1994.

Blumenthal, M., J. Gruenwald, T. Hall, and R.S. Rister, eds. *The Complete German Commission E Monographs: Therapeutic Guide to Herbal Medicine.* Boston: Integrative Medicine Communications, 1998.

Chevallier A. *The Encyclopedia of Medicinal Plants: A Practical Reference Guide to More Than 550 Key Medicinal Plants & Their Uses.* 1st American ed. New York: Dorling Kindersley Publications, 1996.

Leung, A.Y., and S. Foster. *Encyclopedia of Common Natural Ingredients Used in Food, Drugs, and Cosmetics.* 2nd ed. New York: John Wiley & Sons, 1996.

Ody, P. *The Herb Society's Complete Medicinal Herbal.* London: Dorling Kindersley Limited, 1993.

Weiss, R.F. *Herbal Medicine,* trans. A. R. Meuss, from the 6th German edition. Beaconsfield, England: Beaconsfield Publishers, Ltd., 1988.

TEXT CITATIONS:

1. A.Y. Leung and S. Foster, *Encyclopedia of Common Natural Ingredients Used in Food, Drugs, and Cosmetics,* 2nd ed. (New York: John Wiley & Sons, 1996).
2. R.F. Weiss, *Herbal Medicine,* trans. A. R. Meuss, from the 6th German edition (Beaconsfield, England: Beaconsfield Publishers, Ltd., 1988).
3. Leung and Foster, op. cit.
4. M. Blumenthal, J. Gruenwald, T. Hall, and R.S. Rister, eds., *The Complete German*

Commission E Monographs: Therapeutic Guide to Herbal Medicine (Boston: Integrative Medicine Communications, 1998).

5. W. Ramadan et al., *International Journal of Dermatology*, 35(6) (1996): 448–49.
6. M. Reiter and W. Brandt, *Arzneimittel-Forschung*, 35(1A) (1985): 408–14.
7. Weiss, op. cit.
8. Leung and Foster, op. cit. G.L. Mwaiko, *East African Medical Journal*, 69(4) (1992): 223–26. Y. Satoh et al., *Yakugaku Zasshi—Journal of the Pharmaceutical Society of Japan*, 116(3) (1996): 244–50. Y.T. Huang et al., *Life Sciences*, 57(22) (1995): 2011–20.
9. Blumenthal et al., op. cit.
10. Leung and Foster, op. cit.

PRIMARY NAME:
BLACKBERRY

SCIENTIFIC NAME:
Rubus fruticosus L. (European), *Rubus villosus* Ait. (American), and various other *Rubus* species. Family: Rosaceae

COMMON NAMES:
Bramble leaf, dewberry, goutberry, rubus

RATING:
2 = According to a number of well-designed studies and common use, this substance appears to be relatively effective and safe when used in recommended amounts for the indications noted in the "Will It Work for You?" section.

What Is Blackberry?

Virtually all parts of this prickly and vigorous flowering bush, from the dried root bark and palm-shaped leaves to the juicy blue-black berries, have been used medicinally. Blackberry, part of the same botanical family as strawberries and roses, grows wild across most of North America.

What It Is Used For:

Blackberry was once quite popular—particularly in ancient times and in medieval Europe—for treating diarrhea, dropsy (fluid retention and swelling), gout, bleeding wounds, and a host of other conditions. The bark was once officially listed in the *U.S. Pharmacopoeia* and the *National Formulary*. Today, few herbalists recommend blackberry anymore except to treat simple diarrhea and mild inflammation, sores, or infections in the mouth or throat. Some suggest applying a compress soaked with the herb to wounds and hemorrhoids. Blackberry is widely used as a food and beverage flavoring.

Forms Available Include:

Capsule, decoction (made of powdered or whole root bark), infusion (made with leaves or dried or fresh berries), tablet, tea (instant), and tincture. The berries can be purchased fresh.

Dosage Commonly Reported:

An infusion is made using 1 to 2 teaspoons chopped leaves per cup of water and is drunk up to six times per day. A decoction is commonly made using 1 to 2 teaspoons powdered bark per cup of water. A root tea is also used as an astringent for diarrhea; it is taken in dosages of 1,500 milligrams up to three times a day. The tincture is taken in dosages of up to 2 teaspoons per day.

Will It Work for You? What the Studies Say:

Several traditional uses for blackberry appear to be justified owing to the presence of high concentrations of tannin, a widely recognized astringent. Tannins are believed to control or stop diarrhea by calming intestinal inflammation.

German health authorities approve of a (dried) leaf infusion for acute but simple diarrhea (i.e., not caused by an underlying medical condition or bacterial infection), although they recommend consulting a doctor if the diarrhea persists for more than three to four days.[1] The root bark can be used for the same purpose but a decoction (rather than an infusion) should be made to extract adequate amounts of tannins.[2] The berries contain even less tannin than the root bark.

Tannins also constrict (tighten) tissue and control oozing and minor bleeding. German health authorities endorse the use of the berries themselves, or a mouthwash or gargle made from the leaves (usually based on an infusion), for oral lesions, sore throat, or other inflammations or mild infections in the mouth or throat. The herb's astringency also helps explain why generations have used it to treat hemorrhoids.

Although much more research is needed to determine the implications for treating human cancers, a team of researchers report antitumor properties in the tannins of *Rubus odoratus* L.[3]

Will It Harm You? What the Studies Say:

No evidence indicates that medicinal concentrations of blackberry are hazardous in any way, but exercise caution in ingesting large amounts of any tannin-containing plants, given still unresolved concerns about their cancer-causing potential. Some herbalists recommend avoiding large amounts of blackberry tea if you suffer from chronic stomach or intestinal problems.[4] German health authorities, commenting on both blackberry leaf and bark preparations, cite no known side effects, known situations in which the plant should not be used, or known interactions with other remedies.[5]

GENERAL SOURCES:

Bisset, N.E., ed. *Herbal Drugs and Phytopharmaceuticals.* Stuttgart: medpharm GmbH Scientific Publishers, 1994.

Blumenthal, M., J. Gruenwald, T. Hall, and R.S. Rister, eds. *The Complete German Commission E Monographs: Therapeutic Guide to Herbal Medicine.* Boston: Integrative Medicine Communications, 1998.

Castleman, M. *The Healing Herbs: The Ultimate Guide to the Curative Power of Nature's Medicines.* New York: Bantam Books, 1995.

Chevallier, A. *The Encyclopedia of Medicinal Plants: A Practical Reference Guide to More Than 550 Key Medicinal Plants & Their Uses.* 1st American ed. New York: Dorling Kindersley Publications, 1996.

Duke, J.A. *CRC Handbook of Medicinal Herbs.* Boca Raton, FL: CRC Press, 1985.

Leung, A.Y., and S. Foster. *Encyclopedia of Common Natural Ingredients Used in Food, Drugs, and Cosmetics.* 2nd ed. New York: John Wiley & Sons, 1996.

Tierra, M. *The Way of Herbs.* New York: Pocket Books, 1990.

Tyler, V.E. *Herbs of Choice: The Therapeutic Use of Phytomedicinals.* Binghamton, NY: Haworth Press/Pharmaceutical Products Press, 1994.

TEXT CITATIONS:

1. M. Blumenthal, J. Gruenwald, T. Hall, and R.S. Rister, eds, *The Complete German Commission E Monographs: Therapeutic Guide to Herbal Medicine* (Boston: Integrative Medicine Communications, 1998).

2. V.E. Tyler, *Herbs of Choice: The Therapeutic Use of Phytomedicinals* (Binghamton, NY: Haworth Press/Pharmaceutical Products Press, 1994).
3. H.H.S. Fong et al., *Journal of Pharmaceutical Sciences*, 61(11) (1972): 1818.
4. M. Castleman, *The Healing Herbs: The Ultimate Guide to the Curative Power of Nature's Medicines* (New York: Bantam Books, 1995).
5. Blumenthal et al., op. cit.

PRIMARY NAME:
BLACK COHOSH

SCIENTIFIC NAME:
Cimicifuga racemosa (L.)
Nuttall. Family: Ranunculaceae

COMMON NAMES:
Black snakeroot, bugbane, bugwort, cimicifuga, cohosh bugbane, rattleroot, rattleweed, sheng ma, snakeroot, squaw root

RATING:
2 = According to a number of well-designed studies and common use, this substance appears to be relatively effective when used in recommended amounts for the indications noted in the "Will It Work for You?" section. See safety precautions in the "Will It Harm You?" section, however.

What Is Black Cohosh?

The knotty black rhizomes (underground stems) and roots of this flowering perennial, a member of the buttercup family found in East Coast American forests, are used medicinally.

What It Is Used For:

Certain Native Americans drank decoctions made of black cohosh to remedy multiple ailments including sore throat, bronchitis, indigestion, rheumatism, and snakebites. But they primarily relied on it for female discomforts such as painful menstruation. The settlers adopted a number of these practices. Black cohosh featured prominently in a popular nineteenth-century remedy for "female weaknesses" such as menstrual cramps. "Cimicifuga" means "bug repellant" in Latin, and the plant has at times been used this way.

Contemporary herbalists also recommend black cohosh to relax the body, promote fluid loss (as a diuretic, or "water pill"), treat persistent cough, and clear mucus from congested airways. Homeopaths recommend the herb in minute amounts for menstruation and childbirth difficulties. (See page 2 for a discussion of homeopathy.)

Forms Available Include:

Decoction, root (powdered), tincture. Usually flavored with honey or lemon to mask the herb's unpleasant aroma and bitter taste.

Dosage Commonly Reported:

A daily dosage of 40 to 200 milligrams is typical. A decoction is made using 1/2 teaspoon powdered root per cup of water; 2 tablespoons are taken every few hours, up to 1 cup per day. The tincture is taken in dosages of up to 1 teaspoon per day.

Will It Work for You? What the Studies Say:

The few studies done so far indicate that black cohosh contains several active ingredients, but whether they will have an impact on a person's health remains unclear. The FDA did not think so; after reviewing the literature, the agency concluded in 1986 that black cohosh has "no therapeutic value." But Europeans still use the herb extensively. German health authorities have deemed black cohosh root effective for treating premenstrual and menstrual discomfort or pain, and menopause-associated nervousness.[1]

Advocates of black cohosh for "female troubles" point to evidence that it contains substances that perform similarly to the female sex hormone estrogen. One study demonstrated that substances in black cohosh attach to estrogen receptors in the rat uterus.[2] Another study of sixty women under forty who had undergone hysterectomies and suffered from symptoms of ovarian insufficiency found that those treated with various estrogens fared as well as those treated with black cohosh extracts.[3] Researchers have also shown that black cohosh suppresses luteinizing hormone (LH), which regulates the activities of the testes and ovaries. This was demonstrated in rats in 1985[4] and in humans a few years later; an alcoholic extract of black cohosh reduced LH levels in menopausal women and consequently relieved menopause-associated hot flashes.[5] The preparation used in this study—*Remifemin*—is prescribed for German women.

Speculation that black cohosh can help lower blood pressure continues, although no well-designed studies in humans have been done so far. Investigators reporting in the 1960s showed that a steroidal derivative called actein in the plant could lower blood pressure in rabbits and cats and help open up the blood vessels in dog limbs.[6]

Test-tube and animal studies indicate that black cohosh helps counter inflammation, lower blood sugar levels, and fight certain bacteria. Whether the herb will work in these ways in humans has not been tested.

Will It Harm You? What the Studies Say:

Scientists know relatively little about whether black cohosh is safe to use, especially over the long term. Toxicity studies in animals have been inconclusive. German health authorities list stomach discomfort as a potential side effect.[7] A few people who have consumed the leaves or roots have developed nausea, vomiting, and stomach upset, and miscarriages have followed large doses.[8] In 1986, the FDA warned of possible side effects with black cohosh. The agency declined to declare the herb a safe food ingredient. German health authorities warn against taking black cohosh for more than six months (for any purpose) because so little is known about its long-term effects.[9] They do not cite any situations in which the herb should not be taken, although given its estrogen-like component, pregnant and nursing women should probably avoid the herb. Some herbalists extend this warning to women with estrogen-dependent cancer and women who are taking birth control pills or estrogen supplements after menopause.[10] The same precaution applies to individuals with certain types of heart disease or those taking sedatives or blood pressure medications. Anyone who wants to take black cohosh—but particularly the aforementioned individuals—should talk to a doctor first.

GENERAL SOURCES:

American Pharmaceutical Association. *Handbook of Nonprescription Drugs*. 11th ed. Washington, D.C.: American Pharmaceutical Association, 1996.

Bisset, N.E., ed. *Herbal Drugs and Phytopharmaceuticals*. Stuttgart: medpharm GmbH Scientific Publishers, 1994.

Blumenthal, M., J. Gruenwald, T. Hall, and R.S. Rister, eds. *The Complete German Commission E Monographs: Therapeutic Guide to Herbal Medicine*. Boston: Integrative Medicine Communications, 1998.

Castleman, M. *The Healing Herbs: The Ultimate Guide to the Curative Power of Nature's Medicines*. New York: Bantam Books, 1995.

Genazzani, E., and L. Sorrentin. *Nature*. 194 (1962): 544.

Lawrence Review of Natural Products. St. Louis: Facts and Comparisons, September 1992.

Leung, A.Y. *Encyclopedia of Common Natural Ingredients Used in Food, Drugs, and Cosmetics*. New York: John Wiley & Sons, 1980.

TEXT CITATIONS:

1. M. Blumenthal, J. Gruenwald, T. Hall, and R.S. Rister, eds., *The Complete German Commission E Monographs: Therapeutic Guide to Herbal Medicine* (Boston: Integrative Medicine Communications, 1998).
2. H. Jarry, *Planta Medica*, 55 (1985): 316.
3. E. Lehmann-Willenbrock and H.H. Riedel, *Zentrallblatt für Gynakologie*, 110(10) (1988): 611–18.
4. H. Jarry and G. Harnischfeger, *Planta Medica*, 55 (1985): 46–49.
5. E.M. Duker et al., *Planta Medica*, 57(5) (1991): 420–24.
6. E. Genazzani and L. Sorrentin, *Nature*, 194 (1962): 544. S.E. Corsano, *Gazzette Chimica Italiana*, 99 (1969): 9154.
7. Blumenthal et al., op. cit.
8. *Lawrence Review of Natural Products* (St. Louis: Facts and Comparisons, September 1992).
9. Blumenthal et al., op. cit.
10. M. Castleman, *The Healing Herbs: The Ultimate Guide to the Curative Power of Nature's Medicines* (New York: Bantam Books, 1995).

PRIMARY NAME:
BLACK CURRANT

SCIENTIFIC NAME:
Ribes nigrum L. Family: Grossulariaceae

COMMON NAMES:
European black currant, quinsy berries

RATING:
3 = Studies on the effectiveness and safety of this substance are conflicting, or there are not enough studies to draw a conclusion.

What Is Black Currant?

This thornless shrub belongs to the red currant family. It has wrinkly lobed leaves with distinctive yellow dots (glands) on the underside, small bell-shaped flowers, and brownish-black fruits (berries or "seeds") that are widely used in jams, liqueurs, and juices. The leaves and berries are used medicinally.

What It Is Used For:

In European folk medicine, black currant once had a considerable reputation for controlling diarrhea, promoting urine output (as a diuretic, or "water pill"), and reducing arthritic and rheumatic pains. A soothing hot drink was made to induce sweating in cases of cough, flu, and chills. In rare cases the leaves were used topically for wounds. Modern Europeans value black currant juice as a refreshing, nutritious drink. Many take it as a tonic during recovery from an illness. Capsules containing a fixed oil drawn from the seeds—black currant oil—are sold as a source of gamma-linoleic acid (GLA) to treat a wide range of ailments. Most American health food outlets sell black currant in the encapsulated oil form.

Forms Available Include:

Capsule (of seed oil), leaf, infusion (of leaf), juice (of fruit).

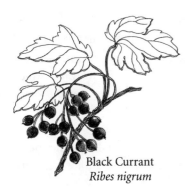

Black Currant
Ribes nigrum

Dosage Commonly Reported:

A daily dosage of 600 to 6,000 milligrams is typical. Capsules containing black currant oil are available in 200- to 400-milligram doses; this oil typically has a fixed oil component containing 14 to 19 percent GLA. For atopic eczema, four 250-milligram capsules are taken twice a day. Diarrhea patients are given a glass of black currant juice several times a day. A tea is made using 1 to 2 teaspoons of chopped leaves per cup of water and is taken several times a day.

Will It Work for You? What the Studies Say:

Scant scientific evidence can be found to support the traditional uses of black currant leaves. Substances such as flavonoids, tannins, and traces of an essential oil have been identified, but researchers have yet to fully characterize their ingredients.[1] One flavonoid has shown antifungal properties.[2] On the basis of empirical evidence, however, a number of European physicians consider black currant leaf a good choice for treating diarrhea, presumably owing to the presence of the astringent tannin and abundant vitamin C.[3] Tannins are believed to control or stop diarrhea by reducing intestinal inflammation. Although the implications for treating inflammatory diseases in humans are still far from clear, an alcoholic extract of the leaves performed very well in a 1989 study using a classic model to test inflammation in rats.[4]

The berries also contain the astringent tannin, as well as potassium, rutin, and a black pigment. German physicians recommend the berry juice as a regular beverage for people who tend to get diarrhea.[5] Some people object to the taste and will drink it only when it is mixed with other juices. The berries pack considerable quantities of vitamin C—about twice as much as lemons or oranges—and their juice (diluted with hot water) is valued for treating flu, colds, and other illnesses associated with chilling.[6] Heating the juice directly would probably destroy the vitamins.

All together, considerably more sound evidence can be found for using the plant's seed (berry) oil than its leaves or whole berries; the seeds yield a fixed oil containing 14 to 19 percent of a potentially important substance, GLA. Research indicates that the body can convert this essential polyunsaturated fatty acid into a precursor of the hormone prostaglandin. Although GLA is a major component in human milk, only small amounts appear in commonly eaten foods. Factors such as high cholesterol, aging, stress, alcohol, diabetes, premenstrual syndrome (PMS), aging, viral infections, and other conditions may interfere with the normal conversion of linoleic acid into GLA.[7] Plant experts contend that people who get little GLA through their diets may benefit from taking GLA-rich supplements like black currant seed oil, as may those whose systems are unable to metabolize linoleic acid into GLA.[8]

Still up for debate, however, is whether GLA can actually ameliorate such conditions as arthritis, PMS, high blood pressure, and heart disease, as some advocates assert. Animal studies and increasing numbers of human studies indicate that some of these claims may be true, although the results are controversial and critics remain skeptical. To confuse matters, most investigations have been carried out on the other two GLA-rich dietary supplements on the American market: **Evening Primrose Oil** and **Borage Oil**. Because of chemical differences in the oils from these plants, the reactions they generate in the body may be different as well, and thus study findings not necessarily relevant.[9] Much remains to be learned about GLA and what it can do for human health.

Will It Harm You? What the Studies Say:

Europeans have long been drinking black currant juice and taking other berry and leaf preparations to no apparent ill effect. German health authorities warn that people with fluid accumulation because of heart or kidney insufficiency should not take the leaf preparations, however.[10] As for black currant oil, no studies appear to have been done to determine its safety over the long term; preliminary findings for other GLA-rich oils suggest that these kinds of supplements are relatively safe.

GENERAL SOURCES:

American Pharmaceutical Association. *Handbook of Nonprescription Drugs*. 11th ed. Washington, D.C.: American Pharmaceutical Association, 1996.

Bisset, N.E., ed. *Herbal Drugs and Phytopharmaceuticals*. Stuttgart: medpharm GmbH Scientific Publishers, 1994.

Bremness, L. *Herbs*. 1st American ed. Eyewitness Handbooks. New York: Dorling Kindersley Publications, 1994.

Duke, J.A. *CRC Handbook of Medicinal Herbs*. Boca Raton, FL: CRC Press, 1985.

Stary, F. *The Natural Guide to Medicinal Herbs and Plants*. Prague: Barnes & Noble, Inc. in arrangement with Aventinum Publishers, 1996.

Tyler, V.E. *Herbs of Choice: The Therapeutic Use of Phytomedicinals*. Binghamton, NY: Haworth Press/Pharmaceutical Products Press, 1994.

Weiss, R.F. *Herbal Medicine*, trans. A. R. Meuss, from the 6th German edition. Beaconsfield, England: Beaconsfield Publishers, Ltd., 1988.

TEXT CITATIONS:

1. N.E. Bisset, ed., *Herbal Drugs and Phytopharmaceuticals* (Stuttgart: medpharm GmbH Scientific Publishers, 1994).
2. B.L. Fitt et al., *Plant Soil*, 66 (1982): 405.
3. R.F. Weiss, *Herbal Medicine*, trans. A. R. Meuss, from the 6th German edition (Beaconsfield, England: Beaconsfield Publishers, Ltd., 1988).
4. C. Declume, *Journal of Ethnopharmacology*, 27(1–2) (1989): 91–98.
5. Weiss, op. cit.
6. Ibid.
7. American Pharmaceutical Association, *Handbook of Nonprescription Drugs*, 11th ed. (Washington, D.C.: American Pharmaceutical Association, 1996).
8. V.E. Tyler, *Herbs of Choice: The Therapeutic Use of Phytomedicinals* (Binghamton, NY: Haworth Press/Pharmaceutical Products Press, 1994). H. Traitler et al., *Lipids*, 19(12) (1984): 923–28.
9. American Pharmaceutical Association, op. cit.
10. Bisset, op. cit.

PRIMARY NAME:
BLACK HAW

SCIENTIFIC NAME:
Viburnum prunifolium L.
Family: Caprifoliaceae

COMMON NAMES:
American sloe, Southern black haw (*Viburnum rufidulum*), stagbrush, stag bush, viburnum

RATING:
3 = Studies on the effectiveness and safety of this substance are conflicting, or there are not enough studies to draw a conclusion.

What Is Black Haw?

This native North American shrub or small tree has wide spreading branches with oval leaves that turn red in autumn. It produces showy clusters of white flowers and blue-black fruit. The reddish-brown bark of its root and stems is used medicinally.

What It Is Used For:

Native American women once took black haw tea to prevent miscarriage, control menstrual pain, stop uterine bleeding, encourage recovery from childbirth, and allay menopausal discomfort. By the nineteenth century, more than a few American women were relying on it as a "uterine tonic." The *U.S. Pharmacopoeia* and the *National Formulary* officially listed it for some time. Now, after a period of lack of interest, many herbalists and dietary supplement distributors are recommending black haw for female reproductive system discomforts and occasionally for other uses that hark back to Native American and folk traditions: diarrhea, asthma, and nervousness (as a nerve tonic and antispasmodic). Black haw contains salicin, the source for the synthesis of the famous pain reliever commonly known as aspirin, inspiring some sources to recommend the herb for general aches and pains, fever, and headache.

Forms Available Include:

Bark, capsule, decoction, infusion, tablet, tincture.

Dosage Commonly Reported:

A decoction is made using 2 teaspoons dried bark per cup of water. The tincture is taken in dosages of up to 2 teaspoons three times per day. Use commercial preparations according to package directions.

Will It Work for You? What the Studies Say:

Little research has been published on black haw since the 1960s, when researchers identified a substance called scopoletin in the root bark. According to test-tube studies at the time, scopoletin exerts antispasmodic actions on the uterine muscle, meaning it relaxes the uterus and may ease the cramping that causes menstrual pains, for example.[1] Experts believe the root bark may contain other uterine-relaxing constituents as well.[2] Because the plant has not been well studied in animals or humans directly, however, there is no way of determining conclusively whether it will in fact help allay menstrual pains or other ailments that involve uterine cramping. Scopoletin's antispasmodic properties may explain the plant's folk use as a calming agent for the whole body, but similarly little is known about this. One German textbook considers black haw "probably" sedative overall and moderately antispasmodic.[3]

The justification for using black haw bark as a pain reliever, based solely on the presence of a close chemical relative of aspirin called salicin, appears to be relatively weak; not only is the concentration of this ingredient hard for the consumer to verify, but no animal or human studies appear to have been done to test the effectiveness or safety of black haw salicin. The presence of astringent tannins in black haw bark may explain why so many people instinctively used it to treat diarrhea, as tannins are widely believed to reduce intestinal inflammation and thus encourage firmer stools.

Will It Harm You? What the Studies Say:

Scientists know relatively little about the safety of black haw. Importantly, no reports of significant adverse reactions survive centuries of use. Because of its potential to relax the uterus, no pregnant women should take black haw without talking to an obstetrician first. Just as aspirin should not be taken during pregnancy because it has been implicated in birth defects, black haw should also be avoided, given its salicin content. Similarly, just as children under sixteen should never be given aspirin if they have flu symptoms or chicken pox because of the risk of a rare but potentially fatal condition called Reye's syndrome, black haw preparations should never be given to children with these symptoms. Do not take this herb if you are allergic to aspirin. The berries may cause unpleasant reactions such as nausea in some individuals.[4]

GENERAL SOURCES:

Castleman, M. *The Healing Herbs: The Ultimate Guide to the Curative Power of Nature's Medicines*. New York: Bantam Books, 1995.

Chevallier, A. *The Encyclopedia of Medicinal Plants: A Practical Reference Guide to More Than 550 Key Medicinal Plants & Their Uses*. 1st American ed. New York: Dorling Kindersley Publications, 1996.

Duke, J.A. *CRC Handbook of Medicinal Herbs*. Boca Raton, FL: CRC Press, 1985.

Foster, S., and J.A. Duke. *The Peterson Field Guide Series: A Field Guide to Medicinal Plants. Eastern and Central North America*. Boston: Houghton Mifflin Company, 1990.

Leung, A.Y., and S. Foster. *Encyclopedia of Common Natural Ingredients Used in Food, Drugs, and Cosmetics*. 2nd ed. New York: John Wiley & Sons, 1996.

Mowrey, D.B. *Proven Herbal Blends: A Rational Approach to Prevention and Remedy*. (Condensed from *The Scientific Validation of Herbal Medicine*.) New Canaan, CT: Keats Publishing, Inc., 1986.

Tierra, M. *The Way of Herbs*. New York: Pocket Books, 1990.

Weiss, R.F. *Herbal Medicine*, trans. A. R. Meuss, from the 6th German edition. Beaconsfield, England: Beaconsfield Publishers, Ltd., 1988.

TEXT CITATIONS:

1. C.H. Jarboe, *Journal of Medicinal Chemistry*, 10 (1967): 488. C.H. Jarboe et al., *Nature.*, 212 (1966): 837.

2. A.Y. Leung and S. Foster, *Encyclopedia of Common Natural Ingredients Used in Food, Drugs, and Cosmetics*, 2nd ed. (New York: John Wiley & Sons, 1996).

3. R.F. Weiss, *Herbal Medicine*, trans. A. R. Meuss, from the 6th German edition (Beaconsfield, England: Beaconsfield Publishers, Ltd., 1988).

4. S. Foster and J.A. Duke, *The Peterson Field Guide Series: A Field Guide to Medicinal Plants. Eastern and Central North America* (Boston: Houghton Mifflin Company, 1990).

PRIMARY NAME:
BLACK WALNUT

SCIENTIFIC NAME:
Juglans nigra L. Family: Juglandaceae

COMMON NAMES:
American walnut, Eastern black walnut

RATING:
3 = Studies on the effectiveness and safety of this substance are conflicting, or there are not enough studies to draw a conclusion.

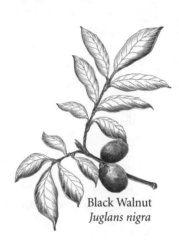

Black Walnut
Juglans nigra

What Is Black Walnut?

The stately black walnut tree boasts a rounded crown of aromatic foliage and deeply furrowed dark brown bark. Small green flowers bloom in spring, and lance-shaped leaves turn yellow in autumn. Sweet edible seeds (nuts) can be found in the irregularly ridged fruits. The tree grows in the woods of eastern North America. The inner bark, husks, leaves, and nuts have all been used medicinally.

What It Is Used For:

This shady tree, so coveted in early America as a source of hardwood for furniture, guns, and other items that it was a target of robbers,[1] offers a valuable source for healing agents, according to some contemporary herbalists. Many of the uses they propose echo traditional Native American ones. Assorted tribes reportedly prepared a juice from the nut husks to treat ringworm, chewed the husks for colic, made a poultice of the husk to control skin inflammation, brewed a tea from the inner bark to treat constipation and induce vomiting, and concocted a leaf tea to fight bed bugs.[2]

Contemporary herbalists continue to highlight the astringent nature of the dried bark, recommending internal preparations as mild laxatives for constipation, improved digestion, and bowel regulation. Many indicate that black walnut can strengthen the body and fight internal fungal, bacterial, and parasitic infections, and some recommend hull extracts to rub into the skin for warts, fungal infections, herpes, eczema, psoriasis, bruising, and other skin ailments. A few suggest sipping a leaf infusion for many of these disorders. The hulls were traditionally boiled to make a wool dye. Generations of Americans have enjoyed the taste of the sweet nuts.

Forms Available Include:

- *For internal use:* Capsule, decoction, extract, infusion, tincture (made with hulls).
- *For external use:* Extract, poultice.

Dosage Commonly Reported:

The extract is taken in dosages of 10 to 20 drops per day. The 495-milligram capsules made from the hulls are taken three times a day. For skin problems, the extract is applied twice a day.

Will It Work for You? What the Studies Say:

There is very little information on black walnut's medicinal properties. No clinical trials are reported in the literature, and apparently very few studies have been done in the laboratory. A substance called juglone has been identified in parts of the plant including the hulls and leaves and is believed to possess astringent properties that aid in shrinking tissues and preventing oozing when applied externally, qualities valuable in treating some wounds, mouth and throat sores, and irritations such as hemorrhoids. In the proper concentration, astringents are also believed to decrease inflammation in the intestines and help control loose stools.

Several sources also assert that juglone contains antifungal properties, which might justify its use for fungal skin infections such as ringworm, for example. Others have shown that juglone fights numerous oral bacteria and may work in combination with other substances to control infectious diseases in the mouth.[3] However, black walnut's ability to do these things has not been verified in animal or human studies, and information on the concentration of juglone in the various parts of the plant is hard to find.

Although implications for treating human disease are far from clear, studies in laboratory mice suggest that extracts of the leaves and fruit hulls have anti-tumor activity,[4] and test-tube experiments indicate that the fruit has the ability to fight dangerous cell changes (mutations) in certain substances.[5] A 1990 German patent contends that extracts (polysaccharides) from the dried nut shells inhibit the HIV virus in the test tube.[6]

Will It Harm You? What the Studies Say:

Not much is known about the potential toxicity of black walnut preparations, although no reports of serious harm appear in the recent medical literature—at least in humans. Horses exposed to black walnut shavings develop laminitis, swelling, fast breathing, and other signs of adverse reactions.[7] This was noted in the late 1980s, and researchers now rely on the ability of a water extract of the tree shavings to induce signs of severe laminaria in horses[8] to study ways to treat the disorder and other ailments. (Laminaria is an inflammatory disease characterized by swelling in the feet, lameness at walk, and refusal to lift the feet.)

Pollen from the tree has caused moderately severe allergic reactions in sensitive individuals.[9]

GENERAL SOURCES:

Balch, J.F., and P.A. Balch. *Prescription for Nutritional Healing: A Practical A to Z Reference to Drug-Free Remedies Using Vitamins, Minerals, Herbs & Food Supplements.* 2nd ed. Garden City Park, NY: Avery Publishing Group, 1997.

Foster, S., and J.A. Duke. *The Peterson Field Guide Series: A Field Guide to Medicinal Plants. Eastern and Central North America.* Boston: Houghton Mifflin Company, 1990.

Little, E.L. *National Audubon Society Field Guide to North American Trees. Eastern Region.* New York: Alfred A. Knopf, Inc., 1980.

Mindell, E. *Earl Mindell's Herb Bible.* New York: Simon & Schuster/Fireside, 1992.

Tierra, M. *The Way of Herbs.* New York: Pocket Books, 1990.

TEXT CITATIONS:

1. E.L. Little, *National Audubon Society Field Guide to North American Trees. Eastern Region* (New York: Alfred A. Knopf, Inc., 1980).
2. S. Foster and J.A. Duke, *The Peterson Field Guide Series: A Field Guide to Medicinal Plants. Eastern and Central North America* (Boston: Houghton Mifflin Company, 1990).
3. N. Didry et al., *Pharmazie*, 49(9) (1994): 681–83.
4. V.A. Bharga and B.A. Westfall, *Journal of Pharmaceutical Sciences*, 1968; 57:1674. M. Yoshihara et al., 1990 German Patent 3,942,638, 8 pages.
5. M.E. Wall et al., *Journal of Natural Products*, 51(5) (1988): 866–73.
6. Yoshihara, op. cit.
7. C. Uhlinger, *Journal of the American Veterinary Medical Association*, 195(3) (1989): 343–44.

8. F.D. Galey et al., *Journal of Comparative Pathology*, 104(3) (1991): 313–26.

9. W.H. Lewis and W.E. Imber, *Annals of Allergy*, 35(2) (1975): 113–19.

PRIMARY NAME:
BLESSED THISTLE

SCIENTIFIC NAME:
Cnicus benedictus L. Family: Asteraceae (Compositae)

COMMON NAMES:
Cnicus, holy ghost herb, holy thistle

RATING:
- *For internal use:* 4 = Research indicates that this herb will not fulfill the claims made for it, but that it is also unlikely to cause any harm.
- *For external use:* 3 = Studies on the effectiveness and safety of this herb are conflicting, or there are not enough studies to draw a conclusion.

What Is Blessed Thistle?

True to its name, this annual looks thistlelike, with distinctive spiny leaves. The upper leaves form cups around singular yellow flowers. It grows in meadows and moist environments across Europe and North America. The aboveground parts of the plant, once dried, are used medicinally.

What It Is Used For:

Blessed thistle featured prominently as a plague cure in the Middle Ages. Believing the herb could stimulate bile production, folk healers also recommended it for liver and gallbladder diseases. But its primary reputation was as an appetite stimulant and soothing agent for digestive upset, stomach discomfort, and excess gas, ailments for which modern herbalists continue to recommend it. Its bitter taste accounts for its inclusion in bitters and liqueurs such as Benedictine.

Long esteemed as a "woman's herb," blessed thistle was also used as a contraceptive and menstruation promoter. Today it appears in contemporary herbal mixtures for controlling menstrual pain or amenorrhea (absence of menstruation), regulating the menstrual cycle, and fulfilling the "nutritional needs of women" during periods of "stress" such as menstruation. Other properties ascribed to blessed thistle over the years include an ability to lower fever, boost a mother's milk production, increase perspiration, dissolve blood clots, control bleeding, and reduce rheumatic pain. It has also been used topically for wounds.

Forms Available Include:

- *For internal use:* Capsule, decoction, fluid extract, infusion, oil, tincture. A common ingredient in herbal tea mixtures.
- *For external use:* Extracts appear in "healing" skin lotions, creams, and salves.

Dosage Commonly Reported:

Many sources recommend a daily dosage of 4 to 6 grams. A decoction is made using 1$\frac{1}{2}$ to 2 teaspoons (1$\frac{1}{2}$ to 2 grams) of finely chopped herb in a cup of water. As an aromatic bitter, a cup is drunk one-half hour before meals. The extract is taken in dosages of 10 to 20 drops in water daily. Two capsules of 360 milligrams each are taken three times a day.

Will It Work for You? What the Studies Say:

The main active ingredient in blessed thistle—a bitter diterpenoid lactone called cnicin—endows the herb with a relatively high "bitter" index, a quality considered valuable in stimulating the appetite and aiding digestion by encouraging the secretion of saliva and gastric juice. Cnicin may also act directly on the stomach and part of the small intestine.[1] German health authorities approve of blessed thistle tea for treating indigestion and appetite loss.[2] Some German doctors prescribe it for chronic stomach conditions.[3] Many experts, however, consider other bitters more potent. Cnicin keeps better in liquid extract than in dried form.[4]

One study found blessed thistle extracts as potent an anti-inflammatory as indomethacin, a powerful prescription drug for such conditions as arthritis and bursitis.[5] No human studies to test the herb's value for such ailments appear to have been done, however. More research is also needed to explore suggested antitumor activity for the herb. Blessed thistle cannot, as was once believed, reduce fever.[6] Nor has anyone ever scientifically shown that it can promote menstruation or affect the female reproductive system in any other way, or aid the liver or gallbladder by stimulating the production of bile.

Overall, research indicates that blessed thistle benefits external ailments more than internal ones. Test-tube analyses show that essential oil extracts contain more than a dozen antibacterial compounds, prompting some experts to consider it potentially useful as an antiseptic for minor wounds.[7] Unfortunately, the herb contains very small amounts of this essential oil. A compound in the herb may help stop bleeding, according to recent research, but whether this applies to humans remains unknown. Japanese investigators have isolated a component that stanches bleeding in laboratory mice.[8]

Will It Harm You? What the Studies Say:

Scientists know as little about the safety of blessed thistle as they do about its effectiveness. Overall, it appears to be harmless, although it can cause allergic reactions. Avoid it if you are sensitive to other members of the daisy family. People with acute stomach inflammation, ulcers, or hyperacidity should not use the herb because it stimulates gastric juices. Injection of cnicin into lab mice caused considerable tissue irritation; never try injecting the herb on your own.[9] Blessed thistle does not appear to interact negatively with other remedies. Given its traditional use as a menstruation promoter—a property not confirmed by scientific studies—pregnant women may want to avoid the herb.

If collecting the plant yourself, wear protective glasses and clothes because it can cause very painful inflammation of the skin, eyes, and mucous membranes. Do not confuse holy thistle with the closely named milk thistle (*Silybum marianum*).

GENERAL SOURCES:

Bisset, N.E., ed. *Herbal Drugs and Phytopharmaceuticals.* Stuttgart: medpharm GmbH Scientific Publishers, 1994.

Blumenthal, M., J. Gruenwald, T. Hall, and R.S. Rister, eds. *The Complete German Commission E Monographs: Therapeutic Guide to Herbal Medicine.* Boston: Integrative Medicine Communications, 1998.

Heinerman, J. *Heinerman's Encyclopedia of Healing Herbs and Spices.* West Nyack, NY: Parker Publishing Co., 1996.

McCalbeb, R. *Better Nutrition.* August 1991.

Mindell, E. *Earl Mindell's Herb Bible.* New York: Simon & Schuster/Fireside, 1992.

Tierra, M. *The Way of Herbs.* Denver, CO: Washington Square Press, 1990.

Tyler, V.E. *Herbs of Choice: The Therapeutic Use of Phytomedicinals.* Binghamton, NY: Haworth Press/Pharmaceutical Products Press, 1994.

Tyler, V.E., L.R. Brady, and J.E. Robbers, eds. *Pharmacognosy.* Philadelphia: Lea & Febiger, 1988.

Weiss, R.F. *Herbal Medicine.*, trans. A. R. Meuss, from the 6th German edition. Beaconsfield, England: Beaconsfield Publishers, Ltd., 1988.

TEXT CITATIONS:

1. S. Wolf and M. Mack, *Drug Standards*, 24 (1956): 98–101.
2. M. Blumenthal, J. Gruenwald, T. Hall, and R.S. Rister, eds., *The Complete German Commission E Monographs: Therapeutic Guide to Herbal Medicine* (Boston: Integrative Medicine Communications, 1998).
3. R.F. Weiss, *Herbal Medicine*, trans. A. R. Meuss, from the 6th German edition (Beaconsfield, England: Beaconsfield Publishers, Ltd., 1988).
4. G. Schneider and I. Lachner, *Planta Medica*, 63(3) (1987): 247–51.
5. Ibid.
6. J. Delphaut et al., *Comptes Rendus Sociologique et Biologique*, 135 (1941): 1458–60.
7. R. Vanhaelen-Fastre, *Planta Medica*, 24(2) (1973): 165–75. E.M. Cobb, 1973 British Patent Number 1,335,181; also in *Chemical Abstracts* 8348189j, 1973.
8. Y. Ito and H. Kato, Japanese Patent Application Number 86/22,226.
9. Schneider and Luckner, op. cit.

PRIMARY NAME:

BLOODROOT

SCIENTIFIC NAME:
Sanguinaria canadensis L.
Family: Papaveraceae

COMMON NAMES:
Indian plant, Indian red plant, red puccoon, redroot, sanguinaria, tetterwort

RATING:

- *For commercial mouthwashes and toothpastes:* 2 = According to a number of well-designed studies and common use, this substance appears to be relatively effective and safe when used in recommended amounts.
- *For other external uses:* 3 =

What Is Bloodroot?

This perennial wildflower is native to the forests of eastern North America. A solitary, delicate white flower emerges in spring from its singular large leaves. The plant owes its common name to the orange-red, blood-colored juice contained in the root and stout rhizome (underground stem). The dried rhizome is used medicinally.

What It Is Used For:

Several Native American tribes reportedly used bloodroot tea externally for rheumatic pains, sore throat, skin burns, and fungal infections. Some concocted a body paint from the colorful sap. Others valued it as a cancer cure, still others as an insect repellent. American and Russian folk healers treated skin ulcers and cancers, nasal polyps, warts, and other external ailments with topical formulations such as bloodroot powder. The herb was also used internally to treat fever and in large doses to induce vomiting. Bloodroot's popularity as an expectorant to clear congestion associated with coughs and colds developed over time, and small concentrations may still be found in herbal cough remedies. By the mid-1800s, root extracts were being used as a dental analgesic, and a mixture of the herb's alkaloids called "sanguinaria extract" can be found in mouthwashes and toothpastes today. Homeopaths recommend minute amounts of bloodroot for various ailments. (See page 2 for a discussion of homeopathy.)

BLOODROOT *(Continued)*

Studies on the effectiveness and safety of this substance are conflicting, or there are not enough studies to draw a conclusion.

• *For internal use:* 5 = Studies indicate that there is a definite health hazard to using this substance, even in recommended amounts.

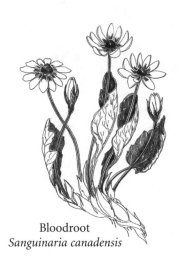

Bloodroot
Sanguinaria canadensis

Forms Available Include:

• *For external use:* Decoction, ointment, powder, tincture. Extracts appear in commercial mouthwashes and toothpastes.
• *For internal use:* Decoction, tincture.

Dosage Commonly Reported:

Caution is recommended with internal formulations; see the "Will It Harm You?" section. Follow package instructions when using commercial preparations for external use.

Will It Work for You? What the Studies Say:

Bloodroot has been most extensively studied as an ingredient in mouthwashes and toothpastes to fight plaque formation and associated gum disease. Research shows that two of the numerous pharmacologically active alkaloids in the underground parts of the plant—sanguinarine and chelerythrine—help inhibit plaque from settling on the tooth enamel, fight oral compounds responsible for bad breath, reduce inflammation, numb pain perception locally (sanguinarine), and work against numerous common bacteria believed to contribute to plaque formation.[1] Although studies report success in these arenas, one scientist who conducted a critical review of the many clinical studies done using sanguinaria extracts reported that the majority actually failed to demonstrate consistent benefits.[2]

Many of the properties discovered in the hunt for an effective toothpaste and mouthwash ingredient may also explain certain folk uses for bloodroot, such as its application to inflamed and painful rheumatic joints. Still, no animal or human studies appear to have been done to determine the herb's effectiveness for such ailments. Researchers have started to look closely at the herb's folk uses for cancer; both sanguinarine and chelerythrine have shown anticancer activity in mice.[3]

Will It Harm You? What the Studies Say:

No reports of irritation or allergic reactions to topical bloodroot formulations appear in the medical literature, and toothpastes and mouthwashes containing bloodroot extracts are very unlikely to cause harm as long as they are not swallowed.[4] With extracts, stick to commercial products with set concentrations.[5]

When it comes to ingesting bloodroot, however, most herbalists and plant experts consider it much safer simply to stay away from the herb. Adverse reactions have been noted anecdotally in humans, as well as in animal studies.[6] Large doses in particular can cause nausea, vomiting, dangerous slowing down of the central nervous system, low blood pressure, shock, coma, and death.[7] The USDA placed bloodroot on its 1977 list of unsafe herbs. Pregnant women should definitely avoid it.

GENERAL SOURCES:
American Pharmaceutical Association. *Handbook of Nonprescription Drugs.* 11th ed. Washington, D.C.: American Pharmaceutical Association, 1996.

Bremness, L. *Herbs*. 1st American ed. Eyewitness Handbooks. New York: Dorling Kindersley Publications, 1994.

Duke, J.A. *CRC Handbook of Medicinal Herbs*. Boca Raton, FL: CRC Press, 1985.

Hallowell, M. *Herbal Healing: A Practical Introduction to Medicinal Herbs*. Garden City Park, NY: 1994.

Lawrence Review of Natural Products. St. Louis: Facts and Comparisons, July 1992.

Leung, A.Y., and S. Foster. *Encyclopedia of Common Natural Ingredients Used in Food, Drugs, and Cosmetics*. 2nd ed. New York: John Wiley & Sons, 1996.

Tierra, M. *The Way of Herbs*. New York: Pocket Books, 1990.

Tyler, V.E. *Herbs of Choice: The Therapeutic Use of Phytomedicinals*. Binghamton, NY: Haworth Press/Pharmaceutical Products Press, 1994.

Weiner, M.A., and J.A. Weiner. *Herbs That Heal: Prescription for Herbal Healing*. Mill Valley, CA: Quantum Books, 1994.

TEXT CITATIONS

1. K.C. Godowski, *Journal of Clinical Dentistry*, 1(4) (1989): 96–101. J.L. Dzink and S.S. Socransky, *Antimicrobic Agents and Chemotherapy*, 27 (1985): 663. A.D. Eisenberg et al., *Journal of Dental Research*, 64 (1985): 341. G.L. Southgard et al., *Journal of the American Dental Association*, 108 (1984): 338. A.Y. Leung and S. Foster, *Encyclopedia of Common Natural Ingredients Used in Food, Drugs, and Cosmetics*, 2nd ed. (New York: John Wiley & Sons, 1996).

2. T.E. Balanyk, *Clinical Preventive Dentistry*, 12(3) (1990): 18–25. American Pharmaceutical Association, *Handbook of Nonprescription Drugs*, 11th ed. (Washington, D.C.: American Pharmaceutical Association, 1996).

3. Leung and Foster, op. cit. M.J. Shear and J.L. Hartwell, *Cancer Chemotherapy Report*, July 19 (1960).

4. *Lawrence Review of Natural Products* (St. Louis: Facts and Comparisons, July 1992).

5. V.E. Tyler, *Herbs of Choice: The Therapeutic Use of Phytomedicinals* (Binghamton, NY: Haworth Press/Pharmaceutical Products Press, 1994).

6. P.J. Becci et al., *Journal of Toxicology & Environmental Health*, 20(1–2) (1987): 199–208.

7. J.A. Duke, *CRC Handbook of Medicinal Herbs* (Boca Raton, FL: CRC Press, 1985).

PRIMARY NAME:
BLUEBERRY

SCIENTIFIC NAME:
Vaccinium corymbosum L.
Family: Ericaceae

COMMON NAME:
N/A

RATING:
2 = According to a number of well-designed studies and common use, this substance appears to be relatively effective and safe when used in

What Is Blueberry?

The delicate blue-purple berry found nestling among the leaves of this native American shrub in late summer is no challenge for the average American to identify. The plant's European counterpart is the **Bilberry** (*Vaccinium myrtillus* L.). Blueberry's dried fruits and leaves are used medicinally.

What It Is Used For:

Dried blueberry fruits and leaves have a considerable reputation among plant medicine experts as diarrhea remedies. Europeans are even more familiar with this practice.

Forms Available Include:

Decoction (of dried berries), dried blueberries (to chew and swallow), fresh blueberries, infusion (of finely cut leaf), tea bag.

recommended amounts for the indication(s) noted in the "Will It Work for You?" section.

Dosage Commonly Reported:

To treat diarrhea, 3 tablespoons dried berries are chewed. Alternatively, a decoction is made using the crushed fruits. An infusion tea is made by macerating 1 to 2 teaspoons chopped leaves per cup of cold water and drunk up to three times a day.

Will It Work for You? What the Studies Say:

Dried blueberries and blueberry leaf tea are effective for treating simple diarrhea because they contain astringent substances called tannins, as well as pectin. The leaves contain as much as 10 percent tannins, which is considered moderately high.[1] Tannins are believed to control or stop diarrhea by reducing inflammation in the intestines. This type of remedy is appropriate only for simple diarrhea not caused by an underlying disease. Pectin is a high-fiber substance that adsorbs water and expands into a gelatinous clump as it travels through the stomach and intestines, thus moisturizing dry, hard stools and making them easier to pass. The sheer bulk provided by the fiber also stimulates bowel contractions and ultimately a bowel movement. Loose stools are likewise endowed with form and substance. Use only dried blueberries, however, as the fresh ones may well do the opposite of what you want when treating diarrhea: promote a bowel movement.[2]

Astringent properties also make blueberry leaf teas and infusions a good choice for treating sore throat and other inflammations of the mouth or mucous membranes of the throat.[3] Astringents constrict (tighten) tissue and help reduce oozing.

Will It Harm You? What the Studies Say:

Much remains to be learned about the risk of adverse reactions from dried blueberry fruits or leaves, although the evidence collected so far indicates that they are safe to take in typically recommended amounts. However, no tannin-rich drug should be used over long periods of time given the potential, still not fully understood, of an increased risk of cancerous changes. If you suffer from persistent diarrhea, see a doctor.

GENERAL SOURCES:

Stary, F. *The Natural Guide to Medicinal Herbs and Plants.* Prague: Barnes & Noble, Inc., in arrangement with Aventinum Publishers, 1996.

Tyler, V.E. *Herbs of Choice: The Therapeutic Use of Phytomedicinals.* Binghamton, NY: Haworth Press/Pharmaceutical Products Press, 1994.

TEXT CITATIONS:

1. D. Frohne, *Zeitschrift für Phytotherapie,* 11 (1990): 209–13.
2. V.E. Tyler, *Herbs of Choice: The Therapeutic Use of Phytomedicinals* (Binghamton, NY: Haworth Press/Pharmaceutical Products Press, 1994).
3. Ibid.

PRIMARY NAME:
BLUE COHOSH

SCIENTIFIC NAME:
Caulophyllum thalictroides (L.)
Michx. Family: Berberidaceae

COMMON NAMES:
Blueberry root, blue ginseng,
caulophyllum, papoose root,
squaw root, yellow ginseng

RATING:
5 = Studies indicate that there
is a definite health hazard to
using this herb, even in
recommended amounts.

What Is Blue Cohosh?

This perennial grows in damp woods of eastern North America, sending up its namesake blue-purple stem and single large leaf in early spring. The plant's dark blue berries contribute to the name as well. In summer it produces small clusters of yellow-green or green-purple flowers that develop into seeds. The thick and crooked rhizome (underground stem) and roots are used medicinally. Despite the common last name, blue cohosh is not related to black cohosh (*Cimicifuga racemosa*); see **Black Cohosh**.

What It Is Used For:

Native American tribes familiar with blue cohosh reportedly brewed a root tea to promote menstruation, aid labor, and treat disorders ranging from rheumatism to urinary tract infections, epilepsy, and colic.[1] Early settlers adopted it for similar purposes, but especially to trigger and hasten labor. They also used it to promote fluid loss (as a diuretic, or "water pill"), clear mucus from congested airways, and reduce fever by inducing sweating. Blue cohosh has held official drug status at certain times, being listed in the *U.S. Pharmacopoeia* and the *National Formulary*.

In line with their nineteenth-century colleagues, herbalists today describe blue cohosh as a uterine stimulant and antispasmodic, recommending it for uterine inflammation and to normalize menstrual irregularities (typically to promote menstruation or ease painful periods) and ease childbirth pains. Some also suggest taking it for intestinal worms, muscle spasms, anxiety, memory problems, arthritis, cough, asthma, high blood pressure, and other ailments.

Forms Available Include:

Capsule, decoction, liquid extract, tablet, tincture. The herb tastes very bitter.

Dosage Commonly Reported:

Blue cohosh should not be used medicinally.

Will It Work for You? What the Studies Say:

Investigators have identified chemicals in blue cohosh that can provoke strong uterine contractions, indicating it may well induce labor and promote menstruation as legend implies. Experts hold the glycosides caulosaponin and caulophyllosaponin responsible for these properties.[2] Potentially serious adverse reactions to the plant limit its use, however.

Investigators have uncovered a number of other interesting properties in blue cohosh that may one day prove useful if the toxic element can be removed, although all require much more research. For example, investigators in India have found that low doses of blue cohosh extract inhibit ovulation in test rats, suggesting a contraceptive potential.[3] A specially treated extract of the tops (aerial parts) showed anti-inflammatory activity in a rat study, but much remains unknown about its value for inflammatory ailments such as arthritis in humans.[4] Similarly, the practical value of antimicrobial activity seen in other studies for wounds and other infections must still be explored.[5]

Will It Harm You? What the Studies Say:

On the basis of its chemical constituents, blue cohosh poses considerable risk of harm; the same chemicals that stimulate the uterus may also cause heart damage by dangerously narrowing the arteries that supply blood to the heart (the coronary blood vessels). Animal studies have also shown that they can provoke intestinal spasms.[6] Another chemical in the herb, an alkaloid called N-methylcytisine (caulophylline), stimulates the small intestines, lowers blood sugar levels, and increases blood pressure.[7] It bears some resemblance to nicotine but is far less potent (about one-fortieth as toxic) according to animal research done in the 1940s.[8] Mucous membrane irritation may develop after using the powdered or dried form of blue cohosh.[9] The raw, bitter-tasting seeds have caused serious poisonings after being swallowed.[10] Ingesting the leaves and seeds may induce severe stomach pain. The berries and roots can cause cell death.[11]

Given the unpredictable reaction to the plant and the risk for serious side effects, never attempt to induce labor or stimulate menstruation with blue cohosh. Pregnant women should avoid it through all three trimesters, especially given its still poorly understood mechanism of action on the uterus and its unpredictable effects.

GENERAL SOURCES:

Balch, J.F., and P.A. Balch. *Prescription for Nutritional Healing: A Practical A to Z Reference to Drug-Free Remedies Using Vitamins, Minerals, Herbs & Food Supplements.* 2nd ed. Garden City Park, NY: Avery Publishing Group, 1997.

Benoit, P.S. *Lloydia.* 39 (1976): 160.

Castleman, M. *The Healing Herbs: The Ultimate Guide to the Curative Power of Nature's Medicines.* New York: Bantam Books, 1995.

Chandrasekhar, K., and G.H.R. Sarma. *Journal of Reproduction and Fertility.* 38 (1974): 236.

Lawrence Review of Natural Products. St. Louis: Facts and Comparisons, October 1992.

Leung, A.Y., and S. Foster. *Encyclopedia of Common Natural Ingredients Used in Food, Drugs, and Cosmetics.* 2nd ed. New York: John Wiley & Sons, 1996.

Tierra, M. *The Way of Herbs.* New York: Pocket Books, 1990.

Tyler, V.E. *The Honest Herbal.* Binghamton, NY: Haworth Press/Pharmaceutical Products Press, 1993.

Weiner, M.A., and J.A. Weiner. *Herbs That Heal: Prescription for Herbal Healing.* Mill Valley, CA: Quantum Books, 1994.

TEXT CITATIONS:

1. A.Y. Leung and S. Foster, *Encyclopedia of Common Natural Ingredients Used in Food, Drugs, and Cosmetics,* 2nd ed. (New York: John Wiley & Sons, 1996). *Lawrence Review of Natural Products* (St. Louis: Facts and Comparisons, October 1992).

2. *Lawrence Review of Natural Products,* op. cit. C.T. Che, *Dissertation Abstracts Int. B.* 43 (1982): 1049. Leung and Foster, op. cit.

3. K. Chandrasekhar and G.H.R. Sarma, *Journal of Reproduction and Fertility,* 38 (1974): 236.

4. P.S. Benoit, *Lloydia,* 39 (1976): 160.

5. M.M. Anisimov et al., *Antibiotiki i Khimioterapiia (Moskva),* 17 (1972): 834.

6. H.C. Ferguson and L.D. Edwards, *Journal of the American Pharmaceutical Association,* 43 (1954): 16. J. McShefferty and J.B. Stenlake, *Journal of the Chemical Society,* (1956): 2314–16.

7. Leung and Foster, op. cit.

8. C.C. Scott and K.K. Chen, *Therapeutics,* 79 (1943): 334.

9. *Lawrence Review of Natural Products*, op. cit.
10. J.A. Duke, *CRC Handbook of Medicinal Herbs* (Boca Raton, FL: CRC Press, 1985). K.E. Lampe and M.A. McCann, *AMA Handbook of Poisonous and Injurious Plants* (Chicago: American Medical Association, 1985).
11. Ferguson and Edwards, op. cit.

PRIMARY NAME:
BOGBEAN

SCIENTIFIC NAME:
Menyanthes trifoliata L. Family: Menyanthaceae

COMMON NAMES:
Buckbean, marsh trefoil

RATING:
2 = According to a number of well-designed studies and common use, this substance appears to be relatively effective and safe when used in recommended amounts for the indications noted in the "Will It Work for You?" section.

What Is Bogbean?

As its name suggests, this perennial favors bogs and other wet environments. It grows in temperate regions of the northern hemisphere, including many parts of North America. The large, three-part ("trefoil"), grayish-green leaves emerge off a jointed, creeping underground stem. Spikelike clusters of dense pink and white flowers appear in late spring. The dried leaves and occasionally the dried roots are used medicinally.

What It Is Used For:

Traditional healers have recommended this classic bitter digestive tonic since the seventeenth century to stimulate the appetite, increase the secretion of gastric juices and bile, and soothe digestive system upset. In some parts of Europe today, bogbean preparations are given to people suffering from exhaustion after an operation or infectious illness in the belief that the herb will soothe, stimulate, and strengthen not only the stomach but the entire body.

Folk healers once considered bogbean an important fever-reducer and treatment for worms, skin diseases, bleeding, malaria, and liver ailments. Although most of these uses have largely disappeared, the herb and occasionally extracts from its bitter principles still appear in herbal mixtures to control rheumatism, boost health in the aged, and treat a number of other conditions. Large doses are considered laxative.

Forms Available:

Decoction, dried leaves, extract, infusion. A common component in herbal blends.

Dosage Commonly Reported:

A tea is made using ½ to 1 teaspoon finely chopped dried leaves and is drunk one-half hour before meals.

Will It Work for You? What the Studies Say:

Scientists have apparently not studied bogbean in animals or humans, although they have identified its chemical constituents. On the basis of an understanding of these, many experts contend that the herb will effectively stimulate the appetite and serve as a soothing digestive tonic, but generally prefer more proven and powerful bitters such as **Gentian**.[1] On a "bitter" index, bogbean ranks low. It contains several bitter attributes (secoridoid glycosides), which stimulate saliva and gastric juices. One has even been shown to help digestive tract spasms.[2] Because tannins (7 percent) in the herb can actually irritate the stomach and because of the bitter taste of the leaves, bogbean is usually prepared as part of an herbal blend.[3] German health authorities approve of bogbean preparations to treat indigestion and appetite loss.[4]

Chemicals in bogbean such as the coumarins scoparone and scopoletin may also help protect the liver and stimulate its production of bile, fight inflammation, and reduce stomach spasms, according to recent research.[5] But since tests of these properties using bogbean per se have not yet been conducted in humans or laboratory animals, their implications remain unclear.

Will It Harm You? What the Studies Say:

Science offers very little information about the potential toxicity of bogbean. It is significant that many people have reportedly used it over the centuries to no apparent ill effect. German health authorities cite no known side effects or situations in which the herb should not be used. However, British health authorities recommend that people suffering from diarrhea (including infectious diarrhea) or colitis (bowel inflammation) avoid it.[6] Use the dried leaves or root, as the fresh plant can cause vomiting.[7]

GENERAL SOURCES:

Bisset, N.E., ed. *Herbal Drugs and Phytopharmaceuticals.* Stuttgart: medpharm GmbH Scientific Publishers, 1994.

Blumenthal, M., J. Gruenwald, T. Hall, and R.S. Rister, eds. *The Complete German Commission E Monographs: Therapeutic Guide to Herbal Medicine.* Boston: Integrative Medicine Communications, 1998.

Bradley, P.C., ed. *British Herbal Compendium: A Handbook of Scientific Information on Widely Used Plant Drugs,* vol. 1. Bournemouth (Dorset), England: British Herbal Medicine Association, 1992.

Foster, S., and J.A. Duke. *The Peterson Field Guide Series: A Field Guide to Medicinal Plants. Eastern and Central North America.* Boston: Houghton Mifflin Company, 1990.

Huang, C., et al. *Yao Hsueh Pao—Acta Pharmaceutica Sinica.* 30(8) (1995): 621–26.

Stary, F. *The Natural Guide to Medicinal Herbs and Plants.* Prague: Barnes & Noble, Inc., in arrangement with Aventinum Publishers, 1996.

Weiss, R.F. *Herbal Medicine,* trans. A.R. Meuss, from the 6th German edition. Beaconsfield, England: Beaconsfield Publishers, Ltd., 1988.

TEXT CITATIONS:

1. R.F. Weiss, *Herbal Medicine,* trans. A. R. Meuss from the 6th German edition. (Beaconsfield, England: Beaconsfield Publishers, Ltd., 1988).
2. N.E. Bisset, ed., *Herbal Drugs and Phytopharmaceuticals* (Stuttgart: medpharm GmbH Scientific Publishers, 1994).
3. Weiss, op. cit.
4. M. Blumenthal, J. Gruenwald, T. Hall, and R.S. Rister, eds., *The Complete German Commission E Monographs: Therapeutic Guide to Herbal Medicine* (Boston: Integrative Medicine Communications, 1998).
5. U. Adamczyk et al., *Plantes Med Phytother,* 24 (1990):73–78. Bisset, op. cit. C. Huang et al., *Yao Hsueh Hsueh Pao—Acta Pharmaceutica Sinica,* 30(8) (1995): 621–26.
6. Blumenthal et al., op. cit. P.C. Bradley, ed., *British Herbal Compendium: A Handbook of Scientific Information on Widely Used Plant Drugs,* vol. 1 (Bournemouth [Dorset], England: British Herbal Medicine Association, 1992).
7. S. Foster and J.A. Duke, *The Peterson Field Guide Series: A Field Guide to Medicinal Plants. Eastern and Central North America* (Boston: Houghton Mifflin Company, 1990).

BOLDO

SCIENTIFIC NAME:
Peumus boldus Mol. Also referred to as *Boldu boldus* [Mol.] Lyons and *Boldea fragrans* Gay. Family: Monimiaceae

COMMON NAMES:
Boldea, boldoa, boldus

RATING:
2 = According to a number of well-designed studies and common use, this substance appears to be relatively effective and safe when used in recommended amounts for the indication(s) noted in the "Will It Work for You?" section. However, see the safety warnings in the "Will It Harm You?" section.

What Is Boldo?

The pungently spicy dried leaves of this native Chilean evergreen shrub (or small tree) are used medicinally. Boldo is naturalized in Europe.

What It Is Used For:

In South American regions where boldo has grown for years, traditional healers have turned to their plant for help with numerous ailments, although the emphasis reportedly has always been on treating digestive, liver, and biliary disorders. European and Canadian herbalists now use boldo similarly,[1] as well as for cramplike stomach upset, indigestion, rheumatism, intestinal worms, gout, and numerous other maladies.[2] Many consider boldo diuretic (able to increase urine output), laxative, sedative, and antispasmodic. Homeopaths recommend minute amounts for similar ailments. (See page 2 for a discussion of homeopathy.)

Forms Available Include:

Dried leaves, extracts, infusion, tablet, tincture. Boldo leaves frequently appear in prepared herbal cholagogue and biliary tea remedies. (Cholagogues purportedly control indigestion by promoting the flow and discharge of bile from the liver.) Formulations standardized for a critical ingredient called boldine, which may dissipate if the infusion is not properly prepared, may be the wisest choice.[3]

Dosage Commonly Reported:

An infusion is made with 1 to 2 teaspoonsful (1.5 to 3.0 grams) of the dried leaves. Choose commercial preparations standardized for boldine when available; follow package instructions.

Will It Work for You? What the Studies Say:

The widespread use of boldo as a diuretic, laxative, stomach soother, and component in "liver tonic" teas may be justified by the presence of an alkaloid called boldine. Research indicates that boldine stimulates the liver to secrete more bile and the kidneys to boost urine output.[4] Definitive human studies do not appear to have been done, however. Recent findings indicate that one of the herb's other numerous alkaloids may be responsible for some of these actions. A 1991 rat study found that the plant displayed notable liver-protectant actions as well as anti-inflammatory properties evidently unrelated to boldine.[5] Apparently on the basis of these findings as well as evidence that the herb can increase the secretion of gastric juices and help relieve muscle spasms,[6] German health authorities endorse boldo leaf preparations for treating dyspepsia (indigestion) and mild, cramplike stomach and intestinal upset.[7]

Although boldo was never formally tested against other diuretics, increased urination has been observed in humans following ingestion of boldo.[8] In a dog study, boldine appeared to increase urine output by 50 percent.[9] There is evidence that boldo, unlike a "true" diuretic, increases urination by promoting blood flow in the kidneys.[10] Large doses may be necessary to get a diuretic effect.[11] Boldo also contains volatile oils (about 2 percent) believed to perform similarly to boldine[12] and to account for the herb's strong aromatic odor.

Scientists have recently started to focus on boldine and other boldo extracts as antioxidants that could help prevent or treat certain cancers, atherosclerosis, autoimmune and inflammatory diseases, and other disorders.[13] Antioxidants are believed to help scavenge toxic by-products that may contribute to cancer cell formation.

Will It Harm You? What the Studies Say:

Use boldo with care. The volatile oils contain high levels (about 40 percent) of ascaridole, a somewhat toxic substance.[14] Ascaridole accounts for boldo's folk use for fighting worms. No long-term studies on the effect of boldo in humans appear to have been done, but large oral doses have been reported to cause exaggerated reflexes, excitement, cramps, convulsions, and even death from respiratory paralysis in severe cases.[15] An oral dose of 15 grams caused fatal intoxication in dogs.[16] Although communities in South America have been using the herb for some time, they are also known to handle the herb with extreme caution.[17]

Given the dearth of long-term testing in humans, some experts recommend that pregnant women avoid the herb altogether and that no one should use it for prolonged periods.[18] Because of ascaridole, German health authorities warn against using distillates or the essential oil of boldo.[19] They also advise people with gallstones to consult their doctors before taking it and individuals with a serious liver condition or bile duct obstruction to avoid it altogether.

GENERAL SOURCES:

Bisset, N.E., ed. *Herbal Drugs and Phytopharmaceuticals.* Stuttgart: medpharm GmbH Scientific Publishers, 1994.

Blumenthal, M., J. Gruenwald, T. Hall, and R.S. Rister, eds. *The Complete German Commission E Monographs: Therapeutic Guide to Herbal Medicine.* Boston: Integrative Medicine Communications, 1998.

Duke, J.A. *CRC Handbook of Medicinal Herbs.* Boca Raton, FL: CRC Press, 1985.

Lawrence Review of Natural Products. St. Louis: Facts and Comparisons, May 1991.

Leung, A.Y., and S. Foster. *Encyclopedia of Common Natural Ingredients Used in Food, Drugs, and Cosmetics.* 2nd ed. New York: John Wiley & Sons, 1996.

Tyler, V.E. *Herbs of Choice: The Therapeutic Use of Phytomedicinals.* Binghamton, NY: Haworth Press/Pharmaceutical Products Press, 1994.

Weiss, R.F. *Herbal Medicine*, trans. A.R. Meuss, from the 6th German edition. Beaconsfield, England: Beaconsfield Publishers, Ltd., 1988.

TEXT CITATIONS:

1. *Lawrence Review of Natural Products* (St. Louis: Facts and Comparisons, May 1991).
2. J.A. Duke, *CRC Handbook of Medicinal Herbs* (Boca Raton, FL: CRC Press, 1985). N.E. Bisset, ed., *Herbal Drugs and Phytopharmaceuticals* (Stuttgart: medpharm GmbH Scientific Publishers, 1994).
3. C. Van Hulle et al., *Journal de Pharmacie de Belgique*, 38 (1983): 97.
4. D.W. Hughes et al., *Journal of Pharmaceutical Sciences*, 57 (1968): 1023.
5. M.C. Lanher et al., *Planta Medica*, 57 (1991): 110.
6. H. Speisky et al., *Planta Medica*, 57 (1991): 519–22.
7. M. Blumenthal, J. Gruenwald, T. Hall, and R.S. Rister, eds., *The Complete German Commission E Monographs: Therapeutic Guide to Herbal Medicine* (Boston: Integrative Medicine Communications, 1998).
8. *Lawrence Review of Natural Products*, op. cit.

9. H. Kreitmar, *Pharmazie*, 7 (1952): 507.

10. V.E. Tyler, *Herbs of Choice: The Therapeutic Use of Phytomedicinals* (Binghamton, NY: Haworth Press/Pharmaceutical Products Press, 1994).

11. Speisky, op. cit.

12. *Lawrence Review of Natural Products*, op. cit.

13. H. Speisky and B.K. Cassels, *Pharmacological Research*, 29(1) (1994): 1–12. A.I. Ceberbaum et al., *Biochemical Pharmacology*, 44(9) (1992): 1765–72.

14. Tyler, op. cit.

15. Duke, op. cit.

16. K. Genest and D.W. Hughes, *Canadian Journal of Pharmaceutical Science*, 3 (1965): 85.

17. Duke, op. cit.

18. Ibid.

19. Blumenthal et al., op. cit.

PRIMARY NAME:
BONESET

SCIENTIFIC NAME:

Eupatorium perfoliatum L.
Family: Asteraceae
(Compositae)

COMMON NAMES:

Agueweed, crosswort, eupatorium, feverwort, gravelroot, Indian sage, sweating plant, thoroughwort, vegetable antimony

RATING:

3 = Studies on the effectiveness and safety of this substance are conflicting, or there are not enough studies to draw a conclusion. However, see the safety warning in the "Will It Harm You?" section.

What Is Boneset?

This distinctive-looking perennial has grown for centuries along the shores and in the marshes and swamps of North America. The unusual tapering leaves appear to be pierced through the center by the hairy stem. The dried leaves and dried white flowering tops are used medicinally.

What It Is Used For:

Various Native American tribes treated colds, flu, rheumatism, and a number of other ailments with this herb. Above all, they valued it for bringing down fevers caused by diseases such as typhoid and dengue (at one time commonly referred to as "breakbone fever," hence the name "boneset"). Settlers adopted this folk wisdom, for decades turning to boneset to break fevers by inducing sweating. They picked up a number of other Native American practices as well, treating such ailments as indigestion and appetite loss with the herb. At one point, boneset came to be regarded as a general tonic and cure-all.

The official medical establishment in America recognized boneset for some time; the *U.S. Pharmacopoeia* listed it as a treatment for fevers from 1820 through 1916, as did the *National Formulary* from 1926 through 1950. But with the surging popularity of safer and more effective fever-reducers such as aspirin, the demand for boneset dwindled.[1] Modern-day herbalists recommend boneset, especially in a hot drink, to stimulate sweating and alleviate the aches and pains of arthritis, colds, flu, and other minor inflammatory, viral, and bacterial illnesses. Some recommend it in the form of a cold infusion for indigestion, loss of appetite, and mild constipation. Boneset has a bitter taste and can be nauseating, especially when added to a hot liquid. Homeopaths prescribe minute amounts of boneset for various conditions. (See page 2 for a discussion of homeopathy.) Notwithstanding the suggestive name, no one—at least in recent times—has reportedly tried to set a broken bone with boneset.

Forms Available Include:

Dried leaves, extracts, infusion, tincture.

Dosage Commonly Reported:

An infusion is made using 1 to 2 teaspoons chopped dried leaves per cup of water and is drunk up to three times per day. The tincture is taken in dosages of $1/2$ to 1 teaspoon up to three times per day. Consult the labels on extracts for dosage information.

Will It Work for You? What the Studies Say:

Many plant experts fail to see any medicinal value in boneset. Even when health authorities in the United States officially sanctioned its use, apparently few doctors actually prescribed it, and the editors of the 1955 *U.S. Dispensatory* recommended it not be used.[2] No well-designed clinical trials have been done to test whether boneset is safe or effective for human use.

But boneset has its advocates. They point to test-tube studies indicating several active ingredients in the herb. Many who recommend it for boosting resistance to infection cite the presence of a bitter-tasting compound, eupatorin. Antibacterial properties were demonstrated in a test-tube study in which an extract of the plant (combined with other herbs) stimulated phagocytes, white blood cells that help engulf and destroy disease-causing agents.[3]

Boneset's most widely held reputation—as a fever-breaker—remains unsubstantiated. No studies have ever shown that the herb significantly relieves dengue fever, malaria, or other feverish conditions for which it was once enthusiastically recommended. Of course, a person may start to sweat more and even become nauseated while drinking boneset tea, especially if it is hot.

In times past, boneset was occasionally combined with hops to battle tumors. Scientists have identified cell-destroying and tumor-fighting (antineoplastic) properties in boneset and related species, but the researchers themselves note that much more research is needed before the herb can be recommended as a cancer-fighter.[4] The arthritis-relieving implications of a study showing that a boneset extract can function as a weak anti-inflammatory in rats are likewise unclear.[5] Researchers are still investigating whether boneset contains compounds that enhance blood coagulation, protect the liver, or increase bile output by the liver.[6]

Will It Harm You? What the Studies Say:

Early American medical sources indicate that small doses of boneset may promote urination (as a diuretic, or "water pill") and exert a mild laxative effect. But large amounts may cause vomiting and potentially severe diarrhea.[7] Fresh boneset in particular must be avoided, as it contains a chemical—tremerol—that can produce nausea, vomiting, muscle tremors, increased respiration, and, at high doses, death in some cases.[8] As the plant dries, this chemical dissipates, eliminating the risk of poisoning.

There is scant evidence that anyone has suffered harm directly as a result of using recommended doses of boneset. By the same token, no controlled studies in humans can be cited to demonstrate that it is safe, and there is considerable information to cause concern. The FDA has classified boneset as an herb of "undefined safety." Scientists have discovered that *Eupatorium* species contain dangerous chemicals—pyrrolizidine alkaloids (PAs)—that can cause liver damage and even liver cancer if taken over long periods of time. Even very low levels of certain types, when taken for long periods, may cause considerable harm. Given this hazard, German health authorities at one point advised consumers to ingest no more than 1 microgram of PAs a day, a challenging proposition for American consumers, who have no way of ascertaining the PA content of the product they buy unless the herb manufacturer decides to note it. In contrast, German consumers can monitor their intake because authorities have established "safe" minimums. So far, no one appears to have actually suffered such liver damage from taking boneset, but the potential risk has led some experts to recommend against using any plant that contains these alkaloids.[9] Others simply warn against using the herb for more than two weeks at a time, and recommend that anyone with liver problems or a history of alcoholism talk to a doctor before taking it.[10]

Contact dermatitis from this member of the daisy family is a risk.

GENERAL SOURCES:

Bisset, N.E., ed. *Herbal Drugs and Phytopharmaceuticals.* Stuttgart: medpharm GmbH Scientific Publishers, 1994.

Castleman, M. *The Healing Herbs: The Ultimate Guide to the Curative Power of Nature's Medicines.* New York: Bantam Books, 1995.

Der Marderosian, A., and L. Liberti. *Natural Product Medicine: A Scientific Guide to Foods, Drugs, Cosmetics.* Philadelphia: George F. Stickley, 1988.

Duke, J.A. *CRC Handbook of Medicinal Herbs.* Boca Raton, FL: CRC Press, 1985.

Hall, Jr., T.B. *Missouri Medicine.* 71(9) (1974): 527–28.

Lawrence Review of Natural Products. St. Louis: Facts and Comparisons, February 1993.

Leung, A.Y., *Encyclopedia of Common Natural Ingredients Used in Food, Drugs, and Cosmetics.* New York: John Wiley & Sons, 1980.

Tyler, V.E. *The Honest Herbal.* Binghamton, NY: Haworth Press/Pharmaceutical Products Press, 1992.

Zhao, X.L., et al. *American Journal of Chinese Medicine.* 17(1–2) (1989): 71–78.

TEXT CITATIONS:

1. A. Der Marderosian and L. Liberti, *Natural Product Medicine: A Scientific Guide to Foods, Drugs, Cosmetics* (Philadelphia: George F. Stickley, 1988).
2. A. Osol et al., *United States Dispensatory, 25th Edition* (Philadelphia: J.B. Lippincott Co., 1955).
3. H. Wagner and K. Jurcic, *Arzneimittel-Forschung,* 41(10) (1991): 1072–76.
4. M. Tsuda, *Canadian Journal of Chemistry,* 8 (1963): 1919. S.M. Kupchan et al., *Tetrahedron,* 25(8) (1969): 1603–15. J.A. Duke, *CRC Handbook of Medicinal Herbs* (Boca Raton, FL: CRC Press, 1985. Duke, 1985).
5. A.Y. Leung, *Encyclopedia of Common Natural Ingredients Used in Food, Drugs, and Cosmetics* (New York: John Wiley & Sons, 1980).
6. T. Triratana et al., *Journal of the Medical Association of Thailand,* 74 (1991): 283. A. Lexa et al., *Planta Medica,* 55(2) (1989): 127–32.
7. Duke, op. cit. Leung, op. cit.
8. M. Castleman, *The Healing Herbs: The Ultimate Guide to the Curative Power of Nature's Medicines* (New York: Bantam Books, 1995).

9. Der Marderosian and Liberti, op. cit.
10. Castleman, op. cit.

PRIMARY NAME:
BORAGE

SCIENTIFIC NAME:
Borago officinalis L. Family:
Boraginaceae

COMMON NAMES:
Beebread, bee plant, borrage,
burrage, common borage,
common bugloss, cool tankard,
ox's tongue, starflower

RATING:
- *For borage:* 4 = Research indicates that this substance will not fulfill the claims made for it, but that it is also unlikely to cause any harm.
- *For borage seed oil:* 3 = Studies on the effectiveness and safety of this substance are conflicting, or there are not enough studies to draw a conclusion. However, see the safety warning in the "Will It Harm You?" section.

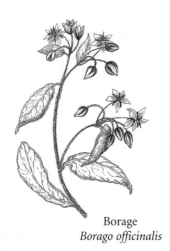

Borage
Borago officinalis

What Is Borage?

From the bristly stems to the blue star-shaped flowers, virtually all parts of this robust annual have been used as a medicine and food flavoring. An oil is made from the seeds. The plant grows across Europe and North America.

What It Is Used For:

Europeans turned to borage as a refreshing tea and herbal remedy centuries ago, soaking the leaves and flowers in wine to dispel melancholy and boredom. Convinced of the herb's soothing and astringent qualities, herbalists have recommended borage preparations for colds, bronchitis, rheumatisms, kidney stones, corns, diarrhea, and many other ailments. Some have promoted borage as a diuretic ("water pill") and a breast milk stimulant. Borage once held official drug status in Spain, Portugal, Romania, Germany, Brazil, Venezuela, and Mexico.

Modern herbalists recommend borage for relieving nervous tension, alleviating the discomforts of premenstrual syndrome, fighting inflammation, and restoring adrenal function. Many point to the high concentration of gamma-linoleic acid (GLA) in the seed oil as a reason for using the herb. Fresh borage has a mildly salty, cucumberlike flavor and qualifies as a common kitchen herb in parts of Europe.

Forms Available Include:

Extracts, fresh herb, seed oil capsules, tea.

Dosage Commonly Reported:

One 300-milligram softgel containing the seed oil (24 percent GLA) is taken daily. The liquid leaf extract is taken in doses of 2 to 4 milliliters.

Will It Work for You? What the Studies Say:

Research indicates that, with the possible exception of the seed oil, borage exerts negligible or no therapeutic effects. The presence of tannin may explain the plant's astringent qualities and constipating actions, but these are in fact mild; one small-animal study found that except for a minimal constipating effect, borage was virtually inert.[1] Malic acid and potassium nitrate may generate a slight diuretic effect,[2] but most experts agree that conditions requiring a diuretic usually merit more rigorous treatment. Evidence that a soothing gelatinous substance called mucilage appears in concentrations large enough to clear congested airways and prove effective in cold remedies is nowhere to be found.[3] Nor has the plant's reputation as a mood-enhancer been proved.[4]

The seed oil may tell a different story because it contains a rich store (20 to 26 percent) of a possibly important substance, GLA. Advocates say GLA has potential for ameliorating such conditions as arthritis, inflammatory skin diseases, premenstrual syndrome, and heart disease. Animal studies and a growing number of human studies support some of these claims, although the results are controversial and critics remain skeptical.

A 1993 study involving thirty-seven individuals suffering from painful rheumatoid arthritis and active inflammation around the joints found that those randomly selected to take borage seed oil daily over a period of twenty-four weeks experienced notable improvements in disease indicators such as the number of joints that felt tender and swollen. Those given a placebo, on the other hand, experienced no change or an actual worsening of their condition.[5] Importantly, none of the subjects taking the borage seed oil withdrew from the study because of unwanted side effects. But the dosage used—1.4 grams a day—was much higher than most herbalists typically recommend, and the authors note the need for more research before treating any disease with this herb. In an earlier study, six of seven individuals with active rheumatoid arthritis who took borage seed oil capsules daily (totaling 1.1 grams a day of GLA) for twelve weeks both felt better and experienced improvements in laboratory indications of inflammation.[6] However, the subjects knew they were being given borage seed oil, so the possibility that they imagined they were improving even if they were not cannot be ruled out.

Researchers are investigating whether GLA can reduce symptoms of skin inflammation in humans as it has been able to do in numerous small-animal studies. In a 1992 study, the condition of five out of seven atopic dermatitis sufferers randomly chosen to take borage oil improved, while that of only one out of five who took a placebo improved.[7] This was a very small study, however. Much remains to be learned about GLA and what it can do for human health.

Will It Harm You? What the Studies Say:

People have been using borage as a folk remedy for centuries without suffering any notable ill effects. In the mid-1980s, however, disturbing reports indicated that potentially poisonous substances—toxic unsaturated pyrrolizidine alkaloids (PAs) such as lycopasamine and amabiline—appear in the plant, albeit at very low concentrations.[8] Scientists are exploring what this means for people interested in taking this herb or its seed oil medicinally. PAs have been implicated in liver damage and primary liver cancer. Even very low levels of certain types, when taken for long periods, may cause considerable harm. Given this hazard, German health authorities at one point advised consumers to ingest no more than 1 microgram of PAs a day, a challenging proposition for American consumers, who have no way of ascertaining the PA (or GLA) content of the borage product they buy unless the herb manufacturer decides to note it. In contrast, German consumers can monitor their intake because authorities have established "safe" minimums for medicinal plants such as borage. Ultimately, however, the German authorities declined to approve of the herb for any medicinal use.[9] Certainly, caution would dictate that no borage product—especially a seed oil—be used on a long-term basis unless a physician is overseeing your case, at least until experts can soundly establish its safety.[10]

GENERAL SOURCES:

Awang, D.V.C. *Canadian Pharmaceutical Journal.* 123 (1990): 121–26.

Bahmer, F.A., and J. Schafer. *Kinderarztliche Praxis.* 60(7) (1992): 199–202.

Bisset, N.E., ed. *Herbal Drugs and Phytopharmaceuticals.* Stuttgart: medpharm GmbH Scientific Publishers, 1994.

Blumenthal, M., J. Gruenwald, T. Hall, and R.S. Rister, eds. *The Complete German Commission E Monographs: Therapeutic Guide to Herbal Medicine.* Boston: Integrative Medicine Communications, 1998.

Hallowell, M. *Herbal Healing: A Practical Introduction to Medicinal Herbs.* Garden City Park, NY: 1994.

Lawrence Review of Natural Products. St. Louis: Facts and Comparisons, August 1992.

Mayell, M. *Off-the-Shelf Natural Health: How to Use Herbs and Nutrients to Stay Well.* New York: Bantam Books, 1995.

Tyler, V.E. *Herbs of Choice: The Therapeutic Use of Phytomedicinals.* Binghamton, NY: Haworth Press/Pharmaceutical Products Press, 1994.

———. *The Honest Herbal.* Binghamton, NY: Haworth Press/Pharmaceutical Products Press, 1993.

Weiss, R.F. *Herbal Medicine,* trans. A.R. Meuss, from the 6th German edition. Beaconsfield, England: Beaconsfield Publishers, Ltd., 1988.

TEXT CITATIONS:

1. E. Hannig, *Die Pharmazie,* 5 (1995): 35.
2. V.E. Tyler, *The Honest Herbal* (Binghamton, NY: Haworth Press/Pharmaceutical Products Press, 1993).
3. *Lawrence Review of Natural Products* (St. Louis: Facts and Comparisons, August 1992).
4. R.F. Weiss, *Herbal Medicine,* trans. A. R. Meuss, from the 6th German edition (Beaconsfield, England: Beaconsfield Publishers, Ltd., 1988).
5. L.J. Leventhal et al., *Annals of Internal Medicine,* 119(9) (1993): 867–73.
6. S. Pullman-Mooar et al., *Arthritis & Rheumatism,* 33(10) (1990): 1526–33.
7. F.A. Bahmer and J. Schafer, *Kinderarztliche Praxis,* 60(7) (1992): 199–202.
8. K.M. Larson et al., *Journal of Natural Products,* 47(4) (1984): 747–48. J. Luethy et al., *Pharmaceutica Acta Helvetiae,* 59(9–10) (1984): 242–46.
9. M. Blumenthal, J. Gruenwald, T. Hall, and R.S. Rister, eds., *The Complete German Commission E Monographs: Therapeutic Guide to Herbal Medicine* (Boston: Integrative Medicine Communications, 1998).
10. V.E. Tyler, *Herbs of Choice: The Therapeutic Use of Phytomedicinals* (Binghamton, NY: Haworth Press/Pharmaceutical Products Press, 1994).

PRIMARY NAME:

BOSWELLIN

SCIENTIFIC NAME:

Boswellia serrata. Family: Burseraceae

COMMON NAMES:

Boswellic acids, Indian frankincense, Indian olibanum

What Is Boswellin?

The gummy resin called boswellin is found under the bark of *Boswellia serrata,* a moderately large branching tree that grows in India. The resin is extracted and purified for medicinal use.

What It Is Used For:

Traditional Indian (Ayurvedic) healers have long considered boswellin a valuable anti-inflammatory and rheumatic disease remedy. American herbal outlets now sell boswellin tablets to treat rheumatic disorders, and boswellin-containing skin creams to relieve minor arthritis-associated aches and pains temporarily, moisturize dry skin, and shrink wrinkles. Ayurvedic healers reportedly also treat diarrhea, fungal infections such as ringworm, boils, and other conditions with the resin. Western sources often refer to boswellin as "Indian frankincense." Its essential oil appears in oriental perfumes.

Forms Available Include:

- *For internal use:* Capsule and tablet, often standardized for boswellic acids.
- *For external use:* Extracts in creams and various cosmetics.

Dosage Commonly Reported:

Boswellin in 195-milligram-capsule form is taken three times a day. Tablets standardized for boswellic acids should be taken according to package instructions.

Will It Work for You? What the Studies Say:

Numerous test-tube and small-animal studies, the majority of them carried out in India and a handful done in Europe, have identified the active ingredients in boswellin—four triterpene acids referred to as "boswellic acids" (BAs)—that support boswellin's traditional standing as an inflammatory disease remedy. BA injected into rats significantly lessened inflammation in the classic model to test a substance's anti-inflammatory properties, the chemically induced swollen rat paw.[1] It also markedly reduced certain chemical markers of inflammatory activity (complement). Injected into rabbits, BA significantly curtailed the movement of inflammatory white cells (leukocytes) into damaged tissue.[2] According to a 1993 European patent application, BA also inhibits inflammation resulting from the formation of leukotrienes, chemicals critical to the inflammatory process in disorders such as Crohn's disease and ulcerative colitis.[3] In a 1991 study, boswellic acid showed protective activity against chemically induced hepatitis in mice.[4] No analgesic or fever-reducing actions were noted in animal studies, however.[5]

While intriguing, these properties have not been tested in well-designed human trials. Some sources cite human trials in which boswellin was one of several ingredients given to the subjects, making its specific contribution difficult to discern.[6] Most of the promising animal studies also involved injecting boswellin (or BA); tablets to swallow and creams to apply to the skin are the formulations available in America today.

According to preliminary studies, salai guggal, a product prepared from the plant's gum resin exudate and BAs, may prove more potent as an anti-inflammatory than BAs alone.[7]

Will It Harm You? What the Studies Say:

Boswellin has been used for centuries in traditional Indian medicine; in addition, none of the scientific evidence collected so far indicates that boswellin poses significant risk of harm. None of the animals appeared to suffer from stomach irritation or ulcer development, both risks with standard nonsteroidal anti-inflammatory medicines commonly taken to control arthritis pain. On the other hand, most of the animals were not at such risk for stomach upset, given the fact that they were injected with the substance.

GENERAL SOURCES:

Balch, J.F., and P.A. Balch. *Prescription for Nutritional Healing: A Practical A to Z Reference to Drug-Free Remedies Using Vitamins, Minerals, Herbs & Food Supplements.* 2nd ed. Garden City Park, NY: Avery Publishing Group, 1997.

Bremness, L. *Herbs.* 1st American ed. Eyewitness Handbooks. New York: Dorling Kindersley Publications, 1994.

Singh, G.B., et al. *Drugs Today.* 32(2) (1996): 109–12.

TEXT CITATIONS:

1. A. Kapil, *International Journal of Inflammopharmocology*, 2(4) (1994): 361–67.
2. M.L. Sharma et al., *International Journal of Immunopharmacology*, 11(6) (1989): 674–752.
3. H.P.T. Ammon et al., European Patent Application EP 552,657.
4. H. Safayhi et al., *Biochemical Pharmacology*, 41(10) (1991): 1536–67.
5. G.B. Singh and C.K. Atal, *Agents & Actions*, 18(3–4) (1986): 407–12.
6. R.R. Kulkarni et al., *Journal of Ethnopharmacology*, 33(1–2) (1991): 91–95.
7. G. Kesava Reddy and S.C. Dhar, *Italian Journal of Biochemistry*, 36(4) (1987): 205–17.

PRIMARY NAME:

BROMELAIN

SCIENTIFIC NAME:
N/A

COMMON NAME:
N/A

RATING:
3 = Studies on the effectiveness and safety of this substance are conflicting, or there are not enough studies to draw a conclusion.

What Is Bromelain?

Bromelain is a naturally occurring enzyme found in the pineapple plant (*Ananas comosus*), the well-known tropical succulent perennial. Its fruit is eaten in many parts of the world. There are two types of bromelain; that taken from the fruit, called fruit bromelain; and that taken from the stem, called stem bromelain. Commercial bromelain is typically made with stem bromelain and also contains other enzymes and calcium.[1]

What It Is Used For:

Commercial manufacturers extract bromelain, one of the pineapple plant's enzymes, for use as a meat tenderizer. Introduced in 1957 and intensively studied since then,[2] this enzyme has been promoted for a number of medicinal purposes as well, including encouraging good digestion, for example, by helping to break down food more completely. Some sources recommend bromelain for removing dead tissue from skin burns; for treating inflammation and edema (fluid retention or swelling) caused by surgery, trauma, allergies, arthritis, and infections; and for easing diarrhea due to digestive enzyme deficiency. Others still promote it for respiratory tract infections, painful menses, vein inflammation (thrombophlebitis) and varicose veins, wound healing, pain and swelling in sports injuries, and ulcer prevention, and as an adjunct to cancer therapy. Bromelain appears in cosmetics such as facial cleansers and bath preparations, and in food as an agent to chillproof and modify dough. Bromelain often serves as a substitute for the more costly proteolytic enzyme called papain, derived from the unripe papaya fruit (see **Papaya**). See also **Pineapple**.

Forms Available Include:

Extract, tablet. The tablet usually carries an indication of potency based on enzyme units established by the supplier. The extract also appears in vitamin and herbal blends. When used as a digestive aid, bromelain should ideally be taken on an empty stomach.[3]

Dosage Commonly Reported:

Tablets of 250 milligrams to 500 milligrams are taken three times per day between meals. As a digestive aid, bromelain is taken with meals.

Will It Work for You? What the Studies Say:

Studies on bromelain indicate a broad spectrum of action, but the American medical community no longer prescribes it because clinical trials failed to prove that it was effective for most ailments when taken by human beings.[4]

Will It Harm You? What the Studies Say:

Bromelain is not generally associated with adverse reactions, although nausea, vomiting, diarrhea, skin rash, and excessive menstrual flow have been reported in people taking medicinal doses.[5] It can also cause allergic reactions if you have been sensitized to it or are exposed to it over long periods of time.[6] An odd reaction among pineapple cutters has been noted: repeated exposure to the bromelain destroys their fingerprints.[7]

GENERAL SOURCES:

Duke, J.A. *CRC Handbook of Medicinal Herbs.* Boca Raton, FL: CRC Press, 1985.
Lawrence Review of Natural Products. St. Louis: Facts and Comparisons, July 1993.
Leung, A.Y., and S. Foster. *Encyclopedia of Common Natural Ingredients Used in Food, Drugs, and Cosmetics.* 2nd ed. New York: John Wiley & Sons, 1996.
Mayell, M. *Off-the-Shelf Natural Health: How to Use Herbs and Nutrients to Stay Well.* New York: Bantam Books, 1995.
Murray, M.T. *The Healing Power of Herbs: The Enlightened Person's Guide to the Wonders of Medicinal Plants.* Revised and expanded 2nd ed. Rocklin, CA: Prima Publishing, 1995.
Mayell, M. *Off-the-Shelf Natural Health: How to Use Herbs and Nutrients to Stay Well.* New York: Bantam Books, 1995.
Weiss, R.F. *Herbal Medicine,* trans. A.R. Meuss, from the 6th German edition. Beaconsfield, England: Beaconsfield Publishers, Ltd., 1988.

TEXT CITATIONS:

1. A.Y. Leung and S. Foster, *Encyclopedia of Common Natural Ingredients Used in Food, Drugs, and Cosmetics,* 2nd ed. (New York: John Wiley & Sons, 1996).
2. M.T. Murray, *The Healing Power of Herbs: The Enlightened Person's Guide to the Wonders of Medicinal Plants,* Revised and expanded 2nd ed. (Rocklin, CA: Prima Publishing, 1995).
3. Ibid.
4. *Lawrence Review of Natural Products* (St. Louis: Facts and Comparisons, July 1993).
5. Leung and Foster, op. cit.
6. Murray, op. cit.
7. J.A. Duke, *CRC Handbook of Medicinal Herbs* (Boca Raton, FL: CRC Press, 1985).

PRIMARY NAME:
BROOM

SCIENTIFIC NAME:
Cytisus scoparius (L.) Link, occasionally referred to as *Sarothamnus scoparius* (L.) Wimm., *Sarothamnus vulgaris* Wimm., or *Spartium scoparium* L. Family: Leguminosae (Fabaceae)

COMMON NAMES:
Bannal, besom, broom tops, hogweed, Irish broom, scoparius, Scotch broom, Scottish broom

RATING:
3 = Studies on the effectiveness and safety of this substance are conflicting, or there are not enough studies to draw a conclusion. However, see the safety warnings in the "Will It Harm You?" section.

What Is Broom?

In early summer, the golden-yellow butterflylike flowers of this large shrub, a native of Europe, bloom across the Atlantic and Pacific Northwest coasts of America. For medicinal purposes, the tops are picked and dried just before flowering. Other parts of the plant are occasionally used as well.

What It Is Used For:

Broom has an established reputation in traditional American and European medicine as a diuretic ("water pill") and laxative. Larger doses have been used to induce vomiting. Europeans have also long considered broom tea an excellent choice for improving cardiac circulation. A purified compound of the herb (sparteine) has been used to treat arrhythmias (abnormal heart rhythms) and extrasystole, a type of extra heartbeat. Veterinarians have treated animals with sparteine for its diuretic and heart tonic effects. Some manufacturers tout broom as a general tonic. Topical forms have been applied to swellings, abscesses, and sore muscles, and to lighten the hair. Various parts of the plant were once included in antitumor formulas. For a time in the 1970s, people smoked the moldy, dried blossoms in the hope of getting a legal high. Homeopaths recommend broom in minute amounts for various ailments. (See page 2 for a discussion of homeopathy.)

Forms Available Include:

Infusion (of flower tops). In Europe particularly, a liquid extract of broom containing the critical ingredient sparteine appears in a number of ready-made preparations.

Dosage Commonly Reported:

Not recommended for self-administration.

Will It Work for You? What the Studies Say:

Broom contains a complex mixture of chemicals, the most potent one being the volatile alkaloid sparteine, which appears in concentrations up to 1.5 percent and resembles nicotine in certain ways. Studies show that sparteine can slow the heart and inhibit arrhythmias and extrasystoles by damping overstimulation of the system responsible for conducting nerve impulses through the heart.[1] Studies also show that it can correct abnormally low blood pressure.[2] Other broom alkaloids may affect the heart as well.

The *U.S. Pharmacopeia* listed sparteine and broom tops for several decades until the early 1900s. In 1978, the FDA withdrew approval of sparteine for heart problems because it deemed the health risks too high. Meanwhile, health agencies in other countries have endorsed the herb for certain heart ailments.[3] German health authorities approve of broom for functional heart and circulation disorders and abnormally low blood pressure, usually as a supportive (secondary) treatment.[4] Many German experts consider broom on a par with the well-known drug quinidine for arrhythmias, but at the same time gentler and less toxic.[5]

Experimental and clinical studies indicate that sparteine stimulates uterine

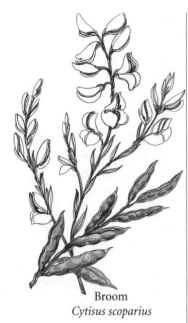

Broom
Cytisus scoparius

contractions.[6] Women in some countries today reportedly still take broom to induce labor. But American and other medical establishments have deemed it unsafe and its use for gynecologic problems unjustifiable.

Research indicates that the herb's flowers in particular are diuretic, and that the glycoside scoparoside is probably responsible.[7] Broom reportedly also functions as a laxative and emetic.[8] But no clinical studies on these subjects in humans appear to have been done, at least recently. Nor has the value of broom in topical formulations been adequately tested.

Numerous investigators have questioned the validity of claims made by broom smokers who assert that just one cigarette will produce two hours of euphoria and calm with no unwanted side effects such as hallucinations.[9]

Will It Harm You? What the Studies Say:

Consensus on the safety of broom appears unlikely anytime soon. The FDA considers the herb unsafe and warns of adverse reactions such as nausea, diarrhea, vertigo, fast heartbeat with circulatory collapse, and stupor.[10] In contrast, German experts have deemed it relatively nontoxic and say that long-term treatment poses few risks and overdosage is unlikely.[11] Still, German and other national health authorities warn that people should not self-medicate themselves with broom (or purified sparteine) because it is so potent. They caution that pregnant women and individuals with high blood pressure should avoid it altogether, and that simultaneous treatment with drugs called monoamine oxidase (MAO) inhibitors could cause sudden blood pressure changes.[12] Certain heart conditions, such as absolute arrhythmias, are apparently never treated with the herb.[13] Smoking broom tops poses the risk of heart problems, uterine contractions, headaches, serious infection with fungi from moldy material, and other adverse reactions.[14]

GENERAL SOURCES:

Bisset, N.E., ed. *Herbal Drugs and Phytopharmaceuticals*. Stuttgart: medpharm GmbH Scientific Publishers, 1994.

Blumenthal, M., J. Gruenwald, T. Hall, and R.S. Rister, eds. *The Complete German Commission E Monographs: Therapeutic Guide to Herbal Medicine*. Boston: Integrative Medicine Communications, 1998.

Duke, J.A. *CRC Handbook of Medicinal Herbs*. Boca Raton, FL: CRC Press, 1985.

Kagen, S.L., et al. *New England Journal of Medicine*. 304 (1981): 483–84.

Lawrence Review of Natural Products. St. Louis: Facts and Comparisons, February 1996.

Leung, A.Y., *Encyclopedia of Common Natural Ingredients Used in Food, Drugs, and Cosmetics*. New York: John Wiley & Sons, 1980.

Tyler, V.E. *The Honest Herbal*. Binghamton, NY: Haworth Press/Pharmaceutical Products Press, 1993.

Weiss, R.F. *Herbal Medicine*, trans. A.R. Meuss, from the 6th German edition. Beaconsfield, England: Beaconsfield Publishers, Ltd., 1988.

TEXT CITATIONS:

1. V.M. Raschack, *Arzneimittel-Forschung*, 24(5) (1974): 753.

2. *Lawrence Review of Natural Products* (St. Louis: Facts and Comparisons, February 1996).

3. V.E. Tyler, *The Honest Herbal* (Binghamton, NY: Haworth Press/Pharmaceutical Products Press, 1993).

4. M. Blumenthal, J. Gruenwald, T. Hall, and R.S. Rister, eds., *The Complete German Commission E Monographs: Therapeutic Guide to Herbal Medicine* (Boston: Integrative Medicine Communications, 1998).

5. R.F. Weiss, *Herbal Medicine*, trans. A. R. Meuss, from the 6th German edition (Beaconsfield, England: Beaconsfield Publishers, Ltd., 1988).

6. K. DeVoe et al., *American Journal of Obstetrics & Gynecology*, 105(3) (1969): 304–8. A.Y. Leung, *Encyclopedia of Common Natural Ingredients Used in Food, Drugs, and Cosmetics* (New York: John Wiley & Sons, 1980).

7. E. Steinegger and R. Hansel, *Lehrbuch der Pharmakognosie*, 3rd ed. (Berlin: Springer-Verlag, 1972, pp. 291–92).

8. Leung, op. cit.

9. *Lawrence Review of Natural Products*, op. cit. Tyler, op. cit.

10. *Lawrence Review of Natural Products*, op. cit.

11. Weiss, op. cit.

12. N.E. Bisset, ed., *Herbal Drugs and Phytopharmaceuticals* (Stuttgart: medpharm GmbH Scientific Publishers, 1994).

13. Weiss, op. cit.

14. J.K. Brown and M.H. Malone, *Pacific Information Service on Street Drugs*, 5(3–6) (1977): 21. Tyler, op. cit.

PRIMARY NAME:

BUCHU

SCIENTIFIC NAME:

Barosma betulina (Berg.) Bartl. & Wendl., *Barosma serratifolia* (Curt.) Willd., *Barosma crenulata* (L.) Hook. Family: Rutacea

COMMON NAMES:

Bookoo, bucco, bucku, buku, diosma

RATING:

4 = Research indicates that this substance will not fulfill the claims made for it, but that it is also unlikely to cause any harm.

What Is Buchu?

Buchu commonly refers to three species of the barosma plant: *Barosma betulina*, *Barosma crenulata*, and *Barosma serratifolia*. These low flowering shrubs are native to South Africa and do not grow in the United States. The leaves have a spicy odor and pungent, minty taste and are dried for medicinal use. Take care not to confuse the Barosma species with Indian buchu (*Myrtus communis* L.), which does not have the same effects.

What It Is Used For:

Long before the plant was introduced into Europe in the first part of the nineteenth century, southern Africans were using buchu for urinary problems and various other ailments. Through the decades, the herb has been hailed as a cure-all and general stimulant.[1] In the mid-1800s, an American entrepreneur—"Helmbold, the Buchu King"—made a fortune with Helmbold's Compound Extract of Buchu. He declared it a remedy for assorted ills including kidney stones, venereal disease, and urinary difficulties.

Although the *National Formulary* once listed buchu as a diuretic ("water pill") and urinary antiseptic (disinfectant), physicians in the United States no longer prescribe the herb. Herbalists, however, continue to recommend it as a diuretic for such conditions as high blood pressure and congestive heart failure. The herb appears in herbal blends for premenstrual bloating and prostate problems. Some people sip an infusion as a stomach tonic. German herbal manufacturers market buchu for irritable bladder and as an antiseptic for mild inflammation and infections of the kidneys and urinary tract. One American herbalist suggests applying washcloths soaked in buchu tea to bruises,[2] a practice Africans still follow, using buchu-flavored brandy instead of tea. Buchu appears as a flavoring agent in beverages and foods, often as artificial black currant flavor.

Forms Available Include:

Capsule, dried leaves, essential oil, extracts, infusion. Buchu is also available in commercial herbal teas.

Dosage Commonly Reported:

An infusion is made using 1 teaspoon dried, crushed leaves and is drunk several times per day. A common dosage of the extract is 10 to 30 drops in water or juice. Commercial formulations such as capsules and oil are labeled with dosages.

Will It Work for You? What the Studies Say:

Buchu's volatile oil contains a substance, diosphenol (barosma camphor), thought to be responsible for its purported diuretic and urinary cleansing properties. But one team of investigators found that the tea's diuretic action matches that of common tea and coffee, not a resounding endorsement by any measure.[3] Researchers conducting test-tube studies have also reported that the plant fails to inhibit or kill the bacteria commonly responsible for urinary tract infections.[4] Anyone considering taking buchu for its diuretic or urinary antiseptic properties may well have a condition that merits more vigorous, proven treatment.

German health authorities declined to endorse buchu for any medicinal use because of its lack of proven effectiveness.[5] After a more limited examination, an FDA review panel decided against approving buchu for use in over-the-counter preparations for premenstrual discomforts. However, both countries allow buchu leaves to be used in foods or as a taste or aroma enhancer.

Will It Harm You? What the Studies Say:

Buchu preparations appear to be safe. No cases of poisoning have been reported, and according to German health authorities, no side effects are likely to develop with typically recommended amounts.[6] British authorities suggest taking the herb with food, given reports that it can occasionally cause gastrointestinal upset.[7] They also recommend that pregnant women stay away from buchu. If you have kidney problems (or pain while urinating or blood in the urine), avoid the herb, given the risk of kidney irritation, a possibility with nearly all herbal diuretics containing a volatile oil.

GENERAL SOURCES:

Bisset, N.E., ed. *Herbal Drugs and Phytopharmaceuticals.* Stuttgart: medpharm GmbH Scientific Publishers, 1994.

Blumenthal, M., J. Gruenwald, T. Hall, and R.S. Rister, eds. *The Complete German Commission E Monographs: Therapeutic Guide to Herbal Medicine.* Boston: Integrative Medicine Communications, 1998.

Bradley, P.C., ed. *British Herbal Compendium: A Handbook of Scientific Information on Widely Used Plant Drugs. Vol.* 1. Bournemouth (Dorset), England: British Herbal Medicine Association, 1992.

Castleman, M. *The Healing Herbs: The Ultimate Guide to the Curative Power of Nature's Medicines.* New York: Bantam Books, 1995.

Duke, J.A. *CRC Handbook of Medicinal Herbs.* Boca Raton, FL: CRC Press, 1985.

Gentry, H.S. *Economic Botany.* 15 (1961): 326–31.

Heinerman, J. *Heinerman's Encyclopedia of Healing Herbs and Spices.* West Nyack, NY: Parker Publishing Co., 1996.

Lawrence Review of Natural Products. St. Louis: Facts and Comparisons, May 1990.

Leung, A.Y. *Encyclopedia of Common Natural Ingredients Used in Food, Drugs, and Cosmetics.* New York: John Wiley & Sons, 1980.

Mindell, E. *Earl Mindell's Herb Bible.* New York: Simon & Schuster/Fireside, 1992.

TEXT CITATIONS:

1. J.M. Watt and M.G. Breyer-Brandwijk, *The Medicinal and Poisonous Plants of Southern and Eastern Africa,* 2nd ed. (Edinburgh: E. & S. Livingstone, 1962).
2. J. Heinerman, *Heinerman's Encyclopedia of Healing Herbs and Spices* (West Nyack, NY: Parker Publishing Co., 1996).
3. *The Medical Letter,* 21 (1979): 29.
4. R. Kaiser et al., *Journal of Agricultural and Food Chemistry,* 23 (1975): 943. P.C. Bradley, ed., *British Herbal Compendium: A Handbook of Scientific Information on Widely Used Plant Drugs,* vol. 1 (Bournemouth [Dorset], England: British Herbal Medicine Association, 1992).
5. M. Blumenthal, J. Gruenwald, T. Hall, and R.S. Rister, eds., *The Complete German Commission E Monographs: Therapeutic Guide to Herbal Medicine* (Boston: Integrative Medicine Communications, 1998).
6. Ibid.
7. Bradley, op. cit.

PRIMARY NAME:

BUGLEWEED

SCIENTIFIC NAME:

Lycopus virginicus L. (North American) or *Lycopus europaeus* L. (European). Family: Labiateae (Lamiaceae)

COMMON NAMES:

Bugleweed; *Lycopus virginicus:* Virginia water hound; *Lycopus europaeus:* gypsywort

RATING:

2 = According to a number of well-designed studies and common use, this substance appears to be relatively effective and safe when used in recommended amounts for the indication(s) noted in the "Will It Work for You?" section.

What Is Bugleweed?

The closely related, square-stemmed *Lycopus* perennials have lance-shaped leaves that grow in pairs. In late summer they produce whorls of small whitish flowers with purple dots inside. The leaves and preflowering tops are used medicinally. Bugleweed favors stream banks and other damp environments.

What It Is Used For:

Legend has it that Gypsies dyed their skin with the dark juice of this plant to impersonate Egyptians.[1] More conclusive evidence can be found for the juice's effectiveness as a fabric dye. Herbalists through the years have considered bugleweed a fever-reducer, sedative, heart tonic for anxiety and palpitations, and tonic astringent for controlling mucus production. In recent years, the herb has been enlisted primarily to treat the symptoms of hyperthyroidism, a common endocrine disorder involving an overactive thyroid gland. When the condition becomes more severe, it is sometimes referred to as Graves' disease or thyrotoxicosis. Characteristic symptoms include weight loss, weakness, fast heartbeat, nervousness, and goiter.

Forms Available Include:

Infusion, liquid herb extract.

Dosage Commonly Reported:

Bugleweed should be taken only under a doctor's supervision. (No dosage information is available.)

Will It Work for You? What the Studies Say:

Studies indicate that bugleweed has potential for alleviating mild cases of hyperthyroidism.[2] It appears to prevent stimulation of the thyroid by binding to and weakly blocking receptors on the gland called thyroid-stimulating hormone receptors.[3] Bugleweed may also interfere with normal pituitary influence on the human gonadal system through a similar mechanism.[4] The gonadal system is responsible for healthy reproductive function. Experts have yet to identify the substances that exert these effects.[5] One German textbook advises that bugleweed be reserved for less severe cases of hyperthyroidism, as there are more powerful synthetic drugs to treat this serious condition.[6]

Test-tube studies indicate that bugleweed has notable antioxidant activities.[7] Antioxidants control the formation of dangerous substances called free radicals that can damage cells through oxidation, in some cases even causing cancerous changes.

Will It Harm You? What the Studies Say:

No reports of serious harm have been linked to this herb, but it clearly has a profound impact on the body and should be taken with care. Avoid it during pregnancy. If you suspect you suffer from hyperthyroidism, see a doctor and talk to him or her about using this herb. Such a complex disease with potentially serious complications demands close monitoring. German health authorities recommend that people with an enlarged thyroid (and no functional disorder) avoid this herb.[8] They report that in rare cases, extended use of high dosages of bugleweed has caused an enlargement of the thyroid gland, and suddenly stopping the herb can precipitate an increase in thyroid disorder symptoms. They cite no known interactions with other medicines, although they warn that the herb may interfere with nuclear imaging studies of the gland, such as thyroid uptake scan.

GENERAL SOURCES:

Blumenthal, M., J. Gruenwald, T. Hall, and R.S. Rister, eds. *The German Complete Commission E Monographs: Therapeutic Guide to Herbal Medicine.* Boston: Integrative Medicine Communications, 1998.

Bremness, L. *Herbs.* 1st American ed. Eyewitness Handbooks. New York: Dorling Kindersley Publications, 1994.

Chevallier, A. *The Encyclopedia of Medicinal Plants: A Practical Reference Guide to More Than 550 Key Medicinal Plants & Their Uses.* 1st American ed. New York: Dorling Kindersley Publications, 1996.

Tyler, V.E. *Herbs of Choice: The Therapeutic Use of Phytomedicinals.* Binghamton NY: Haworth Press/Pharmaceutical Products Press, 1994.

Weiss, R.F. *Herbal Medicine,* trans. A.R. Meuss, from the 6th German edition. Beaconsfield, England: Beaconsfield Publishers, Ltd., 1988.

TEXT CITATIONS:

1. L. Bremness, *Herbs,* 1st American ed., Eyewitness Handbooks (New York: Dorling Kindersley Publications, 1994).

2. R.F. Weiss, *Herbal Medicine*, trans. A. R. Meuss, from the 6th German edition. (Beaconsfield, England: Beaconsfield Publishers, Ltd., 1988).

3. H. Winterhoff et al., *Arzneimittel-Forschung*, 44(1) (1994): 41–45. M. Auf'mkolk et al., *Endocrinology*, 116(5) (1985): 1687–93. M. Auf'mkolk et al., *Endocrinology*, 115(2) (1985): 527–34.

4. M. Auf'mkolk et al., *Hormone & Metabolic Research*, 16(4) (1984): 188–92.

5. V.E. Tyler, *Herbs of Choice: The Therapeutic Use of Phytomedicinals* (Binghamton, NY: Haworth Press/Pharmaceutical Products Press, 1994).

6. Weiss, op. cit.

7. J.L. Lamaison et al., *Pharmaceutica Acta Helvetiae*, 66(7) (1991): 185–88.

8. M. Blumenthal, J. Gruenwald, T. Hall, and R.S. Rister, eds., *The Complete German Commission E Monographs: Therapeutic Guide to Herbal Medicine* (Boston: Integrative Medicine Communications, 1998).

PRIMARY NAME:
BURDOCK ROOT

SCIENTIFIC NAME:
Arctium lappa L. (great burdock) and *Arctium minus* (Hill) Bernh. (common burdock). Family: Asteraceae (Compositae)

COMMON NAMES:
Bardana, beggar's buttons, burr, clotbur, common burdock, edible burdock, great bur, great burdock, gobo, lappa, niu bang zi

RATING:
3 = Studies on the effectiveness and safety of this substance are conflicting, or there are not enough studies to draw a conclusion.

What Is Burdock Root?

Burdock root consists of the dried roots of *Arctium lappa*, a large biennial with wrinkled leaves and purple flowers that mature into hooked burrs. It grows in many parts of Europe and the United States. *Arctium minus*, a smaller version of the plant, is also used. A similar-appearing plant, deadly nightshade (*Atropa belladonna*), is extremely poisonous.

What It Is Used For:

Although the herb's popularity has waned in recent decades, burdock root once featured prominently in the repertoires of European and American folk healers. Europeans started using it heavily in the Middle Ages. They and their predecessors were perhaps most committed to the herb's role as a diuretic ("water pill") that could "purify blood" by flushing toxins out of the body, including the microorganism that causes syphilis. Today it is touted as a body "cleanser." Over the centuries, burdock root was also enlisted to break up kidney and bladder stones, alleviate constipation, remedy stomach and intestinal disorders, promote sweating, control arthritis and gout pains, and ease childbirth. Traditional Chinese and Indian doctors often select this herb for treating colds, flu, and other throat and chest conditions.

Many contemporary herbalists continue to promote burdock root in internal form as a diuretic and remedy for such ailments as urinary tract infections, ulcers, backache, arthritis, and sciatica pain. Some consider it a potential cancer-fighter. They also carry on the long-standing tradition of recommending external forms for canker sores, warts, poorly healing wounds, and chronic skin conditions such as psoriasis and eczema. A number of hair growth formulations contain the herb. Homeopaths add minute amounts to their formulations for pain, rheumatism, stomach upset, and other ailments. (See page 2 for a discussion of homeopathy.) Asians consider burdock root a food. The young leaves are also eaten as greens.

Forms Available Include:

- *For internal use:* Capsule, decoction, extract, powdered root, tea, tincture. Burdock root appears mostly in herbal blends.
- *For external use:* Oil, tincture.

Dosage Commonly Reported:

A decoction is made using 1¼ teaspoons chopped or coarsely powdered root in a cup of water. The tincture is taken in dosages of ½ to 1 teaspoon up to three times per day. Three capsules of 475 milligrams each are taken three times a day.

Will It Work for You? What the Studies Say:

Despite centuries of use, none of the many claims made for burdock root has been substantiated. German health authorities found no evidence to justify treating any ailment with it.[1] Even long-standing assertions that the herb will work as a diuretic appear to be ill-founded, as are claims that it can stimulate hair growth or ameliorate chronic skin ailments such as psoriasis or eczema.[2]

Chemicals in the root called polyacetylenes fight disease-causing bacteria and fungi, but a team of investigators found that once the root is dried to be sold commercially, only trace amounts of such infection-fighting chemicals remain.[3] Investigators have also shown that burdock root can stimulate liver and bile function and reduce blood-sugar levels (important for treating diabetes) in rats, and that root infusions may help dissolve bladder stones.[4] Reports indicate that the herb may reduce the number of mutations in cells exposed to mutation-causing chemicals, inhibit experimental tumor growth,[5] and suppress chromosome aberrations in rat bone marrow cells.[6] Unfortunately, no one has ever demonstrated that any of these properties can help treat disease in humans. Reports that burdock extract fights HIV (the virus that causes AIDS) in the test tube were later refuted.[7]

Will It Harm You? What the Studies Say:

As a food, burdock root is generally considered safe. But very spotty information is available on its potential toxicity when used in medicinal concentrations. The FDA classifies it as an herb of "undefined safety." Contact with the plant itself can cause irritation and dermatitis. If you are pregnant or diabetic, you may want to avoid the herb; evidence that it may stimulate the uterus raises concerns about miscarriage (although miscarriage has never been documented), and studies in mice indicate that it can aggravate a diabetic condition.[8]

In the 1970s, commercially packaged burdock-root tea was implicated in a number of atropine poisonings in the United States and Europe. But further investigation revealed that the herb had been adulterated with the similar-appearing but toxic **Deadly Nightshade**.[9] Buy burdock root only from a reliable source.

GENERAL SOURCES:

Bisset, N.E., ed. *Herbal Drugs and Phytopharmaceuticals.* Stuttgart: medpharm GmbH Scientific Publishers, 1994.

Blumenthal, M., J. Gruenwald, T. Hall, and R.S. Rister, eds. *The Complete German Commission E Monographs: Therapeutic Guide to Herbal Medicine.* Boston: Integrative Medicine Communications, 1998.

Castleman, M. *The Healing Herbs: The Ultimate Guide to the Curative Power of Nature's Medicines.* New York: Bantam Books, 1995.

Der Marderosian, A., and L. Liberti. *Natural Product Medicine. A Scientific Guide to Foods, Drugs, Cosmetics.* Philadelphia: George F. Stickley, 1988.

Dombradi, C.A., and S. Foldeak. *Tumori.* 52(3) (1966): 173–75.

Duke, J.A. *CRC Handbook of Medicinal Herbs.* Boca Raton, FL: CRC Press, 1985.

Heinerman, J. *Heinerman's Encyclopedia of Healing Herbs and Spices.* West Nyack, NY: Parker Publishing Co., 1996.

Lawrence Review of Natural Products. St. Louis: Facts and Comparisons, July 1991.

Leung, A.Y., *Encyclopedia of Common Natural Ingredients Used in Food, Drugs, and Cosmetics.* New York: John Wiley & Sons, 1980.

Mindell, E. *Earl Mindell's Herb Bible.* New York: Simon & Schuster/Fireside, 1992.

Rhoads, P.M., et al. *Journal of Toxicology-Clinical Toxicology,* 22 (1985): 581–84.

Tyler, V.E. *Herbs of Choice: The Therapeutic Use of Phytomedicinals.* Binghamton, NY: Haworth Press/Pharmaceutical Products Press, 1994.

———. *The Honest Herbal.* Binghamton, NY: Haworth Press/Pharmaceutical Products Press, 1993.

Tyler, V.E., L.R. Brady, J.E. Robbers, eds. *Pharmacognosy.* Philadelphia: Lea & Febiger, 1988.

Weiss, R.F. *Herbal Medicine,* trans. A.R. Meuss, from the 6th German edition. Beaconsfield, England: Beaconsfield Publishers, Ltd., 1988.

TEXT CITATIONS:

1. Blumenthal, M., J. Gruenwald, T. Hall, and R.S. Rister, eds., *The Complete German Commission E Monographs: Therapeutic Guide to Herbal Medicine* (Boston: Integrative Medicine Communications, 1998).

2. V.E. Tyler, *Herbs of Choice: The Therapeutic Use of Phytomedicinals* (Binghamton, NY: Haworth Press/Pharmaceutical Products Press, 1994).

3. K.E. Schulte et al., *Arzneimittel-Forschung,* 17 (1967): 829–33.

4. Grases et al., *International Urology & Nephrology,* 26(5)(1994): 507–11.

5. G. Dombradi, *Chemotherapy,* 15 (1970): 250. K. Morita et al., *Mutation Research,* 129 (1984): 25.

6. Y. Ito et al., *Mutation Research,* 172(1) (1986): 55.

7. *Bulletin of the World Health Organization.* 67(6) (1989): 613–18. X.J. Yao et al., *Virology,* 187(1) (1992): 56–62.

8. M. Castleman, *The Healing Herbs: The Ultimate Guide to the Curative Power of Nature's Medicines* (New York: Bantam Books, 1995). S.K. Swanston-Flatt, *Diabetes Research,* 10(2) (1989): 69.

9. P.D. Bryson et al., *Journal of the American Medical Association,* 239 (1978): 2157.

PRIMARY NAME:
BUTCHER'S BROOM

SCIENTIFIC NAME:
Ruscus aculeatus L. Family: Liliaceae

What Is Butcher's Broom?

Butcher's broom consists of the fleshy rootstock of *Ruscus aculeatus,* a relatively common evergreen shrub native to Mediterranean countries and now found in many parts of the world, including the southern United States. It belongs to the same plant subgroup as asparagus, and years ago people consumed it as a vegetable.

BUTCHER'S BROOM
(Continued)

COMMON NAMES:

Box holly, knee holly, pettigree

RATING:

3 = Studies on the effectiveness and safety of this substance are conflicting, or there are not enough studies to draw a conclusion.

What It Is Used For:

Although the history of butcher's broom as a folk remedy dates back to the dawn of the first millennium, its immense current popularity was born with the discovery in the 1950s that an extract of the underground stems could constrict (narrow) blood vessels in small animals.[1] Soon, companies were manufacturing capsules for conditions believed to benefit from this property: hemorrhoids and poor leg circulation, such as varicose vein syndrome. Formulations for these purposes are popular in Europe.

Earlier uses as a laxative and broken bone remedy have not survived, but contemporary herbalists do continue to recommend butcher's broom for reducing water retention and related swelling in the hands and feet, improving circulation in these areas, and bringing down inflammation due to arthritis and rheumatism.

Forms Available Include:

- *For internal use:* Capsule, tablet.
- *For external use* (hemorrhoids): Rectal ointment and suppositories.

Dosage Commonly Reported:

Tablets typically contain about 300 milligrams dried extract; follow the package instructions when using the tablets or commercial ointments containing butcher's broom.

Will It Work for You? What the Studies Say:

After establishing that steroidal-type compounds in the herb (ruscogenin and neuroscogenin primarily) constrict veins in dogs and hamsters as well as increase their strength and tone,[2] scientists were able to point to studies showing that the herb can help alleviate the signs and symptoms of certain venous disorders in humans. For example, in a double-blind trial involving forty individuals with chronic venous insufficiency affecting the lower limbs, those randomly selected to take an extract of butcher's broom combined with hesperidin and ascorbic acid for two months noticed a general improvement in their condition.[3] They reported a drop in swelling, numbness and tingling, itching, and sensations of heaviness and cramping. Significantly, patients reported no such improvements during the two months they took a placebo.

The same type of general improvement in varicose-vein problems was noted in a similarly randomized, placebo-controlled, and double-blind study of fifty individuals done a year earlier. The improvements were not dramatic, however, possibly because the study lasted only two weeks.[4] While promising, these data fall short of being conclusive. The FDA was not sufficiently impressed with these and other findings—in terms of either efficacy or safety—to approve of butcher's broom as a treatment for venous disorders.[5] But Europeans continue to use it widely. German health authorities approve of the herb as a supportive therapy for discomforts of chronic venous insufficiency such as pain and heaviness, as well as cramps in the legs, itching, and swelling.[6] Hemorrhoidal itching and burning may also be treated with it.

Whether topical ointments and suppositories made from butcher's broom extracts will help shrink hemorrhoids has yet to be clearly demonstrated. Scientists know that, in test tubes at least, a number of ingredients in butcher's broom can inhibit inflammation and constrict vessels, certainly useful qualities when it comes to dilated veins. According to one study in rats with chemically induced swollen paws, an injected form of the herb helped bring the swelling down.[7] But no clinical trials to explore the value of these formulations in humans appear to have been done so far.

Will It Harm You? What the Studies Say:

Scientists know relatively little about the safety of butcher's broom. It is notable that the forty subjects in the study described above did not suffer any adverse reactions while taking the herb. No toxicity has been reported in other people taking it. Circulation problems that might be treated with butcher's broom are often quite serious, however, and should always be treated by a doctor.

GENERAL SOURCES:

Blumenthal, M., J. Gruenwald, T. Hall, and R.S. Rister, eds. *The Complete German Commission E Monographs: Therapeutic Guide to Herbal Medicine.* Boston: Integrative Medicine Communications, 1998.

Lawrence Review of Natural Products. St. Louis: Facts and Comparisons, September 1991.

Mindell, E. *Earl Mindell's Herb Bible.* New York: Simon & Schuster/Fireside, 1992.

Salzmann, P., et al. *Fortschritte der Medizin.* 95(21) (1977): 1419–22.

Tyler, V.E. *Herbs of Choice: The Therapeutic Use of Phytomedicinals.* Binghamton, NY: Haworth Press/Pharmaceutical Products Press, 1994.

———. *The Honest Herbal.* Binghamton, NY: Haworth Press/Pharmaceutical Products Press, 1993.

Weiss, R.F. *Herbal Medicine*, trans. A.R. Meuss, from the 6th German edition. Beaconsfield, England: Beaconsfield Publishers, Ltd., 1988.

TEXT CITATIONS:

1. F. Caujolle et al., *Annales Pharmaceutiques Françaises*, 11 (1953): 109–20.
2. C. Sannie and H. Lapin, *Bulletin de la Société Chemique de France* (1957): 1237–1241. G. Rubanyi et al., *General Pharmacology*, 15(5) (1984): 431–34. G. Marcelon et al., *General Pharmacology*, 14 (1983): 103. E. Bouskela et al., *Journal of Cardiovascular Pharmacology*, 22(2) (1993): 221–24.
3. R. Cappelli et al., *Drugs Under Experimental and Clinical Research*, 14 (1988): 277–84.
4. N. Weindorf and U. Schultz-Ehrenburg, *Zeitschrift für Hautkrankeheiten*, 62 (1987): 28–30, 35–38.
5. V.E. Tyler, *The Honest Herbal* (Binghamton, NY: Haworth Press/Pharmaceutical Products Press, 1993).
6. M. Blumenthal, J. Gruenwald, T. Hall, and R.S. Rister, eds., *The Complete German Commission E Monographs: Therapeutic Guide to Herbal Medicine* (Boston: Integrative Medicine Communications, 1998).
7. J.P. Tarayre and H. Lauressergues, *Annales Pharmaceutiques Françaises*, 37(5–6) (1979): 191–98.

CALAMUS

SCIENTIFIC NAME:
Acorus calamus L. Family:
Araceae

COMMON NAMES:
Acorus, rat root, sweet
cinnamon, sweet flag, sweet
myrtle, sweet root, sweet sedge

RATING:
5 = Studies indicate that there
is a definite health hazard to
using this substance, even in
recommended amounts.

What Is Calamus?

This fragrant perennial grows in damp environments throughout North America, Europe, and Asia. The rhizomes (underground stems) and occasionally the roots are used medicinally. Steam distillation of the rhizomes yields an essential oil.

What It Is Used For:

Calamus has been used since ancient times for stomach upset, gas, digestive disorders, and childhood colic. Fever, jangled nerves, rheumatoid arthritis, appetite loss, epilepsy, and a variety of other ailments have also been treated with it. It has held "wonder drug" status in some areas. Traditional Chinese healers have used calamus for more than two thousand years. Contemporary herbalists recommend it for a similarly broad variety of ailments, with an emphasis on its purported indigestion- and gas-relieving properties. Calamus oil or spirits are commonly added to baths or rubbed into the skin to stimulate blood circulation and heal such ailments as varicose veins. Some herbalists suggest chewing the leaves to facilitate digestion or suppress a craving for tobacco. German parents give teething children bits of the rhizome wrapped in a small piece of cloth to gnaw on. In many countries calamus is used as a flavoring. Calamus oil serves as a fragrance in many commercial products.

Four subtypes of calamus have been identified, each native to a different part of the world. Only one of the four—the one that grows in the United States, type 1 —is apparently safe to use. The oil in two others contains significant amounts of a toxic, cancer-promoting compound (beta-asarone; isoasarone), and the fourth contains lesser but still significant amounts.

Forms Available Include:

Bath formula, decoction, extract, infusion, leaf, oil, powdered rhizome, spirit, tincture. Calamus extracts commonly appear in European herbal mixtures.

Dosage Commonly Reported:

In cases in which sources offer dosage information despite health concerns, recommendations have included a decoction made using ½ teaspoon finely chopped or powdered rhizome, which is drunk at mealtime as an aromatic bitter. The tincture is taken in dosages of 20 to 30 drops, three times a day.

Will It Work for You? What the Studies Say:

According to continuing scientific research, calamus may indeed have sedative, antispasmodic, and indigestion-relieving properties. Small animals injected with calamus oil move around less spontaneously than those injected with a placebo, for example; and the higher the dose, the less they move.[1] In other animal studies, extracts of the herb and its oil have shown anticonvulsant and blood-pressure-lowering properties.[2] Experts hold isoasarone and other ingredients in the essential oil responsible for many of these actions.

Unfortunately, isoasarone is also toxic. The hope is that isoasarone-free type 1 calamus will prove as medicinally potent as the other types—if not more so. In one test-tube experiment, type 1 calamus oil showed antispasmodic properties on a par with a standard antihistamine, while the other types were devoid of this property altogether.[3] Although such findings suggest that type 1 calamus has potential as a remedy for indigestion and similar spasm-associated ailments, much more research is needed.[4]

Will It Harm You? What the Studies Say:

Isoasarone can apparently induce dangerous cell mutations and has been shown to cause cancer in small animals.[5] Rats fed a certain variety of calamus oil developed malignant tumors and abnormalities in major organs such as the liver and heart.[6] Those fed dietary amounts for two years grew more slowly and experienced slight but potentially serious organ changes.

While the North American type of calamus—type 1—contains no isoasarone and would therefore be considered nontoxic, it often gets mixed together with other types during commercial processing. The United States government has therefore banned calamus from the marketplace as a food or food additive, placing the herb in the small category of long-used herbs now condemned for safety reasons.[7]

Health authorities in some other countries are not as critical of calamus, however. Numerous German experts have concluded that as long as the concentration of isoasarone can be controlled and people avoid taking it for long stretches, even the type of calamus that contains low levels of this toxic chemical can be safely used.[8] Other sources point to the lack of evidence that anyone has ever developed cancer as a result of using the herb.[9] German health authorities do not, however, approve of the use of calamus baths, given the "unavoidable" absorption of isoasarones.[10]

GENERAL SOURCES:

Abel, G. *Planta Medica.* 53 (1987): 251.

Bisset, N.G., ed. *Herbal Drugs and Phytopharmaceuticals.* Stuttgart: medpharm GmbH Scientific Publishers, 1994.

Blumenthal, M., J. Gruenwald, T. Hall, and R.S. Rister, eds. *The Complete German Commission E Monographs: Therapeutic Guide to Herbal Medicine.* Boston: Integrative Medicine Communications, 1998.

Goggelmann, W., and O. Schimmer. *Mutation Research.* 121(3–4) (1983): 191–94.

Haberman, R.T. *Project P 153–70, Report of the FDA.* 1971.

Lawrence Review of Natural Products. St. Louis: Facts and Comparisons, March 1996.

Leung, A.Y. *Encyclopedia of Common Natural Ingredients Used in Food, Drugs, and Cosmetics.* New York: John Wiley & Sons, 1980.

Menon, M.K., and P.C. Dandiya. *Journal of Pharmacy & Pharmacology.* 19(3) (1967): 170–75.

Tyler, V.E. *Herbs of Choice: The Therapeutic Use of Phytomedicinals.* Binghamton, NY: Haworth Press/Pharmaceutical Products Press, 1994.

———. *The Honest Herbal.* Binghamton, NY: Haworth Press/Pharmaceutical Products Press, 1993.

Tyler, V.E., L.R. Brady, and J.E. Robbers, eds. *Pharmacognosy.* Philadelphia: Lea & Febiger, 1988.

Weiss, R.F. *Herbal Medicine,* trans. A.R. Meuss, from the 6th German edition. Beaconsfield, England: Beaconsfield Publishers, Ltd., 1988.

TEXT CITATIONS:

1. N.S. Dhalla and I.C. Bhattacharya, *Archives Internationales de Pharmacodynamie et de Therapie*, 172(2) (1968): 356. G.M. Panchal et al., *Indian Journal of Experimental Biology*, 27(6) (1989): 561–67.
2. A.Y. Leung, *Encyclopedia of Common Natural Ingredients Used in Food, Drugs, and Cosmetics* (New York: John Wiley & Sons, 1980).
3. K. Keller et al., *Planta Medica*, 1 (1995): 6–9.
4. V.E. Tyler, *The Honest Herbal* (Binghamton, NY: Haworth Press/Pharmaceutical Products Press, 1993).
5. S.N. Sivaswamy et al., *Indian Journal of Experimental Biology*, 29(8) (1991): 730–37.
6. J.M. Taylor et al., *Toxicology and Applied Pharmacology*, 10 (1967): 405.
7. Ibid.
8. N.G. Bisset, ed., *Herbal Drugs and Phytopharmaceuticals* (Stuttgart: medpharm GmbH Scientific Publishers, 1994).
9. R.F. Weiss, *Herbal Medicine*, trans. A.R. Meuss (Beaconsfield, England: Beaconsfield Publishers, Ltd., 1988).
10. M. Blumenthal, J. Gruenwald, T. Hall, and R.S. Rister, eds., *The Complete German Commission E Monographs: Therapeutic Guide to Herbal Medicine* (Boston: Integrative Medicine Communications, 1998).

PRIMARY NAME:

CALENDULA

SCIENTIFIC NAME:

Calendula officinalis L. Family: Asteraceae (Compositae)

COMMON NAMES:

Garden marigold, goldblood, mary-bud, pot marigold

RATING:

- *For internal use:* 4 = Research indicates that this herb will not fulfill the claims made for it, but that it is also unlikely to cause any harm.
- *For external use:* 2 = According to a number of well-designed studies and common use, this herb appears to be relatively effective and safe when used in recommended amounts for the indication(s) noted in the "Will It Work for You?" section.

What Is Calendula?

The yellow-red flowers of the native European *Calendula officinalis* dot gardens and parks throughout the world. Most people call the plant garden marigold. The florets (flower tops) are used medicinally.

What It Is Used For:

The ancients were the first to recognize the antiseptic and healing properties of this herb. It was enormously popular in medieval Europe for treating blemishes, bedsores, and skin infections. Contemporary herbalists continue to highlight its value in topical form for inflamed or damaged skin: poorly healing wounds and ulcers, burns (including sunburn), boils, rashes, bruises, chapped hands, infectious sores such as herpes zoster (shingles), and varicose veins. Gargles and rinses are used for mouth and throat inflammation. Calendula tea, once quite popular, is still recommended to promote sweating and lower fever, help heal painful stomach ulcers, reduce menstrual cramping, calm gallbladder inflammation, and damp stomach and intestinal spasms. Many herbal mixtures contain fiery orange flecks of calendula to brighten them. And it is not uncommon to see the leaves tossed into a salad and the dried florets mixed into dishes as seasoning and coloring.

Forms Available Include:

- *For external use:* Essential oil, extracts, gargle, infusion, mouth rinse, tincture. Calendula appears in many skin lotions, ointments, cosmetics, and other commercial products.
- *For internal use:* Dried flowers, extracts, infusion, tincture.

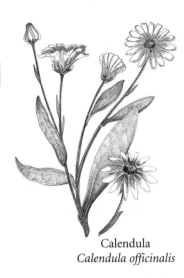

Calendula
Calendula officinalis

Dosage Commonly Reported:

A mouthwash, gargle, or lotion is made using 1 to 2 teaspoons tincture per ¼ to ½ liter water. Ointments are used in concentrations of 2 to 5 grams calendula per 100 grams ointment. A tea is made for use as a gargle or compress using 1 to 2 teaspoons herb per cup of water.

Will It Work for You? What the Studies Say:

Studies indicate that calendula will soothe inflamed skin and help wounds heal. An anti-inflammatory action, believed to be largely due to constituents called triterpenoids,[1] has been demonstrated in animal studies. Calendula ointment (plus allantoin) placed on laboratory-inflicted wounds in rats significantly increased the presence of cells important to wound healing.[2] In another rat study, chronic inflammatory eye conditions subsided with calendula treatment.[3] The herb also contains a volatile oil, mucilage, resins, and virus- and bacteria-fighting chemicals, among others. The latter constituents, identified in test-tube studies, possibly explain calendula's reputation as a wound-healer.[4] The herb may also offer immune-system-stimulating properties[5] and holds hope as an ulcer remedy.[6] Well-designed trials to test these properties in humans do not appear to have been done so far. German health authorities endorse the use of external formulations for reducing skin and mucous membrane inflammation and promoting wound healing.[7] Gargles and rinses (made from an infusion) are approved for treating mouth and throat inflammations.

Laboratory analyses have failed to detect any other calendula components with unique medicinal value, but even now, after decades of intensive investigation, new discoveries about the plant's constituents continue to be made.[8]

Limited animal studies indicate that calendula extracts taken internally may counter high lipid levels, produce sedation and trigger other central nervous system changes, influence bile output and help treat hepatitis, encourage sunburn healing, exert a tonic effect on the uterus, and reduce signs of systemic inflammation.[9] Test-tube studies indicate that calendula extracts may have potential as spermicides.[10] Some animal studies indicate that calendula actually possesses few important healing properties.[11] None of the properties have been confirmed in human studies. Drinking calendula tea may be pleasant, but it offers no clear therapeutic benefit.

Will It Harm You? What the Studies Say:

No toxic reactions have been reported in the Western literature after centuries of use as a culinary and medicinal herb, although the plant can certainly cause an allergic reaction if you are sensitive to this or other plants of the daisy family. German health authorities identify no side effects or dangerous interactions with other remedies or any situations in which a person should not use the herb medicinally.[12] Some herbalists caution against using the herb during pregnancy, although the basis for this warning is unclear.[13]

GENERAL SOURCES:

Bisset, N.G., ed. *Herbal Drugs and Phytopharmaceuticals.* Stuttgart: medpharm GmbH Scientific Publishers, 1994.

Blumenthal, M., J. Gruenwald, T. Hall, and R.S. Rister, eds. *The Complete German Commission E Monographs: Therapeutic Guide to Herbal Medicine.* Boston: Integrative Medicine Communications, 1998.

Fleischner, A.M. *Cosmetic Toiletries.* 100(10) (1985): 45–46, 48–51, 54–55, 58.

Lawrence Review of Natural Products. St. Louis: Facts and Comparisons, January 1995.

Mayell, M. *Off-the-Shelf Natural Health: How to Use Herbs and Nutrients to Stay Well.* New York: Bantam Books, 1995.

Mindell, E. *Earl Mindell's Herb Bible.* New York: Simon & Schuster/Fireside, 1992.

Tyler, V.E. *Herbs of Choice: The Therapeutic Use of Phytomedicinals.* Binghamton, NY: Haworth Press/Pharmaceutical Products Press, 1994.

———. *The Honest Herbal.* Binghamton, NY: Haworth Press/Pharmaceutical Products Press 1993.

TEXT CITATIONS:

1. R.D. Loggia et al., *Planta Medica,* 60(6) (1994): 516–20.
2. E. Klouchek-Popava et al., *Acta Physiologica et Pharmacologica Bulgarica,* 8 (1982): 63.
3. V.N. Marinchev et al., *Oftalmologicheskii Zhurnal,* 26 (1971): 196.
4. G. Dumenil et al., *Annales Pharmaceutiques Françaises,* 38(6) 1980: 493–99.
5. H. Wagner et al., *Arzneimittel-Forschung,* 35 (1985): 1069.
6. *Lawrence Review of Natural Products* (St. Louis: Facts and Comparisons, January 1995).
7. M. Blumenthal, J. Gruenwald, T. Hall, and R.S. Rister, eds., *The Complete German Commission E Monographs: Therapeutic Guide to Herbal Medicine* (Boston: Integrative Medicine Communications, 1998).
8. J.J.C. Scheffer, *Pharmaceutisch Weekblad,* 114 (1979): 1149–57.
9. N.G. Bisset, ed., *Herbal Drugs and Phytopharmaceuticals* (Stuttgart: medpharm GmbH Scientific Publishers, 1994). I.P. Ubeeva et al., *Farmakologiai Toksikologia,* 50(1) (1987): 66–71. M.F. Aubin, French Patent Application number 76/13,599, 06, 1976.
10. R.M. Parkhurst and S.J. Stolzenberg, 1975 United States Patent Application Number 3844,101.
11. A.L. Iatsyno et al., *Farmakologiai Toksikologia,* 41 (1978): 556.
12. Blumenthal et al., op. cit.
13. E. Mindell, *Earl Mindell's Herb Bible* (New York: Simon & Schuster/Fireside, 1992).

PRIMARY NAME:

CAMPHOR

SCIENTIFIC NAME:

Cinnamomum camphora L.
Family: Lauraceae

COMMON NAMES:

Gum camphor, laurel camphor, zhang nao

What Is Camphor?

This volatile, aromatic compound is obtained through steam distillation of parts of a tall flowering east Asian tree called *Cinnamomum camphora.* Camphor is typically used in the form of an oil ("camphorated oil"). As much as 75 percent of camphor used in the United States is now produced synthetically.[1]

What It Is Used For:

Camphor can be found in topical products to cool and soothe muscle aches and pains, reduce pain from inflamed arthritic joints and chilblains, relieve acute and chronic cough and other upper respiratory congestion and irritation, lessen mild itches, and minimize the pain from cold sores by softening and protecting them. It

CAMPHOR (Continued)

also appears in sprays and other products to "cool" and "refresh" aching or smelly feet. More than a few families still use camphorated oil in home cough remedies. Some hot steam vaporizer solutions, as well as some over-the-counter eardrops, contain camphor blended along with other ingredients such as menthol. Camphor appears in nail polish and a number of other commercial products.

Forms Available Include:

- *For external use:* Diluted in a gel, drops, oil, ointment, or other formulation for use on the skin, and in hot steam vaporizer solutions. In the United States, commercial topical preparations contain concentrations of up to 11 percent camphor.
- *For internal use:* Camphor should not be used internally.

Dosage Commonly Reported:

As a counterirritant, camphor is used in topical preparations in concentrations of 3 to 11 percent, applied no more than four times per day. In burn products and for external use with hemorrhoids, camphor is typically used in similar concentrations, or 3 to 10.8 percent if combined with a light mineral oil.

Will It Work for You? What the Studies Say:

Camphor (in concentrations from 3 to 11 percent) is a scientifically proven and widely used counterirritant; by slightly and superficially irritating the skin and stimulating nerve endings, it causes redness and produces a sensation similar to coolness. This masks underlying pain signals, bringing relief to aching muscles, for example. Concentrations below 3 percent are effective in topical analgesic, anti-itch, and pain-numbing formulations because the camphor depresses skin receptors.[2] Studies show that camphor also fights certain bacteria, albeit weakly.

The significant anticough properties of camphor in the form of an aromatic vapor (as used in a steam vaporizer, for example) were demonstrated in a 1994 study involving guinea pigs.[3] The vapors probably control cough by producing a local anesthetic action.[4] Topical camphor-containing products (up to 11 percent camphor) are considered safe and effective in reducing cough in young children (over age two) when applied externally to the chest and throat.[5] German health authorities approve of the external and internal use of camphor for respiratory tract congestion (catarrh).[6] They also endorse external formulations for muscular rheumatism and cardiac symptoms (they do not define these well) and consider internal formulations beneficial to circulation disorders, contending that they act as a tonic. The Germans presumably have safe commercial formulations for these purposes.

Will It Harm You? What the Studies Say:

When used as recommended in topical products, camphor is very unlikely to cause an adverse reaction, although in rare cases it can produce a skin rash in sensitive individuals. Do not apply a camphor-containing formula more than three to four times a day. Overuse may cause tissue irritation or damage, and even poses the risk of absorption into the body.

Never ingest camphor, as it is extremely poisonous and can cause seizures. Take care that children in particular do not misuse any camphor-containing product; reports of serious poisonings from camphorated oil in children continue to appear.[7] To avoid accidental ingestion in children especially, do not apply the camphor-containing product near the mouth or nose. Some experts consider the risk of misuse and poisoning with camphorated oil so high and its benefits so readily obtainable from other sources that it should be removed from the market, especially in Canada, where concentrations of up to 20 percent camphorated oil are sold.[8] Serious burns have been associated with the use of hot steam vaporizers, a number of which contain camphor. No sound research has ever shown that camphor is safe or effective in nonprescription eardrop formulations.[9]

GENERAL SOURCES:

American Pharmaceutical Association. *Handbook of Nonprescription Drugs.* 11th ed. Washington, D.C.: American Pharmaceutical Association, 1996.

Blumenthal, M., J. Gruenwald, T. Hall, and R.S. Rister, eds. *The Complete German Commission E Monographs: Therapeutic Guide to Herbal Medicine.* Boston: Integrative Medicine Communications, 1998.

Chevallier, A. *The Encyclopedia of Medicinal Plants: A Practical Reference Guide to More Than 550 Key Medicinal Plants & Their Uses.* 1st American ed. New York: Dorling Kindersley Publications, 1996.

Leber, M.R., et al. *Handbook of Over-the-Counter Drugs and Pharmacy Products.* Berkeley, CA: Celestial Arts Publishing, 1994.

Tierra, M. *The Way of Herbs.* New York: Pocket Books, 1990.

Tyler, V.E. *Herbs of Choice: The Therapeutic Use of Phytomedicinals.* Binghamton, NY: Haworth Press/Pharmaceutical Products Press, 1994.

TEXT CITATIONS:

1. American Pharmaceutical Association, *Handbook of Nonprescription Drugs*, 11th ed. (Washington, D.C.: American Pharmaceutical Association, 1996).
2. Ibid.
3. E.A. Laude et al., *Pulmonary Pharmacology*, 7(3) (1994): 179–84.
4. American Pharmaceutical Association, op. cit.
5. Ibid.
6. M. Blumenthal, J. Gruenwald, T. Hall, and R.S. Rister, eds., *The Complete German Commission E Monographs: Therapeutic Guide to Herbal Medicine* (Boston: Integrative Medicine Communications, 1998).
7. American Pharmaceutical Association, op. cit.
8. J.G. Theis and G. Koren, *Canadian Medical Association Journal*, 152(11) (1995): 1821–24.
9. American Pharmaceutical Association, op. cit.

PRIMARY NAME:
CARAWAY

SCIENTIFIC NAME:
Carum carvi L., sometimes referred to as *Apium carvi* Crantz. Family: Apiaceae (Umbelliferae)

What Is Caraway?

This very common member of the carrot family has feathery, doubly divided leaves that end in clusters of small, umbrella-shaped flowers. The grayish-brown, crescent-shaped ribbed fruits, commonly referred to as "seeds," are gathered just before they fully ripen in summer. For medicinal purposes these aromatic seeds are used after being dried. Steam distillation yields an essential oil.

COMMON NAMES:
Carraway, carum

What It Is Used For:

Since ancient Grecian times or possibly even earlier, people have celebrated the aromatic and mildly spicy kick that caraway seeds can give to breads, liqueurs, and other foods and drinks. For apparently just as long, they have valued the seeds for promoting good digestion, expelling excess gas, controlling stomach spasms and colic, boosting the appetite, allaying menstrual discomforts, controlling incontinence, countering spasms, and tempering the effects of laxative herbs.

Modern herbalists echo their predecessors in also recommending the seeds in tea form for clearing congestion in coughs and colds, encouraging breast milk production, and combating nausea. The oil appears in various herbal mouthwashes and commercial European gastrointestinal remedies.[1] In foods from rye bread to cheese, the seeds and even the oil still find widespread use as a spice and flavoring. The oil appears in various "digestive" liqueurs such as Scandinavian aquavit, and serves as a fragrance in many lotions, mouthwashes, and cosmetics.

Forms Available Include:

Infusion, liquid extract, oil, seed (whole, crushed, or pulverized for infusions, to chew, to mix into foods), tincture.

Dosage Commonly Reported:

An infusion is made using 1 to 2 teaspoons of freshly crushed seeds and is drunk two to four times per day between meals. The extract is taken in dosages of 3 to 4 drops in liquid three to four times per day. The seeds are chewed a teaspoon at a time three to four times a per day. The tincture is taken in dosages of ½ to 1 teaspoon up to three times per day.

Will It Work for You? What the Studies Say:

As with other essential-oil-containing herbs, caraway is believed to stimulate the appetite by promoting the secretion of gastric juices.[2] The main constituents of the seed oil—carvole and d-limonene (carvene)—are held responsible for its apparent soothing action on the digestive tract and ability to help expel gas. Researchers have demonstrated in animal organs tested in the laboratory dish muscle-spasm-reducing properties that may affect the digestive system as well, although this has never been proved.[3]

In fact, disagreement over caraway's effectiveness for easing digestion and relieving gas and griping (sharp stomach pains) persists, with one German textbook citing it as one of the "most reliable and powerful" carminatives[4] while an American plant expert classifies it as a "minor" carminative herb.[5] German health authorities decided to endorse caraway seeds and caraway's essential oil for treating dyspeptic upset such as bloating, gas, and mild colicky upset (gastrointestinal spasms).[6] Germans sometimes add a teaspoonful of caraway infusion to the bottles of infants or small children suffering from digestive system upset.[7]

Caraway oil possesses notable antifungal, antibacterial, and larvicidal properties, according to various studies, although whether this means the plant will help treat wounds or infections remains largely unexplored.[8] Some enthusiasts point to an antihistamine property in the herb to support treatment of respiratory tract problems, but in practical terms, caraway's effect appears to be minimal.[9]

The ingredient carvene has demonstrated intriguing cancer-fighting properties.[10] In one study, caraway oil (particularly when applied topically) delayed the appearance of skin tumors in mice, retarded tumor development, and caused apparent tumors to regress.[11] The cancer-fighting element has not yet been tested in humans.

Caraway tea may have a role to play in preventing or treating such conditions as iron-deficiency anemia in children and adults, according to the authors of a 1990 study, who found that it notably increased intestinal iron absorption in laboratory rats.[12]

Will It Harm You? What the Studies Say:

People have used caraway as a food and medicine for centuries without incident, and both the seeds and their oil appear to be very safe.[13] German health authorities cite no known side effects, dangerous interactions with other remedies, or situations in which a person should not use caraway medicinally, although the plant can certainly cause an allergic reaction if you are sensitive to it or have an allergy to other members of the daisy family.[14] Some herbalists recommend that pregnant women avoid medicinal concentrations of caraway, given evidence of its antispasmodic—and potentially uterine-relaxing—properties, although the herb has been used for generations to promote menstruation.[15] No reports of miscarriage can be found in the medical literature.

GENERAL SOURCES:

Bisset, N.G., ed. *Herbal Drugs and Phytopharmaceuticals.* Stuttgart: medpharm GmbH Scientific Publishers, 1994.

Blumenthal, M., J. Gruenwald, T. Hall, and R.S. Rister, eds. *The Complete German Commission E Monographs: Therapeutic Guide to Herbal Medicine.* Boston: Integrative Medicine Communications, 1998.

Castleman, M. *The Healing Herbs: The Ultimate Guide to the Curative Power of Nature's Medicines.* New York: Bantam Books, 1995.

Duke, J.A. *CRC Handbook of Medicinal Herbs.* Boca Raton, FL: CRC Press, 1985.

Foster, S., and J.A. Duke. *The Peterson Field Guide Series: A Field Guide to Medicinal Plants. Eastern and Central North America.* Boston: Houghton Mifflin Company, 1990.

Leung, A.Y., and S. Foster. *Encyclopedia of Common Natural Ingredients Used in Food, Drugs, and Cosmetics.* 2nd ed. New York: John Wiley & Sons, 1996.

Mindell, E. *Earl Mindell's Herb Bible.* New York: Simon & Schuster/Fireside, 1992.

Stary, F. *The Natural Guide to Medicinal Herbs and Plants.* Prague: Barnes & Noble, Inc. in arrangement with Aventinum Publishers, 1996.

Tyler, V.E. *Herbs of Choice: The Therapeutic Use of Phytomedicinals.* Binghamton, NY: Haworth Press/Pharmaceutical Products Press, 1994.

Weiss, R.F. *Herbal Medicine,* trans. A.R. Meuss, from the 6th German edition. Beaconsfield, England: Beaconsfield Publishers, Ltd., 1988.

TEXT CITATIONS:

1. N.G. Bisset, ed., *Herbal Drugs and Phytopharmaceuticals* (Stuttgart: medpharm GmbH Scientific Publishers, 1994).

2. Ibid.

3. A.Y. Leung and S. Foster, *Encyclopedia of Common Natural Ingredients Used in Food, Drugs, and Cosmetics,* 2nd ed. (New York: John Wiley & Sons, 1996). M. Reiter and W. Brandt, *Arzneimittel-Forschung,* 35(1A) (1985): 408–14.

4. R.F. Weiss, *Herbal Medicine*, trans. A.R. Meuss, from the 6th German edition (Beaconsfield, England: Beaconsfield Publishers, Ltd., 1988).

5. V.E. Tyler, *Herbs of Choice: The Therapeutic Use of Phytomedicinals* (Binghamton, NY: Haworth Press/Pharmaceutical Products Press, 1994).

6. M. Blumenthal, J. Gruenwald, T. Hall, and R.S. Rister, eds., *The Complete German Commission E Monographs: Therapeutic Guide to Herbal Medicine* (Boston: Integrative Medicine Communications, 1998).

7. Bisset, op. cit.

8. G.G. Ibragimov and O.D. Vasilev, *Azerbaidzhanskii Meditsinskii Zhurnal*, 62 (1985): 44. Leung and Foster, op. cit.

9. Weiss, op. cit.

10. Leung and Foster, op. cit. G.Q. Zheng et al., *Planta Medica*, 58(4) (1992): 338–41. L.W. Wattenberg, *Basic Life Sciences*, 52 (1990): 155–66. T. Kinouschi et al., *Kankyo Hen'igen Kenkyu*, 17(1) (1995): 99–105.

11. M.H. Shwaireb, *Nutrition & Cancer*, 19(3) (1993): 321–25.

12. F.A. el-Shobaki et al., *Zeitschrift fur Ernahrungswissenschaft*, 29(4) (1990): 264–69.

13. Leung and Foster, op. cit. D.L.J. Opdyke, *Food and Cosmetic Toxicology*, 11 (1973): 1051.

14. Blumenthal et al., op. cit. A. Niinimaki and M. Hannuksela, *Allergy*, 26(7) (1981): 487–93.

15. M. Castleman, *The Healing Herbs: The Ultimate Guide to the Curative Power of Nature's Medicines* (New York: Bantam Books, 1995).

PRIMARY NAME:
CARDAMOM

SCIENTIFIC NAME:
Elettaria cardamomum (L.)
Maton. Family: Zingiberaceae

COMMON NAMES:
Cardamom seed, cardamon,
elaci

RATING:
2 = According to a number of well-designed studies and common use, this substance appears to be relatively effective and safe when used in recommended amounts for the indication(s) noted in the "Will It Work for You?" section.

What Is Cardamom?

This tropical perennial bears violet-marked white flowers and long, lance-shaped leaves that emerge off tapering stems. Harvesters handpick the aromatic seed pods just before they begin to open in autumn. The pods are sold in fresh (green), bleached, or sun-dried form. The dried ripe fruits (pods) and seeds are used medicinally. They yield an essential oil through steam distillation.

What It Is Used For:

Modern herbalists carry on an ancient Indian (Ayurvedic) tradition in recommending this aromatic and pungent spice for soothing indigestion, gas and bloating, and other digestive system upsets. Many Indians enjoy a warming, stimulant tea made of cardamom. The Ayurvedic tradition reportedly considers the spice valuable for treating asthma, fatigue, and a host of other ailments and symptoms. Traditional Chinese healers have turned to cardamom for similar ills, particularly digestive system upset and occasionally urinary problems; they prefer to use the cardamom variety *Amomum cardamomom* L.[1] Contemporary Western herbalists also extoll cardamom's breath-sweetening and aphrodisiac qualities. Aromatherapists recommend the essential oil to stimulate and tone the digestive system.

As a spice, fragrance, and flavoring, both cardomom seeds and oil appear in many baked goods, sweets, traditional Indian curries and spice mixtures (including pan masala), and beverages. This expensive spice is vital to world trade.

Forms Available Include:

Fruit, infusion (of crushed seeds), oil, seeds, tea bags, tincture. Cardamom appears in some commercial laxative, carminative (antigas), and stomach-soothing preparations.

Dosage Commonly Reported:

A tea is made using fifteen crushed seeds per ½ cup water and is drunk up to five times per day.

Will It Work for You? What the Studies Say:

In the 1960s, researchers reported that cardamom's volatile oil (present in concentrations of approximately 3 to 8 percent) exerts strong antispasmodic actions on mouse intestines in the laboratory dish.[2] Numerous herbalists took this as confirmation that the oil could effectively soothe the stomach as well as ease stomach pain, cramps, colic, gas, and griping (sharp stomach pains). Although clinical trials are lacking, centuries of use for such ills may be taken into consideration. German health authorities, satisfied with the available evidence, endorse the use of cardamom (fruit) for dyspeptic (indigestion) disorders.[3]

Cardamom contains no caffeine, but many plant experts and herbalists consider it a mild stimulant,[4] presumably because of the presence of other ingredients and its spicy flavor. Several preliminary test-tube studies cite cardamom as one of several potentially effective spice oils with anticancer properties.[5] As for cardamom's breath-sweetening features, you may want to try the remedy for yourself.

Will It Harm You? What the Studies Say:

On the basis of centuries of use and the little data available, cardamom poses essentially no risk of toxicity, although allergic skin reactions have developed in spice factory workers exposed to cardamom powder.[6]

GENERAL SOURCES:

Blumenthal, M., J. Gruenwald, T. Hall, and R.S. Rister, eds. *The Complete German Commission E Monographs: Therapeutic Guide to Herbal Medicine.* Boston: Integrative Medicine Communications, 1998.

Leung, A.Y., and S. Foster. *Encyclopedia of Common Natural Ingredients Used in Food, Drugs, and Cosmetics.* 2nd ed. New York: John Wiley & Sons, 1996.

Mayell, M. *Off-the-Shelf Natural Health: How to Use Herbs and Nutrients to Stay Well.* New York: Bantam Books, 1995.

Mindell, E. *Earl Mindell's Herb Bible.* New York: Simon & Schuster/Fireside, 1992.

TEXT CITATIONS:

1. A.Y Leung and S. Foster, *Encyclopedia of Common Natural Ingredients Used in Food, Drugs, and Cosmetics,* 2nd ed. (New York: John Wiley & Sons, 1996).
2. J. Haginiwa et al., *Yakugaku Zasshi,* 83 (1963): 624. Leung and Foster, op. cit.
3. M. Blumenthal, J. Gruenwald, T. Hall, and R.S. Rister, eds. *The Complete German Commission E Monographs: Therapeutic Guide to Herbal Medicine* (Boston: Integrative Medicine Communications, 1998).
4. Leung and Foster, op. cit.
5. S. Hashim et al., *Nutrition & Cancer,* 21(2) (1994): 169–75.

6. Leung and Foster, op. cit. D.L.J. Opdyke, *Food and Cosmetics Toxicology*, 12(Suppl) (1974): 837. B. Meding, *Contact Dermatitis*, 29(4) (1993): 202–5. A. Dooms-Goosens et al., *Dermatologic Clinics*, 8(1) (1990): 89–93. H. Mobacken and S. Fregert, *Contact Dermatitis*, 1(3) (1975): 175–76.

PRIMARY NAME:
L-CARNITINE

SCIENTIFIC NAME:
N/A

COMMON NAMES:
Carnitine, DL-carnitine

RATING:
3 = Studies on the effectiveness and safety of this substance are conflicting, or there are not enough studies to draw a conclusion.

What Is L-Carnitine?

L-carnitine is an essential nutrient stored in the body's muscle tissue. It is often referred to as a vitamin-like molecule because it is synthesized in the liver and kidneys from the amino acid lysine and other nutrients. Many sources classify carnitine as a nonessential amino acid. At a basic cellular level, carnitine plays a critical role in the metabolism of fat, contributing to the oxidation of fatty acids and transporting long-chain fatty acids to the place in the cells (mitochondria) where they are processed to help provide energy, among other things. Most people get adequate amounts of carnitine through their body's own synthesis of it or through foods such as dairy products and meat.

What it is Used For:

The government has not established a Recommended Daily Allowance (RDA) for L-carnitine, although a deficiency in the compound can occur. Often such cases are due to an uncommon, inherited defect in L-carnitine synthesis. Signs and symptoms of the illness include muscle weakness, abnormal liver function, heart disease (specifically, cardiomyopathy), and hypoglycemia (low blood sugar) during fasting. Some newborns are also at risk for L-carnitine deficiency because their bodies are not as good at synthesizing it. Those given only soy formulas or fed intravenously must be given supplemental carnitine.

In recent years, a number of health food outlets, supplement manufacturers, and others have contended that excessive exercise, illness, and advancing age can cause L-carnitine deficiency. Some argue that men need more L-carnitine than women because men tend to have more muscle mass. Many recommend that athletes and others take L-carnitine to maximize fat burning, boost strength and endurance, reduce the risk of heart disorders and promote better heart function, encourage weight loss by preventing fatty buildup, bolster the body's capacity to create energy by encouraging the metabolization of stored fat, inhibit alcohol-induced fatty liver, and lower cholesterol levels.

Forms Available Include:

Capsule, liquid, tablet. Often found in multi-ingredient formulations. Most supplements are sold as L-carnitine.

Dosage Commonly Reported:

Capsules and tablets are typically sold in units of 250 to 500 milligrams. A common daily dose for continuous use is 500 milligrams.

Will It Work for You? What the Studies Say:

Enthusiasts make often clever-sounding arguments for why people should take L-carnitine supplements, frequently basing their explanations on convenient but ultimately misleading interpretations of how the body uses this molecule. Many recklessly imply that the results of studies involving individuals with specific and often serious medical conditions such as angina pectoris (chest pain) or kidney disease apply to the general population. The word *fatty* also inspires mixed emotions in modern consumers; keep in mind that fatty acids are building blocks of the human body and are necessary for normal functioning.

Consider carefully the studies on which claims are being based. Studies have shown that oral L-carnitine supplements increase exercise tolerance and reduce signs of dangerous heart function changes in men with chronic, stable angina pectoris (chest pain),[1] and that carnitine supplements may significantly improve various heart measurements, such as arrhythmias (abnormal heart rhythms) in diabetes sufferers with high blood pressure.[2] Some trials indicate that intravenous L-carnitine supplementation benefits individuals with inherited carnitine-deficiency syndrome and heart attack victims suffering from a dangerous accumulation of fatty acids in muscle cells.[3] Keep in mind that in most healthy people, this kind of dangerous fatty acid accumulation does not occur.

Studies exploring the capacity of carnitine supplementation to improve athletic endurance and performance have yielded mixed results. In one small double-blind trial, young elite cyclists who supplemented their diets with protein and oral carnitine tablets tested significantly better on measurements of strength, lean body mass, and fat mass than those given a placebo.[4] But another well-designed study in healthy nonathletes found only a minimal and inconsistent increase in exercise performance (e.g., reduced heart rate, reduced metabolic concentrations).[5]

Oral carnitine supplementation for lowering cholesterol levels in individuals on hemodialysis has shown mixed results, with some people showing no benefits at all.[6] No recent clinical trials on carnitine supplementation and cholesterol levels in otherwise healthy individuals have been reported in the medical literature.

Acetyl-L-carnitine, a substance closely related to L-carnitine, is now available as a dietary supplement from some sources. Clinical trials indicate that it offers promise in improving memory function (constructional thinking) and emotional state[7] in mildly impaired elderly people or individuals suffering from Alzheimer's disease, and according to one case study, in chronic alcoholics.[8]

There are reports indicating that many carnitine supplements do not contain what they claim; a survey by the National Organization for Rare Disorders found that two of twelve brands of L-carnitine they tested contained no detectable carnitine and that the concentrations in other brands varied from as much as 20 percent to 85 percent.[9]

Will It Harm You? What the Studies Say:

The medical literature contains no reports of significant adverse reactions to L-carnitine supplementation, and most people who took the supplements in clinical trials seemed to tolerate them well. The health risks of normal individuals who take large doses over long periods of time are not known, however.

GENERAL SOURCES:

American Pharmaceutical Association. *Handbook of Nonprescription Drugs.* 11th ed. Washington, D.C.: American Pharmaceutical Association, 1996.

Balch, J.F., and P.A. Balch. *Prescription for Nutritional Healing: A Practical A to Z Reference to Drug-Free Remedies Using Vitamins, Minerals, Herbs & Food Supplements.* 2nd ed. Garden City Park, NY: Avery Publishing Group, 1997.

Mayell, M. *Off-the-Shelf Natural Health: How to Use Herbs and Nutrients to Stay Well.* New York: Bantam Books, 1995.

Text Citations:

1. A. Cherchi et al., *International Journal of Clinical Pharmacology, Therapy, & Toxicology,* 23(10) (1985): 569–72.
2. V. Digiesi et al., *Minerva Medica,* 80(3) (1989): 227–31.
3. P. Rizzon et al., *European Heart Journal.* 10(6) (1989): 502–8.
4. G.I. Dragan et al., *Physiologie,* 25(3) (1988): 129–32.
5. C. Grieg et al., *European Journal of Applied Physiology & Occupational Physiology,* 56(4) (1987): 457–60.
6. K.B. Yderstraede et al., *Nephrology, Dialysis, Transplantation,* 1(4) (1987): 238–41.
7. C. Cipolli and G. Chiari, *Clinica Terapeutica,* (1990): 479–510.
8. E. Tempesta et al., *International Journal of Clinical Pharmacology Research,* 10(1–2) (1990): 101–7.
9. *Consumer Reports* (November 1995): 702.

PRIMARY NAME:
CARROT

SCIENTIFIC NAME:
Garden carrot: *Daucus carota* L. Subsp. *sativus* (Hoffm.) Arcang. Wild carrot: *Daucus carota* L. subsp. *carota.* Family: Umbelliferae (Apiaceae)

COMMON NAMES:
Wild carrot: daucus, Queen Anne's lace

What Is Carrot?

The well-known, commonly cultivated garden carrot (*Daucus carota* L. subsp. *sativus* [Hoffm.] Arcang.) has a distinctive, edible orange root. The whitish root of the closely related wild carrot (*Daucus carota* L. subsp. *carota*), on the other hand, is too tough to eat. This flowering plant grows freely in North America. An extraction of the garden carrot's orange root yields a root oil, and steam distillation of the dried fruits ("seeds") of both types produces a seed oil. These oils, as well as the garden carrot's fleshy orange root, have been used medicinally.

Take care not to confuse the wild carrot with the similar-appearing poison hemlock (*Conium maculatum*), which is extremely poisonous and can be fatal.

What It Is Used For:

After singing the praises of the garden carrot's rich fiber and nutrient content, contemporary herbalists add that it can also be used to promote healthy eyes, soothe indigestion, lower cholesterol, and help prevent cancer. In parts of Europe today, people sip brews made from the root or dried aboveground parts

RATING:

4 = Research indicates that this herb will not fulfill the claims made for it, but that it is also unlikely to cause any harm.

of the wild carrot to promote urination (as a mild diuretic, or "water pill"), prevent worms, and break up bladder stones. The seeds have been used in traditional medicine as a diuretic and to stimulate menstruation, prevent conception (as a "morning after" pill), and relieve gas. Although the seed oil is primarily used as a fragrance and flavoring today, in years past it was enlisted as a treatment for such wide-ranging ailments as worms, diabetes, and kidney disease, and was even considered an aphrodisiac.[1] The root oil finds use in sunscreens and as a yellow food color, and is valued as a source of vitamin A and beta-carotene.[2]

Forms Available Include:

Juice, raw vegetable, root oil (of garden carrot), seed oil (of both types).

Dosage Commonly Reported:

A common daily dose is 1 to 2 cups carrot juice or 1 to 2 raw carrots.

Will It Work for You? What the Studies Say:

Few sources dispute the nutritional richness of the edible garden carrot (and the root oil), which contains plentiful stores of beta-carotene, a plant form of vitamin A that the body relies on in many important ways. (See **Beta-Carotene** for more information on the nutritional value of this substance.) Many of the claims for carrot appear to be based on the presence of vitamin A, including its cancer-preventing potential. Of course, few American children have not been informed of the importance of carrots—actually beta-carotene—to healthy eyesight.

Most medicinal claims for both garden and wild carrots demand more research. Investigators are following several interesting leads, however. According to reports, carrot extracts dilate vessels and relax smooth muscles of animal organs isolated in the laboratory, slow heart activity in frog and dog hearts, and lower blood pressure by relaxing the heart and smooth muscle in rats.[3] The implications for treating liver, heart, or other diseases in humans still require extensive research. Some German physicians recommend a one- to two-day diet of coarsely or finely grated carrot for treating threadworms in children,[4] but scientific justification for this purpose cannot be traced.

No evidence can be found to confirm (or refute) the proposed diuretic action of wild carrot. Scientists are exploring the contraceptive potential of its seed extracts; they showed promise in preventing implantation of fertilized eggs in mice studies.[5] According to a 1995 study, an extract of the garden carrot may merit investigation as a liver protectant; in mice it helped to shield the organ from carbon tetrachloride poisoning.[6] This solvent, commonly used in dry cleaning fluids, has caused complications in people working in the dry cleaning industry.

Will It Harm You? What the Studies Say:

Evidence indicates that both the vegetable and the oils are safe to consume in moderation. Too much of either may be unwise, however. Carrot seeds contain a psychoactive agent called myristicin, which, if taken in large amounts, raises the risk for neurologic reactions.[7] Skin irritation and blisters can develop after handling the leaves, especially if they are wet and you are then exposed to the sun.

GENERAL SOURCES:

Bradley, P.C., ed. *British Herbal Compendium: A Handbook of Scientific Information on Widely Used Plant Drugs*, vol. 1. Bournemouth (Dorset), England: British Herbal Medicine Association, 1992.

Duke, J.A. *CRC Handbook of Medicinal Herbs*. Boca Raton, FL: CRC Press, 1985.

Foster, S., and J.A. Duke. *The Peterson Field Guide Series: A Field Guide to Medicinal Plants. Eastern and Central North America*. Boston: Houghton Mifflin Company, 1990.

Lawrence Review of Natural Products. St. Louis: Facts and Comparisons, June 1996.

Leung, A.Y., and S. Foster. *Encyclopedia of Common Natural Ingredients Used in Food, Drugs, and Cosmetics*. 2nd ed. New York: John Wiley & Sons, 1996.

Mindell, E. *Earl Mindell's Herb Bible*. New York: Simon & Schuster/Fireside, 1992.

Weiss, R.F. *Herbal Medicine*, trans. A. R. Meuss, from the 6th German edition. Beaconsfield, England: Beaconsfield Publishers, Ltd., 1988.

TEXT CITATIONS:

1. *Lawrence Review of Natural Products*. St. Louis: Facts and Comparisons, June 1996.

2. A.Y. Leung and S. Foster, *Encyclopedia of Common Natural Ingredients Used in Food, Drugs, and Cosmetics*, 2nd ed. (New York: John Wiley & Sons, 1996).

3. Ibid. A.H. Gilani et al., *Archives of Pharmacologic Research*, 17(3) (1994): 150. A. Bishayee et al., *Journal of Ethnopharmacology*. 47(2) (1995): 69.

4. Weiss, R.F. *Herbal Medicine*, trans. A. R. Meuss, from the 6th German edition (Beaconsfield, England: Beaconsfield Publishers, Ltd., 1988).

5. S. Foster and J.A. Duke, *The Peterson Field Guide Series: A Field Guide to Medicinal Plants. Eastern and Central North America* (Boston: Houghton Mifflin Company, 1990).

6. Bishayee, op. cit.

7. *Lawrence Review of Natural Products*, op. cit.

PRIMARY NAME:

CASCARA SAGRADA

SCIENTIFIC NAME:
Rhamnus purshiana D.C., sometimes referred to as *Frangula purshiana* (D.C.) (A. Gray ex J.C. Cooper) Family: Rhamnaceae

COMMON NAMES:
Buckthorn (European version), chittem bark, sacred bark

What Is Cascara Sagrada?

This small- to medium-sized wild tree grows in the American Northwest. It has thin and pointy dark green leaves that fall in autumn, small purplish-black fruits, and a reddish-brown bark with gray or white lichen patches. The bark is used medicinally.

What It Is Used For:

Mexican and Spanish priests living in frontier California reportedly discovered Native Americans using the bark of this indigenous tree as a laxative. The tree's European and western Asian counterpart, the buckthorn shrub (*Rhamnus frangula*), has been similarly used since the Middle Ages. By the 1870s, the American medical establishment began to integrate cascara sagrada into its repertoire,[1] and the bark earned official and enduring status in the *U.S. Pharmacopoeia* in 1890. Today it may well be the leading laxative in many parts of the world.

Herbalists and others through the years have also recommended cascara sagrada (or buckthorn) for fighting cancer (it even appeared in Harry Hoxsey's controversial cancer formula up through the 1950s), arthritis, gallstones, jaundice, and liver problems, among other ailments. Commercial sunscreens sometimes contain cascara sagrada.

Forms Available Include:

Capsule, decoction (traditionally mixed with other herbs in certain parts of the world), liquid extract, powdered bark, tablet, tincture. Appears in numerous commercial laxative products, including Milk of Magnesia-Cascara.

Dosage Commonly Reported:

Commercial laxative products—capsules, powders, and tablets—offer specific dosage instructions. A decoction is made using ½ teaspoon powdered bark per cup of water and is drunk morning and/or night, only for short periods. The tincture is taken in dosages of ½ teaspoon. The fluid extract is taken in dosages of 2 to 6 milliliters.

Will It Work for You? What the Studies Say:

Cascara sagrada is a proven laxative. In fact, it works so well that it is most accurately classified as a "cathartic" or "drastic purgative." After taking a typically recommended dose, expect a bowel movement in six to eight hours. The soft stool should ease pain or other discomfort associated with hemorrhoids, anal fissures, or similar conditions. Substances called anthraquinones (in concentrations of about 8 percent) are responsible for the herb's laxative effect; they stimulate a bowel movement by increasing the volume of the bowel and initiating peristalsis, the wavelike contractions of the large intestine that we experience as "the urge."[2] Anthraquinones are also responsible for the effectiveness of laxatives such as senna (see **Senna**) and aloe (see **Aloe Vera**). German health authorities endorse the use of buckthorn in laxative formulations.[3] Mainstays of good bowel function include exercise, a fiber-rich diet, and high fluid intake. If constipation nonetheless develops, first try a bulk-forming laxative such as psyllium (see **Psyllium**). Turn to a stronger laxative such as cascara sagrada (and consult your doctor) only if this strategy fails.

Scientists have found that a component in cascara sagrada (the anthraquinone aloe-emodin) actively fights a type of mouse leukemia,[4] but much more research is needed before this notably toxic substance can be considered seriously for treating human cancers. Test-tube studies also indicate that aloe-emodin can inactivate the herpes simplex virus (types 1 and 2), the varicella-zoster virus (which causes chicken pox and shingles), the influenza virus (which causes flu), and the pseudorabies virus,[5] but methods for actually treating these types of infections with cascara sagrada in humans have apparently not been developed.

Will It Harm You? What the Studies Say:

Fresh cascara bark is very irritating and can cause severe vomiting, so the formulation you purchase should have been stored for at least twelve months (or specially heat-treated) to allow critical, natural chemical changes that eliminate this toxicity to take place. As long as this aging or heating has been properly carried out and you take the proper dosage, you are unlikely to experience any adverse reactions.

Take a stimulant laxative such as this only for short periods (a maximum of ten days); if taken for longer periods or abused, cascara sagrada can cause chronic diarrhea and cramps, laxative dependence, pigment deposits (melanin) in the colon's mucous membranes, and a loss of critical fluids and salts (including potassium) that may lead to weakness and possibly other complications. Do not take this herb if you suffer from any kind of intestinal obstruction. If you are pregnant or nursing, do not use it or any other laxative except under the advice of a doctor.

GENERAL SOURCES:

American Pharmaceutical Association. *Handbook of Nonprescription Drugs.* 11th ed. Washington, D.C.: American Pharmaceutical Association, 1996.

Balch, J.F., and P.A. Balch. *Prescription for Nutritional Healing: A Practical A to Z Reference to Drug-Free Remedies Using Vitamins, Minerals, Herbs & Food Supplements.* 2nd ed. Garden City Park, NY: Avery Publishing Group, 1997.

Bisset, N.G., ed. *Herbal Drugs and Phytopharmaceuticals.* Stuttgart: medpharm GmbH Scientific Publishers, 1994.

Blumenthal, M., J. Gruenwald, T. Hall, and R.S. Rister, eds. *The Complete German Commission E Monographs: Therapeutic Guide to Herbal Medicine.* Boston: Integrative Medicine Communications, 1998.

Bradley, P.C., ed. *British Herbal Compendium: A Handbook of Scientific Information on Widely Used Plant Drugs,* vol. 1. Bournemouth (Dorset), England: British Herbal Medicine Association, 1992.

Castleman, M. *The Healing Herbs: The Ultimate Guide to the Curative Power of Nature's Medicines.* New York: Bantam Books, 1995.

Lawrence Review of Natural Products. St. Louis: Facts and Comparisons, May 1996.

Leung, A.Y., and S. Foster. *Encyclopedia of Common Natural Ingredients Used in Food, Drugs, and Cosmetics.* 2nd ed. New York: John Wiley & Sons, 1996.

Mindell, E. *Earl Mindell's Herb Bible.* New York: Simon & Schuster/Fireside, 1992.

Tyler, V.E. *Herbs of Choice: The Therapeutic Use of Phytomedicinals.* Binghamton, NY: Haworth Press/Pharmaceutical Products Press, 1994.

Weiner, M.A., and J.A. Weiner. *Herbs That Heal: Prescription for Herbal Healing.* Mill Valley, CA: Quantum Books, 1994.

Weiss, R.F. *Herbal Medicine,* trans. A.R. Meuss, from the 6th German edition. Beaconsfield, England: Beaconsfield Publishers, Ltd., 1988.

TEXT CITATIONS:

1. *Lawrence Review of Natural Products* (St. Louis: Facts and Comparisons, May 1996).
2. F.H.L. Os, *Pharmacology,* 14 (Suppl.1) (1976): 18–29.
3. M. Blumenthal, J. Gruenwald, T. Hall, and R.S. Rister, eds., *The Complete German Commission E Monographs: Therapeutic Guide to Herbal Medicine* (Boston: Integrative Medicine Communications, 1998).
4. S.M. Kupchan and A. Karim, *Lloydia,* 39 (1976): 223–24.
5. R.J. Sydiskis et al., *Antimicrobial Agents & Chemotherapy,* 35(12) (1991): 2463–66.

PRIMARY NAME:
CASTOR OIL

SCIENTIFIC NAME:
Ricinus communis L. Family:
Euphorbiaceae

COMMON NAME:
Castor seed oil

RATING:
2 = According to a number of
well-designed studies and
common use, this substance
appears to be relatively
effective and safe when used in
recommended amounts for the
indication(s) noted in the "Will
It Work for You?" section.
However, see the warnings in
the "Will It Harm You?"
section.

What Is Castor Oil?

In temperate zones, this common and extensively cultivated ornamental annual
bears flowers that eventually turn into seed-bearing pods. Upon drying, these
pods explode and eject the oval seeds ("beans") within. Castor oil is extracted
from the ripe beans. In warm climates, *Ricinus* is a perennial, and many varieties grow as a broad-leafed shrub or tree.

What It Is Used For:

Over the centuries, generations of Egyptians, Indians, Chinese, and other
peoples have used castor oil as a cathartic (strong laxative).[1] Countless American children were coaxed to take a teaspoon of the acrid-tasting oil to ease
constipation. In Algiers the seeds are reportedly used as an oral contraceptive.[2] A 1994 survey of Ghanian women found that nearly 30 percent treated
acute respiratory infections in their children with castor oil and enemas.[3]
Numerous other conditions have been treated with the plant and oil. Doctors still recommend castor-oil-containing preparations to prepare the bowel
or rectum for X-ray examination or surgery. External preparations have been
applied to sores and abcesses. A handful of contemporary herbalists recommend castor oil internally as a laxative and treatment for food poisoning,
and externally for dissolving warts, cysts, and other skin growths.[4] Castor oil
can be found in lubricants, lipsticks and other cosmetics, and a variety of
other commercial preparations.

Forms Available Include:

Capsule, liquid (flavored), oil.

Dosage Commonly Reported:

Castor seeds are highly toxic and should be used only in commercial products.
A common dosage of castor oil is 15 to 60 milliliters. Because a laxative effect
occurs within two to six hours, do not take castor oil at bedtime. Plain castor
oil can be sweetened with fruit juice or soda to mask its disagreeable taste.

Will It Work for You? What the Studies Say:

Castor oil is a proven laxative that is most accurately described as a "cathartic"
or "drastic purgative," given its potency. After taking a typically recommended
dose, expect a major bowel movement within 2 to 6 hours. Very few sources still
recommend it for chronic constipation, however, partly because of the risk of
excessive loss of important fluids, salts, and nutrients. Continued use may also
cause the colon to become "lazy" and fail to function well. Gentler laxatives can
be found for even acute constipation.

No sound research can be found to justify or verify the value of castor oil for
treating warts or other skin growths, although the oil does have emollient (softening and soothing) properties and the protein, ricin, has shown some promise as a
pain reliever. The subject demands further study.[5] In 1970, researchers reported
success in treating mouse leukemia with ricin, but no further studies (or human
investigations) appear to have been done.[6] A preliminary 1988 *Science* article

reported intriguing evidence that a component of ricin may be active against HIV, but nothing more on the subject appears to have been reported since then.[7]

Will It Harm You? What the Studies Say:

All parts of the castor plant contain the poison ricin, although none remains in properly processed commercial oil made from the beans. Chewing the beans or ingesting any other part of the plant directly is dangerous, however. Ricin is so potent that the FBI considers it the third most poisonous substance known. It took only a few hundred millionths of a gram of the substance on the tip of an umbrella for Soviet agents to kill a Bulgarian defector at a London bus stop in 1978.[8] Although recent anecdotal evidence suggests its toxicity is not so extreme, wisdom still dictates handling it with great care.[9] One or two chewed beans can kill a human, although if swallowed whole they may pass through the body intact and cause no harm. Ricin rapidly disrupts the functioning of healthy cells in the body, efficiently killing them. Ingestion, inhalation, or intravenous administration causes severe mouth and throat irritation, nausea, vomiting, diarrhea, severe stomach pains, thirst, dimmed vision, kidney failure, and ultimately death.[10]

The oil, which is officially listed in the *U.S. Pharmacopoeia*, has been approved for food use. The oil in wart removers causes contact dermatitis in some people.[11]

GENERAL SOURCES:

American Pharmaceutical Association. *Handbook of Nonprescription Drugs*. 11th ed. Washington, D.C.: American Pharmaceutical Association, 1996.

Balch, J.F., and P.A. Balch. *Prescription for Nutritional Healing: A Practical A to Z Reference to Drug-Free Remedies Using Vitamins, Minerals, Herbs & Food Supplements*. 2nd ed. Garden City Park, NY: Avery Publishing Group, 1997.

Der Marderosian, A., and L. Liberti. *Natural Product Medicine: A Scientific Guide to Foods, Drugs, Cosmetics*. Philadelphia: George F. Stickley, 1988.

Lawrence Review of Natural Products. St. Louis: Facts and Comparisons, November 1992.

Leung, A.Y., and S. Foster. *Encyclopedia of Common Natural Ingredients Used in Food, Drugs, and Cosmetics*. 2nd ed. New York: John Wiley & Sons, 1996.

Tierra, M. *The Way of Herbs*. New York: Pocket Books, 1990.

TEXT CITATIONS:

1. A.Y. Leung and S. Foster, *Encyclopedia of Common Natural Ingredients Used in Food, Drugs, and Cosmetics*, 2nd ed. (New York: John Wiley & Sons, 1996).
2. V.J. Brondegaard, *Planta Medica*, 23 (1973): 167.
3. D.E.M. Denno et al., *Annals of Tropical Paediatrics*, 14(4) (1994): 293–301.
4. M. Tierra, *The Way of Herbs* (New York: Pocket Books, 1990).
5. C.C. Chen et al., *Journal of the Formosan Medical Association*, 75 (1976): 239.
6. J. Lin et al., *Nature*, 227 (1970): 292.
7. *Science.* 242 (1988): 1166–68. *HerbalGram*, 20 (1989): 22.
8. *HerbalGram*, 37:10.
9. *Lawrence Review of Natural Products* (St. Louis: Facts and Comparisons, November 1992).
10. P.A. Kinamore et al., *Clinical Toxicology*, 17 (1980): 401.
11. A.I. Tabar et al., *Contact Dermatitis*, 29(1) (1993): 49–50. A. Lodi et al., *Contact Dermatitis*, 26(4) (1992): 266–67.

CATNIP

SCIENTIFIC NAME:
Nepeta cataria L. Family:
Labiatae (Lamiaceae)

COMMON NAMES:
Catmint, catswort, field balm

RATING:
3 = Studies on the effectiveness
and safety of this herb are
conflicting, or there are not
enough studies to draw a
conclusion.

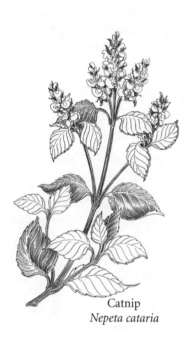

Catnip
Nepeta cataria

What Is Catnip?

The aromatic, fuzzy gray-green leaves and white flowering tops of this member of the mint family are famous for exciting cats. The perennial grows wild in many parts of the world, including parts of the United States and Canada. Its dried leaves and flowering tops are used medicinally.

What It Is Used For:

While acclaimed for its power to project some cats into a euphoric frenzy, this herb has a reputation for *sedating*—not stimulating—human beings. People from Siberia to North America have used it extensively as a traditional remedy, and for a time it appeared as a stomach-soothing agent in the *U.S. Pharmacopoeia* and the *National Formulary*. Catnip tea continues to be recommended by herbalists and regularly brewed in some regions of the country, such as Appalachia, to promote sleep (especially in children), remedy infant colic, relax and calm jangled nerves, soothe the digestive tract and control diarrhea, reduce gas, induce perspiration to lower fever, counteract hives, ease the discomfort of menstrual cramps, promote menstruation, and control a cold or bronchitis.[1] Poultices have been applied to swellings and corns, and there are reports of people smoking the dried leaves for respiratory ailments. In the 1960s, many took up smoking catnip for its supposed euphoric and hallucinogenic properties. Many people consider the herb a good insect repellant.

Forms Available Include:

- *For internal use:* Capsule, dried leaves, liquid extracts, infusion (made from dried leaves or extract in some cases; do not boil), oil, tincture.
- *For external use:* Bath formulations, poultice.

Dosage Commonly Reported:

Commercial preparations such as capsules and extracts are accompanied by dosage information. An infusion is made using 2 teaspoons dried herb per cup of water and is drunk up to three times per day. The tincture is taken in dosages of ½ to 1 teaspoon three times per day.

Will It Work for You? What the Studies Say:

The obvious kick some domestic and even large cats such as lions and jaguars get on contact with this herb—from joyful licking and rolling to body rubbing—is attributed to a substance in the herb's essential oil (present at 70 to 90 percent in the leaves) called nepetalactone. Some people have reported success in their attempts to get the same sort of mood boost and intoxication by smoking the dried leaves or tobacco soaked in catnip brews.[2] A 1969 article published in the distinguished *Journal of the American Medical Association* fueled the enthusiasm, but was later found to contain references to the marijuana plant, not catnip.[3] No evidence indicates that humans will respond as cats do to this herb.

Likewise, no sound studies have been done to test the theory that a cup of hot catnip tea can induce sleepiness and help ensure a good night's sleep in humans, although much anecdotal evidence suggests it can. Expectation may play a large role, and many people continue to enjoy catnip tea as a calmative and sleep aid. Some enthusiasts note that the herb's essential oil contains a form of nepetalactone structurally similar to the sedative compounds (valepotriates) found in another "sedative" herb, valerian (see **Valerian**). Others point to studies done in the 1980s indicating that catnip (especially a treated hot-water extract) positively influences sleep behavior in chicks when given to them in low or moderate doses.[4] A 1995 study similarly reported increased sleeping time and catalepsy in mice fed large amounts of catnip over several days.[5] Interestingly, high doses of the herb caused fewer chicks in the first study to sleep, and when given over a short period of time, decreased sleeping time and induced an amphetamine-like response in the mice in the second study. Both regimens increased the susceptibility to seizures. The reactions in humans may be very different.

Generations have reached for a mug of lemon-minty catnip tea to soothe the stomach and relieve gas or griping, but no studies have conclusively proven that it will have these effects. The best arguments for the herb's effectiveness may be its soothing flavor, the apparent antispasmodic properties in nepetalactone,[6] and possibly the actions of the herb's volatile oil.

Will It Harm You? What the Studies Say:

There are no reports of serious adverse reactions to catnip tea or other preparations, although smoking the herb may cause a sore throat, a headache, or a feeling of general malaise. Excessive amounts of the tea may cause vomiting.[7]

GENERAL SOURCES:

Balch, J.F., and P.A. Balch. *Prescription for Nutritional Healing: A Practical A to Z Reference to Drug-Free Remedies Using Vitamins, Minerals, Herbs & Food Supplements.* 2nd ed. Garden City Park, NY: Avery Publishing Group, 1997.

Castleman, M. *The Healing Herbs: The Ultimate Guide to the Curative Power of Nature's Medicines.* New York: Bantam Books, 1995.

Der Marderosian, A., and L. Liberti. *Natural Product Medicine: A Scientific Guide to Foods, Drugs, Cosmetics.* Philadelphia: George F. Stickley, 1988.

Duke, J.A. *CRC Handbook of Medicinal Herbs.* Boca Raton, FL: CRC Press, 1985.

Lawrence Review of Natural Products. St. Louis: Facts and Comparisons, January 1991.

Leung, A.Y., and S. Foster. *Encyclopedia of Common Natural Ingredients Used in Food, Drugs, and Cosmetics.* 2nd ed. New York: John Wiley & Sons, 1996.

Mindell, E. *Earl Mindell's Herb Bible.* New York: Simon & Schuster/Fireside, 1992.

Tierra, M. *The Way of Herbs.* New York: Pocket Books, 1990.

Tyler, V.E. *Herbs of Choice: The Therapeutic Use of Phytomedicinals.* Binghamton, NY: Haworth Press/Pharmaceutical Products Press, 1994.

———. *The Honest Herbal.* Binghamton, NY: Haworth Press/Pharmaceutical Products Press 1993.

Tyler V.E., L.R. Brady, and J.E. Robbers, eds. *Pharmacognosy.* Philadelphia: Lea & Febiger, 1988.

Weiss, R.F. *Herbal Medicine,* trans. A. R. Meuss, from the 6th German edition. Beaconsfield, England: Beaconsfield Publishers, Ltd., 1988.

TEXT CITATIONS:

1. *Lawrence Review of Natural Products* (St. Louis: Facts and Comparisons, January 1991). J.A. Duke, *CRC Handbook of Medicinal Herbs* (Boca Raton, FL: CRC Press, 1985).
2. *Lawrence Review of Natural Products*, op. cit.
3. B. Jackson and A. Reed, *Journal of the American Medical Association*, 207 (1969): 1349. J. Poundstone, *Journal of the American Medical Association*, 208 (1969): 360.
4. V.E. Tyler, *Herbs of Choice: The Therapeutic Use of Phytomedicinals* (Binghamton, NY: Haworth Press/Pharmaceutical Products Press, 1994). C.J. Sherry and J.P. Mitchell, *International Journal of Crude Drug Research*, 21 (1983): 89–92. C.J. Sherry and P.S. Hunter, *Experientia*, 35(2) (1979): 237–38.
5. C.O. Massoco et al., *Veterinary & Human Toxicology*, 37(6) (1995): 530–33.
6. A.Y. Leung and S. Foster, *Encyclopedia of Common Natural Ingredients Used in Food, Drugs, and Cosmetics*, 2nd ed. (New York: John Wiley & Sons, 1996).
7. *Lawrence Review of Natural Products*, op. cit.

PRIMARY NAME:

CAT'S CLAW

SCIENTIFIC NAME:

Uncaria tomentosa (Willd.) DC and *Uncaria guianensis* (Aubi.) (Gmel.) Family: Rubiaceae

COMMON NAMES:

Life-giving vine of Peru, samento, una de gato

RATING:

3 = Studies on the effectiveness and safety of this substance are conflicting, or there are not enough studies to draw a conclusion.

What Is Cat's Claw?

Cat's claw is a twining, woody vine that grows throughout the tropics of South America and the Asian continent. There are dozens of known species of *Uncaria*. Formulations of the species native to Peru—*Uncaria tomentosa*—can now be found in most American health food outlets. Primarily the dried root bark is used medicinally.

What It Is Used For:

Peruvian Indian tribes have brewed cat's claw tea for centuries to treat a myriad of conditions from arthritis to intestinal ailments, weakened immune systems, ulcers, asthma, allergies, tumors, gonorrhea, yeast infections, and inflammatory ailments such as arthritis. Many consider it a cure-all. European reports that cat's claw taken with AZT can benefit AIDS patients stimulated demand for the plant in North America; consumers buy it for this and other purposes, including to treat peptic ulcers, gastritis, and hemorrhoids.[1]

Forms Available Include:

Capsule, decoction, extract, liquid, tablet.

Dosage Commonly Reported:

One to two 500-milligram bark capsules are taken three times a day.

Will It Work for You? What the Studies Say:

Although scientists have identified a number of interesting chemicals in the *Uncaria* species over the past few years, evidence that the plant will benefit humans remains largely anecdotal and untested in clinical trials. Scientists have identified alkaloids and other substances in *Uncaria tomentosa* believed to stimulate the immune system by increasing phagocytosis, the process in which white blood cells engulf abnormal cells, bacteria, and other unwanted matter.[2]

This property was demonstrated in test-tube studies. A patent application describes increased immunoglobulin levels in melanoma patients after being administered a cat's claw extract.[3] Some reports also indicate that the plant has antimutagenic properties—at least in the test tube—meaning that it helped inhibit or fight potentially dangerous, cancer-causing cell mutations.[4] The same team reported that the urine of two smokers who drank a decoction of *Uncaria tomentosa* for fifteen days became less mutagenic (less likely to cause potentially dangerous cell mutations) in certain bacteria. But whether these immune-stimulating and antimutagenic properties can converge to boost the prospects of cancer sufferers or AIDS patients remains to be verified in animal studies and clinical trials.

Anti-inflammatory properties have also been identified in *Uncaria tomentosa*,[5] but questions as to their ability to translate into relief from inflammatory diseases in humans remain unanswered. At most, studies have shown that a glycoside in the plant exerts anti-inflammatory actions in the classic rat-paw inflammation test.[6] Test-tube studies indicate antiviral activity for several glycosides.[7] The implications of properties reportedly found during test-tube or animal studies of other *Uncaria* species, from an ability to lower blood pressure[8] to reducing blood cholesterol and heart rate, are still unclear.

Will It Harm You? What the Studies Say:

The medical literature contains no reports of major toxic reactions to cat's claw. Some communities have used it consistently over decades or longer. Keep in mind, however, that no large clinical trials have been done to fully assess its safety profile, particularly over the long term. The author of a popular book on the herb recommends avoiding it if you have undergone organ transplantation or take ulcer medications.[9]

GENERAL SOURCES:
Foster, S. *Health Food Business.* June (1995): 24.
Lawrence Review of Natural Products. St. Louis: Facts and Comparisons, April 1996.
Steinberg, P.N. *Cat's Claw: The Wondrous Herb from the Peruvian Rain Forest.* New York: Healing Wisdom Publications, 1996.

TEXT CITATIONS:
1. *Lawrence Review of Natural Products* (St. Louis: Facts and Comparisons, April 1996).
2. H. Wagner et al., *Planta Medica,* (1985): 419–23.
3. K. Keplinger, 1982 International Patent Application Number WO-82 01,130. K. Keplinger and D. Keplinger, U.S. Patent 5,302,611. 1994.
4. R. Rizzi et al., *Journal of Ethnopharmacology,* 38(1) (1993): 63–77.
5. A. Senatore et al., *Bollettino-Societa Italiana Biologia Sperimentale,* 65(5) (1989): 517–20.
6. R. Aquino et al., *Journal of Natural Products,* 54(2) (1991): 453–59. K. Keplinger, 1982 International Patent Application Number WO-82 01, 130.
7. R. Aquino et al., *Journal of Natural Products,* 52(4) (1989): 679–85.
8. K. Endo et al., *Planta Medica,* 49 (1983): 188.
9. P.N. Steinberg, *Cat's Claw: The Wondrous Herb from the Peruvian Rain Forest* (New York: Healing Wisdom Publications, 1996).

PRIMARY NAME:

CEDAR, EASTERN RED

SCIENTIFIC NAME:

Juniperus virginiana L. Family: Pinaceae

COMMON NAMES:

Cedar, red juniper

RATING:

- *For internal use:* 5 = Studies indicate that there is a definite health hazard to using this substance, even in recommended amounts.
- *For external use:* 3 = Studies on the effectiveness and safety of this substance are conflicting, or there are not enough studies to draw a conclusion.

What Is Eastern Red Cedar?

The aromatic eastern red cedar qualifies as one of America's most widely distributed eastern conifers. It has a narrow, columnar crown, reddish-brown bark, and overlapping scalelike leaves. The leaves, the blue-green fruit, the wood, and the wood oil have been used medicinally. Other cedar species have been enlisted in healing as well, including *Cedrus libani* (cedar of Lebanon) and *Thuja occidentalis* L. (northern white cedar).

What It Is Used For:

More than a century ago, Native Americans brewed a tea from the fruits to control coughs, colds, rheumatism, and intestinal worms, and to induce sweating. Some dealt with canker sore pain by chewing the fruit. Many inhaled the smoke or steam from the leaves (and sometimes other parts of the tree) to relieve such ills as bronchitis and rheumatic pain. The smoke or steam was used in purification rituals. Others made berry infusions as diuretics, or "water pills."

Modern herbalists tout cedar oil's antiviral and antifungal properties, claiming it can cleanse the urine and lymph system, clear congestion, stimulate the immune system, and boost blood flow. External formulations are placed on warts. Aromatherapists use cedar wood in liquid form.

The essential oil of the cedar leaf also appears in various commercial products, including steam vaporizer solutions. Its distinctive, vigorous fragrance is put to work in aftershave lotions and other men's products. Dandruff products sometimes contain cedar extracts to control greasy hair. The wood oil was once a common ingredient in insect repellents. The hard wood, treasured by early settlers for making furniture, log cabins, fence posts, and pencils, still commands great respect in manufacturing industries. The tree is a popular Christmas tree.

Forms Available Include:

- *For internal use:* Capsule (from berries). However, eastern red cedar is not recommended for internal use.
- *For external use:* Liquid (from wood, for use in aromatherapy), oil.

Dosage Commonly Reported:

For topical use and for use in steam inhalations, use commercial formulations and follow the package instructions. Not recommended for internal use.

Will It Work for You? What the Studies Say:

Many sources ascribe antiseptic, expectorant, astringent, and antifungal properties to cedar extracts, which, if true, would explain a number of the traditional uses. Studies on various *Juniperus* species, most of them in the test tube, indicate that a number of the claims are valid. Parts of the eastern red cedar may also contain the antitumor compound podophyllotoxin. (See **Mayapple, American,** for more information on podophyllotoxin.) The *U.S. Pharmacopoeia* and *National Formulary* once listed the wood as a diaphoretic (an agent that induces sweating).[1]

Even if these claims are proved true, however, they are somewhat irrelevant—at least for internal use—given the tree's toxicity. The wisest approach may be to stick to commercial formulations for use on the skin or for inhalation. *Never ingest the essential oil.* To confuse matters, many herbalists fail to specify which cedar tree they are referring to when recommending the plant, making it hard to verify the accuracy of their claims. Evidence indicates that the wood oil is probably not effective as an insect repellent.[2]

Will It Harm You? What the Studies Say:

The limited information available indicates that all parts of the tree are toxic,[3] but that recommended amounts of the essential oil are probably safe to use in topical form or in commercial steam vaporizers. Watch out for skin irritation with these as well, however. Pregnant women should avoid eastern red cedar altogether.

GENERAL SOURCES:

American Pharmaceutical Association. *Handbook of Nonprescription Drugs.* 11th ed. Washington, D.C.: American Pharmaceutical Association, 1996.

Balch, J.F., and P.A. Balch. *Prescription for Nutritional Healing: A Practical A to Z Reference to Drug-Free Remedies Using Vitamins, Minerals, Herbs & Food Supplements.* 2nd ed. Garden City Park, NY: Avery Publishing Group, 1997.

Chevallier, A. *The Encyclopedia of Medicinal Plants: A Practical Reference Guide to More Than 550 Key Medicinal Plants & Their Uses.* First American Edition. New York: Dorling Kindersley Publications, 1996.

Foster, S. *Forest Pharmacy: Medicinal Plants in American Forests.* Durham, NC: Forest History Society, 1995.

Foster, S., and Duke, J.A. *The Peterson Field Guide Series: A Field Guide to Medicinal Plants. Eastern and Central North America.* Boston: Houghton Mifflin Company, 1990.

Little, E.L. *National Audubon Society Field Guide to North American Trees: Eastern Region.* New York: Alfred A. Knopf, Inc., 1980.

TEXT CITATIONS:

1. S. Foster, *Forest Pharmacy: Medicinal Plants in American Forests* (Durham, NC: Forest History Society, 1995).

2. American Pharmaceutical Association, *Handbook of Nonprescription Drugs,* 11th ed. (Washington, D.C.: American Pharmaceutical Association, 1996).

3. S. Foster and J.A. Duke, *The Peterson Field Guide Series: A Field Guide to Medicinal Plants. Eastern and Central North America* (Boston: Houghton Mifflin Company, 1990).

PRIMARY NAME:
CELERY SEED

SCIENTIFIC NAME:
Apium graveolens L. Family: Umbelliferae (Apiaceae)

COMMON NAMES:
Apium, celery fruit, marsh parsley, smallage fruit, wild celery

What Is Celery Seed?

Spicy and somewhat bitter fruits ("seeds") develop on the white flowers of the widely recognized, pale green biennial celery plant. There are multiple varieties of celery, a carrot-family member. Once ripened, the seeds are collected and dried. Steam distillation of the seeds produces an essential oil.

What It Is Used For:

This extensively cultivated plant and its seeds have been used for centuries as a seasoning and medicine. Celery wine was bestowed on victorious athletes in ancient Greece. Several ancient healing traditions, including the Indian (Ayurvedic) and oriental, considered celery seeds valuable in many ways, recommending them to treat fluid retention (as a diuretic, or "water pill"), colds, arthritis, indigestion, and liver disease. Europeans have used celery-seed preparations medicinally for several centuries. Commercial celery elixirs and tonics made with the crushed seeds figured prominently in American and European pharmacies of the nineteenth century. Modern herbalists recommend celery seed preparations for many of the same ailments as their predecessors did, especially as a diuretic to shed water weight, treat bladder and kidney disorders, or even manage more serious ailments such as congestive heart failure. Many consider it an excellent tonic for nervous restlessness, an anti-inflammatory for rheumatic complaints and gout, and a potentially effective remedy for treating diabetes, stomach upset, obesity, delayed menstruation, and high blood pressure. More than fifty British anti-inflammatory remedies contain celery seed.[1]

Forms Available Include:

Infusion (made of crushed seeds), seeds, tincture.

Dosage Commonly Reported:

Use the seeds in infusions and tinctures. An infusion is made using 1 to 2 teaspoon freshly crushed seeds per cup of water. The tincture is taken in dosages of $\frac{1}{2}$ to 1 teaspoon up to three times per day.

Will It Work for You? What the Studies Say:

Overall, little conclusive evidence can be found to substantiate the use of celery seed for any ailment; no human clinical trials are found in the (recent) medical literature. German health authorities have declined to endorse the seeds or any other part of the plant for proposed traditional uses.[2]

According to animal studies, celery seeds increase urine production. But particularly given the often serious nature of ailments treated with this class of medicines, much more well-designed and thorough research is needed to confirm that the diuretic action is potent enough to benefit humans. Responsible sources do not recommend diuretics as diet aids, as any lost weight represents transitory fluid loss.

The implications for human health of other intriguing findings are likewise hazy. In one study, celery oil injected into rabbits and dogs notably reduced blood pressure over several weeks, and fourteen of sixteen individuals who drank celery juice in another study done in China experienced a drop in their blood pressure.[3] But confirmatory studies are needed given various limitations of these studies. Rodent studies indicate that substances called phthalides in the oil have sedative and anticonvulsant properties,[4] but whether this translates into an ability to calm anxiety, nervous restlessness, or insomnia in humans remains far from clear. Similarly undetermined are the implications for treating high cholesterol based on preliminary recent evidence that a liquid extract of celery significantly reduces certain lipid (fat) levels in laboratory rats.[5] Hints of potential anticancer properties in phthalides and other components of this plant, some of which were shown to reduce stomach tumors in mice, remain to be more fully explored,[6] as do indicators of significant liver-protectant properties in rats administered an alcoholic extract of the seeds.[7] Reports from the early 1970s that celery-seed preparations may benefit diabetes sufferers by reducing blood sugar levels await exploration and confirmation from clinical trials.[8]

Other parts of the celery plant have shown some intriguing properties as well. Liquid extracts of celery stems exert a significant anti-inflammatory action in animals, indicating a potential for treating inflammatory diseases such as arthritis in humans, but no clinical trials on the subject have been published so far.[9]

Will It Harm You? What the Studies Say:

The seeds and other parts of the celery plant appear to be safe to consume, although allergic reactions can occur and become serious in some cases; hives, swelling, breathing trouble, and anaphylaxis have been reported.[10] Skin reactions after handling the plant and mild to potentially severe system-wide allergic reactions have occurred. A substance called bergapten (a type of furocoumarin) in celery can cause sun sensitivity, inciting contact dermatitis in individuals who have handled the plant and are then exposed to ultraviolet rays such as sunlight. Sunscreen apparently protects against this.[11] Bergapten apparently does not remain in the blood after eating celery, although recent reports indicate that individuals who ingest large amounts of the roots and are then exposed to intensive PUVA therapy may develop a skin reaction.[12] One woman who ate a lot of celery root and then visited a suntan parlor suffered a serious phytotoxic burn.[13] Furocoumarins may be carcinogenic (cancer-causing).[14]

Various European authorities, including the British, advise pregnant women and people with kidney disorders not to use celery medicinally. Do not use seeds sold for cultivation as medicinal agents. Limit the medicinal use of celery seed oil to situations in which a doctor oversees your case. Toxic reactions possibly including central nervous system depression can occur with large amounts of the oil, although this is not well understood.[15] Consult your doctor first if you want to use celery seeds as a diuretic.

The FDA classifies celery and celery seeds as safe for food use.

GENERAL SOURCES:

Bisset, N.G., ed. *Herbal Drugs and Phytopharmaceuticals.* Stuttgart: medpharm GmbH Scientific Publishers, 1994.

Blumenthal, M., J. Gruenwald, T. Hall, and R.S. Rister, eds. *The Complete German Commission E Monographs: Therapeutic Guide to Herbal Medicine.* Boston: Integrative Medicine Communications, 1998.

Castleman, M. *The Healing Herbs: The Ultimate Guide to the Curative Power of Nature's Medicines.* New York: Bantam Books, 1995.

Chevallier, A. *The Encyclopedia of Medicinal Plants: A Practical Reference Guide to More Than 550 Key Medicinal Plants & Their Uses.* First American Edition. New York: Dorling Kindersley Publications, 1996.

Lawrence Review of Natural Products. St. Louis: Facts and Comparisons, January 1996.

Leung, A.Y., and S. Foster. *Encyclopedia of Common Natural Ingredients Used in Food, Drugs, and Cosmetics.* 2nd ed. New York: John Wiley & Sons, 1996.

TEXT CITATIONS:

1. N.G. Bisset, ed., *Herbal Drugs and Phytopharmaceuticals* (Stuttgart: medpharm GmbH Scientific Publishers, 1994).

2. M. Blumenthal, J. Gruenwald, T. Hall, and R.S. Rister, eds., *The Complete German Commission E Monographs: Therapeutic Guide to Herbal Medicine* (Boston: Integrative Medicine Communications, 1998).

3. A.Y. Leung and S. Foster, *Encyclopedia of Common Natural Ingredients Used in Food, Drugs, and Cosmetics*, 2nd ed. (New York: John Wiley & Sons, 1996).

4. L.F. Bjeldanes and I. Kim, *Journal of Organic Chemistry*, 42 (1977): 2333. R.P. Kohli et al., *Indian Journal of Medical Research*, 55 (1967): 1099. S.R. Yu et al., *Acta Pharmacol Sin*, 9 (1988): 385.

5. D. Tsi et al., *Planta Medica*, 61(1) (1995): 18–21.

6. G.Q. Zheng et al., *Nutrition & Cancer*, 19(1) (1993): 77–86. S. Hashim et al., *Nutrition & Cancer*, 21(2) (1994): 169.

7. A. Singh and S.S. Handa, *Journal of Ethnopharmacology*, 49(3) (1995): 119–26.

8. *Lawrence Review of Natural Products* (St. Louis: Facts and Comparisons, January 1996). N.R. Farnsworth and A.B. Segelman, *Tile and Till* (Eli Lilly and Company), 57(3) (1971): 52.

9. M.K. Al-Hindawi et al., *Journal of Ethnopharmacology*, 26(2) (1989): 163–68. Leung and Foster, op. cit. D.A. Lewis et al., *International Journal of Crude Drug Research*, 23(1) (1985): 27.

10. Zheng, op. cit.

11. *Lawrence Review of Natural Products*, op. cit.

12. N. Gral et al., *Annales de Dermatologie et de Venereologie*, 120(9) (1993): 599–603.

13. B. Ljunggren, *Archives of Dermatology*, 126(10) (1990): 1334–36.

14. B.N. Ames, *Science*, 221(4617) (1983): 1256.

15. *Lawrence Review of Natural Products*, op. cit.

PRIMARY NAME:

CHAMOMILE, GERMAN

SCIENTIFIC NAME:

Matricaria chamomilla L., also referred to as *Matricaria recutita* and *Chamomilla recutita* (L.) Rauschert. Family: Asteraceae (Compositae)

COMMON NAMES:

Genuine chamomile or Hungarian chamomile

RATING:

2 = According to a number of well-designed studies and common use, this substance appears to be relatively

What Is German Chamomile?

Of the two major types of chamomile—German or Hungarian, and Roman or English—only the former is discussed here. It is more widely available on the North American and world market and is chemically distinct from Roman chamomile (*Chamaemelum nobile* L., synonymous with *Anthemis nobilis* L.),[1] which is mostly used in Britain. The daisylike, yellow flower heads of the fragrant *Matricaria chamomilla*, an annual, are dried before being used medicinally. Steam distillation produces a blue-colored volatile oil.

What It Is Used For:

It seems that few human ills have escaped treatment with a cup of German chamomile tea at some point over the centuries. Since ancient Roman times, the herb has perhaps been known best as a soothing and relaxing warm drink to savor or to treat digestive upset (stomach cramps, gas), stimulate digestion, calm anxiety or stress, encourage sleep, reduce fever, control ulcers, resolve menstrual cramps or other spasms, fight infections from minor illness, and lessen rheumatic pain. Today it may well rank as America's best-selling herbal tea. Europeans consider chamomile a panacea.[2] Compresses, lotions, and other external formulations have also been recommended for encouraging wounds to

CHAMOMILE. GERMAN
(Continued)

effective and safe when used in recommended amounts for indication(s) noted in the "Will It Work for You?" section.

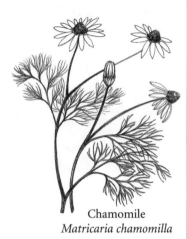

Chamomile
Matricaria chamomilla

heal and reducing inflammation in skin irritations such as eczema and hemorrhoids. Many a blond over the centuries has rinsed his or her hair with chamomile to maintain its luster and highlight golden tones. The essential oil can be found in many hair rinses, bath oils, skin creams, and other cosmetics, and as a flavoring in foods and drinks.

Forms Available Include:

- *For internal use:* Capsule, extract, infusion (made with dried flowers), tincture.
- *For external use:* Bath formulations, compress (made with a strong infusion), extract, lotion, ointment.

Dosage Commonly Reported:

A tea is made using 2 to 3 heaping teaspoons dried flowers per cup of water and is used as a compress as well as a beverage. The tincture is taken in dosages of ½ to 1 teaspoon up to three times per day. A gargle is made using 10 drops of fluid extract per glass of water.

Will It Work for You? What the Studies Say:

Intensive research over the decades indicates that several of the traditional uses for chamomile make scientific sense. Of the herb's various active constituents, the most important is probably a complex, blue-colored essential oil made up largely of a sesquiterpene alcohol called alpha-bisabolol ("bisabolol") and small amounts of a critical ingredient called chamazulene. Flower heads contain about 0.5 percent of the oil.

Antispasmodic and anti-inflammatory properties have been identified in bisabolol, which probably explains why the herb helps soothe stomach upset; it probably relaxes the smooth muscle lining of the stomach or intestines and calms inflamed tissue. These properties have been demonstrated in classic animal tests for inflammation[3] and test-tube experiments for spasms.[4] Enhancing bisabolol's actions are chemicals called flavonoids in the dried flower heads, which likewise exert antispasmodic and anti-inflammatory actions,[5] and chamazulene, which in animals demonstrates anti-inflammatory and even anti-allergenic properties.[6] Chamomile products sold in Germany are often standardized for chamazulene and bisabolol content.[7] Rat experiments indicate that bisabolol fights fever,[8] often a component of inflammatory diseases. German health authorities endorse the use of chamomile flower teas and other preparations for gastrointestinal spasms and inflammatory diseases such as arthritis.[9] The antispasmodic properties may help explain why the plant has traditionally been used as a calming sedative, but little information on this can be found, and it does not appear to have been tested for this purpose.

German authorities also endorse chamomile tea for peptic ulcers. Rat studies indicate that bisabolol both inhibits the development of gastric ulcers and speeds healing in ulcers that have already developed.[10]

Chamomile may also help prevent infections and speed wound healing by fighting certain disease-causing microbes, including bacteria such as *Staphylococcus aureus* and fungi such as *Candida albicans* (commonly implicated in vaginal yeast infections).[11] The polysaccharides stimulate the immune system, according to a 1985 study of various plants.[12] Bisabolol's anti-inflammatory properties may also contribute to wound healing; it helps attract cells that contribute to building new tissue and scar formation (technically, tissue regeneration and granulation).[13] One small double-blind clinical trial found that chamomile significantly decreased the surface area of wounds and helped them to dry out.[14] In a guinea pig study, bisabolol applied to burns reduced the time it took them to heal.[15] Eczema has responded to creams made with the flower extract.[16] On the basis of these and other findings, German health authorities endorse topical chamomile products for treating bacterial skin diseases and mouthwashes (made with infusions) for soothing inflammatory mouth and gum problems.[17]

Limitations to using chamomile should be noted, however. The critical essential oil is not very water-soluble, so even when you prepare a strong tea properly, only about 10 to 15 percent of this oil is extracted into the liquid.[18] Whole extracts and other high-concentration preparations are hard to find in the United States, although drinking chamomile regularly over extended periods of time may produce the wanted results.[19] To ensure that you are getting the highest-quality chamomile, buy formulations that contain whole flower heads from a reputable source.[20] Avoid pulverized or powdered formulations or ones full of stems or other parts of the plant.

Will It Harm You? What the Studies Say:

Chamomile is widely considered safe to use in typically recommended amounts, both internally and externally.[21] The FDA has placed chamomile on its list of herbs generally considered safe for food use. However, if you are allergic to other members of the aster family such as ragweed, carefully avoid chamomile, given the risk of cross-reactions and the potential for adulteration with other potential allergens.[22] So far, only about five cases of allergy to chamomile plants worldwide (between 1887 and 1982) have been directly attributed to *Matricaria recutita*.[23] Ingesting large amounts of the dried flowers may cause vomiting.[24]

GENERAL SOURCES:

American Pharmaceutical Association. *Handbook of Nonprescription Drugs.* 11th ed. Washington, D.C.: American Pharmaceutical Association, 1996.

Balch, J.F., and P.A. Balch. *Prescription for Nutritional Healing: A Practical A to Z Reference to Drug-Free Remedies Using Vitamins, Minerals, Herbs & Food Supplements.* 2nd ed. Garden City Park, NY: Avery Publishing Group, 1997.

Blumenthal, M., J. Gruenwald, T. Hall, and R.S. Rister, eds. *The Complete German Commission E Monographs: Therapeutic Guide to Herbal Medicine.* Boston: Integrative Medicine Communications, 1998.

Bradley. P.C., ed. *British Herbal Compendium: A Handbook of Scientific Information on Widely Used Plant Drugs.* vol. 1. Bournemouth (Dorset), England: British Herbal Medicine Association, 1992.

Castleman, M. *The Healing Herbs: The Ultimate Guide to the Curative Power of Nature's Medicines.* New York: Bantam Books, 1995.

Der Marderosian, A., and L. Liberti. *Natural Product Medicine: A Scientific Guide to Foods, Drugs, Cosmetics.* Philadelphia: George F. Stickley, 1988.

Duke, J.A. *CRC Handbook of Medicinal Herbs.* Boca Raton, FL: CRC Press, 1985.

Foster, S. *Chamomile: Matricaria recutita & Chamaemelum nobile.* American Botanical Council Botanical Series 307.

Lawrence Review of Natural Products. St. Louis: Facts and Comparisons, March 1991.

Leung, A.Y., and S. Foster. *Encyclopedia of Common Natural Ingredients Used in Food, Drugs, and Cosmetics.* 2nd ed. New York: John Wiley & Sons, 1996.

Tyler, V.E. *Herbs of Choice: The Therapeutic Use of Phytomedicinals.* Binghamton, NY: Haworth Press/Pharmaceutical Products Press, 1994.

———. *The Honest Herbal.* Binghamton, NY: Haworth Press/Pharmaceutical Products Press 1993.

Weiss, R.F. *Herbal Medicine*, trans. A.R. Meuss, from the 6th German edition. Beaconsfield, England: Beaconsfield Publishers, Ltd., 1988.

TEXT CITATIONS:

1. American Pharmaceutical Association, *Handbook of Nonprescription Drugs*, 11th ed. (Washington, D.C.: American Pharmaceutical Association, 1996).

2. V.E. Tyler, *The Honest Herbal* (Binghamton, NY: Haworth Press/Pharmaceutical Products Press 1993).

3. V. Jakovlev et al., *Planta Medica*, 35 (1979): 125.

4. H.B. Forster et al., *Planta Medica*, 40 (1980): 309.

5. American Pharmaceutical Association, op. cit.

6. P. Stern and R. Milin, *Arzneimittel-Forschung*, 6 (1956): 445.

7. Forster, op. cit.

8. A. Der Marderosian and L. Liberti, *Natural Product Medicine: A Scientific Guide to Foods, Drugs, Cosmetics* (Philadelphia: George F. Stickley, 1988).

9. M. Blumenthal, J. Gruenwald, T. Hall, and R.S. Rister, eds., *The Complete German Commission E Monographs: Therapeutic Guide to Herbal Medicine* (Boston: Integrative Medicine Communications, 1998).

10. I. Szelenyi et al., *Planta Medica*, 35 (1979): 218.

11. A.Y. Leung and S. Foster, *Encyclopedia of Common Natural Ingredients Used in Food, Drugs, and Cosmetics*, 2nd ed. (New York: John Wiley & Sons, 1996).

12. H. Wagner et al., *Arzneimittel-Forschung*, 35 (1985): 1069–75.

13. P.C. Bradley, ed., *British Herbal Compendium: A Handbook of Scientific Information on Widely Used Plant Drugs*, vol. 1 (Bournemouth [Dorset], England: British Herbal Medicine Association, 1992).

14. H.J. Glowania et al., *Zeitschrift fur Hautkrankheiten*, 62 (1987): 1262–71.

15. O. Isaac, *Planta Medica*, 35 (1979): 118.

16. Bradley, op. cit.

17. Blumenthal et al., op. cit.

18. N.R. Farnsworth and B.M. Morgan, *Journal of the American Medical Association*, 221 (1972): 410. *Lawrence Review of Natural Products* (St. Louis: Facts and Comparisons, March 1991).

19. Tyler, *The Honest Herbal*, op. cit.

20. V.E. Tyler, *Herbs of Choice: The Therapeutic Use of Phytomedicinals* (Binghamton, NY: Haworth Press/Pharmaceutical Products Press, 1994).

21. S. Habersang et al., *Planta Medica*, 37 (1979): 115.

22. S. Foster, *Chamomile: Matricaria recutita & Chamaemelum nobile.* American Botanical Council Botanical Series 307.

23. Tyler, *Herbs of Choice*, op. cit.

24. Der Marderosian and Liberti, op. cit.

PRIMARY NAME:
CHAPARRAL

SCIENTIFIC NAME:
Larrea divaricata Cov., sometimes referred to as *Larrea tridentata* (DC) Cov. or *Larrea glutinosa* Engelm. Family: Zygophyllacea

COMMON NAMES:
Creosote bush, greasewood, hediondillal, stinkweed

RATING:
5 = Studies indicate that there is a definite health hazard to using this substance, even in recommended amounts.

What Is Chaparral?

Chaparral refers to a group of wild shrubs that grow throughout much of the arid western United States and parts of Mexico. Most health food outlets sell chaparral products containing twigs and leaflets of *Larrea divaricata* Cov. Like other chaparrals, this olive green or yellow shrub has strong-smelling (some say foul-smelling), resinous leaves.

What It Is Used For:

More than a century ago, Native American tribes familiar with these evergreen shrubs reportedly made a tea from the leaves and twigs to remedy a broad spectrum of ailments including colds, bronchitis, rheumatism, cancer, and snakebites. They applied the resin to burns. Settlers adopted and expanded on many of these applications, including the treatment of various cancers, parasitical and other infections, pain, diarrhea, and venereal diseases. The *U.S. Pharmacopoeia* listed chaparral for nearly a century.

Modern herbalists have focused on the herb's purported cancer-fighting and antiaging qualities and its potential for fighting infection, "purifying" the blood (often a euphemism for combating venereal disease), treating colds, encouraging weight loss, helping in withdrawal from alcohol, and controlling acne. Some recommend external formulations to prevent wound infections. Although the FDA now prohibits it, the United States Department of Agriculture still endorses the use of an ingredient in chaparral called nordihydroguaiaretic acid (NDGA) as an animal fat preservative.[1]

Forms Available Include:

- *For internal use:* Capsule, extract, infusion. Appears in herbal blends.
- *For external use:* Extract.

Dosage Commonly Reported:

Chaparral should not be used medicinally. In past times, an infusion or mouthwash was made using 1 tablespoon dried leaves and stems per quart of water.

Will It Work for You? What the Studies Say:

Chaparral leaves contain relatively large amounts of NDGA, a potent antioxidant valued for preserving certain animal fats. It is sold commercially in the United States. In human beings, antioxidants are believed to help scavenge toxic by-products that may contribute to cancer cell formation. Apparently spurred by anecdotal reports that individuals with cancers such as malignant melanoma, lymphosarcoma, and metastatic choriocarcinoma experienced regressions of their disease with chaparral tea, the National Cancer Institute undertook test-tube studies of NDGA and found potent anticancer properties.[2] Unfortunately, this quality failed to persist in studies that involved living creatures such as mice, and subsequent reports from more than thirty cancer patients treated with the herb indicated that NDGA actually propagates more malignancies than it helps to regress.[3] No statistically significant anticancer activity was noted in a 1968–69 study involving fifty-nine individuals with advanced malignancies who were treated with the herb.[4]

Some proponents assert that antioxidants such as NDGA may help retard the aging process by preventing damaging free radicals from forming. In one study, the average life span of mosquitoes jumped from twenty-nine days to forty-five days when they were fed NDGA.[5] But much remains to be learned about the potential of NDGA—or any antioxidant, for that matter—to prolong human life.

Some traditional uses for chaparral may be explained by research indicating that the herb (specifically, NDGA) has antimicrobial, antiyeast, and anti-inflammatory properties[6] and can kill certain larvae and fatally poison the American cockroach. But no human clinical trials have been done to examine its value for infections, inflammatory conditions such as arthritis, or any illness other than cancer. Nor are the implications clear of mid-1990s studies showing that lignans from *Larrea tridentata* inhibit HIV-1 activity in the test tube,[7] or of another study done the same year indicating that chaparral contains estrogenic (female hormone) compounds.[8] More important, perhaps, the health risks of proceeding with these kinds of trials are prohibitive.

Will It Harm You? What the Studies Say:

Chaparral has been linked to the development of acute liver damage (hepatitis) in several North Americans. Most of these individuals developed signs and symptoms of liver damage after taking the herb for several weeks or more. One sufferer required a liver transplant.[9] In another case, a thirty-three-year-old woman took up to fifteen chaparral-leaf tablets a day for about five months in the hope that the herb would help clear up a benign breast lump. She developed symptoms of hepatitis three months after starting to take the pills, and recovered from the illness only after stopping the herb and being hospitalized for supportive care.[10] In another report, a seventy-one-year-old man and a forty-two-year-old woman both developed hepatitis after taking chaparral for several weeks but recovered after stopping the herb.[11] A 1994 report cites the development of kidney disease and cancer (cystic renal cell carcinoma and renal cystic disease) in a woman who consumed chaparral tea for a long period of time.[12]

In 1992 the FDA issued a warning about the risks of hepatitis that prompted many herbal catalogs and health food stores to remove the herb from circulation.[13] The agency removed NDGA from its list of substances generally regarded as safe (GRAS) for consumption as long ago as 1970, when studies showed that rats fed NDGA for seventy-four weeks developed suspicious lesions on their lymph nodes and kidneys.

Contact with the plant itself can cause contact dermatitis.[14]

GENERAL SOURCES:

Castleman, M. *The Healing Herbs: The Ultimate Guide to the Curative Power of Nature's Medicines.* New York: Bantam Books, 1995.

Der Marderosian, A., and L. Liberti. *Natural Product Medicine: A Scientific Guide to Foods, Drugs, Cosmetics.* Philadelphia: George F. Stickley, 1988.

Duke, J.A. *CRC Handbook of Medicinal Herbs.* Boca Raton, FL: CRC Press, 1985.

Lawrence Review of Natural Products. St. Louis: Facts and Comparisons, August 1993.

Leung, A.Y., and S. Foster. *Encyclopedia of Common Natural Ingredients Used in Food, Drugs, and Cosmetics*. 2nd ed. New York: John Wiley & Sons, 1996.

Mindell, E. *Earl Mindell's Herb Bible*. New York: Simon & Schuster/Fireside, 1992.

Stashower, M.E., and R.Z. Torres. *Journal of the American Medical Association*. 274(11) (1995): 8712.

Tyler, V.E. *The Honest Herbal*. Binghamton, NY: Haworth Press/Pharmaceutical Products Press, 1993.

Tyler, V.E., L.R. Brady, and J.E. Robbers, eds. *Pharmacognosy*. Philadelphia: Lea & Febiger, 1988.

TEXT CITATIONS:

1. A.Y. Leung and S. Foster, *Encyclopedia of Common Natural Ingredients Used in Food, Drugs, and Cosmetics*, 2nd ed. (New York: John Wiley & Sons, 1996).
2. D. Burk and M. Woods, *Radiation Research Supplement*, 3 (1963): 212.
3. *Unproven Methods of Cancer Management*, American Cancer Society, 1970. *Lawrence Review of Natural Products* (St. Louis: Facts and Comparisons, August 1993).
4. C.R. Smart et al., *Cancer Chemotherapy*, Rep Pt 1. 53 (1969):147. C.R. Smart et al., *Rocky Mountain Medical Journal*. 1970: 7. Leung and Foster, op. cit.
5. S. Boxer, *Discover*, 8(i) (1987): 13–14.
6. M.A. Verastegui et al., *Journal of Ethnopharmacology*, 52(3) (1996): 175–77. Leung and Foster, op. cit.
7. J.N. Gnabre et al., *Journal of Chromatography A*, 719(2) (1996): 353–64. J.N. Gnabre et al., *Proceedings of the National Academy of Sciences of the United States of America*, 92(24) (1995): 11239–43.
8. W.R. Obermeyer et al., *Proceedings of the Society for Experimental Biology & Medicine*, 208(1) (1995): 6–12.
9. D.W. Gordon et al., *Journal of the American Medical Association*, 273(6) (1995): 489–90.
10. M. Katz and F. Saibil, *Journal of Clinical Gastroenterology*, 12 (1990): 203–6.
11. W.B. Batchelor et al., *American Journal of Gastroenterology*, 90(5) (1995): 831–33.
12. A.Y. Smith et al., *Journal of Urology*, 152(6 pt 1) (1994): 2089–91.
13. *Morbidity & Mortality Weekly Report*, 43 (1992): 812–14.
14. K.F. Lampe and M.A. McCann, *AMA Handbook of Poisonous and Injurious Plants* (Chicago: American Medical Association, 1985). D.R. Shasky, *Journal of the American Academy of Dermatology*, 15(2 Pt 1) (1986): 302.

PRIMARY NAME:

CHASTE TREE BERRY

SCIENTIFIC NAME:
Vitex agnus-castus L. Family: Verbenaceae

COMMON NAMES:
Chasteberry, cloister pepper, hemp tree, monk's pepper, vitex

What Is Chaste Tree Berry?

Vitex agnus-castus is a shrub or small deciduous tree that bears slender spikes of violet flowers and aromatic, peppery reddish-black fruit ("berries"). Once ripened, these berries are dried and used medicinally. Chaste tree berry, native to southwestern Europe and western Asia, can now be found in southeastern parts of North America.

What It Is Used For:

Since antiquity, European healers have relied on this herb for female reproductive tract disorders such as painful or absent menstrual periods. It purportedly helps flush out the placenta after birth. Given its common name, it comes as little surprise that the "chaste tree" berry was once trumpeted as a key to sup-

CHASTE TREE BERRY
(Continued)

RATING:

2 = According to a number of well-designed studies and common use, this substance appears to be relatively effective and safe when used in recommended amounts.

pressing female sexual desires. Although long used in Europe, the herb has only recently appeared on the American herbal market.[1]

Forms Available Include:

Capsule, decoction, dried fruit, extract, tincture.

Dosage Commonly Reported:

A common daily dosage is 20 milligrams crude fruit, usually taken in the form of a tincture.

Will It Work for You? What the Studies Say:

Chaste tree fruit contains a complex mixture of chemicals, including a volatile oil that accounts for its peppermint-like odor. The herb may positively influence certain menstrual and menopausal disorders by altering the output of female hormones. Women who experience absent menstrual cycles (amenorrhea) or irregular cycles are sometimes found to have elevated levels of prolactin, a peptide hormone produced by the pituitary gland at the base of the brain. Although scientists still do not fully understand the mechanism involved, animal studies indicate that chaste tree berry preparations reduce prolactin levels by acting on the pituitary gland. This in turn allows for the increased luteinizing hormone levels so critical to the normal functioning and length of the second part of the menstrual cycle, the luteal phase.[2] Interestingly, amenorrhea often responds to reductions in prolactin concentrations through the use of other drugs.[3] Chaste tree berry should be used only for these types of problems once the specific cause has been determined, and it should not be taken along with other hormonal therapies.[4]

Much remains to be learned about the impact these hormonal changes have on abnormal or painful menstrual cycles, premenstrual syndrome (PMS), and menopause, but research so far is quite promising. There are reports that chaste tree berry can increase milk production in women who are nursing (when taken over an extended period of time),[5] but more research is needed before it can be recommended. There is also evidence that it can reduce fluid in the knee joints associated with PMS.[6] According to a German study, chaste tree fruit can significantly lessen PMS discomforts. In the study, 90 percent of more than 1,500 women who regularly suffered from PMS reported a complete relief of symptoms after an average of 25.3 days of taking a commercial extract of the plant (Agnolyt).[7] Both the patients and their doctors reported the results. German health authorities endorse the use of chaste tree fruit for a variety of problems caused by corpus luteum insufficiency, including PMS, mastalgia, inadequate milk production in nursing mothers, and menopausal symptoms.[8]

Researchers have also identified antibacterial, anti-inflammatory, and antifungal (against *Candida albicans*, frequently implicated in vaginal yeast infections) properties.[9] The practical use of these properties has not yet been established.

Will It Harm You? What the Studies Say:

No reports of significant adverse reactions have been associated with the use of this herb, although some individuals develop an itchy rash or stomach discomfort.[10] In the PMS study noted above, the most common complaint was gastrointestinal upset.[11] But very few—seven of 1,542—women stopped taking the drug because of unwanted side effects. A team of investigators warned that chaste tree berry should not be used to promote normal ovarian function in women, given the risk of ovarian hyperstimulation syndrome (excessive stimulation of the ovaries). One woman developed this potentially dangerous condition while taking the herb during in-vitro fertilization treatment.[12] Chaste tree berry may interfere with the actions of oral contraceptives, hormone replacement medicines, and other endocrine therapies and should probably not be taken simultaneously with them.

Pregnant women should stay away from the herb, and researchers have yet to examine its safety in children.[13] Individuals taking drugs classified as dopamine-receptor antagonists may want to avoid the drug, given animal-study findings indicating that chaste tree berries may interfere with their metabolism.[14]

GENERAL SOURCES:

American Pharmaceutical Association. *Handbook of Nonprescription Drugs.* 11th ed. Washington, D.C.: American Pharmaceutical Association, 1996.

Balch, J.F., and P.A. Balch. *Prescription for Nutritional Healing: A Practical A to Z Reference to Drug-Free Remedies Using Vitamins, Minerals, Herbs & Food Supplements.* 2nd ed. Garden City Park, NY: Avery Publishing Group, 1997.

Blumenthal, M., J. Gruenwald, T. Hall, and R.S. Rister, eds. *The Complete German Commission E Monographs: Therapeutic Guide to Herbal Medicine.* Boston: Integrative Medicine Communications, 1998.

Lawrence Review of Natural Products. St. Louis: Facts and Comparisons, December 1994.

Leung, A.Y., and S. Foster. *Encyclopedia of Common Natural Ingredients Used in Food, Drugs, and Cosmetics.* 2nd ed. New York: John Wiley & Sons, 1996.

Tierra, M. *The Way of Herbs.* New York: Pocket Books, 1990.

Tyler, V.E. *Herbs of Choice: The Therapeutic Use of Phytomedicinals.* Binghamton, NY: Haworth/Press Pharmaceutical Products Press, 1994.

Weiss, R.F. *Herbal Medicine,* trans. A.R. Meuss, from the 6th German edition. Beaconsfield, England: Beaconsfield Publishers, Ltd., 1988.

TEXT CITATIONS:

1. V.E. Tyler, *Herbs of Choice: The Therapeutic Use of Phytomedicinals* (Binghamton, NY: Haworth Press/Pharmaceutical Products Press, 1994).
2. G. Sluitz et al., *Hormone and Metabolism Research,* 25 (1993): 253. *Lawrence Review of Natural Products* (St. Louis: Facts and Comparisons, December 1994).
3. Tyler, op. cit.
4. C.A. Newall et al., *Herbal Medicines: A Guide for Health-Care Professionals* (London: The Pharmaceutical Press, 1996).
5. R.F. Weiss, *Herbal Medicine,* trans. A.R. Meuss, from the 6th German edition (Beaconsfield, England: Beaconsfield Publishers, Ltd., 1988).
6. *Lawrence Review of Natural Products,* op. cit. D. Propping, *Therapiewoche,* 38 (1988): 2992.
7. A. Milewicz et al., *Arzneimittel-Forschung,* 43 (1993): 752. American Pharmaceutical Association, *Handbook of Nonprescription Drugs,* 11th ed. (Washington, D.C.: American Pharmaceutical Association, 1996).

8. American Pharmaceutical Association, op. cit.
9. A.Y. Leung and S. Foster, *Encyclopedia of Common Natural Ingredients Used in Food, Drugs, and Cosmetics*, 2nd ed. (New York: John Wiley & Sons, 1996).
10. American Pharmaceutical Association, op. cit.
11. D.J. Brown, *Quarterly Review of Natural Medicine*, Summer (1994): 111.
12. D.J. Cahill et al., *Human Reproduction*, 9(8) (1994): 1469–70.
13. *Lawrence Review of Natural Products*, op. cit.
14. M. Blumenthal, J. Gruenwald, T. Hall, and R.S. Rister, eds., *The Complete German Commission E Monographs: Therapeutic Guide to Herbal Medicine* (Boston: Integrative Medicine Communications, 1998).

PRIMARY NAME:
CHICKWEED

SCIENTIFIC NAME:
Stellaria media (L.) Vill. Family:
Caryophyllaceae

COMMON NAMES:
Mouse-ear, satinflower, starweed, starwort, tongue grass, white bird's-eye, winterweed

RATING:
4 = Research indicates that this substance will not fulfill the claims made for it, but that it is also unlikely to cause any harm.

What Is Chickweed?

In North America and many other parts of the world, this common, low-growing annual rates as a pesky wayside weed at best. Primarily its oval leaves and thin stems, and occasionally its star-shaped white flowers, are used medicinally.

What It Is Used For:

Over the centuries, people have enjoyed chickweed as a pot herb for salads and greens. Compresses and other external formulations were smoothed onto rashes, sores, itches, ulcers, abscesses, boils, and other skin irritations. Although less popular, internal formulations were taken to soothe sore throats and other mucous membrane inflammations, encourage weight loss, and to treat fever, bronchial asthma, constipation, lung diseases, and blood disorders. Many outlets today sell chickweed as a source for vitamins and other nutrients. Homeopaths prescribe it in minute doses for psoriasis and rheumatic pains.[1] (See page 2 for a discussion of homeopathy.)

Forms Available Include:

- *For external use:* Compress, extract, cream, oil, poultice, salve, tincture.
- *For internal use:* Capsule, decoction, infusion, tincture.

Dosage Commonly Reported:

Three 389-milligram capsules are taken three times a day.

Will It Work for You? What the Studies Say:

Scientists have identified low levels of vitamin C and other constituents in chickweed, but overall, the herb has not been well studied except in regard to controlling its weedlike growth.[2] None of its ingredients—rutin (a flavonoid glycoside), saponins, steroids, various plant acids—are considered valuable in treating skin rashes or any other ailments, given that they are present in such low concentrations, although the vitamin C may have at one time played a role in preventing and treating scurvy.[3] A German textbook notes a lack of success in treating rheumatic pain with the herb.[4] No human studies of chickweed appear in the medical literature.

Will It Harm You? What the Studies Say:

Animals grazing on chickweed have suffered nitrate poisoning, and sketchy anecdotal reports suggest that paralysis developed in individuals who drank large amounts of chickweed infusions.[5] Given its known ingredients, however, and the fact that many people have used it without incident over the centuries, chickweed appears to be a relatively safe herb to use in moderation.

GENERAL SOURCES:

Lawrence Review of Natural Products. St. Louis: Facts and Comparisons, February 1992.

Leung, A.Y., and S. Foster. *Encyclopedia of Common Natural Ingredients Used in Food, Drugs, and Cosmetics.* 2nd ed. New York: John Wiley & Sons, 1996.

Ody, P. *The Herb Society's Complete Medicinal Herbal.* London: Dorling Kindersley Limited, 1993.

Tierra, M. *The Way of Herbs.* New York: Pocket Books, 1990.

Tyler, V.E. *The Honest Herbal.* Binghamton, NY: Haworth Press/Pharmaceutical Products Press, 1993.

Weiss, R.F. *Herbal Medicine,* trans. A.R. Meuss, from the 6th German edition. Beaconsfield, England: Beaconsfield Publishers, Ltd., 1988.

TEXT CITATIONS:

1. *Lawrence Review of Natural Products* (St. Louis: Facts and Comparisons, February 1992).
2. A.Y. Leung and S. Foster, *Encyclopedia of Common Natural Ingredients Used in Food, Drugs, and Cosmetics,* 2nd ed. (New York: John Wiley & Sons, 1996). *Lawrence Review of Natural Products,* op. cit.
3. V.E. Tyler, *The Honest Herbal* (Binghamton, NY: Haworth Press/Pharmaceutical Products Press, 1993).
4. R.F. Weiss, *Herbal Medicine,* trans. A.R. Meuss, from the 6th German edition (Beaconsfield, England: Beaconsfield Publishers, Ltd., 1988).
5. *Lawrence Review of Natural Products,* op. cit.

PRIMARY NAME:

CHICORY

SCIENTIFIC NAME:

Cichorium intybus L. Family: Asteraceae (Compositae)

COMMON NAMES:

Blue sailor's succory, succory, wild succory

RATING:

3 = Studies on the effectiveness and safety of this substance are conflicting, or there are not enough studies to draw a conclusion. Safety seems to depend on proper use, however; see the "Will It Harm You?" section.

What Is Chicory?

This tall perennial, a member of the daisy family, bears striking blue flowers. Not only are many chicory varieties cultivated, but the plant also grows freely as a weed in many parts of the world, including North America, India, and its native Europe. Chicory was introduced into North America in the late nineteenth century. The dried root and herb are used medicinally.

What It Is Used For:

Chicory root is roasted for use as a caffeine-free coffee substitute or additive. Many people enjoy its rich and mellow taste. The leaves are eaten raw, blanched, or boiled depending on their maturity. Some people eat the boiled root as well. In European, American, and other folk medicine cultures, chicory has a reputation as a digestive aid, bile stimulant (choleretic), appetite booster, mild laxative, diuretic ("water pill"), liver and heart remedy, cancer treatment, and mildly sedating tonic. A poultice made of bruised leaves is applied to skin inflammations and swellings. Homeopaths recommend minute doses for a variety of conditions. (See page 2 for a discussion of homeopathy.)

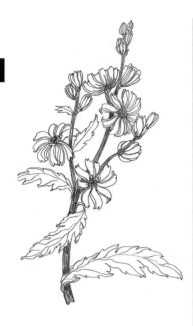

Chicory
Cichorium intybus

Forms Available Include:

Fresh plant, infusion, poultice, root (roasted).

Dosage Commonly Reported:

The bruised leaves are applied as a poultice. The roasted root is substituted for coffee beans.

Will It Work for You? What the Studies Say:

German health authorities approve of chicory root and herb preparations to soothe stomach upset and increase the appetite.[1] Their decision appears to have been based on the mild bile stimulation produced by bitter-tasting compounds such as lactucin and lactucopicrin in the plant, which are also believed to stimulate gastric juices, as well as the presence of pentosans and a white starchy substance called inulin. No studies to confirm these actions in humans can be found in the medical literature, however.

Chicory's renown as a sedative has little scientific support, although adding the caffeine-free substance to coffee will obviously reduce the relative amount of caffeine in the beverage. In one study, coffee and chicory mixtures on average contained 3.18 milligrams per fluid ounce of caffeine, compared with 12.61 in the same amount of pure instant coffee, and about 8 in a Ceylon tea blend steeped for one minute.[2] The contention that chicory will actually calm you or counter "coffee nerves," however, appears to be based largely on small-animal studies done in 1940, which require confirmatory updating and human testing.[3] The distinctive aroma and taste that chicory contributes are due to its contained inulin (up to nearly 60 percent in cultivated plants), a polysaccharide that exudes a coffeelike aroma upon roasting. Chicory is an industrial source of the sweetener fructose and a sugar-enhancer called maltol.

In 1973, Egyptian researchers exploring the traditional use of chicory for heart irregularities discovered a digitalis-like principle in the dried and roasted roots that markedly slowed the rate and amplitude of the heartbeat in toad hearts in a laboratory dish.[4] Though this is intriguing, much more research is needed to determine the potential for chicory extracts to benefit disorders such as tachycardia (fast heartbeat) and arrhythmias (irregular heartbeats).[5]

Investigators have uncovered a number of other interesting properties in chicory that may one day prove useful, although they all require more research. For example, studies of alcoholic extracts indicate that the herb has anti-inflammatory properties in rats,[6] but whether this means that chicory will reduce swelling or inflammation when placed on human skin, a popular folk practice, is far from clear. The implications of a test-tube study suggesting that the plant has strong to moderate antimutagenic properties and may therefore help inhibit the formation of potentially cancer-causing cells are likewise hard to determine,[7] as are indications of liver-protective principles in the plant.[8]

Will It Harm You? What the Studies Say:

Chicory has been consumed by millions of people over the years without any reports of serious harm, although rare allergic reactions have occurred from both handling and ingesting the plant. Avoid chicory if you are allergic to it or any other member of the daisy family. German health authorities warn that anyone with gallstones should consult a doctor before using chicory preparations, given its possible bile-stimulating properties.[9]

GENERAL SOURCES:

Blumenthal, M., J. Gruenwald, T. Hall, and R.S. Rister, eds. *The Complete German Commission E Monographs: Therapeutic Guide to Herbal Medicine.* Boston: Integrative Medicine Communications, 1998.

Foster, S., and J.A. Duke. *The Peterson Field Guide Series: A Field Guide to Medicinal Plants. Eastern and Central North America.* Boston: Houghton Mifflin Company, 1990.

Lawrence Review of Natural Products. St. Louis: Facts and Comparisons, March 1996.

Leung, A.Y., and S. Foster. *Encyclopedia of Common Natural Ingredients Used in Food, Drugs, and Cosmetics.* 2nd ed. New York: John Wiley & Sons, 1996.

Stary, F. *The Natural Guide to Medicinal Herbs and Plants.* Prague: Barnes & Noble, Inc., in arrangement with Aventinum Publishers, 1996.

Tyler, V.E. *The Honest Herbal.* Binghamton, NY: Haworth Press/Pharmaceutical Products Press, 1993.

Weiss, R.F. *Herbal Medicine,* trans. A.R. Meuss, from the 6th German edition. Beaconsfield, England: Beaconsfield Publishers, Ltd., 1988.

TEXT CITATIONS:

1. M. Blumenthal, J. Gruenwald, T. Hall, and R.S. Rister, eds., *The Complete German Commission E Monographs: Therapeutic Guide to Herbal Medicine* (Boston: Integrative Medicine Communications, 1998).
2. G.T. Galasko et al., *Food & Chemical Toxicology,* 27(1) (1989): 49–51.
3. V.E. Tyler, *The Honest Herbal* (Binghamton, NY: Haworth Press/Pharmaceutical Products Press, 1993).
4. S.I. Balboa et al., *Planta Medica,* 24 (1973): 133–44.
5. Tyler, op. cit.
6. P.S. Benoit et al., *Lloydia,* 39 (1976): 160.
7. R. Edenharder et al., *Food & Chemical Toxicology,* 32(5) (1994): 443–59.
8. S. Sultana et al., *Journal of Ethnopharmacology,* 45(3) (1995): 189–92.
9. Blumenthal et al., op. cit.

PRIMARY NAME:
CHIVE

SCIENTIFIC NAME:
Allium schoenoprasum L.
Family: Liliaceae

COMMON NAME:
N/A

RATING:
4 = Research indicates that this herb will not fulfill the claims made for it, but that it is also unlikely to cause any harm.

What Is Chive?

The tender, hollow green spear grows in bunches from white bulbous roots. It's a perennial and belongs to the lily family, which also includes leeks, garlic, onion, and shallots. Chives are native to Asia and enjoy popularity as a winter kitchen herb.

What It Is Used For:

In addition to the mild but distinctively oniony flavor they lend foods, chives have developed a lesser reputation for stimulating the appetite and encouraging smooth digestion, particularly of fatty foods. Some sources suggest including plentiful amounts of chives in the diet to ward off iron-deficiency anemia.

Forms Available Include:

Fresh spears.

Dosage Commonly Reported:

The fresh, chopped herb is commonly used in cooking.

Will It Work for You? What the Studies Say:

Chives have an aroma and taste that piques the appetite for many, but evidence for any direct appetite-stimulating properties cannot be found. Chives have always been considered a weaker sibling in the stellar lily family, unable to compete with the flavor or medicinal might of members such as garlic and onion. **Garlic** in particular has been shown to help improve digestion, and may well prove more effective for this purpose.

Though chives contain iron, it would pose a challenge to consume enough of them to reverse a case of iron-deficiency anemia. Such a deficiency should be treated more vigorously in any case, with chives being one of many foods or supplements to boost iron intake.

Will It Harm You? What the Studies Say:

No reports of significant adverse reactions have been associated with the use of chives. Their mild onion odor does not seem to linger on the breath for very long.

GENERAL SOURCES:

Hylton, W.H., ed. *The Rodale Herb Book: How to Use, Grow, and Buy Nature's Miracle Plants.* Emmaus, PA: Rodale Press, Inc., 1974.

Mindell, E. *Earl Mindell's Herb Bible.* New York: Simon & Schuster/Fireside, 1992.

Weiss, R.F. *Herbal Medicine,* trans. A.R. Meuss, from the 6th German edition. Beaconsfield, England: Beaconsfield Publishers, Ltd., 1988.

PRIMARY NAME:
CHLORELLA

SCIENTIFIC NAME:
Chlorella vulgaris, Chlorella pyrenoidosa, and other *Chlorella* species

COMMON NAME:
N/A

RATING:
4 = Research indicates that this substance will not fulfill the claims made for it, but that it is also unlikely to cause any harm.

What Is Chlorella?

Chlorella is a seaweed—a type of algae that grows in water. It is tiny, consisting of single-celled algae. Various species of chlorella are used to make dietary supplements. The substance is valued as a rich source of chlorophyll, the pigment responsible for collecting energy from sunlight and turning plants green. The whole plant is used medicinally. It must be specially processed for medical use; do not try to collect it on your own. Most chlorella sold in the United States is imported from Japan or Taiwan, where it is cultivated in tanks.

What It Is Used For:

Numerous sources have touted chlorella as a nutritious source of chlorophyll, and as such it is promoted as an effective treatment for various diseases, fighting bacteria and other infectious organisms, reducing odors, and accelerating "cleansing of the bloodstream," among other things. Many hail chlorella as a "green food supplement" worth taking for its nutritional value. It is also billed as a protective agent against the effects of ultraviolet radiation and as a valuable source of vitamin B. In some regions of the world, such as southern Formosa, people use it to treat skin cancer of the foot.[1]

Forms Available Include:

Capsule, extracts, juice, liquid concentrate, powder. Chlorella may also be found in "nutrient" blends and "whole-food" concentrates.

Dosage Commonly Reported:

Two to three 414-milligram capsules are taken three times a day. Commercial preparations, including extracts, juice, liquid concentrate, and powder, are labeled with dosage instructions.

Will It Work for You? What the Studies Say:

Chlorella is indeed nutritious, containing significant amounts of protein, lipid, carotenoids, minerals, vitamins, and unique pigments.[2] According to various studies, including one in which the nutritional efficacy of long-term uncooked vegan diets was examined, chlorella qualifies as one of the seaweeds that supply adequate amounts of vitamin B when consumed in sufficient amounts.[3] But whether this qualifies chlorella as a superior (and cost-effective) source for these substances is questionable.

Scientists have isolated substances in chlorella that show antitumor properties in test-tube experiments,[4] immune-system-enhancing actions in tumor-bearing mice,[5] and virus-fighting activity. However, the practical value of these properties in treating disease has apparently never been shown in well-designed human trials.

Chlorella also contains notable amounts of **Chlorophyll**, a substance which, despite considerable hype, has never been shown to help fight any type of disease. Apparently no study has been done to soundly demonstrate or refute an anticancer or immune-system effect. Although antibiotic properties have been shown in test-tube studies, no evidence can be found to support the theory that chlorella is a practical agent for fighting infection in humans.

Other than a few specialized situations, no evidence can be found to support the theory that chlorophyll taken orally can reduce normal body or urinary odors.[6] The exceptions may include unpleasant colostomy- and ileostomy-related fecal odors when a particular chlorophyll component (chlorophyllin) and bismuth sugallate are taken in combination. A 1989 double-blind, crossover trial reported that the fecal odor in colostomy patients did not differ when they were given a chlorophyll tablet and when they took a placebo, at least according to the subjects themselves.[7]

Will It Harm You? What the Studies Say:

The major risk associated with the use of chlorella is an allergic reaction. Some reactions are severe and even involve anaphylaxis.[8] Allergic reactions have been reported in people working with the substance, such as pharmacists,[9] as well as in children.[10] One report describes sun sensitivity in the sun-exposed areas of five individuals who had taken chlorella; analysis identified pheophorbide-a (and its ester) as the photosensitizing component.[11] Laboratory research bears out chlorella's potential as an allergic substance, as it contains components that specifically bind to IgE antibodies in the human body.[12]

As a substance high in vitamin K, chlorella may inhibit the coagulation activity of anticlotting medicines such as warfarin, according to a case in which a seventy-five-year-old man on warfarin experienced a disturbance in his clotting mechanisms after taking chlorella.[13]

GENERAL SOURCES:

American Pharmaceutical Association. *Handbook of Nonprescription Drugs.* 11th ed. Washington, D.C.: American Pharmaceutical Association, 1996.

Balch, J.F., and P.A. Balch. *Prescription for Nutritional Healing: A Practical A to Z Reference to Drug-Free Remedies Using Vitamins, Minerals, Herbs & Food Supplements.* 2nd ed. Garden City Park, NY: Avery Publishing Group, 1997.

Barrett, S., and V. Herbert. *The Vitamin Pushers: How the Health Food Industry Is Selling America a Bill of Goods.* Amherst, NY: Prometheus Books, 1994.

Mayell, M. *Off-the-Shelf Natural Health: How to Use Herbs and Nutrients to Stay Well.* New York: Bantam Books, 1995.

Weiner, M.A., and J.A. Weiner. *Herbs That Heal: Prescription for Herbal Healing.* Mill Valley, CA: Quantum Books, 1994.

TEXT CITATIONS:

1. S. Ichimura, *Nippon Eiseigaku Zasshi—Japanese Journal of Hygiene,* 30(1) (1975): 66.
2. R.A. Kay, *Critical Reviews in Food Science & Nutrition,* 30(6) (1991): 555–73.
3. A.L. Rauma et al., *Journal of Nutrition,* 125(10) (1995): 2511–15.
4. T. Morimoto et al., *Phytochemistry,* 40(5) (1995): 1433–37.
5. Y. Miyazawa et al., *Journal of Ethnopharmacology,* 24(2–3) (1988): 135–46.
6. American Pharmaceutical Association, *Handbook of Nonprescription Drugs,* 11th ed. (Washington, D.C.: American Pharmaceutical Association, 1996).
7. S.B. Christiansen et al., *Ugeskrift for Laeger,* 151(27) (1989): 753–54.
8. I. Pukhova et al., *Kosmicheskaia Biologiia I Meditsina,* 6(1) (1972): 23–28.
9. T.P. Ng et al., *Respiratory Medicine,* 88(7) (1994): 555–57.
10. E. Tiberg et al., *Journal of Allergy & Clinical Immunology,* 96(2) (1995): 257–59.
11. K. Jitsukawa et al., *International Journal of Dermatology,* 23(4) (1984): 263–68.
12. E. Tiberg and R. Einarsson, *International Archives of Allergy & Applied Immunology,* 90(3) (1989): 301–6.
13. S. Ohkawa et al., *Rinsho Shinkeigaku—Clinical Neurology,* 35(7) (1995): 806–7.

PRIMARY NAME:
CHLOROPHYLL

SCIENTIFIC NAME:
N/A

COMMON NAME:
Green food

RATING:
4 = Research indicates that this substance will not fulfill the claims made for it, but that it is also unlikely to cause any harm.

What Is Chlorophyll?

This naturally occurring pigment is found in the chloroplasts (parts of the cell structure) of all green plants. It is responsible for collecting energy from sunlight and turning plants green. Chlorophyll appears in other organisms that perform photosynthesis as well, and in certain bacteria.

What It Is Used For:

Numerous sources have attributed medicinal properties to chlorophyll, from an ability to fight cancer to boosting immune system function and scavenging the bloodstream for potentially cell-damaging substances called free radicals. Others have claimed that it has deodorant properties.

Forms Available Include:

In "green-food concentrates" such as **Chlorella** and **Spirulina**, or in young cereal plant grasses such as **Alfalfa** and **Barley Grass**. These substances are typically available in extract, liquid concentrate, powder, and tablet forms.

Dosage Commonly Reported:

Chlorophyll is found in "green-food" concentrates; follow the package instructions.

Will It Work for You? What the Studies Say:

Despite considerable publicity, chlorophyll has never been shown to help fight any type of disease. No study has been done to demonstrate an anticancer or immune-system effect, and no evidence indicates that it reduces normal human body or urinary odors. See **Chlorella** for more information.

Will It Harm You? What the Studies Say:

The recent medical literature contains no reports of serious harm resulting from the use of chlorophyll directly. See the label on the "green food" you decide to take for information on the associated risks, however.

GENERAL SOURCES:

American Pharmaceutical Association. *Handbook of Nonprescription Drugs.* 11th ed. Washington, D.C.: American Pharmaceutical Association, 1996.

Barrett, S., and V. Herbert. *The Vitamin Pushers: How the "Health Food" Industry Is Selling America a Bill of Goods.* Amherst, NY: Prometheus Books, 1994.

Leber, M.R., et al. *Handbook of Over-the-Counter Drugs and Pharmacy Products.* Berkeley: Celestial Arts Publishing, 1994.

Mayell, M. *Off-the-Shelf Natural Health: How to Use Herbs and Nutrients to Stay Well.* New York: Bantam Books, 1995.

Weiner, M.A., and J.A. Weiner. *Herbs That Heal: Prescription for Herbal Healing.* Mill Valley, CA: Quantum Books, 1994.

CHROMIUM PICOLINATE

SCIENTIFIC NAME:
N/A

COMMON NAME:
N/A

RATING:
4 = Research indicates that this substance will not fulfill the claims made for it. Its safety, even in recommended amounts, remains unclear. See the "Will It Harm You?" section.

What Is Chromium Picolinate?

Chromium is an essential trace mineral. Chromium picolinate is a patented, synthetic form of chromium.

What It Is Used For:

Chromium helps the body maintain normal metabolic function. It is a critical component of "glucose tolerance factor," which is believed to encourage insulin to bind to insulin receptors. Insulin plays a key role in regulating the body's metabolism of carbohydrates, proteins, and fats. Small amounts of chromium are normally present in the healthy adult and are ingested through certain foods. As an industrial metal, chromium is a key additive in the manufacture of steel alloys.

Chromium picolinate is a new, patented form of chromium that some sources suggest represents the best way to get chromium into your system.[1] Promoters recommend taking it as a dietary supplement to help shed body fat, promote weight loss, increase muscle mass, speed up metabolism, help control blood-glucose levels and prevent diabetes, enhance normal insulin function, reduce food cravings, enhance the senses, reduce cholesterol, and improve strength and endurance, among other things. Some have suggested taking it as an "insurance-level" multivitamin and multimineral supplement.[2] Body builders and dieters take it to burn fat.

Forms Available Include:

Capsule, liquid, tablet. Chromium appears in many multivitamin and multimineral supplements.

Dosage Commonly Reported:

A typical dosage of chromium picolinate is up to 300 micrograms a day.

Will It Work for You? What the Studies Say:

Humans require chromium, and a deficiency may contribute to atherosclerosis and adult-onset diabetes mellitus.[3] In reality, however, few Americans suffer from a deficiency. People who do run a risk for this include those who eat primarily processed (or highly refined) foods and those being fed through an intravenous line.[4] A balanced diet that includes such chromium-rich foods as whole-grain products, potatoes (with skin), fish, beef, milk, fresh fruit, eggs, organ meats, whole grains, and brewer's yeast is likely to provide adequate amounts of this element.

Chromium picolinate is a different subject, however. So many "deceptive" and "unsubstantiated" claims were being made for this hot-selling dietary supplement, according to the Federal Trade Commission (FTC), that the agency decided to take action. In 1997 the company with exclusive rights to market chromium picolinate in the United States—Nutrition 21 in San Diego—and two of the many companies that sell it signed a "consent agreement" with the FTC to make no more unsubstantiated claims for their products.[5] Nutrition 21 will probably make only one claim from now on, pending the collection of more substantiating data: that chromium picolinate may help moderately obese individuals improve body composition, though not necessarily lose weight.[6] In other words, the companies concede there is no scientific evidence to substantiate claims that chromium picolinate will lead to weight loss, for example (remember that fat loss is different from weight loss), or that supplements will lower blood-sugar levels in individuals who do not suffer from blood-sugar-regulating problems.[7]

Numerous independent placebo-controlled, double-blind studies have found supplemental chromium picolinate no more effective than a placebo in reducing body weight or body fat, boosting lean body mass, or increasing strength in normal adults. This conclusion was reached after analyzing data from a 1995 sixteen-week study at the Naval Health Research Center involving seventy-six men and sixteen women, half of whom took 400 milligrams of chromium picolinate a day.[8] In another study, football players who took 200 milligrams of chromium picolinate daily for nine weeks experienced no more notable changes in body composition or strength during their intensive weight-lifting training than those taking a placebo.[9]

Will It Harm You? What the Studies Say:

Dietary supplementation with chromium has generally not been linked to serious adverse reactions, although a case of chronic kidney failure has been reported in a forty-nine-year-old woman who took three times the recommended dose for dietary supplementation of chromium picolinate, the equivalent of twelve to forty-five times the usual intake of dietary chromium.[10] The safe dose for chromium in healthy adults is 50 to 200 milligrams a day.[11]

Relatively little is known about the effects of long-term or high-dosage use of chromium in any form. The FDA says that it has "safety concerns" and that reports of adverse reactions such as irregular heartbeats have been noted. Recently published research also raises some concerns. Common wisdom held that excess chromium was simply flushed out of the body in urine, but authors of a 1995 investigation warn that chromium is likely to accumulate in human tissue with long-term use or large doses, posing the risk of chromosome (DNA) damage similar to that seen in laboratory animals and test-tube studies.[12] They based this conclusion on pharmacokinetic models used to test how a drug is taken up, metabolized, and excreted. Chromosome damage raises the risk for cancer development.

In a 1996 review, an investigator warns that individuals prone to behavioral disorders should be particularly cautious about using chromium picolinate supplements, given data indicating that analogues of picolinic acids cause notable changes in certain brain chemicals (serotonin, dopamine, norepinephrine).[13] If you suffer from any type of behavioral disorder, or if you have diabetes or take insulin, talk to a doctor before using chromium picolinate supplements.

The types of chromium that people are sometimes exposed to in the workplace (hexavalent forms of chromium; this does not include chromium picolinate) can be toxic and carcinogenic; skin reactions such as ulceration and severe eczematous dermatitis have been reported following exposure to chromium and chromate salts.[14]

GENERAL SOURCES:

American Pharmaceutical Association. *Handbook of Nonprescription Drugs*. 11th ed. Washington, D.C.: American Pharmaceutical Association, 1996.

Balch, J.F., and P.A. Balch. *Prescription for Nutritional Healing: A Practical A to Z Reference to Drug-Free Remedies Using Vitamins, Minerals, Herbs & Food Supplements*. 2nd ed. Garden City Park, NY: Avery Publishing Group, 1997.

Barrett, S., and V. Herbert. *The Vitamin Pushers: How the "Health Food" Industry Is Selling America a Bill of Goods*. Amherst, NY: Prometheus Books, 1994.

Lawrence Review of Natural Products. St. Louis: Facts and Comparisons, June 1992.

Leber, M.R., et al. *Handbook of Over-the-Counter Drugs and Pharmacy Products*. Berkeley: Celestial Arts Publishing, 1994.

Mayell, M. *Off-the-Shelf Natural Health: How to Use Herbs and Nutrients to Stay Well*. New York: Bantam Books, 1995.

TEXT CITATIONS:

1. J.F. Balch and P.A. Balch, *Prescription for Nutritional Healing: A Practical A to Z Reference to Drug-Free Remedies Using Vitamins, Minerals, Herbs & Food Supplements*, 2nd ed. (Garden City Park, NY: Avery Publishing Group, 1997).

2. M. Mayell, *Off-the-Shelf Natural Health: How to Use Herbs and Nutrients to Stay Well* (New York: Bantam Books, 1995).

3. F. Dubois and F. Belleville, *Pathologie et Biologie*, 39(8) (1991): 801.

4. *Lawrence Review of Natural Products* (St. Louis: Facts and Comparisons), June 1992.

5. M. Burros, *The New York Times*, January 29 (1997): C3.

6. Ibid.

7. *AMA Drug Evaluations Annual 1991*, American Medical Association, 1990.

8. L.K. Trent, *Journal of Sports Medicine & Physical Fitness*, 35(4) (1995): 273–80.

9. S.P. Clancy et al., *International Journal of Sport Nutrition*, 4(2) (1994): 142–53.

10. W.G. Wasser and N.S. Feldman, *Annals of Internal Medicine*, 126(5) (1997): 410.

11. American Pharmaceutical Association, *Handbook of Nonprescription Drugs*, 11th ed. (Washington, D.C.: American Pharmaceutical Association, 1996).

12. D.M. Stearns et al., *FASEB Journal*, 9(15) (1995): 1650–57.

13. S.A. Reading, *Journal of the Florida Medical Association*, 83(1) (1996): 29–31.

14. *Lawrence Review of Natural Products*, op. cit.

PRIMARY NAME:

CINNAMON (and CASSIA)

SCIENTIFIC NAME:

Multiple *Cinnamomum* species including *Cinnamomum zeylanicum* Blume and *Cinnamomum cassia*. Family: Lauraceae

What Is Cinnamon?

There are many species of cinnamon. Most North Americans are familiar with the type derived from the dried bark of exotic evergreen *Cinnamomum* trees found in the West Indies and Asia primarily. This is the same source for the distinctive spice found domestically on most kitchen shelves around the world. Sometimes pharmaceutical manufacturers use the similar-tasting *Cinnamomum cassia*, known as Chinese cinnamon or simply cassia, interchangeably. Overall, however, *Cinnamomum zeylanicum* and its oils are considered superior in flavor. Essential oils from the leaves, bark, stems, and roots of all of these species are extracted through steam distillation and used in many ways, including medicinally.

CINNAMON (and CASSIA)
(Continued)

COMMON NAMES:

Ceylon, cinnamomon, Saigon cinnamon

RATING:

1 = Years of use and extensive, high-quality studies indicate that this substance is very effective and safe when used in recommended amounts for the indication(s) noted in the "Will It Work for You?" section. However, see the warnings in the "Will It Harm You?" section.

What It Is Used For:

From the ancient Egyptians and Chinese healers down through the centuries, traditional healers around the world have revered cinnamon as a spice, taste enhancer, and incense. They have also coveted it as a healing aid for stomach upset and gas, chronic diarrhea, rheumatism, kidney ailments, and abdominal pain, among other ills. Cinnamon "drops" consisting of the essential oil of cinnamon and cassia are similarly famous for treating stomach upset, gas, painful menstruation, and bleeding.

Contemporary herbalists continue to recommend cinnamon enthusiastically for many of these same ailments, from enhancing digestion to relieving nausea, diarrhea, appetite loss, bloating, and colicky indigestion. Some contend that cinnamon calms the uterus (interestingly, others claim the opposite) and boosts peripheral blood circulation. A number of herbal healing preparations contain cinnamon to spice up their flavor and enhance their aroma.

Forms Available Include:

Capsule, infusion, essential oil ("drops"), powder, tea bags, tincture. Extracts appear in various Chinese herbal blends.

Dosage Commonly Reported:

An infusion is made using 1 scant teaspoon of cinnamon per cup of water and is drunk two or three times per day during meals. Capsules of the dried herbs are taken in 2-gram doses one or two times a day with food or beverage. Take other commercial preparations according to package directions.

Will It Work for You? What the Studies Say:

Cinnamon not only titillates the palate; its volatile oil (4 percent in cinnamon bark and 1 to 2 percent in cassia oil) may actually help you digest food by breaking down fats in the digestive tract.[1] The essential oil has been found to stimulate movement in the gastrointestinal tract.[2] Test-tube and in some cases animal studies show that cinnamon's essential oil also has carminative (gas-relieving) powers. The bark of both cinnamon and cassia boasts carminative and astringent properties. Aromatherapists contend that cinnamon's enticing aroma stimulates salivation and in this way encourages good digestion.

Cassia may aid digestion in other ways as well. Research in laboratory rats has shown that it may stimulate bile production and help reduce pain.[3] Its essential oil demonstrates antidiarrheal properties in the test tube,[4] and water and ether extracts show antidiarrheic actions in laboratory mice.[5] In one study, cassia tea helped protect against ulcers in rats and mice.[6] Whether any of these activities occur in humans remains to be properly examined. German health authorities approve of cassia and cinnamon bark for treating dyspeptic discomfort such as mild gastrointestinal spasms.[7] They have also been approved for appetite loss.

The essential oil in cinnamon contains a substance that fights and in some cases kills disease-causing microbes and fungi,[8] possibly explaining the logic behind its use in mouthwashes and toothpastes. Test-tube studies show that cinnamon oil, probably from the bark, fights fungi, viruses, bacteria, and larvae.[9] A liquid extract of the bark suppressed the growth of common infection-causing organisms such as *Candida albicans* (a fungus responsible for yeast infections), *Escherichia coli*, and *Staphylococcus aureus*.[10] In one study, three of five HIV-infected individuals experienced an improvement in their oral candidiasis (a fungal infection) after taking a commercial cinnamon preparation for one week.[11]

A chemical called eugenol, which appears in other oils such as clove and allspice and can be found in various types of cinnamon bark extracts and oils, as well as the leaves of *Cinnamomum zeylanicum*, has proven local anesthetic (numbing) properties. It is not found in cassia bark, however.[12] Studies show that eugenol also has antiseptic and irritant actions.[13] These properties help explain the herb's traditional use for painful minor cuts and abrasions.

According to German health authorities, evidence that cinnamon-flower (*Cinnamomum aromaticum* or *Cinnamomum cassia*) preparations work as a "blood purifier" is weak or nonexistent and indicates that such preparations should not be used for this purpose.[14]

Cassia lowers blood pressure and has sedative effects in laboratory animals, according to Chinese and Japanese studies.[15] The implications of this for humans remain to be explored.

Will It Harm You? What the Studies Say:

Cinnamon is generally safe to use in medicinal concentrations, although allergic skin and mucous membrane reactions are always a possibility and a particularly high risk with cinnamon-flower preparations.[16] There are reports of people experiencing allergic reactions to cinnamon in chewing gums,[17] and of asthma and dermatitis symptoms such as skin itching and irritation developing in spice factory workers and others who have frequent and heavy contact with cinnamon powder.[18]

If you take very large doses of cinnamon bark, you risk developing unpleasant symptoms such as a fast heartbeat and increased breathing, sweating, and intestinal function, ultimately followed by sedation and other signs of central nervous system slowdown.[19] Moderate amounts of cinnamon oil may cause the same reaction. German health authorities warn that pregnant women and people with stomach or intestinal ulcers should avoid medicinal concentrations of cinnamon.[20] People who are allergic to cinnamon or even balsam of Peru should probably avoid it altogether.

Avoid ingesting cinnamon oil, which is highly concentrated; it can cause nausea, vomiting, and even kidney damage in certain cases.[21] Sometimes applying it to the skin causes redness and burning sensations.

GENERAL SOURCES:

Balch, J.F., and P.A. Balch. *Prescription for Nutritional Healing: A Practical A to Z Reference to Drug-Free Remedies Using Vitamins, Minerals, Herbs & Food Supplements.* 2nd ed. Garden City Park, NY: Avery Publishing Group, 1997.

Bensky, D., and A. Gamble, eds. *Chinese Herbal Medicine: Materia Medica.* Seattle: Eastland Press, Inc., 1986.

Bisset, N.G., ed. *Herbal Drugs and Phytopharmaceuticals.* Stuttgart: medpharm GmbH Scientific Publishers, 1994.

Blumenthal, M., J. Gruenwald, T. Hall, and R.S. Rister, eds. *The Complete German Commission E Monographs: Therapeutic Guide to Herbal Medicine.* Boston: Integrative Medicine Communications, 1998.

Castleman, M. *The Healing Herbs: The Ultimate Guide to the Curative Power of Nature's Medicines.* New York: Bantam Books, 1995.

Duke, J.A. *CRC Handbook of Medicinal Herbs.* Boca Raton, FL: CRC Press, 1985.

Lawrence Review of Natural Products. St. Louis: Facts and Comparisons, December 1995.

Leung, A.Y. *Chinese Healing Foods and Herbs.* Glen Rock, NJ: AYSL Corp, 1984.

Leung, A.Y., and S. Foster, *Encyclopedia of Common Natural Ingredients Used in Food, Drugs, and Cosmetics.* 2nd ed. New York: John Wiley & Sons, 1996.

Mayell, M. *Off-the-Shelf Natural Health: How to Use Herbs and Nutrients to Stay Well.* New York: Bantam Books, 1995.

Weiner, M.A., and J.A. Weiner. *Herbs That Heal: Prescription for Herbal Healing.* Mill Valley, CA: Quantum Books, 1994.

TEXT CITATIONS:

1. G. Paulet et al., *Revue Française des Corps Gras,* 21 (1974): 415. E. Halbert and D.G. Weeden, *Nature* (London), 212 (1966): 1603.

2. M. Blumenthal, J. Gruenwald, T. Hall, and R.S. Rister, eds., *The Complete German Commission E Monographs: Therapeutic Guide to Herbal Medicine* (Boston: Integrative Medicine Communications, 1998).

3. *Lawrence Review of Natural Products* (St. Louis: Facts and Comparisons, December 1995).

4. A.Y. Leung and S. Foster, *Encyclopedia of Common Natural Ingredients Used in Food, Drugs, and Cosmetics.* 2nd ed. (New York: John Wiley & Sons, 1996).

5. *Lawrence Review of Natural Products,* op. cit.

6. T. Akira et al., *Planta Medica,* 52 (1986): 440. Z.P. Zhu et al., *Chung-Kuo Chung Yao Tsa Chih—China Journal of Chinese Materia Medica,* 18(9) (1993): 553–57, 514–15.

7. Blumenthal et al., op. cit.

8. S. Morozumi, *Applied and Environmental Microbiology,* 4 (1973): 54.

9. Leung and Foster, op. cit.

10. J.A. Duke, *CRC Handbook of Medicinal Herbs* (Boca Raton, FL: CRC Press, 1985).

11. J.M. Quale et al., *American Journal of Chinese Medicine,* 24(2) (1996): 103–9.

12. Leung and Foster, op. cit.

13. Ibid.

14. Blumenthal et al., op. cit.

15. A.Y. Leung, *Chinese Healing Foods and Herbs* (Glen Rock, NJ: AYSL Corp, 1984).

16. Blumenthal et al., op. cit.

17. R.C. Mihail, *Journal of Otolaryngology,* 21(5) (1992): 366.

18. B. Meding, *Contact Dermatitis,* 29(4) (1993): 202. C.G. Uragoda, *British Journal of Industrial Medicine,* 41(2) (1984): 224–27.

19. N.G. Bisset, ed., *Herbal Drugs and Phytopharmaceuticals* (Stuttgart: medpharm GmbH Scientific Publishers, 1994).

20. Ibid.

21. *Lawrence Review of Natural Products,* op. cit.

PRIMARY NAME:

CLEAVERS

SCIENTIFIC NAME:
Galium aparine L. Family:
Rubiaceae

COMMON NAMES:
Bedstraw, catchweed, cleavers
herb, clivers herb, goosegrass

RATING:
3 = Studies on the effectiveness
and safety of this substance are
conflicting, or there are not
enough studies to draw a
conclusion.

What Is Cleavers?

This persistent weed can be found in rich, moist soils throughout North America. Small whitish flowers appear in spring. Its raspy, sticky stems and bristly mature fruit have earned it the names cleavers or catchweed herb. Whorls of lance-shaped leaves and often other aboveground parts are dried and used medicinally.

What It Is Used For:

The most prominent use for this herb through the centuries has been as a diuretic ("water pill"). As such it has been hailed as a treatment for cystitis, venereal disease, kidney stones, and other bladder, kidney, and reproductive tract inflammation. Shoots were prepared in teas as "cleansing" spring tonics for the blood and entire body. Other internal uses have included the treatment of swollen or enlarged lymph glands, fever, psoriasis, vitamin C deficiency (and scurvy), and jaundice. Powders and compresses have been applied to bleeding wounds and used to encourage healing in scalds, burns, ulcers, psoriasis, and skin inflammations. Various cancers have been treated with the herb. The cooked plant can be eaten like a vegetable and the seeds roasted to make a coffee substitute.

Forms Available Include:

- *For internal use:* Infusion, juice, tincture.
- *For external use:* Compress, cream, hair rinse (infusion), powder.

Dosage Commonly Reported:

A tincture is taken in 5- to 10-milliliter doses three times a day. The infusion is made with one ounce of leaves and a pint of water and is taken three times a day.

Will It Work for You? What the Studies Say:

What minimal data are available indicate that this herb increases urine output, albeit mildly, probably by acting directly on the kidneys. According to animal studies, substances called iridoid glycosides are probably responsible for this property as well as for exerting a mild laxative action.[1] The presence of astringent substances called tannins (2.5 to 4 percent) may help explain why folk healers have recommended it for skin inflammations, burns, and abrasions, although no great effect would be expected considering the relatively low concentration of these tannins. (Astringents help skin heal by drawing together and protecting tissue.) The herb fails to fight most bacteria, according to a 1985 report, except possibly *Staphylococcus aureus*, a common culprit in skin infections.[2] Cleavers also demonstrates strong larvacidal properties and fights certain yeasts.

The herb has a folk reputation for treating cancers, but recent studies in mice indicated that it has no notable tumor-fighting actions.[3]

Researchers have identified blood-pressure-lowering substances in a related species,[4] *Galium triflorum*, but more research is needed to determine the implications for hypertension in humans.

Will It Harm You? What the Studies Say:

No reports of significant adverse reactions associated with cleavers appear in the medical literature, and it is probably safe for most people to use. Common sense dictates that anyone with kidney problems avoid ingesting the herb, however, given that it may increase urination by irritating the kidneys.

GENERAL SOURCES:

Bradley, P.C. ed. *British Herbal Compendium: A Handbook of Scientific Information on Widely Used Plant Drugs*, vol. 1. Bournemouth (Dorset), England: British Herbal Medicine Association, 1992.

Dobelis, I.N., ed. *The Magic and Medicine of Plants: A Practical Guide to the Science, History, Folklore, and Everyday Uses of Medicinal Plants.* Pleasantville, NY: Reader's Digest Association, 1986.

Foster, S., and J.A. Duke. *The Peterson Field Guide Series: A Field Guide to Medicinal Plants. Eastern and Central North America.* Boston: Houghton Mifflin Company, 1990.

Mowrey, D.B. *Proven Herbal Blends: A Rational Approach to Prevention and Remedy.* (Condensed from *The Scientific Validation of Herbal Medicine.*) New Canaan, CT: Keats Publishing, Inc., 1986.

Ody, P. *The Herb Society's Complete Medicinal Herbal.* London: Dorling Kindersley Limited, 1993.

Tierra, M. *The Way of Herbs.* New York: Pocket Books, 1990.

TEXT CITATIONS:

1. P.C. Bradley, ed., *British Herbal Compendium: A Handbook of Scientific Information on Widely Used Plant Drugs*, vol. 1. (Bournemouth [Dorset], England: British Herbal Medicine Association, 1992).
2. J.D. Chesney and R.P. Adams, *Economic Botany*, 39(1) (1985): 74–86.
3. T. Kosuge et al., *Yakugaku Zasshi.* 105(8) (1985): 791–95.
4. R.P. Knott and R.X. McCutcheon, *Journal of Pharmaceutical Sciences*, 50(11) (1961): 963–65.

PRIMARY NAME:

CLEMATIS

SCIENTIFIC NAME:

Clematis virginiana L. and occasionally other *Clematis* species. Family: Ranunculeae

What Is Clematis?

This perennial vine, a member of the buttercup family boasting more than two hundred species worldwide, bears heavy clusters of graceful, sweet-smelling flowers that eventually turn into fruit with feathery plumes. The leaves consist of three sharply toothed leaflets. The leaves and occasionally other parts of the plant have been used medicinally. Related species include the Chinese *Clematis chinensis* and Europe's *Clematis recta*.[1]

What It Is Used For:

Both traditional healers and physicians in North America at one time recommended clematis, now recognized as a toxic plant, in liquid preparations to apply to skin disorders such as sores, cuts, itches, and venereal eruptions. In folk

CLEMATIS (Continued)

COMMON NAMES:
Devil's darning needle, old-man's beard, traveler's joy, vine bower, virgin's bower, woodbine. *Clematis chinensis:* wei ling xian

RATING:
5 = Studies indicate that there is a definite health hazard to using this substance, even in recommended amounts.

medicine, a tea was brewed to treat nervousness, twitching, insomnia, headache, cancers, ulcers, and other ailments. Homeopaths have used clematis to treat various conditions. (See page 2 for a discussion of homeopathy.)

Forms Available Include:

Leaf, infusion.

Dosage Commonly Reported:

Clematis should not be used medicinally. It may appear in Chinese herbal blends.

Will It Work for You? What the Studies Say:

Recent studies on other *Clematis* species and shared components indicate not only that *Clematis virginiana* has various active ingredients, but that a number of them may explain folk uses; it may have blood-pressure-lowering, liver-protectant, and central-nervous-stimulant properties.[2] These findings are irrelevant, however, given the risks involved in using this very toxic plant. Researchers have even found anti-inflammatory properties in the related *Clematis chinensis,*[3] which is ironic given the often notable skin irritation seen with *Clematis virginiana.*

Will It Harm You? What the Studies Say:

All parts of this plant are toxic, particularly when fresh. Animal and human studies show that when applied to the skin or mucous membranes, the poisonous element—protoanemonin—can cause severe irritation. If swallowed, it can bring about intense pain in the mouth, blistering, profuse salivation, abdominal cramping, severe diarrhea, bloody vomiting, kidney irritation with pain and excessive urination as well as blood in the urine, dizziness, fainting, and convulsions in severe cases.[4] Protoanemonin appears to lose some of its toxicity when dried or cooked.[5]

GENERAL SOURCES:
Duke, J.A. *CRC Handbook of Medicinal Herbs.* Boca Raton, FL: CRC Press, 1985.
Foster, S., and J.A. Duke. *The Peterson Field Guide Series: A Field Guide to Medicinal Plants. Eastern and Central North America.* Boston: Houghton Mifflin Company, 1990.
Lampe, K.E., and M.A. McCann. *AMA Handbook of Poisonous and Injurious Plants.* Chicago: American Medical Association, 1985.
Review of Natural Products. St. Louis: Facts and Comparisons, October 1996.

TEXT CITATIONS:
1. *Review of Natural Products* (St. Louis: Facts and Comparisons, October 1996).
2. Ibid.
3. M.J. Wei et al., *Acta Pharma Sinica,* 26(10) (1991): 772.
4. K.E. Lampe and M.A. McCann, *AMA Handbook of Poisonous and Injurious Plants* (Chicago: American Medical Association, 1985). *Review of Natural Products,* op. cit.
5. *Review,* op. cit.

PRIMARY NAME:

CLOVE

SCIENTIFIC NAME:
Syzygium aromaticum (L.)
Merr. & TM Perry. Also referred
to as *Caryophyllum aromaticus*
L., and *Eugenia caryophyllus*
Thnub. Family: Myrtaceae

COMMON NAMES:
Caryophyllum, ding xiang

RATING:
1 = Years of use and extensive,
high-quality studies indicate
that this substance is very
effective and safe when used in
recommended amounts for the
indication(s) noted in the "Will
It Work for You?" section.
However, see the warnings in
the "Will It Harm You?"
section.

What Is Clove?

Cloves are the dried, unexpanded flower buds of the *Syzygium aromaticum* tree, a stately evergreen found in tropical countries. The dark brown nuggets are used as a spice. They also contain a volatile oil, which is extracted through steam distillation. Occasionally the oil is drawn from the stems and leaves as well.

What It Is Used For:

Few curries, pumpkin pies, or mugs of mulled wine go untouched by this aromatic, sweet-hot spice, and countless soaps, perfumes, insect repellents, and other products contain the essential oil. Clove's status as a medicinal remedy is no less impressive. Its oil in particular boasts antiseptic and anesthetic (numbing) properties, both of which have been put to use in soothing mouthwashes and toothache remedies. Clove tea, made with a few drops of oil, claims wide renown as a nausea-reliever. Herbalists have for years recommended this tea and other clove preparations for stomach upset, gas, coughs, congestion, and sore throat. Some recommend clove oil as an infection preventive and painkiller for cuts and bites. Others have touted the herb as a general tonic and aphrodisiac.

Traditional Chinese healers, familiar with clove for more than two thousand years, extend the repertoire to include the treatment of such ailments as nasal polyps, diarrhea, bad breath, and hernia. Aromatherapists consider clove oil a balm for the digestive system. Sucking on whole cloves is said to curb alcohol cravings temporarily. Ground cloves appear in clove cigarettes or "kreteks" from Indonesia that make crackling sounds when smoked. Cloves are used as a spice in cooking.

Forms Available Include:

Cigarettes, clove (whole or ground), mouthwashes and other oral preparations, oil, tea.

Dosage Commonly Reported:

Clove tea is made with a few drops of the oil. In mouthwashes, the oil is used in concentrations of 1 to 5 percent. For toothache pain, the undiluted oil is applied to the affected area, but use cautiously, especially for children. See the "Will It Harm You?" section.

Will It Work for You? What the Studies Say:

Studies indicate that both cloves and clove oil have great medicinal potential, particularly in terms of fighting infection and numbing pain. Eugenol, the component primarily responsible for these properties, appears in high concentrations (85 to 95 percent) in the essential oil. Numerous test-tube studies have shown that eugenol vigorously fights certain bacteria, viruses, fungi, parasites, and larvae, including certain strains of *Staphylococcus aureus* and *Pseudomonas bacteria* (organisms that commonly cause skin infections), as well as the fungus *Candida albicans*, which can cause skin and vaginal yeast infections.[1] As an anesthetic, eugenol apparently depresses the sensory receptors critical to perceiving pain. These properties help explain why people have instinctively chosen clove preparations for treating insect bites, abrasions, and other skin irritations.

No controlled trials to test these properties in humans have been done so far, but German health authorities have endorsed clove oil as a local antiseptic and anesthetic. They also approve of using clove mouthwashes for soothing mucous membrane inflammations in the mouth and throat. Dentists around the world, likewise convinced of clove's potency, use the oil widely in dental cements, fillings, and dry socket preparations. Clove oil rubbed on aching gums should offer several hours of pain relief. Traveler's diarrhea and intestinal infections may succumb to the antibacterial elements in clove tea, although studies to prove they are potent enough to accomplish this in humans have not been done.

Investigators have uncovered a number of other interesting properties in cloves that may one day prove useful, although they all require more research. Clove extracts and oil appear to have antioxidative properties and cancer-fighting potential.[2] (Antioxidants help prevent the formation of free radicals, chemicals capable of becoming toxic, possibly leading to cancerous changes in cells.) Cloves may help heal stomach ulcers.[3] The oil boasts antiplatelet properties and has demonstrated a capacity to break up blood clots in small animals.[4]

Will It Harm You? What the Studies Say:

No reports of serious illness survive centuries of use. Clove and clove oil appear in many foods and commercial products (at FDA-approved concentrations). Problems arise, however, with high concentrations of clove, especially its oil. Consuming the oil in anything but minute amounts may cause stomach upset and other irritation. Although toxic reactions are not well documented, a number of infants and small children have suffered serious complications after accidentally swallowing clove oil, including blood abnormalities and central nervous system depression.[5]

Although it can cause skin irritation or allergic sensitivity reactions in certain people, clove oil for external use boasts an admirable safety record.[6] Smoking clove cigarettes qualifies as unwise at best, however. They contain approximately 40 percent ground cloves and 60 percent tobacco, which is packed with cancer-causing substances.[7] Animal studies indicate that smokers run the risk of pulmonary edema.[8] More than a dozen people have suffered toxic lung reactions.[9] Some smokers have coughed up blood-tinged sputum.[10] Allergic reactions are also a risk. By numbing the throat, cloves may cause smokers to inhale more deeply and for longer than they normally would, allowing toxins greater access to the throat and lungs. The American Lung Association strongly warns against smoking these cigarettes.

GENERAL SOURCES:

Abraham, S.K., and P.C. Kesavan. *Indian Journal of Experimental Biology.* 16(4) (1978): 518.

Bisset, N.G., ed. *Herbal Drugs and Phytopharmaceuticals.* Stuttgart: medpharm GmbH Scientific Publishers, 1994.

Castleman, M. *The Healing Herbs: The Ultimate Guide to the Curative Power of Nature's Medicines.* New York: Bantam Books, 1995.

Duke, J.A. *CRC Handbook of Medicinal Herbs.* Boca Raton, FL: CRC Press, 1985.

Federal Register. 42(146) (1997): 38613.

Guidotti, T.L. *Archives of Toxicology*. 63(1) (1989): 7–12.

Guidotti, T.L., and L. Laing. *Western Journal of Medicine*. 156(5) (1992): 537–38.

Lane, B.W., et al. *Human & Experimental Toxicology*. 10(4) (1991): 291–94.

Leung, A.Y., *Encyclopedia of Common Natural Ingredients Used in Food, Drugs, and Cosmetics*. New York: John Wiley & Sons, 1980.

Mayell, M. *Off-the-Shelf Natural Health: How to Use Herbs and Nutrients to Stay Well*. New York: Bantam Books, 1995.

Mindell, E. *Earl Mindell's Herb Bible*. New York: Simon & Schuster/Fireside, 1992.

Morbidity & Mortality Weekly Report. 34(21) (1985): 297–99.

Pediatrics. 88(2) (1991): 395–96.

Tyler, V.E. *Herbs of Choice: The Therapeutic Use of Phytomedicinals*. Binghamton, NY: Haworth Press/Pharmaceutical Products Press, 1994.

TEXT CITATIONS:

1. M.A. el-Naghy et al., *Zentralblatt für Mikrobiologie*, 147(3–4) (1992): 214–20. D.L.J. Opdyke, *Food & Cosmetics Toxicology*, 13 (1975): 761. K. Oishi et al., *Nippon Suisan Gakkaishi*, 40 (1974): 1241. W.J. Zhang, *China Journal of Chinese Materia Medica*, 19(9) (1994): 532–34, 574. J. Briozzo et al., *Journal of Applied Bacteriology*, 66(1) (1989): 69–75.

2. G.Q. Zheng et al., *Journal of Natural Products*, 55(7) (1992): 999–1003. M.V. Kumari, *Cancer Letters*, 60(1) (1991): 67–73. A.Y. Leung, *Encyclopedia of Common Natural Ingredients Used in Food, Drugs, and Cosmetics* (New York: John Wiley & Sons, 1980).

3. S.H. Zaidi, *Indian Journal of Medical Research*, 46 (1958): 732.

4. S.A. Saeed and A.H. Gilani, *Journal of the Pakistan Medical Association*, 44(5) (1994): 112–15. K.C. Srivastava, *Prostaglandins, Leukotrienes, and Essential Fatty Acids*, 48(5) (1993): 363–72.

5. S.A. Brown et al., *Blood Coagulation and Fibrinolysis*, 3(5) (1992): 665–68.

6. E. Rudzki and Z. Grzywa, *Contact Dermatitis*, 9(1) (1983): 40–45. A.S. Rothenstein et al., *Food & Chemical Toxicology*, 21(6) (1983): 727–33.

7. T.L. Guidotti, *Archives of Toxicology*, 63(1) (1989): 7–12.

8. J.W. McDonald and J.E. Heffner, *American Review of Respiratory Disease*, 143 (4 Part 1) (1991): 806–9.

9. *Journal of the American Medical Association*, 260 (1988): 3461.

10. A. Rasheed et al., *New England Journal of Medicine*, 310(1) (1984): 50.

PRIMARY NAME:
CLUB MOSS

SCIENTIFIC NAME:
Lycopodium clavatum L. Family: Lycopodiaceae

COMMON NAMES:
Common club moss, ground pine, running club moss, running pine, stag's horn club moss

What Is Club Moss?

The trailing stems of this mosslike evergreen herb send out upright branches that taper off into sets of elongated cones. The cones, composed of tight formations of yellowish green leaves, contain ripe yellow spores that are used medicinally. Sometimes the moss is used as well. The plant grows in North America, Europe, China, and elsewhere, although it is a protected plant in some countries, including Germany.

What It Is Used For:

Club moss was once widely used in folk medicine (as a diuretic, or "water pill") for bladder and kidney ailments, to increase urine production.[1] Years ago, Native Americans reportedly made a plant tea for fever and postpartum pain,

CLUB MOSS *(Continued)*

sprinkled a prepared powder on bleeding cuts and other minor skin wounds, and sniffed it to control nosebleeds. The fluffy yellow powder from the spores was once commonly used to coat pills and suppositories and was included in baby powders and remedies for eczema, herpes sores, and other skin problems. Some contemporary herbalists still recommend club moss externally for minor skin wounds. Today the spores are found in dusting agents for condoms, surgical gloves, and other materials. When set on fire, the spores explode. They appear in some fireworks.[2] In the United States, homeopathic formulations appear to be the most common use of club moss. Homeopaths recommend it in minute amounts for various ailments. (For more information on homeopathy, see page 2.)

Forms Available Include:

- *For internal use:* Decoction, extract.
- *For external use:* Powder.

Dosage Commonly Reported:

Club moss is no longer widely recommended. Follow package instructions for formulations designed for external use on skin wounds.

Will It Work for You? What the Studies Say:

On the basis of the identified ingredients, club moss probably exerts some diuretic action; several of the more than one hundred alkaloids are believed to stimulate urine production, as do the contained flavonoids.[3] Researchers have also isolated strong laxative and emetic (vomiting) properties,[4] and documented fever-reducing action in rats,[5] painkilling activity in mice (injected with an extract),[6] antibacterial and antifungal actions (in the test tube)[7] and anti-inflammatory activity (with an alcoholic extract of the entire plant).[8] The alkaloid lycopine stimulates peristalsis (the wavelike movement that moves intestinal contents forward), which encourages bowel movements. Estrogenic activity has been identified in female rats,[9] and lycopine in particular has caused uterine contractions in rodents.[10] No investigations into the plant's ability to stop bleeding can be found.

Will It Harm You? What the Studies Say:

There are significant health hazards associated with the use of this herb, especially in oral form and when used over extended periods of time. Many of the herb's alkaloids are known mucous membrane irritants, and some may stimulate urine production by irritating the kidneys.[11] This type of diuretic is not considered ideal by any measure. Asthma has developed in workers exposed to club moss spores used to dust rubber condoms and other products.[12]

GENERAL SOURCES:

Bisset, N.G., ed. *Herbal Drugs and Phytopharmaceuticals.* Stuttgart: medpharm GmbH Scientific Publishers, 1994.

Bremness, L. *Herbs.* 1st American ed. Eyewitness Handbooks. New York: Dorling Kindersley Publications, 1994.

Foster, S., and J.A. Duke. *The Peterson Field Guide Series: A Field Guide to Medicinal Plants. Eastern and Central North America.* Boston: Houghton Mifflin Company, 1990.

Hylton, W.H., ed. *The Rodale Herb Book: How to Use, Grow, and Buy Nature's Miracle Plants.* Emmaus, PA: Rodale Press, Inc., 1974.

Mindell, E. *Earl Mindell's Herb Bible.* New York: Simon & Schuster/Fireside, 1992.

Weiner, M.A., and J. Weiner. *Weiner's Herbal: A Guide to Herb Medicine.* Mill Valley, CA: Quantum Books, 1991.

TEXT CITATIONS:

1. N.G. Bisset, ed., *Herbal Drugs and Phytopharmaceuticals* (Stuttgart: medpharm GmbH Scientific Publishers, 1994).

2. L. Bremness, *Herbs*, 1st American ed., Eyewitness Handbooks (New York: Dorling Kindersley Publications, 1994).

3. Bisset, op. cit.

4. Ibid.

5. W.M. Nikonorow, *Acta Poloniae Pharmaceutica*, 3 (1939): 23–56.

6. S.Y. Chow et al., *Journal of the Formosa Medical Association*, 75 (1976): 349–57.

7. A.R. McCutcheon et al., *Journal of Ethnopharmacology*, 44(3) (1994): 157–69.

8. B.H. Han et al., *Korean Journal of Pharmacology*, 4(3) (1972): 205–9.

9. A. Nobelli, *Anales de Farmacia y Bioquimica (Buenos Aires)*, 21(2) (1954): 80.

10. Bisset, op. cit.

11. Ibid.

12. P. Cullinan et al., *Thorax*, 48(7) (1993): 774–75. S. Nakamura et al., *Arerugi—Japanese Journal of Allergology*, 18(4) (1969): 258–62.

PRIMARY NAME:

COCOA

SCIENTIFIC NAME:
Theobroma cacao L. subsp. *cacao*. Family: Stericuliaceae

COMMON NAMES:
Cacao, chocola, theobroma

RATING:
4 = Research indicates that this substance will not fulfill the claims made for it, but that it is also unlikely to cause any harm.

What Is Cocoa?

Several varieties of the tall *Theobroma cacao* tree, an evergreen with leathery leaves and scented flowers, grow in the tropics. Berrylike fruits containing seeds commonly referred to as cacao "beans" grow straight off the trunk and branches. Once cacao beans have been dried, roasted, ground, and further processed, they are referred to as cocoa products: powder, butter, and extracts.[1] These are in turn used to make cocoa liquor (made with ground cacao nibs) and, of course, chocolate.

Do not confuse cocoa (or cacao) with coca, the source of cocaine.

What It Is Used For:

As every schoolchild learns, the Spanish conquistador Hernando Cortés spirited the recipe for a delicious drink he tasted at Mexico's glittering Aztec court back to Spain, from where it eventually spread to the rest of Europe and the world despite fervent attempts to keep it at home. Northern Europeans artfully endowed the concoction with sugar and milk to blunt its bitter taste, creating the drink now enjoyed as hot chocolate. Cacao beans were literally worth their weight in gold on commercial markets. It was only in the 1800s that chocolate as we know it was fashioned into blocks and made into candies.

For centuries before Cortés's arrival, Central Americans were using cacao beans to treat a variety of conditions including coughs, fever, and pregnancy and childbirth complications. They smoothed soothing cocoa butter onto irritated skin, chapped lips, burns, and the sore breasts of nursing mothers. Traditional European healers learned to value cocoa in similar ways, considering it an effective treatment (sometimes in combination with other substances) for asthma, bronchial congestion, cough, endocrine gland dysfunction, diarrhea, infectious intestinal diseases, and other ailments.[2] They dabbed the butter around the eyes, mouth, and neck to reduce wrinkles.[3]

Some modern herbalists continue to extoll cocoa as a remedy for asthma and chest congestion, and a few tout it as a stimulant, mild diuretic ("water pill"), digestive aid, and aphrodisiac, among other things. Cocoa is found extensively in commercial foods and medicines as a flavoring. Cocoa butter appears in multiple creams, massage lotions, ointments, suppositories, soaps, and other commercial products.[4]

Forms Available Include:

Cocoa butter, extract, liquor, powder, syrup, and other products, some of which go into making chocolate.

Dosage Commonly Reported:

Hot cocoa is made with 1 to 2 heaping teaspoons cocoa per cup of water or milk. Cocoa butter is used liberally in creams and lotions as an emollient. In the treatment of minor burns, cocoa butter is applied in concentrations of 50 to 100 percent.

Will It Work for You? What the Studies Say:

Like coffee and tea, cocoa is a stimulant, albeit a milder one, given its lower caffeine content. As a result, it is less likely to cause the jitteriness and other often unwanted side effects of larger caffeine doses. The average cup (8 ounces) of cocoa contains 10 milligrams of caffeine, notably less than the approximately 100 milligrams found in a cup of coffee. Another important substance in cocoa—the alkaloid theobromine (0.5 to 2.7 percent)—also mildly stimulates the central nervous system[5] and heart, and possesses other caffeine-like properties; it dilates the coronary vessels, increases urine production, and relaxes smooth muscles.[6] But putting cocoa to practical use for related ailments appears to be impractical. For example, while it increases urine output, the increase is only mild and short-lived. To reduce fluid retention would require so much cocoa or chocolate that side effects such as a fast heartbeat would probably develop before any benefit could be seen.[7]

The same holds true for enlisting cocoa as an asthma remedy; even though its caffeine and theobromine have important similarities to the standard drug for opening up the bronchial tubes—theophylline—too much cocoa would have to be consumed. Moreover, asthma attacks can be life-threatening, so counting on cocoa is risky at best. Some herbalists still consider cocoa or chocolate a viable candidate for cold- or flu-related chest congestion, however, asserting it is powerful enough in palatable doses to open the bronchial passages in the lungs.[8] No human trials to test this theory can be found in the medical literature. Because there is a lack of substantiating evidence, German health authorities do not recommend cocoa beans for any ailment, although they do (thankfully!) allow it as a flavoring.

Cocoa butter, while a bit greasy, effectively soothes, softens, and protects skin. Cocoa and cocoa butter both hold promise as sources of natural antioxidants, although the subject demands more research.[9] Antioxidants are believed to help scavenge toxic by-products that may contribute to cancer cell formation.

Chinese researchers have identified antibacterial activity (to a penicillin-resistant strain of *Staphylococcus aureus*) in extracts of cacao seed bark,[10] but practical applications for this property have not been identified so far.

Will It Harm You? What the Studies Say:

Cocoa has been safely consumed by millions over the centuries, and the FDA classifies both cocoa and chocolate as safe for food use. Be aware, however, that if you are sensitive to caffeine even the relatively small amount in cocoa may make you irritable, jittery, have trouble falling asleep, or suffer from other unwanted side effects. Children may be particularly susceptible. In the mid-1980s, reports appeared of a dog who had a toxic reaction to the caffeine and theobromine in cocoa after eating two pounds of chocolate chips; he became extremely excited, suffered convulsions and collapse, and died.[11]

Substances called tyramines in chocolate—also found in red wine, hard cheese, and certain other foods—trigger headaches in some people. Cocoa powders produced by the Dutch process often contain notable amounts of sodium, an important factor for people on sodium-restricted diets to consider. Avoid cocoa-containing products if you suffer from irritable bowel syndrome.[12] Allergic skin reactions to cocoa butter can occur,[13] and in animal tests the butter clogs pores, causing blackheads.[14] Evidence cannot be found, however, to support the theory that cocoa or chocolate causes acne, kidney stones, or infant colic.[15]

GENERAL SOURCES:

Bremness, L. *Herbs*. 1st American ed. Eyewitness Handbooks. New York: Dorling Kindersley Publications, 1994.

Castleman, M. *The Healing Herbs: The Ultimate Guide to the Curative Power of Nature's Medicines*. New York: Bantam Books, 1995.

Duke, J.A. *CRC Handbook of Medicinal Herbs*. Boca Raton, FL: CRC Press, 1985.

Lawrence Review of Natural Products. St. Louis: Facts and Comparisons, January 1992.

Leung, A.Y., and S. Foster. *Encyclopedia of Common Natural Ingredients Used in Food, Drugs, and Cosmetics*. 2nd ed. New York: John Wiley & Sons, 1996.

Tyler, V.E. *Herbs of Choice: The Therapeutic Use of Phytomedicinals*. Binghamton, NY: Haworth Press/Pharmaceutical Products Press, 1994.

TEXT CITATIONS:

1. A.Y. Leung and S. Foster, *Encyclopedia of Common Natural Ingredients Used in Food, Drugs, and Cosmetics*, 2nd ed. (New York: John Wiley & Sons, 1996).

2. Ibid.

3. Ibid. J.A. Duke, *CRC Handbook of Medicinal Herbs* (Boca Raton, FL: CRC Press, 1985).

4. Leung and Foster, op. cit.

5. V.E. Tyler, *Herbs of Choice: The Therapeutic Use of Phytomedicinals* (Binghamton, NY: Haworth Press/Pharmaceutical Products Press, 1994).

6. Leung and Foster, op. cit.

7. Tyler, op. cit.

8. M. Castleman, *The Healing Herbs: The Ultimate Guide to the Curative Power of Nature's Medicines* (New York: Bantam Books, 1995).

9. Leung and Foster, op. cit.

10. C. Perez and C. Anesini, *American Journal of Chinese Medicine*, 22(2) (1994): 169–74.

11. *Medical Sciences Bulletin*, 7(11) (1985): 4.

12. G. Friedman, *Gastroenterology Clinics of North America*, 20(2) (1991): 313.

13. Duke, op. cit.

14. O.H. Mills et al., *British Journal of Dermatology*, 98 (1978): 145.

15. Castleman, op. cit.

PRIMARY NAME:
COD-LIVER OIL

SCIENTIFIC NAME:
N/A

COMMON NAME:
N/A

RATING:
2 = According to a number of well-designed studies and common use, this substance appears to be relatively effective and safe when used in recommended amounts for the indication(s) noted in the "Will It Work For You?" section.

What Is Cod-Liver Oil?

The cold-water codfish yields this concentrated oil. Many sources import it from Norway. It contains the fat-soluble vitamins A and D and is relatively low in saturated fatty acids. See page 00 for a discussion of fish oils in general.

What It Is Used For:

Some sources promote the use of cod-liver oil as a good source for essential fatty acids (EFAs) such as omega-3s like eicosapentaenoic acid (EPA) and docosahexaenoic acid (DHA). EFAs are substances that enthusiasts assert can do several things: lower blood fats and cholesterol and thus help reduce the risk of certain kinds of cardiovascular disease, reduce inflammation and thus benefit such illnesses as arthritis and allergies, and thin the blood to help prevent potentially hazardous clots. Cod-liver oil appears (typically combined with other substances) in topical products for prickly heat, diaper rash, and hemorrhoids and forms a physical barrier on the skin to prevent irritation.

Forms Available Include:

- *For internal use:* Capsule.
- *For external use:* A component in various topical products.

Dosage Commonly Reported:

Cod-liver oil supplements are often taken in dosages of 20 milliliters daily. Follow package instructions when using commercial cod-liver oil capsules.

Will It Work for You? What the Studies Say:

While fish-rich diets have been shown to reduce the risk of death from heart attack and other ischemic heart disease in some studies, results of trials involving supplement forms of cod-liver oil are not as promising. In one study, for example, no significant changes in the twenty-four-hour prevalence of irregular heart rhythms or ventricular extrasystoles (extra heartbeats) were observed in heart attack victims who took cod-liver oil supplements (20 milliliter) for six weeks.[1] Trials indicate that cod-liver oil supplements reduce platelet aggregation and may therefore lower the risk for blood clots; these clots can cause heart attacks and strokes, among other complications. Cod-liver oil apparently has little or no effect on the body's mechanism for breaking down blood clots (fibrinolysis), however.[2]

High cholesterol is considered a risk factor for cardiovascular disease. Cod-liver oil supplements may have small beneficial effects on cholesterol levels, but definitive conclusions are still lacking. One study found no benefit of daily cod-liver oil supplementation in men who had suffered a heart attack.[3] Measurements such as total cholesterol and high-density-lipoprotein (HDL) cholesterol did not significantly change in the subjects involved in this randomized, crossover study who took 20 milliliters daily for shifts of six weeks each. Another study reported that cholesterol levels and platelets responded differently to cod-liver oil supplementation in men and women, with minor and relatively insignificant changes in cholesterol levels in both.[4]

Although cod-liver oil supplements (and their EFAs) have been promoted as arthritis "cures," a well-designed twenty-four-week trial involving eighty-six osteoarthritis sufferers found no benefit to the supplement in terms of joint pain or inflammation, interference with activities, and other parameters, as judged by their doctors at four-week visits.[5]

There have been some positive findings with cod-liver oil supplements. They may reduce musculoskeletal pain such as backache, strains, and joint pain, particularly in individuals with musculoskeletal disease, according to an examination of data taken from the 1985 Norwegian Health Survey and published in 1996.[6] No other trials on the subject appear in the medical literature.

Investigators have also found that dietary supplementation with cod-liver oil may help prevent a marker of advancing renal (kidney) failure in non-insulin-dependent diabetes (NIDD): protein (albumin) loss through leakage from tiny blood vessels. This was the conclusion of a 1989 double-blind study involving eighteen individuals who took cod-liver oil supplements for eight weeks, and then a placebo (olive oil) for the same amount of time, or vice versa.[7] A more recent trial determined that giving pure EPA-E (eicosapentaenoic acid) from cod-liver oil to NIDD sufferers with kidney disease could lower the secretion of urinary protein (albumin) for sustained periods.[8]

Cod-liver oil is probably effective as a protectant in hemorrhoidal products, but whether it will encourage wound healing is unclear.[9] Investigators are reportedly testing its ability to help prevent toxemia, a complication of pregnancy.[10]

Will It Harm You? What the Studies Say:

The potential risks of taking any fish oil supplement in large doses or over extended periods of time are not known.[11] Most clinical trials report no adverse reactions to cod-liver oil supplements, but some sources recommend finding another source of EFAs because you would have to take so much fish oil that toxic amounts of vitamins A and D might build up in your system.

GENERAL SOURCES:

American Pharmaceutical Association. *Handbook of Nonprescription Drugs.* 11th ed. Washington, D.C.: American Pharmaceutical Association, 1996.

Balch, J.F., and P.A. Balch. *Prescription for Nutritional Healing: A Practical A to Z Reference to Drug-Free Remedies Using Vitamins, Minerals, Herbs & Food Supplements.* 2nd ed. Garden City Park, NY: Avery Publishing Group, 1997.

Mayell, M. *Off-the-Shelf Natural Health. How to Use Herbs and Nutrients to Stay Well.* New York: Bantam Books, 1995.

TEXT CITATIONS:

1. T. Hardarson et al., *Journal of Internal Medicine*, 226(1) (1989): 33–37.
2. G. Hellsten et al., *Current Medical Research & Opinion*, 13(3) (1993): 133–39.
3. G.V. Skuladottir et al., *Journal of Internal Medicine*, 228(6) (1990): 563–68.
4. J.B. Hansen et al., *European Journal of Clinical Nutrition*, 47(2) (1993): 123–31.
5. T. Stammers et al., *Annals of the Rheumatic Diseases*, 51(1) (1992): 128–29.
6. W. Eriksen et al., *European Journal of Clinical Nutrition*, 50(10) (1996): 689–93.
7. T. Jensen et al., *New England Journal of Medicine*, 321(23) (1989): 1572–77.
8. H. Shimizu et al., *Diabetes Research & Clinical Practice*, 28(1) (1995): 35–40.
9. American Pharmaceutical Association, *Handbook of Nonprescription Drugs*, 11th ed. (Washington, D.C.: American Pharmaceutical Association, 1996).
10. G. Boog, *Revue Française de Gynecologie et de Obstetrique*, 88(2) (1993): 63–68.
11. American Pharmaceutical Association, op. cit.

PRIMARY NAME:

CODONOPSIS

SCIENTIFIC NAME:
Codonopsis pilosula (Franch.) Nannf. and numerous other *Codonopsis* species. Family: Campanulaceae

COMMON NAMES:
Bastard ginseng, bonnet bellflower, dangshen

RATING:
2 = According to a number of well-designed studies and common use, this substance appears to be relatively effective and safe when used in recommended amounts for the indication(s) noted in the "Will It Work for You?" section.

What Is Codonopsis?

This small twining perennial, a native of Asia now cultivated in the United States and many other parts of the world, bears distinctive bell-shaped, greenish purple flowers. The dried root is used medicinally.

What It Is Used For:

Since its relatively recent debut in the Chinese materia medica several centuries ago, the odiferous and sweet-tasting codonopsis root has earned a widespread reputation as a gentle *qi* (vital energy) tonic on a par with such age-old standbys as **Astragalus** and **Ginseng**, and is even referred to as the "poor man's ginseng" because it is so frequently substituted for that ancient tonic.[1] Herbalists recommend codonopsis root for replenishing a weakened immune system, rejuvenating a weakened or fatigued body, treating appetite loss and digestive system upset (chronic diarrhea, vomiting), improving stamina, building "strong blood," and alleviating respiratory ailments such as asthma and shortness of breath. Some herbalists recommend it for people looking for something milder and shorter-lasting than ginseng.[2]

Forms Available Include:

Capsule, decoction, dried root, liquid, tablet, tincture.

Dosage Commonly Reported:

The dried root is often used in a decoction; up to 25 grams are commonly taken per day. To use commercial codonopsis capsules or tablets, follow the package instructions. Commercially prepared tinctures and liquids are labeled with dosage information.

Will It Work for You? What the Studies Say:

Although few if any controlled human studies appear to have been done so far, scientists in the 1980s and 1990s, mostly in China, have begun to learn a lot about the chemical constituents of codonopsis root and its actions in mice and other small laboratory animals. In these types of experiments, codonopsis root and certain extracts frequently help boost stamina, enhance tolerance to stress such as high temperatures and lack of oxygen, protect against ulcers, stimulate the central nervous system, increase red and white blood cell counts along with other blood parameters, prolong life and inhibit detrimental antibody production (in mice with chemically induced systemic lupus erythematosus), and fortify the immune system on the cellular level.[3] Many of these and other reactions parallel those seen with ginseng, but the plants are in fact chemically quite different.[4] Studies in humans have been done to explore the value of codonopsis in treating coronary heart disease[5] and bronchitis,[6] among other conditions, but findings are inconclusive so far.

Will It Harm You? What the Studies Say:

No reports of serious illness survive centuries of use in China. Because clinical trials to test its safety in humans do not appear to have been done, however, the conclusion that it is safe for long-term use particularly should be considered premature.

GENERAL SOURCES:

Chevallier, A. *The Encyclopedia of Medicinal Plants: A Practical Reference Guide to More Than 550 Key Medicinal Plants & Their Uses.* 1st American ed. New York: Dorling Kindersley Publications, 1996.

Leung, A.Y., and S. Foster. *Encyclopedia of Common Natural Ingredients Used in Food, Drugs, and Cosmetics.* 2nd ed. New York: John Wiley & Sons, 1996.

Tang, W., and G. Eisenbrand. *Chinese Drugs of Plant Origin: Chemistry, Pharmacology, and Use in Traditional and Modern Medicine.* Berlin: Springer-Verlag, 1992.

TEXT CITATIONS:

1. A.Y. Leung and S. Foster, *Encyclopedia of Common Natural Ingredients Used in Food, Drugs, and Cosmetics*, 2nd ed. (New York: John Wiley & Sons, 1996).

2. A. Chevallier, *The Encyclopedia of Medicinal Plants: A Practical Reference Guide to More Than 550 Key Medicinal Plants & Their Uses*, 1st American ed. (New York: Dorling Kindersley Publications, 1996).

3. Leung and Foster, op. cit. S.M. Wang and Y. Yang, *Shanxi Zhongyi*, 5(1) (1989): 37. X.L. Mao et al., *Chinese Journal of Integrated Traditional Western Medicine*, 5(12) (1985): 739. C.Q. Ling, *Henan Zhongyi*, 13 (1993): 94. M.X. Zhuang et al., *Zhongguo Yaoxue Zazhi*, 27 (1992): 653. J.C. Cui et al., *Zhongcaoyao*, 19(8) (1988): 21. W. Li et al., *Jilin Zhongyiyao*, 6 (1990): 33. J.P. Chen et al., *American Journal of Chinese Medicine.* 21(3–4) (1993): 257–62.

4. M.P. Wong et al., *Planta Medica*, 49 (1983): 60.
5. X. Xu et al., *Chung-Kuo Chung Hsi I Chieh Ho Tsa Chih*, 15(7) (1995): 398–400. Liao et al., *Journal of Traditional Chinese Medicine*, 8(1) (1988): 1–8.
6. S.L. Feng and C.S. Song, *Chinese Journal of Modern Developments in Traditional Medicine*, 5(2) (1985): 102–4, 68–69.

PRIMARY NAME:
COENZYME Q10

SCIENTIFIC NAME:
N/A

COMMON NAMES:
Mitoquinone, ubidecarenone, ubiquinone

RATING:
3 = Studies on the effectiveness and safety of this substance are conflicting, or there are not enough studies to draw a conclusion.

What Is Coenzyme Q10?

Coenzyme Q10 is one in a series of ubiquinones, naturally occurring compounds produced in nearly every cell of the body, and was discovered as recently as 1957. Coenzyme Q10 helps convert food into energy at a very basic, cellular level. It is also an antioxidant.

What It Is Used For:

Coenzyme Q10 is sold as a dietary supplement in the United States. Currently there is no Recommended Daily Allowance (RDA) for it. Manufacturers and others recommend taking it to prevent or treat a dizzying variety of conditions. Many claim that it can protect and strengthen the heart; help treat congestive heart failure, cardiac arrhythmias, high blood pressure, and other cardiovascular diseases; counteract the aging process; strengthen muscles and improve physical performance and endurance; stimulate the immune system; help reduce the adverse effects of chemotherapy; promote weight loss; and benefit the treatment of diabetes, obesity, and Alzheimer's disease.

Many sources note that Japanese, Russian, and European practitioners have administered coenzyme Q10 as a medicinal agent for various illnesses, including cardiovascular and periodontal disease.[1] Some recommend taking it as a supplement because inherent amounts decline with age and physical activity. One source cites coenzyme Q10 as one of several nutritional substances shown "to play a significant role in optimal health."[2]

Forms Available Include:

Capsule, liquid, oil.

Dosage Commonly Reported:

A daily intake of 15 to 30 milligrams is commonly reported.

Will It Work for You? What the Studies Say:

As an antioxidant, coenzyme Q10 is believed to control the formation of dangerous substances called free radicals that can damage cells through oxidation. In so doing, and possibly also by stabilizing membranes, coenzyme Q10 may help keep atherosclerotic plaque from forming, thus preventing or encouraging healing in certain types of cardiovascular heart disease such as congestive heart failure, ischemic heart disease, and possibly high blood pressure. This is particularly relevant in situations in which the body tissue is deprived of blood (and thus oxygen) for periods of time.[3] Preliminary evidence of coenzyme Q10's antioxidant properties were observed in animal studies in the 1980s. A protective effect was seen in rat livers transplanted into other rats; the recipients survived longer and showed other notable improvements when the donor had been treated with coenzyme Q10.[4] Evidence that antioxidants can retard the aging process, as some sources claim, is built on shaky scientific ground.

A team of investigators reviewing the medical literature on coenzyme Q10 and heart failure in 1994 found "promising" results overall from the eight clinical trials published up to that point. They deemed these trials well-designed (placebo-controlled, double-blind), but also reported that their results were inconsistent and that a few relied on questionable methodological approaches.[5] The small size of most also limited their value. The authors conclude that more trials are needed before any conclusions can be made about coenzyme Q10's potential as a heart-failure treatment. Studies on the effectiveness of coenzyme Q10 for cardiomyopathy (a type of heart failure typically caused by an enlarged heart) have been mixed, with a well-designed 1989 trial involving twenty-five individuals showing no effect at all,[6] but a 1988 trial with eighty-eight individuals found statistically significant improvements in two parameters of heart function.[7] Coenzyme Q10's value in treating periodontal disease remains unclear despite the several studies that have been done. A 1995 *British Dental Journal* review of the limited English-language literature on treating periodontal disease with coenzyme Q10 reported no sound evidence to support its use, concluding that supplements have "no place" in modern periodontal treatment.[8]

Little evidence can be found to support the use of coenzyme Q10 for any of the myriad other ailments it has been recommended for. Still up for debate is whether the supplements work when swallowed, as some evidence suggests that they are destroyed during the digestive process.

Will It Harm You? What the Studies Say:

Coenzyme Q10 appears to be a relatively safe dietary supplement, although in rare cases stomach upset, diarrhea, appetite loss, and nausea can develop.[9] The effects of prolonged use or high doses have yet to be carefully examined in humans, as does its safety for pregnant or nursing women.

GENERAL SOURCES:

Balch, J.F., and P.A. Balch. *Prescription for Nutritional Healing: A Practical A to Z Reference to Drug-Free Remedies Using Vitamins, Minerals, Herbs & Food Supplements.* 2nd ed. Garden City Park, NY: Avery Publishing Group, 1997.

Barrett, S., and V. Herbert. *The Vitamin Pushers: How the "Health Food" Industry Is Selling America a Bill of Goods.* Amherst, NY: Prometheus Books, 1994.

Lawrence Review of Natural Products. St. Louis: Facts and Comparisons, May 1988.

Mayell, M. *Off-the-Shelf Natural Health: How to Use Herbs and Nutrients to Stay Well.* New York: Bantam Books, 1995.

TEXT CITATIONS:

1. *Lawrence Review of Natural Products* (St. Louis: Facts and Comparisons, May 1988).
2. M. Mayell, *Off-the-Shelf Natural Health: How to Use Herbs and Nutrients to Stay Well* (New York: Bantam Books, 1995).

3. *Lawrence Review of Natural Products,* op. cit. S.M. Greenberg and W.H. Firshman, *Medical Clinics of North America,* 72 (1987): 243.
4. K. Sumimoto et al., *Surgery,* 102 (1987): 821.
5. O. Spigest, *Tidsskrift for Den Norske Laegeforening,* 114(8) (1994): 939–42.
6. B. Permanetter et al., *Zeitschrifft für Kardiologie,* 78(6) (1989): 360–65.
7. P.H. Langsjoen et al., *Klinische Wochenschrift,* 66(13) (1988): 583–90.
8. T.L. Watts, *British Dental Journal,* 178(6) (1995): 209–13.
9. *Lawrence Review of Natural Products,* op. cit.

PRIMARY NAME:
COLLISONIA

SCIENTIFIC NAME:
Collisonia canadensis L. Family: Labiatae (Lamiaceae)

COMMON NAMES:
Horse-balm, horseweed, ox balm, pilewort, richweed, stone root

RATING:
4 = Research indicates that this substance will not fulfill the claims made for it, but that it is also unlikely to cause any harm.

What Is Collisonia?

This square-stemmed perennial, a member of the mint family, is native to the damp woods of eastern North America. It has large, oval leaves and bears branched clusters of greenish-yellow flowers that converge and exude a lemony scent. Primarily the dried rhizome (underground stem) and roots are used medicinally.

What It Is Used For:

Among Native Americans and early settlers on the East Coast, collisonia enjoyed a reputation as a sweat-inducer (typically to lower fevers), antispasmodic, sedative, and tonic. In the years since then, many folk healers have recommended it as a diuretic ("water pill") to increase urine production and flow in cases of fluid retention and bladder and kidney stones. The root's purported astringent properties have been enlisted in the form of a tea to control diarrhea, shrink varicose veins, and soothe digestive system ailments such as irritable bowel syndrome. But the most enduring use of this herb—various nonprescription herbal products still contain it—may be as a hemorrhoid treatment. Just consider one of its common names: pilewort. Some contemporary herbalists also recommend poultices and washes of the fresh leaves or roots to treat cuts, bruises, burns, and sores.

Forms Available Include:

- *For internal use:* Decoction, extract, tincture.
- *For external use:* Poultice, wash.

Dosage Commonly Reported:

The liquid root extract is taken in doses of 1 to 4 milliliters, and the tincture is taken in doses of 2 to 8 milliliters. Commercial preparations—poultices and washes—are labeled with dosage instructions.

Will It Work for You? What the Studies Say:

Very little scientific data can be found on this plant. Most popular sources cite the presence of a volatile oil, saponins, mucilage, resin, alkaloids, and tannins, all of which have medicinal potential in adequate concentrations. Tannins, for example, may help explain the root tea's reputation as an astringent. But without specific information on relative concentrations, collisonia's potency is difficult to determine. Even more important, the plant has apparently never been tested in animals or humans, or even in the test tube. Its use in nonprescription hemorrhoid products is outdated,[1] particularly given the availability of safer and more effective products.

Will It Harm You? What the Studies Say:

While no reports of toxic reactions to collisonia appear in the modern medical literature, so little scientific information is available that moderation may be the best approach. *Do not ingest preparations made with fresh leaves, as even very small doses may cause vomiting.*[2]

GENERAL SOURCES:

American Pharmaceutical Association. *Handbook of Nonprescription Drugs.* 11th ed. Washington, D.C.: American Pharmaceutical Association, 1996.

Chevallier, A. *The Encyclopedia of Medicinal Plants: A Practical Reference Guide to More Than 550 Key Medicinal Plants & Their Uses.* 1st American ed. New York: Dorling Kindersley Publications, 1996.

Dobelis, I.N., ed. *The Magic and Medicine of Plants: A Practical Guide to the Science, History, Folklore, and Everyday Uses of Medicinal Plants.* Pleasantville, NY: Reader's Digest Association, 1986.

Duke, J.A. *Handbook of Northeastern Indian Medicinal Plants.* Lincoln, MA: Quarterman Publications, Inc., 1986.

Foster, S., and J.A. Duke. *The Peterson Field Guide Series: A Field Guide to Medicinal Plants. Eastern and Central North America.* Boston: Houghton Mifflin Company, 1990.

Tierra, M. *The Way of Herbs.* New York: Pocket Books, 1990.

TEXT CITATIONS:

1. American Pharmaceutical Association, *Handbook of Nonprescription Drugs,* 11th ed. (Washington, D.C.: American Pharmaceutical Association, 1996).
2. S. Foster and J.A. Duke, *The Peterson Field Guide Series: A Field Guide to Medicinal Plants. Eastern and Central North America* (Boston: Houghton Mifflin Company, 1990).

PRIMARY NAME:
COLTSFOOT

SCIENTIFIC NAME:
Tussilago farfara L. Family: Compositae

COMMON NAMES:
Cough plant, coughwort, horse-foot, horse-hoof, kuan dong hua

What Is Coltsfoot?

This native European perennial, a member of the daisy family, grows wild in the United States and southern Canada. Both its yellow flowers and its hoof-shaped, woolly leaves (and the roots on occasion) are used medicinally.

What It Is Used For:

Coltsfoot may be the world's oldest cough remedy. For centuries traditional European and Asian doctors recommended it to suppress dry coughs and hoarseness, soothe throat and mouth irritations, and lessen cold-related congestion. Many still do, and numerous proprietary European cough and respiratory remedies feature this herb. Eighteenth-century French apothecary shop owners signaled the presence of their shop by painting an image of coltsfoot on the shingle hanging outside. Sometimes people try fighting a cough or wheeze

COLTSFOOT (Continued)

RATING:

- *For leaf preparations:* 2 = According to a number of well-designed studies and common use, this substance appears to be relatively effective and safe when used in recommended amounts for the indication(s) noted in the "Will It Work for You?" section. See warnings in the "Will It Harm You?" section, however.

- *For plant parts other than the leaf:* 5 = Studies indicate that there is a definite health hazard to using this substance, even in recommended amounts.

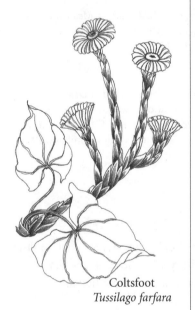

Coltsfoot
Tussilago farfara

by inhaling the vapors from coltsfoot leaves simmering in water or smoking coltsfoot along with other herbs. Traditional Indian doctors recommend the herb in powdered form (to snuff) for nasal stuffiness and cough.

Contemporary herbalists, including traditional Chinese doctors, also recommend coltsfoot for chronic respiratory problems such as asthma. The Chinese have prescribed coltsfoot for lung cancer. The fresh leaf, crushed and wetted, is sometimes placed directly on burns, bites, and skin inflammations.

Forms Available Include:

Extract, infusion (often mixed with honey for sweetening), juice, leaves, ointment, powder, tincture.

Dosage Commonly Reported:

The fresh leaf is used in a poultice. A tea is made using 2 teaspoons crushed leaves per cup of water. To use commercial coltsfoot preparations, follow the package instructions. The daily dose of coltsfoot should not contain more than 1 gram of pyrrolizidine alkaloids.

Will It Work for You? What the Studies Say:

Research indicates that the thousands if not millions of people around the world who still use coltsfoot are not misguided when it comes to certain ailments. Coltsfoot contains a substance called mucilage that coats and soothes the delicate mucous membranes of the airways (including the mouth), shielding them from irritants and lessening the impulse to cough. It also helps clear mucus from the airways, as was shown in a study in which the activity of the cilia, the microscopic hairs in the breathing tubes responsible for propelling mucus outward, increased in frogs fed coltsfoot tea.[1] When smoked, however, the plant will not work because heat will make the all-valuable mucilage disintegrate. In fact, smoking coltsfoot will probably exacerbate rather than alleviate any respiratory tract problems.[2] Inhaling vapors from leaves simmering in water will also fail—the medicinal part of the vapor will probably never reach the ailing tissue.

According to recent research, coltsfoot buds suppress a compound—a platelet-activating-factor antagonist—involved in triggering asthma attacks and other inflammatory airway diseases.[3] In a 1989 study, Chinese investigators found that coltsfoot helped reduce airway obstruction in sixty-six asthmatics.[4] Other preliminary studies indicate that another chemical—the pyrrolizidine alkaloid (PA) tussilagone—may stimulate the cardiovascular system and affect the respiratory system. Dogs injected with tussilagone in one study experienced a short but significant increase in blood pressure and started to breathe more quickly.[5] Implications for treating human disease are not clear.

German health authorities approve of using coltsfoot leaf (fresh or dried) preparations for dry coughs, hoarseness, and acute but mild mouth and throat inflammation, but remain unconvinced of the value of other applications.[6]

Will It Harm You? What the Studies Say:

Serious health risks are not usually associated with an herb tested by centuries of use, but coltsfoot may be one of the exceptions. Experts believe all parts of the herb—the flowers, the leaves, the roots—contain varying amounts of toxic pyrrolizidine alkaloids (PAs), which research indicates can damage the liver and cause liver cancer if ingested over time. More than 65 percent of rats fed relatively high concentrations of dried young coltsfoot flower (higher than 4 percent) in a Japanese study developed cancerous liver tumors.[7] In another study, cancerous liver tumors developed in two-thirds of rats fed meal containing 8 percent of the PA senkirkine over two years.[8] PAs can also cause a grave condition in which the blood vessels of the liver become dangerously narrow (hepatic veno-occlusive disease), seriously compromising the ability of this major organ to function properly.

On the basis of these findings, the FDA has classified coltsfoot as an herb of "undefined safety." Some critics are calling for an outright ban. Canadian authorities have instituted one. A number of American herbalists say it is "highly unadvisable" to use any coltsfoot preparations. In Germany, restrictions and warnings are not so stringent, probably because minimum allowable amounts of toxic PAs have been established for commercial herbs such as coltsfoot. In the United States, such precise information on PA levels is very hard to come by, which means consumers have no way of knowing the risk they are exposing themselves to.[9] German authorities point to evidence that the concentration of the alkaloids in coltsfoot tea is probably quite low.[10] But they do warn that the coltsfoot-leaf preparations should be used only as prescribed and that no one should take them for more than four to six weeks a year. The daily dose of coltsfoot tea and mixed teas should not contain more than 1 gram of PAs.[11]

Pregnant and nursing women should avoid the herb,[12] and given the potential action on the liver, some herbalists advise that people with liver disease or those who drink heavily should avoid it, as should those allergic to other members of the daisy family.

GENERAL SOURCES:

Bisset, N.G., ed. *Herbal Drugs and Phytopharmaceuticals*. Stuttgart: medpharm GmbH Scientific Publishers, 1994.

Blumenthal, M., J. Gruenwald, T. Hall, and R.S. Rister, eds. *The Complete German Commission E Monographs: Therapeutic Guide to Herbal Medicine*. Boston: Integrative Medicine Communications, 1998.

Castleman, M. *The Healing Herbs: The Ultimate Guide to the Curative Power of Nature's Medicines*. New York: Bantam Books, 1995.

Hirono, I., et al., *Journal of the National Cancer Institute*, 63 (1979): 469.

Lawrence Review of Natural Products. St. Louis: Facts and Comparisons, June 1996.

Smith, L.W., and C.C.J. Culvenor. *Journal of Natural Products (Lloydia)*, 44 (1981): 129–52.

Tyler, V.E. *Herbs of Choice: The Therapeutic Use of Phytomedicinals*. Binghamton, NY: Haworth Press/Pharmaceutical Products Press, 1994.

———. *The Honest Herbal*. Binghamton, NY: Haworth Press/Pharmaceutical Products Press, 1993.

TEXT CITATIONS:

1. W. Muller-Limmroth and H.H. Frohlich, *Fortschritte der Medizin*, 98(3) (1980): 95–101.

2. *Lawrence Review of Natural Products* (St. Louis: Facts and Comparisons, June 1996).

3. S.B. Hwang et al., *European Journal of Pharmacology*, 141(2) (1987): 269.

4. J.X. Fu, *Chung Hsi I Chieh Ho Tsa Chih*, 9(11) (1989): 658.

5. Y.P. Li and Y.M. Wang, *General Pharmacology*, 19(2) (1988): 261.

6. M. Blumenthal, J. Gruenwald, T. Hall, and R.S. Rister, eds., *The Complete German Commission E Monographs: Therapeutic Guide to Herbal Medicine* (Boston: Integrative Medicine Communications, 1998).

7. I. Hirono et al., *Gann*, 67 (1976): 125–29.

8. E. Roder et al., *Planta Medica*, 43 (1981): 99.

9. V.E. Tyler, *Herbs of Choice: The Therapeutic Use of Phytomedicinals* (Binghamton, NY: Haworth Press/Pharmaceutical Products Press, 1994).

10. F.C. Czygan, *Zeitschrift für Phytotherapie*, 4 (1983): 630.

11. Blumenthal et al., op. cit.

12. Ibid.

COMFREY

SCIENTIFIC NAME:

Symphytum officinale L., *Symphytum asperum* Lepechin, or a hybrid of these two, *Symphtum* x *uplandicum* Nym. (Russian comfrey). Family: Boraginaceae

COMMON NAMES:

Blackwort, bruisewort, common comfrey, knitback, knitbone, prickly comfrey, Russian comfrey, slippery root

RATING:

5 = Studies indicate that there is a definite health hazard to using this substance, even in recommended amounts.

What Is Comfrey?

This stout perennial has rough, hairy stems and lance-shaped leaves, and bears clusters of bell-shaped purplish to pale yellow flowers. It can be seen blooming in moist grasslands in eastern parts of North America and most of Europe from May to September. The leaves and thick root and rhizome (underground stem) are used medicinally.

Do not confuse it with the similar-appearing and highly toxic herb **Foxglove**.

What It Is Used For:

Comfrey has been used as an herbal healer since the time of the ancient Greeks, who reportedly applied it to wounds and swollen tissue around broken bones, hence the common name "knitbone." Wounds of other types were eventually treated with it as well, from sprains to bruises and burns, and ultimately internal formulations were recommended for "internal" wounds. Some herbalists continue to recommend taking comfrey internally for such ailments as digestive upset, internal bleeding and bleeding gums, bronchial congestion, and ulcerative colitis. Gargles and mouthwashes have been used to treat sore throats, bleeding gums, and hoarseness. The young shoots and leaves were even eaten as a food.[1]

Given now-well-recognized health hazards, however, most herbalists recommend limiting the use of comfrey to topical formulations for soothing and promoting speedy healing in everything from skin wounds to leg ulcers, insect bites, ulcerative lesions, bedsores, dry or chapped skin, rashes, sunburn, itchy skin, and bruises.

Forms Available Include:

- *For external use:* Compress (made with leaves or a root decoction), powder. Leaf and root extracts appear in balms, ointments, lotions, creams, salves, and cosmetics.
- *For internal use:* Decoction, infusion, tincture.

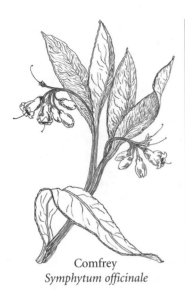

Comfrey
Symphytum officinale

Dosage Commonly Reported:

For external use, commercial ointments and other formulations are commonly available; follow the directions on the package.

Will It Work for You? What the Studies Say:

Comfrey's reputation as a wound healer probably has to do with the presence of substances called allantoin and mucilage. Allantoin promotes the growth of new cells and has recognized healing properties that have been put to work in commercial ointments for psoriasis and other skin disorders. The root contains much higher concentrations of allantoin than the leaves, although the leaves contain higher amounts of an astringent substance called tannin,[2] which helps wounds heal by constricting (tightening) tissue and reducing oozing and bleeding. Comfrey's popularity no doubt belongs in part to its high mucilage content; mucilage expands into a gooey mass when it comes into contact with liquids, softening, soothing, and protecting irritated skin and mucous membranes. Finally, animal studies have shown that the plant has significant anti-inflammatory activity, most likely due to allantoin and other ingredients.[3]

German health authorities approve of comfrey externally for treating bruises, strains, and sprains; they cite the herb's ability to inhibit inflammation and promote the formation of callus.[4]

Will It Harm You? What the Studies Say:

Many sources strongly recommend against taking comfrey because it contains pyrrolizidine alkaloids (PAs), chemicals that can cause liver damage and even promote liver cancer. The risk of this develops over time, as the effect of the PAs is cumulative.[5] There have been several documented cases of liver disease caused by comfrey. Hepato-occlusive disease, a disorder in which veins leading into the liver become blocked and starve liver tissue of oxygen, has been linked to long-term use of comfrey in several cases.[6] It was diagnosed in one woman who took a comfrey-pepsin concoction for four months,[7] and in a vegetarian who died of liver failure due to the disease after consuming comfrey as part of his diet.[8] These represent just a few of the cases reported so far.[9] Rats fed comfrey root or leaves developed signs of liver toxicity within 180 days, and liver and urinary adenomas eventually developed in all of the animals.[10] Roots caused more cancer than leaves.

Topical formulations appear to be much safer, although several sources warn that only preparations with mature leaves should be used.[11] German health authorities advise the use of comfrey for no more than four to six weeks a year.[12] They likewise warn that topical formulations should be used only on intact skin, and that it should be used during pregnancy only after consulting a doctor.[13] One study indicated that when applied to the skin of rats, comfrey alkaloids were subsequently detected in the urine, which suggests that they passed through the skin and into the body.[14] The researcher also reported detecting the toxic alkaloids in the breast milk of rats. What this means for human beings who apply the herb topically requires further examination.

Young children and pregnant or lactating women should never take comfrey.

GENERAL SOURCES:

Balch, J.F., and P.A. Balch. *Prescription for Nutritional Healing: A Practical A to Z Reference to Drug-Free Remedies Using Vitamins, Minerals, Herbs & Food Supplements.* 2nd ed. Garden City Park, NY: Avery Publishing Group, 1997.

Blumenthal, M., J. Gruenwald, T. Hall, and R.S. Rister, eds. *The Complete German Commission E Monographs: Therapeutic Guide to Herbal Medicine.* Boston: Integrative Medicine Communications, 1998.

Bradley, P.C., ed. *British Herbal Compendium: A Handbook of Scientific Information on Widely Used Plant Drugs,* vol. 1. Bournemouth (Dorset), England: British Herbal Medicine Association, 1992.

Castleman, M. *The Healing Herbs: The Ultimate Guide to the Curative Power of Nature's Medicines.* New York: Bantam Books, 1995.

Lawrence Review of Natural Products. St. Louis: Facts and Comparisons, October 1995.

Leung, A.Y., and S. Foster. *Encyclopedia of Common Natural Ingredients Used in Food, Drugs, and Cosmetics.* 2nd ed. New York: John Wiley & Sons, 1996.

Mindell, E. *Earl Mindell's Herb Bible.* New York: Simon & Schuster/Fireside, 1992.

Newall, C.A., et al., *Herbal Medicines: A Guide for Health-Care Professionals.* London: The Pharmaceutical Press, 1996.

Stary, F. *The Natural Guide to Medicinal Herbs and Plants.* Prague: Barnes & Noble, Inc. in arrangement with Aventinum Publishers, 1996.

Tierra, M. *The Way of Herbs.* New York: Pocket Books, 1990.

Tyler, V.E. *Herbs of Choice: The Therapeutic Use of Phytomedicinals.* Binghamton, NY: Haworth Press/Pharmaceutical Products Press, 1994.

————. *The Honest Herbal.* Binghamton, NY: Haworth Press/Pharmaceutical Products Press, 1993.

Weiss, R.F. *Herbal Medicine,* trans. A. R. Meuss, from the 6th German edition. Beaconsfield, England: Beaconsfield Publishers, Ltd., 1988.

TEXT CITATIONS:

1. A.Y. Leung and S. Foster, *Encyclopedia of Common Natural Ingredients Used in Food, Drugs, and Cosmetics,* 2nd ed. (New York: John Wiley & Sons, 1996).

2. V.E. Tyler, *The Honest Herbal* (Binghamton, NY: Haworth Press/Pharmaceutical Products Press, 1993).

3. N. Mascolo et al., *Phytotherapy Research,* 1 (1987): 28–31. *Lawrence Review of Natural Products* (St. Louis: Facts and Comparisons, October 1995).

4. M. Blumenthal, J. Gruenwald, T. Hall, and R.S. Rister, eds., *The Complete German Commission E Monographs: Therapeutic Guide to Herbal Medicine* (Boston: Integrative Medicine Communications, 1998).

5. K.S. Winship, *Adverse Drug Reactions and Toxicological Reviews,* 10 (1991): 47–59.

6. P.M. Ridker and W.V. McDermott, *The Lancet,* I (1989): 657–58. R.J. Huxtable et al., *New England Journal of Medicine,* 315 (1986): 1095.

7. P.M. Ridker et al., *Gastroenterology,* 88 (1985): 1050.

8. M.L. Yeong et al., *Journal of Gastroenterology and Hepatology,* 5(2) (1990): 211.

9. *Lawrence Review of Natural Products,* op. cit.

10. I. Hirono et al., *Journal of the National Cancer Institute,* 61(5) (1978): 865–69.

11. V.E. Tyler, *Herbs of Choice: The Therapeutic Use of Phytomedicinals* (Binghamton, NY: Haworth Press/Pharmaceutical Products Press, 1994).

12. Blumenthal et al., op. cit.

13. Ibid.

14. R. Schoenta, *Toxicology Letters,* 10 (1982): 323.

CORIANDER

SCIENTIFIC NAME:
Coriandrum sativum L. Family: Umbelliferae (Apiaceae)

COMMON NAMES:
Chinese parsley, cilantro

RATING:
2 = According to a number of well-designed studies and common use, this substance appears to be relatively effective and safe when used in recommended amounts for the indication(s) noted in the "Will It Work for You?" section.

What Is Coriander?

Coriander refers to the small ribbed brown fruit ("seeds") of the delicate, bright green *Coriandrum sativum*; its leaves are best known as cilantro or Chinese parsley. Both the seeds and the leaves are used medicinally, as is an essential oil extracted from the seeds. The strong-smelling, flowering annual is widely cultivated in the United States and other countries.

What It Is Used For:

Coriander is used primarily as a culinary herb. The warm, spicy fragrance and flavor of the dried ripe fruit (as opposed to the "bedbug" smell of the unripe fruit and herb) have long been celebrated in digestive liqueurs and spirits, and the essential oil is widely used as a flavoring. Contemporary herbalists also carry on a tradition, thousands of years old in some parts of the world, of recommending coriander seed preparations to stimulate a flagging appetite, ease indigestion, fight diarrhea, and relieve gas pains. Traditional Chinese healers have used the seeds—and in certain cases the whole herb—as a digestive aid as well as a remedy for dysentery, hemorrhoids, measles, toothaches, bad breath, unwanted female genital odors, and nausea.[1] Seed preparations have been used externally to prevent wound infections and added to rubs and salves to reduce muscle and joint pains. The many other folk applications for coriander around the world from southeast Asia to the Middle East include use as an aphrodisiac, nerve pain remedy, worm-killer, fever-reducer, and eyewash.

Forms Available Include:

Decoction, infusion, liquid extract, seed (crushed, powdered, whole).

Dosage Commonly Reported:

A decoction is made using 1 to 2 teaspoons bruised or crushed seeds per cup of water and is drunk up to three times per day between meals. The liquid extract is taken in doses of 0.5 to 2 milliliters, and the powder in doses of 0.3 to 1 gram.

Will It Work for You? What the Studies Say:

An enormous amount of research has been done on coriander, particularly in the test tube. But the implications for treating human disease are for the most part still quite unclear. Perhaps most convincing are findings indicating effectiveness in treating stomach upset. The seeds contain small amounts (about 0.4 to 1 percent) of an aromatic volatile oil that explains why a tea made with the seeds has for so long been used to help relieve gas and settle an upset stomach, albeit mildly. German health authorities officially approve of seed preparations for indigestion and related complaints, including appetite loss.[2] The leaves also contain the volatile oil, but less than the seeds.

Researchers have found a rich supply of other biologically active constituents, including vitamins and minerals, in the herb's seeds and to a lesser extent in its leaves.[3] Extensive test-tube experiments in laboratories worldwide indicate that the essential oil fights certain fungi,[4] bacteria,[5] and larvae (weakly), and has smooth-muscle-relaxant activity in rabbits[6] and antiswelling actions in mice.[7] These findings may help explain why people in different parts of the globe instinctively turned to coriander for such infectious conditions as dysentery, for example.

Similarly, more advanced research in small animals such as dogs indicates that coriander may have blood-sugar-lowering, blood-pressure-reducing, antiinflammatory, contraceptive (anti-implantation),[8] and antimutagenic (meaning it inhibits potentially cancerous cell changes)[9] properties. A study of the dried seed in humans indicated a diuretic ("water pill") effect,[10] and animal experiments suggest that this property can be quite strong.[11] Overall, however, none of these actions has been well studied in humans and it is hard to say whether any will actually translate into reliable or effective treatment. To confuse matters, some research findings are contradictory.

Will It Harm You? What the Studies Say:

Coriander poses little apparent risk of an adverse reaction when used in typically recommended amounts. According to studies done so far, it does not cause any adverse reactions or pose particular hazards for people with other medical conditions,[12] although allergic reactions and in some cases sun-sensitivity reactions are a risk for some.[13] The FDA considers coriander generally safe to use as a food.

GENERAL SOURCES:

Bisset, N.G., ed. *Herbal Drugs and Phytopharmaceuticals*. Stuttgart: medpharm GmbH Scientific Publishers, 1994.

Blumenthal, M., J. Gruenwald, T. Hall, and R.S. Rister, eds. *The Complete German Commission E Monographs: Therapeutic Guide to Herbal Medicine*. Boston: Integrative Medicine Communications, 1998.

Castleman, M. *The Healing Herbs: The Ultimate Guide to the Curative Power of Nature's Medicines*. New York: Bantam Books, 1995.

Farnsworth, N.R., and A.B. Seligman. *Tile and Till*. 57 (1971): 52.

Heinerman, J. *Heinerman's Encyclopedia of Healing Herbs and Spices*. West Nyack, NY: Parker Publishing Co., 1996.

Leung, A.Y. *Chinese Healing Foods and Herbs*. Glen Rock, NJ: AYSL Corp, 1984.

Leung, A.Y., and S. Foster. *Encyclopedia of Common Natural Ingredients Used in Food, Drugs, and Cosmetics*. 2nd ed. New York: John Wiley & Sons, 1996.

Mascolo, N., et al. *Phototherapy Research*. 1 (1987): 28.

Stary, F. *The Natural Guide to Medicinal Herbs and Plants*. Prague: Barnes & Noble, Inc. in arrangement with Aventinum Publishers, 1996.

Tyler, V.E. *Herbs of Choice: The Therapeutic Use of Phytomedicinals*. Binghamton, NY: Haworth Press/Pharmaceutical Products Press, 1994.

Weiss, R.F. *Herbal Medicine*, trans. A. R. Meuss, from the 6th German edition. Beaconsfield, England: Beaconsfield Publishers, Ltd., 1988.

TEXT CITATIONS:

1. A.Y. Leung and S. Foster, *Encyclopedia of Common Natural Ingredients Used in Food, Drugs, and Cosmetics*, 2nd ed. (New York: John Wiley & Sons, 1996).

2. M. Blumenthal, J. Gruenwald, T. Hall, and R.S. Rister, eds., *The Complete German Commission E Monographs: Therapeutic Guide to Herbal Medicine* (Boston: Integrative Medicine Communications, 1998).

3. Leung and Foster, op. cit.

4. S.K. Sharma and V.P. Singh, *Indian Drugs and Pharmaceuticals Industry*, 14(1) (1979): 3–6.

5. M.R. Meena and V. Sethi, *Journal of Food Science Technology*, 31(1) (1994): 68–70.

6. D. Mehin et al., *Acta Pharmaceutica Hungarica*, 56(3) (1986): 109–13.

7. K. Yasukawa et al., *Phytotherapy Research*, 7(2) (1993): 185–89.

8. M.S. Al-Said et al., *Journal of Ethnopharmacology*, 21(2) (1987): 165–73.

9. W. Goggelmann and O. Schimmer, *Mutation Research*, 12(3/4) (1983): 191–94.

10. M. Udupihille and M.T.M. Jiffry, *Indian Journal of Physiology and Pharmacology*, 30(1) (1986): 91–97.

11. A. Caceres et al., *Journal of Ethnopharmacology*, 19(3) (1987): 233–45.

12. Blumenthal et al., op. cit.

13. N.G. Bisset, ed., *Herbal Drugs and Phytopharmaceuticals* (Stuttgart: medpharm GmbH Scientific Publishers, 1994). K. Seetharam and J.S. Pasricha, *Indian Journal of Dermatology, Venereology and Leprology*, 53(6) (1987): 325–28.

PRIMARY NAME:

CORN SILK

SCIENTIFIC NAME:

Zea mays L. Family: Gramineae

COMMON NAME:

In China, referred to as *Stigmata maydis*, yu mi xu

RATING:

4 = Research indicates that this substance will not fulfill the claims made for it, but that it is also unlikely to cause any harm.

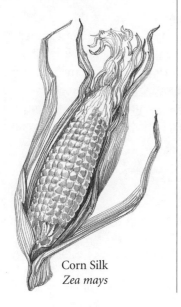

Corn Silk
Zea mays

What Is Corn Silk?

The fine silk, or tassel, of the seedhead (popularly called an ear) of this universally recognized annual grass is used medicinally.

What It Is Used For:

Modern Western herbalists carry on a long-standing folk tradition in recommending corn silk tea as a diuretic ("water pill") to reduce inflammation and painful symptoms related to urinary tract infections, cystitis, bladder stones, prostate disorders, premenstrual syndrome, fluid retention, obesity, gout, dropsy, rheumatism, and various other disorders. It was once quite popular for treating gonorrhea. Corn silk's popularity as a diuretic endures in parts of Europe, Asia, and other regions of the world.

Forms Available Include:

Extract, infusion (of fresh or dried silk), tincture.

Dosage Commonly Reported:

An infusion made using 1 teaspoon corn silk per cup of water is drunk several times per day. Commercially prepared liquid corn silk extract or tincture is taken according to package directions.

Will It Work for You? What the Studies Say:

Corn silk's diuretic properties have not been well investigated. The one study that appears in the recent literature—a 1992 Vietnamese trial—calls its effectiveness into question.[1] As one of four traditional Vietnamese diuretics tested in the placebo-controlled, double-blind study, corn silk failed to influence twelve- and twenty-four-hour urine output. Without a diuretic action, corn silk cannot be expected to alleviate many of the ailments for which people have been using it, such as fluid retention.

Will It Harm You? What the Studies Say:

No reports of serious adverse reactions can be found in the medical literature. Given how much remains unknown about corn silk's diuretic action, however, people with kidney problems may want to avoid it.

GENERAL SOURCES:

Balch, J.F., and P.A. Balch. *Prescription for Nutritional Healing: A Practical A to Z Reference to Drug-Free Remedies Using Vitamins, Minerals, Herbs & Food Supplements.* 2nd ed. Garden City Park, NY: Avery Publishing Group, 1997.

Foster, S., and J.A. Duke. *The Peterson Field Guide Series: A Field Guide to Medicinal Plants. Eastern and Central North America.* Boston: Houghton Mifflin Company, 1990.

Mowrey, D.B. *Proven Herbal Blends: A Rational Approach to Prevention and Remedy.* (Condensed from *The Scientific Validation of Herbal Medicine.*) New Canaan, CT: Keats Publishing, Inc., 1986.

Tierra, M. *The Way of Herbs.* New York: Pocket Books, 1990.

Weiner, M.A., and J.A. Weiner. *Herbs That Heal: Prescription for Herbal Healing.* Mill Valley, CA: Quantum Books, 1994.

TEXT CITATIONS:

1. D.D. Doan et al., *Journal of Ethnopharmacology*, 36(3) (1992): 225–31.

PRIMARY NAME:

COUCH GRASS

SCIENTIFIC NAME:

Agropyron repens (L.) Beauv., sometimes referred to as *Elymus repens* (L.) Gould or *Triticum repens* L. Family: Poaceae

COMMON NAMES:

Dog grass, quack grass, wheat grass, witchgrass

RATING:

3 = Studies on the effectiveness and safety of this substance are conflicting, or there are not enough studies to draw a conclusion.

What Is Couch Grass?

This vigorous and unwelcome weed introduced from Europe years ago has spread to the central and northern parts of the United States and to Canada. Spikelets with tiny, single purplish flowers bloom on this coarse grass from May to September. The slender, yellow-white rhizomes (underground stems), roots, and short pieces of the stem are used medicinally.

What It Is Used For:

Cattle eagerly consume the nutritious underground stems of this plant, as do humans when desperate for a coffee or flour substitute in times of famine.[1] As a folk medicine, couch grass tea has long been recommended as a diuretic ("water pill") for such urinary tract ailments as cystitis, prostate inflammation, and kidney and bladder stones. The other primary folk use for couch grass has been as a cough remedy and bronchial decongestant, and less commonly for skin conditions, gout, and rheumatic disorders. Most sources ascribe soothing, demulcent properties to the herb.

Forms Available Include:

Decoction, infusion, root.

Dosage Commonly Reported:

A decoction is made using 2 to 3 teaspoons finely chopped root and is drunk up to four times per day.

Will It Work for You? What the Studies Say:

Little research has been published on this herb's medicinal potential. Scientists know that it contains a substance called mucilage, which swells when it comes into contact with liquid, creating a gooey mass that coats and protects the lining of the delicate mucous membranes that can get so raw and inflamed with a cough or bronchial irritation. For this reason, its traditional use for cough and even for chronic skin conditions may be justified. However, no studies appear to have been done to test couch grass's effectiveness for these disorders.

Apparently on the basis of common experience more than extensive testing, a number of sources cite the ability of infusions and other drinks made with couch grass to exert a mild but pronounced diuretic action, slightly increasing the output of urine. Some sources attribute this action to the presence of substances called saponins.[2] German health authorities endorse the use of couch grass for increasing urination and thus reducing urinary tract inflammation.[3] They also consider it valuable for preventing kidney stones; increased irrigation of the kidneys is thought to aid this disorder.

The plant's essential oil also fights certain bacteria, but what this means for its medicinal value is unclear.

Will It Harm You? What the Studies Say:

Scientists have not learned much about the potential toxicity of couch grass, although its history as a cattle fodder and famine food point to a relatively benign safety profile. German health authorities cite no known side effects or known interactions with other medicines, although they do warn that extra fluids should be taken while on a diuretic such as this.[4] They also advise that such diuretics should not be used in cases of edema (swelling) caused by heart or kidney insufficiency.

GENERAL SOURCES:

Bisset, N.G., ed. *Herbal Drugs and Phytopharmaceuticals.* Stuttgart: medpharm GmbH Scientific Publishers, 1994.

Blumenthal, M., J. Gruenwald, T. Hall, and R.S. Rister, eds. *The Complete German Commission E Monographs: Therapeutic Guide to Herbal Medicine.* Boston: Integrative Medicine Communications, 1998.

Dobelis, I.N., ed. *The Magic and Medicine of Plants: A Practical Guide to the Science, History, Folklore, and Everyday Uses of Medicinal Plants.* Pleasantville, NY: Reader's Digest Association, 1986.

Weiner, M.A., and J.A. Weiner. *Herbs That Heal: Prescription for Herbal Healing.* Mill Valley, CA: Quantum Books, 1994.

Weiss, R.F. *Herbal Medicine,* trans. A.R. Meuss, from the 6th German edition. Beaconsfield, England: Beaconsfield Publishers, Ltd., 1988.

TEXT CITATIONS:

1. I.N. Dobelis, ed., *The Magic and Medicine of Plants: A Practical Guide to the Science, History, Folklore, and Everyday Uses of Medicinal Plants* (Pleasantville, NY: Reader's Digest Association, 1986).

2. R.F. Weiss, *Herbal Medicine,* trans. A.R. Meuss, from the 6th German edition (Beaconsfield, England: Beaconsfield Publishers, Ltd., 1988).

3. M. Blumenthal, J. Gruenwald, T. Hall, and R.S. Rister, eds., *The Complete German Commission E Monographs: Therapeutic Guide to Herbal Medicine* (Boston: Integrative Medicine Communications, 1998).

4. Ibid.

PRIMARY NAME:
COWSLIP, EUROPEAN

SCIENTIFIC NAME:
Primula veris L., sometimes referred to as *Primula officinalis* (L.) Hill. Family: Primulaceae

COMMON NAMES:
Cowslip, fairy cup, keyflower, key of heaven, paigle, primrose

RATING:
3 = Studies on the effectiveness and safety of this substance are conflicting, or there are not enough studies to draw a conclusion.

What Is European Cowslip?

The dried roots and rhizomes (underground stems) as well as the sweet-smelling, golden yellow flowers that grow in clusters hanging off the stalk of this perennial are used medicinally. The plant is native to Eurasia but now grows in many parts of the world including temperate regions of North America.

What It Is Used For:

A tea made from the cowslip flower has long been appreciated in Europe as a mild sedative for anxiety-related sleeplessness, restlessness, nervous excitability, and headache. Herbalists commonly recommend the flowers and root as expectorants for clearing congestion related to colds, coughs, bronchitis, and other bronchopulmonary disorders. A skin-cleansing lotion prepared with the flowers is quite popular in some places. The flowers have also been ascribed painkilling, laxative, heart tonic, and mild diuretic ("water pill") properties, while the roots have traditionally been used to treat asthma, whooping cough, nerve-related problems (neuralgia), and gout.

Forms Available Include:

Infusion, dried flowers, liquid extract, syrup, tincture. Appears in herbal tea mixtures and extracts for cough and congestion.

Dosage Commonly Reported:

The dried flowers are taken in the form of an infusion in doses of 1 to 2 grams, three times a day. The liquid extract is taken in doses of 1 to 2 milliliters three times a day.

Will It Work for You? What the Studies Say:

Science has revealed relatively little about the chemical makeup and pharmacologic properties of cowslip. It contains tannins, which are astringent and may explain the herb's traditional use in skin creams, although the tannin content is quite low. Astringents aid skin healing by constricting tissue and reducing oozing and bleeding if it is present.

Constituents called saponins have been reported in the roots but not the flowers. These saponins have been shown to have an interesting effect in anesthetized laboratory animals: an initial lowering of blood pressure followed by a long-lasting rise in blood pressure.[1] They also show slight anti-inflammatory, analgesic, and antigranulation (antiscar-formation and antiwound-healing) properties in test-tube studies.[2] Constituents called flavonoids are typically recognized as exerting antispasmodic and anti-inflammatory effects. The actions of these ingredients as they appear in cowslip in particular have never been tested in humans, however.

The one property of saponins that appears to be widely accepted is the ability to help liquefy and loosen sticky secretions and thus encourage clearing of congestion in coughs, colds, and other respiratory disorders. German health authorities approve of both flower and root preparations for treating respiratory tract congestion, recommending that an infusion of the flowers in particular be drunk as hot as possible to achieve the desired effect.

Will It Harm You? What the Studies Say:

Science has revealed relatively little about the potential toxicity of cowslip. The saponins—detected only in root preparations—may irritate the stomach and intestines. Both stomach upset and nausea develop in some people.[3] Given animal-study findings indicating that the saponins affect blood pressure, individuals with blood pressure problems may want to avoid root preparations.[4] Contact dermatitis with skin reddening and blistering has also occurred after direct (skin) contact with the flowers.[5]

GENERAL SOURCES:

Bisset, N.G., ed. *Herbal Drugs and Phytopharmaceuticals.* Stuttgart: medpharm GmbH Scientific Publishers, 1994.

Dobelis, I.N., ed. *The Magic and Medicine of Plants: A Practical Guide to the Science, History, Folklore, and Everyday Uses of Medicinal Plants.* Pleasantville, NY: Reader's Digest Association, 1986.

Newall, C.A., et al. *Herbal Medicines: A Guide for Health-Care Professionals.* London: The Pharmaceutical Press, 1996.

TEXT CITATIONS:

1. B. Cebo et al., *Herba Polonica,* 22 (1976): 154–62. C.A. Newall et al., *Herbal Medicines: A Guide for Health-Care Professionals* (London: The Pharmaceutical Press, 1996).
2. Cebo, op. cit.
3. N.G. Bisset, ed., *Herbal Drugs and Phytopharmaceuticals* (Stuttgart: medpharm GmbH Scientific Publishers, 1994).
4. Newall, op. cit.
5. B.M. Hausen, *Archives of Dermatology Research,* 261 (1978): 311–21.

PRIMARY NAME:

CRAMP BARK

SCIENTIFIC NAME:
Viburnum opulus L. Family: Caprifoliaceae

COMMON NAMES:
Guelder rose, highbush cranberry, pembina, pimbina, snowball tree, whitten tree

What Is Cramp Bark?

The bark of this North American shrub or tree is used medicinally. Its seasonal white flowers, lobed leaves, and bright red oval fruit ("berries") may have been used at one time as well. It also grows in parts of Europe.

What It Is Used For:

Native American tribes in the Northeast reportedly used the bark and leaves of *Viburnum opulus* as a diuretic ("water pill") and to treat swollen glands, mumps, and eye disorders.[1] The *National Formulary* listed it as an antispasmodic for asthma and a sedative for nervous conditions for many years. A number of contemporary herbalists advocate these uses, and some continue a practice begun in the mid-1800s of recommending the aptly named cramp bark for menstrual cramps and other uterine discomforts, and to reduce the risk of miscarriage. Many also consider it useful for spasm-related conditions such as colic and muscle tension.

Forms Available Include:

Decoction, lotion, tincture. Cramp bark often appears in herbal blends.

Dosage Commonly Reported:

The tincture is taken in dosages of 1 teaspoon with water up to three times per day. It is also used as a rub. A decoction is made with 15 grams bark per 750 milliliters of water.

Will It Work for You? What the Studies Say:

Limited scientific data are available to determine the value of cramp bark for any ailment. Many herbalists cite the findings of researchers at the University of Louisville School of Medicine, who conducted a series of experiments in the 1960s and early 1970s showing that alcoholic and water extracts of the bark could counteract spasms and relax an artificially stimulated rat uterus placed in a chemical bath, probably owing to substances identified as scopoletin and viopudial.[2] While intriguing, these findings fall far short of proving that cramp bark will ease discomfort associated with uterine cramping in humans or in any way prevent a miscarriage.

The Louisville team also reported that viopudial (and possibly other components) could lower blood pressure, slow the heartbeat, and decrease the contractile strength of the heart muscle in laboratory rats, cats, and dogs,[3] possibly explaining—but again, not proving—the bark's traditional use as an antispasmodic and calming agent. Cramp bark also contains small amounts of astringent tannins.

Will It Harm You? What the Studies Say:

There is no way to determine conclusively the health risks involved in taking cramp bark preparations, given the lack of research on the herb. However, no reports of serious adverse reactions to the bark appear in recent medical literature. Because of its possible effects on the uterus and heart, however, pregnant women and people with heart conditions may want to take the findings of the Louisville researchers into account.

GENERAL SOURCES:

Balch, J.F., and P.A. Balch. *Prescription for Nutritional Healing: A Practical A to Z Reference to Drug-Free Remedies Using Vitamins, Minerals, Herbs & Food Supplements.* 2nd ed. Garden City Park, NY: Avery Publishing Group, 1997.

Chevallier, A. *The Encyclopedia of Medicinal Plants: A Practical Reference Guide to More Than 550 Key Medicinal Plants & Their Uses.* 1st American ed. New York: Dorling Kindersley Publications, 1996.

Tierra, M. *The Way of Herbs.* New York: Pocket Books, 1990.

TEXT CITATIONS:

1. J.A. Nicholson et al., *Proceedings of the Society of Experimental Biology and Medicine.* 140(2) (1972): 457–61.
2. C.H. Jarboe et al., *Nature,* 212 (1966): 837. J.A. Nicholson et al., op. cit. C.H. Jarboe et al., *Journal of Medical Chemistry,* 10 (1967): 488.
3. Nicholson, op. cit.

CRANBERRY

SCIENTIFIC NAME:
Vaccinium macrocarpon Ait.
Family: Ericaceae

COMMON NAME:
Trailing swamp cranberry

RATING:
1 = Years of use and extensive, high-quality studies indicate that this substance is very effective and safe when used in recommended amounts for the indication(s) noted in the "Will It Work for You?" section.

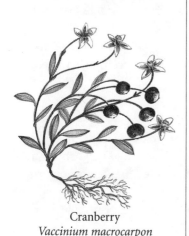

Cranberry
Vaccinium macrocarpon

What Is Cranberry?

Cranberry is the well-known red acidic fruit or berry of a small evergreen shrub. A number of species are cultivated throughout the United States, especially in Washington and Massachusetts. The medicinal part of cranberry is the juice from the berries.

What It Is Used For:

More than a century ago, American Indians consumed crushed cranberries to prevent and treat urinary tract infections. Many women around the country subsequently turned to this home remedy, often drinking cranberries in the form of a cranberry cocktail. Even today, long after the introduction of antibiotics capable of eradicating the bacteria responsible for this common and often chronic condition, many women still swear by this remedy. Some women also drink cranberry juice to treat inflammation of the urinary bladder, known as cystitis. The juice is also reported to help deodorize urine.

Forms Available Include:

Berry, capsule, juice (available in many forms, including unsweetened and in cranberry juice cocktail). A 90-milliliter glass of cranberry juice cocktail, which consists of about one-third pure juice, is reportedly equivalent to six capsules of dried cranberry powder.[1]

Dosage Commonly Reported:

To prevent urinary tract infections, 3 fluid ounces (90 milliliters) cranberry juice cocktail or the equivalent is drunk daily. To treat an existing infection, 12 to 32 ounces is drunk daily. Two to four 505 milligrams (fruit) capsules each are taken three times a day for infections.

Will It Work for You? What the Studies Say:

Many doctors, most herbalists, and countless women who suffer from recurrent urinary tract infections believe that cranberry juice effectively prevents urinary tract infections. Disagreement about how much is necessary to achieve this effect persists, however, and some skeptics say more randomized clinical trials need to be done before a definitive statement can be made.[2] Many of the earlier studies were small and inconsistent and did not involve women without urinary tract infections for comparison. Also, some of the studies may have been tainted by reliance on urine that had been freely voided, for example, rather than taken directly from the urinary tract, where vaginal bacteria would not corrupt the specimen.

No one is exactly sure how cranberry works. Scientists first took a good look at cranberries as a urinary-tract-infection remedy in the early 1920s when a team discovered that the urine of subjects who drank a lot of cranberry juice cocktail became more acidic.[3] In theory, this would make the urinary tract inhospitable to bacteria, which flourish in alkaline environments. Recent research indicates that the benefits are more likely due to cranberry's ability to make the urinary tract unfavorable to these bacteria in another way: by inhibiting them from sticking to the wall of the bladder, so that they simply get flushed out before they can do any damage.[4]

An important 1994 study reported in the *Journal of the American Medical Association* found that cranberry juice was more effective in treating than preventing urinary bacterial infections.[5] It was also notable for being the first placebo-controlled, large-scale clinical trial to show that cranberry juice does in fact reduce bacteria levels in the urine as well as the attendant influx of white blood cells to fight the infection. Of the 153 elderly women given a placebo to drink every day over six months, far fewer experienced a reduction in these levels compared with those who drank 300 milliliters of cranberry juice cocktail a day. These and other findings indicate that the old remedy probably does work, although critics of the study are not hard to find.[6] Currently, the *U.S. Pharmacopeia* lists cranberry juice as an effective remedy for preventing urinary tract infections.

Recent findings suggest that cranberry juice can affect urine in another way as well: it can lessen the urinary odor of incontinent individuals by slowing the activity of bacteria (*Escherichia coli* in particular) that contribute to it, primarily by reducing the urine's acidity.[7] A 6-ounce glass of cranberry juice twice a day may also reduce the risk of urinary stone recurrence and relieve symptoms of chronic kidney infection (pyelonephritis), at least according to anecdotal reports.[8]

Will It Harm You? What the Studies Say:

No problems have been reported with the use of cranberry juice for medicinal purposes. Of course, some people may be allergic to it, and pregnant or nursing women and people taking medications that affect the kidney or urinary tract should talk to their doctors before using cranberry juice as medicine. Drinking very large amounts of the juice may cause diarrhea and stomach upset.[9] Most important, no one should self-medicate a urinary tract infection; antibiotics are almost always warranted. Left untreated, a urinary tract infection can cause serious complications.

GENERAL SOURCES:

American Pharmaceutical Association. *Handbook of Nonprescription Drugs.* 11th ed. Washington, D.C.: American Pharmaceutical Association, 1996.

Castleman, M. *The Healing Herbs: The Ultimate Guide to the Curative Power of Nature's Medicines.* New York: Bantam Books, 1995.

Lawrence Review of Natural Products. St. Louis: Facts and Comparisons, July 1994.

Nursing Times. 87(48) (1991): 36–37.

Tyler, V.E. *Herbs of Choice: The Therapeutic Use of Phytomedicinals.* Binghamton, NY: Haworth Press/Pharmaceutical Products Press, 1994.

———. *The Honest Herbal.* Binghamton, NY: Haworth Press/Pharmaceutical Products Press, 1993.

TEXT CITATIONS:

1. V.E. Tyler, *Herbs of Choice.: The Therapeutic Use of Phytomedicinals* (Binghamton, NY: Haworth Press/Pharmaceutical Products Press, 1994).

2. W.J. Hopkins et al., *Journal of the American Medical Association* (Letter), 272(8) (1994): 588–89.
3. N.R. Blatherwich and M.L. Long, *Journal of Biological Chemistry*, 57 (1923): 815–18.
4. I. Ofek et al., *New England Journal of Medicine*, 324 (1991): 1599. M.S. Soloway and R.A. Smith, *Journal of the American Medical Association*, 260 (1988): 1465. A.E. Sabota, *Journal of Urology*, 131 (1984): 1013–16.
5. J. Avor et al., *Journal of the American Medical Association*, 271 (1994): 751.
6. R. Goodfriend, *Journal of the American Medical Association*, 72(8) (1992): 588.
7. *Lawrence Review of Natural Products* (St. Louis: Facts and Comparisons, July 1994).
8. Ibid. H.H. Zinsser et al., *New York State Journal of Medicine*, 68 (1968): 3001.
9. *Lawrence Review of Natural Products*, op. cit.

PRIMARY NAME:

CUCUMBER, CHINESE

SCIENTIFIC NAME:

Trichosanthes kirilowii Maxim.
Family: Cucurbitaceae

COMMON NAMES:

Chinese snake gourd, compound Q, gua-lou, tian-hya-fen

RATING:

3 = Studies on the effectiveness and safety of this substance are conflicting, or there are not enough studies to draw a conclusion. Safety is a major concern, however; see the "Will It Harm You?" section.

What Is Chinese Cucumber?

Many parts of this plant, a member of the gourd family, have been used for centuries in traditional Chinese medicine. Other *Trichosanthes* species are occasionally used as well. Do not confuse Chinese cucumber with the common green cucumber (*Cucumis sativus*) found in American supermarkets. The fruit, peel, stems, seeds, and root of the Chinese cucumber are used medicinally. "Compound Q" appears to refer to one of two trichosanthins (ribosome-inactivating proteins): alpha-trichosanthin.[1]

What It Is Used For:

Traditional Chinese healers have relied on *Trichosanthes kirilowii* preparations for centuries to treat fever, constipation, cough and congestion, and inflammation, among other things. In China, a specially prepared root extract called trichosanthin (a protein) has been used to induce abortions in early pregnancy, treat diabetes, fight certain kinds of tumors, and help regulate the immune system. Scientists are carefully examining whether a highly purified form of trichosanthin, GLQ-223, can benefit HIV-infected individuals.

Forms Available Include:

Not for home use.

Dosage Commonly Reported:

Not for home use.

Will It Work for You? What the Studies Say:

Test-tube and animal studies indicate that certain Chinese cucumber extracts—and particularly trichosanthin—have wide-ranging biological and pharmacological abilities,[2] including an ability to inhibit blood sugar increases in rats (possibly valuable for treating diabetes),[3] kill (or inhibit) certain tumor cells (including melanoma cells),[4] fight certain bacteria,[5] and inhibit (suppress) inflammation.[6] Their capacity to modify aspects of immune system activity has sparked interest in testing for treatment of diseases such as systemic lupus erythematosus, HIV infection and AIDS, and even some types of lymphoma and leukemia.[7]

Clinical trials to determine whether trichosanthin's (or GLQ-223's) power to inhibit replication of the HIV virus in the test tube extends to infected humans are under way in the United States, with mixed results so far. A 1989 study sparked intense interest in the subject: GLQ-223 appeared to stop the virus from replicating in monocytes and macrophages in blood samples drawn from three HIV-infected individuals.[8] The blood was exposed to GLQ-233 for three hours, and the effect lasted at least five days. Significantly, it also killed HIV-infected macrophages, but not uninfected ones.

A 1994 trial in HIV-infected individuals, some who had AIDS and in whom antiretroviral treatment was failing, found that trichosanthin therapy significantly increased the concentration of important immune system cells (CD4+ T lymphocytes) in the eighty-five patients whose condition was ultimately evaluated. However, fevers, muscle pain, liver changes, anaphylactic (mild to moderate) reactions, and mental changes developed in some of the subjects.[9] A 1992 European trial of twenty individuals found evidence that trichosanthin therapy could reduce viral activity and improve certain symptoms in asymptomatic but HIV-positive individuals as well as in those who had started to show signs of AIDS.[10] Subjects with advanced disease did not respond as well.

Critics continue to question the value of this highly toxic substance for HIV infection and AIDS. Much remains to be learned about trichosanthin's capacity to fight the virus and the disease, including which formulations may be effective (an oral form may have no impact at all), and whether there is any safe way to use the compound in humans. In 1991, researchers reported finding another protein in *Trichosanthes kirilowii*, TAP 29, with anti-HIV properties that, according to the authors, may be stronger and safer for treating HIV infection and AIDS.[11]

Numerous chemical, animal, and human studies confirm the ability of trichosanthin—the active principle in the plant's root—to induce abortion. A 1995 report from China describes a 90 percent success rate in terminating tubal pregnancies in twenty women.[12] The extract's enormous health hazards require its use to be carefully monitored by a qualified medical professional. Only certain forms and extracts are effective at particular stages of pregnancy.[13]

Will It Harm You? What the Studies Say:

Careful administration by a qualified medical professional is required, owing to the potential for severe and even fatal reactions to extracts of Chinese cucumber, especially when administered by injection or intravenously. Trichosanthin can cause bleeding in the brain, heart damage, and other complications. Coma and various neurological problems have developed in HIV-infected patients who had no neurologic symptoms before taking trichosanthin, and there is evidence that individuals who already have disease-related dementia may experience a deterioration in their neurologic condition.[14] Pregnant women should never take Chinese cucumber in any form, given the evidence that it can cause birth defects (in mice)[15] and terminate pregnancies at certain stages. Women injected with trichosanthin to induce abortion often become very sensitized to the extract and can experience severe and even fatal allergic reactions to the herb more than a decade after the first exposure. Flulike symptoms, seizure, and coma can also develop. Trichosanthin may be toxic to liver cells, according to a 1994 test-tube rat study.[16]

GENERAL SOURCES:

Balch, J.F., and P.A. Balch. *Prescription for Nutritional Healing: A Practical A to Z Reference to Drug-Free Remedies Using Vitamins, Minerals, Herbs & Food Supplements.* 2nd ed. Garden City Park, NY: Avery Publishing Group, 1997.

Lawrence Review of Natural Products. St. Louis: Facts and Comparisons, April 1990.

Leung, A.Y. *Chinese Healing Foods and Herbs.* Glen Rock, NJ: AYSL Corp, 1984.

Shaw, P.C., et al. *Life Sciences.* 55(4) (1994): 253–62.

Tang, W., and G. Eisenbrand. *Chinese Drugs of Plant Origin: Chemistry, Pharmacology, and Use in Traditional and Modern Medicine.* Berlin: Springer-Verlag, 1992.

TEXT CITATIONS:

1. *Lawrence Review of Natural Products* (St. Louis: Facts and Comparisons, April 1990).
2. P. Shaw et al., *Life Sciences*, 55(4) (1994): 253–62.
3. Y.B. Chung and C.C. Lee, *Yakhak Hoechi*, 39(5) (1995): 528–34.
4. R. Zhang et al., *Zhongguo Miznyixue Zazhi*, 9(6) (1993): 348–51. S.H. Lee et al., *Archives of Pharmacologic Research*, 17(5) (1994): 348–53. H. Qiu et al., *Shengwu Huaxue Yu Shengwu Wuli Xuebao*, 25(1) (1993): 39–43.
5. M. Harit and P.S. Rathee, *Asian Journal of Chemistry*, 7(4) (1995): 909–11.
6. T. Akihisa et al., *Chemical and Pharmaceutical Bulletin*, 42(5) (1994): 1101–6.
7. L.Q. Bi et al., *Chung-Kuo Chung Hsi I Chieh Ho Tsa Chih*, 14(1) (1994): 3–4, 18–20. Y.T. Zheng et al., *Immunopharmacology & Immunotoxicology*, 17(1) (1995): 69–79.
8. M.S. McGrath et al., *Proceedings of the National Academy of Science*, 86 (1989): 2844–48.
9. V.S. Byers et al., *AIDS Research & Human Retroviruses*, 10(4) (1994): 413–20.
10. R.A. Mayer et al., *European Journal of Clinical Investigation*, 22(2) (1992): 113–22.
11. S. Lee-Huang et al., *Proceedings of the National Academy of Sciences of the United States*, 88(15) (1991): 6570–74.
12. H.P. Zhong et al., *Chung-Kuo Chung Hsi I Chieh Ho Tsa Chih*, 15(2) (1995): 90–91.
13. W. Tang and G. Eisenbrand, *Chinese Drugs of Plant Origin: Chemistry, Pharmacology, and Use in Traditional and Modern Medicine* (Berlin: Springer-Verlag, 1992).
14. P.A. Garcia et al., *Neuropathology & Applied Neurobiology*, 19(5) (1993): 402–5. Mayer, op. cit. L. Pulliam et al., *AIDS*, 5(10) (1991): 1237–42.
15. W.Y. Chan et al., *Teratogenesis, Carcinogenesis, & Mutagenesis*, 13(2) (1993): 47–57.
16. T.B. Ng et al., *Journal of Ethnopharmacology*, 43(2) (1994): 81–87.

PRIMARY NAME:

CUCURBITA

SCIENTIFIC NAME:

Cucurbita pepo L. convar. citrullinina GREB var. styriaca

What Is Cucurbita?

The huge, edible *Cucurbita* fruits grow on vinelike stems and produce large yellow flowers and flattened, oval seeds. These are typically dried and have a sweetish taste. Many varieties of this native North American plant are cultivated around the world. The seeds are used medicinally.

CUCURBITA (Continued)

GREB and occasionally
Cucurbita maxima Duchesne,
Cucubita moschata [Duchesne]
Poir. Family: Cucurbitaceae

COMMON NAMES:
Varieties of *Cucurbita* include
autumn squash, butternut
squash, China squash,
crookneck squash, nan guazi,
pepo, pumpkin, pumpkin seed,
summer squash

RATING:
3 = Studies on the effectiveness
and safety of this substance are
conflicting, or there are not
enough studies to draw a
conclusion.

What It Is Used For:

The seeds of certain *Cucurbita* species once commanded global renown as a cure for intestinal worms, and some people still eat a few seeds every day as a protective measure. Some European herbalists recommend the seeds when other intestinal remedies are not appropriate because of their harshness, for example.[1] An updated and trendier use for the seeds (coarsely ground or chewed and taken with a fluid) involves the prevention and treatment of benign prostatic hypertrophy (BPH). This condition affects millions of men worldwide but interestingly, far fewer men on average in Balkan countries such as Bulgaria, Ukraine, and Turkey, where men are in the custom of chewing a handful of these seeds every day.[2] Various prostatic and urologic remedies containing cucurbita seeds are sold in Europe.

Forms Available:

Emulsion (made from seeds beaten with sugar or honey and milk or water), infusion, oil, seed (ground or whole).

Dosage Commonly Reported:

For treating intestinal worms an emulsion is made with the ground seeds mixed with sugar or honey and milk or water and taken in three daily doses totaling a dosage of 60 to as much as 500 grams. Often this is taken in conjunction with castor oil. To treat benign prostatic hypertrophy, a handful of the seeds is eaten daily.

Will It Work for You? What the Studies Say:

Researchers have shown that an ingredient in cucurbita seeds—an unusual amino acid called cucurbitin found only in certain species—kills worms in the test tube. In adequate doses, this substance is also believed to paralyze worms in a person's intestines, enabling the body to flush them out naturally.[3] Tapeworms and roundworms in particular are susceptible. At least one patent has been granted for cucurbita worm treatment (a liquid extract).[4]

Getting a high enough concentration of the herb to expel worms can be challenging, however, partly because the concentration of cucurbitin varies widely among *Cucurbita* plants. The concentration of cucurbitin in *Cucurbita pepo* (pumpkin) can range as much as 5 percent.[5] Such variations may explain why some investigators have declared the herb ineffective for intestinal worms; there may not have been enough cucurbitin in their samples, or possibly in the variety they were testing.[6] In fact, no one seems quite sure how many cucurbita seeds (or how much cucurbitin) it takes to vanquish worms. These unknowns make it difficult to endorse or dismiss this traditional remedy.

Still more remains unresolved about the value of cucurbita seeds for treating symptoms of prostate enlargement. Even German health authorities, who have approved of cucurbita seeds for treating irritable bladder and symptoms associated with early (stages I and II) prostate enlargement (adenoma),[7] concede that the evidence is largely empirical and not supported by pharmacologic findings. At the same time, sources note that the seeds contain ingredients that suggest it may work, that random samplings of men who take it report improvements in their symptoms, and that an increasing number of reliable clinical reports indicate the regimen works. For example, the seeds contain a large amount of a fatty oil (45 percent; made of various fatty acids) which may mildly increase urine flow (as a diuretic). But whether this or any other property actually helps resolve prostate enlargement symptoms is unclear.[8] Other ingredients such as betasitosterol, cucurbitacins, and tocopherols may play an even larger role, one German expert contends, although nothing definitive is known.[9] German health authorities note that the regimen would have to be followed for weeks or possibly months before a man would notice any improvement in symptoms.

Seeds from your ordinary Halloween pumpkin will undoubtedly do nothing for an ailing prostate, as they contain none of the main active principle. Double-blind trials reinforce the finding of an investigator who reported that the variety of cucurbita referred to as *Cucurbita pepo* L. convar. citrullinina GREB var. styriaca GREB should be used because it has been widely tested and has demonstrated a notable impact on the prostate gland.[10] But other experts remain unimpressed with the scanty evidence.[11]

Will It Harm You? What the Studies Say:

Research has shed as little understanding on the effectiveness of cucurbita seeds as it has on their safety. The medical literature contains no reports of toxic or undesirable reactions, however, and no adverse reactions were noted in an experiment that involved giving rats and swine extracts of dried *Cucurbita maxima* seeds.[12] One German physician's textbook refers to the herb as so safe that it should be considered for pregnant women, children, or people with liver disease, hepatitis, or other ailments.[13] Again, because the concentration of active ingredients varies so widely, it is virtually impossible to determine if concentrations above a certain level will cause problems.[14]

GENERAL SOURCES:

Bisset, N.G., ed. *Herbal Drugs and Phytopharmaceuticals.* Stuttgart: medpharm GmbH Scientific Publishers, 1994.

Lawrence Review of Natural Products. St. Louis: Facts and Comparisons, May 1990.

Tyler, V.E. *The Honest Herbal.* Binghamton, NY: Haworth Press/Pharmaceutical Products Press, 1993.

Tyler, V.E., L.R. Brady, and J.E. Robbers, eds. *Pharmacognosy.* Philadelphia: Lea & Febiger, 1988.

Weiss, R.F. *Herbal Medicine,* trans. A.R. Meuss, from the 6th German edition. Beaconsfield, England: Beaconsfield Publishers, Ltd., 1988.

TEXT CITATIONS:

1. R.F. Weiss, *Herbal Medicine,* trans. A.R. Meuss, from the 6th German edition (Beaconsfield, England: Beaconsfield Publishers, Ltd., 1988).

2. K.W. Donsbach, *Your Prostate* (Huntington Beach, CA: International Institute of Natural Health Sciences, 1976) 2–4.

3. V.E. Tyler, *The Honest Herbal* (Binghamton, NY: Haworth Press/Pharmaceutical Products Press, 1993).

4. *Lawrence Review of Natural Products* (St. Louis: Facts and Comparisons, May 1990).

5. V.H. Mihranian and C.I. Abou-Chaar, *Lloydia*, 31 (1968): 23.

6. V.E. Tyler, L.R. Brady, and J.E. Robbers, eds., *Pharmacognosy* (Philadelphia: Lea & Febiger, 1988).

7. N.G. Bisset, ed., *Herbal Drugs and Phytopharmaceuticals* (Stuttgart: medpharm GmbH Scientific Publishers, 1994).

8. Donsbach, op. cit.

9. Weiss, op. cit.

10. H. Schlicher, *Zeitschrift für Angewande Phytotherapie*, 2 (1981) and 14 (1986): 7 and 19. Weiss, op. cit.

11. Tyler, op. cit.

12. A. de Queiroz-Neto et al., *Journal of Ethnopharmacology*, 43(1) (1994): 45–51.

13. Weiss, op. cit.

14. Tyler, op cit.

PRIMARY NAME:
DAMIANA

SCIENTIFIC NAME:
Turnera diffusa Willd., and possibly other *Turnera* species. Family: Turneraceae

COMMON NAMES:
Mexican damiana, old woman's broom

RATING:
4 = Research indicates that this substance will not fulfill the claims made for it, but that it is also unlikely to cause any harm.

What Is Damiana?

Damiana consists of the aromatic, dried yellow-brown leaves of the subtropical *Turnera diffusa* shrub, a fruit-bearing plant native to Mexico and the southern United States. The dried branches are sometimes used medicinally as well.

What It Is Used For:

Damiana has a long but checkered history as an aphrodisiac, sexual stimulant, and tonic that dates back to the early Mexican Indians. Despite cries of fraud, a North American pharmacist in the late 1800s rather successfully promoted an alcoholic extract of the herb as a sexual stimulant and panacea for the "enfeebled and aged."[1] It reappeared on the North American market in the 1960s as a vehicle for a "high" described by enthusiasts as a sixty- to ninety-minute state of relaxation and mild sexual stimulation. This was said to be induced by smoking or drinking the herb.[2]

Some contemporary herbalists promote damiana as an aphrodisiac, mild euphoric, potency enhancer, energy booster, anxiety reliever, and general tonic to enhance overall body function. Other folk uses for damiana include the treatment of constipation, diabetes, cough, asthma, kidney inflammation, headache, and menstrual disorders. Homeopaths prescribe minute amounts for various ailments. (See page 2 for a discussion of homeopathy.) The *National Formulary* listed the herb until the late 1940s. Damiana is used to flavor various foods and beverages, including liqueurs.

Forms Available Include:

Capsule, concentrated drops, extracts, tea, tincture. Often appears in herbal blends.

Dosage Commonly Reported:

One or two 400-milligram capsules or 1 dropperful of tincture or concentrated drops is taken daily.

Will It Work for You? What the Studies Say:

According to the scientific evidence collected so far, those seeking sexual stimulation or any other reaction to damiana woo only disappointment. None of the ingredients identified through chemical analyses—including a volatile oil likely to be responsible for the herb's distinctive odor and taste—qualify as aphrodisiac. Not even reports that the herb contains caffeine, which is a central nervous system stimulant that might explain its popularity as an energy enhancer, have been substantiated. Perhaps the love-hungry were feeling the effects of the alcoholic base in which many damiana formulations were once offered, or the irritating effects of the herb's volatile oil on the genitourinary tract (urethral membranes).[3] A similar lack of evidence applies to its purported hallucinogenic properties. Citing this dearth of evidence, German and various other European health authorities have declined to approve of damiana as an herbal stimulant or remedy for any ailment.[4]

Will It Harm You? What the Studies Say:

There is no evidence that damiana has ever caused anyone significant harm. It has been used by various cultures for generations. However, no long-term clinical trials have been conducted to confirm that it is risk-free.

The FDA approves of damiana for food use.

GENERAL SOURCES:

Blumenthal, M., J. Gruenwald, T. Hall, and R.S. Rister, eds. *The Complete German Commission E Monographs: Therapeutic Guide to Herbal Medicine.* Boston: Integrative Medicine Communications, 1998.

Bradley, P.C., ed. *British Herbal Compendium: A Handbook of Scientific Information on Widely Used Plant Drugs,* vol. 1. Bournemouth (Dorset), England: British Herbal Medicine Association, 1992.

Dominguez, X.A., and M. Hinojosa. *Planta Medica.* 30(1) (1976): 68–71.

Duke, J.A. *CRC Handbook of Medicinal Herbs.* Boca Raton, FL: CRC Press, 1985.

Lawrence Review of Natural Products. St. Louis: Facts and Comparisons, July 1996.

Leung, A.Y. *Encyclopedia of Common Natural Ingredients Used in Food, Drugs, and Cosmetics.* New York: John Wiley & Sons, 1980.

Lowry, T.P. *Journal of Psychoactive Drugs.* 16(3) (1984): 267–68.

Mayell, M. *Off-the-Shelf Natural Health: How to Use Herbs and Nutrients to Stay Well.* New York: Bantam Books, 1995.

Mindell, E. *Earl Mindell's Herb Bible.* New York, NY: Simon & Schuster/Fireside, 1992.

Tyler, V.E. *The Honest Herbal.* Binghamton, NY: Haworth Press/Pharmaceutical Products Press, 1993.

———. *Pharmacy in History.* 25(2) (1983): 55.

Tyler, V.E., L.R. Brady, and J.E. Robbers, eds. *Pharmacognosy.* Philadelphia: Lea & Febiger, 1988.

TEXT CITATIONS:

1. V.E Tyler, L.R. Brady, and J.E. Robbers, eds., *Pharmacognosy* (Philadelphia: Lea & Febiger, 1988).
2. V.E. Tyler, *The Honest Herbal* (Binghamton, NY: Haworth Press/Pharmaceutical Products Press, 1993).
3. *Lawrence Review of Natural Products* (St. Louis: Facts and Comparisons, July 1996). Tyler, op. cit.
4. P.C. Bradley, ed., *British Herbal Compendium: A Handbook of Scientific Information on Widely Used Plant Drugs,* vol. 1 (Bournemouth [Dorset], England: British Herbal Medicine Association, 1992).

PRIMARY NAME:
DANDELION

SCIENTIFIC NAME:
Taraxacum officinale Weber and other *Taraxacum* species.
Family: Asteraceae
(Compositae)

What Is Dandelion?

Few Americans would fail to recognize this perennial, which grows like a weed across meadows and roadsides in North America and many other parts of the world, including its native Europe. Its bright yellow flowers bloom through most of the year, opening and closing depending on the light and weather. A seed-filled puffball develops upon maturation, primed to drift in the wind. Typically the root and the rosette of grooved leaves are used medicinally. There are dozens of specialized varieties of dandelion.

COMMON NAMES:

Blowball, canker wort, fairy clock, Irish daisy, lion's tooth, piss-in-bed, priest's crown, puffball, swine's snout, wet-a-bed, taraxacum, white endive, wild endive

RATING:

3 = Studies on the effectiveness and safety of this substance are conflicting, or there are not enough studies to draw a conclusion.

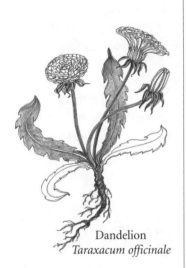

Dandelion
Taraxacum officinale

What It Is Used For:

The dandelion has a long and complex history of folk use in such parts of the world as Europe, China, and India. The most prominent uses in Western folk medicine include the treatment of stomach upset and liver and kidney disorders. Dandelion teas and other preparations have been used to promote the elimination of bile and encourage good digestion, stimulate the appetite, prevent and treat gallstones, ease constipation (as a laxative), remedy skin diseases, alleviate rheumatic conditions, and prompt the kidneys to produce more urine (as a diuretic, or "water pill") for weight loss, premenstrual syndrome (PMS), heart failure, and other problems sometimes related to fluid retention. The dried rhizome and roots were official in the *U.S. Pharmacopoeia* from 1831 to 1926.

Many traditional medicine cultures around the world, including those in India and Russia, focus on dandelion's purported value as a liver tonic. In China, where they commonly rely on *Taraxacum mongolicum*, traditional healers prescribe the herb for colds, bronchitis, mastitis, chronic gastritis, urinary tract infections, skin sores, and various kinds of infections, often as part of complex herbal blends.

The bitter-tasting, aromatic young leaves are mixed into salad greens, and a coffeelike nonstimulating beverage is made of the roasted roots. The flowers have been used to make wine and schnapps. The roots are also cooked and eaten as a vegetable.

Forms Available Include:

Capsule, decoction (typically of dried or powdered root), flower, fluid extract, infusion (typically of dried leaf), juice (of root), leaf (dried fresh in salads or as a vegetable), root (dried, fresh powdered, or roasted), tincture.

Dosage Commonly Reported:

An infusion is made with ½ ounce dried leaves per cup of water; a decoction, with 1 to 3 teaspoons chopped or powdered root. The dried root is taken in doses of 3 to 5 grams three times a day, or in infusion or decoction form. The tincture is taken at a dosage of 1 to 2 teaspoons up to three times per day. A tablespoon of dandelion juice in water is taken morning and evening.

Will It Work for You? What the Studies Say:

On the basis of extensive research done primarily in test tubes and rodents, dandelion preparations may affect certain conditions mildly. But evidence is shaky overall, and promoters and critics part ways on how to interpret studies.

Dandelion leaves and roots contain bitters (sesquiterpene lactones, particularly taraxacin), inulin, essential oils, and other substances that may help explain their popularity for stimulating the appetite and aiding digestion, as they probably stimulate gastric juices and increase the liver's secretion of bile. In a frequently cited 1959 study, an alcoholic extract of the root increased bile secretion in rats by more than 40 percent.[1] But skeptics question whether this age-old theory does not rest on the outdated belief that the appearance of a plant reflects its healing powers. As a liver disorder characterized by yellowing of the skin, jaundice would call for treatment with a yellow flower such as this. Nonetheless, German and other European health commissions officially approved of dandelion root and herb for treating disturbances of bile flow, appetite loss, indigestion, and gas.[2]

Rodent experiments indicate that fluid extracts such as infusions of the leaves (and roots, to a lesser extent) have a diuretic effect, comparable in one test to the commonly used diuretic furosemide.[3] Diuretics are prescribed for fluid retention, PMS, and sometimes very serious conditions such as congestive heart failure. Responsible sources do not promote diuretics as weight reducers, as any lost weight simply represents a transitory loss of fluids. The active ingredient remains a mystery, however, and the diuretic action in humans poorly documented. Many plant experts contend it is quite weak. Proponents point out that dandelion's potassium content reduces the risk of a deficiency in this mineral, a risk with other diuretics. German health authorities consider all parts of the plant diuretic.[4]

Critics and skeptics agree, however, that a bitter substance such as taraxacin will increase gastric juices and salivation and thus boost the appetite.[5] Dandelion root preparations appear to have a mild laxative effect, although the responsible ingredient has yet to be identified.[6] Researchers have also found evidence that the root may help fight inflammation, possibly explaining its traditional use for rheumatism, for example.[7] This is considered a very preliminary finding, however, as are indications that the herb reduces blood sugar levels in animals[8] and may therefore have a role to play in controlling diabetes. Chinese researchers have reportedly had success in treating bronchitis and upper respiratory infections with the root.[9]

All sources agree that dandelions are an excellent source for vitamin A (they have even more than carrots).

Will It Harm You? What the Studies Say:

Dandelion is considered very safe and virtually free of risks for adverse reactions other than possible hyperacidity in the stomach. In rare cases a skin rash (dermatitis) develops in sensitized individuals.[10] German health authorities warn that people with intestinal blockages or inflammation or occlusion of the bile duct (ileus or gallbladder empyema) should not use dandelion preparations.[11] They also recommend taking dandelion preparations in moderation for limited stretches of time (i.e., four to six weeks).

The FDA lists dandelion as Generally Recognized As Safe (GRAS) for food use.

GENERAL SOURCES:

Blumenthal, M., J. Gruenwald, T. Hall, and R.S. Rister, eds. *The Complete German Commission E Monographs: Therapeutic Guide to Herbal Medicine.* Boston: Integrative Medicine Communications, 1998.

Bradley, P.C., ed. *British Herbal Compendium: A Handbook of Scientific Information on Widely Used Plant Drugs*, vol. 1. Bournemouth (Dorset), England: British Herbal Medicine Association, 1992.

Castleman, M. *The Healing Herbs: The Ultimate Guide to the Curative Power of Nature's Medicines.* New York: Bantam Books, 1995.

Lawrence Review of Natural Products. St. Louis: Facts and Comparisons, December 1987.

Leung, A.Y. *Chinese Healing Foods and Herbs.* Glen Rock, NJ: AYSL Corp, 1984.

Leung, A.Y., and S. Foster. *Encyclopedia of Common Natural Ingredients Used in Food, Drugs, and Cosmetics.* 2nd ed. New York: John Wiley & Sons, 1996.

Mindell, E. *Earl Mindell's Herb Bible.* New York: Simon & Schuster/Fireside, 1992.

Murray, M.T. *The Healing Power of Herbs: The Enlightened Person's Guide to the Wonders of Medicinal Plants.* Revised and expanded 2nd ed. Rocklin, CA: Prima Publishing, 1995.

Tierra, M. *The Way of Herbs.* New York: Pocket Books, 1990.

Tyler, V.E. *The Honest Herbal.* Binghamton, NY: Haworth Press/Pharmaceutical Products Press, 1993.

———. *Herbs of Choice. The Therapeutic Use of Phytomedicinals.* New York: Pharmaceutical Products Press, 1994.

Weiner, M.A., and J.A. Weiner. *Herbs That Heal: Prescription for Herbal Healing.* Mill Valley, CA: Quantum Books, 1994.

Weiss, R.F. *Herbal Medicine,* trans. A.R. Meuss, from the 6th German edition. Beaconsfield, England: Beaconsfield Publishers, Ltd., 1988.

TEXT CITATIONS:

1. K. Bohm, *Arzneimittel-Forschung,* 9 (1959): 376–78.

2. P.C. Bradley, ed., *British Herbal Compendium: A Handbook of Scientific Information on Widely Used Plant Drugs,* vol. 1. (Bournemouth [Dorset], England: British Herbal Medicine Association, 1992). M. Blumenthal, J. Gruenwald, T. Hall, and R.S. Rister, eds., *The Complete German Commission E Monographs: Therapeutic Guide to Herbal Medicine* (Boston: Integrative Medicine Communications, 1998).

3. Bohm, op. cit.

4. Blumenthal et al., op. cit.

5. T. Kuusi et al., *Lebensmittel-Wissenschaft und Technologie,* 18 (1985): 347–49.

6. V.E. Tyler, *The Honest Herbal* (Binghamton, NY: Haworth Press/Pharmacautical Products Press, 1993).

7. N. Mascolo, *Phytotherapy Research,* 1 (1987): 28.

8. K. Yamashita et al., *Nutrition Research,* 4 (1984): 491–96.

9. A.Y. Leung and S. Foster, *Encyclopedia of Common Natural Ingredients Used in Food, Drugs, and Cosmetics,* 2nd ed. (New York: John Wiley & Sons, 1996).

10. *Lawrence Review of Natural Products* (St. Louis: Facts and Comparisons, December 1987).

11. Blumenthal et al., op. cit.

PRIMARY NAME:

DEADLY NIGHTSHADE

SCIENTIFIC NAME:

Atropa belladonna L. Family: Solanaceae

COMMON NAMES:

Belladonna, black cherry root, dwale, fair lady

What Is Deadly Nightshade?

This poisonous perennial is cultivated worldwide and also grows wild. In autumn, glossy black berries replace the drooping, bell-shaped purple-brown to greenish flowers. It is the dull green leaves, however, and occasionally the creeping root, that are used medicinally.

What It Is Used For:

The botanical name of this native Eurasian plant refers to Atropos, one of the three Fates famous in Greek mythology for having severed the thread of life.[1] The second part of the name—"belladonna," meaning "beautiful woman"—is believed to refer to its use by women of another era to beautify themselves by dilating their pupils. Today, eye doctors apply a chemical from the plant—atropine—to dilate the pupils for examination and surgery of the retina. Other

DEADLY NIGHTSHADE
(Continued)

RATING:

5 = Studies indicate that there is a definite health hazard to using this herb in crude form, even in recommended amounts.

extracts from the plant such as hyoscyamine and scopolamine are also considered sedative, antispasmodic, and capable of relaxing smooth muscles. They appear in conventional prescription and over-the-counter remedies for such disorders as intestinal colic, peptic ulcers, diarrhea, stomach acidity, seasickness, urinary tract spasms, irritable colon, constipation, asthma, cold, and hay fever, and in sedatives for nervous disorders. Scopolamine was used in the form of a "truth serum" to loosen the tongues of World War II soldiers and spies.

Deadly nightshade has been enlisted to treat Parkinson's disease symptoms such as tremors, rigidity, speech problems, and difficulty moving. Because of the plant's toxicity, however, most traditional uses of the herb (the root in particular) have been reserved for external complaints such as rheumatism, gout, neuralgia (nerve pain), and sciatica. Atropine is given in emergency settings to stimulate cardiac electrical activity.

Forms Available Include:

Injection, ointment (for external use), tincture. Most formulations consist of active ingredients such as atropine that have been extracted from the plant.

Dosage Commonly Reported:

To use commercial ointments and other formulations containing deadly nightshade, follow the package instructions.

Will It Work for You? What the Studies Say:

The leaves and root of this plant contain important substances—tropane alkaloids—such as atropine and hyoscyamine. Typically, these substances are extracted for medicinal use. But not all herbalists agree with this practice, and some argue that the whole drug rather than these derivatives be prescribed.[2] In any case, few sources question the activity of the compounds. They inhibit the parasympathetic nervous system responsible for controlling involuntary body functions; intestinal, bronchial, gastric, and saliva secretions are reduced. The bladder, intestines, and urinary system slow down. The heart rate increases at certain doses. The central nervous system, after an initial period of stimulation, eventually slows down.

These properties are thought to help resolve spasm-related stomach, intestinal, and bile duct disorders, among other conditions.[3] German physicians apparently prescribe the herb for gastrointestinal conditions such as ulcers and gastritis, severe chronic colitis, and persistent constipation.[4] Given the toxicity risks associated with all parts of this plant and its extracts, however, most United States plant experts do not recommend the plant as a home remedy.

No information can be found on the herb's relative value for treating skin complaints.

Will It Harm You? What the Studies Say:

All parts of the aptly named deadly nightshade are extremely poisonous. Use the plant only under the direction of qualified medical supervision, as the beneficial dosage is very close to the toxic dosage. Even relatively small doses can cause such adverse reactions as excitation, dryness of the mouth, dilated pupils, intense thirst, burning sensations in the throat, double vision, nausea, and even palpitations, hallucinations, delirium, coma, and death in some cases.

Children should be warned to avoid the sweet-tasting but extremely toxic ripe berries, which can be fatal to this age group in as small a quantity as three fruits.[5] Handling the plant can cause dermatitis, vesiculo-pustular eruptions on the face, and visual problems.[6]

The FDA placed deadly nightshade on its former list of "Unsafe Herbs," which the agency no longer maintains.

GENERAL SOURCES:

Bremness, L. *Herbs.* 1st American ed. Eyewitness Handbooks. New York: Dorling Kindersley Publications, 1994.

Chevallier, A. *The Encyclopedia of Medicinal Plants: A Practical Reference Guide to More Than 550 Key Medicinal Plants & Their Uses.* 1st American ed. New York: Dorling Kindersley Publications, 1996.

Dobelis, I.N., ed. *The Magic and Medicine of Plants: A Practical Guide to the Science, History, Folklore, and Everyday Uses of Medicinal Plants.* Pleasantville, NY: Reader's Digest Association, 1986.

Duke, J.A. *CRC Handbook of Medicinal Herbs.* Boca Raton, FL: CRC Press, 1985.

Weiss, R.F. *Herbal Medicine,* trans. A.R. Meuss, from the 6th German edition. Beaconsfield, England: Beaconsfield Publishers, Ltd., 1988.

TEXT CITATIONS:

1. I.N. Dobelis, ed., *The Magic and Medicine of Plants: A Practical Guide to the Science, History, Folklore, and Everyday Uses of Medicinal Plants* (Pleasantville, NY: Reader's Digest Association, 1986).
2. R.F. Weiss, *Herbal Medicine,* trans. A.R. Meuss, from the 6th German edition (Beaconsfield, England: Beaconsfield Publishers, Ltd., 1988).
3. Ibid.
4. Ibid.
5. J.A. Duke, *CRC Handbook of Medicinal Herbs* (Boca Raton, FL: CRC Press, 1985).
6. Ibid.

PRIMARY NAME:

DEER ANTLER

SCIENTIFIC NAME:
Cervus nippon

COMMON NAME:
Lu rong

RATING
4 = Research indicates that this substance will not fulfill the claims made for it, but that it is also unlikely to cause any harm.

What Is Deer Antler?

The traditional healing substance known as deer antler consists of a cross-section of the antler taken from the Sika red deer of northern China, reportedly from antlers that have been shed naturally by mature deer or from the tips of antlers of young deer, cut in a way that causes no pain and so that new tips can be grown.[1] The antler tissue is taken as an alcoholic extract.

What It Is Used For:

Deer antler reportedly holds an esteemed position in traditional Chinese medicine as a *qi* (vital energy) tonic valuable for stimulating the libido of both sexes and for curing impotence. Some sources also say that it can prevent stress-related problems, boost physical strength and performance, and improve athletic skill.

Forms Available Include:

Alcoholic extract, antler pieces (to make a tea or tincture), decoction, tablet. Appears in some Chinese herbal blends.

Dosage Commonly Reported:

A standard dosage is 1 to 3 grams. Follow package instructions on commercial deer-antler tablets, tinctures, and combination products.

Will It Work for You? What the Studies Say:

Scientific evidence to demonstrate that deer antler stimulates the libido, eradicates impotence, or in any other way affects the human body does not appear in the recent medical literature, at least that which is accessible in the West. Claims that it contains sterols with potential testosterone-like properties could not be confirmed.

Researchers are examining the effect on aging in mice of repeatedly administering deer antler extract.[2]

Will It Harm You? What the Studies Say:

No reports of significant adverse reactions to deer antler appear in the medical literature. Essentially very little is known about its potential toxicity, however.

General Sources:

Bensky, D., and A. Gamble. *Chinese Herbal Medicine: Materia Medica.* Rev. ed. Seattle: Eastland Press, Inc., 1993.
Mayell, M. *Off-the-Shelf Natural Health: How to Use Herbs and Nutrients to Stay Well.* New York: Bantam Books, 1995.
Tierra, M. *The Way of Herbs.* New York: Pocket Books, 1990.

TEXT CITATIONS:

1. M. Tierra, *The Way of Herbs* (New York: Pocket Books, 1990).
2. B.X. Wang et al., *Chemical & Pharmaceutical Bulletin,* 36(7) (1988): 2587–92.

PRIMARY NAME:
DEVIL'S CLAW

SCIENTIFIC NAME:
Harpagophytum procumbens
DC. Family: Pedaliaceae

COMMON NAMES:
Grapple plant, wood spider

What Is Devil's Claw?

Devil's claw grows wild in the deserts and steppes of southern Africa. The fruit tips bear small and menacing-looking barbs or "claws." Only the secondary roots (or "storage tubers") appear to possess any medicinal properties.

What It Is Used For:

Africans have used devil's claw for many ailments, including rheumatism, stomach upset, indigestion, appetite loss, headache, cancerous growths, blood disorders, fever, and pregnancy and labor pains. Increasing numbers of European and North American herbalists, first introduced to the herb in the 1950s and 1960s, recommend it for a number of these and other conditions. Devil's claw has at times been regarded as a wonder drug. Particularly, it has a reputa-

DEVIL'S CLAW (Continued)

tion for promoting flexibility in painful arthritic joints; many Europeans take it for this purpose.

Forms Available Include:

Capsule, decoction, liquid extract, root (chopped, powdered).

Dosage Commonly Reported:

A common daily dosage is 4.5 grams, taken in the form of capsules, extracts, or a decoction made with 1 teaspoon powdered or finely chopped root per 2 cups of water and drunk throughout the day.

Will It Work for You? What the Studies Say:

According to clinical studies with humans and laboratory tests with small animals, devil's claw fails to live up to its most widespread claim: that it can remedy the pain and discomfort of arthritis. So far, only one study indicates that the herb can noticeably reduce inflammation in humans; individuals in the 1976 study who took devil's claw experienced anti-inflammatory activity comparable to that of another group of subjects who took the common arthritis drug phenylbutazone.[1] Those who took devil's claw experienced some pain relief. Tests also showed a reduction of abnormally high levels of cholesterol and uric acid. But follow-up studies have failed to produce similarly optimistic results. In a 1981 study, the signs and symptoms of arthritis did not improve significantly in subjects given devil's claw for six weeks.[2] A group of healthy individuals who took devil's claw capsules for twenty-one days in a 1992 study did not experience the important blood changes that would normally be seen with nonsteroidal anti-inflammatory drugs like Ibuprofen.[3] Rodent studies have yielded similarly conflicting results.

Despite such uneven findings, many European herbalists continue to enthusiastically recommend devil's claw tea preparations as anti-inflammatories. They point to test-tube evidence that the plant has slight painkilling and anti-inflammatory properties, primarily due to the actions of the main chemical component in the herb, the iridoid glycoside harpagoside.[4] A number of rat studies have shown that the plant can minimally damp inflammation and swelling when compared with a dummy drug, a standard anti-inflammatory drug like indomethacin, or aspirin, for example. German and other European health authorities stop short of endorsing devil's claw as a remedy for arthritis symptoms, however.

In Germany, devil's claw extracts are sometimes injected under the skin around an arthritic joint to ease swelling, albeit with the warning that other measures should be used to control the condition as well. There may be some logic to this approach; a 1994 report indicates that injected forms of the herb may pack more punch, as oral forms appear to lose some potency during the long trek to the stomach.[5]

Devil's claw contains bitter-tasting substances that explain its enduring popularity as an appetite stimulant and indigestion remedy. Some sources consider a decoction of the plant one of the strongest bitter tonics known, and South

African folk healers recommend it highly.[6] When drunk over several days, devil's claw tea helps relieve functional problems involving the first part of the small intestine and the pancreas.[7] German health authorities approve of taking a devil's claw root tea or other root preparations for appetite loss, peptic discomforts, and degenerative motor system conditions.[8]

Devil's claw may affect the heart. An extract administered to isolated hearts of rabbits and rats, for example, significantly reduced irregular heartbeat activity, heart rate, and blood pressure.[9] What this means for humans has yet to be carefully examined. As for the many other claims made for devil's claw, none appears to have been put to the test of clinical trials, and chemical analysis does not suggest it would work.

Not all devil's claw products are made alike; French analysts found considerable variability in the quality of devil's claw capsules in a 1995 investigation.[10]

Will It Harm You? What the Studies Say:

Conservative herbalists warn that devil's claw has yet to prove itself a safe and effective medicine. Studies in humans done so far, however, indicate that adverse reactions are rare. The few reactions that have been reported include loss of appetite, ringing in the ears, and headache.[11] Trials that involved giving extracts of devil's claw to rats over short periods of time (such as three weeks) likewise indicated that the substance was safe and nontoxic. Little is known about the plant's interaction with other medicines, including other commonly used anti-inflammatory drugs. Individuals with ulcers, gallstones, or heart problems should probably avoid devil's claw unless a doctor approves of it.[12]

GENERAL SOURCES:

Abramowicz, M. *Medical Letter on Drugs and Therapeutics.* 21(7) (1979): 30.

Bisset, N.G., ed. *Herbal Drugs and Phytopharmaceuticals.* Stuttgart: medpharm GmbH Scientific Publishers, 1994.

Blumenthal, M., J. Gruenwald, T. Hall, and R.S. Rister, eds. *The Complete German Commission E Monographs: Therapeutic Guide to Herbal Medicine.* Boston: Integrative Medicine Communications, 1998.

Duke, J.A. *CRC Handbook of Medicinal Herbs.* Boca Raton, FL: CRC Press, 1985.

Lawrence Review of Natural Products. St. Louis: Facts and Comparisons. March 1996.

Tyler, V.E. *The Honest Herbal.* Binghamton, NY: Haworth Press/Pharmaceutical Products Press, 1993.

Weiss, R.F. *Herbal Medicine,* trans. A.R. Meuss, from the 6th German edition. Beaconsfield, England: Beaconsfield Publishers, Ltd., 1988.

TEXT CITATIONS:

1. R. Kampf, *Schweitzer Apotheker Zeitung,* 114 (1976): 337.

2. R. Grahame and B.V. Robinson, *Annals of Rheumatic Disease,* 40(6) (1981): 632.

3. C. Moussard, D. Alber, M.M. Toubin, N. Thevenon, and J.C. Henry, *Prostaglandins, Leukotrienes and Essential Fatty Acids,* 46(4) (1992): 283–86.

4. M.C. Lanhers et al., *Planta Medica,* 58(2) (1992): 117–23.

5. R. Soulimani et al., *Canadian Journal of Physiology and Pharmacology,* 72(12) (1994): 1532–36.

6. R.F. Weiss, *Herbal Medicine*, trans. A.R. Meuss, from the 6th German edition (Beaconsfield, England: Beaconsfield Publishers, Ltd., 1988). N.G. Bisset, ed., *Herbal Drugs and Phytopharmaceuticals* (Stuttgart: medpharm GmbH Scientific Publishers, 1994).

7. W. Zimmerman, *Physikaliske Medizin Rehabilitationsmedizin Kurortmedizin*, 18 (1977): 317–19.

8. M. Blumenthal, J. Gruenwald, T. Hall, and R.S. Rister, eds., *The Complete German Commission E Monographs: Therapeutic Guide to Herbal Medicine* (Boston: Integrative Medicine Communications, 1998).

9. C.R. de Pasquale et al., *Journal of Ethnopharmacology*, 13(2) (1983): 193–99. C. Circosta et al., *Journal of Ethnopharmacology*, 11(3) (1984): 259–74. *Lawrence Review of Natural Products* (St. Louis: Facts and Comparisons, March 1996).

10. O. Mestadagh and M. Torck, *Annales Pharmaceutiques Françaises*, 53(3) (1995): 135–37.

11. Grahame and Robinson, op. cit.

12. Blumenthal et al., op. cit.

PRIMARY NAME:
DEVIL'S DUNG

SCIENTIFIC NAME:

Ferula assafoetida L. and certain other *Ferula* species, including *Ferula rubricaulis* Boiss. and *Ferula foetida* Regel. Family: Umbilliferae (Apiaceae)

COMMON NAMES:

Asafetida, asafoetida, asant, gum asafedita

RATING:

3 = Studies on the effectiveness and safety of this substance are conflicting, or there are not enough studies to draw a conclusion.

What Is Devil's Dung?

Harvesters reap this substance, a gum resin, by slashing the roots and rhizomes (underground stems) of a colorful perennial found growing wild in Iran and Afghanistan.

What It Is Used For:

Ironically, the putrid odor and objectionable, acrid taste of this resin actually work to its advantage: it makes a strong statement when used as a spice and garlic substitute in Indian, Chinese, and other Asian cuisines. Without it, Worcestershire sauce as we know it would not exist. The resin's reputation as a food preservative is long-standing. In Western countries today, devil's dung is used primarily as a fragrance component in perfumes,[1] despite its strong odor, which is manipulated to appeal to rather than disgust the sense of smell. Special preparations have been used to repel cats, dogs, and wildlife.[2]

Devil's dung appears in a well-known Indian (Ayurvedic) digestive formula.[3] In North American folk medicine it continues to find use, particularly in African-American communities,[4] as a remedy for gas and griping (sharp stomach pains), an expectorant to clear congestion in chronic bronchitis and other conditions, and a treatment for irritable colon. Rectal formulations have been used to control colic. Years ago, the plant was reportedly given to people with epilepsy. In addition to a number of these traditional practices, some sources today consider devil's dung a valuable nerve tonic for hysteria and mood swings, a treatment for low blood sugar and food sensitivities, and an effective stimulant (even aphrodisiac), sedative, antifungal, and abdominal tumor treatment.[5]

Forms Available Include:

Capsule, gum resin, powdered solution. Because of the way in which the plant is selected, collected, and stored, the quality of commercial devil's dung products varies widely.[6] Some samples contain large amounts of other material.

Dosage Commonly Reported:

The gum resin is taken in doses of 0.3 to 1 gram.

Will It Work for You? What the Studies Say:

Evidence to support any of the traditional or proposed uses for devil's dung is sparse. At most, its relatively high volatile oil content (6 to 17 percent) explains a carminative action and suggests that it may well help treat gas and griping, and possibly chronic bronchitis and asthma through a related expectorant action.[7] Its offensive odor may help alleviate certain types of neuroses, according to British authorities.[8] Clinical trials on its potential for treating high cholesterol have produced conflicting results.[9] Test-tube studies examining the spice's anticancer and antitumor properties have also yielded mixed results, although a number are quite positive.[10] An alcoholic extract proved somewhat effective in fighting tumor cells in a laboratory dish[11]—garlic, ginger, and other spices fared better—but studies in mice have indicated that the substance is devoid of anticancer-causing (anticarcinogenic) properties.[12] Researchers have looked into its value for treating irritable colon.[13]

Will It Harm You? What the Studies Say:

Adverse reactions to devil's dung in adults appear to be rare, although no systematic evaluation of its safety has been done. Never give devil's dung to an infant (up to one year old); in test-tube studies with fetal blood it causes dangerous changes in the part of the red blood cells called hemoglobin, the component responsible for transporting oxygen through the body.[14] A five-week-old child given an over-the-counter solution containing devil's dung developed severe methemoglobinemia, a potentially fatal condition in which the hemoglobin is abnormally formed.[15] Adult hemoglobin does not appear to be at risk. The FDA considers devil's dung safe to use in small amounts as a spice. Topical formulations may cause skin irritation in sensitive individuals.[16]

GENERAL SOURCES:

Bradley, P.C., ed. *British Herbal Compendium: A Handbook of Scientific Information on Widely Used Plant Drugs*, vol. 1. Bournemouth (Dorset), England: British Herbal Medicine Association, 1992.

Der Marderosian, A., and L. Liberti. *Natural Product Medicine: A Scientific Guide to Foods, Drugs, Cosmetics*. Philadelphia: George F. Stickley, 1988.

Lawrence Review of Natural Products. St. Louis: Facts and Comparisons, January 1993.

Tierra, M. *The Way of Herbs*. New York: Pocket Books, 1990.

Weiss, R.F. *Herbal Medicine*, trans. A.R. Meuss, from the 6th German edition. Beaconsfield, England: Beaconsfield Publishers, Ltd., 1988.

TEXT CITATIONS:

1. *Lawrence Review of Natural Products* (St. Louis: Facts and Comparisons, January 1993).
2. Ibid.
3. M. Tierra, *The Way of Herbs* (New York: Pocket Books, 1990).
4. *Lawrence Review of Natural Products*, op. cit.
5. J.A. Duke, *CRC Handbook of Medicinal Herbs* (Boca Raton, FL: CRC Press, 1985). Tierra, op. cit.

6. P.C. Bradley, ed., *British Herbal Compendium: A Handbook of Scientific Information on Widely Used Plant Drugs*, vol. 1 (Bournemouth [Dorset], England: British Herbal Medicine Association, 1992).

7. *United States Dispensatory*, 1937.

8. Bradley, op. cit.

9. V.S. Kamanna and N. Chandrasekhara, *Lipids*, 17 (1982): 483. A. Bordia and S.K. Arora, *Indian Journal of Medical Research*, 63 (1975): 707–11.

10. M.C. Unnikrishnan and R. Kuttan, *Cancer Letters*, 51(1) (1990): 85–89. K. Aruna and V.M. Sivaramakrishnan, *Indian Journal of Experimental Biology*, 28(11) (1990): 1008–11.

11. M.C. Unnikrishnan and R. Kuttan, *Nutrition & Cancer*, 11 (1988): 251–57.

12. K. Aruna and V.M. Sivaramakrishnan, *Food & Chemical Toxicology*, 30(11) (1992): 953–56.

13. V.W. Rahlfs and P. Mossinger, *Deutsche Medizinische Wochenschrift*, 104 (1978): 140–43.

14. A. Der Marderosian and L. Liberti, *Natural Product Medicine: A Scientific Guide to Foods, Drugs, Cosmetics* (Philadelphia: George F. Stickley, 1988).

15. K.J. Kelly et al., *Pediatrics*, 73 (1984): 717.

16. *Lawrence Review of Natural Products*, op. cit.

PRIMARY NAME:
DHEA

SCIENTIFIC NAME:
N/A

COMMON NAME:
N/A

RATING:
3 = Studies on the effectiveness and safety of this substance are conflicting, or there are not enough studies to draw a conclusion.

What Is DHEA?

Dehydroepiandosterone (DHEA) is a hormone produced by the adrenal glands located on top of the kidneys. The body converts DHEA into the hormones testosterone and estrogen.

What It Is Used For:

The body uses DHEA in multiple ways, many of them still poorly understood. Dietary supplement makers and numerous other sources have made a dizzying array of claims for the benefits of taking DHEA in supplement form. Their claims echo many of those made in the early to mid-1980s, when the FDA banned the hormone from over-the-counter sale. The 1994 Dietary Supplement and Health Education Act effectively canceled out this ruling, and sales of DHEA have skyrocketed since then.

Because body levels of DHEA decline with age,[1] proponents reason, lack of this hormone can be linked to the development of aging-related ailments, sickness in general, and even death. Many sources recommend taking the supplements to slow the aging process, strengthen the immune system, reduce the symptoms of lupus, fend off heart disease, forestall cancer and diabetes, and prevent or retard the progression of Alzheimer's and Parkinson's diseases. Others claim that it can improve mood, burn fat, and jog the libido.

Forms Available Include:

Capsule, liquid spray, tablet.

Dosage Commonly Reported:

A common daily dosage is 30 to 90 milligrams. To use commercial DHEA formulations, follow package instructions.

Will It Work for You? What the Studies Say:

Currently, the scientific evidence for DHEA is based on several studies in animals and a handful in humans, most of them small and short-term. In fact, not one of the benefits claimed for DHEA has been demonstrated in a properly designed—large, randomized, and placebo-controlled—human trial.[2] Despite often intriguing findings, many established scientists assert that this is the type of study needed before any firm conclusions can be made about the benefits or safety of taking DHEA, clearly a powerful hormone.

Small human trials have shown promising results for various ailments. In one, DHEA significantly improved depression symptoms in three men and three women suffering from major depression. The subjects ranged in age from fifty-one to seventy-two, and knew they were being given a substance to affect their mood; they took 30 to 90 milligrams of DHEA a day for four weeks.[3]

Diabetes sufferers may benefit from DHEA supplementation, according to a small study that still needs confirmation from larger trials. In that three-week double-blind trial in fifteen older (postmenopausal) women with non-insulin-dependent diabetes, insulin sensitivity was significantly enhanced in the subjects given 50 milligrams of DHEA daily compared with those given a placebo.[4]

Population studies indicate that higher DHEA levels may offer some protection against the development of heart disease. In a unique, nineteen-year study of 1,029 men (ranging in age from thirty to eighty-two) and 942 women (ranging in age from fifty to eighty-eight) in San Diego, men who had higher DHEA levels in their bloodstream were found to have a modestly reduced risk for death from cardiovascular disease.[5] The risk for fatal cardiovascular disease was actually higher in women, however, although not significantly so. Another study reported that DHEA may aid heart conditions by inhibiting platelet aggregation, meaning that it makes the blood less sticky and thus less likely to clot in dangerous ways.

Of all the claims made for DHEA, the one most thoroughly substantiated is that supplements of the hormone may help control the symptoms of systemic lupus erythematosus, an autoimmune disease characterized by fatigue, joint pain, skin rashes, and blood abnormalities.[6]

Will It Harm You? What the Studies Say:

No one knows what long-term effects DHEA supplements have on the human body, and the only way to assess this properly is through long-term studies in humans. More than a few scientists have expressed grave concern that so many people are taking a clearly potent hormone without assurance that it will not harm them. A number of scientifically reliable sources have warned against taking the supplements, including the Center for Science in the Public Interest.

In fact, there are warning signs already. Some animal and population studies have found that higher-than-normal levels of DHEA may be linked to an increased risk of cancer. One investigator detected an increased risk of ovarian cancer among 20,000 individuals in a prospective community survey who had increased levels of DHEA in their bloodstreams.[7]

Purity and potency remain unknown factors as well. One expert recommends protecting yourself by only ordering from large and well-known sources that can be sued in case of adverse reactions.[8] Store the original bottle with the last five pills in a dark, cool place so that you know what you have taken should an adverse reaction occur.

The same furor surrounding estrogen replacement therapy in postmenopausal women could theoretically apply here as well, since DHEA is converted into potent sex hormones in the body. Regimens to replace these sex hormones, such as estrogen replacement therapy, are carefully evaluated and intensively studied. Even with the massive amounts of data collected so far, controversy regarding their risks and benefits persists.

Many experts recommend that you at least tell your doctor that you are taking DHEA, partly because its interactions with other drugs are still unknown. A number of experts also suggest that people under age thirty not take the hormone because it could interfere with the body's natural production of it.[9] An individual's serum DHEA level should be tested before starting on replacement therapy.

GENERAL SOURCES:

Balch, J.F., and P.A. Balch. *Prescription for Nutritional Healing: A Practical A to Z Reference to Drug-Free Remedies Using Vitamins, Minerals, Herbs & Food Supplements.* 2nd ed. Garden City Park, NY: Avery Publishing Group, 1997.

Burros, M. "Eating Well." *The New York Times.* April 23 (1997): C7.

"Dehydroepiandosterone (DHEA)." *Medical Letter on Drugs & Therapeutics.* 38 (985) (1996): 91–92.

Kellog, G.J., et al. "Clinical Development Plan: DHEA analog 8354." *Journal of Cellular Biochemistry—Supplement.* 20 (1994): 141–46.

Skolnick, A.A. "Scientific Verdict Still Out on DHEA." *Journal of the American Medical Association.* 276(17) (1996): 1365–67.

TEXT CITATIONS:

1. *Annals of the New York Academy of Sciences.* 774 (1995): 121–27.
2. A.A. Skolnick. *Journal of the American Medical Association,* 276 (17) (1996): 1365–67.
3. *Annals of the New York Academy of Sciences,* op. cit.
4. Ibid.
5. Ibid.
6. *Arthritis & Rheumatism,* 37 (1994): 1305–10.
7. K.J. Helzlsouer, *Journal of the American Medical Association,* 274 (1995): 1926–30.
8. Skolnick, op. cit.
9. Ibid.

PRIMARY NAME:
DILL

SCIENTIFIC NAME:
Anethum graveolens L. Family:
Umbelliferae (Apiaceae)

COMMON NAME:
N/A

RATING:
3 = Studies on the effectiveness
of this substance are conflicting,
or there are not enough studies
to draw a conclusion. Safety is
not a concern.

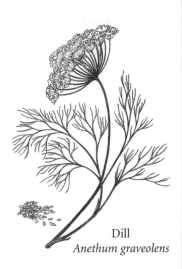

Dill
Anethum graveolens

What Is Dill?

Both the dried ripe fruit ("seeds") and fine, needlelike leaves of this common, fragrant herb are used medicinally. Dill is cultivated in many parts of the world.

What It Is Used For:

The medicinal use of this popular kitchen herb and food preservative dates back to early civilizations. Traditional Chinese healers reportedly considered it a gentle digestive aid and remedy for stomachache, colic, gas, appetite loss, and bloating. American colonists were known to give colicky infants and children mild dill-seed infusions (called "dillwater") for sour stomach and cough.

Drawing on these and other traditional uses, modern Western herbalists recommend dill to soothe colicky stomach pain and uncomfortable gas in children especially, and many consider it an effective appetite stimulant and antispasmodic for countering spasm-related gastrointestinal upset, jangled nerves, and insomnia. Some recommend it as a diuretic ("water pill") to treat kidney and urinary tract disorders and to soothe hemorrhoid pain (including using the infusion as a retention enema). Others say that a nursing mother who drinks dill tea will increase her breast milk. Chewing the seeds is said to dispel bad breath.

Forms Available Include:

Herb (leaf and upper stem, fresh or dried), infusion (of crushed or bruised seeds), oil (of seeds or herb, the latter being referred to as dillweed oil), pills, powder, seeds, tincture.

Dosage Commonly Reported:

To freshen the breath, ½ to 1 teaspoon of seeds is chewed. An infusion is made with 2 teaspoons bruised seeds per cup of water; weaker infusions are given to children under two.

Will It Work for You? What the Studies Say:

The oil in dill seeds fights certain bacteria in the test tube, including those known to cause intestinal tract havoc. Although this finding helps explain some of its traditional uses for infectious conditions, the subject has apparently never been well studied in animals or humans.[1] German health authorities approve of dill seed preparations for dyspeptic disorders (e.g., indigestion), particularly those related to certain bacteria.[2] They also consider it an effective antispasmodic for intestinal upset. Smooth-muscle-relaxing properties have been observed in cats injected with an emulsion containing dill seed oil.[3] Increased urination occurred in dogs given alcoholic extracts of dill seeds, as well as its volatile oil, but whether the same diuretic actions occur in humans remains untested.[4]

An infusion of the herb (leaves or upper stems) injected into laboratory animals lowers blood pressure, stimulates respiration, slows the heart rate, and exerts various other actions, according to research findings, but whether any of these properties carry over into humans who simply drink the infusion is far from clear.[5] German health authorities, citing a lack of proven effectiveness, declined to approve of medicinal preparations made with dill herb (as opposed to the seeds) for proposed treatment of gastrointestinal upset, sleep disorders, and kidney and urinary tract disorders.[6]

Will It Harm You? What the Studies Say:

When used in typically recommended amounts, dill leaf, seed, and seed oil are not considered toxic in any way.[7] The FDA considers dill safe for use as a food.

GENERAL SOURCES:

Blumenthal, M., J. Gruenwald, T. Hall, and R.S. Rister, eds. *The Complete German Commission E Monographs: Therapeutic Guide to Herbal Medicine.* Boston: Integrative Medicine Communications, 1998.

Castleman, M. *The Healing Herbs: The Ultimate Guide to the Curative Power of Nature's Medicines.* New York: Bantam Books, 1995.

Hylton, W.H., ed. *The Rodale Herb Book: How to Use, Grow, and Buy Nature's Miracle Plants.* Emmaus, PA: Rodale Press, Inc., 1974.

Leung, A.Y., and Foster S. *Encyclopedia of Common Natural Ingredients Used in Food, Drugs, and Cosmetics.* 2nd ed. New York: John Wiley & Sons, 1996.

Stary, F. *The Natural Guide to Medicinal Herbs and Plants.* Prague: Barnes & Noble, Inc., in arrangement with Aventium Publishers, 1996.

Tierra, M. *The Way of Herbs.* New York: Pocket Books, 1990.

Weiss, R.F. *Herbal Medicine,* trans. A.R. Meuss, from the 6th German edition. Beaconsfield, England: Beaconsfield Publishers, Ltd., 1988.

TEXT CITATIONS:

1. F.M. Ramadan et al., *Chemie Mikrobiologie, Technologie der Lebensmittel,* 1 (1972): 96.
2. M. Blumenthal, J. Gruenwald, T. Hall, and R.S. Rister, eds., *The Complete German Commission E Monographs: Therapeutic Guide to Herbal Medicine* (Boston: Integrative Medicine Communications, 1998).
3. A.Y. Leung and S. Foster, *Encyclopedia of Common Natural Ingredients Used in Food, Drugs, and Cosmetics,* 2nd ed. (New York: John Wiley & Sons, 1996).
4. G.H. Mahran et al., *Phytotherapy Research,* 5 (1992): 169.
5. Leung and Foster, op. cit.
6. Blumenthal et al., op. cit.
7. *Federal Register,* 39 (1974): 34211.

PRIMARY NAME:
DONG QUAI

SCIENTIFIC NAME:
Angelica polymorpha Max. var. *sinensis* Oliv., sometimes referred to as *Angelica sinensis* (Oliv.) Diels. Family: Apiaceae

COMMON NAME:
Dong gui

What Is Dong Quai?

The dried, yellowish-brown, thick-branched root of this fragrant perennial found growing at high altitudes in China, Korea, and Japan is used medicinally. The plant has smooth, purplish stems and bears umbels (umbrella-shaped clusters) of white flowers. Distinctive, winged fruits appear in July and August.

Refer to **Angelica** for information on American, European, and other *Angelica* species such as *Angelica archangelica* L., as none of the following information applies to these herbs.

RATING:

2 = According to research and common use, this substance appears to be relatively effective and safe when used properly and in recommended amounts for the indication(s) noted in the "Will It Work for You?" section. However, see safety warning in the "Will It Harm You?" section.

What It Is Used For:

Dong quai can claim centuries of use as a spice, tonic, and drug in Chinese and other traditional Far Eastern medicines. It has been used primarily for ensuring a healthy pregnancy and delivery and to treat gynecologic problems such as irregular periods, menstrual cramps, menstrual-related weakness, stomachache after childbirth, infertility, and vaginal infection discharges. Contemporary Western herbalists recommend dong quai for similar purposes, as well as to allay menopausal symptoms.

Dong quai has also been used traditionally as an antispasmodic, and to prevent and treat allergy symptoms, control anemia and allay headaches due to blood deficiency, manage high blood pressure, reduce ulcers, allay constipation, control rheumatism, and "purify" the blood.[1]

According to one source, dong quai ranks as one of the best-selling Chinese traditional herbal products outside of China, as well as one of the most widely used medicinal herbs in China.[2]

Forms Available Include:

Capsule, decoction, injection formulation (possibly used exclusively in China), liquid extract, powder, root, tincture.

Dosage Commonly Reported:

A standard daily dosage for dong quai is from 3 to 15 grams. It is predominantly used in traditional Chinese medicine combinations. It is also a common ingredient in Chinese soups.

Will It Work for You? What the Studies Say:

Through test-tube and small-animal studies, researchers have documented a number of active properties for dong quai, although most if not all may be irrelevant, given the toxicity risks associated with the plant (see "Will It Harm You?" below).

Dong quai contains as many as seven active ingredients, called coumarin derivatives, including psoralen and bergapten,[3] and an essential oil containing safrole. Coumarins are widely accepted active substances, many of them capable of dilating (opening up) vessels, stimulating the central nervous system, and fighting spasms, among other things.[4] Experiments have shown that the root affects the uterus, possibly explaining its long-standing use for gynecologic ailments; it appears to contract as well as relax this muscle in anesthetized cats, dogs, and rabbits.[5] Tests also demonstrate that the root may suppress allergic symptoms by altering immune system reactions; an extract given orally and by injection has been shown to inhibit substances critical to immune system reactions (IgE titers).[6] Animal and test-tube studies have found an impact on the cardiovascular and central nervous systems (inhibiting the latter slightly), and revealed an ability to slightly increase urine output (as a mild diuretic, or "water pill") and inhibit platelet function. Many plant experts consider dong quai mildly laxative.

Will It Harm You? What the Studies Say:

Traditional Chinese healers note that dong quai should not be used during pregnancy (particularly during the first three months) or by women with a history of spontaneous abortion.[7] They also advise that it not be taken in the case of a cold or flu, nor by diarrhea sufferers, given the root's mild laxative effect.

Dong quai contains substances called psoralens and bergapten (furocoumarins) that can incite a severe sunburn, rash, or other signs of a sensitivity reaction after a person uses it—internally or externally—and is then exposed to the sun or another source of ultraviolet rays. According to animal studies, furocoumarins can also cause cancer and instigate dangerous cell changes without exposure to light.[8] To put things in perspective, however, these substances are also found in celery, carrots, and other members of the carrot family. Problems with toxicity tend to be associated with the use of purified compounds of this herb, not crude dong quai.

Dong quai's essential oil contains another potentially hazardous substance as well—safrole—*when taken in purified form.* This is a widely recognized carcinogenic substance[9] and the ingredient responsible for the banning of **Sassafras** in the United States.[10]

GENERAL SOURCES:

Castleman, M. *The Healing Herbs: The Ultimate Guide to the Curative Power of Nature's Medicines.* New York: Bantam Books, 1995.

Duke, J.A. *CRC Handbook of Medicinal Herbs.* Boca Raton, FL: CRC Press, 1985.

Lawrence Review of Natural Products. St. Louis: Facts and Comparisons, April 1990.

Tyler, V.E. *The Honest Herbal.* Binghamton, NY: Haworth Press/Pharmaceutical Products Press, 1993.

Weiner, M.A., and J.A. Weiner. *Herbs That Heal: Prescription for Herbal Healing.* Mill Valley, CA: Quantum Books, 1994.

TEXT CITATIONS:

1. C.P. Sung et al., *Journal of Natural Products*, 45 (1982): 398. *Lawrence Review of Natural Products* (St. Louis: Facts and Comparisons, April 1990). S. Foster and C. Yue, *Herbal Emissaries: Bringing Chinese Herbs to the West* (Rochester, VT: Healing Arts Press, 1992).
2. Foster and Yue, op. cit.
3. K. Hata et al., *Yakugaku Zasshi*, 87 (1967): 464–65.
4. *Lawrence Review of Natural Products*, op. cit.
5. D. Bensky and A. Gamble, *Chinese Herbal Medicine: Materia Medica* (Seattle WA: Eastland Press, 1986). D.P.Q. Zhu, *American Journal of Chinese Medicine*, 3–4 (1987): 117–25.
6. C.P. Sung et al., *Journal of Natural Products*, 45: 398.
7. Zhu, op. cit.
8. G.W. Ivie et al., *Science*, 213 (1981): 909–10.
9. *Lawrence Review of Natural Products*, op. cit.
10. J.A. Duke, *CRC Handbook of Medicinal Herbs* (Boca Raton, FL: CRC Press, 1985).

SCIENTIFIC NAME:
Echinacea angustifolia DC (Rudbeckia and Bruneria), as well as the closely related *Echinacea purpurea* Moench and *Echinacea pallida* (Nutt.) Britton. Family: Asteraceae (Compositae)

COMMON NAMES:
American coneflower, black Sampson, black susan, comb flower, coneflower, Indian head, Kansas snakeroot, narrow-leaved purple coneflower, niggerhead, purple coneflower, Sampson root, scurvy root

RATING:
2 = According to a number of well-designed studies and common use, this substance appears to be relatively effective and safe when used in recommended amounts for the indication(s) noted in the "Will It Work for You?" section.

What Is Echinacea?

Echinacea angustifolia, a member of the daisy family, is native to the American Midwest. It has thick narrow leaves and bears a single flower distinguished by purple rays emanating from a cone-shaped center. The black rootstock is used medicinally. Nine species of *Echinacea* grow in American soil, including those noted at the left, but *Echinacea purpurea* probably ranks as the most commonly used commercially.[1] Confusion over the identity of the herb, such as misidentification of *E. angustifolia* as *E. pallida*, has interfered with its proper study and use over the decades, and results of many earlier trials must be dismissed because of this.

What It Is Used For:

Echinacea has been used for generations to treat a variety of ailments. Native Americans of the Great Plains recognized the plant's antiseptic properties and placed it on insect bites, skin wounds, and snakebites (particularly rattlesnake bites). They calmed toothaches and sore gums with the herb, and reportedly drank it in the form of a tea to treat colds, mumps, arthritis, and a variety of other conditions. Early settlers picked up on many of these uses. In the early 1870s, a Nebraska doctor—a patent-medicine purveyor—promoted echinacea as a "blood purifier" (often a euphemism for a venereal disease remedy) and agent for treating a myriad of conditions including migraine headache, rheumatism, pain, indigestion, sore eyes, tumors, rattlesnake bite, malaria, and hemorrhoids. The herb was very much in vogue over the following decades, until the introduction of potent antibiotics in the 1930s, when it rapidly fell out of favor. The *National Formulary* listed it from 1916 until 1950.

Interest in echinacea perked up again as part of the herbal revival of the 1970s. Modern herbalists recommend it highly as an immune-system stimulant to boost resistance to colds and flu, yeast and bladder infections, and other infectious conditions. Some suggest putting it on the skin to help heal wounds and boils, cuts, burns, psoriasis and eczema, cold sores, and genital herpes sores. Still others promote it as a digestive aid. German investigators report success in treating bronchitis, tonsillitis, meningitis, tuberculosis, abscesses, whooping cough, arthritis, and ear infections.

Forms Available Include:

Capsules, concentrated drops, decoction (of coarsely powdered herb), extracts of various types, injection (not available in the United States), root (dried), tincture. Commercial preparations may contain more than one echinacea species. Store extracts in solution and roots whole.[2]

To take advantage of the benefits of echinacea, try to get the highest-quality herb available; buy it from a well-known manufacturer or source. In times past, many batches were adulterated with a substance known as Missouri snakeroot or prairie dock. The rootstock should not be used once it has lost its odor.

Dosage Commonly Reported:

The herb is taken three times daily in the form of a decoction made with 2 teaspoons root material per cup of water. One to two droppersful of tincture or

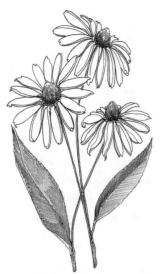

Echinacea
Echinacea purpurea
Echinacea angustifolia

concentrated drops are taken, or 300 to 400 milligrams of solid extract. Two or three of the 455-milligram root capsules are taken two to three times a day; two 125-milligram root-extract capsules containing 3.2 to 4.8 percent echinacoside are taken two to three times a day. After taking echinacea for six to eight weeks, a break of one to four weeks is often recommended, to rest the immune system.

Will It Work for You? What the Studies Say:

So much has been written about echinacea over the years, and so many claims made, that the truth might take some time to float to the surface. Many experts warn that more human trials are needed before any recommendations can be made with confidence. In previous decades, many research studies involved the use of impure (adulterated) or misidentified *Echinacea* species, making it difficult to draw firm conclusions from them today. So far, scientists have not identified a particular compound in echinacea to which they can ascribe the herb's medicinal benefits.[3] Controversy persists over the relative effectiveness of echinacea when taken orally.

Most studies involving humans so far have involved small numbers of subjects and were not soundly designed, meaning they were not randomized, placebo-controlled, or double-blind. The majority used the trademarked commercial preparation called Echinacin (the fresh juice of the aerial parts) or Esberitox, an herbal blend.[4] The bulk of the studies done in Germany have involved injectable preparations not available in the United States. A 1994 critical review of the human trials done to date reported that of the twenty-six placebo-controlled studies identified, only six tested extracts of echinacea alone, so that results could not be attributed to the herb directly. Some of these studies were not well designed.[5]

Still, significant pharmacologic potential has been documented in both test-tube and animal studies for the expressed juice of the upper parts of *Echinacea purpurea* and for alcoholic extracts of the roots of the three *Echinacea* species noted above.[6] Test-tube studies indicate that alcohol and water extracts of the plant fight certain viruses, including influenza and herpes[7]; these experiments show that cells immersed in echinacea can fend off infection from influenza and herpes viruses better than those that are not. But more research is needed to determine whether these actions will help fight related infections in humans. Echinacea specifically has not been shown to kill bacteria, but still-unidentified compounds in the plant appear to stimulate the immune system to fight certain invading organisms. It appears to boost the immune system by promoting the potency of infection-fighting cells such as macrophages, natural killer cells, and T lymphocytes. It may also increase the mobility of infection-fighting leukocytes (white blood cells) and stimulate phagocytosis, the process in which white blood cells consume invading organisms. Results have not been consistent, with some animal studies supporting the value of echinacea extracts in stimulating phagocytosis,[8] but others detecting no such actions.[9] The herb also appears to stimulate the production of other important immune system components, including a group of inflammatory mediators called tumor necrosis factor (TNF) and interferon.

These and possibly other properties come into play when you attempt to prevent or treat a common cold, sore throat, or other related symptoms with the herb. One study found good evidence for the effectiveness of 180 drops a day of *Echi-*

nacea purpurea tincture for helping to control the symptoms of upper respiratory tract infections, but no benefit over a placebo for lesser amounts, such as 90 drops a day.[10] German health authorities endorse the use of preparations made from the fresh aboveground parts of *Echinacea purpurea* and the root of *Echinacea pallida* (along with other substances) for helping to treat recurring respiratory and urinary tract infections. Interestingly, echinacea may work best when taken sparingly. One study found that a single dose stimulated the immune system in humans, but that taking the herb repeatedly over a period of days actually suppressed it.[11]

Laboratory findings have also confirmed the value of echinacea in treating superficial, poorly healing wounds such as cuts, cold sores, and psoriasis lesions. The polysaccharide extract echinacin appears to be responsible for this wound-healing property.[12] German health authorities approve of *Echinacea purpurea* preparations for these purposes.

A 1992 study involving fifteen individuals with very advanced colorectal cancer found that a formula of immune-system boosters including echinacea extracts (echinacin in particular) was not only well tolerated but beneficial in increasing the life expectancy of the subjects.[13] Similar results were seen with individuals suffering from advanced hepatocellular carcinoma.[14]

While laboratory studies suggest that echinacea stimulates the immune system, documentation to support the claims that it actually fights cancer, AIDS, or numerous other conditions is still weak or nonexistent.[15] It is also still too early to determine whether anticancer activity, as seen in a few animal tumors,[16] will translate into something meaningful for humans.

Clinical studies in Germany indicate that echinacea holds promise as a treatment for yeast infection and rheumatoid arthritis. If you suffer from either of these conditions, talk to your doctor about your interest in using echinacea to treat them.

Will It Harm You? What the Studies Say:

No significant side effects have been reported with the use of echinacea, although its toxicity has yet to be carefully examined in long-term clinical trials. The FDA placed echinacea on its formerly maintained list of "Herbs of Undefined Safety." German health authorities recommend that no one take echinacea either internally or externally for more than eight weeks in a row.[17] According to these authorities and several plant experts, echinacea should not be taken if you suffer from severe systemic illnesses such as multiple sclerosis, tuberculosis, AIDS, collagen vascular diseases, or other autoimmune diseases.[18] Theoretically, echinacea could interfere with other immunosuppressive therapy, so talk to your doctor before mixing medicines.[19]

Echinacea may cause allergic reactions in some people, particularly in those allergic to other members of the daisy family, such as ragweed, but this is not common. Some people feel a strange tingling sensation on their tongue, but this is harmless.

Some sources have questioned the wisdom of taking echinacea, given its apparent stimulation of a group of inflammatory mediators called tumor necrosis factor (TNF) and interferon,[20] which has a far-reaching and not completely understood role in the body's immune system.

GENERAL SOURCES:

Bauer, R. "Echinacea Drugs—Effects and Active Ingredients. Review." *Zeitschrift für Arztliche Fortbildung.* 90(2) (1996): 111–15.

Blumenthal, M., J. Gruenwald, T. Hall, and R.S. Rister, eds. *The Complete German Commission E Monographs: Therapeutic Guide to Herbal Medicine.* Boston: Integrative Medicine Communications, 1998.

Bradley, P.C., ed. *British Herbal Compendium: A Handbook of Scientific Information on Widely Used Plant Drugs,* vol. 1. Bournemouth (Dorset), England: British Herbal Medicine Association, 1992.

Castleman, M. *The Healing Herbs: The Ultimate Guide to the Curative Power of Nature's Medicines.* New York: Bantam Books, 1995.

Foster, S. *Forest Pharmacy: Medicinal Plants in American Forests.* Durham, NC: Forest History Society, 1995.

Lawrence Review of Natural Products. St. Louis: Facts and Comparisons, May 1995.

Murray, M.T. *The Healing Power of Herbs: The Enlightened Person's Guide to the Wonders of Medicinal Plants.* Rev. 2nd ed. Rocklin, CA: Prima Publishing, 1995.

Newall, C.A., et al. *Herbal Medicines: A Guide for Health-Care Professionals.* London: The Pharmaceutical Press, 1996.

Tyler, V.E. *Herbs of Choice: The Therapeutic Use of Phytomedicinals.* Binghamton, NY: Haworth Press/Pharmaceutical Products Press, 1994.

———. *The Honest Herbal.* Binghamton, NY: Haworth Press/Pharmaceutical Products Press, 1993.

TEXT CITATIONS:

1. V.E. Tyler, *The Honest Herbal* (Binghamton, NY: Haworth Press/Pharmaceutical Products Press, 1993).
2. P.C. Bradley, ed., *British Herbal Compendium: A Handbook of Scientific Information on Widely Used Plant Drugs,* vol. 1 (Bournemouth [Dorset], England: British Herbal Medicine Association, 1992).
3. *Lawrence Review of Natural Products* (St. Louis: Facts and Comparisons, May 1995).
4. Bradley, op. cit.
5. D. Melchart et al., *Phytomedicine,* 1 (1994): 245–54.
6. R. Bauer, *Zeitschrift für Arztliche Fortbildung,* 90(2) (1996): 111–15.
7. A. Wacker and W. Hilbig, *Planta Medica,* 33 (1978): 89–102.
8. R. Bauer et al., *Arzneimittel-Forschung,* 38 (1988): 276–81.
9. Bradley, op. cit. A. Schumacher and K.D. Friedberg, *Arzneimittel-Forschung,* 41 (1991): 141–47.
10. Melchart, op. cit.
11. E.G. Coeugniet and E. Elek, *Onkologie,* 10(Suppl 3) (1987): 27–33.
12. K. Busing, *Arzneimittel-Forschung,* 2 (1952): 467–69.
13. C. Lersch et al., *Cancer Investigation,* 10(5) (1992): 343–48.
14. C. Lersch et al., *Archiv für Geschwulstforschung,* 60(5) (1990): 379–83.
15. V.E. Tyler, *Herbs of Choice: The Therapeutic Use of Phytomedicinals* (Binghamton, NY: Haworth Press/Pharmaceutical Products Press, 1994).
16. D.J. Voaden and M. Jacobson, *Journal of Medical Chemistry,* 15 (1972): 619–23.
17. M. Blumenthal, J. Gruenwald, T. Hall, and R.S. Rister, eds., *The Complete German Commission E Monographs: Therapeutic Guide to Herbal Medicine* (Boston: Integrative Medicine Communications, 1998).
18. Tyler, op. cit. Blumenthal et al., op. cit.
19. Bradley, op. cit.
20. Ibid.

PRIMARY NAME:
ELDER

SCIENTIFIC NAME:
Sambucus canadensis L.
(American elder) and *Sambucus nigra* L. (European elder)
Family: Caprifoliaceae.

COMMON NAMES:
Common elder, elderberry, sambucus, sweet elder

RATING:
- *Flowers:* 2 = According to a number of well-designed studies and common use, this substance appears to be relatively effective and safe when used in recommended amounts for the indication(s) noted in the "Will It Work for You?" section.
- *Berries:* 4 = Research indicates that this fruit will not fulfill the claims made for it, but that it is also unlikely to cause any harm.

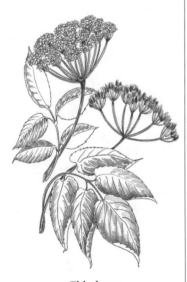

Elderberry
Sambucus canadensis

What Is Elder?

American elder is a shrub native to the eastern part of North America. European elder, a somewhat taller shrub or tree, can now be found in this country as well. Both are deciduous. The small cream-colored flowers, blue-black fruit ("berries"), roots, and inner bark have been used medicinally.

What It Is Used For:

Elder is steeped in folklore, the flowers and dried fruit ("berries") having been variously used since ancient times as flavorings, food colorings, and ingredients in perfumes, wines, preserves, and other foods. Both the flowers and the berries have also been valued as healing agents to induce perspiration for feverish chills, promote urination as a diuretic ("water pill"), dispel constipation, fight rheumatic inflammation, and control coughs, colds, flus, and associated fevers. External formulations have been enlisted as astringents, pain relievers, and gargles.

Forms Available Include:

- *Dried flowers:* Cream, flowers, infusion, liquid extract (including flower water), tablet, tea bag, tincture.
- *Dried berries:* Capsule, decoction, liquid extract, lozenge, ointment, tea bag.

Dosage Commonly Reported:

Elder-flower tea is made with 2 teaspoons dried flowers per cup of water and is drunk several times per day. To use commercial ointments and teas containing elder, follow the package instructions.

Will It Work for You? What the Studies Say:

Despite a general lack of clinical research into elder, a number of reliable sources accept that elder-flower preparations increase perspiration, a property traditionally considered valuable in treating symptoms of the common cold, flu, and other feverish conditions. Scientists are uncertain as to why it promotes this diaphoretic reaction, although drinking the infusion while it is still quite hot certainly helps and may be critical (as with any hot drink) in loosening mucus so that it is then easier to cough up, not to mention giving the user a mini steam bath. More data are needed to verify that chemicals in the plant called flavonoids and phenolic acids help encourage perspiration as well.[1] German health authorities officially approve of elder-flower preparations for treating symptoms of the common cold and feverish conditions.[2]

Studies also indicate that elder-flower preparations stimulate increased urination, which, if true, no doubt aids in the recovery from a feverish cold or flu as well, just as drinking a lot of fluids would. The flavonoids have been held responsible for this. No clinical trials to test these diuretic actions in humans appear to have been done, however. A diuretic effect would explain the widespread use of elder flower in "slimming" pills and other dieting formulas; it may produce a transitory loss of fluid weight from the body. Scientists attribute a laxative effect to elder flower as well,[3] which, if true, may explain its traditional use for constipation.

Some herbalists base their advice to use elder-flower preparations for arthritic and other rheumatic conditions on the premise that a diaphoretic and diuretic will promote the "removal of waste products" from the body.[4] This shaky theory does not appear to be substantiated by any research, although one animal study reported moderately strong anti-inflammatory actions in elder flowers.[5] No European regulatory agency recognizes this proposed antirheumatic action.

While elder berries are rich in vitamin C, evidence for any healing properties—laxative, diaphoretic, anti-inflammatory—is slim at best. Recently identified compounds (certain lectins) may prove valuable in blood typing and tests.[6]

Will It Harm You? What the Studies Say:

Primarily on the basis of years of folk use, elder-flower preparations appear to be safe to consume. German authorities report that they cause no known side effects or negative reactions with other medicines.[7] The raw berries are edible but may cause nausea and vomiting; once properly cooked, however, they pose no risk, as any lover of elderberry jam knows. The leaves and stems contain the potentially fatal poison cyanide; carefully avoid them.

GENERAL SOURCES:

Bisset, N.G., ed. *Herbal Drugs and Phytopharmaceuticals.* Stuttgart: medpharm GmbH Scientific Publishers, 1994.

Blumenthal, M., J. Gruenwald, T. Hall, and R.S. Rister, eds. *The Complete German Commission E Monographs: Therapeutic Guide to Herbal Medicine.* Boston: Integrative Medicine Communications, 1998.

Bradley, P.C., ed. *British Herbal Compendium: A Handbook of Scientific Information on Widely Used Plant Drugs,* vol. 1. Bournemouth (Dorset), England: British Herbal Medicine Association, 1992.

Chevallier, A. *The Encyclopedia of Medicinal Plants: A Practical Reference Guide to More Than 550 Key Medicinal Plants & Their Uses.* 1st American ed. New York: Dorling Kindersley Publications, 1996.

Duke, J.A. *CRC Handbook of Medicinal Herbs.* Boca Raton, FL: CRC Press, 1985.

Lawrence Review of Natural Products. St. Louis: Facts and Comparisons, July 1992.

Leung, A.Y., and S. Foster. *Encyclopedia of Common Natural Ingredients Used in Food, Drugs, and Cosmetics.* 2nd ed. New York: John Wiley & Sons, 1996.

Lin, C.N., and W.P Tome. *Planta Medica.* 54(3) (1988): 223.

Mindell, E. *Earl Mindell's Herb Bible.* New York: Simon & Schuster/Fireside, 1992.

Morbidity & Mortality Weekly Report. 33(13) (1984): 173.

Shibuya, N., et al. *Journal of Biochemistry.* 105(6) (1989): 1099.

TEXT CITATIONS:

1. P.C. Bradley, ed., *British Herbal Compendium: A Handbook of Scientific Information on Widely Used Plant Drugs,* vol. 1 (Bournemouth [Dorset], England: British Herbal Medicine Association, 1992).

2. M. Blumenthal, J. Gruenwald, T. Hall, and R.S. Rister, eds., *The Complete German Commission E Monographs: Therapeutic Guide to Herbal Medicine* (Boston: Integrative Medicine Communications, 1998).

3. A.Y. Leung and S. Foster, *Encyclopedia of Common Natural Ingredients Used in Food, Drugs, and Cosmetics,* 2nd ed. (New York: John Wiley & Sons, 1996).

4. Chevallier, A. *The Encyclopedia of Medicinal Plants: A Practical Reference Guide to More Than 550 Key Medicinal Plants & Their Uses,* 1st American ed. (New York: Dorling Kindersley Publications 1996).

5. N. Mascolo et al., *Phytotherapy Research*, 1(1987): 28–31.
6. Leung and Foster, op. cit.
7. Blumenthal et al., op. cit.

PRIMARY NAME:

ELECAMPANE

SCIENTIFIC NAME:
Inula helenium L. Family:
Asteraceae (Compositae)

COMMON NAMES:
Elf dock, horseheal, scabwort,
velvet dock, wild sunflower

RATING:

3 = Studies on the effectiveness
and safety of this substance are
conflicting, or there are not
enough studies to draw a
conclusion. Safety is a concern,
however; see the "Will It Harm
You?" section.

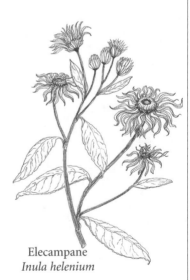

Elecampane
Inula helenium

What Is Elecampane?

The striking, golden-yellow flowers that bloom on this robust, hairy perennial reveal it as a member of the daisy family. Although indigenous to Asia, it is now cultivated worldwide as an ornamental. Its hefty rhizomes (underground stems) and roots are used medicinally.

What It Is Used For:

Folk healers have recommended this herb since ancient times as a digestive tonic, stomach soother, intestinal worm agent, menstrual pain remedy, and diuretic ("water pill") for such ills as kidney and urinary tract disease, and congestive heart failure. Traditional Indian (Ayurvedic) and Chinese doctors prescribe it for respiratory ailments such as asthma, congestion, and chronic bronchitis. The *U.S. Pharmacopoeia* once listed the dried root as a remedy for digestive, liver, and respiratory disorders. Elecampane-soaked bandages have reportedly been used to treat skin irritations and infections.

Modern Western herbalists generally limit their recommendations to respiratory ailments such as cough, bronchitis, and emphysema, although the herb can sometimes be found in gastrointestinal remedies, parasite cures, kidney and urinary tract treatments, laxatives, and arthritis preparations.

Forms Available Include:

Decoction, pill, powdered root, tea, tincture. Elecampane appears in numerous herbal blends.

Dosage Commonly Reported:

A decoction is made using ¼ teaspoon powdered root per cup of water. To use commercial elecampane preparations, follow the package instructions.

Will It Work for You? What the Studies Say:

Plant experts hold responsible a substance called alantolactone (a sesquiterpene lactone) in elecampane's volatile oil for the herb's activity in various studies. In animal studies, alantolactone has blood-pressure-lowering and blood-sugar-lowering effects,[1] although large doses actually increase blood sugar levels. Human studies suggest that it can fight intestinal parasites.[2] Test-tube and animal studies indicate that it and another lactone, isoalantolactone, vigorously fight bacteria and fungi[3] and have antitumor activity.[4] An assortment of other experiments have found that alantolactone may stimulate the immune system,[5] increase urination (as a diuretic), stimulate the flow of bile, and possibly even help break up secretions that may contribute to congestion in coughs and colds.[6]

Elecampane's volatile oil content (1 to 4 percent) helps explain its use in cough, bronchitis, and other respiratory remedies; these oils are believed to encourage clearing of congestion.[7] Its value as an anticough or asthma remedy has not been well substantiated, however.[8] Its bitter-tasting substances may explain why people turned to it to soothe stomach upset and gas. Mice fed an infusion of the herb became sedated,[9] and this points to a possible sedative action in humans that still demands investigation.

Ultimately, however, elecampane's health risks may outweigh its still-unclear benefits for most people. German health authorities concluded not only that evidence for the herb's effectiveness in treating gastrointestinal, respiratory, or lower urinary tract ailments is poorly substantiated, but that the risk of an allergic reaction is too high to justify its use.[10]

The root also contains a sweet-tasting substance called inulin, which has been used as a sugar substitute for diabetics. Anyone with blood-sugar-regulating problems should note, however, that large doses of an extract in elecampane actually increased blood sugar levels in animals.

Will It Harm You? What the Studies Say:

The substances probably responsible for rendering elecampane potentially effective—the sesquiterpene lactones—are also blamed for its hazardous effects. The sesquiterpene lactones irritate mucous membranes. Allergic reactions and contact dermatitis have occurred in people previously sensitized to it and who have skin contact with the herb or its oil.[11] It may also cause an allergic reaction if you are sensitive to other members of the daisy family.

If taken in large amounts, elecampane can cause vomiting, diarrhea, vertigo, abdominal cramps, and symptoms of paralysis.[12] Although no complications have been documented in pregnant women, they may want to avoid it, given its past folk use for stimulating the uterus. Largely on the basis of these types of apparent health risks, German health authorities declined to approve the herb for any medicinal purpose. The FDA has concluded that as a food, elecampane rhizome and root are generally recognized as safe, but it has made no statement regarding their safety in medicinal concentrations.

GENERAL SOURCES:

Bisset, N.G., ed. *Herbal Drugs and Phytopharmaceuticals*. Stuttgart: medpharm GmbH Scientific Publishers, 1994.

Blumenthal, M., J. Gruenwald, T. Hall, and R.S. Rister, eds. *The Complete German Commission E Monographs: Therapeutic Guide to Herbal Medicine*. Boston: Integrative Medicine Communications, 1998.

Bradley, P.C., ed. *British Herbal Compendium: A Handbook of Scientific Information on Widely Used Plant Drugs*, vol. 1. Bournemouth (Dorset), England: British Herbal Medicine Association, 1992.

Castleman, M. *The Healing Herbs. The Ultimate Guide to the Curative Power of Nature's Medicines*. New York: Bantam Books, 1995.

Leung, A.Y., and S. Foster. *Encyclopedia of Common Natural Ingredients Used in Food, Drugs, and Cosmetics*. 2nd ed. New York: John Wiley & Sons, 1996.

Stary, F. *The Natural Guide to Medicinal Herbs and Plants*. Prague: Barnes & Noble, Inc., in arrangement with Aventinum Publishers, 1996.

Tierra, M. *The Way of Herbs*. New York: Pocket Books, 1990.

Weiner, M.A., and J.A. Weiner. *Herbs That Heal: Prescription for Herbal Healing*. Mill Valley, CA: Quantum Books, 1994.

Weiss, R.F. *Herbal Medicine*, trans. A.R. Meuss, from the 6th German edition. Beaconsfield, England: Beaconsfield Publishers, Ltd., 1988.

TEXT CITATIONS:

1. A.Y. Leung and S. Foster. *Encyclopedia of Common Natural Ingredients Used in Food, Drugs, and Cosmetics*, 2nd ed. (New York: John Wiley & Sons, 1996).

2. Ibid.

3. Ibid.

4. N.G. Bisset, ed., *Herbal Drugs and Phytopharmaceuticals* (Stuttgart: medpharm GmbH Scientific Publishers, 1994).

5. H. Wagner and A. Proksch, *Economic and Medicinal Plant Research*, vol. 1., N. Farnsworth et al., eds. (New York: Academic Press, 1985).

6. Bisset, op. cit.

7. R.F. Weiss, *Herbal Medicine*, trans. A.R. Meuss, from the 6th German edition (Beaconsfield, England: Beaconsfield Publishers, Ltd., 1988).

8. Ibid.

9. R. Kieswetter and M. Müller, *Pharmazie*, 13 (1958): 777.

10. M. Blumenthal, J. Gruenwald, T. Hall, and R.S. Rister, eds., *The Complete German Commission E Monographs: Therapeutic Guide to Herbal Medicine* (Boston: Integrative Medicine Communications, 1998).

11. J.C. Mitchell et al., *Journal of Investigative Dermatology*, 54 (1970): 233.

12. Bisset, op. cit.

PRIMARY NAME:

ENGLISH WALNUT LEAF

SCIENTIFIC NAME:
Juglans regia L. Family: Juglandaceae

COMMON NAME:
N/A

RATING:
2 = According to a number of well-designed studies and common use, this substance appears to be relatively effective and safe when used in recommended amounts for the indication(s) noted in the "Will It Work for You?" section.

What Is English Walnut Leaf?

The dried, lance-shaped leaves of the English walnut, a stately tree cultivated throughout North America and many other parts of the world, are used medicinally. They taste harsh and rather bitter. The flowering trees also bear a smooth, nutlike fruit.

What it Is Used For:

Traditional healers consider the English walnut leaf a classic astringent substance for skin disorders ranging from chronic eczema to acne, eczema, ulcers, scrofula (a form of tuberculosis), inflammation of the eyelids, fungal infections, and the redness and inflammation of dermatitis. A German textbook cites it as a good choice for children's skin complaints.[1] Although no longer commonly recommended, infusions of the leaves were once taken internally for diarrhea, worms, and fungal infections.

Forms Available Include:

Bath, decoction, dressing, eyewash, lotion, poultice, rinse, wash.

Dosage Commonly Reported:

A decoction for external use is made with 5 teaspoons chopped leaf in 200 milliliters (about 1 cup) water and is applied three or four times per day.

Will It Work for You? What the Studies Say:

Walnut leaves contain abundant amounts (about 10 percent) of an astringent substance called tannin, which explains and justifies the plant's traditional use for skin inflammations and wounds; tannins are known to constrict (tighten) tissue, reducing oozing, weeping, and bleeding, and protecting the skin. German health authorities endorse the use of English walnut leaves externally for mild, superficial inflammation of the skin as well as excessive sweating of the hands, feet, and other parts of the body.[2]

Several sources also assert that the chemical juglone[3] and the plant's essential oil[4] are astringent, possibly justifying walnut leaf's use for fungal skin infections such as ringworm, for example. Others have shown that juglone fights numerous oral bacteria and may work in combination with other substances to control infectious diseases in the mouth.[5] Juglone appears to inhibit certain types of tumors when injected into mice.[6] What this means for treating tumors in humans remains unclear.

Will It Harm You? What the Studies Say:

The recent medical literature contains no references to serious adverse reactions to English walnut leaf preparations. German health authorities cite no side effects, situations in which the herb should not be used, or interactions with other medicines.

GENERAL SOURCES:

Bisset, N.G., ed. *Herbal Drugs and Phytopharmaceuticals.* Stuttgart: medpharm GmbH Scientific Publishers, 1994.

Blumenthal, M., J. Gruenwald, T. Hall, and R.S. Rister, eds. *The Complete German Commission E Monographs: Therapeutic Guide to Herbal Medicine.* Boston: Integrative Medicine Communications, 1998.

Ody, P. *The Herb Society's Complete Medicinal Herbal.* London: Dorling Kindersley Limited, 1993.

Tyler, V.E. *Herbs of Choice: The Therapeutic Use of Phytomedicinals.* Binghamton, NY: Haworth Press/Pharmaceutical Products Press, 1994.

Weiss, R.F. *Herbal Medicine,* trans. A.R. Meuss, from the 6th German edition. Beaconsfield, England: Beaconsfield Publishers, Ltd., 1988.

TEXT CITATIONS:

1. R.F. Weiss, *Herbal Medicine,* trans. A.R. Meuss from the 6th German edition (Beaconsfield, England: Beaconsfield Publishers, Ltd., 1988).
2. M. Blumenthal, J. Gruenwald, T. Hall, and R.S. Rister, eds., *The Complete German Commission E Monographs: Therapeutic Guide to Herbal Medicine* (Boston: Integrative Medicine Communications, 1998).
3. N.G. Bisset, ed., *Herbal Drugs and Phytopharmaceuticals* (Stuttgart: medpharm GmbH Scientific Publishers, 1994).
4. A. Nahrstedt et al., *Planta Medica,* 42 (1981): 313.
5. N. Didry et al., *Pharmazie,* 49(9) (1994): 681–83.
6. U.C. Bhargava and B.A. Westfall, *Journal of Pharmacy and Parmacology,* 57 (1968): 1674. T.A. Okada et al., *Proceedings of the Society of Experimental Biology and Medicine,* 126 (1967): 583.

EPHEDRA

SCIENTIFIC NAME:

Ephedra sinica Stapf., *Ephedra intermedia* Shrenk et C.A. Mey, and *Ephedra equisetina* Bge. Family: Ephedraceae (Gnetaceae)

COMMON NAMES:

Cao mahaung, Chinese ephedra, epitonin, ma-huang gen

RATING:

5 = Studies indicate that there is a definite health hazard to using this substance, even in recommended amounts.

What Is Ephedra?

Ephedra species found around the world, including *Ephedra sinica*, are typically short and nearly leafless evergreen shrubs that favor dry, sandy or rocky environments. They bear minute, yellow-green flowers and fruits. The herbaceous green stems and the root are used medicinally. Most species emit a strong odor of pine.

There are numerous *Ephedra* species. For information on the type that grows in North America, see **Mormon Tea** (*Ephedra nevadensis*), which contains none of ephedra's active ingredients.

What It Is Used For:

For years, most Americans took over-the-counter cold and allergy remedies containing ephedrine and pseudoephedrine (a closely related compound) without realizing that they were partaking in an herbal tradition many millennia old. The Chinese had been relying on the plant that these substances were derived from—ephedra—in similar ways as a decongestant for common colds as well as a treatment for asthma, bronchitis, hay fever, and other upper respiratory ailments. Western medicine first showed interest in this ancient Chinese herb in the early 1920s, when researchers discovered that it contained an alkaloid, ephedrine, directly responsible for these properties.

Traditional Chinese healers have also valued ephedra for treating arthritis, fever, hives, lack of perspiration, headache, aching joints and bones, wheezing, and low blood pressure, among other things. Traditional healers in Pakistan, India, and other parts of the world had been turning to their respective ephedra species for treating many of the same ailments.

Standardized ephedrine and pseudoephedrine drugs can be found on the shelves of every American drugstore today. But contemporary herbalists carry on in the tradition of the ancients, touting the whole herb as the key to relieving nasal and chest congestion due to colds and flu and improving respiratory function impaired by asthma and hay fever. Many sources also promote ephedra's stimulant properties in "energy" formulas, hailing it as a source for a "natural high." Numerous herbal weight-loss and body-building formulas feature the herb, as do formulas promoted for increasing sexual sensations and heightening awareness.

Forms Available Include:

Capsule, decoction, dried herb, tablet, tincture. Many states have banned the sale of ephedra-containing dietary supplements, owing to health concerns.

Dosage Commonly Reported:

A decoction is made with 2 grams (1 heaping teaspoon) herb in 240 milliliters (½ pint) water, and provides about 15 to 30 milligrams ephedrine. The National Foods Association in California recommends that tablets, capsules, and other solid-dosage forms contain a maximum of 10 milligrams of total ephedra alkaloids; that no more than 20 milligrams of these alkaloids be ingested in one dose; and that no more than 60 milligrams be taken in one day.

Will It Work for You? What the Studies Say:

Ephedra contains a critical mixture of alkaloids (1 to 2 percent) composed of ephedrine and pseudoephedrine. The crude drug, often sold in dietary supplements, can have the same effects on the body that the extracted ephedrine used in standard cold and asthma remedies can. At typically recommended (conventional) doses, ephedrine constricts peripheral blood vessels, relieving nasal congestion in mucous tissues; and opens up bronchial tubes, making it easier for allergy and asthma sufferers to breathe. The chemically related compound pseudoephedrine does not have as powerful an effect as ephedrine on the heart, although it has a stronger ability to induce urine secretion.[1] Ephedrine and pseudoephedrine have also shown anti-inflammatory properties in laboratory animals,[2] and antiallergy actions have been demonstrated in test-tube studies.[3] German health authorities endorse the use of the crude drug, ephedra, for treating respiratory tract diseases with mild bronchospasms in adults.[4]

Ephedra can rightfully be called an "energizer," although this stimulant effect comes at a price. It is the contained ephedrine, an amphetamine-like stimulant, that is responsible for this sensation at certain dosages. It works by revving up the central nervous system and stimulating the heart, increasing the heart rate and often elevating blood pressure. This can be hazardous; see the "Will It Harm You?" section for more information. Ephedra tea, as well as the volatile oil, induces sweating in humans.

No evidence has ever shown that ephedra—or its constituents—will burn fat, reduce appetite, or result in weight loss. A number of herbalists contend that ephedrine, in combination with caffeine, will be thermogenic (produce body heat) and thus burn certain types of body fat—brown adipose tissue, specifically. This does not, however, represent a large percentage of adult body fat.

Will It Harm You? What the Studies Say:

Ephedra is a potent medicine that must be used with care. Failure to do so has proved not only uncomfortable but fatal in some cases. Like amphetamine, ephedrine at certain dosages stimulates the heart and central nervous system, increasing blood pressure (both systolic and diastolic),[5] and it can cause palpitations, dizziness, skin flushing, headache, nervousness, sleeplessness, tingling, vomiting, anxiety, high blood pressure, glaucoma, urinary problems, impaired brain circulation, and other problems.[6] Individuals who suffer from heart conditions, high blood pressure, thyroid disorders, difficulty urinating due to an enlarged prostate, or diabetes should be particularly careful in taking ephedra or its constituents. Those taking blood pressure medicines or antidepressants should also exercise great care.

So far, seventeen deaths have been attributed to dietary supplements containing ephedrine. The FDA has received hundreds of reports regarding adverse reactions to the herb, and many more have been reported on the state level. As of mid-1997, the federal government was considering requiring that all dietary supplements containing ephedrine carry safety warning labels. The FDA also expressed a desire to ban the marketing of ephedrine-containing bodybuilding and weight-loss agents. Many states have already restricted sales of ephedra.

Sensitive individuals have developed skin reactions to ephedrine.[7]

GENERAL SOURCES:

American Pharmaceutical Association. *Handbook of Nonprescription Drugs*. 11th ed. Washington, D.C.: American Pharmaceutical Association, 1996.

Castleman, M. *The Healing Herbs: The Ultimate Guide to the Curative Power of Nature's Medicines*. New York: Bantam Books, 1995.

Lawrence Review of Natural Products. St. Louis: Facts and Comparisons, November 1995.

Leung, A.Y., and S. Foster. *Encyclopedia of Common Natural Ingredients Used in Food, Drugs, and Cosmetics*. 2nd ed. New York: John Wiley & Sons, 1996.

Mindell, E. *Earl Mindell's Herb Bible*. New York: Simon & Schuster/Fireside, 1992.

Murray, M.T. *The Healing Power of Herbs: The Enlightened Person's Guide to the Wonders of Medicinal Plants*. Revised and expanded 2nd ed. Rocklin, CA: Prima Publishing, 1995.

Tyler, V.E. *Herbs of Choice: The Therapeutic Use of Phytomedicinals*. Binghamton, NY: Haworth Press/Pharmaceutical Products Press, 1994.

———. *The Honest Herbal*. Binghamton, NY: Haworth Press/Pharmaceutical Products Press, 1993.

Weiner, M.A., and J.A. Weiner. *Herbs That Heal: Prescription for Herbal Healing*. Mill Valley, CA: Quantum Books, 1994.

TEXT CITATIONS:

1. A.Y. Leung and S. Foster, *Encyclopedia of Common Natural Ingredients Used in Food, Drugs, and Cosmetics*, 2nd ed. (New York: John Wiley & Sons, 1996).
2. Ibid.
3. Ibid.
4. Ibid.
5. V.E. Tyler, *The Honest Herbal* (Binghamton, NY: Haworth Press/Pharmaceutical Products Press, 1993).
6. Leung and Foster, op. cit. P. Kalix, *Journal of Ethnopharmacology*, 32(1–3) (1991): 201.
7. Kalix, P., op. cit.

PRIMARY NAME:

EUCALYPTUS

SCIENTIFIC NAME:
Eucalpytus globulus Labill.
Family: Myrtaceae

COMMON NAMES:
Blue gum, fever tree, gum tree, Tasmanian blue gum

What Is Eucalyptus?

Few trees in the world are larger and faster-growing than this native Australian evergreen. They are cultivated worldwide and have a smooth bluish-white bark and a distinctive smell. A special steaming process extracts a strongly aromatic essential oil from the fresh, bluish-green leaves. Medicinal preparations are made from the leaves and this oil.

What It Is Used For:

Schoolchildren learn that koala bears like to munch on eucalyptus leaves, but they probably do not get briefed on the many uses the Australian Aborigines had for this tree. When the outback got scorched, they chewed on the water-clogged leaves for liquid. They also counted on the leaves and the oil to reduce

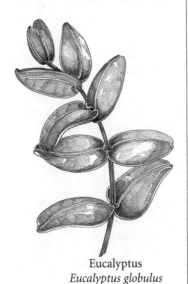

Eucalyptus
Eucalyptus globulus

fevers, control coughs and asthma, and treat arthritis, stomach disorders, and skin sores. European settlers picked up on a number of these practices, also turning to the abundant tree for cleaning wounds and fighting ulcers and cancers. European and American hospitals started to sterilize surgical equipment, including catheters, with the oil. This explains the once-popular term for eucalyptus oil: catheter oil.

Thousands of miles away, traditional Chinese doctors recommended parts of the eucalyptus tree for many of the same ailments. Folk healers through the ages have also used the leaves in the form of decoctions and liquid extracts to treat ringworm, dysentery, sore muscles, and scores of other ailments. At one time, eucalyptus was referred to as the "Australian fever tree" because a tea made from the leaves seemed to quash epidemics involving high fevers.

Today, eucalyptus appears in popular American trademarked medicines such as Listerine, Dristan Nasal Decongestant Spray, Hall's Mentho-Lyptus Cough Suppressants, and Vicks VapoRub, not to mention numerous herbal cough and other remedies. The herb can claim fame as a topical antiseptic, a soothing skin rub for arthritic and other rheumatic pains, and an ingredient in steam inhalation for nasal stuffiness caused by cold or flu, asthma, bronchitis, or croup. Herbalists enthusiastically recommend eucalyptus leaf tea as a gargle for sore throats and bronchitis. Aromatherapists say eucalyptus relaxes and soothes the body. Small amounts of eucalyptus oil and its extracts appear in foods, alcohol, toothpastes, candies, dentistry agents, soaps and detergents (as a fragrance), and other commercial products.

Forms Available Include:

Leaves (for teas, herbal wraps, and other preparations), oil (not to be used for teas), tincture. The oil appears in numerous commercially prepared steam vaporizer products, skin rubs (ointments and balms), antiseptics, mouthwashes, herbal baths, cough lozenges and syrups, and other medicinal products.

Dosage Commonly Reported:

A steam inhalation is made using a handful of leaves or a few drops essential oil. The drops can also be added to a vaporizer. An infusion is made using 1 to 2 teaspoons leaves. Follow package instructions on commercial preparations.

Will It Work for You? What the Studies Say:

According to centuries of use and scientific findings, eucalyptus is an herbal winner. Much of this can be attributed to the primary ingredient in the volatile oil, eucalyptol, which boasts a number of medicinal qualities. As a decongestant and expectorant, it loosens sticky phlegm (mucus) in the chest so that it is easier to cough up. To be effective, the leaf oil must be derived from *E. globulus*, *E. polybractea*, *E. smithii*, or *E. australiana* and contain at least 70 to 85 percent of eucalyptol (not all species of the tree do). German health authorities approve of eucalyptus preparations for treating congested airways.[1]

Cough lozenges with eucalyptol suppress coughs by boosting saliva production. Once the person swallows more frequently to contend with this increased saliva, the tendency to cough is lessened. A number of lozenges with similar volatile oils work this way as well.[2]

Scientifically proven antibacterial and antiviral properties in eucalyptus make the herb effective in preventing infection in minor cuts or scrapes and help explain why people turned to it in the days before antibiotics. The antiseptic properties have been demonstrated in test tubes and to a limited extent in animals.[3] Always wash a wound well before applying a few drops of the oil or liquid extracts of the herb, and see a doctor if an infection develops.

When eucalyptus tea is slowly sipped, ingredients called tannins in the plant have an astringent, soothing effect on inflammation in the mouth and throat.[4] Astringents constrict (tighten) tissue and reduce oozing. Scientists now know that the "Australian fever tree" was powerless against the organism that caused the scourge—malaria—but was nevertheless effective in abolishing it: The eucalyptus tree soaks up so much moisture that swampy areas promptly dry out. As a result, malaria-carrying mosquitoes are squeezed out of their boggy habitats.

A number of eucalyptus oils and ointments are billed as sore muscle balms. Research shows that the herb does increase the flow of blood to the area, generating a sensation of warmth. Whether this actually eases the uncomfortable feeling of muscle soreness is probably pretty subjective.

Eucalyptus boasts a number of other intriguing properties as well. In one test-tube study, constituents in the herb demonstrated antitumor properties.[5] Extracts have shown promise as antidiabetic agents in test animals.[6] In a randomized, placebo-controlled trial reported in 1994, a mixture of eucalyptus, peppermint, and ethanol oils did not reduce headache pain in thirty-two subjects, but when applied to the forehead and temples it had mental- and muscle-relaxing effects and reportedly increased cognitive performance.[7]

Will It Harm You? What the Studies Say:

When used as recommended, eucalyptus tea and commercial preparations are very safe. Not surprisingly, however, large doses of any eucalyptus product can cause nausea, vomiting, or diarrhea or other reactions. Children under two years old should probably not be given any eucalyptus product, including topical ones (see below). German health authorities caution that people who have serious liver problems or who suffer from inflammation of the stomach, intestines, or biliary tract should not use any other internal eucalyptus preparations, including tea.[8] Pregnant women should not take eucalyptus.

Cough drops and other commercial products contain so little eucalyptus oil that they pose no risk. *But avoid ingesting the oil in anything other than prepared products because high doses can be very toxic.* Eucalyptus-oil poisoning in children can cause vomiting, loss of consciousness, lung disease, and other serious complications, including death in some cases. Extremely dangerous depression of consciousness can occur after an infant or small child has ingested 5 milliliters or more of pure oil.[9] As little as a teaspoonful (3.5 milliliters) has been fatal to both children and adults. Some investigators contend that the oil is actually much less toxic than believed, however, and that a child who has been poisoned but has gotten prompt and adequate care (including having his or her stomach pumped out) will probably have a good outcome.

Topical preparations of the oil pose very little risk. Except in the few individuals who are sensitive to the plant and might develop a rash, it is not likely to irritate the skin. Never apply eucalyptus preparations to the face of a baby or very young child; the area around the nose may be especially sensitive and eucalyptus could cause a gagging reaction.

GENERAL SOURCES:

Bisset, N.G., ed. *Herbal Drugs and Phytopharmaceuticals.* Stuttgart: medpharm GmbH Scientific Publishers, 1994.

Blumenthal, M., J. Gruenwald, T. Hall, and R.S. Rister, eds. *The Complete German Commission E Monographs: Therapeutic Guide to Herbal Medicine.* Boston: Integrative Medicine Communications, 1998.

Castleman, M. *The Healing Herbs: The Ultimate Guide to the Curative Power of Nature's Medicines.* New York, NY: Bantam Books, 1995.

Heinerman, J. *Heinerman's Encyclopedia of Healing Herbs and Spices.* West Nyack, NY: Parker Publishing Co., 1996.

Leung, A.Y. *Encyclopedia of Common Natural Ingredients Used in Food, Drugs, and Cosmetics.* New York: John Wiley & Sons, 1980.

Marzuella, J.C., and P.A. Henry. *Journal of the American Pharmaceutical Association.* 47 (1958): 294.

Mindell, E. *Earl Mindell's Herb Bible.* New York: Simon & Schuster/Fireside, 1992.

Opdyke, D.L.J. *Food & Cosmetics Toxicology.* 13 (1975): 105, 107.

Schaller, M., and H.C. Korting. *Clinical and Experimental Dermatology.* 20(2) (1995): 143–45.

Trease, G. E, and W. C. Evans *Trease and Evans' Pharmacognosy.* 13th ed. Philadelphia: Bailliere Tindall, 1989.

Tyler, V.E. *Herbs of Choice: The Therapeutic Use of Phytomedicinals.* Binghamton, NY: Haworth Press/Pharmaceutical Products Press, 1994.

Webb, N.J., and W.R. Pitt. *Journal of Paediatrics and Child Health.* 29(5) (1993): 368–71.

Weiss, R.F. *Herbal Medicine*, trans. A.R. Meuss, from the 6th German edition. Beaconsfield, England: Beaconsfield Publishers, Ltd., 1988.

TEXT CITATIONS:

1. M. Blumenthal, J. Gruenwald, T. Hall, and R.S. Rister, eds., *The Complete German Commission E Monographs: Therapeutic Guide to Herbal Medicine* (Boston: Integrative Medicine Communications, 1998).

2. V.E. Tyler, *Herbs of Choice: The Therapeutic Use of Phytomedicinals* (Binghamton, NY: Haworth Press/Pharmaceutical Products Press, 1994).

3. A.Y. Leung, *Encyclopedia of Common Natural Ingredients Used in Food, Drugs, and Cosmetics* (New York: John Wiley & Sons, 1980).

4. N.G. Bisset, ed., *Herbal Drugs and Phytopharmaceuticals* (Stuttgart: medpharm GmbH Scientific Publishers, 1994).

5. M. Takasaki et al., *Biological and Pharmaceutical Bulletin*, 18(3) (1995): 435–38.

6. S.K. Swanston-Flatt et al., *Diabetologia*, 33(8) (1990): 462–64. J. Boufek et al., *Plantes Medicinales et Phytotherapie*, 10 (1976): 119.

7. H. Gobel et al., *Cephalalgia*, 14(3) (1994): 228–34.

8. Blumenthal et al., op. cit.

9. J. Tibballs, *Medical Journal of Australia*, 163(4) (1995): 177–80.

PRIMARY NAME:
EVENING PRIMROSE OIL

SCIENTIFIC NAME:
Oenothera biennis L. Family: Onagraceae

COMMON NAME:
King's cure-all

RATING:
2 = According to a number of well-designed studies and common use, this substance appears to be relatively effective and safe when used in recommended amounts for the indication(s) noted in the "Will It Work for You?" section.

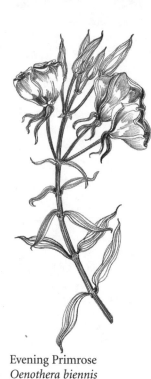

Evening Primrose
Oenothera biennis

What Is Evening Primrose Oil?

The large, delicate evening primrose is a wildflower native to eastern North America. The small, reddish seeds contain an oil rich in an important substance called gamma-linoleic acid (GLA). The seeds are cultivated in many parts of the world, and the oil from them is sold as a nutritional supplement or ingredient in specialty foods in more than thirty countries. The United States and Canada alone produce more than three hundred to four hundred tons of the seeds annually. The bright yellow flowers usually bloom in the evening and remain open only through the following day. Although a member of the primrose family, this plant is not a true primrose.

What It Is Used For:

Native American tribes regarded evening primrose as a food and remedy for various ailments long before Europeans were introduced to it in the seventeenth century. In the centuries since then, folk healers have recommended an infusion made with the entire plant as an astringent and sedative and as a treatment for stomach and intestinal disorders, asthmatic cough, and whooping cough. Poultices prepared from these infusions were used to encourage wound healing. Many herbalists still recommend the whole herb for treating anxiety and helping to keep skin healthy.

The oil is the star feature of evening primrose. It contains abundant amounts of essential fatty acids (EFAs), especially GLA and *cis*-linoleic acid, that are converted into important hormones inside the body. Both are important to normal physiologic function. Experts contend that many disorders may be caused by insufficient amounts of EFAs in the body or an inability to metabolize them properly. Advocates say GLA has the potential to ameliorate such conditions as arthritis, inflammatory skin diseases (e.g., eczema), premenstrual syndrome (PMS), hair loss, breast pain, infertility (in men especially), weak immune-system function, and heart disease. Animal studies and a growing number of human studies support some of these claims, although the results are controversial and critics remain skeptical. The oils of **Black Currant** and **Borage** also contain EFAs and are similarly used.

Forms Available:

Capsule (liquid-filled), liquid, oil, tablet.

Dosage Commonly Reported:

Dosages vary, depending on the type of ailment being treated. A common dosage is 250 milligrams taken up to three times a day. For PMS, the oil is taken two to three days before the expected onset of symptoms. About 270 to 720 milligrams a day of evening primrose oil (EPO), equivalent to 1 to 2 grams of GLA, may be needed for inflammatory and cardiovascular disorders. More modest doses are typically recommended for atopic eczema, equivalent to about 250 to 500 milligrams of GLA a day.

Will It Work for You? What the Studies Say:

The seeds of this plant contain about 14 percent of a fixed oil—evening primrose oil (EPO)—that contains about 7 to 10 percent GLA (an essential polyunsaturated fatty acid) and *cis*-linoleic acid (about 50 to 70 percent). Research indicates that by ingesting this oil, the body can convert the contained GLA into a precursor form of the hormone prostaglandin. Although GLA is a major component in human milk, only small amounts of it appear in commonly eaten foods. Factors such as high cholesterol, aging, stress, alcohol, diabetes, PMS, aging, viral infections, and other conditions may also interfere with the normal conversion of linoleic acid into GLA.[1] Plant experts contend that people who get little GLA through their diets may benefit from taking GLA-rich supplements like evening primrose oil, as may those whose systems are unable to metabolize *cis*-linoleic acid into GLA.[2]

Still up for debate, however, is whether GLA can ameliorate such conditions as arthritis, PMS, high blood pressure, and heart disease, as some advocates assert. Animal studies and increasing numbers of human studies indicate that some of these claims may be true, although the results are controversial and critics remain skeptical. When considering the value of any of these studies, bear in mind that in almost all cases capsules were used. Buy them from a reliable source, as cheap oil substitutes such as safflower oil have been found in a number of products.[3]

Studies indicate that GLA may help prevent or treat heart disease and stroke by lowering blood cholesterol levels and reducing the stickiness of blood platelets (platelet aggregation) that can lead to blood clots.[4] In a 1983 study, significant drops in serum cholesterol (31.5 percent) were documented in 179 subjects who took an evening primrose oil product for three months, while no such reductions were seen in a small group of subjects who took a placebo.[5] No other human trials on this subject appear in the recent medical literature.

A mounting body of research indicates that people who suffer from atopic eczema have a disorder of EFAs (specifically, a defect in the function of a crucial enzyme that GLA helps to metabolize).[6] Results of clinical trials testing EPO's (and thus, GLA's) ability to control itching and other symptoms associated with atopic eczema and other skin disorders have been mixed, with some showing modest improvements and others showing no changes at all. Oral dietary supplement forms of GLA not only have proved effective in improving atopic eczema in various studies,[7] including one involving children who experienced "dramatic" improvements after four weeks of treatment,[8] but have also been shown to be significantly superior to a placebo in relieving itching and reducing the need for steroid medications in these situations.[9] Not all trials have reported such positive results, however.[10] Topical EPO formulations for treating atopic eczema are officially approved of and commonly used in England.[11]

Mixed results have also been seen in tests of EPO's ability to help control rheumatoid arthritis. The oil has been intensively studied as a treatment for this often debilitating condition,[12] with several studies reporting significant improvement over placebos in reducing such factors as the number of tender and swollen joints.[13] In an apparently well-designed double-blind trial reported in 1988, EPO capsules significantly improved the condition of rheumatoid arthritis sufferers compared with a placebo, as reported by the subjects themselves.[14] The same positive results held true for subjects given EPO along with fish oil. In fact, the improvement was so notable in some of the subjects that they could consider stopping treatment with nonsteroidal anti-inflammatory drugs.

Intriguing findings have also been reported for such ailments as ulcerative colitis (limited success in a placebo-controlled study),[15] diabetes (potential to reverse neurologic damage has been reported, as well as normalization of certain lipid metabolism factors),[16] multiple sclerosis (slight improvements in human trials),[17] breast pain caused by such conditions as polycystic breast disease (notable improvements in human trials),[18] and alcohol withdrawal symptoms (as well as speed of liver healing).[19] Researchers report that EPO can kill certain tumor cells both in the test tube and in living animals, but the implications for treating human cancers remain unclear.[20] EPO injections have significantly reduced tumors in animal studies when compared with a placebo.[21]

In a handful of studies, breast tenderness and other PMS symptoms such as irritability, depression, and bloating improved significantly in women taking EPO as compared with those taking a placebo.[22] Not all such studies have reported positive results,[23] however, and this application remains a subject of debate.[24]

Will It Harm You? What the Studies Say:

Evening primrose oil qualifies favorably in terms of safety when taken in typically recommended amounts. The medical literature contains no references to serious adverse reactions despite widespread use. A commercial supplier of the oil who carried out animal toxicity studies reported a sound safety profile.[25]

GENERAL SOURCES:
American Pharmaceutical Association. *Handbook of Nonprescription Drugs.* 11th ed. Washington, D.C.: American Pharmaceutical Association, 1996.
Lawrence Review of Natural Products. St. Louis: Facts and Comparisons, November 1993.
Leung, A.Y., and S. Foster. *Encyclopedia of Common Natural Ingredients Used in Food, Drugs, and Cosmetics.* 2nd ed. New York: John Wiley & Sons, 1996.
Mindell, E. *Earl Mindell's Herb Bible.* New York: Simon & Schuster/Fireside, 1992.
Trease, G. E., and W.C. Evans *Trease and Evans' Pharmacognosy.* 13th ed. Philadelphia: Bailliere Tindall, 1989.
Weiss, R.F. *Herbal Medicine,* trans. A.R. Meuss, from the 6th German edition. Beaconsfield, England: Beaconsfield Publishers, Ltd., 1988.

TEXT CITATIONS:
1. American Pharmaceutical Association, *Handbook of Nonprescription Drugs*, 11th ed. (Washington, D.C.: American Pharmaceutical Association, 1996).
2. V.E. Tyler, *Herbs of Choice: The Therapeutic Use of Phytomedicinals* (Binghamton, NY: Haworth Press/Pharmaceutical Products Press, 1994). H. Traitler et al., *Lipids*, 19(12) (1984): 923–28.
3. *Lawrence Review of Natural Products* (St. Louis: Facts and Comparisons, November 1993).

4. J. Poulaka et al., *Journal of Reproductive Medicine*, 30 (1985): 149. *Lawrence Review of Natural Products*, op. cit.

5. D.F. Horrobin and M.S. Manku, Paper presented at the annual meeting of the International Conference on Oils, Fats, and Waxes, Auckland, 1983. *Lawrence Review of Natural Products*, op. cit.

6. American Pharmaceutical Association, op. cit.

7. S. Wright, *Acta Dermato-Venereologica. Supplementum*, 114 (1985): 143–45. M.J. Kerscher and H.C. Korting, *Clinical Investigator*, 70(2) (1992): 167–71.

8. P.L. Biagi et al., *Drugs Under Experimental & Clinical Research*, 14(4) (1988): 285–90.

9. *Lawrence Review of Natural Products*, op. cit.

10. J. Berth-Jones and R.A. Graham-Brown, *The Lancet*, 341(8860) (1993): 1557–60.

11. American Pharmaceutical Association, op. cit.

12. L.A. Joe and L.L. Hart, *Annals of Pharmacotherapy*, 27(12) (1993): 1475–77.

13. L.J. Leventhal et al., *Annals of Internal Medicine*, 119(9) (1993): 867–73.

14. J.J. Belch et al., *Annals of the Rheumatic Diseases*, 47(2) (1988): 96–104.

15. S.M. Greenfield et al., *Alimentary Pharmacology and Therapeutics*, 7(2) (1993): 159–66.

16. G.A. Jamal, *The Lancet*, 1 (1986): 1098. R. Takahashi et al., *Prostaglandins, Leukotrienes, and Essential Fatty Acids*, 49(2) (1993): 569–71.

17. E.F. Field, *The Lancet*, 1 (1978): 780. D.F. Horrobin, *Medical Hypotheses*, 5 (1979): 365. *Lawrence Review of Natural Products*, op. cit.

18. C.A. Gately and R.E. Mansel, *British Medical Bulletin*, 47 (1991): 284.

19. I. Glen et al., *Alcoholism, Clinical & Experimental Research*, 11 (1987): 37–41.

20. G. Ramesh et al., *Nutrition*, 8(5) (1992): 343–47.

21. T. Ghayor and D.F. Horrobin, *IRCS Medical Science*, 9 (1981): 582.

22. D.F. Horrobin, *Journal of Reproductive Medicine*, 28(7) (1983): 465–68.

23. *Lawrence Review of Natural Products*, op. cit.

24. A. Stewart, *Journal of Reproductive Medicine*, 32(6) (1987): 435–41.

25. *Lawrence Review of Natural Products*, op. cit.

PRIMARY NAME:
EYEBRIGHT

SCIENTIFIC NAME:
Euphrasia officinalis L. Family: Scrophulariaceae

COMMON NAMES:
Augentrost, eufrasia, meadow eyebright, red eyebright

RATING:
- *For use in the eyes:* 5 = Studies indicate that there is a definite health hazard to using this substance, even in recommended amounts.

What Is Eyebright?

This delicate herb yields a profusion of small white or purplish flowers once a year. Some of the blossoms are tinged with red; all bear a single yellow spot. The resemblance to bloodshot eyes inspired the name "eyebright." A plant ascribed powers based on its physical appearance reflects what is known as the "doctrine of signatures." Eyebright grows in parts of North America. All parts of the plant have been used to make such medicinal preparations as eye compresses and teas.

What It Is Used For:

In the Middle Ages, eyebright was believed to cure "all evils of the eye." Contemporary herbalists recommend the herb for many of the medical conditions their predecessors did: to relieve fatigued, inflamed, or bloodshot eyes. Styes, black eyes, and inflammation of the eyelids and conjunctiva (blepharitis and conjunctivitis) have all been treated with eyebright. So have eyes that are runny

- *For internal use:* 4 = Research indicates that this substance will probably not fulfill the claims made for it, but that it is unlikely to cause any harm.

or itchy as a result of colds or allergies such as hay fever. Supporters say the herb improves vision. It appears in many herbal eyewash mixtures.

Some herbalists carry on the tradition of their seventeenth-century counterparts in recommending that eyebright be taken internally to keep eyes and vision "bright," and the entire body rigorous and healthy. A few recommend very warm eyebright tea for coughs, hoarseness and other throat irritations, and nasal congestion. The herb appears in British Herbal Tobacco, a concoction smoked for chronic bronchial colds. Homeopaths prescribe minute amounts of eyebright diluted in a liquid to treat conjunctivitis and other eye problems. (See page 2 for a discussion of homeopathy.)

Forms Available Include:

- *For use in the eyes:* Compress, drop, eyewash, lotion, poultice (hot, for styes), tincture.
- *For internal use:* Capsule, tea.

Dosage Commonly Reported:

For the eyes, *use only commercially sterilized eyebright solutions*; follow package instructions. For internal use, one to two 44-milligram capsules of the herb are taken three times a day.

Will It Work for You? What the Studies Say:

Researchers have identified a number of chemicals in eyebright, but few if any are believed to offer any healing qualities. One, tannin, has anti-inflammatory and astringent properties, but experts doubt that it has much of an effect on the human eye. Even those who recommend eyebright concede that any active ingredients remain a mystery and that other herbs are probably more potent. No well-designed studies have been done to shed more light on the subject. The bottom line for scientists and a good share of herbalists is that eyebright fails to fulfill any of the claims made for it. German health authorities declined to approve of its use for eye conditions, citing hygiene concerns and a lack of substantiating evidence.[1] The value of commercial, sterilized eyewash products that do not contain eyebright has not been proved, but they do not pose the same type of health hazard as those that do.

Will It Harm You? What the Studies Say:

Eyebright does not appear to be toxic when taken internally, although the subject has not been well studied. The tincture, however, may cause numerous adverse reactions when applied to the eye, according to German studies. They indicate that 10 to 60 drops of the tincture may cause itching and other discomfort of the lids, dim vision, sensitivity to light, confusion, and sensations of eye pressure with tearing, nausea, constipation, sweating, and numerous other reactions.[2] Consider the fundamentals of hygiene whenever you put foreign material in your eye; if it is not sterile, it could irritate your eye even more. Homemade solutions are particularly risky.

GENERAL SOURCES:

Bisset, N.G., ed. *Herbal Drugs and Phytopharmaceuticals.* Stuttgart: medpharm GmbH Scientific Publishers, 1994.

Blumenthal, M., J. Gruenwald, T. Hall, and R.S. Rister, eds. *The Complete German Commission E Monographs: Therapeutic Guide to Herbal Medicine.* Boston: Integrative Medicine Communications, 1998.

Dobelis, I.N., ed. *The Magic and Medicine of Plants: A Practical Guide to the Science, History, Folklore, and Everyday Uses of Medicinal Plants.* Pleasantville, NY: Reader's Digest Association, 1986.

Duke, J.A. *CRC Handbook of Medicinal Herbs.* Boca Raton, FL: CRC Press, 1985.

Harkiss, K.J., and P. Timmins. *Planta Medica.* 23(4) (1973): 342–47.

Lawrence Review of Natural Products. St. Louis: Facts and Comparisons, September 1996.

Leung, A.Y., and S. Foster. *Encyclopedia of Common Natural Ingredients Used in Food, Drugs, and Cosmetics.* 2nd ed. New York: John Wiley & Sons, 1996.

Mindell, E. *Earl Mindell's Herb Bible.* New York: Simon & Schuster/Fireside, 1992.

Tyler, V.E., *The Honest Herbal.* Binghamton, NY: Haworth Press/Pharmaceutical Products Press, 1993.

Weiss, R.F. *Herbal Medicine*, trans. A.R. Meuss, from the 6th German edition. Beaconsfield, England: Beaconsfield Publishers, Ltd., 1988.

TEXT CITATIONS:

1. A.Y. Leung and S. Foster, *Encyclopedia of Common Natural Ingredients Used in Food, Drugs, and Cosmetics*, 2nd ed. (New York: John Wiley & Sons, 1996).

2. *Lawrence Review of Natural Products* (St. Louis: Facts and Comparisons, September 1996).

PRIMARY NAME:
FALSE UNICORN ROOT

SCIENTIFIC NAME:
Chamaelirium luteum L. Gray.
Family: Liliaceae

COMMON NAMES:
Chamaelirium, colic root, devil's bit, fairywand, helonias

RATING:
4 = Extremely limited information on this substance makes both efficacy and safety nearly impossible to determine.

What Is False Unicorn Root?

This perennial herb is native to North America east of the Mississippi. Its tall, slender stem emerges from a rosette of basal leaves and ends in a crowded spike of small whitish flowers that turn yellow over time. The dried rhizomes (underground stems) and roots are used medicinally. Do not confuse this plant with *Aletris farinosa* L., another member of the lily family native to the eastern United States and commonly referred to as "true" unicorn root. It resembles *Chamaelirium luteum* only in its common name, not in appearance.

What It Is Used For:

Native American tribes reportedly used this root as a cure-all for cough, colic, stomach upset, intestinal worms, fever, and pain. They considered it a diuretic ("water pill") and effective for inducing vomiting and cleaning out the bowels at certain doses. Many nineteenth-century Americans considered it a liver remedy. But the most enduring reputation for false unicorn root is that of a remedy for male and female reproductive organ ailments, from painful menstrual symptoms and amenorrhea (absent menstrual cycles) to threatened miscarriage, menopausal complaints, infertility, and prostate disorders. Some herbalists also consider it an effective tonic for the genitourinary tract as a whole.

Forms Available:

Decoction, infusion, liquid extract, tincture. Extracts appear in numerous herbal blends.

Dosage Commonly Reported:

The liquid extract is taken in 2- to 4-milliliter doses.

Will It Work for You? What the Studies Say:

The lack of scientific data on this herb makes it difficult to determine its effectiveness or safety. Scientists long ago established that it contains steroidal saponins (including the diosgenin glycosides, chamaelirin and helonin). Sometimes these exert hormonal activity and affect parts of the body such as the female reproductive system, but whether this holds true in the case of false unicorn root remains unclear.

Will It Harm You? What The Studies Say:

False unicorn root has not been associated with any reports of serious harm. Avoid excessive doses, however, as they may cause nausea and vomiting.[1] Although no firm evidence indicates that it is a risk, pregnant women may want to avoid the herb, given its traditional use as a uterine tonic to promote menstruation and hasten childbirth.

GENERAL SOURCES:
Balch, J.F., and P.A. Balch. *Prescription for Nutritional Healing: A Practical A to Z Reference to Drug-Free Remedies Using Vitamins, Minerals, Herbs & Food Supplements.* 2nd ed. Garden City Park, NY: Avery Publishing Group, 1997.

Bradley, P.C., ed. *British Herbal Compendium: A Handbook of Scientific Information on Widely Used Plant Drugs*, vol. 1. Bournemouth (Dorset), England: British Herbal Medicine Association, 1992.

Dobelis, I.N., ed. *The Magic and Medicine of Plants: A Practical Guide to the Science, History, Folklore, and Everyday Uses of Medicinal Plants.* Pleasantville, NY: Reader's Digest Association, 1986.

Duke, J.A. *Handbook of Northeastern Indian Medicinal Plants.* Lincoln, MA: Quarterman Publications, Inc., 1986.

Foster, S., and J.A. Duke. *The Peterson Field Guide Series: A Field Guide to Medicinal Plants. Eastern and Central North America.* Boston: Houghton Mifflin Company, 1990.

Tierra, M. *The Way of Herbs.* New York: Pocket Books, 1990.

Weiner, M.A., and J.A. Weiner. *Herbs That Heal: Prescription for Herbal Healing.* Mill Valley, CA: Quantum Books, 1994.

TEXT CITATIONS:

1. P.C. Bradley, ed., *British Herbal Compendium: A Handbook of Scientific Information on Widely Used Plant Drugs*, vol. 1 (Bournemouth [Dorset], England: British Herbal Medicine Association, 1992).

PRIMARY NAME:

FENNEL

SCIENTIFIC NAME:

Foeniculum vulgare Mill. Also referred to as *Foeniculum officinale* All. and *Anethum foeniculum* L. Family: Umbelliferae (Apiaceae)

COMMON NAMES:

Bitter fennel, carosella, common fennel, finocchio, Florence fennel, garden fennel, large fennel, sweet fennel, wild fennel, xiao hui xiang

RATING:

1 = Years of use and extensive, high-quality studies indicate that this substance is very effective and safe when used in recommended amounts for the indication(s) noted in the "Will It Work for You?" section. However, see the "Will It Harm You?" section for warnings regarding fennel oil.

What Is Fennel?

This tall, aromatic perennial belongs to the same plant family as caraway, and the fruit has a flavor reminiscent of licorice and anise. Its numerous varieties are cultivated worldwide. Medicinal preparations are made from the ripe fruit, which when dried forms tiny yellowish-brown crescents and is commonly referred to as "seeds," and the seeds' essential oil.

What It Is Used For:

Since the earliest times, people have relied on fennel as a scent, vegetable, food flavoring, and folk remedy. The seeds were used to help digest food, especially when stomach upset or gas spoiled the enjoyment of a meal. They also have a long-standing reputation for counteracting the effects of poisons, boosting milk production in nursing mothers, promoting menstruation, increasing urination (in the form of a diuretic, or "water pill"), and suppressing appetite, a use once highly valued by the poor. Demand for fennel was high during the Middle Ages and in the New England colonies. An official drug in the Chinese pharmacopoeia, fennel has been valued there since the sixth century to calm the stomach and treat bleeder ailments, hernia (of the small intestine), nausea, vomiting, painful menstrual periods, and bedwetting.[1]

Fennel has long been used externally as well. Loose compresses soaked in fennel tea or water are placed over the eye to treat conjunctivitis and other eye ailments. Sometimes the liquid is used to bathe the eye directly. Certain German experts consider this a gentle approach to reducing inflammation, but value it most for soothing and "strengthening" the eyes.[2] Chinese healers mix fennel into a poultice for poorly healing snakebites.

Today, people around the world continue to use fennel in many of the same

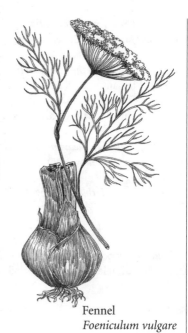

Fennel
Foeniculum vulgare

ways, both internally and externally. Some even recommend considering the herb for treating prostate cancer, as long as a physician is overseeing care. Manufacturers have added fennel to laxatives to counteract cramping. More recently fennel and its oil have appeared as flavoring agents in candies.

Forms Available Include:

Capsules, compress, decoction, oil, powder, seeds, tincture. Fennel-flavored syrups and honey may also be available.

Dosage Commonly Reported:

A decoction is made using 1 to 2 teaspoons bruised seeds per cup of water; weaker infusions made with crushed seeds are given to children under the age of two. A tincture is taken in dosages of ½ to 1 teaspoon up to three times per day. Fennel in syrup or honey is taken in dosages of 10 to 20 grams. Two to three of the 455-milligram seed capsules are taken three times a day. Take commercial preparations according to package directions.

Will It Work for You? What the Studies Say:

The traditional use of fennel for stomach upset and gas makes sense, according to animal research demonstrating the ability of the volatile oil in the seeds (2 to 6 percent) to reduce stomach spasms in smooth muscles and therefore relax areas such as the digestive tract lining.[3] This quality helps explain why people have for generations turned to fennel to soothe stomach upset and dispel excess gas or cramplike stomach pains.[4] German health authorities approve of fennel for treating mild stomach upset, indigestion, bloating, gas, and cramplike pains. The standard recommendation is to add an infusion of crushed fennel to milk or soft food for infants and young children suffering from such conditions as colic or diarrhea. One German textbook suggests giving fennel to children in this way to calm them; the dried fruits may have mild narcotic properties.[5]

Fennel oil contains a substance—estragole—that appears to act like the female hormone estrogen. In the 1930s, the herb was considered a source for producing synthetic estrogens. An extract of the seeds given to rats produces reactions in the genital organs of both males and females similar to what one would expect with estrogen.[6] Such findings lend substance to fennel's traditional use for promoting menstruation, boosting a nursing mother's milk secretion, increasing the female sex drive, and moderating the male climax. The subject still awaits verification through human testing, however.

German health authorities also approve of using fennel in various forms, including fennel-flavored syrup and honey, for upper respiratory congestion.[7] They cite evidence that the herb can dissolve mucus secretions in the respiratory tract and has mild expectorant properties.[8] Numerous European cough medicines include fennel seeds to help loosen and expel chest phlegm (mucus). Test-tube studies also indicate that fennel fights certain bacteria, but whether this validates its traditional use as a diarrhea remedy has yet to be determined.[9]

Will It Harm You? What the Studies Say:

Neither the research done so far nor years of experience suggest that using fennel seeds in typically recommended amounts poses any health risk. But to be safe, German health authorities recommend that no one take the herb for longer than several weeks without seeing a doctor or consulting a pharmacist.[10] No evidence suggests that fennel interacts negatively with any other remedies. In unusual cases, sensitive individuals have suffered allergic reactions, photo-dermatitis (sun sensitivity), and contact dermatitis.

The risks associated with using pure fennel oil—as opposed to the seeds—are far more considerable. Even small amounts (as little as 1 to 5 milliliters) taken orally have caused nausea, vomiting, seizures, and respiratory problems.[11] German health authorities warn that infants and young children run the risk of shortness of breath, spasms of the larynx, and excitement. One investigator found that when fed to rats, the purified oil worsened liver damage.[12]

The mild estrogen-like effects attributed to the estragole in fennel oil raise concerns as well, as studies indicate that estragole can cause tumors in animals.[13] German health authorities have recommended that pregnant women not use fennel preparations that are stronger than an infusion (or the equivalent amount of volatile oil).[14] Women who have had breast cancer or who have been told not to take the birth-control pill should probably avoid fennel in any form, or at least discuss with a doctor using medicinal amounts of the plant.[15] Because of still poorly understood effects on the liver, people with liver disease, hepatitis, or problems with alcoholism may want to avoid medicinal concentrations.

Evidence for the effectiveness and safety of treating eye ailments with fennel cannot be found. Keep in mind that introducing anything other than sterilized substances into the eyes raises the risk of infection.

In the form of a fragrance, culinary herb, or vegetable, fennel is probably harmless. The FDA categorizes it as Generally Recognized As Safe (GRAS) to consume as a food. Contamination with disease-causing bacteria is a risk, although probably small; investigators surveying samples of fennel in Italy found a number of bacteria such as *streptococci* and *salmonella*, which can cause stomach and intestinal illnesses.[16]

GENERAL SOURCES:

Albert-Puleo, M. *Journal of Ethnopharmacolgy.* 2(4) (1980): 337–44.

Bisset, N.G., ed. *Herbal Drugs and Phytopharmaceuticals.* Stuttgart: medpharm GmbH Scientific Publishers, 1994.

Blumenthal, M., J. Gruenwald, T. Hall, and R.S. Rister, eds. *The Complete German Commission E Monographs: Therapeutic Guide to Herbal Medicine.* Boston: Integrative Medicine Communications, 1998.

Castleman, M. *The Healing Herbs: The Ultimate Guide to the Curative Power of Nature's Medicines.* New York: Bantam Books, 1995.

Lawrence Review of Natural Products. St. Louis: Facts and Comparisons, August 1994.

Leung, A.Y. *Chinese Healing Foods and Herbs.* Glen Rock, NJ: AYSL Corp, 1984.

Leung, A.Y. *Encyclopedia of Common Natural Ingredients Used in Food, Drugs, and Cosmetics.* New York: John Wiley & Sons, 1980.

Sekizawa, J., and T. Shibamoto. *Mutation Research.* 101 (1982): 127.

Tyler, V.E. *The Honest Herbal.* Binghamton, NY: Haworth Press/Pharmaceutical Products Press, 1993.

Weiss, R.F. *Herbal Medicine,* trans. A.R. Meuss, from the 6th German edition. Beaconsfield, England: Beaconsfield Publishers, Ltd., 1988.

TEXT CITATIONS:

1. A.Y. Leung, *Chinese Healing Foods and Herbs* (Glen Rock, NJ: AYSL Corp, 1984).

2. R.F. Weiss, *Herbal Medicine*, trans. A.R. Meuss, from the 6th German edition (Beaconsfield, England: Beaconsfield Publishers, Ltd., 1988).

3. T. Shipochliev, *Veterinarno Meditsinski Nauki*, 5 (1968): 63. M. Reiter and W. Brandt. *Arzneimittel-Forschung*, 35(1A) (1985): 408.

4. M. Blumenthal, J. Gruenwald, T. Hall, and R.S. Rister, eds., *The Complete German Commission E Monographs: Therapeutic Guide to Herbal Medicine* (Boston: Integrative Medicine Communications, 1998).

5. Weiss, op. cit.

6. T. Malini et al., *Indian Journal of Physiology & Pharmacology*, 29 (1985): 21.

7. Blumenthal et al., op. cit.

8. Ibid.

9. F.M. Ramadan et al., *Chemie, Mikrobiologie, Technologie der Lebensmittel,* 2 (1972): 51.

10. Blumenthal et al., op. cit.

11. V.E. Tyler, *The Honest Herbal* (Binghamton, NY: Haworth Press/Pharmaceutical Products Press, 1993). C. Marcus and E.P. Lichtenstein, *Journal of Agricultural & Food Chemistry*, 27 (1979): 1217.

12. L.L. Gershbein *Food & Cosmetics Toxicology*, 15 (1977): 173.

13. A.Y. Leung, *Encyclopedia of Common Natural Ingredients Used in Food, Drugs, and Cosmetics* (New York: John Wiley & Sons, 1980).

14. N.G. Bisset, ed., *Herbal Drugs and Phytopharmaceuticals* (Stuttgart: medpharm GmbH Scientific Publishers, 1994).

15. Castleman, M. *The Healing Herbs: The Ultimate Guide to the Curative Power of Nature's Medicines* (New York: Bantam Books, 1995).

16. G.L. Ercolani, *Applied & Environmental Microbiology*, 31 (1976): 847. G. Cavazzini et al., *Annali di Igiene*, 1(5) (1989): 1279–89.

PRIMARY NAME:

FENUGREEK

SCIENTIFIC NAME:
Trigonella foenum-graecum L.
Family: Leguminosae

COMMON NAMES:
Bird's foot, Greek hayseed, hu lu ba, trigonella

RATING:
2 = According to a number of well-designed studies and common use, this substance appears to be relatively effective and safe when used in recommended amounts for the indication(s) noted in the "Will It Work for You?" section.

What Is Fenugreek?

This small flowering annual bears smooth, very hard, irregularly shaped seeds that, once ripened, are dried for use as a spice and drug. The seeds have a characteristic odor and somewhat bitter taste. Fenugreek, a native of Asia and southeastern Europe, is cultivated in many parts of the world, but not North America.

What It Is Used For:

The seeds of this ancient herb have been treasured for millennia as both a spice and an herbal remedy in the Middle East, India, and Egypt, and for a slightly shorter time in Europe, China, and other parts of the world. As a folk medicine fenugreek has been commonly used as a digestive aid and to treat intestinal gas, diarrhea and other stomach upsets, chronic cough, bronchitis, tuberculosis, fever, sore throat, mouth ulcers, and diabetes. Poultices and other external formulations have been smoothed onto wounds, skin irritations, and areas afflicted by nerve pain. Traditional Chinese healers use both unroasted and roasted seeds for such problems as abdominal pain, hernias, kidney disorders, and rheumatism, and male problems such as impotence.[1]

Contemporary herbalists in the United States tend to focus on fenugreek as an

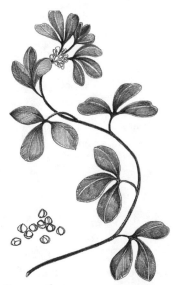

Fenugreek
Trigonella foenum-graecum

agent for clearing upper respiratory tract congestion, soothing ulcers, relieving stomach upset and related inflammation in the stomach and intestines, encouraging a flagging appetite (including more serious manifestations such as anorexia), promoting soft stools, lowering blood sugar in diabetes, alleviating a sore throat (as a gargle), and controlling skin inflammations in the form of a skin-softening agent (an emollient). A chemical component called diosgenin, a steroidal sapogenin, is used to synthesize hormones and related medicines. Fenugreek appears in curries and numerous spice blends. Extracts are commonly used to flavor imitation maple syrup and other foods, and appear in a number of commercial products including detergents and lotions.[2]

Forms Available:

- *For internal use:* Capsule, decoction, seed (whole, crushed, powdered and roasted).
- *For external use:* Gargle (made with infusion), ointment, paste, poultice.

Dosage Commonly Reported:

A gargle is made with 1 tablespoon pulverized seeds in 8 ounces water and used up to three times per day. One 626-milligram seed capsule is taken two to three times a day. The powdered or pulverized seeds are mixed with water to make a paste used as a poultice.

Will It Work for You? What the Studies Say:

Fenugreek's rich chemical store includes vitamins, minerals, alkaloids, saponins, a fixed oil, and flavonoids. Considerable amounts (up to 50 percent) of a substance called mucilage that swells quickly into a gooey mass upon contact with liquid explain the logic behind many of the medicinal uses for the seeds, from skin ointments to sore throat gargles and internal preparations for upset stomach, especially gas pains. German health authorities approve of fenugreek poultices for treating local skin inflammations.[3] They also endorse the use of fenugreek seeds internally for appetite loss.[4] A 1995 study showed that the herb's steroid saponins significantly encouraged food consumption and motivation to eat in laboratory rats.[5]

Scientists continue to examine the capacity of fenugreek seeds to lower cholesterol levels as well as help manage diabetes. In several investigations, both serum cholesterol and glucose levels dropped in rats, dogs, and other animals fed the seeds.[6] One study recorded significant reductions in both parameters in both normal and diabetic dogs who had high cholesterol to begin with.[7] Future research may explain whether this action should be attributed to the fiber in the seeds, to their mucilage content, or to a particular ingredient such as steroidal saponins.[8] The most recent research indicates that the steroid saponins are responsible.[9] Small studies in humans indicate that extracts of the whole seeds lower blood sugar levels in otherwise healthy individuals.[10] Other findings are also promising but still inconclusive.[11]

Liquid and alcoholic extracts of fenugreek stimulate the guinea pig uterus in a chemical bath,[12] indicating potential usefulness in treating delayed labor. This property has never been formally studied in human beings, however.

Although much more research is needed, numerous small-animal studies indicate that fenugreek seeds and their extracts hold promise as treatments for inflammation, water retention, cancer, baldness, infections, and hazardous calcium oxalate deposits in the kidneys.[13] Extracts have been shown to stimulate both the uterus and the intestines, and to accelerate the heartbeat in animal organs placed in chemical baths,[14] raising the possibility of treating various disorders.

Will It Harm You? What the Studies Say:

Fenugreek seed is safe to use in culinary concentrations, and no reports of serious adverse reactions to medicinal concentrations survive millennia of common use. Given the still poorly understood actions of the herb's many ingredients, however, it may be wise to practice moderation. This is especially true for individuals on diabetes drugs, MAO inhibitors, or heart, hormonal, or blood-thinning medicines.[15] Pregnant women may also want to exercise caution. Some of the ingredients, such as coumarins and estrogens, can be toxic in overdose.[16] Fenugreek has caused myopathy in certain mammals (ruminants) who graze on it.[17]

Although it is generally not irritating or sensitizing to human skin,[18] prolonged or excessive use of external preparations may cause unwanted skin reactions.

The FDA places fenugreek on its Generally Recognized As Safe (GRAS) list for food use.

GENERAL SOURCES:

Bisset, N.G., ed. *Herbal Drugs and Phytopharmaceuticals*. Stuttgart: medpharm GmbH Scientific Publishers, 1994.

Blumenthal, M., J. Gruenwald, T. Hall, and R.S. Rister, eds. *The Complete German Commission E Monographs: Therapeutic Guide to Herbal Medicine*. Boston: Integrative Medicine Communications, 1998.

Dobelis, I.N., ed. *The Magic and Medicine of Plants: A Practical Guide to the Science, History, Folklore, and Everyday Uses of Medicinal Plants*. Pleasantville, NY: Reader's Digest Association, 1986.

Duke, J.A. *CRC Handbook of Medicinal Herbs*. Boca Raton, FL: CRC Press, 1985.

Lawrence Review of Natural Products. St. Louis: Facts and Comparisons, July 1996.

Leung, A.Y., and S. Foster. *Encyclopedia of Common Natural Ingredients Used in Food, Drugs, and Cosmetics*. 2nd ed. New York: John Wiley & Sons, 1996.

Mindell, E. *Earl Mindell's Herb Bible*. New York: Simon & Schuster/Fireside, 1992.

Newall, C.A., et al. *Herbal Medicines: A Guide for Health-Care Professionals*. London: The Pharmaceutical Press, 1996.

Tyler, V.E. *The Honest Herbal*. Binghamton, NY: Haworth Press/Pharmacentical Products Press, 1993.

TEXT CITATIONS:

1. A.Y. Leung and S. Foster, *Encyclopedia of Common Natural Ingredients Used in Food, Drugs, and Cosmetics*, 2nd ed. (New York: John Wiley & Sons, 1996).

2. Ibid.

3. M. Blumenthal, J. Gruenwald, T. Hall, and R.S. Rister, eds., *The Complete German Commission E Monographs: Therapeutic Guide to Herbal Medicine* (Boston: Integrative Medicine Communications, 1998).

4. Ibid.
5. P.R. Petit et al., *Steroids*, 60(10) (1995): 674–80.
6. G. Ribes et al., *Annals of Nutrition and Metabolism*, 28 (1984): 37. *Lawrence Review of Natural Products* (St. Louis: Facts and Comparisons, July 1996).
7. G. Valette et al., *Atherosclerosis*, 50(1) (1984): 105–11.
8. *Lawrence Review of Natural Products*, op. cit. N.G. Bisset, ed., *Herbal Drugs and Phytopharmaceuticals* (Stuttgart: medpharm GmbH Scientific Publishers, 1994).
9. P.R. Petit et al., op. cit.
10. R.D. Sharma et al., *European Journal of Clinical Nutrition*, 44(4) (1990): 301–6.
11. C.A. Newall et al., *Herbal Medicines: A Guide for Health-Care Professionals* (London: The Pharmaceutical Press, 1996).
12. Leung and Foster, op. cit.
13. V.E. Tyler, *The Honest Herbal* (Binghamton, NY: Haworth Press/Pharmaceutical Products Press, 1993). S.K. Ahsan et al., *Journal of Ethnopharmacology*, 26(3) (1989): 249. J. Totte and A.J. Vlietinck, *Farmaceutisch Tijdschrift voor Belgie*, 60 (1983): 203.
14. Bisset, op. cit. M.S. Abdo and A.A. Al-Kafawi, *Planta Medica*, 17 (1969): 14.
15. Newall, op. cit.
16. J.A. Duke *CRC Handbook of Medicinal Herbs* (Boca Raton, FL: CRC Press, 1985).
17. A. Shlosberg and M.N. Egyed, *Archives of Toxicology*, Supplement. 6 (1983): 194–96.
18. D.L.J. Opdyke, *Food & Cosmetics Toxicology*, 16(Suppl. 1) (1978): 755.

PRIMARY NAME:
FEVERFEW

SCIENTIFIC NAME:
Tanacetum parthenium (L.) Schultz-Bip. Occasionally referred to as *Chrysanthemum parthenium* (L.) Bernh. or *Matricaria parthenium* L. Family: Asteraceae (Compositae)

COMMON NAMES:
Altamisa, featherfoil, febrifuge plant, midsummer daisy, nosebleed, Santa Maria, wild chamomile, wild quinine

RATING:
2 = According to a number of well-designed studies and common use, this substance appears to be relatively effective and safe when used in recommended amounts for the indication(s) noted in the "Will It Work for You?" section.

What Is Feverfew?

Feverfew is a short, bushy perennial found in fields, along roadsides, and in waste places across North America. The plant has daisylike yellow and white flowers and closely resembles chamomile. The yellow-green leaves are used medicinally.

What It Is Used For:

Early Europeans and Greeks valued feverfew for fevers, headaches, arthritis, menstrual problems, and other aches and pains. They treated wounds with external preparations of the plant. The name's Latin root—*febrifuga*—illustrates the respect it was given as a fever-reducer: it literally means to drive a fever away. Heavy opium users were once given feverfew as an antidote. North Americans followed the lead of their European cousins, cultivating the herb as an ornamental as well as a medicinal plant, although over time fewer and fewer people used the herb.

In 1978 a report that it could control migraines lifted feverfew out of the virtual obscurity it had sunk into. Continuing reports of success have produced a dedicated following among migraine sufferers. Europeans in particular take it both to prevent these scorching headaches and to control associated nausea, vomiting, and other symptoms. Many just chew a few of the fresh leaves every day.

Feverfew extracts also have a reputation for relieving ailments commonly treated with aspirin, such as asthma, menstrual pain, arthritis, and dermatitis. Herbal catalogs promote feverfew for general well-being. Some herbalists even recommend it for relieving nervous tension. Mexicans and others rely on the herb to repel insects. Some consider the strong-smelling plant an air purifier.[1]

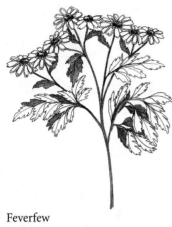

Feverfew
Tanacetum parthenium

Forms Available Include:

Capsule, leaf (fresh and freeze- or heat-dried), liquid extract, tablet, tisane. Many people mask the herb's bitter taste with sweeteners.

Dosage Commonly Reported:

To prevent migraines, two leaves are chewed, or two 400-milligram tablets are taken three times a day. The quality of the tablets varies; a quantity containing 250 micrograms of parthenolide is considered an adequate daily dosage. The liquid leaf extract is taken in doses of 4 to 8 milliliters.

Will It Work for You? What the Studies Say:

Feverfew apparently has no fever-reducing powers, although the subject has yet to be carefully examined. Those intrigued by reports that it can ease arthritis pains may be disappointed. A 1989 double-blind and placebo-controlled study of forty-one subjects showed that it failed to significantly improve rheumatoid arthritis symptoms in those who took 70 to 86 milligrams a day for six weeks.[2] The subjects were allowed to continue taking their regular nonsteroidal anti-inflammatory drugs throughout the study. Scientists attributed positive findings in animal arthritis studies to the way that feverfew inhibits the release of damaging materials from white blood cells in inflamed joints and skin.[3] With the exception of headache relief, other traditional uses have apparently not yet been put to the test of clinical trials.

Migraine sufferers appear to be on to something, however, with positive findings in extensive test-tube and animal trials and two human trials conducted over the past few decades. Evidence indicates that when taken on a regular basis, relatively small amounts of the dried leaves (about 60 to 82 milligrams) can help reduce the frequency, severity, and annoying symptoms such as nausea and vomiting often associated with migraine headaches.[4] Feverfew apparently has no impact on migraine headaches that have already begun. These properties were demonstrated in clinical trials comparing the plant with a placebo. One, reported in 1985, involved seventeen individuals who had independently been eating a few fresh leaves daily to prevent migraine attacks.[5] When nine of the subjects were switched (unknowingly) with a placebo, they experienced a significant increase in the frequency and severity of migraine symptoms such as headache, nausea, and vomiting. On the other hand, those who (unknowingly) were continuing to receive feverfew in capsules experienced no significant change in their condition.

The other clinical trial—a well-designed, two-year study reported in 1988—found that the mean number of migraine headaches during feverfew treatment dropped by nearly a quarter compared with placebo treatment in the fifty-nine subjects who normally suffered from a migraine at least once a month.[6] The subjects were not allowed to take any other medicine, except for oral contraceptives, during the study. The degree of vomiting also dropped, although the duration of attacks remained about the same.

Intensive human research into this antimigraine action began when a

British health magazine reported that a longtime migraine sufferer stopped having the debilitating headaches at the age of sixty-eight after ten months of chewing three leaves of feverfew a day. Scientists had first isolated parthenolide, the chemical constituent believed to be primarily responsible for the herb's antimigraine activity, in the late 1950s and early 1960s. Parthenolide is a sesquiterpene lactone. Feverfew research indicates that parthenolide and possibly other sesquiterpene lactones inhibit the release of compounds called serotonin antagonists from blood platelets; serotonin antagonists released during an attack may contribute to migraine pain by constricting blood vessels. The serotonin antagonists are also thought to inhibit prostaglandin release from white blood cells; that is another potential contributing factor to initiating attacks and may be involved in ameliorating arthritis and psoriasis problems, although these aspects demand more study. Some of these sesquiterpene lactones may even have antispasmodic activity, and parthenolide may lower the pain threshold.

Migraine sufferers should be aware that getting the correct dosage can be challenging, particularly given the often poor quality of North American feverfew products. Some samples contain very little of the critical parthenolide. Experts believe that preparation must contain at least 0.2 percent of parthenolide, equivalent to 250 micrograms.[7] A 1991 Canadian study reported that of all the American feverfew products sampled, none contained this minimum.[8] In a sampling of feverfew products sold in a Louisiana health food store, parthenolide could not be detected in two out of the three samples.[9] The potency of fresh feverfew also varies notably from that of dried feverfew.[10] It should be noted that common tension headaches differ from migraine headaches in several ways, including cause; feverfew probably works only for migraine headaches.

Will It Harm You? What the Studies Say:

Feverfew appears to be relatively safe to use in typically recommended amounts, although more long-term trials are needed before any definitive conclusions can be made, particularly regarding long-term use. Approximately 10 to 18 percent of subjects in various trials so far have developed adverse reactions, with the most notable being mouth ulcers (11 to 12 percent). As many as 7 percent of people involved in a study that included chewing the fresh leaves developed such annoying tongue and mouth irritation, along with lip swelling and loss of taste, that they stopped using the drug.[11] A withdrawal syndrome called "postfeverfew syndrome" has been characterized and includes nervousness, tension headaches, joint stiffness, and tiredness.[12]

Do not take feverfew if you are allergic to other plants in the daisy family, such as chamomile or ragweed. Pregnant and nursing women should avoid the herb, given its still poorly understood potential to promote menstrual flow, among other things.[13] Indications that the drug may interact negatively with anticlotting medicines (e.g., the blood thinners heparin and warfarin) also demand further examination.[14]

GENERAL SOURCES:

Bradley, P.C., ed. *British Herbal Compendium: A Handbook of Scientific Information on Widely Used Plant Drugs*, vol. 1. Bournemouth (Dorset), England: British Herbal Medicine Association, 1992.

Castleman, M. *The Healing Herbs: The Ultimate Guide to the Curative Power of Nature's Medicines*. New York, NY: Bantam Books, 1995.

Der Marderosian, A., and L. Liberti. *Natural Product Medicine: A Scientific Guide to Foods, Drugs, Cosmetics*. Philadelphia: George F. Stickley, 1988.

Duke, J.A. *CRC Handbook of Medicinal Herbs*. Boca Raton, FL: CRC Press, 1985.

Hallowell, M. *Herbal Healing: A Practical Introduction to Medicinal Herbs*. Garden City Park, NY: 1994.

Lawrence Review of Natural Products. St. Louis: Facts and Comparisons, September 1994.

Mindell, E. *Earl Mindell's Herb Bible*. New York: Simon & Schuster/Fireside, 1992.

Newall, C.A., et al. *Herbal Medicines: A Guide for Health-Care Professionals*. London: The Pharmaceutical Press, 1996.

Tyler, V.E. *Herbs of Choice: The Therapeutic Use of Phytomedicinals*. Binghamton, NY: Haworth Press/Pharmaceutical Products Press, 1994.

Tyler, V.E., L.R. Brady, and J.E. Robbers, eds. *Pharmacognosy*. Philadelphia: Lea & Febiger, 1988.

Weiner, M.A., and J.A. Weiner. *Herbs That Heal: Prescription for Herbal Healing*. Mill Valley, CA: Quantum Books, 1994.

Weiss, R.F. *Herbal Medicine*, trans. A.R. Meuss, from the 6th German edition. Beaconsfield, England: Beaconsfield Publishers, Ltd., 1988.

TEXT CITATIONS:

1. *Lawrence Review of Natural Products* (St. Louis: Facts and Comparisons, September 1994).
2. M. Pattrick et al., *Annals of the Rheumatic Diseases*, 48 (1989): 547–49.
3. P.C. Bradley, ed., *British Herbal Compendium: A Handbook of Scientific Information on Widely Used Plant Drugs*, vol. 1 (Bournemouth [Dorset], England: British Herbal Medicine Association, 1992). S. Heptinstall et al., *The Lancet*, I (1985): 1071–74.
4. D.V.C. Awang, *HerbalGram*, (Number 29)66 (1993): 34–36.
5. E.S. Johnson et al., *British Medical Journal of Clinical Research Education*, 291(6495) (1985): 569–73.
6. J.J. Murphy et al., *The Lancet*, ii (1988): 189–92.
7. V.E. Tyler, *Herbs of Choice: The Therapeutic Use of Phytomedicinals* (Binghamton, NY: Haworth Press/Pharmaceutical Products Press, 1994).
8. D.V.C. Awang et al., *Journal of Natural Products*, 54 (1991): 1516–21.
9. J. Castaneda-Acosta et al., *Journal of Natural Products*, 56 (1993): 90–98.
10. R.W. Barsby et al., *Planta Medica*, 59(1) (1993): 20–25.
11. D.V.C. Awang, *Canadian Pharmaceutical Journal*, 122(5) (1989): 266–70. E.S. Johnson et al., *British Medical Journal*, 291 (1985): 569.
12. Johnson, op. cit.
13. Awang, *HerbalGram*, op cit.
14. *Lawrence Review of Natural Products*, op. cit.

PRIMARY NAME:
FLAX

SCIENTIFIC NAME:
Linum usitatissimum L. Family:
Linaceae

COMMON NAMES:
Flaxseed, linseed, lint bells,
linum

RATING:
2 = According to a number of
well-designed studies and
common use, this substance
appears to be relatively
effective and safe when used in
recommended amounts.

What Is Flax?

Linum usitatissimum is a slender-stemmed herb that grows abundantly in many parts of the world, including North America. Delicate blue flowers grow off the branches of the tops. Its brown seeds and the oil derived from them—linseed oil—are used medicinally. Flax is related to but significantly different from the potent purgative *Linum catharticum* (mountain or purging flax), which it does not closely resemble.

What It Is Used For:

Humans have cultivated flax for fabric fiber since prehistoric times, and apparently have treasured its seeds and oil as a folk remedy for millennia. The seeds have traditionally been used to prepare soothing solutions for skin irritations, cough, sore throat, and other inflammatory conditions of the mucous membranes, including digestive and urinary tract irritations such as constipation. Linseed oil is highly valued as an emollient for skin burns and scalds.

Contemporary herbalists highlight a number of these folk uses as well as the considerable content of essential fatty acids (EFAs) in the oil. Many sources consider EFAs helpful in lowering cholesterol, relieving the pain and inflammation of arthritis, and exerting a number of other healing actions. The paint, varnish, and fiber industries use flax extensively.

Forms Available Include:

Capsule, infusion (of seeds, hot or warm), oil, poultice (of crushed seeds mixed with hot water), seeds (whole or ground; eaten alone or mixed with other foods).

Dosage Commonly Reported:

As a laxative, 1 tablespoon whole or crushed (not ground) seeds is taken with 150 milliliters of liquid two or three times per day. The 1,300-milligram softgel capsule, containing 740 milligrams of linoleic acid, is taken once a day.

Will It Work for You? What the Studies Say:

Researchers attribute the demulcent and emollient properties of flaxseeds to their thick outer coating of mucilage. This substance swells when it comes into contact with liquid, rendering flaxseed preparations soothing and protective to irritated skin and mucous membranes. Likewise, constipation and digestive-tract irritations recede as the seeds pass through and absorb liquid, forming a jellylike clump. The high concentration of a fixed oil probably also helps. Flaxseeds are a good source of dietary fiber. German health authorities approve of flaxseed both externally for local inflammation and internally for treating chronic constipation, irritable colon, and colon damage caused by laxative abuse.[1] They also consider it soothing and protective for several disorders of the intestinal tract, including irritation of the stomach (commonly due to infection or acid) and diverticular disease.

Research into flaxseeds is ongoing and intense; there is even a professional journal called *Flaxseed and Human Nutrition*. According to preliminary research, people with high cholesterol may be able to reduce serum total and LDL (low-density lipoprotein) cholesterol significantly (but not HDL, high-density lipoprotein) and related atherogenic risk factors (such as blood clotting) by integrating flaxseed into their diets. This scenario was observed in a 1993 study in which individuals with high lipid (blood fat) levels supplemented their diets with a bread containing flaxseed, as well as 15 grams of flaxseed daily for three months.[2] Similar positive results were seen in another study the same year involving individuals who supplemented their diets with 50 grams of ground flaxseed daily for four weeks.[3] The beneficial reductions in blood lipids and cholesterol levels have been observed in small animal studies as well.[4] But not all human trials report positive results with dietary flax supplementation; one study found fish oil superior to flaxseed oil in producing improvements in lipid levels.[5]

Some experts attribute the lipid-lowering action in part to the essential fatty acids (EFAs) in flaxseed oil; it is particularly rich in *alpha*-linoleic acid and also contains *cis*-linoleic acid. Whether such EFAs can indeed lower lipid or cholesterol levels is being investigated. Flaxseed's power to manage arthritis was not supported by a 1995 randomized, placebo-controlled trial involving twenty-two individuals with rheumatoid arthritis.[6] In the study, three-month supplementation with *alpha*-linoleic acid from flaxseed failed to significantly improve disease factors such as joint pain and tenderness, and blood tests.

Likewise intriguing but still vague are the implications for human health of a study in which researchers added flaxseed to the diet of a group of mice with laboratory-induced systemic lupus, an autoimmune disease, for fourteen weeks.[7] Protein in the urine (proteinuria, a sign of kidney dysfunction) and overall mortality were reduced in these mice compared with those who did not get flaxseed. A follow-up study in eight lupus patients with kidney disease (nephritis) also reported promising findings: kidney function, inflammation, and other disease parameters improved in the patients, who took varying dosages (15, 30, and 45 grams) of flaxseed a day at four-week intervals.[8] The *alpha*-linoleic acid and plant lignans (phytochemicals with weakly estrogenic and antiestrogenic properties) have shown promise in treating lupus-related kidney disease in mice.[9] Other studies have examined potential antimalarial effects of flaxseed and flaxseed oil in the human diet.[10]

Flaxseed may alter female hormonal function (sex steroid action), according to a 1993 study in which the second half (the luteal phase) of the menstrual cycle in eighteen healthy, normally cycling women was lengthened when they supplemented their normally low-fiber diet with 10 grams of flaxseed powder a day.[11] These and other hormone-related changes led the researchers to suspect a role for lignans, of which flaxseed contains a considerable amount. The implications of these and other findings regarding flaxseed, lignans, and cancer are being intensively examined.[12] Preliminary rodent studies also suggest that flaxseed may help prevent colon cancer[13] and reduce the growth of mammary tumors.[14] Scientists are still examining the positive and negative role flaxseed oil may play in preventing or causing cancer.[15]

Will It Harm You? What the Studies Say:

Flaxseed preparations taken in recommended amounts are unlikely to cause adverse reactions, at least on the basis of centuries of use and the current understanding of the plant's chemicals. However, excessive doses could cause toxic reactions because of the presence of trace amounts of poisons. This problem has been seen in animals who graze on the plant.[16] A severe allergic reaction (anaphylaxis) has been reported in a woman who ingested flaxseed.[17] *Never take a flax preparation unless it is designed for human consumption.*

German health authorities also warn that taking flaxseed preparations along with other medicines may negatively affect the way the medicines are absorbed,[18] so talk to your doctor before starting on flaxseed if you are already taking another medicine. They also warn that flaxseed should not be taken if you have a bowel obstruction of any type.

GENERAL SOURCES:

Balch, J.F., and P.A. Balch. *Prescription for Nutritional Healing: A Practical A to Z Reference to Drug-Free Remedies Using Vitamins, Minerals, Herbs & Food Supplements.* 2nd ed. Garden City Park, NY: Avery Publishing Group, 1997.

Blumenthal, M., J. Gruenwald, T. Hall, and R.S. Rister, eds. *The Complete German Commission E Monographs: Therapeutic Guide to Herbal Medicine.* Boston: Integrative Medicine Communications, 1998.

Dobelis, I.N., ed. *The Magic and Medicine of Plants: A Practical Guide to the Science, History, Folklore, and Everyday Uses of Medicinal Plants.* Pleasantville, NY: Reader's Digest Association, 1986.

Lawrence Review of Natural Products. St. Louis: Facts and Comparisons, January 1995.

Mayell, M. *Off-the-Shelf Natural Health: How to Use Herbs and Nutrients to Stay Well.* New York: Bantam Books, 1995.

Ody, P. *The Herb Society's Complete Medicinal Herbal.* London: Dorling Kindersley Limited, 1993.

Weiner, M.A., and J.A. Weiner. *Herbs That Heal: Prescription for Herbal Healing.* Mill Valley, CA: Quantum Books, 1994.

TEXT CITATIONS:

1. M. Blumenthal, J. Gruenwald, T. Hall, and R.S. Rister, eds., *The Complete German Commission E Monographs: Therapeutic Guide to Herbal Medicine* (Boston: Integrative Medicine Communications, 1998).
2. M.L. Bierenbaum et al., *Journal of the American College of Nutrition,* 12 (1993): 501.
3. S.C. Cunnane et al., *British Journal of Nutrition,* 69 (1993): 443.
4. N.M. Jeffrey et al., *Lipids,* 31(7) (1996): 737–45.
5. K.S. Layne et al., *Journal of Nutrition,* 126(9) (1996): 2130–40.
6. D.E. Nordstrom et al., *Rheumatology International,* 14(6) (1995): 231–34.
7. A.V. Hall et al., *American Journal of Kidney Diseases,* 22 (1993): 326.
8. W.F. Clark et al., *Kidney International,* 48(2) (1995): 475–80.
9. W.P. Clarke and A. Parbtani, *American Journal of Kidney Diseases,* 23(5) (1994): 644–47.
10. O.A. Levander and A.L. Ager, Jr., *Flaxseed and Human Nutrition,* (1995): 237–43.
11. W.R. Phipps et al., *Journal of Clinical Endocrinology and Metabolism,* 77 (1993): 1215.
12. L.U. Thompson, *Flaxseed and Human Nutrition,* (1995): 219–36.
13. M. Jenab and L.U. Thompson, *Carcinogenesis,* 17(6) (1996): 1343–48.
14. L.U. Thompson et al., *Carcinogenesis,* 17(6) (1996): 1373–76.
15. P. Johnston, *Flaxseed and Human Nutrition,* (1995): 207–18.
16. *Lawrence Review of Natural Products* (St. Louis: Facts and Comparisons, January 1995).

17. L. Alonso et al., *Journal of Allergy & Clinical Immunology*, 98(2) (1996): 469–70.
18. Blumenthal et al., op. cit.

PRIMARY NAME:

FORSKOLIN (and COLEONOL)

SCIENTIFIC NAME:

Coleus forskohlii and other *Coleus* species. Family: Labiatae (Lamiaceae)

COMMON NAME:

N/A

RATING:

3 = Studies on the effectiveness and safety of this substance are conflicting, or there are not enough studies to draw a conclusion.

What Is Forskolin?

Forskolin is contained in the rootstock of a small, perennial mint-family member, *Coleus forskohlii*, found in tropical and subtropical regions of the Indian subcontinent. Other *Coleus* species are reportedly used as well. The plants are commonly grown as garden annuals or potted plants for their colorful foliage.

What It Is Used For:

Forskolin qualifies as a classic remedy in the Indian (Ayurvedic) and Hindu healing traditions, having long been used for respiratory disorders such as asthma and to treat heart disease, painful urination, insomnia, convulsions, chest pain, and skin disorders such as eczema and psoriasis. Researchers are examining forskolin as a potential treatment for high blood pressure and glaucoma. A substance in the plant closely related to forskolin, called coleonol, has also been used medicinally.

Forms Available Include:

Capsule. Select products with a standardized concentrated forskolin content.

Dosage Commonly Reported:

The extract standardized to contain 18 percent forskolin is commonly taken in a capsule with a dosage of 50 milligrams (totaling 9 milligrams of forskolin) two to three times per day.

Will It Work for You? What the Studies Say:

It was only when a drug research institute in India set out to screen traditional medicinal plants in the mid-1970s that the chemically active compound, forskolin, as well as the closely related antispasmodic and blood-pressure-lowering component coleonol, was first identified.[1] By the mid-1990s, second-generation derivatives of forskolin were being produced for drug treatment.[2]

Forskolin directly activates an enzyme in cell membranes, adenylate cyclase, to boost production of a critical cell-regulating substance called cyclic adenosine monophosphate (AMP).[3] It may also amplify the effects of certain hormones. A number of diseases are characterized by a low level of intracellular AMP and may therefore be helped by forskolin. So far, dozens of test-tube and small animal studies have been conducted on forskolin, and to a lesser extent on coleonol, to examine their disease-fighting potential. Promising findings have been reported for numerous ailments, although human studies are still needed to confirm many of them.

In the case of asthma, for example, notable improvements in bronchodilation and respiratory function were noted among sixteen subjects given single inhalation doses of a standard asthma medicine, fenoterol, or forskolin in capsule form.[4] Metered-dose inhalation forms of forskolin have also shown favorable results comparable to fenoterol in opening up the bronchial tubes, at least in the first few minutes of an asthma attack.[5]

Forskolin eyedrops have shown promise in lowering the intraocular pressure associated with the eye disease glaucoma. This has been shown in small-animal studies and humans.[6] The eyedrops are not yet commercially available, however.[7]

Research also indicates that forskolin can lower blood pressure and improve the contractility (squeezing force) of the heart muscle at the same time. Human studies indicate potential benefit in treating congestive heart failure, although effective doses also produced unpleasant side effects such as flushing.[8]

Studies in laboratory animals also indicate that forskolin can help nerves regenerate after a trauma, reduce excessive urination, and stimulate the secretion of electrolytes by the colon and salivary glands.[9] It also inhibits the aggregation of platelets, meaning that it may help in preventing blood clots,[10] and it boosts stomach acid secretions in animals.[11] Derivatives show promise in suppressing organ transplant rejection.[12] Forskolin has also been closely examined as a substance to treat low thyroid levels (hypothyroidism), depression, cancer metastases, certain digestive disorders, and dryness in the mouth.[13]

Coleonol possesses many of the same properties as forskolin, although its primary action appears to be to relax vascular smooth muscle and thus lower blood pressure. While small doses increase the contractile function of the heart, large doses appear to depress (slow down) the central nervous system.[14]

Will It Harm You? What the Studies Say:

Much remains to be learned about the potential toxicity of forskolin and coleonol, although preliminary findings indicate that they are relatively safe. Individuals who have low blood pressure or peptic ulcers or who are on prescription medications for such conditions as asthma should exercise extra care in taking this herb or its derivatives, if not avoid them altogether.[15] Scientists still have to determine whether other *Coleus* species have similar positive or potentially toxic properties.

GENERAL SOURCES:

Ammon, H.P.T., and A.B. Muller. *Planta Medica.* 51 (1985): 473–77.

Der Marderosian, A., and L. Liberti. *Natural Product Medicine: A Scientific Guide to Foods, Drugs, Cosmetics.* Philadelphia: George F. Stickley, 1988.

De Souza, N.J. *Journal of Ethnopharmacology.* 38 (1993): 177–80.

Murray, M.T. *The Healing Power of Herbs: The Enlightened Person's Guide to the Wonders of Medicinal Plants.* Revised and expanded 2nd ed. Rocklin, CA: Prima Publishing, 1995.

TEXT CITATIONS:

1. H.P.T. Ammon and A.B. Muller, *Planta Medica,* 51 (1985): 473–77. M.T. Murray, *The Healing Power of Herbs: The Enlightened Person's Guide to the Wonders of Medicinal Plants,* revised and expanded 2nd ed. (Rocklin, CA: Prima Publishing, 1995).

2. N.J. De Souza, *Journal of Ethnopharmacology,* 38(2–3) (1993): 177–80.

3. S.J. Hershey et al., *Biochimica et Biophysica Acta,* 755 (1983): 293. A. Der Marderosian and L. Liberti, *Natural Product Medicine: A Scientific Guide to Foods, Drugs, Cosmetics* (Philadelphia: George F. Stickley, 1988).

4. K. Bauer et al., *Clinical Pharmacology and Therapeutics,* 53 (1993): 76–83.

5. G. Kaik and P.U. Witte, *Weiner Medizinische Wochenschrift,* 136 (1986): 637–41.

6. C. Seto et al., *Japanese Journal of Ophthalmology,* 30 (1986): 238–44. J. Caprioli and M. Sears, *The Lancet,* (1983): 958–60. B.H. Meyer et al., *South African Medical Journal,* 71(9) (1987): 570–71.

7. Murray, op. cit.

8. M. Schlepper et al., *Basic Research in Cardiology,* 84(Suppl 1) (1989): 197–212.

9. Der Marderosian and Liberti, op. cit.

10. Ibid.

11. M. Bickel and A.W. Herling, *IRCS Medical Science,* 13(1) (1985): 38–39.

12. A. Matsumori, Japanese Patent Application Number 94/106,976, filed May 20, 1994.

13. Murray, op. cit.

14. M.P. Dubey et al., *Journal of Ethnopharmacology,* 3 (1981): 1. Der Marderosian and Liberti, op. cit.

15. Murray, op. cit.

PRIMARY NAME:

FO-TI

SCIENTIFIC NAME:

Polygonum multiforum Thunb. Family: Polygonaceae

COMMON NAMES:

Climbing knotweed, flowering knotweed, he-shou-wu (spelled and pronounced many ways), knotweed

RATING:

2 = According to a number of well-designed studies and common use, this substance appears to be relatively effective and safe when used in recommended amounts for the indication(s) noted in the "Will It Work for You?" section.

What Is Fo-Ti?

The dried tuberous roots of *Polygonum multiforum,* a climbing perennial evergreen vine native to China and occasionally grown elsewhere, are used medicinally. Fo-ti is solely an American term and it is not used in China.

Do not confuse fo-ti with **Fo-Ti-Tieng™,** a trademark herbal blend devoid of *Polygonum multiforum.*

What It Is Used For:

Traditional Chinese healers use fo-ti in two forms: cured and raw. They consider cured fo-ti an invaluable fortifying, revitalizing, and nourishing tonic, particularly for the liver, kidneys, muscles, bones, tendons, and "vital essence."[1] Signs of premature aging, including graying of hair, are treated with it, as are anemia and nerve-related problems such as limb numbness and dizziness with ear ringing and insomnia. Chinese healers consider raw fo-ti, on the other hand, to be a less potent tonic, and it is cheaper than cured fo-ti.[2] It is traditionally used for skin eruptions such as sores, oozing dermatitis, itching, inflammation, abscesses, carbuncles, athlete's foot, and tuberculosis of the lymph glands. It is also esteemed as a powerful and reliable laxative and considered to have allergy-fighting properties. Both types are used to lower high cholesterol.

Contemporary American herbalists, typically making no distinction between cured and raw fo-ti, tend to emphasize the vine's reputation as a cathartic (strong laxative) and rejuvenating tonic for helping to maintain vigor, boost fertility (in men and women), and encourage longevity. It has also been recommended for diabetes, heart disease, and tumors.

Forms Available Include:

Capsule, concentrated drops, decoction, extracts, powder, root, tablet, tincture.

Dosage Commonly Reported:

The concentrated drops are taken in dosages of ½ to 1 dropperful two to three times per day. Take commercial preparations according to package directions.

Will It Work for You? What the Studies Say:

The concentration of active substances and the expected reactions vary considerably depending on whether the root is taken in raw form, in which case it appears in light brown to brown slices, or cured, in which case it takes on a dark to dark reddish-brown tone. Many of the studies done so far fail to specify which type is being used, rendering results unclear. The majority of studies have been conducted on *Polygonum* species other than *Polygonum multiforum*.[3] In the United States it is often impossible to determine whether you are getting cured or raw fo-ti.

Raw fo-ti contains substances (anthraquinone compounds) that can stimulate a bowel movement, making it a powerful laxative.[4] Whether the plant (in either form) also qualifies as a "rejuvenating tonic" is much harder to determine. Test-tube and small-animal studies conducted in China indicate that it has a number of effects. Cured fo-ti extracts, researchers have found, can enhance immunity in mice, lower cholesterol levels and raise "good" high-density lipoprotein (HDL) cholesterol levels (possibly because of the presence of a fatty compound called lecithin), help protect the liver, inhibit the hepatitis B virus, boost resistance to cold, exert an antiaging effect (observed in mice), and counter the effects of aging on the cellular level.[5] Claims that well-designed human studies have been conducted to test any of these properties could not be verified.

Investigators are also looking into assertions that there are antitumor properties in some of the anthraquinone compounds (emodin and rhein).[6] Other *Polygonum* species contain substances (not consistently found in *Polygonum multiforum*) that fight inflammation, reduce the coagulability ("stickiness") of the blood (which may help in reducing the risk of blood clots), and positively influence the cardiovascular system.[7] Whether fo-ti has the potential to do any of these things in the human body is still unclear.

Will It Harm You? What the Studies Say:

There are scattered reports of allergic reactions, gastrointestinal upset, skin rashes, and numbness of the extremities in reaction to fo-ti,[8] but overall the herb appears to be relatively safe for healthy adults as long as they are not pregnant. To avoid dependence and other complications, do not take any laxative too frequently or in large amounts.

GENERAL SOURCES:

Chevallier, A. *The Encyclopedia of Medicinal Plants: A Practical Reference Guide to More than 550 Key Medicinal Plants & Their Uses.* 1st American ed. New York: Dorling Kindersley Publications, 1996.

Duke, J.A. *CRC Handbook of Medicinal Herbs*. Boca Raton, FL: CRC Press, 1985.

Lawrence Review of Natural Products. St. Louis: Facts and Comparisons, April 1992.

Leung, A.Y., and S. Foster. *Encyclopedia of Common Natural Ingredients Used in Food, Drugs, and Cosmetics*. 2nd ed. New York: John Wiley & Sons, 1996.

Mayell, M. *Off-the-Shelf Natural Health: How to Use Herbs and Nutrients to Stay Well*. New York: Bantam Books, 1995.

Mindell, E. *Earl Mindell's Herb Bible*. New York: Simon & Schuster/Fireside, 1992.

Tang, W., and G. Eisenbrand. *Chinese Drugs of Plant Origin: Chemistry, Pharmacology, and Use in Traditional and Modern Medicine*. Berlin: Springer-Verlag, 1992.

Tierra, M. *The Way of Herbs*. New York: Pocket Books, 1990.

Tyler, V.E. *The Honest Herbal*. Binghamton, NY: Haworth Press/Pharmaceutical Products Press, 1993.

Weiner, M.A., and J.A. Weiner. *Herbs That Heal: Prescription for Herbal Healing*. Mill Valley, CA: Quantum Books, 1994.

TEXT CITATIONS:

1. A.Y. Leung and S. Foster. *Encyclopedia of Common Natural Ingredients Used in Food, Drugs, and Cosmetics*. 2nd ed. New York: John Wiley & Sons, 1996.
2. Ibid.
3. Ibid.
4. V.E. Tyler, *The Honest Herbal* (Binghamton, NY: Haworth Press/Pharmaceutical Products Press, 1993).
5. Leung and Foster, op. cit. X. Pei-Gen et al., *Journal of Ethnopharmacology*, 38 (1993): 167–75. X.G. Chen et al., *Chinese Traditional and Herbal Drugs*, 22 (1991): 357–59.
6. J.A. Duke, *CRC Handbook of Medicinal Herbs* (Boca Raton, FL: CRC Press, 1985).
7. *Lawrence Review of Natural Products* (St. Louis: Facts and Comparisons, April 1992).
8. Leung and Foster, op. cit.

PRIMARY NAME:

FO-TI-TIENG™

SCIENTIFIC NAME:

Reportedly contains gotu kola (*Centella asiatica* [L.] Urban var. *minor*. Family: Umbelliferae), and kola (cola; *Cola nitida* or related species)

COMMON NAME:

N/A

RATING:

4 = Research indicates that this combination herbal product will not fulfill the claims made for it. Its safety is undetermined.

What Is Fo-Ti-Tieng?

This trademark herbal blend contains the herbs noted under "Scientific Name." Do not confuse it with fo-ti (*Polygonum multiforum*); (See **Fo-Ti**.)

What It Is Used For:

This herbal blend enjoyed popularity in the years after World War II and, perhaps more important, kindled interest in the contained herb **Gotu Kola**. Western consumers were told that Fo-Ti-Tieng could promote longevity.[1] The blend, the origin of which is unknown, is said to have enabled a Chinese herbalist to enjoy twenty-three wives over a 256-year lifespan. Its formula has changed over time. Gotu Kola is still widely promoted as an agent to promote longevity, induce calm, and help heal wounds, among other things. Fo-Ti-Tieng is also said to contain a substance called vitamin X, capable of reviving endocrine and brain cells. Note that the components of the Chinese blends may differ considerably from the registered trademark blend sold in the United States.

Forms Available Include:

Proprietary formulations are available from specialized herbal outlets.

Dosage Commonly Reported:

To use commercial Fo-Ti-Tieng formulations, follow the package instructions.

Will It Work for You? What the Studies Say:

Studies specific to this herbal blend do not appear in the recent medical literature. However, the herbs it reportedly contains—particularly gotu kola[2]—have potential healing properties. Check with the manufacturer to determine the relative concentrations of the herbal components, and then see the individual monographs in this book.

Will It Harm You? What the Studies Say:

No information on the potential toxicity of this herbal blend can be found in the recent medical literature; see **Gotu Kola** or other relevant monographs for more information. Given that it contains kola, it has the potential to cause caffeine-related nervousness and other problems, just as coffee does.

GENERAL SOURCES:

Castleman, M. *The Healing Herbs. The Ultimate Guide to the Curative Power of Nature's Medicines.* New York: Bantam Books, 1995.

Lawrence Review of Natural Products. St. Louis: Facts and Comparisons, April 1992.

Tyler, V.E., L.R. Brady, and J.E. Robbers, eds. *Pharmacognosy.* Philadelphia: Lea & Febiger, 1988.

TEXT CITATIONS:

1. M. Castleman, *The Healing Herbs: The Ultimate Guide to the Curative Power of Nature's Medicines*, (New York: Bantam Books, 1995).
2. V.E. Tyler, L.R. Brady, and J.E. Robbers, eds., *Pharmacognosy* (Philadelphia: Lea & Febiger, 1988).

FOXGLOVE

SCIENTIFIC NAME:
Digitalis purpurea L., *Digitalis lanata* Ehrh., and certain related *Digitalis* species. Family: Scrophulariaceae

COMMON NAMES:
Deadmen's bells, digitalis, fairy cap, fairy finger, lady's thimble, lion's mouth, purple foxglove,

What Is Foxglove?

Foxglove, of which there are numerous species, is grown as a biennial or perennial ornamental flower worldwide. Spires of tubular, bell-shaped flowers of various colors hang off a thick and downy stem that can grow two to five feet tall. The plant's long, woolly leaves are dried and made into a powder that is used medicinally. Foxglove should not be misidentified as **Comfrey** (Symphytum officinale), which has a similar appearance.

What It Is Used For:

In the Middle Ages, Europeans used the plant to treat a spectrum of ailments including tuberculosis, madness, and epilepsy. In other parts of the world, traditional medicine cultures treat asthma with the powdered leaves and wounds with

FOXGLOVE (Continued)

scotch mercury, throatwort, witch's bells, woolly foxglove

an ointment made from foxglove. But today foxglove's critical contribution to medicine has been as a treatment for fluid retention caused by congestive heart failure, once commonly referred to as dropsy. An English physician, William Withering, first described this application in a paper published in 1785; two centuries later, medical historians celebrated his seminal finding in professional journals.

Compounds in the leaves called cardiac glycosides, especially digitoxin from both *Digitalis purpurea* and *Digitalis lanata*, as well as digoxin from the latter, increase the ability of the heart to contract forcefully and with a regular rhythm. These glycosides have also been used for other heart disorders. Some strains of the plant typically have higher concentrations of the critical compounds than others; *Digitalis purpurea*, so popular as an ornamental, usually contains low concentrations of the cardiac glycosides.[1]

Forms Available Include:

Standardized digitalis preparations can be obtained only by prescription in the United States.

Dosage Commonly Reported:

Standardized digitalis preparations are available by prescription only.

Will It Work for You? What the Studies Say:

Congestive heart failure is a serious but relatively common condition that has affected millions of people through the ages and worldwide. Many of them have been kept alive by this cardiac stimulant. Scientists have studied foxglove and its derivatives intensively over the decades.

Foxglove components are standard medicines in the United States and many other parts of the world today, particularly for controlling a fast and irregular heart rhythm in individuals with atrial fibrillation. Increasingly in the United States, however, new medicines are being introduced to supplant foxglove and its glycosides as heart disorder treatments.[2] The reason for this is that the amount necessary to take to help control a disorder such as congestive heart failure is very close to the amount that can cause severe side effects, most notably irregular or potentially fatal heart rhythms.

The lower development of new cases of cancer among individuals being treated with digitalis glycosides has prompted curiosity among scientists.[3] One team of investigators noted numerous characteristics in tumors in breast cancer patients taking this medicine compared with those not taking it, including smaller tumors and less likelihood of cancer spreading to distant parts of the body.[4]

Will It Harm You? What the Studies Say:

All parts of this lovely plant are extremely poisonous, from the leaves to the seeds and flowers. Foxglove is a common cause of plant poisoning,[5] and chewing and swallowing a leaf can lead to blurred vision, nausea, constricted pupils, dizziness, convulsions, abnormal heart rhythms, and stupor. These are just a few of the signs of poisoning that can result from ingesting the plant or taking improper doses of the purified drug. One investigator theorizes that the painter

Vincent Van Gogh may have suffered from chronic digitalis intoxication, with yellowing of objects in the visual field and visual halos making their way into his masterpieces.[6] Medicines made from the plant can also cause serious harm if improperly used, as the glycosides accumulate in the body and must be carefully monitored. People have died after drinking a tea made from the plant, which they had misidentified as comfrey.[7]

GENERAL SOURCES:

Dobelis, I.N., ed. *The Magic and Medicine of Plants: A Practical Guide to the Science, History, Folklore, and Everyday Uses of Medicinal Plants.* Pleasantville, NY: Reader's Digest Association, 1986.

Duke, J.A. *CRC Handbook of Medicinal Herbs.* Boca Raton, FL: CRC Press, 1985.

Lawrence Review of Natural Products. St. Louis: Facts and Comparisons, October 1993.

Marullaz, P.D. *Journal of Ethnopharmacology.* 32(1–3) (1991): 111–15.

Poole-Wilson, P.A. *Cardiology.* 75 Suppl 1 (1988): 103–9.

Tyler, V.E. *Herbs of Choice: The Therapeutic Use of Phytomedicinals.* Binghamton, NY: Haworth Press/Pharmaceutical Products Press, 1994.

TEXT CITATIONS:

1. *Lawrence Review of Natural Products* (St. Louis: Facts and Comparisons, October 1993).
2. Ibid.
3. A.G. Goldin and A.R. Safa, *The Lancet,* 8386 (1984): 1134. *Lawrence Review of Natural Products,* op. cit.
4. B. Stenkvist et al., *Analytical and Quantitative Cytology,* 2 (1980): 49.
5. E. Geehr, *Emergency Medicine Clinics of North America,* 2(3) (1984): 553–62.
6. T.C. Lee, *Journal of the American Medical Association,* 245(7) (1981): 1981.
7. J.A. Duke, *CRC Handbook of Medicinal Herbs* (Boca Raton, FL: CRC Press, 1985).

PRIMARY NAME:

FRUIT ACIDS

SCIENTIFIC NAME:

N/A

COMMON NAMES:

Individual acids: citric acid, gluconic acid, gluconolactone, glycolic acid, lactic acid, malic acid, tartaric acid

RATING:

3 = Studies on the effectiveness of these substances are conflicting, or there are not enough studies to draw a conclusion about it. Safety appears to depend on cautious and judicious use; see the "Will They Harm You?" section.

What Are Fruit Acids?

Fruit acids, or alphahydroxy acids, are derived from fruits such as grapes (tartaric acid), citrus fruits (citric acid from oranges and lemons, for example), and apples (malic acid). The term "fruit acid" is also used to apply to lactic acid, which is from milk, and glycolic and gluconic acids, which are from sugarcane. A particular chemical structure—a hydroxyl group at the alpha-carbon position—can be identified in all of these naturally occurring acids and accounts for their similar medicinal properties and the word *fruit* in their name.

What They Are Used For:

For a number of years, dermatologists and other medical professionals have turned to high-concentration fruit-acid products (30 percent or higher), to help debride (remove) dead skin cells associated with scars and age spots, as well as to moisturize top skin layers. These acids also show promise in treating acne.

Recognizing the ability of these acids to slough off dead skin from top layers, some cosmetics companies have started to incorporate lower levels (typically 4 to 10 percent) of these acids into skin creams and other products, claiming that they can rejuvenate skin and counter the effects of aging, as well as improve skin texture and tone, eliminate age spots, and moisturize the skin.

Forms Available Include:

Fruit acids appear in many herbal and conventional over-the-counter skin cleansers, acne treatments, and other skin care products.

Dosage Commonly Reported:

To use commercial products containing fruit acids, follow the package instructions. Limit or discontinue use if irritation develops; see "Will They Harm You?" section for more information.

Will They Work for You? What the Studies Say:

When used properly and in moderation, fruit acids play an important role in conventional medicine for treating various skin conditions. For example, one of the acid components called gluconolactone proved as effective in reducing the total number of acne lesions (inflamed and noninflamed) as benzoyl peroxide (5 percent lotion), a common antiacne medicine, and more effective than a placebo in a twelve-week double-blind study involving 150 acne sufferers.[1] The subjects treated themselves with a 14 percent solution of this fruit acid. They reported less dryness than those who applied the benzoyl peroxide, and fewer adverse reactions overall. The gluconolactone appears to work by loosening the cohesion of certain cells,[2] thereby increasing the rate at which cells slough off from the skin.[3]

Lactic acid in particular has proved valuable in treating dry skin, featuring moisturizing properties that may actually thicken the top skin layers.[4] Concentrations of 2 to 5 percent are most commonly used.

The antiaging, antiwrinkle, and moisturizing properties advertised by cosmetic companies can be attributed to an exfoliant effect; top dead skin cell layers may be removed and fine wrinkles seem to disappear as the skin becomes moisturized. The fundamental aging or wrinkling process is unaffected, however.[5] More important, there are serious limitations to the use of fruit acids in cosmetics because the acids can potentially irritate the skin if the concentration is too high.[6]

Will They Harm You? What the Studies Say:

Fruit acids can severely irritate the skin if applied in high concentrations, possibly causing redness and burning among other reactions. These are also a risk if the products are left on the skin for longer than recommended. Proceed very carefully—if at all—if you have very sensitive or already irritated skin.[7] Take particular care in applying any of these substances to sensitive areas such as the eyes.

GENERAL SOURCES:

American Pharmaceutical Association. *Handbook of Nonprescription Drugs.* 11th ed. Washington, D.C.: American Pharmaceutical Association, 1996.

Lawrence Review of Natural Products. St. Louis: Facts and Comparisons, April 1995.

Mayell, M. *Off-the-Shelf Natural Health: How to Use Herbs and Nutrients to Stay Well.* New York: Bantam Books, 1995.

TEXT CITATIONS:

1. M.J. Hunt and R.S. Barnetson, *Australasian Journal of Dermatology*, 33 (1992): 131. *Lawrence Review of Natural Products* (St. Louis: Facts and Comparisons, April 1995).
2. E.J. Van Scott and R.J. Yu, *Journal of the American Academy of Dermatology*, 11 (1984): 867.
3. *Lawrence Review of Natural Products,* op. cit.
4. American Pharmaceutical Association, *Handbook of Nonprescription Drugs*, 11th ed. (Washington, D.C.: American Pharmaceutical Association, 1996).
5. *Lawrence Review of Natural Products,* op. cit.
6. Ibid.
7. Ibid.

PRIMARY NAME:
FUMITORY

SCIENTIFIC NAME:
Fumaria officinalis L. Family: Fumariaceae

COMMON NAMES:
Common fumitory, earth-smoke, hedge fumitory, wax dolls

RATING:
3 = Studies on the effectiveness of this herb are conflicting, or there are not enough studies to draw a conclusion about it.

What Is Fumitory?

This limp-branched annual bears delicate bluish-green leaves, clusters of tubular, small fruits, and crimson-tipped flowers. It is native to Europe and Asia and can be found growing wild along roadsides and waste places in parts of North America as well. The leaves, stems, and flowers are used medicinally.

What It Is Used For:

Fumitory is an old standard of European herbals that continues to find use today, often in many of the same ways. For centuries it has been used as a diuretic ("water pill") to increase urination, a laxative for constipation, and a balm for skin eruptions. Recent findings indicate that the herb may benefit high blood pressure and heart conditions. But the primary use of fumitory today is for cramplike, spastic biliary (liver) pains and constipation.

Forms Available Include:

Infusion, liquid herbal extract.

Dosage Commonly Reported:

An average daily dosage is 6 grams. An infusion is made using 1¼ to 2 teaspoons (about 2 to 3 grams) of the herb and is drunk up to twice per day. German sources recommend drinking the freshly prepared, still-warm infusion 30 minutes before meals. The liquid herbal extract is taken in 2- to 4-milliliter doses.

Will It Work for You? What the Studies Say:

Research indicates that fumitory reduces spasms in the upper part of the gastrointestinal tract,[1] with the alkaloid protopine exerting a normalizing action on bile output, promoting its secretion when needed,[2] and possibly accounting for fumitory's value as an antispasmodic. According to German textbooks, clinical trials have confirmed that fumitory can alleviate acute biliary colic and even chronic dyskinesia (movement disorders).[3] Pain in the abdominal area dissipates; symptoms such as nausea, vomiting, and headache resolve; and rich foods are better tolerated. German health authorities approve of fumitory for cramplike complaints in the biliary and gastrointestinal tracts.[4]

The presence of fumaric acid, a synthetic drug commonly used for psoriasis today, may explain the herb's traditional use for skin eruptions.[5]

Will It Harm You? What the Studies Say:

No reports of serious adverse reactions to this herb appear in the recent medical literature. According to European sources, the herb is well tolerated in clinical trials.[6] German health authorities cite no known situations in which it should not be used or known interactions with other medicines,[7] and indicate that it is safe to take over a period of several weeks.[8] However, large doses may cause diarrhea and stomachache, according to an American source.

GENERAL SOURCES:

Bisset, N.G., ed. *Herbal Drugs and Phytopharmaceuticals.* Stuttgart: medpharm GmbH Scientific Publishers, 1994.

Blumenthal, M., J. Gruenwald, T. Hall, and R.S. Rister, eds. *The Complete German Commission E Monographs: Therapeutic Guide to Herbal Medicine.* Boston: Integrative Medicine Communications, 1998.

Dobelis, I.N., ed. *The Magic and Medicine of Plants: A Practical Guide to the Science, History, Folklore, and Everyday Uses of Medicinal Plants.* Pleasantville, NY: Reader's Digest Association, 1986.

Weiss, R.F. *Herbal Medicine*, trans. A.R. Meuss, from the 6th German edition. Beaconsfield, England: Beaconsfield Publishers, Ltd., 1988.

TEXT CITATIONS:

1. M. Blumenthal, J. Gruenwald, T. Hall, and R.S. Rister, eds., *The Complete German Commission E Monographs: Therapeutic Guide to Herbal Medicine* (Boston: Integrative Medicine Communications, 1998). N.G. Bisset, ed., *Herbal Drugs and Phytopharmaceuticals* (Stuttgart: medpharm GmbH Scientific Publishers, 1994).
2. Bisset, op. cit. R.F. Weiss, *Herbal Medicine*, trans. A.R. Meuss, from the 6th German edition (Beaconsfield, England: Beaconsfield Publishers, Ltd., 1988).
3. Weiss, op. cit.
4. Blumenthal et al., op. cit.
5. Bisset, op. cit. H. Kretimair, *Pharmazie*, 4 (1949): 242.
6. Weiss, op. cit.
7. Blumenthal et al., op. cit.
8. Bisset, op. cit.

PRIMARY NAME:
GARLIC

SCIENTIFIC NAME:
Allium sativum L. Family:
Liliaceae

COMMON NAMES:
Allium, camphor of the poor, nectar of the gods, poor man's treacle, rustic treacle, stinking rose

RATING:
1 = Years of use and extensive, high-quality studies indicate that this substance is very effective and safe when used in recommended amounts for the indication(s) noted in the "Will It Work for You?" section.

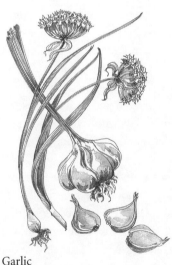

Garlic
Allium sativum

What Is Garlic?

The bulb of the tall, flowering *Allium sativum* serves as the famous food and medicine the world knows as garlic. Pink to purple flowers bloom on this powerhouse of the lily family—a family that also includes onions, leeks, and scallions—from July to September.

What It Is Used For:

Humans have been cultivating garlic for more than five thousand years. The Egyptian pharaohs treasured it, as did ancient Chinese emperors. Egyptian slaves received a daily ration.[1] The bulb has been handed down through the centuries as a preventive medicine and cure-all that many medieval folk healers claimed could even ward off vampires, witches, and other unwanted imaginary creatures. The French scientist Louis Pasteur noted its antibiotic properties in the mid-1800s, and the physician Albert Schweitzer treated amebic dysentery with it in Africa,[2] while physicians in other parts of the world were prescribing garlic inhalation for tuberculosis. Widely used as an antiseptic for generations, garlic became known as "Russian penicillin" in the days of penicillin shortages during World War II, when people resorted to applying the juice to infected wounds.[3]

Specific ailments for which herbalists both modern and ancient recommend garlic include colds (particularly recurrent ones), coughs, flu, chronic bronchitis, whooping cough, ringworm, asthma, intestinal worms, fever, and digestive, gallbladder, and liver disorders. Of particular interest in recent years has been garlic's purported ability, in addition to relieving stomach and intestinal upset, to treat atherosclerosis and heart disease risk factors such as high blood pressure, high cholesterol, and blood clots.

Forms Available Include:

Bulb (fresh, dried), capsule, extract, infusion, juice, liquid, oil, syrup, tablet, tincture. Commercial garlic preparations vary widely in the way they are prepared and the level of active ingredient—alliin, converted by the body into allicin—they contain. Select enteric-coated dried garlic tablets or capsules so that they can survive the trip to the small intestine, where the conversion to allicin can occur.[4] Oil-based garlic preparations are of questionable value because allicin does not always remain intact in oil. Many sources question the medicinal quality of so-called "deodorized" garlic formulations, asserting that the healing benefits are linked to the smell of the garlic, which is, after all, caused by the active ingredient.

Dosage Commonly Reported:

The equivalent of one to five fresh cloves a day is commonly recommended. One clove (4 grams) of garlic yields about 10 milligrams alliin and a total allicin potential of 4,000 micrograms. Aged garlic extract is taken in dosages of 10 to 20 grams daily.

Will It Work for You? What the Studies Say:

An impressive array of healing properties has been found in garlic: an ability to fight bacteria and fungi, prevent blood clots, lower blood pressure, reduce inflammation, reduce high blood sugar, soothe the digestive tract, lower cholesterol levels, and help treat colds and flu. Some of these properties have been more fully substantiated than others, but all have some scientific evidence to support them.

The key ingredient in garlic, the odorless amino acid derivative alliin, converts into a substance called allicin when the garlic bulb is crushed or injured in any way. Chemists first isolated these components in the 1940s, and the amount of interest and research in garlic has been intensive since then, with no fewer than 1,000 papers being reported over recent decades alone.[5]

Research indicates that fresh garlic, at relatively high doses (5 cloves or more a day), can reduce heart disease and atherosclerosis risk factors by lowering cholesterol levels, increasing fibrinolytic activity, and inhibiting blood from clotting.[6] This was the conclusion of an examination of nearly twenty controlled trials on the subject reviewed by Dutch investigators.[7] Commercial garlic preparations, doubtless mixed in their concentration of active ingredients, yielded much more variable results, a problem with all studies on garlic.

Recent studies indicate that in most cases, garlic reduces total cholesterol and low-density-lipoprotein (LDL; the "bad" cholesterol) levels more significantly than a placebo can, in addition to increasing levels of the "good," high-density-lipoprotein (HDL) cholesterol.[8] In a sixteen-week study of 261 individuals with high cholesterol, garlic powder standardized to contain 1.3 percent allicin reduced cholesterol levels by an average of 12 percent and triglyceride levels by 17 percent.[9] Another placebo-controlled study found that garlic tablets reduced total cholesterol levels by 6 percent and LDL cholesterol by 11 percent.[10] In a study of twenty healthy individuals who took garlic in oil twice a day for six months, mean serum cholesterol and triglyceride levels fell significantly, while HDL levels rose.[11]

Other studies indicate that garlic may benefit certain heart conditions, possibly by lowering blood pressure,[12] and especially if blood pressure is already high.[13] The herb may also help reduce the risk of blood clots by inhibiting platelet aggregation.[14] This has been shown not only in test-tube and animal studies, but in humans who eat fresh garlic and then have blood clotting values tested.[15] Garlic also activates fibrinolysis, the body's natural system for breaking down clots.[16] German health authorities approve of 4 grams of minced fresh garlic or 8 milligrams of the essential oil to help dietary attempts to reduce blood lipids (fats) and prevent age-related vessel changes (arteriosclerosis).[17]

Garlic may possess other healing powers as well, showing promise as a treatment for various types of infections, cancers, and digestive ailments, for example. Its antibacterial powers have been well demonstrated in test-tube and animal studies,[18] and even antiviral properties have been detected.[19] Scientists are examining its potential to help treat yeast infections (both oral and vaginal).[20] Anti-inflammatory and worm-fighting properties have also been documented.

Will It Harm You? What the Studies Say:

Although most people tolerate (and even enjoy) garlic in hefty doses, some develop digestive tract discomfort. A burning sensation in the mouth as well as nausea, vomiting, and diarrhea can also occur.[21] Allergic reactions are rare.

Because of the active ingredients in garlic, medicinal doses of the herb may interfere with blood-sugar-lowering medicines and anticoagulants such as warfarin and aspirin.[22] Although there are no recent reports of harm for pregnant women taking medicinal doses of garlic, it has been used as an abortion-inducing agent in some cultures and may affect the menstrual cycle or uterus.[23] Test-tube studies have documented uterine contractions in tissue exposed to garlic.[24] For these reasons, pregnant women may want to avoid medicinal doses of the herb.

The unmistakable odor of garlic on the skin and breath will certainly not harm *you*.

GENERAL SOURCES:

American Pharmaceutical Association. *Handbook of Nonprescription Drugs.* 11th ed. Washington, D.C.: American Pharmaceutical Association, 1996.

Blumenthal, M., J. Gruenwald, T. Hall, and R.S. Rister, eds. *The Complete German Commission E Monographs: Therapeutic Guide to Herbal Medicine.* Boston: Integrative Medicine Communications, 1998.

Bradley, P.C., ed. *British Herbal Compendium: A Handbook of Scientific Information on Widely Used Plant Drugs*, vol. 1. Bournemouth (Dorset), England: British Herbal Medicine Association, 1992.

Castleman, M. *The Healing Herbs: The Ultimate Guide to the Curative Power of Nature's Medicines.* New York: Bantam Books, 1995.

Lawrence Review of Natural Products. St. Louis: Facts and Comparisons, April 1994.

Leung, A.Y., and S. Foster. *Encyclopedia of Common Natural Ingredients Used in Food, Drugs, and Cosmetics.* 2nd ed. New York: John Wiley & Sons, 1996.

Murray, M.T. *The Healing Power of Herbs: The Enlightened Person's Guide to the Wonders of Medicinal Plants.* Revised and expanded 2nd ed. Rocklin, CA: Prima Publishing, 1995.

Newall, C.A., et al. *Herbal Medicines: A Guide for Health-Care Professionals.* London: The Pharmaceutical Press, 1996.

Tyler, V.E. *Herbs of Choice: The Therapeutic Use of Phytomedicinals.* Binghamton, NY: Haworth Press/Pharmaceutical Products Press, 1994.

———. *The Honest Herbal.* Binghamton, NY: Haworth Press/Pharmaceutical Products Press, 1993.

Weiss, R.F. *Herbal Medicine*, trans. A.R. Meuss, from the 6th German edition. Beaconsfield, England: Beaconsfield Publishers, Ltd., 1988.

TEXT CITATIONS:

1. M. Castleman, *The Healing Herbs. The Ultimate Guide to the Curative Power of Nature's Medicines* (New York: Bantam Books, 1995).
2. M.T. Murray, *The Healing Power of Herbs: The Enlightened Person's Guide to the Wonders of Medicinal Plants*, revised and expanded 2nd ed. (Rocklin, CA: Prima Publishing, 1995).
3. Castleman, op. cit.
4. V.E. Tyler, *Herbs of Choice: The Therapeutic Use of Phytomedicinals* (Binghamton, NY: Haworth Press/Pharmaceutical Products Press, 1994).
5. Ibid.
6. B.S. Kendler, *Preventive Medicine,* 16 (1987): 670–85. P. Mansell and J.P.D. Reckless, *British Medical Journal,* 303 (1991): 379–80.
7. Tyler, op. cit. J. Kleijnen et al., *British Journal of Clinical Pharmacology,* 28 (1989): 535–44.

8. E. Ernst, *Pharmatherapeutica*, 5 (1987): 83–89.

9. F.H. Mader, *Arzneimittel-Forschung*, 40(II) (1990): 1111–16.

10. A.K. Jain et al., *American Journal of Medicine*, 94 (1993): 632.

11. *Lawrence Review of Natural Products* (St. Louis: Facts and Comparisons, April 1994).

12. F.G. McMahon et al., *Pharmacotherapy*, 13(4) (1993): 406.

13. W. Auer et al., *British Journal of Clinical Practice*, 44(Suppl. 69) (1990): 3–6.

14. H. Kiesewetter et al., *International Journal of Clinical Pharmacology, Therapy and Toxicology*, 29 (1991): 151–55.

15. D.J. Boullin, *The Lancet*, I (1981): 776.

16. J. Harenberg et al., *Atherosclerosis*, 74 (1988): 247–49.

17. A.Y. Leung and S. Foster, *Encyclopedia of Common Natural Ingredients Used in Food, Drugs, and Cosmetics*, 2nd ed. (New York: John Wiley & Sons, 1996).

18. E.I. Elnima et al., *Pharmazie*, 38 (1983): 747–48.

19. Y. Tsai et al., *Planta Medica*, 51 (1985): 460–61.

20. *Lawrence Review of Natural Products*, op. cit.

21. S. Fulder, *Cardiology in Practice*, 7 (1989): 30–35.

22. C.A. Newall et al., *Herbal Medicines: A Guide for Health-Care Professionals* (London: The Pharmaceutical Press, 1996). W. Sunter, *Pharmaceutical Journal*, 246 (1991): 722.

23. Newall, op. cit.

24. D.J. Joshi et al., *Phytotherapy Research*, 1 (1987): 140–41.

PRIMARY NAME:

GENTIAN

SCIENTIFIC NAME:

Gentiana lutea L. Family: Gentianaceae

COMMON NAMES:

Bitterroot, gall weed, gentiana, pale gentian, stemless gentian, yellow gentian

RATING:

2 = According to a number of well-designed studies and common use, this substance appears to be relatively effective and safe when used in recommended amounts for the indication(s) noted in the "Will It Work for You?" section.

What Is Gentian?

The dried rhizomes (underground stems) and roots of this perennial herb are used medicinally. The plant, native to western Asia and the mountains of central and southern Europe, has large, sturdy oval leaves and bears clusters of orange-yellow flowers. Grown today primarily in Europe, it is occasionally cultivated in the United States as well.

What It Is Used For:

Gentian qualifies as a classic bitter tonic. Many Americans who have tried bitter aperitifs such as Campari or Angostura Bitters will recognize the flavor. Europeans have enjoyed gentian-containing aperitifs and liqueurs for centuries, and not only because the flavor appeals to them; bitters have a reputation for stimulating the appetite and improving digestion. Powers to dispel heartburn, stomachache, vomiting, diarrhea, and other gastrointestinal upsets have also been ascribed to them. Many cases of anorexia and appetite loss, especially when related to indigestion, have been treated with gentian.

Less common uses for gentian include the treatment of sore throat, jaundice, and arthritic inflammations. Topical formulations have been used to treat wounds. Small amounts are allowed as food flavorings in most Western countries, and extracts have been added to antismoking products.

Forms Available Include:

Decoction, extract, powdered dried rhizome, tea, tincture. Gentian appears in many herbal blends.

Dosage Commonly Reported:

A decoction is made using 1 teaspoon powdered dried rhizome and root for every 3 cups of water; 1 tablespoon is drunk about thirty minutes before meals. The tincture is taken in dosages of 20 to 40 drops in water before meals. The extract is taken in dosages of 0.5 to 4 grams per day.

Will It Work for You? What the Studies Say:

Gentian is a time-tested, classic bitter. It contains several bitter-tasting compounds, including amargogentin, which ranks among the most bitter substances known. As salivation is stimulated in reaction to the taste, gastric juices and bile are said to stream into the system, priming the appetite and easing the passage and processing of food. Digestive system problems are purportedly likewise alleviated, although not all research studies have borne this out. German health authorities approve of gentian for treating digestive complaints such as appetite loss, bloating, and flatulence.[1]

Animal studies indicate that gentian may help treat stomach ulcers,[2] although German health authorities consider the presence of stomach or duodenal ulcers to be among the few reasons not to take the herb. Extracts of the herb show bile-stimulating properties (which may aid dyspeptic symptoms) as well as anti-inflammatory actions in laboratory animals.[3] Whether similar reactions occur in humans and help in any way has not yet been determined.

The presence of astringent substances called tannins in gentian may explain its traditional use for treating wounds externally, although other herbs appear be much more popular for this purpose.

Not all gentian preparations are made alike; the highest-quality gentian is dried quickly and remains white (at least for the first few months) instead of turning reddish.[4]

Will It Harm You? What the Studies Say:

No reports of serious adverse reactions to gentian have been handed down through centuries of use. In terms of scientific analysis, however, relatively little is known about the herb. Practical experience indicates that not everyone tolerates it well. For example, although gentian is normally taken to dispel stomach upset and ease digestion, in some cases it actually irritates the stomach lining and can cause nausea and vomiting. It may also trigger a headache in predisposed individuals.[5] Researchers have observed mutagenic (mutation-promoting) activity in classic animal experiments,[6] although what this means—if anything—for humans who ingest gentian is still unclear.

German health authorities warn against taking gentian if you suffer from stomach or duodenal ulcers. Another source indicates that pregnant women and people with very high blood pressure should avoid gentian.[7]

GENERAL SOURCES:

Bisset, N.G., ed. *Herbal Drugs and Phytopharmaceuticals.* Stuttgart: medpharm GmbH Scientific Publishers, 1994.

Blumenthal, M., J. Gruenwald, T. Hall, and R.S. Rister, eds. *The Complete German Commission E Monographs: Therapeutic Guide to Herbal Medicine.* Boston: Integrative Medicine Communications, 1998.

Bradley, P.C., ed. *British Herbal Compendium: A Handbook of Scientific Information on Widely Used Plant Drugs,* vol. 1. Bournemouth (Dorset), England: British Herbal Medicine Association, 1992.

Castleman, M. *The Healing Herbs: The Ultimate Guide to the Curative Power of Nature's Medicines.* New York: Bantam Books, 1995.

Lawrence Review of Natural Products. St. Louis: Facts and Comparisons, April 1993.

Leung, A.Y., and S. Foster. *Encyclopedia of Common Natural Ingredients Used in Food, Drugs, and Cosmetics.* 2nd ed. New York: John Wiley & Sons, 1996.

Newall, C.A., et al. *Herbal Medicines: A Guide for Health-Care Professionals.* London: The Pharmaceutical Press, 1996.

Tyler, V.E. *Herbs of Choice: The Therapeutic Use of Phytomedicinals.* Binghamton, NY: Haworth Press/Pharmaceutical Products Press, 1994.

———. *The Honest Herbal.* Binghamton, NY: Haworth Press/Pharmaceutical Products Press, 1993.

Weiss, R.F. *Herbal Medicine,* trans. A.R. Meuss, from the 6th German edition. Beaconsfield, England: Beaconsfield Publishers, Ltd., 1988.

TEXT CITATIONS:

1. M. Blumenthal, J. Gruenwald, T. Hall, and R.S. Rister, eds., *The Complete German Commission E Monographs: Therapeutic Guide to Herbal Medicine* (Boston: Integrative Medicine Communications, 1998).
2. S. Tanaka et al., *Iryo,* 42 (1988): 591–95.
3. *Lawrence Review of Natural Products* (St. Louis: Facts and Comparisons, April 1993). F. Sadritdinov, *Farmakol Alkaloidov Serdechnykha Glikozidov,* (1971): 146. A.Y. Leung and S. Foster, *Encyclopedia of Common Natural Ingredients Used in Food, Drugs, and Cosmetics,* 2nd ed. (New York: John Wiley & Sons, 1996).
4. V.E. Tyler, *Herbs of Choice: The Therapeutic Use of Phytomedicinals* (Binghamton, NY: Haworth Press/Pharmaceutical Products Press, 1994).
5. Ibid. Blumenthal et al., op. cit.
6. I. Morimoto et al., *Mutation Research,* 116 (1983): 103–17.
7. V.E. Tyler, *The Honest Herbal* (Binghamton, NY: Haworth Press/Pharmaceutical Press, 1993).
8. R. Garnier et al., *Annales de Medicine Interne,* 136 (1985): 125.

PRIMARY NAME:
GINGER

SCIENTIFIC NAME:
Zingiber officinale Roscoe and occasionally other species. Family: Zingiberaceae

COMMON NAMES:
Based on its site of origin: African ginger, black ginger, Chochin (Asian) ginger, gan jiang, Jamaican ginger, race ginger.

What Is Ginger?

Ginger is a perennial plant native to southeast Asia and cultivated in other tropical regions such as Jamaica. The spicy sweet, knotty underground stems (rhizomes) are highly treasured in cooking and as a medicine. The plant produces spikes of green-purple flowers.

What it Is Used For:

Ginger is a powerhouse of Far Eastern traditional medicine, in which it has been used for millennia as a digestive aid and to remedy stomach upset, gassy indigestion, bloating, and cramping. It has also been used to relieve headaches (including migraine), calm inflammation and rheumatic pains, treat kidney ailments, soothe sore throats, and ease other cold symptoms such as cough,

RATING:
1 = Years of use and extensive, high-quality studies indicate that this substance is very effective and safe when used in recommended amounts for the indication(s) noted in the "Will It Work for You?" section.

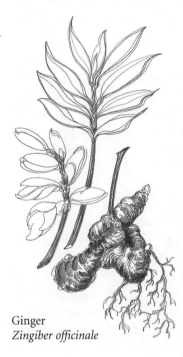

Ginger
Zingiber officinale

among many other things. Ginger tea or tincture taken hot is said to cleanse the system through perspiration and to suppress menstruation.

Contemporary herbalists recommend ginger for many of these traditional purposes, especially for cold and flu symptoms and digestive and menstrual irregularities. A number also consider it potentially valuable for preventing liver damage and treating peptic ulcers, impotence, rheumatic disorders, and depression. Of particular interest lately has been ginger's purported power to prevent nausea due to seasickness, motion sickness, morning sickness, and gynecologic surgery. Chinese sailors were known to chew on ginger root to keep seasickness at bay.

External formulations of ginger juice have traditionally been placed on minor burns and skin inflammations to soothe and heal them. Some sources claim that ginger is useful in combination with olive oil to treat dandruff and that a few drops of the warmed oil will help soothe an earache.

Forms Available Include:

Capsule, decoction, extract, root (fresh and dried; candied, crystallized, whole, grated, ground), tea, tincture (weak and strong).

Dosage Commonly Reported:

3 to 10 grams of fresh ginger, or 2 to 4 grams of dry ginger, are taken daily; a nubbin of ginger may range from 5 to 10 grams. A one-inch-square piece of ginger candy is equivalent to about 500 milligrams ginger. To prevent motion sickness, 1,000 milligrams in capsule form is taken thirty minutes before travel; one to two more 500-milligram capsules are then taken as needed. As a digestive aid, a decoction is made using 2 teaspoons powdered or grated root per cup of water, or three 535-milligram root capsules are taken three times a day.

Will It Work for You? What the Studies Say:

To some extent, time speaks to the medicinal value of ginger. The ancient Greeks and Romans used it as a digestive aid, and it went on to become an important component of the medicinal repertoire of many cultures. The Chinese have reportedly been relying on it as a spice and drug for no less than twenty-five centuries.[1]

Although ginger may be an age-old remedy, researchers have yet to identify its active ingredient or determine exactly how it exerts its effect. It was long believed to act on the central nervous system, but no studies have confirmed this; in fact, they suggest otherwise.[2] Research indicates that ginger functions well as a digestive aid, soothing the gastrointestinal tract and relieving indigestion and abdominal cramping. German health authorities officially approve of ginger for treating indigestion.[3] Current thinking holds that it stimulates saliva flow and acts directly in the stomach, increasing the tone of the intestinal muscle and the involuntary, rhythmic contraction of the esophagus, known as peristalsis, that propels food through the system.

Researchers have identified anti-inflammatory substances in ginger, giving credence to traditional uses for inflammatory conditions such as arthritis. Large-scale clinical trials do not appear to have been carried out to verify this, although a study of seven rheumatoid arthritis sufferers reported that they experienced a decrease in joint pain and an improvement in joint movement with ginger treatment.[4] The same is true for ginger's value in preventing heart disease and stroke; several important studies indicate that it may indirectly help by lowering cholesterol and blood pressure levels and by preventing the formation of hazardous blood clots. But more studies are needed.

Current interest in ginger's antinausea effects is intense, and some investigators are hopeful that it will one day be used regularly in surgery to liberate patients from the unpleasant side effects of other antinausea medications. Several studies have been done on ginger's effect on motion sickness over the past decade or so. In one study of thirty-six college students susceptible to motion sickness, 940 milligrams of ginger powder proved superior to 100 milligrams of the common antinausea drug dimenhydrinate (Dramamine) in keeping nausea at bay while the subjects sat in a computerized rotating chair.[5] Subjects taking ginger tolerated the rotation 57 percent longer than those on dimenhydrinate. Several, but not all, subsequent studies have confirmed such findings.[6] Keep in mind, however, that results from these kinds of trials are often difficult to compare because varying doses and quality levels of ginger were used. In Germany, ginger is endorsed by the authorities as an agent to prevent travel sickness.[7] The antinausea properties have been attributed to substances in ginger called gingerols and shogaols.[8]

Pregnant women suffering from extreme nausea may also benefit from ginger's purported antinausea properties, a 1991 study reports.[9] In this study, a majority of women (70.4 percent) suffering from "morning sickness" preferred ginger treatment to placebo treatment. They took 250 milligrams four times a day or a placebo for four days. Some sources advise that pregnant women not take ginger medicinally, however; see the "Will It Harm You?" section.

Other medicinal properties have been attributed to ginger. The antispasmodic properties that aid digestion may also contribute to its reported value in easing menstrual cramps, for example. Case studies indicate that ginger may help prevent and treat migraine headache, although large-scale trials to verify this have apparently not been done. Chinese studies suggest that ginger helps kill the influenza virus responsible for causing many cases of flu, and the 1 to 3 percent volatile oil in ginger has demonstrated an ability to inhibit the growth of bacteria in test-tube studies.[10] This volatile oil is responsible for ginger's characteristic aroma.

Will It Harm You? What the Studies Say:

The recent medical literature contains no reports of notable adverse reactions to medicinal amounts of ginger, and the spice has certainly been used worldwide for centuries to no apparent ill effect. The FDA includes ginger on its list of foods that are Generally Recognized As Safe (GRAS). Laboratory studies, however, indicate that consuming very large quantities could depress the central nervous system and cause abnormal heart rhythms.[11]

The safety of using ginger to prevent nausea is somewhat unclear; while recommended amounts to prevent motion sickness appear to be harmless, some sources express concern that ginger could cause adverse reactions when used for postoperative nausea or for nausea and vomiting associated with pregnancy. Ginger appears to hinder platelet aggregation—a function crucial to blood clotting—by inhibiting thromboxane synthetase and its action as a prostacylcin agonist. This was observed in a study of seven women who took 5 grams of raw ginger by mouth and then had their blood tested.[12] While this blood alteration is probably dose-related, it has generated considerable concern. Some reassurance can be derived from a randomized, double-blind study of eight healthy male volunteers in which no significant differences in various measures of platelet function were seen when the subjects took 2 grams of dried ginger as compared with a placebo. This does not rule out a hazardous effect with larger doses, however.

Other researchers worry that because ginger is a powerful thromboxane synthetase inhibitor, it may affect testosterone receptor binding in the fetus, possibly influencing sex steroid differentiation of the fetal brain. For these reasons, several sources advise pregnant women to avoid taking ginger in medicinal doses until more research can be done to confirm that this is safe. German health authorities, for example, warn that medicinal amounts of ginger should not be taken for morning sickness.[13] No studies in humans or the laboratory suggest that pregnant women who use small amounts of ginger as a spice could harm their unborn child, however.

According to test-tube and small-animal studies, ginger has properties that may interfere with diabetic, blood-thinning, or heart medicines, so talk to your doctor before starting to take medicinal amounts of ginger.[14] Also, do not use ginger to treat gallstone pain, German health authorities advise, before checking with your doctor.[15] There is confusion over the apparent mutation-promoting and mutation-inhibiting properties of ginger, as seen in some laboratory studies; this requires further exploration.[16]

GENERAL SOURCES:

American Pharmaceutical Association. *Handbook of Nonprescription Drugs.* 11th ed. Washington, D.C.: American Pharmaceutical Association, 1996.

Blumenthal, M., J. Gruenwald, T. Hall, and R.S. Rister, eds. *The Complete German Commission E Monographs: Therapeutic Guide to Herbal Medicine.* Boston: Integrative Medicine Communications, 1998.

Bradley, P.C., ed. *British Herbal Compendium: A Handbook of Scientific Information on Widely Used Plant Drugs*, vol. 1. Bournemouth (Dorset), England: British Herbal Medicine Association, 1992.

Castleman, M. *The Healing Herbs: The Ultimate Guide to the Curative Power of Nature's Medicines.* New York: Bantam Books, 1995.

Lawrence Review of Natural Products. St. Louis: Facts and Comparisons, November 1991.

Leung, A.Y., and S. Foster. *Encyclopedia of Common Natural Ingredients Used in Food, Drugs, and Cosmetics.* 2nd ed. New York: John Wiley & Sons, 1996.

Newall, C.A., et al. *Herbal Medicines: A Guide for Health-Care Professionals.* London: The Pharmaceutical Press, 1996.

Tyler, V.E. *Herbs of Choice: The Therapeutic Use of Phytomedicinals.* Binghamton NY: Haworth Press/Pharmaceutical Products Press, 1994.

———. *The Honest Herbal.* Binghamton, NY: Haworth Press/Pharmaceutical Products Press, 1993.

TEXT CITATIONS:

1. V.E. Tyler, *Herbs of Choice: The Therapeutic Use of Phytomedicinals* (Binghamton, NY: Haworth Press/Pharmaceutical Products Press, 1994).

2. C.A. Newall et al., *Herbal Medicines: A Guide for Health-Care Professionals* (London: The Pharmaceutical Press, 1996).

3. M. Blumenthal, J. Gruenwald, T. Hall, and R.S. Rister, eds., *The Complete German Commission E Monographs: Therapeutic Guide to Herbal Medicine* (Boston: Integrative Medicine Communications, 1998).

4. K. Srivastava et al., *Medical Hypotheses,* 29 (1989): 25–28.

5. D.B. Mowrey and D.E. Clayson, *The Lancet,* I (1982): 655–57.

6. Newall, op. cit. A. Grontved et al., *Acta Otolaryngologica,* 105 (1988): 45–49.

7. Blumenthal et al., op. cit.

8. T. Kawai et al., *Planta Medica,* 60 (1994): 17.

9. W. Fischer-Rasmussen et al., *European Journal of Obstetrics, Gynecology and Reproductive Biology,* 38(1) (1991): 19.

10. S. Inouye et al., *Microbial Biochemistry,* 100 (1984): 232.

11. *Lawrence Review of Natural Products* (St. Louis: Facts and Comparisons, November 1991).

12. K.C. Srivastava, *Prostaglandins, Leukotrienes and Essential Fatty Acids,* 35 (1989): 183–85.

13. Blumenthal et al., op. cit.

14. Newall, op. cit.

15. Blumenthal et al., op. cit.

16. Fischer-Rasmussen, op. cit.

PRIMARY NAME:

GINGKO

SCIENTIFIC NAME:

Gingko biloba L. Family: Gingkoaceae

COMMON NAMES:

Bai guo, gingko biloba, kew tree, maidenhair tree

RATING:

1 = Years of use and extensive, high-quality studies indicate that the widely known extract of this herb, GBE, is very effective and safe when used in recommended amounts for the indication(s) noted in the "Will It Work for You?" section.

What Is Gingko?

During the Ice Age, all members of the *Gingkoaceae* family were wiped out except for one: *Gingko biloba*. It has survived more than 200 million years in China and has since become popular as a stately ornamental tree in parks, gardens, and city streets around the world. The tree is remarkably resistant to insects and disease. Both the male and the female versions have leathery, fan-shaped leaves that turn golden in autumn; the female type bears an inedible, foul-smelling, apricot-size fruit or "seed." The leaves and sometimes the seeds are used medicinally. There are several gingko plantations in the United States, which pick, dry, and process the leaves to a concentrated extract standardized to a potency of 24 percent flavone glycosides and 6 percent terpenes. This type of extract, called GBE, is the only form in which the tree is used medicinally. Individual components called gingkolides are also being tested for various diseases.

What It Is Used For:

While traditional Chinese healers have revered gingko's medicinal properties for millennia, it has been only in the last few decades that Western medicine has shown any interest.[1] Today, gingko constitutes one of the most widely prescribed medicines in numerous European countries, including Germany, where it is sold over the counter.[2]

In Europe and the United States, gingko is sold for ailments including heart disease, asthma, vertigo and tinnitus (ringing in the ears), impotence, cerebral

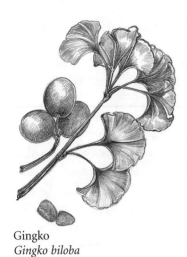

Gingko
Gingko biloba

and vascular insufficiency, eye disorders, neuralgia, peripheral vascular diseases (including intermittent claudication and Raynaud's disease), vascular fragility, improvement of short-term memory, depression-related cognitive problems, brain-trauma injuries, dementia, and a variety of ailments associated with senility. Inhaling a decoction of the leaves is said to help treat asthma.

Extracts of the leaves appear in shampoos, creams, and other cosmetics. Although the practice is not common in the United States (poisoning is a risk unless the seed is processed and administered correctly), traditional Chinese healers use the seeds for asthma, vaginal discharge, bronchitis with asthma, coughs with phlegm, tuberculosis, and other respiratory disorders, and externally for scabies and sores.[3] The seeds are considered a culinary delicacy in Japan and China. Chinese healers also use the root, inner bark, and leaves for certain disorders.

Forms Available Include:

Standardized gingko biloba extract (GBE) in capsule and tablet form, containing either solid or liquid extract. Other forms of the extract, including intravenous ones, are available in other parts of the world. Some cultures use the seeds, leaves, and other parts of the plant in particular ways.

Dosage Commonly Reported:

The leaf extract GBE is taken in doses of 40 milligrams three times a day with meals. The extract should be standardized to 24 percent gingko flavone glycosides and 6 percent terpenes. Alternatively, 10 to 30 drops of the extract standardized to 0.5 percent flavone glycosides are taken three times a day.

Will It Work for You? What the Studies Say:

Most of the research on gingko has involved the use of the standardized extract GBE. This has been necessary because large concentrations of certain gingko substances are needed to demonstrate a meaningful pharmacologic effect. It may also take several weeks or more for the drug to accumulate to levels that produce noticeable results.

While scientists may still have questions about how this herb works, they are increasingly becoming convinced that it does, in fact, work for a variety of conditions. A generous body of pharmacologic and clinical research indicates that it promotes vasodilation—the opening up of blood vessels—and improves the rate of blood flow in capillary vessels and certain small arteries. This reportedly benefits many circulation-related disorders, from varicose veins to short-term memory loss, depression, depression-related cognitive problems, arterial diseases of the lower limbs, postthrombotic syndrome, and inner-ear disorders such as tinnitus and vertigo. Benefits have been particularly notable in studies involving the elderly.

For example, significant relief from the pain associated with a condition called intermittent claudication was noted in a study in which sufferers were given GBE.[4] The disease is caused by hardening of the leg arteries and can cause intense cramping in the calf muscles. Another study found that gingko can help men suffering from impotence (erectile dysfunction) caused by insufficient blood supply to the penis. In a preliminary study, sixty men with this problem took GBE for twelve to eighteen months. By the end, half had regained erections, presumably because of the herb's ability to increase the blood flow through the arteries and veins that are critical to erectile function. This strategy apparently works only with long-term treatment, and more research is needed to confirm study findings.

GBE increases cerebral blood flow in humans, according to a 1973 study that documented a 70 percent increase in men fifty to seventy years old who were injected with the extract.[5] Not as much of an increase was documented in younger men, however: just a 20 percent increase from baseline in those between the ages of thirty and fifty.

Signs and symptoms of chronic cerebral insufficiency in older people are improved by taking a standardized leaf extract of gingko, according a 1985 study.[6] The trial involved 112 individuals with a mean age of 70.5 years who took 120 milligrams of the extract a day. After one year, there was a statistically significant regression of such symptoms as short-term memory loss, headache, vertigo, tinnitus, mood disturbance, and loss of vigilance. Other important parameters, such as heart rate and blood pressure, did not change. A notable shortcoming of the study was that it was not placebo-controlled, meaning that the subjects knew they were being given the gingko extract. According to a critical review of the studies done so far, more double-blind trials in which large numbers of subjects do not know if they are being given GBE or a placebo need to be done before any firm conclusions can be made about aiding cerebral insufficiency.[7] The reviewers identified only eight out of forty published trials on the subject that were free of major methodological flaws. They noted that treatment must last at least six weeks to show any benefit.

Gingko has shown promise in treating senile and presenile dementia, including dementia related to Alzheimer's disease. One study found that elderly men suffering from slight memory loss took less time to process visual information when they were given a gingko supplement.[8] And in a double-blind, crossover study involving eight healthy volunteers (mean age thirty-two), the performance on tests involving memory improved significantly after they took a 600-milligram dose of GBE, as compared with their performance after taking a placebo.[9]

The herb has antiallergic properties, according to test-tube, animal, and human studies. The gingkolides appear to inhibit a key chemical mediator in asthma, allergies, and inflammation—platelet-activating factor—apparently stopping it from latching on to its membrane receptor. In so doing, gingko can often limit the allergic response. This was demonstrated in a study of asthma patients who were given a standardized mixture of mixed gingkolides (40 milligrams three times a day) and a final 120-milligram dose before the challenge test, or a placebo.[10] They were then "challenged" with the substance (the dust or pollen antigen) to which they normally have a response. The findings suggest that gingkolides may help in both the early and the late phases of airway hyperactivity (bronchospasm).[11]

GBE has been shown to improve hearing problems related to poor blood flow to the nerves critical to hearing. This can probably be attributed to increased peripheral blood flow; in one study, hearing test measurements improved about 40 percent in subjects who took an oral extract for two to six months.[12] The extract also was extremely effective in relieving vertigo associated with vestibular dysfunction, a disorder of balance and dizziness involving the inner ear. So far, study results on GBE's effectiveness for treating tinnitus have been mixed.

Research indicates that GBE is an effective free-radical scavenger, meaning that it helps to "mop up" potentially dangerous, cancer-promoting charged particles in body tissues. More research is needed to determine the implications of this finding.

Will It Harm You? What the Studies Say:

Other than minor gastrointestinal problems in nearly 4 percent of individuals, side effects with typically recommended amounts of gingko are relatively uncommon.[13] In rare cases, headache, vertigo, and dizziness develop.[14] Significant adverse reactions were not noted in subjects who took as much as 600 milligrams of leaf extract in single doses.[15]

The pulp and seed are poisonous, and handling the fruit pulp can cause a severe allergic reaction similar to a poison ivy reaction, with possible redness, swelling, itching, and blistering.[16] There may actually be a cross-reactivity between the gingko fruit and poison ivy, oak, and sumac. Children in Asia who ingested as many as fifty gingko seeds have suffered from seizures and loss of consciousness.[17]

Because gingko reduces the rate at which blood clots, people who are taking anticoagulants or who suffer from clotting disorders should proceed with particular care.[18]

GENERAL SOURCES:

American Pharmaceutical Association. *Handbook of Nonprescription Drugs.* 11th ed. Washington, D.C.: American Pharmaceutical Association, 1996.

Castleman, M. *The Healing Herbs: The Ultimate Guide to the Curative Power of Nature's Medicines.* New York: Bantam Books, 1995.

Dobelis, I.N., ed. *The Magic and Medicine of Plants: A Practical Guide to the Science, History, Folklore, and Everyday Uses of Medicinal Plants.* Pleasantville, NY: Reader's Digest Association, 1986.

Lawrence Review of Natural Products. St. Louis: Facts and Comparisons, February 1994.

Leung, A.Y., and S. Foster. *Encyclopedia of Common Natural Ingredients Used in Food, Drugs, and Cosmetics.* 2nd ed. New York: John Wiley & Sons, 1996.

Murray, M.T. *The Healing Power of Herbs: The Enlightened Person's Guide to the Wonders of Medicinal Plants.* Revised and expanded 2nd ed. Rocklin, CA: Prima Publishing, 1995.

Newall, C.A., et al. *Herbal Medicines: A Guide for Health-Care Professionals.* London: The Pharmaceutical Press, 1996.

Tyler, V.E. *Herbs of Choice: The Therapeutic Use of Phytomedicinals.* Binghamton, NY: Haworth Press/Pharmaceutical Products Press, 1994.

———. *The Honest Herbal.* Binghamton, NY: Haworth Press/Pharmaceuticals Products Press, 1993.

TEXT CITATIONS:

1. V.E. Tyler, *The Honest Herbal* (Binghamton, NY: Haworth Press/Pharmaceuticals Press, 1993).

2. Ibid.

3. A.Y. Leung and S. Foster, *Encyclopedia of Common Natural Ingredients Used in Food, Drugs, and Cosmetics*, 2nd ed. (New York: John Wiley & Sons, 1996).

4. V.E. Tyler, *Herbs of Choice: The Therapeutic Use of Phytomedicinals* (Binghamton, NY: Haworth Press/Pharmaceutical Products Press, 1994).

5. G.R. Pistolese, *Minerva Medica*, 79 (1973): 4166.

6. G. Vorberg, *Clinical Trials Journal*, 22 (1985): 149–57.

7. J. Kleijnen and P. Knipschild, *British Journal of Clinical Pharmacology*, 34 (1992): 352–58.

8. H. Allain et al., *Clinical Therapeutics*, 15 (1993): 549–58.

9. S.Z. Hindmarsh, *International Journal of Clinical and Pharmacologic Research*, 4 (1984): 89–93.

10. P. Braquet, *Drugs of the Future*, 12 (1987): 643–99.

11. C.A. Newall et al., *Herbal Medicines: A Guide for Health-Care Professionals* (London: The Pharmaceutical Press, 1996).

12. *Lawrence Review of Natural Products* (St. Louis: Facts and Comparisons, February 1994).

13. American Pharmaceutical Association, *Handbook of Nonprescription Drugs*, 11th ed. (Washington, D.C.: American Pharmaceutical Association, 1996).

14. American Pharmaceutical Association, op. cit.

15. Newall, op. cit.

16. *Lawrence Review of Natural Products*, op. cit.

17. M. Yagi et al., *Yakugaku Zasshi*, 113 (1993): 596.

18. Tyler, *The Honest Herbal*, op. cit.

PRIMARY NAME:

GINSENG, AMERICAN

SCIENTIFIC NAME:

Panax quinquefolius L. Family: Araliaceae

COMMON NAME:

Western ginseng

RATING:

3 = Studies on the effectiveness and safety of this substance are conflicting, or there are not enough studies to draw a conclusion.

What Is American Ginseng?

The root of this unassuming, low-growing perennial is used medicinally. The plant is notoriously difficult to grow and the roots mature slowly, becoming ready for harvesting only every few years. It prospers in the shade and bears bright red berries. The plant was once abundant in parts of eastern North America, particularly in southern Appalachia, but is now considered a rare or endangered species in many regions because of overharvesting. Its harvest and trade are officially restricted. The United States has long been a major exporter of ginseng to Asia.

See also **Ginseng, Siberian** (*Eleutherococcus senticosus*) and **Ginseng, Asian** (*Panax ginseng* L.).

What It Is Used For:

Native American tribes reportedly used this plant in various ways, from treating nosebleeds to treating female infertility, but only scattered information about these uses has survived.[1] For the most part, Americans remained indifferent to (or skeptical of) the plant's healing properties, exporting the bulk of the cultivated crop to Asia, where it is highly valued in traditional Chinese medicine for its "cold" properties. (Asian ginseng, on the other hand, is considered to have "hot" properties.[2]) In Chinese medicine, the concepts of "hot" and "cold" are properties considered to be inherent in both medicines and the diseases they are used to treat. In very gen-

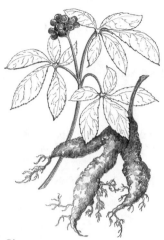

Ginseng
Asian: Panax ginseng
American: Panax quinquefolius

eral terms, Chinese medicine considers "cold" properties valuable for lowering fever, calming respiratory or digestive tract disorders, and quenching the thirst.

In recent years, Westerners have started to regard the herb as a possible "adaptogen" good for increasing the body's resistance to the potentially damaging impact of physical, biological, or chemical stress.[3] The *U.S. Pharmacopoeia* listed American ginseng root for forty years, until 1883, primarily as a stimulant and digestive aid.[4]

Forms Available Include:

Capsule, chewing gum, extract, liquid, root (fresh and dried), soft drink, solution, tablet, tea. Appears in numerous herbal tea blends and cosmetics. American ginseng is sweeter-tasting than Asian ginseng, although many people still dislike the taste.

Dosage Commonly Reported:

The herb is commonly taken in doses of 2 to 9 grams a day. As a stimulant, a typical dosage of capsules standardized for 5 to 9 percent ginsenosides is 500 to 1,000 milligrams. As a tonic, 250 to 500 milligrams is a common recommendation.

Will It Work for You? What the Studies Say:

While thousands of studies have been published on Asian ginseng, scientists have started to examine American ginseng closely only in the past few decades.[5] It is challenging to draw firm conclusions regarding American ginseng's value as a healing agent, given the different standards researchers have used to interpret results, not to mention the often unspecified use of different species, plant parts, purification standards, and dosages.[6]

Researchers have established that American ginseng contains apparently critical saponins called ginsenosides, although not all the ones that Asian ginseng contains. Weak central nervous system activity and adaptogenic properties have been ascribed to the ginsenosides contained in American ginseng.[7] See **Ginseng, Asian**, for a fuller discussion of research findings on ginsenosides. A long-term, controlled human trial may one day elucidate many of the lingering questions regarding American ginseng and whether it offers any healing properties, not to mention whether or not it is safe.[8]

Will It Harm You? What the Studies Say:

The use of American ginseng has not generally been associated with serious adverse reactions. See **Ginseng, Asian**, for more information.

GENERAL SOURCES:

Foster, S. *American Ginseng. Panax quinquefolius.* American Botanical Council's Botanical Series No. 308. 1991.

Lawrence Review of Natural Products. St. Louis: Facts and Comparisons, September 1990.

Leung, A.Y., and S. Foster. *Encyclopedia of Common Natural Ingredients Used in Food, Drugs, and Cosmetics.* 2nd ed. New York: John Wiley & Sons, 1996.

Tyler, V.E. *The Honest Herbal.* Binghamton, NY: Haworth Press/Pharmaceuticals Products Press 1993.

TEXT CITATIONS:

1. S. Foster, *American Ginseng: Panax quinquefolius* (American Botanical Council's Botanical Series No. 308, 1991).
2. A.Y. Leung and S. Foster, *Encyclopedia of Common Natural Ingredients Used in Food, Drugs, and Cosmetics*, 2nd ed. (New York: John Wiley & Sons, 1996).
3. I.I. Brekhman and I.V. Dardymov, *Lloydia*, 32 (1969): 46.
4. Leung and Foster, op. cit.
5. Foster, op. cit.
6. W.H. Lewis, "Ginseng: A Medical Enigma," in N.O. Etkin, ed., *Plants in Indigenous Medicine & Diet: Biobehavioral Approaches* (Bedford Hills, NY: Redgrave Publ. Co., 1986).
7. J.A. Duke, *CRC Handbook of Medicinal Herbs* (Boca Raton, FL: CRC Press, 1985).
8. E.J. Staba, *The Lancet*, 1985: 2 (8467): 1309–10.

PRIMARY NAME:

GINSENG, ASIAN

SCIENTIFIC NAME:

Panax ginseng C.A. Mey., sometimes referred to as *Panax schinseng* Nees. Family: Araliaceae

COMMON NAMES:

Chinese ginseng, Japanese ginseng, Korean ginseng, ren shen (man root)

RATING:

2 = According to a number of well-designed studies and common use, this substance appears to be relatively effective and safe when used in recommended amounts for the indication(s) noted in the "Will It Work for You?" section.

What Is Asian Ginseng?

This low-growing perennial is widely known as difficult to cultivate. The roots mature slowly, becoming ready for harvesting only every sixth autumn or more. The plant favors shade. The roots are typically dried and often cured before medicinal use.

See also **Ginseng, Siberian** (*Eleutherococcus senticosus*) and **Ginseng, American** (*Panax quinquefolius* L.).

What It Is Used For:

"Panax" stems from the Greek word for "all-healing," and in parts of Asia, ginseng has embodied this hope for millennia. Long ago, enthusiasts in China, Japan, Korea, Russia, and other parts of the world noted the curiously human-like shape of the root and started to take it as a "bodywide" tonic and revitalizer to maintain health more than to treat any particular disease. They regard ginseng much the way Americans do vitamin pills.[1]

In traditional Chinese medicine, ginseng root is regarded as tonic, sedating, heart-strengthening, and secretion-promoting. The concepts of "hot" and "cold" are properties believed to be inherent in both medicines and the diseases that these medicines are used to treat. American ginseng is believed to have "cool" properties, while in contrast, Asian ginseng is said to possess "hot" properties good for raising "heat" in the blood or circulatory system. The many conditions Asian ginseng has been taken for, either alone or in combination with other herbs, include bleeding disorders, colitis, headache, fatigue, dizziness, impotence, rheumatism, amnesia, and appetite loss. Symptoms of senility, aging, and cancer have long been treated with ginseng. Interestingly, the leaf of Asian ginseng, which is not used, is said to have properties similar to those of American ginseng root.

In recent times, Western sources have focused primarily on the adaptogenic properties of this treasured Asian root. Adaptogens are believed to strengthen the body, boosting its overall resistance to the potentially damaging impact of physical, biological, or chemical stresses.[2] Ginseng is billed as a key to vitality and longevity, the herb to take in cases of physical or mental exhaustion or lowered resistance to infection. Mild aphrodisiac qualities have been attributed to it.

Forms Available Include:

Capsule, chewing gum, extract, decoction, powder, liquid, root (fresh and dried), soft drink, tablet, tea. There are many types and grades of ginseng. They vary widely in quality, depending on the age of the plant, the source, the part of root used, and the curing method it was subjected to. The highest-quality roots are very expensive, and adulteration with other substances is common. A 1995 survey found that several of fifty some Asian ginseng products on the American market contained no ginseng at all, and another reported "huge variations" in ginseng concentration of the ten different brands tested. To increase the chances of high quality, one source recommends buying ginseng only in root form from a Chinese herb shop.[3]

Dosage Commonly Reported:

A common dosage is 1 to 2 grams per day, although in Chinese medicine the standard is 1 to 9 grams a day. A decoction is made using ½ teaspoon dried, pulverized root per cup of water and is drunk once or twice per day. As a stimulant, a common dose of capsules standardized for 5 to 9 percent ginsenosides is 500 to 1,000 milligrams; as a tonic, 250 to 500 milligrams is common

Will It Work for You? What the Studies Say:

Despite the thousands of studies published on Asian and American ginseng, scientists (and the general public) remain in the dark on how the root works, or even if it works. Separating science from superstition proves formidable indeed. There are several reasons for this. For many years, published studies failed to specify which species of ginseng had been used (Asian, American, Siberian, or other), which root part was administered, how quality and purity were established, and what dosage was given.[4] Standards for interpreting the import of study results also vary dramatically.

A few points have been clarified, however. Asian ginseng contains steroidlike components—saponin glycosides—designated ginsenosides (referred to as panaxosides by Russian scientists),[5] as well as numerous polysaccharides and other components that may well contribute to the root's pharmacologic actions. Interestingly, some of the saponins induce effects that directly oppose those of others.[6]

There are two types of actions cited with relative frequency in regard to ginseng: its adaptogenic properties and its ability to improve physical or mental performance.[7] In a number of stress tests, ginseng extracts increased the resistance of rodents to infection (including elevating natural killer cell activity),[8] boosted their energy metabolism,[9] enabled them to swim longer, protected them against stress-induced ulcers, and improved their learning, memory, and physical powers.[10] Not all animal studies have demonstrated these adaptogenic properties, however.[11] Perhaps most important, the only solid evidence that these adaptogenic properties occur in humans is anecdotal; well-designed human trials have yet to be carried out. Apparently many of the root's adaptogenic and other properties develop only after the root has been taken for some time.[12]

Results of human studies, although these studies are sparse and often small and poorly designed, have been promising nonetheless. Some indicate that ginseng can reduce blood glucose levels, for example; researchers have identified the constituents probably responsible for this.[13] German health authorities approve of ginseng for invigorating and fortifying the body in times of fatigue or debility, convalescence, or poor capacity for work or concentration.[14]

Will It Harm You? What the Studies Say:

Millennia of use certainly testify to the relative safety of Asian ginseng, and serious adverse reactions are not generally reported. It has, however, caused nervousness, agitation, insomnia, diarrhea, and skin eruptions in some people.[15]

Neither a toxic dose nor a reliably effective dose has been described. Although long-term use appears to be safe,[16] it is probably best to avoid taking ginseng continuously for long stretches of time (several months or more), given its documented side effects and pharmacologic activity.[17] Several sources warn against taking ginseng if you have an acute illness, have high blood pressure, or are diabetic (blood-sugar-lowering properties have been reported, which could be dangerous for those taking medicines to lower blood sugar).[18]

A 1979 study describing a "ginseng abuse syndrome," characterized by an agreeable sensation of stimulation but disturbing nervousness, sleeplessness, high blood pressure, and other problems,[19] has largely been discredited because of poor design and quality; the subjects continued to consume caffeine-containing substances, for example. For this reason, however, it would be wise to avoid ginseng if you regularly take another stimulant (including large amounts of caffeine-containing drinks such as coffee).

GENERAL SOURCES:

Blumenthal, M., J. Gruenwald, T. Hall, and R.S. Rister, eds. *The Complete German Commission E Monographs: Therapeutic Guide to Herbal Medicine.* Boston: Integrative Medicine Communications, 1998.

Bradley, P.C., ed. *British Herbal Compendium: A Handbook of Scientific Information on Widely Used Plant Drugs*, vol. 1. Bournemouth (Dorset), England: British Herbal Medicine Association, 1992.

Castleman, M. *The Healing Herbs: The Ultimate Guide to the Curative Power of Nature's Medicines.* New York: Bantam Books, 1995.

Lawrence Review of Natural Products. St. Louis: Facts and Comparisons, September 1990.

Leung, A.Y. *Chinese Healing Foods and Herbs.* Glen Rock, NJ: AYSL Corp, 1984.

Leung, A.Y., and S. Foster. *Encyclopedia of Common Natural Ingredients Used in Food, Drugs, and Cosmetics.* 2nd ed. New York: John Wiley & Sons, 1996.

Newall, C.A., et al. *Herbal Medicines: A Guide for Health-Care Professionals.* London: The Pharmaceutical Press, 1996.

Tyler, V.E. *Herbs of Choice: The Therapeutic Use of Phytomedicinals.* Binghamton, NY: Haworth Press/Pharmaceutical Products Press, 1994.

———. *The Honest Herbal.* Binghamton, NY: Haworth Press/Pharmaceutical Products Press 1993.

TEXT CITATIONS:

1. V.E. Tyler, *The Honest Herbal* (Binghamton, NY: Haworth Press/Pharmaceutical Products Press 1993).
2. I.I. Brekhman and I.V. Dardymov, *Lloydia*, 32 (1969): 46.
3. A.Y. Leung, *Chinese Healing Foods and Herbs* (Glen Rock, NJ: AYSL Corp, 1984).
4. W.H. Lewis, "Ginseng: A Medical Enigma," in N.O. Etkin, ed., *Plants in Indigenous Medicine & Diet: Biobehavioral Approaches* (Bedford Hills, NY: Redgrave Publ. Co., 1986).
5. Brekhman and Dardymov, op. cit.
6. A.Y. Leung and S. Foster, *Encyclopedia of Common Natural Ingredients Used in Food, Drugs, and Cosmetics*, 2nd ed. (New York: John Wiley & Sons, 1996).
7. P.C. Bradley, ed., *British Herbal Compendium: A Handbook of Scientific Information on Widely Used Plant Drugs*, vol. 1 (Bournemouth [Dorset], England: British Herbal Medicine Association, 1992).
8. V.K. Singh, *Planta Medica*, 50 (1984): 462–65.
9. E.V. Avakian et al., *Planta Medica*, 50 (1984): 151–54.
10. V.D. Petkov and A.H. Mosharrof, *American Journal of Chinese Medicine*, 15 (1987): 19–29.
11. W.H. Lewis et al., *Journal of Ethnopharmacology*, 8 (1983): 209.
12. A. Der Marderosian and L. Liberti, *Natural Product Medicine: A Scientific Guide to Foods, Drugs, Cosmetics* (Philadelphia: George F. Stickley, 1988).
13. *Lawrence Review of Natural Products* (St. Louis: Facts and Comparisons, September 1990). C. Kono et al., *Plant Medica*, 50 (1984): 434.
14. M. Blumenthal, J. Gruenwald, T. Hall, and R.S. Rister, eds., *The Complete German Commission E Monographs: Therapeutic Guide to Herbal Medicine* (Boston: Integrative Medicine Communications, 1998).
15. C.A. Baldwin et al., *Pharmaceutical Journal*, 237 (1986): 583–86. T.G. Hammond and J.A. Whitworth, *Medical Journal of Australia*, 1 (1981): 492.
16. R.F. Chandler, *Canadian Pharmaceutical Journal*, 121 (1988): 36–38.
17. C.A. Baldwin et al., *Pharmacy Journal*, 237 (1986): 583–86.
18. Bradley, op. cit. *Lawrence Review of Natural Products*, op. cit.
19. R.K. Siegel, *Journal of the American Medical Association*, 241 (1979): 1614–15.

PRIMARY NAME:

GINSENG, SIBERIAN

SCIENTIFIC NAME:

Eleutherococcus senticosus (Rupr. and Maxim.) Maxim., sometimes referred to as *Acanthopanax senticosus* Harms or *Hedera senticosa*. Family: Ariaceae

What Is Siberian Ginseng?

This deciduous shrub grows abundantly in certain Russian, Chinese, Korean, and Japanese forests. A gray or grayish-brown bark covers its spiny shoots. It has palmate leaves, black oval fruit ("berries"), and violet or yellowish flowers, depending on its sex. Chinese healers traditionally made preparations from the roots, although various cultures today use the leaves, rhizomes (underground stems), and stems as well.

Siberian ginseng belongs to the same plant family (Ariaceae) as other ginsengs but does not belong to the genus *Panax*. See also **Ginseng, Asian** for information on *Panax ginseng* and **Ginseng, American** for information on *Panax quinquefolius*.

What It Is Used For:

Siberian ginseng has held an esteemed position in traditional Chinese medicine for two thousand years, although healers there long regarded its sibling, Asian ginseng, far superior. Siberian ginseng made its global debut in the 1950s, when

GINSENG. SIBERIAN
(Continued)

COMMON NAMES:

Devil's shrub, eleuthera, eleuthero, eleutherococ, shigoka, touch-me-not, Ussarian thorny pepperbush, wild pepper

RATING:

2 = According to a number of well-designed studies and common use, this substance appears to be relatively effective and safe when used in recommended amounts for the indication(s) noted in the "Will It Work for You?" section.

Soviet scientists conducting screening tests on ginseng relatives in the easternmost part of the country discovered the remarkable qualities of this unique herb. In the decades since, Siberian ginseng and its extracts have served as valuable, cheaper alternatives to ginseng, with millions of Russians in particular taking the herb as a stimulant and general tonic. In the 1970s, many herbalists started referring to it as an "adaptogen" capable of reinforcing the body's ability to handle environmental stress and resist disease.[1] Traditional Chinese healers had in fact been using it in similar ways, in addition to turning to it to benefit *qi* (vital energy), normalize body function, stimulate the appetite, promote longevity, and treat fluid retention (in the form of a diuretic, or "water pill"), rheumatoid arthritis, insomnia, and lower back pain.[2]

In addition to its well-known adaptogenic properties, contemporary Western herbalists tout the ability of Siberian ginseng and its extracts to improve overall health and help prevent disease, stimulate the immune system, increase longevity, boost work capacity, fight off fatigue, improve chronic inflammatory conditions, normalize blood pressure, resist depression, shield the body from toxins, shrink tumors, manage atherosclerosis, correct impaired kidney function, and control diabetes. The people of the former Soviet Union, from soldiers and professional athletes to factory workers, reportedly use it extensively.[3]

Forms Available Include:

Capsule, concentrated drops, fluid and other extracts, infusion, powder for mixing with hot water, tablet, tincture. Appears in herbal blends.

Dosage Commonly Reported:

The herb is taken in doses of 250 to 500 milligrams, once or twice per day, or 1 to 2 droppersful of tincture two or three times per day. Two to three 404-milligram root capsules are taken three times a day.

Will It Work for You? What the Studies Say:

Siberian ginseng is related to Asian ginseng (*Panax ginseng*) and shares some of the same chemical compounds, but its mechanism of action is still poorly understood; its contained eleutherosides (A-G) are not unique, for example.[4] Presumably on the basis of clinical trials, however, German health authorities endorse Siberian ginseng as a tonic for invigorating and fortifying the body in times of fatigue, debility, convalescence, or declining capacity for work and concentration.[5]

Intensive research on animals and humans by Russian and former Soviet scientists over the past few decades indicates that Siberian ginseng rightfully qualifies as an "adaptogen." Although still a new word in medical nomenclature and not accepted by all, an adaptogen is defined by most as a substance that is innocuous and has a nonspecific and normalizing action on the body.[6]

Various clinical trials, most of them carried out in the former Soviet Union since the early 1960s and involving more than 2,100 subjects, tested Siberian ginseng's effect on stress in human subjects.[7] Most showed that the herb could improve performance in tests of physical exertion and mental capacity.

Increased work capacity[8] was also observed. A 1985 review of the Soviet studies describes the beneficial effects of Siberian ginseng extracts when given to healthy subjects being tested for their ability to contend with such stressors as exercise, noise, heat, and increased workload. They also note increased mental alertness, athletic performance, and work quality under stressful conditions.[9]

The review also describes studies carried out on more than 2,100 individuals with illnesses such as high blood pressure, rheumatic heart disease, atherosclerosis, and diabetes. Although Siberian ginseng cannot be considered a remedy or cure for these ailments, findings on this herb did indicate notable improvements in test subjects' illnesses and even "normalization" (regardless of the direction of change) in a number of them.[10]

Healthy volunteers (thirty-six in all) injected three times a day with an alcoholic Siberian ginseng extract in one double-blind study experienced dramatic increases in the number of important immune system cells such as T cells and especially helper cells.[11] The implications of this for helping to prevent or fight diseases in which the immune system is crippled, such as chronic fatigue syndrome or HIV infection, remain to be explored. Test-tube studies indicate that extracts of the herb inhibit proliferation of leukemia cells,[12] but what this means for treating leukemia in humans is still unclear. Positive findings have been reported in the immune systems of cancer patients given this herb.[13] Intriguing results have also been described in treating heart conditions (coronary heart disease,[14] heart structure in heart attack,[15] malignant arrhythmias[16]) and diabetes with Siberian ginseng, as well as in helping individuals to recover from radiation damage.[17] Continued research will, it is hoped, elucidate the importance of these findings.

Will It Harm You? What the Studies Say:

Very few adverse reactions to this herb or its extracts were reported by the thousands of people involved in the Soviet studies. In many of these trials the subjects took a 33 percent ethanol root extract in doses ranging from 2 to 16 milliliters, one to three times a day for up to sixty days in a row.[18] Even long-term use appears to be safe, although a number of sources, including British health authorities, recommend limiting intake to occasional one-month rounds followed by at least two-month breaks.[19]

In rare cases people report drowsiness and mild fatigue right after they take the extract, probably due to a slight drop in blood sugar levels.[20] German health authorities cite no known side effects or interactions with other drugs, although they recommend that people with high blood pressure avoid the herb.[21] A number of other sources recommend that people who have a febrile condition, are suffering from a heart attack, or are in a state of advanced dehydration or electrolyte imbalance not take the herb.[22] Given the chemical similarity of Siberian ginseng to *Panax ginseng* root, people who are sensitive to one may want to avoid the other.[23]

GENERAL SOURCES:

Blumenthal, M., J. Gruenwald, T. Hall, and R.S. Rister, eds. *The Complete German Commission E Monographs: Therapeutic Guide to Herbal Medicine.* Boston: Integrative Medicine Communications, 1998.

Bradley, P.C., ed. *British Herbal Compendium: A Handbook of Scientific Information on Widely Used Plant Drugs*, vol. 1. Bournemouth (Dorset), England: British Herbal Medicine Association, 1992.

Foster, S. *Siberian Ginseng: Eleutherococcus senticosus*. American Botanical Council, Botanical Series No. 302, 1991.

Lawrence Review of Natural Products. St. Louis: Facts and Comparisons, June 1988.

Leung, A.Y., and S. Foster. *Encyclopedia of Common Natural Ingredients Used in Food, Drugs, and Cosmetics*. 2nd ed. New York: John Wiley & Sons, 1996.

Mayell, M. *Off-the-Shelf Natural Health: How to Use Herbs and Nutrients to Stay Well*. New York: Bantam Books, 1995.

Murray, M.T. *The Healing Power of Herbs: The Enlightened Person's Guide to the Wonders of Medicinal Plants*. Revised and expanded 2nd ed. Rocklin, CA: Prima Publishing, 1995.

Tierra, M. *The Way of Herbs*. New York: Pocket Books, 1990.

Weiner, M.A., and J.A. Weiner. *Herbs That Heal: Prescription for Herbal Healing*. Mill Valley, CA: Quantum Books, 1994.

Weiss, R.F. *Herbal Medicine*, trans. A.R. Meuss, from the 6th German edition. Beaconsfield, England: Beaconsfield Publishers, Ltd., 1988.

TEXT CITATIONS:

1. S. Foster, *Siberian Ginseng: Eleutherococcus senticosus* (American Botanical Council, Botanical Series No. 302, 1991).

2. A.Y. Leung and S. Foster, *Encyclopedia of Common Natural Ingredients Used in Food, Drugs, and Cosmetics*, 2nd ed. (New York: John Wiley & Sons, 1996). Foster, op. cit.

3. Foster, op. cit.

4. P.C. Bradley, ed., *British Herbal Compendium: A Handbook of Scientific Information on Widely Used Plant Drugs*, vol. 1 (Bournemouth [Dorset], England: British Herbal Medicine Association, 1992). R.J. Collisson, *British Journal of Phytotherapy*, 2 (1991): 61–71.

5. M. Blumenthal, J. Gruenwald, T. Hall, and R.S. Rister, eds., *The Complete German Commission E Monographs: Therapeutic Guide to Herbal Medicine* (Boston: Integrative Medicine Communications, 1998).

6. N.R. Farnsworth et al., "Siberian Ginseng (*Eleutherococcus senticosus*): Current Status as an Adaptogen," in H. Wagner et al., eds., *Economic and Medicinal Plant Research*, vol. 1 (London: Academic Press, 1985).

7. Foster, op. cit.

8. K. Asano et al., *Planta Medica*, 52 (1986): 175–76.

9. Farnsworth, op. cit. Foster, op. cit.

10. Farnsworth, op. cit. Foster, op. cit.

11. B. Bohn et al., *Arzneimittel-Forschung*, 37 (1987): 1193–96.

12. B. Hacker and P.J. Medon, *Journal of Pharmaceutical Science*, 73 (1984): 270–72.

13. *Review of Natural Products* (St. Louis: Facts and Comparisons, June 1988).

14. Y.S. Shang et al., *Chung Hsi I Chih Ho Tsa Chih*, 11(5) (1991): 280.

15. T.N. Afanas'eva and N.P. Lebkova, *Biulleten Eksperimentalnoi Biologii i Meditsiny*, 103(2) (1987): 212.

16. B.J. Tian et al., *Chung Kuo Chung Yao Tsa Chih*, 14(8) (1989): 493.

17. M. Minkova and T. Pantev, *Acta Physiologica et Pharmacologica Bulgarica*, 14(1) (1988): 78.

18. Foster, op. cit.

19. Bradley, op. cit.

20. *Lawrence Review of Natural Products*, op. cit.

21. Blumenthal et al., op. cit.

22. *Lawrence Review of Natural Products*, op. cit.

23. Ibid.

PRIMARY NAME:
GLUCOMANNAN

SCIENTIFIC NAMES:
N/A

COMMON NAME:
Konjac mannan

RATING:
2 = According to a number of well-designed studies and common use, this substance appears to be relatively effective and safe when used in recommended amounts for the indication(s) noted in the "Will It Work for You?" section.

What Is Glucomannan?

Glucomannan is a polysaccharide extracted from the tubers of Konjac (*Amorphophallus konjac,* family Araceae), which is cultivated as a foodstuff in Japan and Indonesia. Enzymes in the human digestive system cannot break down this polysaccharide, which means that it passes through the body largely intact; thus, it is considered a dietary fiber.

What It Is Used For:

Glucomannan swells to many times its size when it comes into contact with water, absorbing as much as sixty times its weight in water. Because of this ability to swell, glucomannan has become popular as a treatment for constipation. Some sources also recommend it as a weight-loss agent, cholesterol-reducer, and agent for normalizing blood sugar in diabetes patients.

Forms Available Include:

Capsule. Glucomannan also appears in some grapefruit diet tablets.[1]

Dosage Commonly Reported:

As a diet aid, two 500-milligram capsules are taken one hour before meals. Follow package instruction for use of commercial preparations for constipation.

Will It Work for You? What the Studies Say:

Scientific evidence for the value of glucomannan as a diet aid is relatively weak. Advocates contend that by swelling in the stomach, glucomannan will promote a sensation of fullness and reduce the desire to eat. But according to clinical trials, dieters do not always respond this way, and actual weight loss is often minimal. In fact, attempts to promote weight loss by producing sensations of satiety with most bulk-producing substances usually fail, perhaps in part because the substances do not linger in the stomach for long; in one experiment, diet tablets such as this had largely passed through the stomach and into the small bowel within thirty minutes.[2]

In a study involving twenty obese individuals who knew a diet aid was being tested, those who took two 500-milligram capsules of purified glucomannan sixty minutes before meals lost an average of 5.5 pounds at the end of eight weeks, compared with a lower average of 1.5 pounds lost in the group taking a placebo.[3] A 1993 study in obese children failed to show any benefit of glucomannan over a placebo.[4] Other studies, however, have indicated some benefit of glucomannan supplementation in encouraging weight loss along with a low-calorie diet.[5]

Several animal and clinical trials have shown that glucomannan may help reduce cholesterol levels, possibly by inhibiting the movement of cholesterol in the middle section of the small intestine and the absorption of bile acids in the last part of the small intestine.[6] For example, total cholesterol fell by 10 percent among sixty-three healthy men who took a daily dose of 3.9 grams of glucomannan for four weeks in a double-blind, crossover trial published in 1995.[7] Blood cholesterol levels dropped as much as 39 percent in some cases—and as little as 0 percent in others—in a study of ten overweight individuals who took 100 milliliters of a 1 percent solution of glucomannan for eleven weeks.[8]

Glucomannan apparently delays the absorption of glucose from the intestines.[9] Mean fasting glucose levels have been shown to drop, reducing the need for blood-sugar-lowering medicines in diabetics, as well as in healthy adults in several studies.[10] Glucomannan has also proved effective in treating constipation in pregnant women,[11] normalizing stools and other intestinal conditions such as gas in healthy adults,[12] and inhibiting lung cancer development in laboratory mice.[13]

Will It Harm You? What the Studies Say:

Although some individuals who take glucomannan develop diarrhea, side effects experienced by subjects in clinical trials have been minimal overall. Be sure to drink plenty of liquids with glucomannan products, however; at least four cases of severe esophageal obstruction have been reported with glucomannan diet tablets,[14] and Australian health authorities have banned tablets containing glucomannan (but not other glucomannan formulations) because of the risk of obstruction lower down in the esophageal tract as well.[15] If the tablets get stuck in these areas, they can expand and cause serious breathing problems.

Diabetes sufferers should exercise extreme care in taking glucomannan because it has been shown to alter glucose levels in the body. Insulin requirements may be altered as well.

GENERAL SOURCES:

American Pharmaceutical Association. *Handbook of Nonprescription Drugs*. 11th ed. Washington, D.C.: American Pharmaceutical Association, 1996.

Balch, J.F., and P.A. Balch. *Prescription for Nutritional Healing: A Practical A to Z Reference to Drug-Free Remedies Using Vitamins, Minerals, Herbs & Food Supplements*. 2nd ed. Garden City Park, NY: Avery Publishing Group, 1997.

Lawrence Review of Natural Products. St. Louis: Facts and Comparisons, August 1995.

Tyler, V.E., L.R. Brady, and J.E. Robbers, eds. *Pharmacognosy*. Philadelphia: Lea & Febiger, 1988.

TEXT CITATIONS:

1. *Lawrence Review of Natural Products* (St. Louis: Facts and Comparisons, August 1995).
2. E.J. Drenck, *Journal of the American Medical Association*, (1975): 234–71.
3. D.E. Walsh et al., *International Journal of Obesity*, 8 (1984): 289–93.
4. L. Vido et al., *Pediatrie und Padologie*, 28(5) (1993): 133–36.
5. M. Cairella and G. Marchini, *Clinica Terapeutica*, 146(4) (1995): 269–74.
6. S. Kiriyama et al., *Journal of Nutrition*, 104(1) (1974): 69.
7. A. Arvill and L. Bodin, *American Journal of Clinical Nutrition*, 61(3) (1995): 585.
8. *Lawrence Review of Natural Products*, op. cit.
9. D.J. Jenkins et al., *British Medical Journal*, 1(6124) (1978): 1392. *Lawrence Review of Natural Products*, op. cit.
10. *Lawrence Review of Natural Products*, op. cit.
11. P. Signorelli et al., *Minerva Ginecologica*, 48(12) (1996): 577–82.
12. L.J. Marsicano et al., *GEN*, 49(1) (1995): 7–14.
13. D.Y. Luo, *Chinese Journal of Oncology*, 14(1) (1992): 48.
14. P. Gaudry, *Medical Journal of Australia*, 14(3) (1985): 204.
15. *Lawrence Review of Natural Products*, op. cit.

PRIMARY NAME:

GLUCOSAMINE

SCIENTIFIC NAMES:
2-Amino-2-deoxyglucose

COMMON NAMES:
Chitosamine, glucosamine sulfate

RATING:
2 = According to a number of well-designed studies and common use, this substance appears to be relatively effective and safe when used in recommended amounts for the indication(s) noted in the "Will It Work for You?" section.

What Is Glucosamine?

Glucosamine is an amino sugar important to the structure of body tissue. It is found in cell membranes, mucopolysaccharides, and chitin, the horny substance in the exoskeleton of crabs, beetles, and various marine invertebrates and microorganisms. The glucosamine sold in dietary supplement outlets is either prepared synthetically or extracted from chitin. Glucosamine sulfate, the most common form, is often sold as N-acetyl-glucosamine, but this form offers no particular advantages over glucosamine.[1]

What It Is Used For:

Glucosamine is sold as a dietary supplement to decrease pain and improve mobility in people suffering from osteoarthritis, a progressive disease of cartilage degeneration. It is also billed as a substance to support healthy joint and connective tissue. Some sources have suggested that it may even help to prevent or postpone the development of osteoarthritis in certain groups, such as the elderly and athletes.[2] Others recommend it for bursitis, tendinitis, asthma, candidiasis, vaginitis, and food allergies.

Forms Available Include:

Capsule, injection.

Dosage Commonly Reported:

To use commercial products containing glucosamine sulfate, follow the package instructions.

Will It Work for You? What the Studies Say:

Osteoarthritis involves a progressive degeneration of cartilage glycosaminoglycans (GAGs), components of cartilage that enable joints to move smoothly. The theory behind taking glucosamine supplements, which are critical to the synthesis of GAGs, is that by flooding the system with them the production of these GAGs will be stimulated.[3] Theoretically, the end result would be cartilage regeneration and joint repair.

Several well-designed studies have shown that glucosamine (taken orally in many cases) does effectively relieve osteoarthritis-related pain and inflammation with minimal side effects. Starting in the early 1980s, several placebo-controlled studies have indicated that injectable and oral glucosamine are significantly superior to placebos in reducing pain and joint tenderness, increasing movement, and speeding up recovery in cases of chronic degenerative articular disorders such as osteoarthritis.[4] Importantly, clinical recovery has lasted beyond the treatment period in some cases—several weeks in one—which does not normally occur when conventional nonsteroidal anti-inflammatory drugs (NSAIDs) are stopped.

In later studies, oral glucosamine proved as effective as such standard NSAIDs as ibuprofen in treating osteoarthritis while proving less likely to cause adverse drug reactions. In one double-blind, placebo-controlled trial, the percentage of subjects suffering from adverse reactions to the drug was 37 percent for those taking ibuprofen, compared with only 7 percent for those taking glucosamine.[6]

In a 1980 study, investigators determined not only that glucosamine therapy helped reduce symptoms and improve mobility better than a placebo in eighty osteoarthritis patients, but that the cartilage of those taking the medication was not dissimilar to healthy cartilage, according to electron microscopy studies. Those taking the placebo, on the other hand, had cartilage in a condition that would be expected with the disease.[7]

Will It Harm You? What the Studies Say:

Clinical studies indicate that most people tolerate glucosamine very well, a particularly important point for those who experience side effects such as stomach upset with conventional medicines for pain and inflammation. Researchers still need to figure out why antirheumatic drugs that include glucosamine among other ingredients have been implicated in bronchopulmonary complications, however.[8]

GENERAL SOURCES:

Balch, J.F., and P.A. Balch. *Prescription for Nutritional Healing: A Practical A to Z Reference to Drug-Free Remedies Using Vitamins, Minerals, Herbs & Food Supplements*. 2nd ed. Garden City Park, NY: Avery Publishing Group, 1997.

Review of Natural Products. St. Louis: Facts and Comparisons, November 1996.

TEXT CITATIONS:

1. *Review of Natural Products* (St. Louis: Facts and Comparisons, November 1996).
2. M. McCarty, *Medical Hypotheses*, 42(5) (1994): 323–27.
3. *Review of Natural Products*, op. cit.
4. E. D'Ambrosia et al., *Pharmatherapeutica*, 2(8) (1981): 504–8. Y. Vajaradul, *Clinical Therapeutics*, 3(5) (1981): 336–43. J.M. Pujalte et al., *Current Medical Research & Opinion*, 7(2) (1980): 110–41.
5. Vajaradul, op cit.
6. L.C. Rovati, *International Journal of Tissue Reactions*, 14(5) (1992): 243–51.
7. A. Drovanti et al., *Clinical Therapeutics*, 3(4) (1980): 260–72.
8. *Review of Natural Products*, op. cit. B. Larget-Piet et al., *Therapiewoche*, 41(4) (1986): 269–77.

PRIMARY NAME:
L-GLUTAMINE

SCIENTIFIC NAME:
N/A

COMMON NAME:
Glutamine

What Is L-Glutamine?

L-glutamine is a nonessential amino acid. "Nonessential" means that the body produces it naturally.

What It Is Used For:

This amino acid is converted into the chemical glutamic acid in the brain and is said to lower undesirable ammonia levels in that organ and in other body tissues. Advocates have taken to describing glutamine as a "brain fuel" capable of boosting clear thinking and mental alertness. They recommend it for bodybuilders and dieters and for people suffering from muscle wasting, arthritis, connective tissue diseases and autoimmune disorders, alcohol addiction recovery, fatigue, schizophrenia, senility, epilepsy, and developmental disabilities.

L-GLUTAMINE (Continued)

RATING:

4 = Research indicates that this substance will not fulfill the claims made for it, but that it is also unlikely to cause any

Forms Available Include:

Capsule, powder, tablet.

Dosage Commonly Reported:

Recommendations vary widely; more liberal sources suggest a daily dosage of 500 to 1,000 milligrams.

Will It Work for You? What the Studies Say:

Little data can be found to support supplementing the diet with L-glutamine. See **L-Tyrosine** for a discussion of amino acid supplementation.

Will It Harm You? What the Studies Say:

Unconfirmed reports indicate that high doses of L-glutamine may cause headaches and other unwanted reactions in some people. Concerns have also been raised about the wisdom of supplementing the diet with any single amino acid; see **L-Tyrosine** for more information.

GENERAL SOURCES:

Balch, J.F., and P.A. Balch. *Prescription for Nutritional Healing: A Practical A to Z Reference to Drug-Free Remedies Using Vitamins, Minerals, Herbs & Food Supplements.* 2nd ed. Garden City Park, NY: Avery Publishing Group, 1997.

Mayell, M. *Off-the-Shelf Natural Health: How to Use Herbs and Nutrients to Stay Well.* New York: Bantam Books, 1995.

PRIMARY NAME:

GOLDENROD

SCIENTIFIC NAME:

Various *Solidago* species, including *Solidago virgaurea* L. (European), *Solidago canadensis* L., *Solidago serotina* Ait. (*Solidago gigantea* Air.). Family: Asteraceae (Compositae)

COMMON NAME:

Woundwort

RATING:

2 = According to a number of well-designed studies and common use, this substance appears to be relatively effective and safe when used in recommended amounts.

What Is Goldenrod?

Dense clusters of mustard-yellow flowers bloom in late summer on this herb, a daisy-family member found in many parts of the world including North America and Europe. The aromatic flowers and long oval leaves emerge off stiff, upright branches. All of the aboveground parts of the plant, once dried, are used medicinally.

What It Is Used For:

Goldenrod has a long-standing reputation, particularly in traditional European medicine, as a diuretic ("water pill") for treating urinary tract inflammation and other disorders and for preventing as well as helping to expel kidney and bladder stones. It has reportedly been used in the form of a douche or mouthwash, or in other external formulations, to treat wounds, combat yeast infections, and control eczema. Native Americans turned to the *Solidago odora* species for many of the same disorders, as well as to stimulate digestion and treat colic, diarrhea, and measles. Goldenrod and its extracts appear in various commercial European diuretic, laxative, and rheumatism remedies.

Forms Available Include:

Decoction, infusion.

Dosage Commonly Reported:

A common daily dosage is 6 to 15 grams. An infusion is made using 3 to 5 grams herb in 240 milliliters water and is drunk several times per day.

Will It Work for You? What the Studies Say:

Despite uncertainty about the responsible ingredients—both flavonoids and saponins have been cited—goldenrod appears to stimulate the elimination of fluid (urination), possibly by directly affecting kidney function,[1] according to studies that have shown significant diuretic activity in rats,[2] the experience and recommendation of European physicians who have observed its effectiveness in patients, and the endorsement of German health authorities.[3] References to published clinical trials cannot be found in the recent medical literature, however. Assuming that goldenrod is an effective diuretic, it will probably help reduce inflammation in the kidneys and lower urinary tract, as well as help to prevent and eliminate kidney and urinary stones and encourage elimination of urinary tract infections.

Some German physicians recommend goldenrod for boosting urine output in cases of acute (not chronic) kidney inflammation (nephritis) involving scanty or absent urination.[4] It may also aid these conditions by reducing spasms,[5] a property observed in several rat studies.[6] German health authorities officially recognize the herb's anti-inflammatory and mildly antispasmodic properties.[7] Animal studies indicate that the chemical leiocarposide reduces inflammation and pain, but whether this translates into any benefit for arthritis remains unclear.[8] A 1995 rat study found the anti-inflammatory action of a goldenrod extract commercially available in Germany to be notable.[9]

Given the presence of astringent tannins, which constrict tissue and reduce oozing and bleeding, goldenrod in external formulations such as oral rinses may help control inflammation in the mouth and throat, as well as encourage wound healing.[10]

Preliminary findings of other studies indicate that constituents in goldenrod may stimulate the immune system, fight certain tumors and fungi (including the *Candida* fungus responsible for most oral thrush and yeast infections), kill sperm (in the test tube), and induce sedation (in mice), but the implication for treating human infections or disease are still very unclear.[11]

Will It Harm You? What the Studies Say:

On the basis of the ingredients identified so far, as well as long-term use, goldenrod appears to be safe for most people to use. Anyone who has a chronic kidney disorder, a urinary tract infection, or another ailment necessitating a diuretic should be seen by a doctor before using this or any other herb with diuretic properties, however. Always drink a lot of fluids when taking an herb with diuretic properties. German health authorities warn that anyone suffering from fluid retention due to kidney or heart insufficiency should not take goldenrod.[12] Avoid the herb if you have ever had an allergic reaction to other members of the daisy family, such as ragweed.

GENERAL SOURCES:

American Pharmaceutical Association. *Handbook of Nonprescription Drugs*. 11th ed. Washington, D.C.: American Pharmaceutical Association, 1996.

Blumenthal, M., J. Gruenwald, T. Hall, and R.S. Rister, eds. *The Complete German Commission E Monographs: Therapeutic Guide to Herbal Medicine*. Boston: Integrative Medicine Communications, 1998.

Bremness, L. *Herbs*. 1st American ed. Eyewitness Handbooks. New York: Dorling Kindersley Publications, 1994.

Chevallier, A. *The Encyclopedia of Medicinal Plants: A Practical Reference Guide to More Than 550 Key Medicinal Plants & Their Uses*. 1st American ed. New York: Dorling Kindersley Publications, 1996.

Foster, S., and J.A. Duke. *The Peterson Field Guide Series: A Field Guide to Medicinal Plants. Eastern and Central North America*. Boston: Houghton Mifflin Company, 1990.

Tyler, V.E. *Herbs of Choice: The Therapeutic Use of Phytomedicinals*. Binghamton NY: Haworth Press/Pharmaceutical Products Press, 1994.

Weiss, R.F. *Herbal Medicine*, trans. A.R. Meuss, from the 6th German edition. Beaconsfield, England: Beaconsfield Publishers, Ltd., 1988.

TEXT CITATIONS:

1. R.F. Weiss, *Herbal Medicine*, trans. A.R. Meuss, from the 6th German edition (Beaconsfield, England: Beaconsfield Publishers, Ltd., 1988).

2. A. Chodera et al., *Acta Poloniae Pharmaceutica*, 42(2) (1985): 199–204. V.E. Tyler, *Herbs of Choice: The Therapeutic Use of Phytomedicinals* (Binghamton, NY: Haworth Press/Pharmaceutical Products Press, 1994).

3. M. Blumenthal, J. Gruenwald, T. Hall, and R.S. Rister, eds., *The Complete German Commission E Monographs: Therapeutic Guide to Herbal Medicine* (Boston: Integrative Medicine Communications, 1998).

4. Weiss, op. cit.

5. N.G. Bisset, ed., *Herbal Drugs and Phytopharmaceuticals* (Stuttgart: medpharm GmbH Scientific Publishers, 1994).

6. J. Leuschner, *Arzneimittel-Forschung*, 45(2) (1995): 165–68.

7. Blumenthal et al., op. cit.

8. J. Metzner et al., *Pharmazie*, 39 (1982): 869.

9. J. Leuschner, op. cit.

10. Bisset, op. cit.

11. Ibid. G. Bader et al., *Pharmazie*, 42 (1987): 140. E. Racz-Kotilla and G. Racz, *Planta Medica*, 33 (1978): 300. B.S. Setty et al., *Contraception*, 14 (1976): 571.

12. Bisset, op. cit.

PRIMARY NAME:
GOLDENSEAL

SCIENTIFIC NAME:

Hydrastis canadensis L. Family: Ranunculaceae

What Is Goldenseal?

This stout perennial grows deep in moist, rich woods along the East Coast of North America. In spring, the small, erect stems produce large hand-shaped leaves, greenish-white flowers, and dark, orange-red berries. The parts of the plant used medicinally are the dried rhizomes (underground stems) and roots. The rhizomes are knotty and yellow-brown and have a bright yellow pulp. Goldenseal is now scarce in the wild, probably because of overharvesting. It earned its name from the appearance of "golden" marks on the yellow rhizome resembling the wax seals once commonly used to seal envelopes.

COMMON NAMES:

Eye balm, eye root, ground raspberry, hydrastine, Indian dye, jaundice root, orange root, tumeric root, yellow Indian paint, yellow puccon, yellowroot

RATING:

3 = Studies on the effectiveness and safety of this substance are conflicting, or there are not enough studies to draw a conclusion.

Do not confuse a shrubby plant also commonly referred to as yellowroot or shrub yellowroot—*Xanthorhiza simplicissima* Marsh synon X. apiifolia—with goldenseal.

What It Is Used For:

Native Americans living on the East Coast introduced this native plant to early settlers. Several tribes had long been using it as a source of brilliant yellow dye. They also collected it for medicinal purposes such as soothing stomach upset, washing the eyes and treating eye ailments, alleviating cough-related congestion, increasing urine output (as a diuretic, or "water pill"), and treating numerous skin conditions such as eczema, psoriasis, ulcers, boils, burn-related scars, and acne. A douche was made from the herb to treat uterine hemorrhage and hemorrhoids. Various cancers were once treated with goldenseal, including those affecting the stomach and uterus.

The settlers picked up a number of these practices, but it was only in the early nineteenth century that goldenseal became quite popular, first as an antiseptic and then as a virtual cure-all and tonic for a dizzying array of ailments. The official medical establishment began to acknowledge and prescribe the herb in the middle of the century; this official recognition lasted until 1960. The *National Formulary* intermittently classified goldenseal as an antiseptic and astringent. Many patent medicines contained the herb, including the popular tonic "Dr. Pierce's Golden Medical Discovery."

With skyrocketing demand in the nineteenth century, goldenseal was collected so intensively that the country's supply was nearly wiped out. The cost of the herb rapidly rose, although many still considered it a "poor man's ginseng."[1] Manufacturers sometimes tried to slip in a less costly herb. Renewed enthusiasm for the herb in recent decades has jacked prices back up again as farmers struggle to meet the demand.[2] Goldenseal has become one of America's most widely sold medicinal plants.[3] The salt of the plant, an alkaloid commonly called hydrastine, is sometimes used independently.

Many contemporary herbalists consider goldenseal antiseptic, tonic, antiinflammatory, and astringent. They recommend it for a multitude of ailments, both external and internal. It has been put to work in preventing infection in wounds; soothing chapped lips; and treating irritated gums, canker sores, and skin ailments such as eczema, acne, dandruff, and fungal infections (e.g., ringworm). Goldenseal mouthwash is said to help prevent gum disease. Many suggest the herb for vaginal infections, menstrual disorders, and postpartum bleeding. Goldenseal also has a reputation for boosting the potency of other herbs. Such broad-ranging internal ills as indigestion and constipation, cold and flu symptoms (nasal congestion, watery eyes), muscular and rheumatic pain, liver disease, and sciatica pain have been treated with it.

Of the many independent uses for hydrastine, perhaps the most popular may be as a component in commercial (sterile) eyewashes, as a local anti-inflammatory, as an antacid, and as a bitter tonic for improved digestion. Homeopaths prescribe minute amounts for such ailments as asthma, alcoholism, indigestion, and constipation. (See page 2 for a discussion of homeopathy.)

Forms Available Include:

- *For internal use:* Capsule, extract, gargle, infusion, powder, rhizome and root, salt (hydrastine), tea, tincture. The bitter taste of the teas can be masked with honey, lemon, or sugar.
- *For external use:* Eyewash, tea.

Select a reliable source; the high cost of goldenseal has inspired some manufacturers to adulterate this herb with a less costly one such as **Barberry**, **Wild Oregon Grape**, **Yellow Dock**, or **Bloodroot**, some of which can cause unwanted reactions when taken in high doses.

Dosage Commonly Reported:

The dried root is taken in dosages of 500 milligrams a day, or 1 dropperful of tincture two to three times a day. An infusion is made with ½ to 1 teaspoon powdered root per cup of water. As a mouthwash or gargle, ½ to 1 teaspoon of goldenseal powder is used per cup of water.

Will It Work for You? What the Studies Say:

Scientists have unveiled the presence of two particularly important ingredients in goldenseal: the alkaloids hydrastine (2 to 4 percent) and berberine (0.5 to 6 percent). Although these important components explain the logic behind several traditional uses, science offers relatively little information about how they directly affect human beings. The last major review of hydrastine and its potential importance as a drug was done in 1950.[4] The recent medical literature contains no references to human studies involving goldenseal directly.

A number of medical establishments around the world—although no longer in the United States—officially recognize hydrastine and berberine as drugs. Both are astringent and have mild antiseptic (specifically, antibiotic) properties, rendering goldenseal valuable in the form of a mouthwash (made of tea) for soothing and healing canker sores and other minor mouth ailments.[5] These are probably the most justifiable uses for the herb. Manufacturers still place goldenseal extracts in eyewashes, but given the risk of introducing other infectious agents into the eye, its value for eye problems in countries with sterilized eye medications is limited indeed.[6]

Hydrastine constricts peripheral blood vessels, which means that it may help stop bleeding, but its once popular use for controlling postpartum bleeding does not appear to be justified; not only is it unreliable, but other drugs have proved more effective for this potentially complicating condition. Researchers doing animal studies have found that the berberine in goldenseal may calm spasms in the uterus, but that it may also stimulate uterine contractions.[7] So whether it will help stop excessive menstrual flow or relieve menstrual pain remains unclear.

Clinical trials done as long ago as the 1950s indicate that the berberine in goldenseal may well work as a weapon against infectious stomach upset by fighting numerous bacteria, including organisms that can cause diarrhea such as *Escherichia coli*, *Shigella dysenteriae*, and the cholera bacteria.[8] Berberine apparently also has stomach-soothing properties, and has been shown to stimulate the secretion of bile in humans, which would also aid digestion of fats especially.[9] There are also indications that goldenseal may reduce stomach inflammation,[10] and it may even help restore digestive function in alcoholics, according to research data.[11]

In times past, goldenseal was enlisted as a cancer-fighter, especially for cancers of the stomach, ovary, and uterus.[12] Interestingly, researchers have discovered that both hydrastine and berberine have tumor-fighting potential, although much more intensive investigation is needed before goldenseal is used to treat humans. The herb may also cause a drop in blood sugar levels, indicating a possible future role in managing diabetes, but much more research is needed to confirm that this property occurs in humans.[13]

A number of traditional uses for goldenseal do not appear to have any hint of scientific justification or are potentially very risky. For example, no studies have been reported to demonstrate that goldenseal in any way affects a urinary tract infection or internal bleeding. Studies have shown that its reputation for masking the presence of illegal substances such as morphine, marijuana, or codeine in urine tests is unfounded.[14]

Will It Harm You? What the Studies Say:

The toxicity of goldenseal has not been carefully examined, although people have certainly used it for generations to no apparent ill effect. The FDA placed the herb on its formerly maintained list of "Herbs of Undefined Safety." The key appears to be to use it with care and moderation. Small, typically recommended amounts are probably safe for most individuals.

Larger doses can be toxic in several ways, however, potentially causing irritation of the mouth and throat, nausea, vomiting, diarrhea, numbness or tingling in the extremities, central nervous stimulation, respiratory failure, and even death. In particular, the hydrastine alkaloid in high doses can cause exaggerated reflexes, high blood pressure, convulsions, and even death from respiratory failure. Topical formulations may cause ulcerations, which can be severe in some cases. Douches may cause vaginal irritation and should not be used.[15]

Pregnant women should not take goldenseal[16] because it is not clear how it affects the uterus; some animal studies indicate that it stimulates uterine contractions, while others suggest that it calms the uterus.[17] Those with high blood pressure, diabetes, glaucoma, a history of stroke, or heart disease should also avoid the herb.

GENERAL SOURCES:

Bradley, P.C., ed. *British Herbal Compendium: A Handbook of Scientific Information on Widely Used Plant Drugs*, vol. 1. Bournemouth (Dorset), England: British Herbal Medicine Association, 1992.

Castleman, M. *The Healing Herbs: The Ultimate Guide to the Curative Power of Nature's Medicines*. New York, NY: Bantam Books, 1995.

Der Marderosian, A., and L. Liberti. *Natural Product Medicine. A Scientific Guide to Foods, Drugs, Cosmetics*. Philadelphia: George F. Stickley, 1988.

Duke, J.A. *CRC Handbook of Medicinal Herbs*. Boca Raton, FL: CRC Press, 1985.

Foster, S. *Goldenseal: Hydrastis canadensis.* American Botanical Council. Botanical Series No. 309. Austin, TX, 1991.

———. *HerbalGram.* 21 (1989): 7.

Genest, K., and D.W. Hughes. *Canadian Journal of Pharmaceutical Sciences* 4 (1969): 41.

Hamon, N.W. *CPJ-RPC.* 11 (1990): 508.

Hartwell, J. *Lloydia.* 34 (1971): 103.

Heinerman, J. *Heinerman's Encyclopedia of Healing Herbs and Spices.* West Nyack, NY: Parker Publishing Co., 1996.

Hobbs, C. *Pharmacy in History.* 32(2) (1990): 79–82.

Lawrence Review of Natural Products. St. Louis: Facts and Comparisons, May 1994.

Leung, A.Y., and S. Foster. *Encyclopedia of Common Natural Ingredients Used in Food, Drugs, and Cosmetics.* 2nd ed. New York: John Wiley & Sons, 1996.

Mayell, M. *Off-the-Shelf Natural Health: How to Use Herbs and Nutrients to Stay Well.* New York: Bantam Books, 1995.

Mindell, E. *Earl Mindell's Herb Bible.* New York: Simon & Schuster/Fireside, 1992.

Newall, C.A., et al. *Herbal Medicines: A Guide for Health-Care Professionals.* London: The Pharmaceutical Press, 1996.

Tyler, V.E. *Herbs of Choice: The Therapeutic Use of Phytomedicinals.* Binghamton, NY: Haworth Press/Pharmaceutical Products Press, 1994.

———. *The Honest Herbal.* Binghamton, NY: Haworth Press/Pharmaceutical Products Press, 1993.

Tyler, V.E., L.R. Brady, and J.E. Robbers, eds. *Pharmacognosy.* Philadelphia: Lea & Febiger, 1988.

TEXT CITATIONS:

1. M. Castleman, *The Healing Herbs: The Ultimate Guide to the Curative Power of Nature's Medicines* (New York: Bantam Books, 1995).
2. S. Foster, *Goldenseal: Hydrastis canadensis* (American Botanical Council, Botanical Series N. 309, Austin, TX, 1991).
3. Ibid. K. Genest and D.W. Hughes, *Canadian Journal of Pharmaceutical Sciences,* 4 (1969): 41.
4. F.E. Shideman, *Committee on the Natural Formulary Bulletin,* 18(102) (1950): 3–19. Foster, op. cit.
5. V.E. Tyler, *The Honest Herbal* (Binghamton, NY: Haworth Press/Phamaceutical Products Press, 1993).
6. A.Y. Leung and S. Foster, *Encyclopedia of Common Natural Ingredients Used in Food, Drugs, and Cosmetics,* 2nd ed. (New York: John Wiley & Sons, 1996).
7. Newall, op. cit.
8. Foster, op. cit.
9. A. Der Marderosian and L. Liberti, *Natural Product Medicine: A Scientific Guide to Foods, Drugs, Cosmetics* (Philadelphia: George F. Stickley, 1988).
10. *Lawrence Review of Natural Products* (St. Louis: Facts and Comparisons, May 1994).
11. J.A. Duke, *CRC Handbook of Medicinal Herbs* (Boca Raton, FL: CRC Press, 1985).
12. S. Farnsworth, *Tile and Till,* 57 (1971): 52.
13. J.A. Ostrenga and D. Perry, *PharmChem Newsletter,* 4(1) (1975): 1.
14. Newall, op. cit.
15. P.C. Bradley, ed., *British Herbal Compendium: A Handbook of Scientific Information on Widely Used Plant Drugs,* vol. 1. (Bournemouth [Dorset], England: British Herbal Medicine Association, 1992).
16. *Lawrence Review of Natural Products,* op. cit.

PRIMARY NAME:
GOTU KOLA

SCIENTIFIC NAME:
Centella asiatica L. Urb., sometimes referred to as *Hydrocotyle asiatica* L. or *Centella coriaca* Nannfd. Family: Umbelliferae (Apiaceae)

COMMON NAMES:
Hydrocotyle, Indian pennywort, marsh penny, sheep rot, talepetrako, water pennywort

RATING:
2 = According to a number of well-designed studies and common use, this substance appears to be relatively effective and safe when used in recommended amounts for the indication(s) noted in the "Will It Work for You?" section.

What Is Gotu Kola?

This creeping perennial favors wet, swampy areas in India, Sri Lanka, South Africa, Madagascar, and other tropical environments. Some of its common names, such as Indian pennywort, refer to the size of its fan-shaped leaves—about that of an old British penny. The leaves are used medicinally. The plant also bears fruits and clusters of small red flowers.

Do not confuse gotu kola with the similarly named **Kola** or cola plant *(Cola nitida),* an herb with stimulant properties.

What It Is Used For:

Traditional Eastern medicines in particular have treasured this plant since ancient times, reportedly using it to treat such ailments as fever, diarrhea, menstrual irregularity, nervous disorders, leprosy, jaundice, rheumatism, wounds, and numerous skin conditions, including psoriasis, eczema, lupus, varicose ulcers, and leprosy.

Sri Lankans were the first to make the connection between the elephants' favorite snack—the leaves of the gotu kola plant—and their longevity. In time, the plant became known in the West as a key to longevity for humans. After decades of uninterest in the West, enthusiasm for gotu kola perked up again in the years after World War II with the popularity of the herbal blend **Fo-Ti-Tieng**™, which was heavily promoted as a longevity balm on the basis of its gotu kola content.[1] The blend is said to have enabled a Chinese herbalist to enjoy twenty-three wives over a 256-year lifespan.

In addition to its famed longevity-promoting qualities, contemporary Western herbalists cite wound-healing actions and the external treatment of varicose veins, cellulite and leg circulation problems, and scleroderma as principal uses for gotu kola. Some have even touted the herb as an aphrodisiac. While small doses are recommended internally as tonic stimulants, large doses are considered sedative. Crushed gotu kola leaves can be found in salads in some parts of the world including Sri Lanka.

Forms Available Include:

- *For internal use:* Concentrated drops, extract (standardized), fluid extract, infusion, injection formulations, leaves (dried), tincture. Bitter and astringent-tasting infusions may benefit from sweetening.
- *For external use:* Compress.

Dosage Commonly Reported:

An infusion is made using ½ teaspoon herb per cup of water and is drunk twice a day or used in a compress. Tincture or concentrated drops are taken in the amount of ½ to 1 dropperful two to three times per day. The standardized extract is taken daily in doses of 60 to 120 milligrams, the crude leaves in doses of 2 to 4 grams, the tincture in doses of 10 to 20 milliliters, and the fluid extract in doses of 2 to 4 milliliters.

Will It Work for You? What the Studies Say:

Gotu kola extracts help wounds heal, according to numerous clinical studies. Chronic lesions appear to benefit the most.[2] The critical ingredients are the glucosides asiaticoside and madecasosside. Asiaticoside stimulates healing, while madecasosside exerts anti-inflammatory actions. Extracts of asiaticoside and a special standardized extract of gotu kola called TECA (titrated extract of *Centella asiatica*) have proved valuable in stimulating scar-free wound healing in surgical wounds, skin ulcers, fistulas, episiotomies, skin grafts, skin tuberculosis, and lupus lesions.[3] In one study, intramuscular injections of TECA over a period of one to three months cured or at least helped to improve 75 percent of cases of bladder lesions with minimal scarring.[4] The herb accelerates the healing of burns while minimizing scarring, according to another study published in 1979.[5]

Painful psoriasis sores responded positively to gotu kola cream (containing oil and water extracts of the leaves) in a small 1973 study.[6] In five of the seven subjects, the welts resolved completely within three to seven weeks. This cream is apparently not commercially available. No other studies on gotu kola in treating psoriasis appear in the recent medical literature.

People suffering from venous insufficiency of the lower limbs may get some relief with TECA, according to a double-blind, placebo-controlled trial reported in 1987.[7] Compared with the subjects treated with a placebo, those taking TECA (12 or 60 milligrams a day) for eight weeks experienced notable improvements in swelling and sensations of pain and heaviness in the legs and reported a sense of overall improvement. TECA appears to have increased the tone of the veins, enabling them to distend more fully.

Study findings support the long-standing tradition of treating leprosy with gotu kola and its extracts in various forms (oral, injection, topical); a chemical, asiaticoside, contained in it, disintegrates the protective coating on the bacteria that causes this disease, enabling the immune system to destroy it.[8]

Researchers reported in 1995 that a cultured extract of gotu kola killed cultured cancer tumor cells in test tubes without causing notable toxic reactions in human lymphocytes.[9] More research on this intriguing finding is needed to determine what it means for enlisting the herb as a cancer-fighter. Although much remains to be learned about the subject, preliminary findings also indicate that oral doses of gotu kola extracts significantly reduced the fertility of test rats,[10] and other studies have shown promise in treating cirrhosis of the liver.[11] Claims that gotu kola will prolong life have not been scientifically substantiated.

Will It Harm You? What the Studies Say:

Gotu kola has a relatively clean safety record, although contact dermatitis has been reported in some cases involving application of the ointment or the plant's fresh or dried parts.[12] The critical ingredient—asiaticoside—may also be weakly cancer-causing, according to a 1972 report citing the development of skin tumors in mice after repeated applications (twice a week for eighteen months) of a concentrated solution.[13] The risk to humans using relatively low doses over shorter periods of time appears to be minimal, but no further research on the subject can be found. Subcutaneous (rather than intramuscular) injections may cause pain at the injection site.[14] Animal studies indicate that gotu kola causes sedation when ingested in large doses.[15]

GENERAL SOURCES:

Castleman, M. *The Healing Herbs: The Ultimate Guide to the Curative Power of Nature's Medicines.* New York: Bantam Books, 1995.

Duke, J.A. *CRC Handbook of Medicinal Herbs.* Boca Raton, FL: CRC Press, 1985.

Lawrence Review of Natural Products. St. Louis: Facts and Comparisons, August 1996.

Leung, A.Y., and S. Foster. *Encyclopedia of Common Natural Ingredients Used in Food, Drugs, and Cosmetics.* 2nd ed. New York: John Wiley & Sons, 1996.

Murray, M.T. *The Healing Power of Herbs: The Enlightened Person's Guide to the Wonders of Medicinal Plants.* Revised and expanded 2nd ed. Rocklin, CA: Prima Publishing, 1995.

Tyler, V.E. *The Honest Herbal.* Binghamton, NY: Haworth Press/Pharmaceutical Products Press, 1993.

TEXT CITATIONS:

1. M. Castleman, *The Healing Herbs: The Ultimate Guide to the Curative Power of Nature's Medicines* (New York: Bantam Books, 1995).
2. *Lawrence Review of Natural Products* (St. Louis: Facts and Comparisons, August 1996).
3. P. Boiteau and A.R. Ratsimamanga, *Therapie,* 11 (1956): 125–49.
4. A. Fam, *International Surgery,* 58 (1973): 451.
5. J.P. Bosse et al., *Annals of Plastic Surgery,* 3 (1979): 1, 13.
6. S. Natarajan and P.P. Paily, *Indian Journal of Dermatology,* 1 8(4) (1973): 82.
7. J.P. Pointel et al., *Angiology,* 38(1 Pt 1) (1987): 46.
8. Boiteau, op. cit.
9. T.D. Babu et al., *Journal of Ethnopharmacology,* 48 (1995): 53.
10. T. Dutta and U.P. Basu, *Indian Journal of Experimental Biology,* 6(3) (1968): 181.
11. F. Damis et al., *Semaine des Hopitaux de Paris,* 55 (1979): 1749–50.
12. H.C. Eun and A.Y. Lee, *Contact Dermatitis,* 13(5) (1985): 310.
13. O.D. Laerum and O.H. Iversen, *Cancer Research,* 32 (1972): 1463–69.
14. Fam, op. cit.
15. A.S. Ramaswamy et al., *Journal of Research in Indian Medicine,* 4 (1970): 160–75. V.E. Tyler, *The Honest Herbal* (Binghamton, NY: Haworth Press/Pharmaceutical Products Press, 1993).

PRIMARY NAME:

GRAPE SEED EXTRACT

SCIENTIFIC NAME:
N/A

COMMON NAME:
Muskat

What Is Grape Seed Extract?

The ground seeds of the common red grapes processed for wine production (*Vitis vinifera* L. and *Vitus coignetiae* Family Vitaceae) are the source of this extract. Sometimes the skins are used as well.

What It Is Used For:

Dietary supplement manufacturers recommend grape seed extract as an antioxidant. Antioxidants (see also **Beta-Carotene**) are said to control the formation of dangerous substances in the body called free radicals, which are believed to damage cells through oxidation and in some cases even contribute

GRAPE SEED EXTRACT
(Continued)

RATING:

3 = Studies on the effectiveness and safety of this substance are conflicting, or there are not enough studies to draw a conclusion.

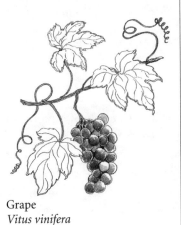

Grape
Vitus vinifera

to cancer cell formation. Taken orally as a dietary supplement for its active components—procyanidolic oligomers (PCOs) or proanthocyanidins—grape seed extract can be used interchangeably with pine bark extract (**Pycnogenol**), which also contains PCOs. Advocates claim that these substances can protect against tumor formation, help fight aging, improve circulation to the benefit of peripheral vascular diseases, reduce inflammation, control diabetes, aid wound healing, treat retinopathy, and fight the breakdown of collagen which can occur with aging and a number of inflammatory collagen diseases. In France, PCOs have been marketed for decades.[1]

Forms Available Include:

Capsule, tablet.

Dosage Commonly Reported:

Capsules or tablets of 75 to 300 milligrams are ingested daily for up to three weeks, followed by a maintenance dose of 40 to 80 milligrams per day.

Will It Work for You? What the Studies Say:

Grape seed oil contains various PCOs, which are condensed tannins. Researchers have shown that these substances are effective antioxidants.

PCOs also inhibit the enzymes responsible for breaking down the chemical substances that compose the supporting structure (collagen, elastin, hyaluronic acid) around blood vessels.[4] This property may be of benefit in maintaining the integrity of the blood vessels and even of skin. Other researchers report evidence to indicate that PCOs can help prevent cavities.[5]

See **Pycnogenol** for more information on PCOs.

Will It Harm You? What the Studies Say:

The recent medical literature contains no reports of significant adverse reactions to grape seed extract. Its toxicity does not appear to have been carefully examined, however.

GENERAL SOURCES:

American Pharmaceutical Association. *Handbook of Nonprescription Drugs.* 11th ed. Washington, D.C.: American Pharmaceutical Association, 1996.

Balch, J.F., and P.A. Balch. *Prescription for Nutritional Healing: A Practical A to Z Reference to Drug-Free Remedies Using Vitamins, Minerals, Herbs & Food Supplements.* 2nd ed. Garden City Park, NY: Avery Publishing Group, 1997.

Lawrence Review of Natural Products. St. Louis: Facts and Comparisons, September 1995.

Mayell, M. *Off-the-Shelf Natural Health: How to Use Herbs and Nutrients to Stay Well.* New York: Bantam Books, 1995.

Murray, M.T. *The Healing Power of Herbs: The Enlightened Person's Guide to the Wonders of Medicinal Plants.* Revised and expanded 2nd ed. Rocklin, CA: Prima Publishing, 1995.

TEXT CITATIONS:

1. M.T. Murray, *The Healing Power of Herbs: The Enlightened Person's Guide to the Wonders of Medicinal Plants,* revised and expanded 2nd ed. (Rocklin, CA: Prima Publishing, 1995).

2. I. Liviero et al., *Fitoterapia,* 65 (1994): 203–9.

3. R. Maffei Facino et al., *Arzneimittel-Forschung*, 44(5) (1994): 592.
4. Ibid.
5. T. Toukairin et al., *Chemical & Pharmaceutical Bulletin*, 39(6) (1991): 1480.

PRIMARY NAME:
GUARANA

SCIENTIFIC NAME:
Paullinia cupana Kunth var.
sorbilis (Mart.) Ducke and
Paullinia sorbilis (L.) Mart.
Family: Sapindaceae

COMMON NAMES:
Brazilian cocoa, guarana gum,
guarana paste, zoom

RATING:
2 = According to a number of
well-designed studies and
common use, this substance
appears to be relatively
effective and safe when used in
recommended amounts for the
indication(s) noted in the "Will
It Work for You?" section.

What Is Guarana?

Guarana consists of a dried paste made from the seeds of climbing evergreen shrubs native to the Amazon, primarily *Paullina cupana* and *Paullina sorbilis*. The seeds can be found in the orange-yellow fruits of these perennials. They are typically dry-roasted, crushed, mixed into a paste with water, molded into bars or cylindrical masses, and dried.

What It Is Used For:

Guarana figures prominently in the social and medicinal culture of Amazonian Indians. Many concoct a hot, caffeine-containing beverage from the paste that offers much the same stimulant and social pleasures as are celebrated by other people around the world who favor tea or coffee. Some boost the intoxicating effect by adding alcohol. South Americans reportedly also treat chronic or infectious diarrhea, headache (including migraine), pain associated with rheumatic or menstrual ailments, water retention (using it as a diuretic, or "water pill"), fevers, malaria, heat stress, and other ailments with guarana. It has a reputation as an aphrodisiac in some regions.

Guarana appears in a carbonated soft drink that is considered the national beverage of Brazil (and is referred to by the name Guarana).[1] Some North American manufacturers promote the herb as a weight-loss aid and as an ingredient in combination herbal "energy" or "upper" products.

Forms Available Include:

Capsule, dried herb, extract, powder, seeds, syrup, tablet, tea. Guarana also appears in soft drinks, in herbal combination products, and in some foods as a flavoring.

Dosage Commonly Reported:

As a stimulant, a common dosage is 500 to 1,000 milligrams of the dried herb. Powdered guarana is taken in doses of 0.5 to 4 grams. Commercial preparations should be used according to package directions.

Will It Work for You? What the Studies Say:

Researchers started taking a close look at the chemical constituents of this herb in the early 1900s. They discovered that guarana is a caffeine-containing stimulant, just as coffee and black tea are. The caffeine concentration averages about 3.5 percent (by dry weight), a higher level than that found in coffee beans (approximately 1 to 2 percent) and dried tea leaves (1 to 4 percent).[2] Of course the amount of caffeine that passes into the body depends in part on the way the beverage or other formulation is prepared. The longer a tea bag steeps, for example, the more caffeine gets extracted into the water.

The caffeine-driven energy boost provided by guarana tablets has earned them the nickname "zoom."[3] In addition to the high caffeine content, the presence of associated alkaloids (theophylline and theobromine) also explains guarana's traditional use in treating migraine headache and suppressing appetite, just as North Americans use coffee or black tea.

Researchers have identified relatively high levels of tannins (5 to 6 percent) in guarana. These astringent substances explain its reputation for alleviating diarrhea; tannins are believed to control or stop diarrhea by reducing inflammation in the intestines. Guarana extracts also inhibit platelet aggregation in laboratory rabbits (after both oral and intravenous administration), which means that they may help inhibit the development of potentially dangerous blood clots. Similar reactions were seen in human blood observed in the test tube.[4] The implications of these findings for treating humans with the herb remain very unclear, however.

On the basis of a urine analysis, alleged psychoactive elements in the essential oils from guarana (estragole and anethole) do not appear to be metabolized in humans, largely ruling out any type of psychoactive effect.[5]

Guarana does not appear to boost "brain power" or alter cognition in humans in any way, as has been claimed according to a 1996 double-blind and placebo-controlled study in which the effects of the long-term use of guarana in forty-five elderly but healthy volunteers were examined.[6]

Will It Harm You? What the Studies Say:

Guarana appears to be relatively safe to use in moderation. Its caffeine content can cause many of the same reactions that some people find distasteful with coffee, tea, cola, and other caffeine-containing drinks: nervousness, shakiness, trouble sleeping, fast or irregular heartbeat, stomach upset. Children, heart disease sufferers, and pregnant women should take caffeine-containing products in moderation or avoid them altogether. The herb has shown some gene-damaging (genotoxic) and mutation-promoting (mutagenesis) properties in test tubes; this 1994 finding demands further exploration to determine its implications for humans who take the herb.[7]

Keep in mind that no tannin-rich drug should be used over long periods of time, given the potential, still not fully understood, of an increased risk of malignant (cancerous) changes. In addition, tannins are nutritionally counterproductive (they interfere with protein use), particularly when used excessively.[8] Drinking guarana with milk may significantly reduce this risk, however. Guarana in cola soda form poses a distinct risk of tooth decay (erosive potential on dental enamel), according to a 1996 study.[9]

GENERAL SOURCES:

Duke, J.A. *CRC Handbook of Medicinal Herbs.* Boca Raton, FL: CRC Press, 1985.

Lawrence Review of Natural Products. St. Louis: Facts and Comparisons, May 1991.

Leung, A.Y., and S. Foster. *Encyclopedia of Common Natural Ingredients Used in Food, Drugs, and Cosmetics.* 2nd ed. New York: John Wiley & Sons, 1996.

Mayell, M. *Off-the-Shelf Natural Health: How to Use Herbs and Nutrients to Stay Well.* New York: Bantam Books, 1995.

Tyler, V.E. *Herbs of Choice: The Therapeutic Use of Phytomedicinals.* Binghamton, NY: Haworth Press/Pharmaceutical Products Press, 1994.

———. *The Honest Herbal.* Binghamton, NY: Haworth Press/Pharmaceutical Products Press, 1993.

Weiner, M.A., and J.A. Weiner. *Herbs That Heal: Prescription for Herbal Healing.* Mill Valley, CA: Quantum Books, 1994.

TEXT CITATIONS:

1. A.Y. Leung and S. Foster, *Encyclopedia of Common Natural Ingredients Used in Food, Drugs, and Cosmetics*, 2nd ed. (New York: John Wiley & Sons, 1996).
2. A. Der Marderosian and L. Liberti, *Natural Product Medicine: A Scientific Guide to Foods, Drugs, Cosmetics* (Philadelphia, PA: George F. Stickley, 1988).
3. *Lawrence Review of Natural Products* (St. Louis: Facts and Comparisons, May 1991).
4. S.P. Bydlowski et al., *Brazilian Journal of Medicine and Biological Research*, 21(3) (1988): 535–38; and 24(4) (1991): 421–24.
5. H. Benoni et al, *Zeitschrift für Lebensmittel-Untersuchung und Forschung*, 203(1) (1996): 95–98.
6. J.C. Galduroz and E.A. Carlini, *Revista Paulista de Medicina* 114(1) (1996): 1073–78.
7. C.A. da Fonesca et al., *Mutation Research*, 321(3) (1994): 165–73.
8. J.F. Morton, *Basic Life Sciences*, 59 (1992): 739–65.
9. L.J. Grando et al., *Caries Research*, 30(5) (1996): 373–78.

PRIMARY NAME:

GUGGUL

SCIENTIFIC NAME:
Commiphora mukul Hook.
Family: Burseraceae

COMMON NAMES:
Guggulipid, guggulu, gum guggul

RATING:
3 = Studies on the effectiveness and safety of this substance are conflicting, or there are not enough studies to draw a conclusion.

What Is Guggul?

Guggul is a gummy, yellowish liquid (an oleo resin) that oozes from cracks or the injured underbark of a small, thorny tree native to India, the *Commiphora mukul*. The closely related *Commiphora molmol* Engl. and other *Commiphora* species represent the source for another gummy medicinal substance, myrrh; for information on that substance, see **Myrrh**.

What It Is Used For:

Guggul is a well-known Indian (Ayurvedic) medicinal remedy. In India, standardized or purified extracts of guggul called guggulipids are commonly produced and sold for the treatment of arthritis and to lower high blood cholesterol and triglyceride levels that pose a risk of heart disease due to atherosclerosis.

Forms Available Include:

Capsule, crude resin, tablet. Most products are standardized for guggulipid or guggulsterone (the steroid component) content, with guggulipid dosage commonly based on guggulsterone concentration. Equally prevalent is the classic compound, yogaraj guggul, which includes guggul.

Dosage Commonly Reported:

A common dosage is 25 milligrams of guggulsterones (or 500 milligrams of a product standardized for 5 percent guggulsterone content) two or three times per day. Yogaraj guggul is taken in dosages of 1 to 3 grams.

Will It Work for You? What the Studies Say:

Interest in guggul as a treatment for heart disease has been mounting, with preliminary findings in animal and human trials indicating a potential value in lowering blood cholesterol and triglyceride levels. Guggul appears to lower lipids by stimulating the thyroid gland, according to both animal and human studies,[1] although other mechanisms may be involved as well. A steroid (a ketosteroid) appears to be the responsible compound.[2]

In one study, guggulipid significantly prevented an increase in cholesterol and triglyceride levels in rats fed a high-cholesterol diet designed to promote atherosclerosis.[3] In one of the few human trials done so far, guggulipid lowered the concentration of blood fats, cholesterol, triglycerides, beta-lipoproteins, and phospholipids in twenty subjects to levels seen with standard lipid-lowering drugs. Similar lipid-lowering activity was demonstrated in a randomized, double-blind trial involving thirty-one subjects taking guggulipid, but not in the thirty subjects taking a placebo; all subjects also followed a sensible, low-cholesterol diet.[5] Other investigators report cholesterol-level reductions of 14 to 27 percent and triglyceride-level reductions of 22 to 30 percent in subjects treated with guggulipid.[6] In 1986, Indian authorities officially approved guggulipid for marketing as a lipid-lowering drug.[7]

Anti-inflammatory properties have also been demonstrated for guggul, but whether these translate into anything meaningful for treating inflammation-related disorders such as arthritis remains to be determined. When given preventively, a steroidal compound effectively reduced inflammation in classic animal models testing effectiveness against acute and chronic inflammation, including the chemically induced swollen rat paw test.[8] In another study, guggul compounds proved effective in decreasing the joint swelling in animals with chemically induced arthritis.[9]

Will It Harm You? What the Studies Say:

Research in animals and experience with humans taking guggul indicate that it is safe and relatively free of side effects, but the subject demands further examination before any definitive statements regarding safety can be made. Animal studies indicate that guggul is not toxic.[10] Side effects such as diarrhea, restlessness, mild nausea, headache, apprehension, and hiccups were reported by subjects in three different trials.[11] The data indicate that people tolerate the standardized extract—guggulipid—much better than the crude oleoresin or other extracts.[12]

GENERAL SOURCES:

Mayell, M. *Off-the-Shelf Natural Health: How to Use Herbs and Nutrients to Stay Well.* New York: Bantam Books, 1995.

Murray, M.T. *The Healing Power of Herbs: The Enlightened Person's Guide to the Wonders of Medicinal Plants.* Revised and expanded 2nd ed. Rocklin, CA: Prima Publishing, 1995.

Newall, C.A., et al. *Herbal Medicines: A Guide for Health-Care Professionals.* London: The Pharmaceutical Press, 1996.

Tierra, M. *The Way of Herbs.* New York: Pocket Books, 1990.

Tyler, V.E. *Herbs of Choice: The Therapeutic Use of Phytomedicinals.* Binghamton, NY: Haworth Press/Pharmaceutical Products Press, 1994.

TEXT CITATIONS:

1. C.A. Newall et al., *Herbal Medicines: A Guide for Health-Care Professionals* (London: The Pharmaceutical Press, 1996). S.N. Tripathi et al., *Indian Journal of Experimental Biology*, 13 (1975): 15–18.

2. Tripathi, op. cit.

3. S. Lata et al., *Journal of Postgraduate Medicine*, 37 (1991): 132.

4. S.C. Malhotra and M.M.S. Ahuja, *Indian Journal of Medical Research*, 59 (1971): 1621–32.

5. R.B. Singh et al., *Cardiovascular Drugs & Therapy*, 8(4) (1994): 659–64.

6. S. Nityanand et al., *Journal of the Association of Physicians in India*, 37 (1989): 321–28. R.C. Agarwal et al., *Indian Journal of Medical Research*, 84 (1986): 626–34. M.T. Murray, *The Healing Power of Herbs: The Enlightened Person's Guide to the Wonders of Medicinal Plants*, revised and expanded 2nd ed. (Rocklin, CA: Prima Publishing, 1995).

7. Murray, op. cit.

8. R.B. Arora et al., *Indian Journal of Medical Research*, 60 (1972): 929–31. M. Duwiejua et al., *Planta Medica*, 59(1)(1993): 12–16.

9. J.N. Sharma and J.N. Sharma, *Arzneimittel-Forschung*, 27(7) (1977): 1455–57.

10. *Drugs Future*, 13 (1988): 618–19.

11. Tripathi, op. cit. Malhotra and Ahuja, op. cit. Singh, op. cit.

12. Murray, op. cit.

PRIMARY NAME:

GYMNEMA

SCIENTIFIC NAME:
Gymnema sylvestre R.Br. Sometimes referred to as *Asclepias geminata* Roxb., *Periploca sylvestris* Willd, and *Gymnema melicida* Edg. Family: Asclepiadaceae

COMMON NAMES:
Gurmar, merasingi, meshashringi

What Is Gymnema?

This tropical plant of the milkweed family, native to India, is now distributed worldwide. The leaves and occasionally the stem are used medicinally.

What It Is Used For:

Traditional Indian (Ayurvedic), African, and other folk medicine cultures have long valued gymnema for managing "honey urine" (diabetes) and other blood sugar disorders, but the herb has appeared only recently in North American and European outlets.[1] Some sources market it for preventing diabetes in individuals at high risk for the disorder or for managing metabolic control in general. Others tout it as a weight-loss agent.

Forms Available Include:

Capsule. Also appears as an ingredient in herbal weight-loss formulas.

Dosage Commonly Reported:

To use commercial gymnema formulations, follow the package instructions.

Will It Work for You? What the Studies Say:

Scientific studies, most of them done in India, indicate that this herb contains substances that can lower blood sugar levels. Of particular interest is a compound of acidic glycosides called gymnemic acid (gymnemin). Most studies have been carried out in small animals artificially induced with diabetes; in the majority of cases, blood sugar levels among the animals administered gymnema dropped and remained lower than in controls not administered the herb.[2] Although the reduction in blood sugar levels did not show up in a group of severely diabetic rats tested in one study, it did prolong their survival time.[3] In a trial of healthy rats, gymnema given orally proved as potent as the standard antidiabetic drug tolbutamide in lowering blood sugar levels and keeping them low for the duration of the one-month study.[4]

Human studies have proved promising as well. In a 1990 study of twenty-seven individuals with insulin-dependent diabetes, a water-soluble extract of the leaves called GS4, appeared to help stimulate the release of (or increase the production of) the subjects' own insulin.[5] Subjects taking GS4 experienced a drop in various blood glucose levels and insulin requirements compared with similarly afflicted subjects not taking the GS4. Whether the herb can likewise help regulate blood sugar levels in healthy individuals has yet to be demonstrated. There is absolutely no evidence, as some herbal manufacturers have claimed, that the herb or its extracts can block the body's ability to absorb or be influenced by sugar in the diet, and therefore help people lose weight.[6]

Some sources have marketed gymnema as an appetite-suppressant, on the basis of a transitory loss of taste observed when chewing the leaves; it appears to block the ability to taste sweet or bitter flavors.[7] The theory is that loss of taste will lead to a decreased desire to eat. The capsule form of the drug would not be expected to have this effect, however, given that the local effect in the mouth would be lost.

Will It Harm You? What the Studies Say:

On the basis of years of use in various countries with no reports of severe adverse reactions, it can be assumed that gymnema is relatively harmless. But keep in mind that well-designed and long-term toxicity studies have not been done. Also, diabetes is a serious condition that requires the care of a qualified physician; people with diabetes should consult their doctor before taking this herb, and always mention it in case it affects the medicines they are presently taking or lowers their blood sugar levels.

GENERAL SOURCES:
Lawrence Review of Natural Products. St. Louis: Facts and Comparisons, August 1993.
Mayell, M. *Off-the-Shelf Natural Health: How to Use Herbs and Nutrients to Stay Well.* New York: Bantam Books, 1995.

TEXT CITATIONS:
1. *Lawrence Review of Natural Products* (St. Louis: Facts and Comparisons, August 1993).
2. Ibid. S.S. Gupta et al., *Indian Journal of Medical Research,* 50 (September 1962): 1.

G

Gymnema

3. Y. Srivastava et al., *International Journal of Crude Drug Research*, 24(4) (1986): 171–76.

4. S.S. Gupta and M.C. Variyar, *Indian Journal of Medical Research*, 52 (February 1964): 200.

5. E.M. Shanmugasundaram et al., *Journal of Ethnopharmacology*, 30(3) (1990): 281–94.

6. M. Mayell, *Off-the-Shelf Natural Health: How to Use Herbs and Nutrients to Stay Well* (New York: Bantam Books, 1995).

7. K.M. Janjua and S. Ali, *Pakistan Journal of Scientific and Industrial Research*, 29(6) (1986): 422–23. R. Suttisri et al., *Journal of Ethnopharmacology*, 47(1) (1995): 9–26.

PRIMARY NAME:
HAWTHORN

SCIENTIFIC NAME:
Crateagus laevigata, Crateagus monogyna Jacquin, and *Crateagus oxyacantha.* Family: Rosaceae

COMMON NAMES:
English hawthorn, haw, may, mayblossom, maybush, mayflower, whitethorn

RATING:
1 = Years of use and extensive, high-quality studies indicate that this substance is very effective and safe when used in recommended amounts for the indication(s) noted in the "Will It Work for You?" section. However, see safety warnings in the "Will It Harm You?" section.

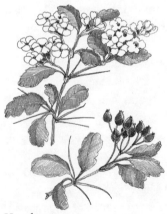

Hawthorn
Crateagus laevigata

What Is Hawthorn?

Hawthorn is a genus of small ornamental trees or bushes that have sharp thorns and yield bunches of aromatic white flowers and bright spherical red fruit ("berries") containing one or several nuts, depending on the species. It belongs to the rose family. Of the hundreds of species of hawthorn, only a few—*Crateagus laevigata* and certain related species—are used medicinally. The dried flowers, leaves, and fruit are used.

What It Is Used For:

In ancient times, people alternated between celebrating hawthorn and regarding it as a symbol of death and illness. By the Middle Ages, folk healers were starting to recommend it for various ills. But hawthorn became a truly popular herbal remedy in Europe and North America only toward the end of the nineteenth century, when its heart-healing properties were discovered. Since then, especially in Europe, both prescription and over-the-counter hawthorn preparations have been used widely to strengthen the heart (as a "heart tonic") and treat heart-related ailments and circulation disorders.

Hawthorn is also billed as a sedative for chronic insomnia. Although this herb is not nearly as well known in the United States as in Europe, an increasing number of American herbalists and even traditional physicians here are now contemplating various other uses for it.

Forms Available Include:

Capsule, dried leaves, elixir, extract, flowers, infusion, injection, liquid extract, tincture. Some may be hard to find in the United States.

Dosage Commonly Reported:

An infusion is made with 1 teaspoon (1.8 grams) of chopped leaves and flowers and is drunk two or three times per day over several weeks. Alternatively, 1 teaspoon of tincture is taken morning and night for several weeks. Two to three 455-milligram capsules containing the flower or fruit are taken two to three times a day.

Will It Work for You? What the Studies Say:

This intensively researched herb is powerful and often effective, but demands considerable care and professional guidance. Findings from test-tube, animal, and a handful of human studies indicate that standardized extracts may help the heart in a number of ways. Perhaps most importantly, they dilate (widen) blood vessels, especially the coronary blood vessels. This lowers resistance to flow, enabling more oxygen-rich blood to get to the heart and potentially reducing the risk that the heart will be deprived of oxygen, possibly causing painful sensations of chest pressure and tightness commonly known as angina pectoris to develop. Dilation of the blood vessels can also improve blood circulation, which can cause related swelling of the legs and feet to subside. By dilating the blood vessels and improving the circulation around the heart, hawthorn may also stabilize blood pressure so that the heart does not have to work as hard to pump blood through the body. Research indicates that hawthorn can even strengthen the heart muscle by making it squeeze (pump) harder. Most of the herb's heart activity is attributed to the presence of chemicals called oligomeric procyanidins. Various flavonoids probably contribute as well.

These kinds of beneficial effects have been observed in numerous, well-designed clinical trials. For example, in a 1993 study, thirty individuals with heart failure (cardiac insufficiency) were randomly selected to take either hawthorn capsules or a placebo two times a day for eight weeks.[1] Various heart-related parameters significantly improved in many of the subjects taking the hawthorn capsules, but not in those taking the placebo. In another important trial, 120 people with mild to moderate congestive heart failure were given a hawthorn tincture or a placebo. The subjects who took hawthorn experienced a significant improvement in heart function and reported considerably fewer palpitations and less shortness of breath than the subjects taking the placebo.[2]

Standardized hawthorn extracts are also occasionally prescribed to normalize heart-rhythm disturbances (arrhythmias). In some parts of the world, including Germany, this kind of regimen is typically recommended for elderly individuals who complain of arrhythmia-related symptoms.[3] German health authorities have approved of taking hawthorn for mild bradyarrhythmias (abnormal, slow heart rhythms), mild heart failure, and angina pectoris.[4] The herb is also given to treat what German texts refer to as "aging" hearts (probably meaning weakened hearts) for which digitalis, a drug commonly given for congestive heart failure and other heart conditions, is not yet needed. Hawthorn is appropriate for preventing only mild and stable angina pectoris.

Some experts contend that people should use hawthorn only as a preventive agent and in certain cases to supplement other more proven, easily standardized drug treatments.[5] Most heart ailments are serious conditions that require a doctor's care in any case.

Research also indicates that hawthorn can prevent increases in, and occasionally actually lower, cholesterol, triglyceride, and blood sugar levels in animals.[6] These findings raise hopes that the herb might help limit cholesterol deposits along artery walls that contribute to atherosclerosis (hardening of the arteries). Much more research is needed, however, before drawing any conclusions about this.

Higher doses of hawthorn can markedly depress (slow down) the central nervous system, which may explain why people have used the herb to treat sleeplessness. Scientists attribute this property to the presence of chemicals in the plant called dehydrocatechins,[7] and have observed this reaction in laboratory mice.[8] Other studies indicate that the herb may function as a mild diuretic ("water pill") and antioxidant[9] but little more data on these subjects are available.

Will It Harm You? What the Studies Say:

Most people tolerate hawthorn well and toxic reactions are uncommon, usually developing only when more than the recommended amount is taken. This was the finding of an investigator who did an extensive review of the literature on hawthorn in the late 1980s.[10] After a rigorous review, German health authorities could likewise identify no side effects or situations in which hawthorn should not be taken.[11]

By the same token, hawthorn is a potent herb that must be used with knowledge and care. It affects such crucial systems as the heart and circulation and is prescribed to treat serious, potentially life-threatening heart conditions. Self-diagnosis and self-treatment of such conditions qualify as unwise at best. For these reasons, most herbalists strongly urge that hawthorn be taken only under the guidance of a doctor. Not surprisingly, this "mild" heart tonic can cause not-so-mild complications if taken in doses substantially higher than recommended. Sedation and dangerously low blood pressure can develop. The FDA placed hawthorn on its formerly maintained list of "Herbs of Undefined Safety."

Do not take hawthorn with other heart medications such as digitalis unless a doctor recommends it. Children and pregnant or nursing women should probably avoid it as well. German health authorities recommend that people not take the herb for more than six weeks at a time.

Remember, hawthorn will not stop an angina attack.

GENERAL SOURCES:

Bisset, N.G., ed. *Herbal Drugs and Phytopharmaceuticals.* Stuttgart: medpharm GmbH Scientific Publishers, 1994.

Blumenthal, M., J. Gruenwald, T. Hall, and R.S. Rister, eds. *The Complete German Commission E Monographs: Therapeutic Guide to Herbal Medicine.* Boston: Integrative Medicine Communications, 1998.

Castleman, M. *The Healing Herbs: The Ultimate Guide to the Curative Power of Nature's Medicines.* New York: Bantam Books, 1995.

Chen, J.D. *Review of Nutrition and Dietetics.* 77 (1995): 147–54.

Heinerman, J. *Heinerman's Encyclopedia of Healing Herbs and Spices.* West Nyack, NY: Parker Publishing Co., 1996.

Lawrence Review of Natural Products. St. Louis: Facts and Comparisons, January 1994.

Li, L.D., et al. *Journal of Traditional Chinese Medicine.* 4(4) (1984): 283–88, 289–92.

Nasa, Y., et al. *Arzneimittel-Forschung.* 43(9) (1993): 945–49.

Mayell, M. *Off-the-Shelf Natural Health: How to Use Herbs and Nutrients to Stay Well.* New York: Bantam Books, 1995.

Mindell, E. *Earl Mindell's Herb Bible.* New York: Simon & Schuster/Fireside, 1992.

Petkov, V. *American Journal of Chinese Medicine.* 7(3) (1979): 197–236.

Rodale, J.I. *The Hawthorn Berry for the Heart.* Emmaus, PA: Rodale Books, 1971.

Shanthi, S., et al. *Indian Journal of Biochemistry and Biophysics.* 31(2) (1994): 143–46.

Schussler, M., et al. *Arzneimittel-Forschung.* 45(8) (1995): 842–45.

Stepka, W., and A.D. Winters. *Lloydia.* 36 (1973): 431.

Thompson, E.B., et al. *Journal of Pharmaceutical Sciences.* 63 (1974): 1936.

Tyler, V.E. *Herbs of Choice: The Therapeutic Use of Phytomedicinals.* Binghamton, NY: Haworth Press/Pharmaceutical Products Press, 1994.

———. *The Honest Herbal.* Binghamton, NY: Haworth Press/Pharmaceutical Products Press, 1993.

Tyler, V.E., L.R. Brady, and J.E. Robbers, eds. *Pharmacognosy.* Philadelphia: Lea & Febiger, 1988.

Wagner, H., and J. Grevel. *Planta Medica.* 45 (1982): 98.

Weiss, R.F. *Herbal Medicine,* trans. A.R. Meuss, from the 6th German edition. Beaconsfield, England: Beaconsfield Publishers, Ltd., 1988.

TEXT CITATIONS:

1. H. Leuchtgens, *Fortschritte der Medizin*, 111(20–21) (1993): 352–54.
2. M. Iwamoto et al., *Planta Medica*, 42 (1981): 1.
3. R.F. Weiss, *Herbal Medicine*, trans. A. R. Meuss, from the 6th German edition (Beaconsfield, England: Beaconsfield Publishers, Ltd., 1988).
4. M. Blumenthal, J. Gruenwald, T. Hall, and R.S. Rister, eds., *The Complete German Commission E Monographs: Therapeutic Guide to Herbal Medicine* (Boston: Integrative Medicine Communications, 1998).
5. V.E. Tyler, *Herbs of Choice: The Therapeutic Use of Phytomedicinals* (Binghamton, NY: Haworth Press/Pharmaceutical Products Press, 1994).
6. G. He, *Chung Hsi I Ho Tsa Chih*, 10 (1990): 361. *Lawrence Review of Natural Products* (St. Louis: Facts and Comparisons, January 1994).
7. W. Rewerski et al., *Arzneimittel-Forschung*, 21 (1971): 886.
8. R. Della Loggia et al., *Rivista di Neurologica*, 51(5) (1981): 297–310.
9. T. Bahorun et al., *Planta Medica*, 60(4) (1994): 323–28.
10. N.W. Hamon, *Canadian Pharmaceutical Journal*, 121 (1988): 708–9, 724.
11. Blumenthal et al., op. cit.

PRIMARY NAME:

HENNA

SCIENTIFIC NAME:
Lawsonia inermis L., sometimes referred to as *Lawsonia inermis* forma alba LAM. Family: Lythraceae

COMMON NAME:
N/A

RATING:
1 = Years of use and extensive, high-quality studies indicate that this substance is very effective and safe when used in recommended amounts for the indication(s) noted in the "Will It Work for You?" section.

What Is Henna?

The crumpled leaves of *Lawsonia inermis*, a plant believed to be indigenous to the Mediterranean region, are used medicinally and as a hair coloring.

What It Is Used For:

Lucille Ball took her cue from the ancients when she borrowed a little "bottled nature"—a paste made from the powdered leaves of *Lawsonia inermis*—to boost her famous red mop. Down through the ages, body parts from nails to beards, palms, and even horse manes have been graced with a reddish tint from henna.

External formulations have also been enlisted to treat eczema, skin sores, and scabies infestations.

Forms Available Include:

Powder. Sometimes mixed with other colorings.

Dosage Commonly Reported:

To use commercial hair-care products containing henna, follow the package instructions.

Will It Work for You? What the Studies Say:

Henna's hair-dying properties can be attributed to a chemical in the herb called lawsone. The ancients were the first to recognize the herb's coloring powers. A paste made with hot water and powdered leaves will color the hair, with deeper colors resulting from the addition of lemon juice or sour milk. The final hair color will depend in part on how long the dye is left on, and how well it is fixed with moist heat.[1]

Without special treatment or other added coloring, henna will turn white hair light blond, ash-blond hair medium red, blond hair to blond hair with reddish shimmers (with weak preparations), brownish hair red, chestnut-brown hair mahogany red, and dark brown hair brown with a reddish sheen.[2] Black hair is not influenced. Natural hair colors are typically produced by adding indigo leaves, which with their blue color neutralize henna's redness.

Henna leaf contains 5 to 10 percent tannins, astringent substances that tighten tissue and possibly explain its folk use for skin disorders such as eczema and sores and for mouth inflammation. Western sources do not recommend the herb for these purposes anymore, however.

Will It Harm You? What the Studies Say:

No reports of serious adverse reactions to external formulations of henna appear in the medical literature.

GENERAL SOURCES:
Bisset, N.G., ed. *Herbal Drugs and Phytopharmaceuticals.* Stuttgart: medpharm GmbH Scientific Publishers, 1994.
Weiner, M.A., and J.A. Weiner. *Herbs That Heal: Prescription for Herbal Healing.* Mill Valley, CA: Quantum Books, 1994.

TEXT CITATIONS:
1. N.G. Bisset, ed. *Herbal Drugs and Phytopharmaceuticals* (Stuttgart: medpharm GmbH Scientific Publishers, 1994).
2. Ibid.

PRIMARY NAME:
HIBISCUS

SCIENTIFIC NAME:
Hibiscus sabdariffa L. Family: Malvaceae

COMMON NAMES:
Jamaica sorrel, karkade, red sorrel, red tea, roselle juice, Sudanese tea

RATING:
4 = Research indicates that this herb will not fulfill the claims made for it, but that it is also unlikely to cause any harm.

What Is Hibiscus?

Striking ruby-red flowers bloom on the *Hibiscus sabdariffa*, an annual native to tropical Africa. Today it grows in tropical climates from Sri Lanka to Mexico. The part of the flower used medicinally—the calyxes, or outer floral envelopes—are picked while still immature, then dried.

What It Is Used For:

African folk healers have long recommended hibiscus for reducing muscle spasms, fighting infections, and encouraging the flow of urine (as a diuretic, or "water pill"), among other things. They apparently use the leaves as a skin emollient. Egyptians treat nerve and heart disorders with the plant.[1] In Western countries, hibiscus is best known for its distinctive red color and refreshing, tart taste in herbal teas. Through the years, countless jams, jellies, beverages, and other foods have been concocted with hibiscus flowers. They even add a special kick to perfumes and sachets.

Forms Available:

Dried herb, infusion (hot or cool), tea bags.

Dosage Commonly Reported:

An infusion is made using 1.5 grams (a scant ¾ teaspoon) dried herb per cup of water. To use the commercial tea bags containing hibiscus, follow the package instructions.

Will It Work for You? What the Studies Say:

Hibiscus may have slight laxative and diuretic effects when drunk in large quantities, according to scientific research, but the other medicinal claims made for it have essentially not been substantiated. Various plant acids—primarily hibiscus acid, although oxalic, malic, citric, and tartaric acids are also present—are held responsible for the mild laxative action, as well as for imparting the tart taste to this thirst-quenching drink.[2] According to various sources, one should not expect much laxative relief from hibiscus tea.[3] One test-tube study indicates that at high concentrations it may even be constipating, inhibiting intestinal motility (movement).[4]

Citing a lack of substantiating evidence, German health authorities declined to approve of hibiscus flower for a variety of proposed uses, including to relieve constipation, stimulate the appetite, clear upper respiratory tract congestion, help treat chills, function as a diuretic, or treat circulation disorders.[5] They do not object to its use in teas for enhancing appearance and taste.

Reports that hibiscus can lower blood pressure are apparently based on 1960s studies in dogs that found a short and transitory drop in pressure upon injection with large amounts of a liquid extract of the herb.[6] The conclusion that drinking hibiscus tea will therefore help reduce blood pressure in humans is far-fetched. Similarly, slight antibacterial and worm-killing properties identified in the plant appear to be of no practical use for human beings.[7]

A 1994 study reported potentially significant findings for people prone to kidney stone formation.[8] The concentration of certain salts in the urine can increase the risk of these stones. In the study, which involved healthy volunteers in Thailand, output of certain salts through the urine decreased significantly with consumption of 16 grams of hibiscus juice a day, actually more than with a higher dose of 24 grams a day.

Will It Harm You? What the Studies Say:

Generations have used hibiscus flowers medicinally to no apparent ill effect. German health authorities cite no known side effects.[9] Mice injected with fluid extracts of hibiscus developed adverse reactions and died within 24 hours; as with many substances, the concerns this may raise probably have no bearing on consuming the herb orally.[10]

If you are taking the antimalarial drug chloroquine and want to use hibiscus, you may want to advise your doctor of a 1994 study that found that a common drink in the Sudan made from hibiscus significantly reduced the effectiveness of this medicine.[11] Do not stop taking the chloroquine without consulting your doctor.

GENERAL SOURCES:

Bisset, N.G., ed. *Herbal Drugs and Phytopharmaceuticals*. Stuttgart: medpharm GmbH Scientific Publishers, 1994.

Blumenthal, M., J. Gruenwald, T. Hall, and R.S. Rister, eds., *The Complete German Commission E Monographs: Therapeutic Guide to Herbal Medicine*. Boston: Integrative Medicine Communications, 1998.

Lawrence Review of Natural Products. St. Louis: Facts and Comparisons, October 1990.

Leung, A.Y., and S. Foster. *Encyclopedia of Common Natural Ingredients Used in Food, Drugs, and Cosmetics*. 2nd ed. New York: John Wiley & Sons, 1996.

Tyler, V.E. *The Honest Herbal*. Binghamton, NY: Haworth Press/Pharmaceutical Products Press, 1993.

Tyler, V.E., L.R. Brady, and J.E. Robbers, eds. *Pharmacognosy*. Philadelphia: Lea & Febiger, 1988.

Weiss, R.F. *Herbal Medicine*, trans. A.R. Meuss, from the 6th German edition Beaconsfield, England: Beaconsfield Publishers, Ltd., 1988.

TEXT CITATIONS:

1. A.M. Osman et al., *Phytochemistry*, 14 (1975): 829.
2. V.E., Tyler, L.R. Brady, and J.E. Robbers, eds., *Pharmacognosy* (Philadelphia: Lea & Febiger, 1988).
3. R.F. Weiss, *Herbal Medicine*, trans. A.R. Meuss, from the 6th German edition (Beaconsfield, England: Beaconsfield Publishers, Ltd., 1988).
4. A. Sharaf, *Planta Medica*, 10 (1962): 48.
5. M. Blumenthal, J. Gruenwald, T. Hall, and R.S. Rister, eds., *The Complete German Commission E Monographs: Therapeutic Guide to Herbal Medicine* (Boston: Integrative Medicine Communications, 1998).
6. Sharaf, op. cit..
7. A. Sharaf and A. Gineidi, *Planta Medica*, 11 (1963): 109. Sharaf, op. cit. *Lawrence Review of Natural Products* (St. Louis: Facts and Comparisons, October 1990).
8. S. Kirdpon et al., *Journal of the Medical Association of Thailand*, 77(6) (1994): 314–21.
9. Blumental et al., op. cit.
10. Sharaf, op. cit.
11. B.M. Mahmoud et al., *Journal of Antimicrobial Chemotherapy*, 33(5) (1994): 1005–9.

PRIMARY NAME:
HONEY

SCIENTIFIC NAME:
N/A

COMMON NAMES:
Clarified, purified, or strained honey; mel

What Is Honey?

Honey is a viscid saccharine substance that bees (*Apis mellifera* L.) regurgitate into honeycombs after collecting the nectar of various flowers and briefly processing it in their systems to form dextrose, fructose, and other sugars. The flavor and color of honey reflect the type of nectar and flowers the bee came into contact with. Honey is purified by melting it, removing impurities, and adding water.

What It Is Used For:

Along with its classic use as a sweetener, honey long ago acquired a reputation for providing important nutrients and having healing properties. Contemporary herbalists who extol the virtues of honey as a soothing remedy for coughs and sore throats, a wound-healing antiseptic, a sleep agent, a diarrhea cure, an asthma remedy, and a treatment for skin ulcers and other skin problems are

HONEY (Continued)

echoing advice given by traditional healers of ancient Egypt. Traditional Chinese healers have used honey in similar ways, also counting on it to help remedy constipation, stomachache, and sinusitis, as well as using it as a binding agent to make pills.[1] Relatively recent proposed uses for honey in the West include boosting energy and treating eye ailments, constipation, and arthritis pain. Honey can be found as a fragrance and additive in many shampoos, bath products, and cosmetics.

Forms Available Include:

Raw and processed (purified or clarified) honey of various origins. Honey in honeycomb sections.

Dosage Commonly Reported:

Honey to taste is added to hot liquids in order to soothe sore throats.

Will It Work for You? What the Studies Say:

This tasty, syrupy liquid contains vitamins C, B_1 and B_2; minerals; and other nutritious components, but all in relatively small amounts.[2] Its fame as an antiseptic and wound healer may be justified in some cases, according to recent research. Investigators have found that honey from the nectar of certain plants may fight common infection-causing bacteria, rendering it a potentially effective antiseptic for wounds.[3] The honeybee may contribute antibacterial substances as well.[4] Other studies have identified antibacterial and antifungal properties in a honey extract.[5]

Probably because of these properties, success has been reported in healing wounds, leg ulcers, burns (treated in the hospital), and skin grafts with honey.[6] Stomach and duodenal ulcers are often caused by a bacteria called *Helicobacter pylori*; several investigators have reported success in eradicating this bacteria using honey and thus helping to heal the ulcer.[7] Chinese and Japanese researchers found beneficial effects in treating several hundred ulcer sufferers with fresh honey three times a day; pain and the associated ulcer resolved in more than 82 percent of individuals, typically within a few weeks.[8] This study was apparently not randomized and the patients knew they were taking honey, possibly inserting bias into the results.

Although a lot of intriguing findings are being published, minimal and in some cases no substantiating information can be found for many of the other claims made for honey, including that it can reduce arthritis pain or cure cancer. For example, a report suggesting anticancer properties in rat and mice tumors remains to be verified by other investigators, and its implications for treating human cancers are far from clear.[9] A 1995 study reported that many people may get a laxative effect with honey—possibly accompanied by stomach upset—because their systems fail to absorb the fructose completely.[10]

Many healing traditions consider honey a soothing agent for sore throats and cough, especially when added to a hot liquid such as tea or lemonade or when used in a gargle or lozenge. No clinical trials have apparently been conducted so far, but your own experience (and enjoyment) may justify its use.

Will It Harm You? What the Studies Say:

Most honey is very safe to consume, gargle, and place on the skin, as well as to administer to (properly cleaned) minor sores and wounds. The risk of poisoning arises, however, if the bee collects nectar from a poisonous plant, such as jimsonweed.[11] In some parts of the world, there has been a rise in these kinds of poisonings as people increasingly buy raw honey straight from the bee-keeper.[12] Some people are also allergic to honey, most likely to the secretions of the honeybee or the pollen proteins contained in the honey.[13] A 1995 report indicated that honey allergy is rare in individuals sensitive to pollens, however.[14] Given the risk for contamination with *Clostridium botulinum* spores, which can cause a serious and sometimes fatal illness called botulism, honey should not be given to infants under one year old;[15] no ill effects appear to develop in older children and adults infected with these spores, however.

GENERAL SOURCES:

Balch, J.F., and P.A. Balch. *Prescription for Nutritional Healing: A Practical A to Z Reference to Drug-Free Remedies Using Vitamins, Minerals, Herbs & Food Supplements.* 2nd ed. Garden City Park, NY: Avery Publishing Group, 1997.

Lawrence Review of Natural Products. St. Louis: Facts and Comparisons, October 1995.

Leung, A.Y. *Chinese Healing Foods and Herbs.* Glen Rock, NJ: AYSL Corp, 1984.

Leung, A.Y., and S. Foster. *Encyclopedia of Common Natural Ingredients Used in Food, Drugs, and Cosmetics.* 2nd ed. New York: John Wiley & Sons, 1996.

Tyler, V.E. *Herbs of Choice: The Therapeutic Use of Phytomedicinals.* Binghamton, NY: Haworth Press/Pharmaceutical Products Press, 1994.

———. *The Honest Herbal.* Binghamton, NY: Haworth Press/Pharmaceutical Products Press, 1993.

Tyler, V.E., L.R. Brady, and J.E. Robbers, eds. *Pharmacognosy.* Philadelphia: Lea & Febiger, 1988.

TEXT CITATIONS:

1. A.Y. Leung and S. Foster. *Encyclopedia of Common Natural Ingredients Used in Food, Drugs, and Cosmetics,* 2nd ed. (New York: John Wiley & Sons, 1996).
2. Ibid.
3. T. Postmes et al., *The Lancet.* 341(8847) (1993): 756–57. D. Greenwood, *The Lancet,* 341 (1993): 191. Leung and Foster, op. cit.
4. P. Casteels et al., *European Journal of Biochemistry,* 187(2) (1990): 381.
5. *Lawrence Review of Natural Products* (St. Louis: Facts and Comparisons, October 1995). S.E. Efem et al., *Infection,* 20(4) (1992): 227. S.S. Radwan et al., *Zentralblatt fuer Mikrobiologie,* 139(4) (1984): 249. E.E. Obaseiki-Ebor and T.C. Afonya, *Journal of Pharmaceutical Pharmacology,* 36(4) (1984): 283.
6. A.Y. Leung, *Chinese Healing Foods and Herbs* (Glen Rock, NJ: AYSL Corp, 1984). *Lawrence Review of Natural Products,* op. cit. Postmes, op. cit. I.H. Bourne, *Journal of the Royal Society of Medicine,* 84(11) (1991): 693. M. Subrahmanyam, *British Journal of Plastic Surgery,* 46(4) (1993): 322. Greenwood, op. cit. M. Subrahmanyam, *Burns,* 22(6) (1996): 491–93. G. Ndayisaba et al., *Revue de Chirurgie Orthopedique et Reparatrice de I Appareil Moteur,* 79(2) (1993): 111–13.
7. N. al Somal et al., *Journal of the Royal Society of Medicine,* 87(1) (1994): 9.
8. Leung, op. cit.
9. N.V. Gribel and V.G. Pashinskii, *Voprosy Onkologii,* 36(6) (1990): 704. *Lawrence Review of Natural Products,* op. cit.
10. S.D. Ladas et al., *American Journal of Clinical Nutrition,* 62(6) (1995): 1212–15.

11. *Lawrence Review of Natural Products,* op. cit.
12. S. Geroulanos et al., *Schweizerische Rundschau für Medizin Praxis*, l81(17) (1992): 535–40.
13. L. Bauer et al., *Journal of Allergy & Clinical Immunology*, 97(Pt 1) (1996): 65–73.
14. R. Kiistala et al., *Allergy*, 50(1) (1995): 844–47.
15. R.A. Mangione, *American Pharmacy*, NS23 (1983): 5. L. Fenicia et al., *European Journal of Epidemiology*, 9(6) (1993): 671–73.

PRIMARY NAME:
HONEYSUCKLE

SCIENTIFIC NAME:
Lonicera japonica Thunb. and other *Lonicera* species. Family: Caprifoliaceae

COMMON NAMES:
Jim yin hua, rendong, shuanghua

RATING:
3 = Studies on the effectiveness and safety of this substance are conflicting, or there are not enough studies to draw a conclusion.

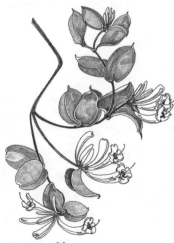

Honeysuckle
Lonicera japonica

What Is Honeysuckle?

The trailing honeysuckle shrub, a native of Asia, now runs wild through many parts of North America. Traditional Chinese healers and Western herbalists most commonly use the Japanese honeysuckle, *Lonicera japonica.* The dried flower buds are used medicinally, as are the leaves and stems on occasion. Pickers collect the fragrant flowers on late spring and early summer mornings after the dew has evaporated.[1]

What It Is Used For:

Traditional Chinese healers have used honeysuckle as a medicinal remedy for hundreds of years for "heat"-associated conditions such as fever, inflammatory diseases like rheumatoid arthritis, acute (as opposed to chronic) infections, and inflamed and itchy skin. Several prominent Chinese cold remedies contain the herb. It is given as a "detoxifying" agent for such "toxic" conditions as poisoning (due to food, drugs, heavy metals, etc.), swellings, and boils. Diarrhea and various cancers have been treated with it as well. Some Chinese skin-care products contain the herb for its purported astringent and antimicrobial actions. Honeysuckle is used far more commonly as a medicinal herb in China than in the West.

Forms Available Include:

Decoction, flower, infusion (for internal or external use), pill, poultice, stem, tincture, vine. In China, there are numerous grades of honeysuckle flower based on purity, location of source, and amount of contained opened flowers. Honeysuckle flower is a common ingredient in Chinese herbal blends.

Dosage Commonly Reported:

An infusion is made with 10 grams of flowers per cup of water. In China a common dosage calls for 9 to 15 grams of dried flowers in decoction, pill, poultice, and other forms.

Will It Work for You? What the Studies Say:

This herb has been studied primarily by Chinese researchers. They have unveiled a number of chemical constituents—chlorogenic acid and luteolin are believed to be critical ones—that may help explain traditional uses. Most of the studies have been done in test tubes or on small animals, with apparently none so far in humans.

Anti-inflammatory properties have been shown in several classic animal tests for inflammation, as well as immune-system-stimulating actions (including activation of phagocytosis in mice), inhibition of tumor formation in animals, prevention of stomach ulcers in test rats, and reduced cholesterol absorption in rabbits on a high-cholesterol diet.[2] Whether these actions explain honeysuckle's traditional use for inflammatory conditions such as arthritis, for example, remains undetermined.

Similarly, honeysuckle flower has proved active against certain viruses including influenza viruses (responsible for colds) and HIV (responsible for causing AIDS)[3] in test-tube studies. It also fights bacteria commonly responsible for various skin and other infections including *Staphylococcus aureus*, *Mycobacterium tuberculosis* (which causes tuberculosis), and *Salmonella typhi* (known to cause food poisoning).[4] In animal studies, the chlorogenic acid in honeysuckle flowers has demonstrated an ability to prevent the formation of cancer-causing compounds.[5]

The flowers contain astringent tannins, which, together with the herb's anti-inflammatory and antibacterial properties, may help explain its long-standing popularity in skin creams and lotions.

Will It Harm You? What the Studies Say:

Very little information on the safety profile of this herb can be found in the medical literature. Plant experts report that its toxicity in mice is low.[6] Its long-standing use in traditional Chinese medicine should be taken into consideration.

GENERAL SOURCES:

Leung, A.Y. *Chinese Healing Foods and Herbs.* Glen Rock, NJ: AYSL Corp, 1984.

Leung, A.Y., and S. Foster. *Encyclopedia of Common Natural Ingredients Used in Food, Drugs, and Cosmetics.* 2nd ed. New York: John Wiley & Sons, 1996.

Ody, P. *The Herb Society's Complete Medicinal Herbal.* London, England: Dorling Kindersley Limited, 1993.

Tierra, M. *The Way of Herbs.* New York: Pocket Books, 1990.

TEXT CITATIONS:

1. A.Y. Leung and S. Foster, *Encyclopedia of Common Natural Ingredients Used in Food, Drugs, and Cosmetics,* 2nd ed. (New York: John Wiley & Sons, 1996).
2. G.Y. Song et al., *Zhongcaoyao,* 16(5) (1985): 37. Leung and Foster, op. cit.
3. Leung and Foster, op. cit.
4. Ibid.
5. A.Y. Leung, *Chinese Healing Foods and Herbs* (Glen Rock, NJ: AYSL Corp, 1984).
6. Ibid.

H

Honeysuckle

PRIMARY NAME:
HOPS

SCIENTIFIC NAME:
Humulus lupulus L. Family:
Cannabaceae (Moraceae)

COMMON NAMES:
Common hops, European hops,
humulus, lupulin

RATING:
3 = Studies on the effectiveness
and safety of this substance are
conflicting, or there are not
enough studies to draw a
conclusion.

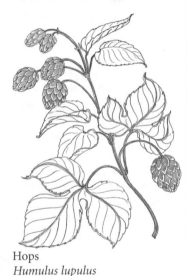

Hops
Humulus lupulus

What Are Hops?

Humulus lupulus is a perennial vine native to North America and Europe and now cultivated around the world. It bears tiny flowers. The hops bitters (bitter acids that function as flavoring agents) are contained in the yellowish glandular hairs that cover the female's pale green conelike fruit. The fruit and the separated glandular hairs (lupulin) are used medicinally.

What They Are Used For:

Hops are best known for the distinctive bitter taste they give to beer; they also help preserve it. Today's beer drinkers may not know, however, that hops have a long history in folk medicine for treating such conditions as restlessness, nervous diarrhea, appetite loss, and intestinal cramping.

Since ancient times, "sleep pillows" or "dream pillows" stuffed with hops were tucked under the heads of insomniacs and restless sleepers to help make them drowsy. The logic behind this gained reinforcement with the observation that hops pickers tend to become unusually tired. Native Americans considered hops a sedative, and the *U.S. Pharmacopeia* classified the herb as a sedative for nearly a century, up until 1916. Contemporary herbalists recommend the herb as a sleep aid and remedy for restlessness, stress, and extreme excitability. German herbalists and some physicians combine it with other sedatives for these purposes as well as to alleviate nervous diarrhea and to control sexual neuroses.

Hops infusions are also recommended to stimulate the appetite and ease digestion. Both Native American and Chinese healers considered the plant a digestive aid. The Chinese also value it as a treatment for pulmonary tuberculosis, leprosy, infectious diarrhea, and bladder inflammation. Hops extracts are occasionally added to skin creams and lotions for their reported skin-softening properties.

Forms Available Include:

Bath additives, concentrated drops, decoction, dried, extract, fruit (fresh or dried), infusion.

Dosage Commonly Reported:

As a sedative, a common dosage is 0.5 grams hops in the form of an infusion or other preparation. The concentrated drops are taken in doses of 1 or 2 droppersful. Use fresh hops as a digestive aid and dried, aged hops as a sedative.

Will They Work for You? What the Studies Say:

The power of hops to promote sedation remains a matter of confusion and dispute. A 1967 German study found that when taken orally, hops resin did not depress (slow down) central nervous system activity;[1] this suggests that it would not be able to cause sedation. But in 1983, scientists identified a sedative chemical in the bitter principle of hops, the volatile chemical dimethylvinyl carbinol (2-methyl-3-butene-2-ol). Although only small amounts were found in the fresh leaves, the concentration of this chemical appears to increase with time.[2] Investigators also found that animals treated with the chemical became notably sleepy. But to confuse matters again, a German investigator reported in 1992 that a lot of hops—150 grams—would be needed to produce a single dose potent enough to make a human being drowsy.[3] In other words, the hops-filled pillow would have to be quite formidable indeed. Clearly, more studies on the subject are needed. German health authorities approve of hops for sleep problems, restlessness, and anxiety, and note that combining hops with other sedative drugs (presumably herbal ones) may be advantageous.[4]

Another ongoing subject of debate is whether hops contain chemicals that function something like the female hormone estrogen. Long ago, it was noted that girls picking hops in the fields tended to get their menstrual periods earlier than expected. Scientists reported detecting a significant level of estrogenic activity in a part of the hops plant.[5] Certain German physicians and herbalists point to such evidence to explain why they prescribe hops (especially very fresh hops) to dampen sexual arousal or control sexual neuroses in men. Other experts disagree, asserting that hops exert no hormonal action at all.[6] In a series of 1973 experiments, animals fed a variety of hops extracts failed to show evidence of estrogenic (or any other hormonal) activity.[7] No well-designed clinical trials have been carried out to determine the potential impact of hops on women's menstrual periods, men's sexual arousal, or any other hormone-related condition.

Hops belong to the same plant family (Cannabaceae) as marijuana. Some people recommend smoking the plant to get a mild high. Whether this works or is safe has yet to be shown scientifically, however. The smoker may accumulate unwanted side effects instead of the desired euphoria—known as being "hopped up"[8] in 1950s terms.

Hops may have merit as a digestive aid. Research indicates that alcoholic extracts of the plant inhibit spasms in the digestive tract and other isolated smooth muscles.[9] Studies to prove this in humans have not been done. The bitter-tasting components also explain, at least in part, the enduring popularity of hops for treating indigestion and stimulating the appetite. Test-tube analyses also show that the bitter acids in hops fight certain bacteria (including *Staphylococcus aureus*) and fungi. The presence of these acids partially explains why hops help preserve beer and possibly why Chinese physicians turn to the plant to fight tuberculosis and other infectious diseases.

Intriguing new research, although very preliminary, indicates that hops may one day be valuable in helping to fight certain kinds of tumors.[10] When considering taking hops for medicinal purposes, it is important to remember that the condition of the active compounds can differ notably from one variety of hops to the next and that the chemicals are quite sensitive to air, light, and time.

Will They Harm You? What the Studies Say:

Hops taken in the amounts typically recommended for medicinal purposes are not likely to cause side effects. German health authorities identify no situations in which a person should not take the herb, although an American herbalist recommends that pregnant women or those with estrogen-dependent breast cancer avoid hops, given that it may contain estrogenlike chemicals.[11] The FDA includes hops on its list of foods "Generally Recognized As Safe" (GRAS). Some sources recommend that individuals with depression not take hops because the herb may accentuate depressive symptoms and that care should be taken in mixing alcohol and any substance that has been reported to cause sedation.[12]

In some regions of the world, hops are considered a significant airborne pollen responsible for respiratory tract allergies. People who pick hops run the risk of a skin reaction (usually a rash) if they develop a sensitivity to them.

GENERAL SOURCES:

Bisset, N.G., ed. *Herbal Drugs and Phytopharmaceuticals.* Stuttgart: medpharm GmbH Scientific Publishers, 1994.

Blumenthal, M., J. Gruenwald, T. Hall, and R.S. Rister, eds. *The Complete German Commission E Monographs: Therapeutic Guide to Herbal Medicine.* Boston: Integrative Medicine Communications, 1998.

Bradley, P.C., ed. *British Herbal Compendium: A Handbook of Scientific Information on Widely Used Plant Drugs,* vol. 1. Bournemouth (Dorset), England: British Herbal Medicine Association, 1992.

Castleman, M. *The Healing Herbs: The Ultimate Guide to the Curative Power of Nature's Medicines.* New York: Bantam Books, 1995.

Langezaal, C.R., et al. *Pharmaceutisch Weekblad Scientific Edition,* 14(6) (1992): 353–56.

Lawrence Review of Natural Products. St. Louis: Facts and Comparisons, May 1991.

Leung, A.Y., and S. Foster. *Encyclopedia of Common Natural Ingredients Used in Food, Drugs, and Cosmetics.* 2nd ed. New York: John Wiley & Sons, 1996.

Newall, C.A., et al. *Herbal Medicines: A Guide for Health-Care Professionals.* London: The Pharmaceutical Press, 1996.

Schmalreck, A.F., et al. *Canadian Journal of Microbiology.* 21 (1975): 205.

Tyler, V.E. *The Honest Herbal.* Binghamton, NY: Haworth Press/Pharmaceutical Products Press, 1993.

Weiss, R.F. *Herbal Medicine,* trans. A.R. Meuss, from the 6th German edition. Beaconsfield, England: Beaconsfield Publishers, Ltd., 1988.

TEXT CITATIONS:

1. R. Hansel and H.H. Wagener, *Arzneimittel-Forschung.* 17 (1967): 79.
2. R. Wolfart et al., *Planta Medica,* 48 (1983): 120.
3. J. Holzl, *Zeitschrift für Phytotherapie,* 13 (1992): 155–61.
4. M. Blumenthal, J. Gruenwald, T. Hall, and R. S. Rister, eds., *The Complete German Commission E Monographs: Therapeutic Guide to Herbal Medicine* (Boston: Integrative Medicine Communications, 1998).
5. A. Zenisek and I.J. Bednar, *American Perfumer and Aromatics,* 75 (1960): 61.
6. *Lawrence Review of Natural Products* (St. Louis: Facts and Comparisons, May 1991).
7. C. Fenselau and P. Talalay, *Food & Cosmetics Toxicology,* 11 (1973): 597.
8. V.E. Tyler, *The Honest Herbal* (Binghamton, NY: Haworth Press/Pharmaceutical Products Press, 1993).
9. F. Caujolle et al., *Agressologie,* 10(5) (1969): 405–10.
10. K. Yasukawa et al, *Oncology,* 52(2) (1995): 156–58.
11. M. Castleman, *The Healing Herbs: The Ultimate Guide to the Curative Power of Nature's Medicines* (New York: Bantam Books, 1995).
12. C.A. Newall et al. *Herbal Medicines: A Guide for Health-Care Professionals* (London: The Pharmaceutical Press, 1996).

PRIMARY NAME:

HOREHOUND

SCIENTIFIC NAME:
Marrubium vulgare (Tourn.) L.
Family: Labiatae (Lamiaceae)

COMMON NAMES:
Common horehound,
hoarhound, marrubium, marvel

RATING:
1 = Years of use and extensive,
high-quality studies indicate
that this substance is very
effective and safe when used in
recommended amounts for the
indication(s) noted in the "Will
It Work for You?" section.

What Is Horehound?

This perennial flowering plant, a European native, grows in many parts of the world including North America. The distinctive woolly leaves are dried and the flowering tops, with their dense whorls of white flowers, are picked to prepare medicinal remedies.

What It Is Used For:

Horehound has been a popular cough and cold remedy since ancient Roman times. For many years in the United States horehound syrup and lozenges were billed as treatments for coughs, colds, and other minor respiratory problems. Users rated the taste so highly—the plant belongs to the mint family and has a fragrance reminiscent of apples—that manufacturers now flavor simple hard candies with the herb and add the extracts to many foods and alcoholic drinks.

Through the centuries, people have also turned to horehound to treat digestive problems, appetite loss, tuberculosis, sore throat, asthma, cancer, and malaria, as well as to encourage sweating and urination, to combat intestinal worms, and to promote menstruation. A number of prepared European cough and expectorant teas contain horehound, as do several liver and bile teas. The "hound" in the common name stems from the herb's reported use by ancient Greeks to treat mad-dog bite, and the "hore" ("hoar") derives from the downy whitish hairs that lend the plant a hoary appearance.

Forms Available Include:

Infusion, liquid extract, lozenge, powder, syrup, tea bag, tincture. Also available as a flavoring in hard candy.

Dosage Commonly Reported:

An infusion made using 1½ teaspoons (1.5 grams) of fresh chopped herb per cup of water is drunk several times per day. The liquid extract is taken in doses of 2 to 4 milliliters, the powdered herb in doses of 1 to 2 grams, and the herb syrup in doses of 2 to 4 milliliters. Numerous lozenges containing horehound are available; follow package instructions.

Will It Work for You? What the Studies Say:

Modern research validates the use of horehound as an expectorant and cough suppressant. Experts believe that a compound in the herb called marrubiin (or possibly its precursor, premarrubiin) stimulates the production of phlegm (mucus) in the airways. Once loosened, these formerly dry secretions are much easier to cough up. The other active component in horehound—a volatile oil—is reported to have expectorant actions as well.

To the confusion and consternation of many scientists and herbalists, the FDA banned horehound from over-the-counter cough remedies in 1989, saying that it did not find evidence supporting the effectiveness of this herb sufficiently convincing. German health authorities, on the other hand, approved the herb a year later for treating not only coughs and colds but indigestion, associated bloating, and appetite loss.[1]

Scattered animal studies offer preliminary information about horehound's value for these and various other uses. One examination in rats showed that a derivative of marrubiin—marrubiinic acid—temporarily encourages the flow of bile.[2] This property may be a key to horehound's value in aiding digestion, but scientists do not know much more about it. As bitters, marrubiin and pre-marrubiin stimulate the appetite by increasing the flow of saliva and gastric juices.[3]

Marrubiin has been reported to help normalize abnormal heart rhythms (cardiac arrhythmias) in animals, but is limited for this purpose because large doses can actually cause abnormal rhythms. The volatile oil may have vessel-expanding (vasodilator) effects, a quality valued for lowering blood pressure, but this property has not been tested in humans.[4]

Scientists have demonstrated blood-sugar-lowering effects with horehound in laboratory rabbits,[5] which means it may have potential as an antidiabetic medicine. More research is needed on this, however.

Will It Harm You? What the Studies Say:

Horehound appears to be safe to use in typically recommended amounts. As many as 5 cups of horehound tea daily do not cause any worrisome side effects.[6] However, very large doses of horehound may cause abnormal heart rhythms, so individuals with heart problems should probably avoid the herb. Large doses are also purgative (strongly laxative).[7]

GENERAL SOURCES:

Bisset, N.G., ed. *Herbal Drugs and Phytopharmaceuticals.* Stuttgart: medpharm GmbH Scientific Publishers, 1994.

Blumenthal, M., J. Gruenwald, T. Hall, and R.S. Rister, eds. *The Complete German Commission E Monographs: Therapeutic Guide to Herbal Medicine.* Boston: Integrative Medicine Communications, 1998.

Bradley, P.C., ed. *British Herbal Compendium: A Handbook of Scientific Information on Widely Used Plant Drugs,* vol. 1. Bournemouth (Dorset), England: British Herbal Medicine Association, 1992.

Castleman, M. *The Healing Herbs: The Ultimate Guide to the Curative Power of Nature's Medicines.* New York: Bantam Books, 1995.

Lawrence Review of Natural Products. St. Louis: Facts and Comparisons, September 1996.

Newall, C.A., et al. *Herbal Medicines: A Guide for Health-Care Professionals.* London: The Pharmaceutical Press, 1996.

Tyler, V.E. *Herbs of Choice: The Therapeutic Use of Phytomedicinals.* Binghamton, NY: Haworth Press/Pharmaceutical Products Press, 1994.

———. *The Honest Herbal.* Binghamton, NY: Haworth Press/Pharmaceutical Products Press, 1993.

TEXT CITATIONS:

1. M. Blumenthal, J. Gruenwald, T. Hall, and R. S. Rister, eds., *The Complete German Commission E Monographs: Therapeutic Guide to Herbal Medicine* (Boston: Integrative Medicine Communications, 1998).

2. I. Krejci and R. Zadina, *Planta Medica,* 7 (1959): 1–7.

3. P.C. Bradley, ed., *British Herbal Compendium: A Handbook of Scientific Information on Widely Used Plant Drugs* vol. 1 (Bournemouth [Dorset], England: British Herbal Medicine Association, 1992).

4. M.O. Karryev et al., *Izvestiya Akademii Nauk Turkmenskoi SRR, Seriy a Biologich-eskikh Nauk,* 3 (1976): 86.
5. R.R. Roman et al., *Archives of Medical Research,* 23(1) (1992): 59.
6. V.E. Tyler, *Herbs of Choice: The Therapeutic Use of Phytomedicinals* (Binghamton, NY: Haworth Press/Pharmaceutical Products Press, 1994).
7. C.A. Newall et al., *Herbal Medicines: A Guide for Health-Care Professionals* (London: The Pharmaceutical Press, 1996).

PRIMARY NAME:

HORSE CHESTNUT

SCIENTIFIC NAME:

Aesculus hippocastanum L.
Family: Hippocastanaceae

COMMON NAME:

Aesculus

RATING:

- *For internal use:* 1 = Years of use and extensive, high-quality studies indicate that this substance is very effective and safe when used in recommended amounts for the indication(s) noted in the "Will It Work for You?" section. Note the warning in the "Will It Harm You?" section, however.

- *For external use:* 3 = Studies on the effectiveness and safety of this substance are conflicting, or there are not enough studies to draw a conclusion.

What Is Horse Chestnut?

The stately horse chestnut tree bursts into bloom in May and June. The tree's fruit contains one to three large shiny brown seeds. These are commonly referred to as the "nuts," and are specially treated to create extracts and purified forms of the active ingredient, aescin. The leaves and bark are occasionally used for medicinal purposes as well. Do not confuse the horse chestnut with the sweet chestnut (*Castanea vesca*), a tree that bears the kind of nonpoisonous edible chestnuts stuffed in holiday turkeys and roasted on winter streets.

What It Is Used For:

For centuries, the fruits and seeds of the horse chestnut have been used to treat such broad-ranging ailments as colds, whooping cough, nerve pain, sunburn, backache, rheumatism, and fever. In Europe today, oral as well as topical horse chestnut seed preparations are sold to reduce inflammation and discomfort from varicose veins and ulcers, hemorrhoids, and similar kinds of vein inflammation (phlebitis). These kinds of preparations are starting to appear in United States health food outlets.

Forms Available Include:

- *For internal use:* Capsule, extract, injection solution, pill. Horse chestnut often appears in herbal blends.
- *For external use:* Gel, lotion, ointment, powder.

Dosage Commonly Reported:

A topical preparation is made with ½ teaspoon powder in 16 ounces water. A common initial internal dosage of the extract is 90 to 150 milligrams of aescin; this is later reduced to 35 to 70 milligrams daily following improvement. One 257-milligram capsule of the extract containing 18 to 22 percent aescin is taken with morning and evening meals. To use commercial gels, lotions, and ointments containing horse chestnut, follow package instructions.

Will It Work for You? What the Studies Say:

Extensive studies in animals and humans indicate that commercial horse chestnut seed extracts taken orally can reduce inflammation and swelling in varicose veins, hemorrhoids, and similar conditions. The most important medicinal substance in the seeds appears to be the saponin aescin, sometimes referred to as escin. It is a member of a class of plant compounds called terpenes. Studies

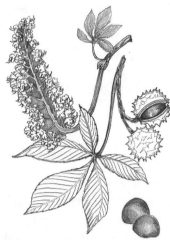

Horse Chestnut
Aesculus hippocastanum

show that aescin reduces the number and diameter of the tiny pores in the capillaries, the small blood vessels that build networks throughout the body. Thus, fluid is inhibited from passing through the capillary membranes, and swelling in surrounding tissues subsides. This "normalizing" effect occurs when the vessel walls are abnormally permeable and susceptible to edema.[1]

Studies in people with chronic venous insufficiency indicate that these properties translate into relief from leg edema and varicose veins.[2] In an important 1996 study, for example, 240 individuals with chronic deep vein incompetence were randomly given either dried horse chestnut seed extract (50 milligrams of aescin twice daily), compression stockings (a standard treatment for this problem), or a placebo over a period of twelve weeks. Compared with the subjects given the placebo, those treated with either active regimen experienced significant improvements in leg swelling by the end of the study. An earlier trial involving forty individuals with swollen leg veins produced similar results.[3] Importantly, subjects taking the horse chestnut seed extract tolerated it well.

Aescin serves another important function as well: it increases the tone and elasticity of the blood vessel walls. In so doing, it improves the blood flow to the heart,[4] and it has therefore been used as a "heart tonic." Little information on this subject is available. In Germany, horse chestnut extracts are sometimes given to prevent blood clots in women—especially those with varicose veins—who are about to undergo gynecologic surgery; varicose veins are a risk factor for blood clots.[5]

The ancient superstition that carrying a seed around in a pocket will ward off or cure arthritis or rheumatism persists, although there is no scientific justification to support it.

Lotions, ointments, and other topical horse chestnut seed preparations widely used in Europe for hemorrhoids and varicose veins have only recently been obtainable in the United States. Occasionally the bark and leaf are used to make these preparations. The FDA does not recommend any horse chestnut extract for hemorrhoids, however. Some plant experts question the value of these topical formulations, noting that no studies have verified that the active ingredient is absorbed into the skin well enough to make a difference.[6]

Will It Harm You? What the Studies Say:

The seeds of the horse chestnut tree are poisonous and must be specially prepared before being used medicinally. Never consume them in any form unless a knowledgeable manufacturer has processed them properly to remove all the toxins. Experts consider a number of the tree's components poisonous, but the glycoside aesculin in the nuts, leaves, twigs, and sprouts causes the most concern. If aesculin is not properly removed, the herb can cause weakness, muscle twitching, dilated pupils, vomiting, diarrhea, paralysis, and stupor.[7] Children have died after ingesting untreated seeds and tea. The seeds are the most toxic part of the plant. The FDA placed horse chestnut on its former list of "Herbs of Undefined Safety."

Once the toxins have been removed, however, oral horse chestnut preparations are relatively safe to use, although some people may develop stomach upset. In rare cases, injection forms have caused severe allergic reactions (anaphylactic shock) and kidney and liver damage.[8] But some of these people may have taken much more than the normally recommended dose. To be safe, use standardized extracts or dosage forms; these started to appear on the American market in the mid-1990s.

A drug for venous diseases (Venocuran) containing horse chestnut extracts has been implicated in causing pseudolupus,[9] a syndrome first described in 1972 that is characterized by muscle and joint pain, fever, and a number of other signs and symptoms. The role horse chestnut plays in the syndrome remains unclear, as the drug also contains cardiac glycosides and phenopyrazone.

External forms of horse chestnut do not pose the same hazards as the internal forms. However, in the early 1990s an investigator warned that potent carcinogens called aflatoxins may appear in certain commercial skin-cleansing products and other cosmetics containing horse chestnut extracts; the manufacturers are responsible for preventing this kind of contamination.[10]

GENERAL SOURCES:

Bisset, N.G., ed. *Herbal Drugs and Phytopharmaceuticals.* Stuttgart: medpharm GmbH Scientific Publishers, 1994.

Diehm, C., et al. *The Lancet.* 347(8997) (1996): 292–94.

Guillaume, M., and F. Padioleau. *Arzneimittel-Forschung.* 44(1) (1994): 25–35.

Lawrence Review of Natural Products. St. Louis: Facts and Comparisons, February 1995.

Leung, A.Y., and S. Foster. *Encyclopedia of Common Natural Ingredients Used in Food, Drugs, and Cosmetics.* 2nd ed. New York: John Wiley & Sons, 1996.

Mindell, E. *Earl Mindell's Herb Bible.* New York: Simon & Schuster/Fireside, 1992.

Newall, C.A., et al. *Herbal Medicines: A Guide for Health-Care Professionals.* London: The Pharmaceutical Press, 1996.

Popp, W., et al. *Allergy.* 47(4 Pt 2) (1992): 380–83.

Rothkopf, M., et al. *Arzneimittel-Forschung.* 27(3) (1977): 598–605.

Tyler, V.E. *Herbs of Choice: The Therapeutic Use of Phytomedicinals.* Binghamton, NY: Haworth Press/Pharmaceutical Products Press, 1994.

TEXT CITATIONS:

1. H. Siering, *Arzneimittel-Forschung,* 12 (1962): 1962.
2. G. Hitzenberger, *Wiener Medizinische Wochenschrift,* 139(17) (1989): 385.
3. C. Diehm et al., *Vasa,* 21(2) (1992): 188–92.
4. V.E. Tyler, *Herbs of Choice: The Therapeutic Use of Phytomedicinals* (Binghamton, NY: Haworth Press/Pharmaceutical Products Press, 1994).
5. J. Endl and W. Auinger, *Wiener Klinische Wochenschrift,* 89(9) (1977): 304–7.
6. Tyler, op. cit.
7. J.W. Hardin, and J.M. Arena, *Human Poisoning from Native and Cultivated Plants,* 2nd ed. (Durham, NC: Duke University Press, 1974).
8. H.J. Wagner, *Archiv für Toxicologie,* 21(2) (1965): 83–88. G. Vogel, *Zeitschfift für Phytotherapie,* 10 (1989): 102–6.
9. P.G. Grob et al., *The Lancet,* 2(7926) (1975): 144–48.
10. S. el-Dessouki, *Food and Chemical Toxicology,* 30(11) (1992): 993–94.

PRIMARY NAME:

HORSERADISH

SCIENTIFIC NAME:

Armoracia rusticana Gaertn., Mey., and Scherb. Also referred to as *Armoracia lapathiofolia* Gilib. and *Cochlearia armoracia.* Family: Cruciferae

COMMON NAME:

N/A

RATING:

3 = Studies on the effectiveness and safety of this substance are conflicting, or there are not enough studies to draw a conclusion.

What Is Horseradish?

The large, white, fleshy root of this flowering perennial is recognized as a condiment around the world. It has been cultivated for about two thousand years and was introduced into North America by the early colonists. Its small white flowers appear in spring. The fresh or dried roots are used medicinally.

What It Is Used For:

The sharp-tasting, bitter root of this enduring condiment was once a traditional medicine for relieving colic, fighting intestinal worms in children, alleviating sciatica pain, and treating a number of other ailments.[1] Although its popularity has waned, some contemporary herbalists recommend it, among other things, for stimulating the appetite, aiding digestion, treating urinary tract infections, increasing urination (as a diuretic, or "water pill"), clearing congestion (as an expectorant), soothing coughs and other respiratory ailments, and helping to fight respiratory tract infections. Some suggest placing horseradish formulations on infected wounds and inflamed joints or tissues.

Forms Available Include:

Juice, poultice, root (cut, whole, grated), tablet.

Dosage Commonly Reported:

A small amount of the grated root is added to hot liquids to help fight respiratory ailments. Fresh horseradish is mixed with cornstarch for use in poultices. To use commercial horseradish tablets, follow the package instructions.

Will It Work for You? What the Studies Say:

Anyone who has ever placed this pungent, bitter herb on the tongue will probably recall a distinct sinus-clearing sensation. German health authorities have actually endorsed the use of horseradish preparations (both internally and externally) for treating respiratory tract inflammation and congestion, such as bronchitis.[2] The herb's stimulating pungency is released upon crushing, which frees chemicals called allylisothiocyanate and butylthiocyanate.[3] German health authorities cite the presence of mustard oil and mustard oil glycosides and their demonstrated antimicrobial actions. No clinical trials conclusively proving that horseradish helps clear respiratory tract congestion appear in the recent medical literature, although you may want to take the subjective experience of millions into account.

German authorities also endorse the use of horseradish as a supportive therapy (along with a primary course of treatment) for urinary tract infections,[4] presumably on the basis of its antimicrobial properties.[5] The antibiotic properties may also explain the herb's reputation as a wound healer.

Horseradish applied to the skin will increase blood flow to the area, reddening it. This property is considered potentially valuable for treating minor muscle aches and pains. German health authorities have approved of it for this purpose.[6]

Will It Harm You? What the Studies Say:

Horseradish is generally considered safe to use in moderate amounts, although it does pose the risk of stomach and intestinal discomfort. Large doses can render this irritation severe or cause diarrhea or unpleasant sweating. Never ingest the essential oil or place it on your skin.[7] Animals have reportedly developed stomach inflammation, excitement, and collapse after ingesting large amounts of horseradish.[8] The FDA includes horseradish on its list of herbs as "Generally Recognized As Safe" (GRAS); it is referring to culinary—not medicinal—amounts of the herb. German health authorities advise people with stomach or intestinal ulcers or kidney disorders to avoid medicinal concentrations of horseradish.[9] Some sources advise against taking the herb if you suffer from hypothyroidism or are taking a drug called thyroxine; the rationale for this warning is not altogether clear, however.[10] Do not give a strong or pungent herb such as horseradish to small children.

Externally, horseradish may harmlessly redden the skin and mucous membranes, although in some cases it can truly irritate the skin or cause blistering, so use it judiciously.

GENERAL SOURCES:

Blumenthal, M., J. Gruenwald, T. Hall, and R.S. Rister, eds. *The Complete German Commission E Monographs: Therapeutic Guide to Herbal Medicine*. Boston: Integrative Medicine Communications, 1998.

Griffith, H.W. *Complete Guide to Vitamins, Minerals, Nutrients & Supplements*. Tucson, AZ: Fisher Books, 1988.

Hylton, W.H., ed. *The Rodale Herb Book: How to Use, Grow, and Buy Nature's Miracle Plants*. Emmaus, PA: Rodale Press, Inc., 1974.

Lawrence Review of Natural Products. St. Louis: Facts and Comparisons, February 1991.

Mindell, E. *Earl Mindell's Herb Bible*. New York: Simon & Schuster/Fireside, 1992.

Newall, C.A., et al. *Herbal Medicines: A Guide for Health-Care Professionals*. London: The Pharmaceutical Press, 1996.

Weiss, R.F. *Herbal Medicine*, trans. A. R. Meuss, from the 6th German edition. Beaconsfield, England: Beaconsfield Publishers, Ltd., 1988.

TEXT CITATIONS:

1. J.W. Courter and A.M. Rhodes, "Historical Notes on Horseradish," *Economic Botany*, (1968): 156.
2. M. Blumenthal, J. Gruenwald, T. Hall, and R.S. Rister, eds., *The Complete German Commission E Monographs: Therapeutic Guide to Herbal Medicine* (Boston: Integrative Medicine Communications, 1998).
3. *Lawrence Review of Natural Products* (St. Louis: Facts and Comparisons, February 1991).
4. Blumenthal et al., op. cit.
5. R.F. Weiss, *Herbal Medicine*, trans. A.R. Meuss, from the 6th German edition (Beaconsfield, England: Beaconsfield Publishers, Ltd., 1988).
6. Blumenthal et al., op. cit.
7. C.A. Newall et al., *Herbal Medicines: A Guide for Health-Care Professionals* (London: The Pharmaceutical Press, 1996).
8. Ibid.
9. Blumenthal et al., op. cit.
10. Newall, op. cit.

HORSETAIL

SCIENTIFIC NAME:
Equisetum arvense L. Family:
Equisetaceae

COMMON NAMES:
Bottle brush, common horsetail,
corncob plant, field horsetail,
horsetail grass, running
clubmoss, scouring rush, shave
brush, shenjincao

RATING:
3 = Studies on the effectiveness
and safety of this substance are
conflicting, or there are not
enough studies to draw a
conclusion.

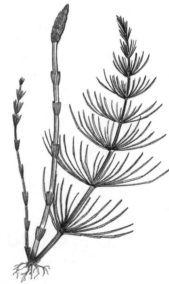

Horsetail
Equisetum arvense

What Is Horsetail?

Horsetail is an ancient nonflowering perennial with hollow, bamboolike stems
and tiny scalelike leaves. It reproduces through the spread of spores from the
brownish cones, which look like horse tails (hence the plant's common names),
and appear at the end of the stems in spring. The sterile green stems that
develop in summer—both fresh and dried—are used medicinally. Horsetail
grows in temperate regions of the northern hemisphere, including North
America and Europe.

What It Is Used For:

Horsetail existed when dinosaurs still roamed the earth. It was once held in
high esteem as a tuberculosis cure. Herbalists today highlight the plant's reputation as an astringent, a wound agent to stanch bleeding, and a diuretic ("water
pill") for edema (swelling), weight loss, and various bladder and kidney problems. Native Americans and traditional European and Indian (Ayurvedic) healers have used it in similar ways for many years.[1] Contemporary herbalists also
note the plant's considerable mineral content (about 15 percent, composed
primarily of silicic acids and silicates) and salt content, asserting that these substances help to increase calcium absorption and thus strengthen bones, hair,
teeth, and nails, as well as enrich the blood and help to heal broken bones and
damaged connective tissue associated with such conditions as arthritis. Homeopaths recommend minute amounts of the herb for various urinary problems.
(See page 2 for more information on homeopathy.)

Herbalists recommend topical formulations to encourage healing and
stanch bleeding in burns and wounds, particularly poorly healing ones, and to
treat fractures, sprains, and rheumatic conditions such as arthritis.

Forms Available Include:

- *For internal use:* Capsule, dried herb, extract, infusion, tablet, tea bag, tincture.
- *For external use:* Bath formulation, compress (from infusion or decoction),
  poultice.

Dosage Commonly Reported:

An infusion is made using 2 to 4 grams (2 to 4 teaspoons) of dried horsetail per
cup of water. Three of the 354-milligram capsules are taken three times a day.
To use commercial tea bags, herbal mixtures, or extracts containing horsetail,
follow the package instructions.

Will It Work for You? What the Studies Say:

Horsetail is weakly diuretic, according to animal studies. This may be due to the
presence of a diuretic chemical, the saponin equisetonin, and flavone glycosides.[2] Many experts contend that conditions meriting a diuretic should usually
be treated with a stronger and more reliable drug.[3] Authors of a 1994 study
reported that horsetail is probably mildly effective for preventing and treating
kidney stone formation, but that more potent and similarly safe substances are
known.[4] Nonetheless, German health authorities recognize horsetail as a mild

diuretic. They endorse its use for increasing urination ("irrigating the system") in cases of posttraumatic and static edema (swelling), and for treating kidney stones and bacterial and inflammatory disorders of the lower urinary tract.[5]

Researchers have also reported that horsetail may help strengthen and regenerate connective tissue, possibly owing to the plant's highly absorbable reserves of silica[6]—the body needs silica to form joint cartilage and connective tissue. Silica once played a role in tuberculosis treatment, but this is no longer true. The plant also contains calcium and other important minerals. The presence of these substances may explain the plant's traditional application in rheumatoid arthritis and connective tissue disorders. A French patent has been awarded for the use of isolated silica compounds from the plant for treating these disorders as well as bone fractures, osteoporosis, and injuries to the teeth or nails.[7] No well-designed studies to prove the value of horsetail in treating any of these ailments in humans have been done, however.

German health authorities also approve of treating poorly healing wounds with compresses soaked in certain horsetail formulations.[8] Horsetail can help stanch bleeding, according to animal studies.[9] A German physician's textbook attributes local stimulant properties to silica, and on this basis recommends horsetail hand, foot, and sitz baths for ankle fractures, chilblains, pelvic disease in women (as long as there is no associated inflammation), rheumatic and neuralgic disorders, chronic eczema, and other disorders in which increased blood circulation would probably be of benefit.[10] No other material can be found to confirm the value of this approach.

Will It Harm You? What the Studies Say:

Horsetail appears to be safe for most people to use in moderation, although much remains to be learned about its safety profile. The FDA once listed it as an "Herb of Undefined Safety." The plant contains very small amounts of nicotine. Ingesting large amounts of the parts other than the stem may cause adverse reactions; livestock that consume horsetail develop toxic reactions similar to nicotine poisoning, with abnormal pulse rates, fever, muscle weakness, weight loss, and other complications.[11] A similar type of toxic reaction has been noted in children who chew the stems.[12] Canadian health authorities require that horsetail preparations contain no thiaminase-like activity, given concerns about irreversible brain damage in individuals deficient in the vitamin thiamine.

German health authorities advise that if you take this herb as a diuretic, you should make sure to get plenty of liquids.[13] They also warn that neither this nor any other diuretic should be used in cases in which swelling is caused by impaired kidney or heart function.[14] They do not report any other situations in which it should not be used, or any known side effects or harmful interactions with other drugs.

GENERAL SOURCES:

Balch, J.F., and P.A. Balch. *Prescription for Nutritional Healing: A Practical A to Z Reference to Drug-Free Remedies Using Vitamins, Minerals, Herbs & Food Supplements.* 2nd ed. Garden City Park, NY: Avery Publishing Group, 1997.

Bisset, N.G., ed. *Herbal Drugs and Phytopharmaceuticals*. Stuttgart: medpharm GmbH Scientific Publishers, 1994.

Blumenthal, M., J. Gruenwald, T. Hall, and R.S. Rister, eds. *The Complete German Commission E Monographs: Therapeutic Guide to Herbal Medicine*. Boston: Integrative Medicine Communication, 1998.

Bradley, P.C., ed. *British Herbal Compendium: A Handbook of Scientific Information on Widely Used Plant Drugs*, vol. 1. Bournemouth (Dorset), England: British Herbal Medicine Association, 1992.

Bremness, L. *Herbs*. 1st American ed. Eyewitness Handbooks. New York: Dorling Kindersley Publications, 1994.

Castleman, M. *The Healing Herbs: The Ultimate Guide to the Curative Power of Nature's Medicines*. New York: Bantam Books, 1995.

Lawrence Review of Natural Products. St. Louis: Facts and Comparisons, October 1991.

Leung, A.Y., and S. Foster. *Encyclopedia of Common Natural Ingredients Used in Food, Drugs, and Cosmetics*. 2nd ed. New York: John Wiley & Sons, 1996.

Mindell, E. *Earl Mindell's Herb Bible*. New York: Simon & Schuster/Fireside, 1992.

Tyler, V.E. *The Honest Herbal*. Binghamton, NY: Haworth Press/Pharmaceutical Products Press, 1993.

Tyler, V.E., L.R. Brady, and J.E. Robbers, eds. *Pharmacognosy*. Philadelphia: Lea & Febiger, 1988.

Weiner, M.A., and J.A. Weiner. *Herbs That Heal: Prescription for Herbal Healing*. Mill Valley, CA: Quantum Books, 1994.

Weiss, R.F. *Herbal Medicine*, trans. A.R. Meuss, from the 6th German edition. Beaconsfield, England: Beaconsfield Publishers, Ltd., 1988.

TEXT CITATIONS:

1. A.Y. Leung and S. Foster, *Encyclopedia of Common Natural Ingredients Used in Food, Drugs, and Cosmetics*, 2nd ed. (New York: John Wiley & Sons, 1996). N.G. Bisset, ed., *Herbal Drugs and Phytopharmaceuticals* (Stuttgart: medpharm GmbH Scientific Publishers, 1994).

2. Bisset, op. cit. Leung and Foster, op. cit. P.C. Bradley, ed., *British Herbal Compendium: A Handbook of Scientific Information on Widely Used Plant Drugs*, vol. 1 (Bournemouth [Dorset], England: British Herbal Medicine Association, 1992). V.E. Tyler, *The Honest Herbal*. (Binghamton, NY: Haworth Press/Pharmaceutical Products Press, 1993).

3. V.E. Tyler, L.R. Brady, and J.E. Robbers, eds., *Pharmacognosy*. (Philadelphia: Lea & Febiger, 1988).

4. F. Grases et al., *International Urology & Nephrology*, 26(5) (1994): 507–11.

5. M. Blumenthal, J. Gruenwald, T. Hall, and R.S. Rister, eds., *The Complete German Commission E Monographs: Therapeutic Guide to Herbal Medicine* (Boston: Integrative Medicine Communications, 1998).

6. Bradley, op. cit. R.F. Weiss, *Herbal Medicine*, trans. A.R. Meuss, from the 6th German edition (Beaconsfield, England: Beaconsfield Publishers, Ltd., 1988).

7. N.W. Hamon and D.V.C. Awang, *Canadian Pharmaceutical Journal* (September 1992): 399.

8. Blumenthal et al., op. cit.

9. Leung and Foster, op. cit. Bradley, op. cit.

10. Weiss, op. cit.

11. *Lawrence Review of Natural Products* (St. Louis: Facts and Comparisons, October 1991). Leung and Foster, op. cit.

12. Leung and Foster, op. cit.

13. Blumenthal et al., op. cit.

14. Bisset, op. cit.

PRIMARY NAME:

HYDRANGEA

SCIENTIFIC NAME:

Hydrangea arborescens L.
Family: Saxifragaceae

COMMON NAMES:

Mountain hydrangea, seven barks, smooth hydrangea, wild hydrangea

RATING:

3 = Studies on the effectiveness of this substance are conflicting, or there are not enough studies to draw a conclusion about it. Safety appears to depend on judicious use; see the "Will It Harm You?" section.

What Is Hydrangea?

This erect, woody-stemmed shrub, a native of eastern North America, typically grows to about ten feet high. It has large oval leaves and heavy clusters of tiny, creamy white flowers. The dried rhizomes (underground stems) and roots are used medicinally.

Do not confuse *Hydrangea arborescens* with other *Hydrangea* species, such as those commonly cultivated in gardens or used in traditional Chinese medicine, as they do not have the same effects.

What It Is Used For:

Native American tribes considered hydrangea a diuretic ("water pill"), cathartic (powerful purgative or laxative), emetic, and topical treatment for wounds, sore muscles, burns, sprains, cancers, and other ailments. Early settlers adopted a number of these uses, adding the treatment of indigestion to the list. Some contemporary herbalists pick up on these traditional uses, recommending hydrangea preparations as diuretics for such ailments as kidney stones and various other genitourinary ailments including bladder stones and infections and prostate disorders.

Forms Available Include:

Liquid extract, tincture. Hydrangea appears in numerous diuretic herbal blends.

Dosage Commonly Reported:

A common dose for the liquid root extract is 2 to 4 milliliters.

Will It Work for You? What the Studies Say:

Science has shed very little light on the chemistry and possible therapeutic properties of *Hydrangea arborescens*; other *Hydrangea* species have been much more intensively examined, particularly those used in traditional Chinese medicine.[1] No ingredient identified so far is particularly notable, although a compound isolated as long ago as the 1880s—hydrangin—does appear to be toxic. Anecdotal reports suggest that hydrangea does have diuretic properties, meaning it increases urination, but this has yet to be scientifically verified. Overall, on the basis of the evidence collected so far, there is no way of determining if this plant will help resolve kidney stones, reduce fluid retention, or exert any other therapeutic influence.[2]

Certain derivatives of the plant display antiallergic properties, but the value of these for treating human allergies remains unclear.[3]

Will It Harm You? What the Studies Say:

Science offers little information about the potential health risks of hydrangea. An extract of hydrangea is reportedly not toxic to animals.[4] However, it is probably wise to avoid consuming hydrangea in large amounts or for long periods of time. Painful stomach upset, dizziness, and vertigo may develop with overdose.[5] The FDA placed hydrangea on its formerly maintained list of "Herbs of

Undefined Safety." Definitely avoid the flower buds, as these contain hydrangin, a cyanide poison.[6] Symptoms of poisoning, which may take several hours to develop, are abdominal pain, vomiting, listlessness, sweating, and possibly more serious reactions. Handling the plant can cause contact dermatitis.

GENERAL SOURCES:

Balch, J.F., and P.A. Balch. *Prescription for Nutritional Healing: A Practical A to Z Reference to Drug-Free Remedies Using Vitamins, Minerals, Herbs & Food Supplements.* 2nd ed. Garden City Park, NY: Avery Publishing Group, 1997.

Chevallier, A. *The Encyclopedia of Medicinal Plants: A Practical Reference Guide to More Than 550 Key Medicinal Plants & Their Uses.* 1st American ed. New York: Dorling Kindersley Publications, 1996.

Duke, J.A. *CRC Handbook of Medicinal Herbs.* Boca Raton, FL: CRC Press, 1985.

Foster, S., and J.A. Duke. *The Peterson Field Guide Series: A Field Guide to Medicinal Plants. Eastern and Central North America.* Boston: Houghton Mifflin Company, 1990.

Lampe, K.E., and M.A. McCann. *AMA Handbook of Poisonous and Injurious Plants.* Chicago: American Medical Association, 1985.

Leung, A.Y., and S. Foster. *Encyclopedia of Common Natural Ingredients Used in Food, Drugs, and Cosmetics.* 2nd ed. New York: John Wiley & Sons, 1996.

Newall, C.A., et al. *Herbal Medicines: A Guide for Health-Care Professionals.* London: The Pharmaceutical Press, 1996.

Tyler, V.E. *The Honest Herbal.* Binghamton, NY: Haworth Press/Pharmaceutical Products Press, 1993.

Tyler, V.E., L.R. Brady, and J.E. Robbers, eds. *Pharmacognosy.* Philadelphia: Lea & Febiger, 1988.

TEXT CITATIONS:

1. A.Y. Leung and S. Foster, *Encyclopedia of Common Natural Ingredients Used in Food, Drugs, and Cosmetics,* 2nd ed. (New York: John Wiley & Sons, 1996).
2. V.E. Tyler, *The Honest Herbal* (Binghamton, NY: Haworth Press/Pharmaceutical Products Press, 1993).
3. Leung and Foster, op. cit.
4. A. Der Marderosian, *Journal of Toxicology and Environmental Health,* 1 (1976): 939–53.
5. J.A. Duke, *CRC Handbook of Medicinal Herbs* (Boca Raton, FL: CRC Press, 1985).
6. K.E. Lampe and M.A. McCann, *AMA Handbook of Poisonous and Injurious Plants* (Chicago: American Medical Association, 1985).

HYSSOP

SCIENTIFIC NAME:
Hyssopus officinalis L. Family: Labiatae (Lamiaceae)

COMMON NAME:
N/A

What Is Hyssop?

The pointed leaves and small blue and violet flowers of *Hyssopus officinalis,* a hardy, stiff-stemmed perennial shrub native to Eurasia and naturalized in North America, are used medicinally. The essential oil distilled from both the leaves and the flowering tops is used medicinally as well. This member of the mint family has a strong camphorlike smell and a rather bitter taste.

Do not confuse *Hyssopus officinalis* with other common North American plants commonly referred to as hyssop, some of which should not be ingested, including hedge hyssop (*Gratiola officinalis*) and giant hyssop (*Agastache foeniculum*).

What It Is Used For:

Although used for centuries in herbal medicine, *Hyssopus officinalis* is probably not related to the hyssop referred to in biblical texts as a cleanser,[1] but it probably was valued as an insect repellent and insecticide and as a healing agent for coughs or colds. Hyssop tea and rubs were renowned for clearing congested airways by loosening sticky phlegm (mucus) and soothing a hoarse or sore throat. Numerous herbal cough and cold preparations contain the herb and its extracts. Many herbalists also consider it a good choice for excess gas, colic, indigestion, fever, asthma, rheumatism, poorly regulated blood pressure, circulation problems, gout, weight problems, and urinary tract infections. Antiseptic properties have been attributed to the herb; poultices made with the fresh green plant are said to heal cuts, and infusions are recommended to help treat cold sores and genital herpes. Hyssop's volatile oil is found in liqueurs and other beverages and foods as a flavoring and in perfumes.

Forms Available Include:

- *For internal use:* Dried leaves and flowers, infusion, liquid extract, oil, tea bag, tincture. Sweeteners are often added to mask the herb's bitter taste.
- *For external use:* Compress, gargle, oil, poultice.

Dosage Commonly Reported:

An infusion made with 1 to 2 teaspoons of hyssop per cup of water is drunk up to three times a day. The infusion is also used as a gargle. A compress is made with 1 ounce of dried herb per pint of water. The liquid extract is taken in doses of 2 to 4 milliliters.

Will It Work for You? What the Studies Say:

Hyssop contains a volatile oil (0.3 to 2.9 percent) responsible for its powerful odor and bitter taste. It also contains camphor-like chemicals and a chemical known for its expectorant actions (marrubiin), and can therefore be expected to soothe a sore throat, help clear chest congestion, and relieve other mild irritations associated with colds.[2]

Do not rely on hyssop as an antiseptic; it will not help prevent infection in wounds or cuts, and it has no apparent antibacterial activity.[3] As many enthusiasts note, the microorganism that produces penicillin (*Penicillium*) grows on hyssop leaves—and millions of other places in the plant kingdom—but in such small amounts that the impact would be insignificant. There is no evidence that any other ingredients in hyssop would fight infection in any significant way.[4] In the test tube, hyssop extracts have inhibited the growth of the herpes simplex virus, the virus responsible for cold sores and genital herpes.[5] This action has apparently not been tested in animals or humans, however, and the experiment found other mint-family members such as *Melissa officinalis* (see **Balm**) far more active. Intriguing test-tube studies indicate that dried hyssop leaves and certain extracts powerfully fight the HIV virus, but much more research is needed to verify their effect or draw any conclusions about the potential for treating HIV infections in humans.[6]

Citing a lack of substantiating evidence, German health authorities do not endorse the use of hyssop or its oil for any ailment, although they do allow tea mixtures to contain less than 5 percent of the herb as a flavoring element.[7]

Will It Harm You? What the Studies Say:

Hyssop is considered a relatively safe herb. It is included on the FDA's list of herbs "Generally Recognized As Safe" (GRAS) for food use. The oil is nonirritating and nonsensitizing to human and animal skin.[8] Moderation may be merited, however. A series of tests by one team of investigators found that commercial essential-oil preparations may pose some risk of central nervous system reactions. In their studies, certain oral dosages of the essential oil led to convulsions in rats.[9]

GENERAL SOURCES:

Balch, J.F., and P.A. Balch. *Prescription for Nutritional Healing: A Practical A to Z Reference to Drug-Free Remedies Using Vitamins, Minerals, Herbs & Food Supplements.* 2nd ed. Garden City Park, NY: Avery Publishing Group, 1997.

Blumenthal, M., J. Gruenwald, T. Hall, and R.S. Rister, eds. *The Complete German Commission E Monographs: Therapeutic Guide to Herbal Medicine.* Boston: Integrative Medicine Communications, 1998.

Castleman, M. *The Healing Herbs: The Ultimate Guide to the Curative Power of Nature's Medicines.* New York: Bantam Books, 1995.

Dobelis, I.N., ed. *The Magic and Medicine of Plants: A Practical Guide to the Science, History, Folklore, and Everyday Uses of Medicinal Plants.* Pleasantville, NY: Reader's Digest Association, 1986.

Foster, S., and J.A. Duke. *The Peterson Field Guide Series: A Field Guide to Medicinal Plants. Eastern and Central North America.* Boston: Houghton Mifflin Company, 1990.

Lawrence Review of Natural Products. St. Louis: Facts and Comparisons, August 1994.

Leung, A.Y., and S. Foster. *Encyclopedia of Common Natural Ingredients Used in Food, Drugs, and Cosmetics.* 2nd ed. New York: John Wiley & Sons, 1996.

Mindell, E. *Earl Mindell's Herb Bible.* New York: Simon & Schuster/Fireside, 1992.

Tyler, V.E. *The Honest Herbal.* Binghamton, NY: Haworth Press/Pharmaceutical Products Press, 1993

Tyler, V.E., L.R. Brady, and J.E. Robbers, eds. *Pharmacognosy.* Philadelphia: Lea & Febiger, 1988.

Weiss, R.F. *Herbal Medicine,* trans. A.R. Meuss, from the 6th German edition. Beaconsfield, England: Beaconsfield Publishers, Ltd., 1988.

TEXT CITATIONS:

1. V.E. Tyler, *The Honest Herbal* (Binghamton, NY: Haworth Press/Pharmaceutical Products Press, 1993).
2. *Lawrence Review of Natural Products* (St. Louis: Facts and Comparisons, August 1994). Tyler, op. cit.
3. M. Felklova, *Ziva,* 7 (1959): 210–11.
4. Tyler, op. cit.
5. E.C. Herrmann and L.S. Kucera, *Proceedings of the Society for Experimental Biology and Medicine,* 124(3) (1967): 874–78.
6. W. Kreis et al., *Antiviral Research,* 14(6) (1990): 323–27. S. Gollapudi et al., *Biochemical & Biophysics Research Communications,* 210(1) (1995): 145.
7. M. Blumenthal, J. Gruenwald, T. Hall, and R.S. Rister, eds., *The Complete German Commission E Monographs: Therapeutic Guide to Herbal Medicine* (Boston: Integrative Medicine Communications, 1998).
8. D.L.J. Opdyke, *Food & Cosmetics Toxicology,* 16(Suppl. 1) (1978): 783.
9. *Lawrence Review of Natural Products,* op. cit. Y. Millet et al., *Revue d'Electroencephalographie et de Neurophysiologie Clinique,* 9(1) (1979): 12. Y. Millet et al., *Clinical Toxicology,* 18(12) (1981): 1485.

ICELAND MOSS

SCIENTIFIC NAME:
Cetraria islandica L. Acharius.
Family: Parmeliaceae

COMMON NAMES:
Consumption moss, Iceland lichen, Islandiches moos

RATING:
2 = According to a number of well-designed studies and common use, this substance appears to be relatively effective and safe when used in recommended amounts for the indication(s) noted in the "Will It Work for You?" section.

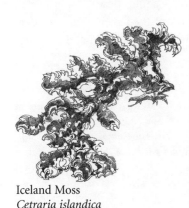

Iceland Moss
Cetraria islandica

What Is Iceland Moss?

Despite the name, Iceland moss is actually a lichen—an alga and a fungus living together—and not a moss. Shrublike clusters of the brownish, leaflike stems can be found on mountainous rocky slopes and in dry woods around the world. For medicinal purposes, the lichen is usually collected in the wild in central Europe and Scandinavia, and then dried and drunk as a tea or mixed into cough remedies.

What It Is Used For:

Iceland moss has a long-standing reputation for alleviating cough and congestion and calming stomach upset. Contemporary herbalists recommend it for the same discomforts, adding that the lichen can also soothe irritation and inflammation in the mouth and throat.

When famine struck certain northern regions of Europe centuries ago, people ate Iceland moss. Interestingly, in some countries today—including Germany—the lichen is drunk in the form of a decoction to stimulate a sagging appetite. Herbalists sometimes mask the disagreeable taste and smell of other medicines by mixing in this lichen. To a lesser degree, Iceland moss has also been used for kidney and bladder problems, lung ailments, and in topical form to encourage healing in lingering wounds.

Forms Available Include:

Decoction or infusion of powdered plant body. Europeans commonly add Iceland moss extracts to cough and cold remedies such as lozenges and instant bronchial teas.

Dosage Commonly Reported:

A tea is made using 1 to 2 teaspoons powdered moss and is drunk several times per day. Iceland moss must be prepared specifically for the type of condition it is intended to treat. For a cough remedy, remove the bitter principle by bringing the water with the lichen in it to a boil, pouring out the hot liquid, and then adding more water and bringing it to a second boil. Unfortunately, this eliminates whatever minor bacteria-fighting constituents are present. To soothe the stomach, steep the lichen in cold water or infuse it in hot water. Either way, the user may want to sweeten the drink.

Will It Work for You? What the Studies Say:

Modern science supports the traditional use of Iceland moss for coughs, colds, respiratory tract problems, and stomach upset. Much of the lichen—about 40 to 50 percent—consists of mucilaginous polysaccharides. Mucilage expands into a gooey mass when it comes into contact with liquid, soothing and protecting the delicate mucous membranes that can get so raw and inflamed from a cough, cold, or chronic bronchitis. It is digested in the intestines, which helps explain why people instinctively turned to Iceland moss to soothe and fill their stomachs when they had nothing else to eat. German health authorities approve of Iceland moss for treating irritations of the mucous membranes of the mouth and throat and the dry cough that often accompanies them.[1]

The other active principle in Iceland moss is a bitter. It stimulates salivation and gastric juices, acting as a tonic on the stomach and stimulating a poor appetite. Iceland moss is officially approved in Germany as an appetite stimulant.[2] The authorities there also consider the lichen a weak antibacterial; it fights certain bacteria in the test tube.

Intriguing research reported in 1995 suggests that a component of Iceland moss (an aliphatic alpha-methylene-gamma-lactone) inhibits a fundamental function of HIV, the virus that causes AIDS.[3] A study published around the same time found that a newly identified component, a polysaccharide, appears to help stimulate the immune system.[4] While such findings are intriguing, an enormous amount still has to be learned about what they might mean for boosting the immune system or potentially preventing HIV infection in human beings.

Will It Harm You? What the Studies Say:

Iceland moss appears to be safe to use as a medicine for short periods of time. German health authorities cite no known side effects, interactions with other remedies, or conditions under which a person should not use it.[5] However, Finnish scientists warned in a 1986 report that using large quantities for long stretches—more than two weeks, for example—could pose a health risk because industrialization has contaminated much of the lichen with considerable amounts of lead.[6] The FDA classifies Iceland moss as "Generally Recognized As Safe" (GRAS) to use as a food.

GENERAL SOURCES:

Bisset, N.G., ed. *Herbal Drugs and Phytopharmaceuticals.* Stuttgart: medpharm GmbH Scientific Publishers, 1994.

Blumenthal, M., J. Gruenwald, T. Hall, and R.S. Rister, eds. *The Complete German Commission E Monographs: Therapeutic Guide to Herbal Medicine.* Boston: Integrative Medicine Communications, 1998.

Kramer, P., et al. *Arzneimittel-Forschung.* 45(6) (1995): 726–31.

Tyler, V.E. *Herbs of Choice: The Therapeutic Use of Phytomedicinals.* Binghamton, NY: Haworth Press/Pharmaceutical Products Press, 1994.

Weiss, R.F. *Herbal Medicine*, trans. A.R. Meuss, from the 6th German edition. Beaconsfield, England: Beaconsfield Publishers, Ltd., 1988.

TEXT CITATIONS:

1. Blumenthal, M., J. Gruenwald, T. Hall, and R.S. Rister, eds., *The Complete German Commission E Monographs: Therapeutic Guide to Herbal Medicine* (Boston: Integrative Medicine Communications, 1998).
2. Ibid.
3. T. Pengsuparp et al., *Journal of Natural Products*, 58(7) (1995): 1024–31.
4. K. Ingolfsdottir et al., *Planta Medica*, 60(6) (1994): 527–31.
5. Blumenthal et al., op. cit.
6. M.M. Airaksinen et al., *Journal of Ethnopharmacology*, 18(3) (1986): 273–96. M.M. Airaksinen, *Archives of Toxicology*, Supplement, 9 (1986): 406–9.

SCIENTIFIC NAME:
Cephaelis ipecacuanha (Brot.)
A. Rich, sometimes referred to
as *Psychotria ipecacuanha*
Stokes, or *Cephaelis acuminata*
Karsten. Sometimes a mixture
of species is used. Family:
Rubiaceae

COMMON NAMES:
Brazilian/Cartagena/Costa Rica/
Matto Grosso/Nicaragua/
Panama/Rio ipecac, Brazilian
root, golden root, ipecacuanha

RATING:
1 = Years of use and extensive,
high-quality studies indicate
that this substance is very
effective and safe when used in
recommended amounts for the
indication(s) noted in the "Will
It Work for You?" section.
However, see the warnings in
the "Will It Harm You?"
section.

What Is Ipecac?

Ipecac is a small evergreen shrub native to tropical parts of South and Central America, and cultivated in regions of southern Asia. It favors shady woods. The dried roots and rhizomes (underground stems) are used medicinally.

What It Is Used For:

Brazilian Indians introduced Europeans to ipecac in the seventeenth century as a remedy for dysentery (infectious diarrhea). Today, the most widely recognized use of ipecac in North America is as a syrup to induce vomiting in selected cases of accidental poisoning, especially in children. Because it brings material back up through the body, however, it should never be used for corrosive poisons such as cleaning fluids, strong acids, and certain other substances. Smaller doses of ipecac in powdered form sometimes appear in commercial formulations to stimulate the appetite, aid digestion, induce sweating in cases of flu, reduce pain, encourage expectoration in cold and cough remedies, and combat nausea (even pregnancy-related nausea, in very small doses).

Forms Available Include:

Fluid extract, powder, syrup, tincture.
WARNING: The fluid extract is far more concentrated than ipecac syrup; do not use the extract for poisonings.

Dosage Commonly Reported:

To induce vomiting, follow instructions for the syrup from a qualified poison control center professional. The root tincture is taken in doses of 0.25 to 1 milliliter, and the powder in doses of 25 to 100 milligrams. To use commercial cough formulations containing ipecac, follow the package instructions. The extract is not commonly available, because of its toxicity.

Will It Work for You? What the Studies Say:

Ipecac syrup, when taken properly in the recommended amount with plenty of fluid, will induce vomiting, usually in fifteen to sixty minutes; take it for poisonings only if instructed to do so by a poison control center agent, however. Ipecac syrup causes vomiting by directly irritating the lining of the stomach and stimulating the vomiting center in the brain.

Much smaller doses of ipecac are useful as expectorants because the irritation of the stomach and intestines also produces a reflexive increase in respiratory tract secretions.[1] Once loosened by these secretions, the sticky phlegm (mucus) is easier to cough up, which is why ipecac is added to some cough and cold remedies. Many sources consider ipecac particularly effective for chronic bronchitis and whooping cough.[2] Only precise amounts of standardized ipecac in commercial preparations should be used for this purpose, however.

The alkaloids emetine and cephaeline are the major active constituents in ipecac root. Researchers have discovered that both (but particularly emetine) can kill amoebas. This goes a long way in explaining ipecac's traditional use for amebic dysentery (infectious diarrhea). Severe side effects limit the practicality of using ipecac for this purpose, however.

Rodent studies indicate that an extract of ipecac has anti-inflammatory properties.[3] The importance of this for treating human illness is unclear.

Will It Harm You? What the Studies Say:

Exercise great caution in using ipecac products; misuse can cause severe and chronic toxicity, and even death. Fluid extract of ipecac is no longer widely available because so many people mistook it for ipecac syrup, often with fatal results; the fluid extract is far more potent than the syrup. Severe complications including major fluid imbalances, muscle weakness, and heart damage have also developed in individuals who abuse ipecac syrup for various reasons, including to lose weight or maintain weight loss through vomiting.[4]

Toxic reactions to the various forms of ipecac and its alkaloids may include stomach and intestinal irritation with accompanying nausea, abdominal pain, or other symptoms; shortness of breath; dizziness; low blood pressure; and fast heartbeat.[5] The value of the purified alkaloid emetine for amebic infections is limited, owing to severe side effects.[6] Ipecac powder has caused severe allergic reactions in individuals who inhaled it.[7]

GENERAL SOURCES:

American Pharmaceutical Association. *Handbook of Nonprescription Drugs*. 11th ed. Washington, D.C.: American Pharmaceutical Association, 1996.

Bradley, P.C., ed. *British Herbal Compendium: A Handbook of Scientific Information on Widely Used Plant Drugs*, vol. 1. Bournemouth (Dorset), England: British Herbal Medicine Association, 1992.

Lawrence Review of Natural Products. St. Louis: Facts and Comparisons, August 1994.

Leung, A.Y., and S. Foster. *Encyclopedia of Common Natural Ingredients Used in Food, Drugs, and Cosmetics*. 2nd ed. New York: John Wiley & Sons, 1996.

Tierra, M. *The Way of Herbs*. New York: Pocket Books, 1990.

Tyler, V.E. *Herbs of Choice: The Therapeutic Use of Phytomedicinals*. Binghamton, NY: Haworth Press/Pharmaceutical Products Press, 1994.

Weiner, M.A., and J.A. Weiner. *Herbs That Heal: Prescription for Herbal Healing*. Mill Valley, CA: Quantum Books, 1994.

Weiss, R.F. *Herbal Medicine*, trans. A.R. Meuss, from the 6th German edition. Beaconsfield, England: Beaconsfield Publishers, Ltd., 1988.

TEXT CITATIONS:

1. E.M. Boyd and L.M. Knight, *Journal of Pharmacy and Pharmacology*, 16 (1964): 118–24.
2. P.C. Bradley, ed., *British Herbal Compendium: A Handbook of Scientific Information on Widely Used Plant Drugs*, vol. 1 (Bournemouth [Dorset], England: British Herbal Medicine Association, 1992).
3. A.Y. Leung and S. Foster, *Encyclopedia of Common Natural Ingredients Used in Food, Drugs, and Cosmetics*, 2nd ed. (New York: John Wiley & Sons, 1996).
4. A.G. Adler et al., *Journal of the American Medical Association*, 243 (1980): 1927. D. Thyagarajan et al., *Medical Journal of Australia*, 56 (1993): 560. R.J. Schiff et al., *Pediatrics*, 78 (1986): 412–16. J. Goebel et al., *Pediatrics*, 92(4) (1993): 601–3. L.P. Dresser et al., *Journal of Neurology, Neurosurgery & Psychiatry*, 56(5) (1992): 560–2.
5. Leung and Foster, op. cit.

6. M.H. Ansari and S. Ahmad, *Fitoterapia*, 62(2) (1991): 171.
7. Leung and Foster, op. cit.

IRISH MOSS

SCIENTIFIC NAME:

Chondrus crispus, Gigartina mamillosa. Family: Gigartinaceae

COMMON NAMES:

Carrageen, carrageenan, carrageenin, carragheen, Fucus irlandicus

RATING:

3 = Studies on the effectiveness and safety of this substance are conflicting, or there are not enough studies to draw a conclusion.

What Is Irish Moss?

Irish moss is the edible, dried thallus (plant body) of two red North Atlantic seaweeds, *Chondrus crispus* and *Gigartina mamillosa*. It contains considerable amounts of an important substance called mucilage.

What It Is Used For:

Irish moss and its extracts have been used in traditional medicine for ulcers, dysentery (infectious diarrhea), and other gastrointestinal disorders. New England colonists reportedly turned to it as a bulk-forming laxative.[1] Some contemporary herbalists consider it a valuable soothing agent (demulcent) for dry coughs, bronchitis, tuberculosis, and other upper respiratory tract ailments. Because it is rich in proteins, iodides, and other substances, many herbalists also consider it an excellent "nutritive tonic." It appears in many herbal drinks.

The manufacturing industry uses Irish moss and its extracts extensively as binders, emulsifiers, stabilizers, and thickening agents in skin lotions, toothpastes, hair rinses, other pharmaceutical and cosmetic substances, milk products, jellies, and other foods.

Forms Available Include:

Decoction. Irish moss appears in capsulated herbal blends and herbal drinks.

Dosage Commonly Reported:

To use commercial herbal blends containing Irish moss, follow the package instructions.

Will It Work for You? What the Studies Say:

Experiments in both animals and humans indicate that Irish moss extracts may help alleviate peptic and duodenal ulcers when taken in a specially prepared commercial form.[2] In Europe especially, an extract of the seaweed (in special "degraded" form) has been used to treat peptic ulcers. In the test tube, carrageenan helps inhibit pepsin activity.[3] The high concentration of mucilage in Irish moss may contribute to its healing properties for ulcers as well as for digestive system upset. Mucilage swells when it comes into contact with liquid, creating a gooey mass that coats and protects the lining of the stomach and intestines, reducing stomach (gastric) secretions and thus helping to form healthy stools and reduce constipation.

The mucilage also protects and soothes the delicate mucous membranes that can get raw and inflamed by a cough, cold, or respiratory ailment. No studies appear to have been done to test Irish moss's effectiveness for these disorders, however. Other herbs are more popular.

Intriguing trials involving injectable forms of Irish moss extract in rodents and other animals indicate that they may have anti-inflammatory, immunosuppressive, blood-pressure-lowering, and other potentially beneficial properties.[4] More research is needed to determine the value of these findings for humans.

Will It Harm You? What the Studies Say:

Irish moss appears to be safe to use in concentrations commonly recommended for food use.[5] Relatively little is known about the risk for toxic reactions with higher medicinal concentrations. Irish moss (carrageenan and its various salts, specifically) are officially listed in the *National Formulary* and are approved for food use.

GENERAL SOURCES:

Balch, J.F., and P.A. Balch. *Prescription for Nutritional Healing: A Practical A to Z Reference to Drug-Free Remedies Using Vitamins, Minerals, Herbs & Food Supplements.* 2nd ed. Garden City Park, NY: Avery Publishing Group, 1997.

Leung, A.Y., and S. Foster. *Encyclopedia of Common Natural Ingredients Used in Food, Drugs, and Cosmetics.* 2nd ed. New York: John Wiley & Sons, 1996.

Tierra, M. *The Way of Herbs.* New York: Pocket Books, 1990.

Weiner, M.A., and J.A. Weiner. *Herbs That Heal: Prescription for Herbal Healing.* Mill Valley, CA: Quantum Books, 1994.

Weiss, R.F. *Herbal Medicine,* trans. A.R. Meuss, from the 6th German edition. Beaconsfield, England: Beaconsfield Publishers, Ltd., 1988.

TEXT CITATIONS:

1. R.F. Weiss, *Herbal Medicine,* trans. A.R. Meuss, from the 6th German edition. (Beaconsfield, England: Beaconsfield Publishers, Ltd., 1988).
2. A.Y. Leung and S. Foster, *Encyclopedia of Common Natural Ingredients Used in Food, Drugs, and Cosmetics,* 2nd ed. (New York: John Wiley & Sons, 1996).
3. Ibid.
4. Ibid.
5. D.J. Stancioff and D.W. Renn, *ACS Symposium Series,* 15 (1975): 282.

PRIMARY NAME:
IVY

SCIENTIFIC NAME:
Hedera helix L. Family: Araliaceae

COMMON NAMES:
English ivy, ivy leaf, true ivy

What Is Ivy?

This climbing plant, which can grow as high as 100 feet, is native to Eurasia and North Africa but can be found across North America. Its dark green, glossy, three- to five-lobed evergreen leaves are used medicinally, either fresh or bruised, macerated (soaked to soften in water), or in the form of a poultice. They have a slightly bitter taste. The plant also bears umbels of green-yellow flowers that give rise to black berries. A resin collected from incisions in the bark, known as ivy gum, has also been used medicinally, as have the berries.

What It Is Used For:

Ivy has an extensive history as a religious and sacred symbol, as well as a medicinal remedy. Standard European herbals once recommended taking the herb internally for various disorders, including to treat upper respiratory tract con-

RATING:

3 = Studies on the effectiveness and safety of this substance are conflicting, or there are not enough studies to draw a conclusion.

gestion, spasm-related coughs, whooping cough, internal parasites, delayed or absent menstruation, and arthritis and rheumatism. Contemporary herbalists recommend the herb for only a few of these uses. Some suggest making a poultice of the leaves or applying the gum resin or another external formulation to sores, burns, skin eruptions, and parasitic conditions such as scabies. The gum resin was once reportedly used to relieve toothache pain.

Forms Available Include:

- *For internal use:* Infusion, leaf (fresh or dried). Ivy leaf appears in some European cough and bronchial teas.
- *For external use:* Decoction, gum resin, poultice.

Dosage Commonly Reported:

An infusion is made by pouring boiling water over about 0.5 grams of ivy leaves, steeping for ten minutes, and straining the brew. This is drunk one to three times a day, sweetened with honey if desired.

Will It Work for You? What the Studies Say:

Ivy leaf preparations are believed to help control symptoms associated with chronic inflammatory bronchial conditions such as whooping cough by means of their antispasmodic, expectorant, and mildly sedative properties.[1] The constituents responsible for these actions are probably saponins and glycosides, and expectorant actions have been speculatively attributed to emetine.[2] German health authorities approve of ivy leaf preparations for inflammatory bronchial conditions, as well as for relieving respiratory tract congestion.[3] As an expectorant, the herb is believed to liquefy and loosen sticky secretions so that they are easier to cough up.

Many Western herbalists no longer recommend ivy leaf for internal use. The reasons for this are not always clear.

A number of traditional external uses for ivy leaf, such as treating skin eruptions and parasitic infestations, may be explained by the discovery that ivy leaf contains antiseptic properties; the contained saponins (hederas) have shown an ability to fight bacteria, worms, protozoa, and fungi,[4] and polyacetylenes demonstrate antibacterial and antifungal properties, as well as painkilling actions.[5]

Will It Harm You? What the Studies Say:

German health authorities cite no known health risks associated with the use of ivy leaf, no situations in which it should not be used, and no known interactions with any other medicines.[6] Avoid the berries, however, and large doses of the whole plant, as they may be toxic.[7] Allergic contact dermatitis can occur after handling the fresh leaves or leaf sap.[8]

GENERAL SOURCES:

Bisset, N.G., ed. *Herbal Drugs and Phytopharmaceuticals.* Stuttgart: medpharm GmbH Scientific Publishers, 1994.

Blumenthal, M., J. Gruenwald, T. Hall, and R.S. Rister, eds., *The Complete German Commission E Monographs: Therapeutic Guide to Herbal Medicine.* Boston: Integrative Medicine Communications, 1998.

Dobelis, I.N., ed. *The Magic and Medicine of Plants: A Practical Guide to the Science, History, Folklore, and Everyday Uses of Medicinal Plants.* Pleasantville, NY: Reader's Digest Association, 1986.

Weiner, M.A., and J.A. Weiner. *Herbs That Heal: Prescription for Herbal Healing.* Mill Valley, CA: Quantum Books, 1994.

Weiss, R.F. *Herbal Medicine,* trans. A.R. Meuss, from the 6th German edition. Beaconsfield, England: Beaconsfield Publishers, Ltd., 1988.

TEXT CITATIONS:

1. R.F. Weiss, *Herbal Medicine,* trans. A.R. Meuss, from the 6th German edition (Beaconsfield, England: Beaconsfield Publishers, Ltd., 1988).
2. Ibid.
3. M. Blumenthal, J. Gruenwald, T. Hall, and R. S. Rister, eds., *The Complete German Commission E Monographs: Therapeutic Guide to Herbal Medicine* (Boston: Integrative Medicine Communications, 1998).
4. N.G. Bisset, ed., *Herbal Drugs and Phytopharmaceuticals* (Stuttgart: medpharm GmbH Scientific Publishers, 1994).
5. S. Tanaka and Y. Ikeshiro, *Arzneimittel-Forschung,* 27 (1977): 2039. Bisset, op. cit.
6. Blumenthal et al., op. cit.
7. I.N. Dobelis, ed., *The Magic and Medicine of Plants: A Practical Guide to the Science, History, Folklore, and Everyday Uses of Medicinal Plants* (Pleasantville, NY: Reader's Digest Association, 1986).
8. J. Boyle and R.H. Harman, *Contact Dermatitis,* 12 (1985): 111.

I

Ivy

PRIMARY NAME:

JASMINE

SCIENTIFIC NAME:

Jasminum grandiflorum L. (sometimes referred to as *Jasminum officinale* L. var. *grandiflorum* Bailey), and other *Jasminum* species, such as *Jasminum sambac.* Family: Oleaceae

COMMON NAMES:

Catalonian jasmine, common jasmine, Italian jasmine, royal jasmine

RATING:

4 = Research indicates that this substance will not fulfill the claims made for it, but that it is also unlikely to cause any harm.

What Is Jasmine?

Various *Jasminum* species native to China, western Asia, and India are now extensively cultivated in Mediterranean countries and other parts of the world as garden plants. The species commonly cultivated for their aroma and medicinal properties are evergreen ramblers with dark green leaves and hefty, fragrant white flowers. These flowers yield a precious essential oil; both the flowers and the oil are used medicinally. The highest-quality essential oil is a pure steam distillation of the flowers.

Do not confuse the *Jasminum* species described above with *Gelsemium sempervirens* (L.) Ait.f., commonly called yellow jessamine, Carolina jasmine, or Carolina jessamine, which does not have the same effects.

What It Is Used For:

Jasmine has been used primarily as a perfume since it was introduced into Europe in the Middle Ages. Generations have savored an infusion made with the flowers for its taste and purported tension-relieving and relaxing properties.

The essential oil distilled from jasmine flowers is used to treat stress, depression, certain skin conditions, and lack of sexual desire. Aromatherapists assert that the oil has powers to lift the spirit and produce feelings of confidence, optimism, and goodwill. Western folklore has also promoted the oil as an aphrodisiac. Some sources say that rubbing the oil onto the body will invoke sexual arousal. Others prefer vaporization of the oil. Still others consider the fragrance in perfume form heady enough. The oil can also be found in cosmetics, in skin creams and lotions to moisturize sensitive or dry skin, and as a flavor ingredient in foods and beverages.

The flowers, leaves, and other parts of *Jasminum* species commonly cultivated in China, such as *Jasminum sambac,* are used medicinally to treat such wide-ranging disorders as hepatitis, infectious diarrhea, pain, insomnia, cancers, and skin ulcers.[1] Chinese jasmine tea is typically made from dried flowers of *Jasminum sambac.*

Forms Available Include:

Infusion, oil (for external use only), tea bag.

Dosage Commonly Reported:

The oil is used in appropriate amounts in vaporization and massage (depending on the container size). The flowers may be used in an infusion according to taste.

Will It Work for You? What the Studies Say:

Apparently no studies have been done in test tubes, on laboratory animals, or on humans to test the ability of jasmine tea to produce sedation or relieve tension. Its ingredients do not suggest that it will, yet many users insist it does. As with so many fragrances, the ability of jasmine to induce sensations of well-being or sexual stimulation probably depends on your personal preference and belief in the powers of aromatherapy. No studies can be found in the recent literature to confirm any mood-altering actions in the herb.

Very preliminary studies indicate that Chinese jasmine tea (along with certain other Chinese teas) may reduce the incidence of esophageal tumors in rats.[2] Much remains to be learned about this property and whether it applies to human beings. Flowers from the same species of jasmine used to make the tea—*Jasminum sambac*—matched the effectiveness of a standard drug (Bromocriptine) in reducing breast engorgement, milk production, and the need for pain relievers in women who had just given birth.[3] This 1988 study did not involve a control group to rule out bias, however.

The purest and most fragrant essential oil is represented by a true distillation of the flowers. Some aromatherapy oils may not contain this pure and relatively expensive form.[4]

Will It Harm You? What the Studies Say:

What little information can be found indicates that jasmine is not toxic or irritating. Allergic reactions to the plant and oil have been reported, however, in some cases involving aromatherapy.[5] Do not swallow the oil. The FDA has placed jasmine on its "Generally Recognized As Safe" (GRAS) list for food consumption.

GENERAL SOURCES:

Chevallier, A. *The Encyclopedia of Medicinal Plants: A Practical Reference Guide to More Than 550 Key Medicinal Plants & Their Uses.* 1st American ed. New York: Dorling Kindersley Publications, 1996.

Leung, A.Y., and S. Foster. *Encyclopedia of Common Natural Ingredients Used in Food, Drugs, and Cosmetics.* 2nd ed. New York: John Wiley & Sons, 1996.

Mayell, M. *Off-the-Shelf Natural Health: How to Use Herbs and Nutrients to Stay Well.* New York: Bantam Books, 1995.

Mindell, E. *Earl Mindell's Herb Bible.* New York: Simon & Schuster/Fireside, 1992.

TEXT CITATIONS:

1. A.Y. Leung and S. Foster, *Encyclopedia of Common Natural Ingredients Used in Food, Drugs, and Cosmetics*, 2nd ed. (New York: John Wiley & Sons, 1996).
2. J. Chen, *Preventive Medicine*, 21(3) (1992): 385–91. J.Q. Zhu et al., *Biomedical & Environmental Sciences*, 4(3) (1991): 225–31. C. Han and Y. Xu, *Biomedical & Environmental Sciences*, 3(1) (1990): 35–42.
3. P. Shrivastav et al., *Australian & New Zealand Journal of Obstetrics & Gynaecology*, 28(1) (1988): 68–71.
4. A. Chevallier, *The Encyclopedia of Medicinal Plants: A Practical Reference Guide to More Than 550 Key Medicinal Plants & Their Uses*, 1st American ed. (New York: Dorling Kindersley Publications, 1996).
5. B.M. Bedi, *Indian Journal of Dermatology*, 16(3) (1971): 61–62. H. Schaller and H.C. Korting, *Clinical & Experimental Dermatology*, 20(2) (1995): 143–45.

PRIMARY NAME:
JEWELWEED

SCIENTIFIC NAME:
Impatiens biflora Walt.,
Impatiens pallida Nutt.,
Impatiens capensis Meerb., and
occasionally one of the other
numerous *Impatiens* species.
Family: Balsaminaceae

COMMON NAMES:
Balsam weed, garden balsam,
jewel balsam weed, speckled
jewels, spotted touch-me-not,
touch-me-not, wild balsam, wild
celandine, yellow jewelweed

RATING:
3 = Studies on the effectiveness
and safety of this substance are
conflicting, or there are not
enough studies to draw a
conclusion.

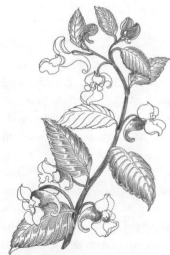

Jewelweed
Impatiens biflora

What Is Jewelweed?

The numerous *Impatiens* species referred to as jewelweed are typically found growing wild in wet and shady soils along the East Coast of North America, or cultivated as bedding or house plants. The flowers are pendantlike with red spots. The oval leaves and stem juice have been used medicinally.

What It Is Used For:

By far the most common folk use for jewelweed is to prevent and treat poison ivy dermatitis, a practice introduced by Native Americans. A poultice made with the crushed leaves has a reputation for alleviating other skin irritations as well—bruises, burns, infections, ringworm, hemorrhoids, sores, warts—but this use is not nearly as widespread. Modern herbalists occasionally recommend jewelweed for mild constipation or liver disorders and as a diuretic ("water pill") for fluid retention.

Forms Available Include:

- *For external use:* Decoction, leaf, undiluted stem sap, poultice (of crushed leaves).
- *For internal use:* Decoction, tisane.

Dosage Commonly Reported:

The sap of the stem is applied externally.

Will It Work for You? What the Studies Say:

Researchers have largely ignored this herb. Its effectiveness in reducing itching, swelling, and other symptoms of poison ivy dermatitis remains unclear. In a 1950s study it fared admirably in a matchup against standard treatments such as topical steroids, relieving symptoms within two or three days in 108 of 115 individuals treated externally with it.[1] But in a follow-up study in 1980, a water extract of jewelweed not only failed to help reduce irritation from poison ivy dermatitis, but appeared to increase it.[2]

A compound in *Impatiens balsamina*—2-methoxynaphthoquinone—has demonstrated antifungal properties, as have glycosides identified in *Impatiens biflora*.[3] These properties explain jewelweed's reputation for treating ringworm. No studies to confirm their effectiveness in animals or humans appear in the recent medical literature, however.

Will It Harm You? What the Studies Say:

There is nothing to indicate that jewelweed will cause any harm when applied to the skin, at least according to the reactions of people in the handful of studies done so far, not to mention years of folk use. Whether it is safe to take internally is less clear, however.[4]

GENERAL SOURCES:

Foster, S., and J.A. Duke. *The Peterson Field Guide Series: A Field Guide to Medicinal Plants. Eastern and Central North America.* Boston: Houghton Mifflin Company, 1990.

Hylton, W.H., ed. *The Rodale Herb Book: How to Use, Grow, and Buy Nature's Miracle Plants.* Emmaus, PA: Rodale Press, Inc., 1974.

Lawrence Review of Natural Products. St. Louis: Facts and Comparisons, March 1995.

Tyler, V.E. *Herbs of Choice: The Therapeutic Use of Phytomedicinals.* Binghamton, NY: Haworth Press/Pharmaceutical Products Press, 1994.

TEXT CITATIONS:

1. R.A. Lipton, *Annals of Allergy*, 16 (1958): 526–67. V.E. Tyler, *Herbs of Choice: The Therapeutic Use of Phytomedicinals* (Binghamton, NY: Haworth Press/Pharmaceutical Products Press, 1994).
2. J.D. Guin and R. Reynolds, *Contact Dermatitis*, 6 (1980): 287–88.
3. *Lawrence Review of Natural Products* (St. Louis: Facts and Comparisons, March 1995).
4. Ibid.

PRIMARY·NAME:

JOJOBA OIL

SCIENTIFIC NAME:

Simmondsia chinensis (Link) C. Schneid., often referred to as *Simmondsia californica* Nutt. Family: Buxaceae

COMMON NAMES:

Deernut oil, goatnut oil, pignut oil

RATING:

3 = Studies on the effectiveness and safety of this substance are conflicting, or there are not enough studies to draw a conclusion.

What Is Jojoba Oil?

This oil is extracted from the seeds enclosed in the leathery, nutlike fruits of this desert shrub native to parts of California, Arizona, and Mexico. Technically it is a liquid wax, not an oil. Animals forage on the woody flowering evergreen and its thick bluish-green leaves. The colorless and odor-free oil can be hydrogenated to a solid wax.

What It Is Used For:

Native Americans and Mexicans long used parts of the jojoba plant as a medicine and survival food. They smoothed the oil onto their hair to condition and restore it. The 1973 ban on the sale of sperm whale oil stimulated the production of jojoba oil for skin and hair conditioners, moisturizers, cleansing products, aftershave products, makeup removers, lipsticks, other cosmetics, and even industrial lubricants.[1] Jojoba oil shampoo is sold for cleaning and moisturizing the hair, often with the claim that it will add luster and shine. Some sources contend that jojoba oil will prevent further hair loss and even restore what has been lost.[2] Skin products are said to clean out clogged pores. Various facial scrubs and other products designed to exfoliate dead skin feature jojoba wax beads. A number of other uses have been proposed, from treating acne and warts to suppressing appetite and lowering cholesterol levels.

Forms Available Include:

Jojoba oil appears in numerous cosmetic products.

Dosage Commonly Reported:

To use commercial products containing jojoba oil, follow the package instructions.

Will It Work for You? What the Studies Say:

Jojoba oil is easily absorbed into the skin, moisturizing, conditioning, softening, and protecting it. It is generally considered nongreasy, although this is a subjective perception, as is its ability to make hair feel soft and look shiny. Whether it will prevent hair loss or rejuvenate hair growth remains unclear. According to a number of sources, jojoba oil chemically and physically resembles sebum, the fatty material secreted by the sebaceous glands on the scalp.[3] Once absorbed into the skin, according to studies, jojoba oil can unclog hair follicles and thereby prevent the natural buildup of sebum, which could cause hair loss.[4] The reasons for hair loss are often more complex than this, however, although signs of flaking such as dandruff may well lessen with lubrication of the scalp.[5]

Preliminary research indicates that jojoba may help alleviate minor skin inflammation and irritation such as chapped or sunburned skin.[6] Investigators have also reported that the oil may help reduce acne and psoriasis, although more data are needed.[7] Other intriguing findings have been reported, including that cholesterol levels dropped in rabbits fed jojoba oil and that the leaves may have antioxidant activity,[8] but all require much more extensive examination before conclusions can be made about their value for treating humans.

Will It Harm You? What the Studies Say:

Except in a few cases of contact dermatitis with characteristic symptoms of redness and swelling, jojoba oil appears to be nontoxic when applied externally.[9] Never swallow it, however, as it contains a potentially toxic substance called erucic acid and has caused toxic reactions in experimental rats.[10]

GENERAL SOURCES:

Lawrence Review of Natural Products. St. Louis: Facts and Comparisons, September 1995.

Leber, M.R., et al. *Handbook of Over-the-Counter Drugs and Pharmacy Products.* Berkeley: Celestial Arts Publishing, 1994.

Leung, A.Y., and S. Foster. *Encyclopedia of Common Natural Ingredients Used in Food, Drugs, and Cosmetics.* 2nd ed. New York: John Wiley & Sons, 1996.

Tyler, V.E. *The Honest Herbal.* Binghamton, NY: Haworth Press/Pharmaceutical Products Press, 1993.

TEXT CITATIONS:

1. *Lawrence Review of Natural Products* (St. Louis: Facts and Comparisons, September 1995).
2. V.E. Tyler, *The Honest Herbal* (Binghamton, NY: Haworth Press/Pharmaceutical Products Press, 1993).
3. G.J. Arndt, *Cosmetic Toiletries,* 102(6) (1987): 68.
4. Tyler, op. cit.
5. T.K. Miwa, *Cosmetics and Perfumery,* 88 (1973): 3941. *Lawrence Review,* op. cit.
6. B. Mosovich, "Proceedings of the 6th International Jojoba Conference," presented at Ben Gurion University, Israel, October 21–26, 1984.
7. J.A. Clarke and D.M. Yermanos, *Biochemical and Biophysical Research Communications,* 102(4) (1981): 1409.
8. J.F. Mallet et al., *Food Chemistry,* 49(1) (1994): 61. M.J. Scott and M.J. Scott, Jr., *Journal of the American Academy of Dermatology,* 6(4 Pt 1) (1982): 545.

9. F. Wantke et al., *Contact Dermatitis*, 34(1) (1996): 71–72. Scott and Scott, op. cit. M. Taguchi and T. Kunimoto, *Cosmetic Toiletries*, 92(9) (1977): 53. A.Y. Leung and S. Foster, *Encyclopedia of Common Natural Ingredients Used in Food, Drugs, and Cosmetics*, 2nd ed. (New York: John Wiley & Sons, 1996).
10. *Lawrence Review of Natural Products,* op. cit. P.M. Verschuren, *Food & Chemical Toxicology*, 27(1) (1989): 35–44.

PRIMARY NAME:
JUJUBE, COMMON

SCIENTIFIC NAME:
Zizyphus jujuba Mill. (sometimes referred to as *Zizyphus jujuba* or *Zizyphus sativa* Gaertn.), *Zizyphus jujuba* Mill. var *inermis* (Bge.) Rehd. (sometimes referred to as *Zizyphus vulgaris* Lam. var. *inermis* Bge.) Family: Rhamnaceae

COMMON NAMES:
Black date, Chinese jujube, da t'sao, da zao, hei zao, jujube date, jujube plum, red date, zao

RATING:
3 = Studies on the effectiveness and safety of this substance are conflicting, or there are not enough studies to draw a conclusion.

What Is Common Jujube?

The whole ripe fruit—the date—of this small shrub or tree is used medicinally once dried, as are the contained seeds and the plant's leaves. Jujube is native to southern Europe and Asia but can be found in the warmer Gulf states of North America. It is widely cultivated. Primarily the red type is available domestically.

What It Is Used For:

Traditional Chinese healers through the ages have regarded the jujube date as a valuable *qi* (energy) tonic, recommending it for fatigue, appetite loss, and diarrhea, and in recent times for such ailments as high blood pressure, insomnia, nervous exhaustion, and anemia. They often put it in herbal blends. Middle Eastern healing traditions have prescribed jujube for wounds and ulcers, fevers, eye diseases, and inflammatory conditions such as asthma, and as a blood "purifier."[1]

In China, the jujube date also qualifies as a taste enhancer in soups, candies, and other foods. Jujube-containing soups and candies eaten in winter are said to keep skin healthy and well-moisturized and to relieve any itching. Liquid and alcoholic extract are popular for use in creams and other skin-care products for their purported moisturizing, soothing, sunburn-relieving, antiwrinkle, and anti-inflammatory properties.[2] Diabetics in parts of Turkey prepare formulations from the leaves to lower their blood sugar levels.

Forms Available Include:

Capsule, date (fresh or dried), decoction, liquid extract, tablet. Jujube date appears as an ingredient in numerous Chinese herbal blends, skin-care products, soup mixes, and candies.

Dosage Commonly Reported:

A common dose is 5 to 10 grams. To use commercial jujube formulations, follow the package instructions.

Will It Work for You? What the Studies Say:

Apparently only test-tube and small-animal studies have been conducted on this nutritious herb, and only a few at that. Painkilling and anti-inflammatory properties have been noted in alcoholic extracts used in a classic animal test for inflammation—chemically induced raw-paw edema[3]—but whether this justifies the herb's use for skin inflammation or such serious inflammatory conditions as asthma remains far from clear.

Extracts of the dates have also been shown to inhibit the growth of a bacteria, *Bacillus subtilis*,[4] which causes certain skin infections and food poisoning, as well as the cavity-causing bacterium *Streptococcus mutans*.[5] The seeds have shown marked blood-pressure-lowering properties in rats and cats,[6] and sedative actions in the test tube (attributed to alkaloids)[7] as well as in mice.[8] Blood-sugar-lowering properties have been documented in rats fed a decoction made with jujube leaves.[9] These and other intriguing findings still require confirmation in human trials.

Will It Harm You? What the Studies Say:

The recent medical literature contains no reports of significant adverse reactions to common jujube, although none appear to test its toxicity specifically. Its popular use by millions of Chinese over the centuries should probably be taken into account, as should its widespread use as an everyday food and flavoring in Asian cuisine. Laboratory animals show no signs of toxic reactions.[10]

GENERAL SOURCES:

Leung, A.Y., and S. Foster. *Encyclopedia of Common Natural Ingredients Used in Food, Drugs, and Cosmetics.* 2nd ed. New York: John Wiley & Sons, 1996.

Tierra, M. *The Way of Herbs.* New York: Pocket Books, 1990.

TEXT CITATIONS:

1. A.H. Shah et al., *Phytotherapy Research*, 3 (1989): 232.
2. A.Y. Leung and S. Foster, *Encyclopedia of Common Natural Ingredients Used in Food, Drugs, and Cosmetics*, 2nd ed. (New York: John Wiley & Sons, 1996).
3. Ibid.
4. Shah, op. cit.
5. Ibid.
6. W. Gu et al., *Journal of Medical Colleges of the People's Liberation Army*, 2(4) (1987): 315–18.
7. B.H. Han and M.H. Park, *Archives of Pharmacological Research*, 10(4) (1987): 203–7.
8. C. Yuan et al., *Zhongyao Tongbao*, 12(9) (1987): 546–48.
9. A. Erenmemisoglu et al., *Journal of Pharmaceutical Pharmacology*, 47(1) (1995): 72–74.
10. Shah, op. cit. Leung and Foster, op. cit.

PRIMARY NAME:

JUNIPER BERRY

SCIENTIFIC NAME:

Juniperus communis L. Family: Cupressaceae

COMMON NAMES:

Geneva, geniver, horse savin

What Is Juniper Berry?

More than seventy species of *Juniperus*, an aromatic evergreen shrub and small tree, populate the northern hemisphere. Small yellow flowers bloom every spring, but it takes two years for the fleshy miniature cones ("berries") to mature to a deep blue-black. At this point they are picked and dried. Steam distillation yields an essential oil.

What It Is Used For:

Juniper berries are most famous for their spicy-sweet contribution to gin. A sixteenth-century Dutch pharmacist inadvertently concocted the beverage while

JUNIPER BERRY *(Continued)*

RATING:

- *For internal and external use:* 3 = Studies on the effectiveness and safety of this substance are conflicting, or there are not enough studies to draw a conclusion. Safety is a major concern, however; see the "Will It Harm You?" section.

- *For use as a diuretic:* 5 = Studies indicate that there is a definite health hazard to using this substance, even in recommended amounts.

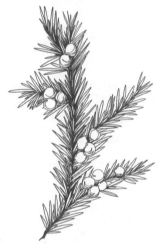

Juniper
Juniperus communis

attempting to make a diuretic ("water pill"); the word *gin* derives from the Dutch word for juniper—*geniver*. Until 1960, United States health authorities officially recognized juniper berries and their extracts as diuretics, a class of medicines sometimes prescribed for fluid retention, for menstrual bloating, and frequently for serious conditions such as congestive heart failure and high blood pressure.

Folk healers have prescribed juniper berry preparations to clear congested airways during a cold, treat arthritis and the painful inflammatory disease called gout, improve digestion, relax intestinal cramping and reduce excess gas, fight intestinal worms, and stimulate the appetite. Numerous laxatives contain juniper. Steam vapors have been used to treat bronchitis. European children are sometimes given juniper berry preparations as a tonic.

United States health authorities long endorsed the age-old tradition of using juniper to disinfect the genitourinary tract. Although that is no longer officially sanctioned, contemporary herbalists hail juniper berries for this purpose. Some consider topical formulations of the berries excellent antiseptics. In Germany, juniper spirits are rubbed into rheumatic joints and body parts aching from nerve pain. In Bulgaria, people suffering from neurasthenia neurosis, a vague ailment characterized by fatigue, are given juniper baths.[1]

Juniper berries and their extracts are added to foods and various alcoholic drinks as a flavoring, and to perfumes, cosmetics, lotions, soaps, and other items as a fragrance.

Forms Available Include:

- *For internal use:* Fruit (dried and ripe), infusion, liquid extract, oil, spirit, syrup, tincture. Because of the presence of a volatile oil that could dissipate with heat, avoid letting the water boil when making an infusion.
- *For external use:* Baths, spirits, tar.

Dosage Commonly Reported:

Juniper syrup is taken in dosages of 1 tablespoon morning and night.

Will It Work for You? What the Studies Say:

Few experts dispute the fact that juniper berries and their volatile oil function as diuretics by irritating the kidneys, not a preferred mechanism of action. A substance called terpinen-4-ol in the oil increases the fluid-filtering rate of these organs.[2] Over the years, many people have apparently benefited from the diuretic activity of juniper. Numerous herbal diuretics contain the plant. But many experts and health authorities consider the potential health risks in irritating the kidneys simply too high.

Juniper berries and their extracts increase intestinal movement and also contain a bitter-tasting substance (juniperin) that stimulates salivation and gastric juices and is believed to soothe stomach upset. German health authorities endorse the use of juniper berry infusions, decoctions, alcoholic extracts, and wine for indigestion and related heartburn, belching, and bloating.[3] The volatile oil and bitter also fight germs, but apparently no studies have been done to show that this helps to remedy bladder infections or that it benefits humans in any other way.

On the basis of a belief in the anti-inflammatory powers of juniper berries, some German doctors prescribe juniper preparations for arthritis and gout.[4] Liquid extracts made from the whole plant show anti-inflammatory activities in the test tube.[5] No clinical trials have verified an anti-inflammatory action or pain reduction in humans, however.

Intriguing new research indicates that juniper berries may hold hope for treating diabetes, although the subject requires further examination in humans. In one study, blood sugar levels and the death rate among mice with chemically induced diabetes dropped significantly after they consumed a decoction of the berries for twenty-four days.[6] This result reinforced earlier research findings that juniper berries could retard the development of chemically induced diabetes.[7]

Will It Harm You? What the Studies Say:

Take care when ingesting preparations of juniper berries. Some experts recommend avoiding the herb altogether or advise consulting a doctor first. A major concern is that excessive doses may seriously irritate and even damage the kidneys. Individuals with impairment of or potentially reduced function in these organs, such as the elderly, are at particularly high risk and may suffer damage even with typically recommended doses.

But even if you have never had kidney problems, avoid extended use. According to a German textbook, no juniper preparation should be taken for more than six weeks in a row.[8] High concentrations of the oil can cause stomach upset or diarrhea, and large doses can result in catharsis or convulsions.[9] If you are a gin drinker, take note that so little juniper oil (not more than 0.006 percent) is present in this and other alcoholic beverages that kidney damage— or any medicinal benefit—is very unlikely.

Never take juniper preparations in place of prescribed diuretics. Pregnant women should avoid the herb altogether, given findings that it can stimulate uterine contractions and thus pose a risk of miscarriage, although this has apparently never been documented. A handful of investigators have found that juniper berries may interfere with implantation of fertilized eggs in rats, but this type of antifertility action has never been demonstrated in humans.[10]

Although it can in some cases cause slight irritation and even allergic reactions, juniper oil appears to be relatively safe to apply to the skin.[11] The story with juniper tar, a type of topical preparation used to treat psoriases in some parts of the world, may be a little different; a recent study in human and mouse tissues found that it can lead to the formation of potentially cancer-causing cell damage.[12]

The pollen from juniper trees and various preparations made from the plant can cause allergic reactions.

GENERAL SOURCES:

Bisset, N.G., ed. *Herbal Drugs and Phytopharmaceuticals.* Stuttgart: medpharm GmbH Scientific Publishers, 1994.

Blumenthal, M., J. Gruenwald, T. Hall, and R.S. Rister, eds. *The Complete German Commission E Monographs: Therapeutic Guide to Herbal Medicine.* Boston: Integrative Medicine Communications, 1998.

Bousquet, J., et al. *Clinical Allergy.* 14 (1984): 249.

Castleman, M. *The Healing Herbs: The Ultimate Guide to the Curative Power of Nature's Medicines.* New York: Bantam Books, 1995.

Duke, J.A. *CRC Handbook of Medicinal Herbs.* Boca Raton, FL: CRC Press, 1985.

Hallowell, M. *Herbal Healing: A Practical Introduction to Medicinal Herbs.* Garden City Park, NY: 1994.

Kaufman, H.S., et al. *Annals of Allergy.* 53 (1984): 135.

Leung, A.Y. *Encyclopedia of Common Natural Ingredients Used in Food, Drugs, and Cosmetics.* New York: John Wiley & Sons, 1980.

Mascolo, N., et al. *Phytotherapy Research.* 1:1 (1987): 28.

Mayell, M. *Off-the-Shelf Natural Health: How to Use Herbs and Nutrients to Stay Well.* New York: Bantam Books, 1995.

Mindell, E. *Earl Mindell's Herb Bible.* New York: Simon & Schuster/Fireside, 1992.

Newall, C.A., et al. *Herbal Medicines: A Guide for Health-Care Professionals.* London: The Pharmaceutical Press, 1996.

Opdyke, D.L.J. *Food & Cosmetics Toxicology.* 14 (1976): 307.

Review of Natural Products. St. Louis: Facts and Comparisons, February 1997.

Takacsova, M., et al. *Nahrung.* 39(3) (1995): 241–43.

Tyler, V.E. *Herbs of Choice: The Therapeutic Use of Phytomedicinals.* Binghamton, NY: Haworth Press/Pharmaceutical Products Press, 1994.

———. *The Honest Herbal.* Binghamton, NY: Haworth Press/Pharmaceutical Products Press, 1993.

Weiss, R.F. *Herbal Medicine,* trans. A.R. Meuss, from the 6th German edition. Beaconsfield, England: Beaconsfield Publishers, Ltd., 1988.

TEXT CITATIONS:

1. S. Jonkov and G. Naidenov, *Folia Medica,* 16 (1974): 291–96.
2. J. Janku et al., *Experientia,* 13 (1957): 255.
3. N.G. Bisset, ed., *Herbal Drugs and Phytopharmaceuticals* (Stuttgart: medpharm GmbH Scientific Publishers, 1994). M. Blumenthal, J. Greenwald, T. Hall, and R. S. Rister, eds., *The Complete German Commission E Monographs: Therapeutic Guide to Herbal Medicine* (Boston: Integrative Medicine Communications, 1998).
4. R.F. Weiss, *Herbal Medicine,* trans. A.R. Meuss, from the 6th German edition (Beaconsfield, England: Beaconsfield Publishers, Ltd., 1988).
5. H. Tunon et al., *Journal of Ethnopharmacology,* 48(2) (1995): 61–76.
6. F. Sanchez de Medina et al., *Planta Medica,* 60(3) (1994): 197–200.
7. S.K. Swanston-Flatt et al., *Diabetologia,* 33(8) (1990): 462–64.
8. Weiss, op. cit.
9. *Review of Natural Products* (St. Louis: Facts and Comparisons, February 1977).
10. A.O. Prakash et al., *Acta Europaea Fertilitatis,* 16(6) (1985): 441–48. O.P. Agrawal et al., *Planta Medica,* Suppl. (1980): 98–101.
11. A.Y. Leung, *Encyclopedia of Common Natural Ingredients Used in Food, Drugs, and Cosmetics* (New York: John Wiley & Sons, 1980).
12. B. Schoket et al., *Journal of Investigative Dermatology,* 94(2) (1990): 241–46.

KAVA

SCIENTIFIC NAME:
Piper methysticum Forst. f.
Family: Piperaceae

COMMON NAMES:
Awa, intoxicating pepper, kava-kava, kew, tonga

RATING:
2 = According to a number of well-designed studies and common use, this substance appears to be relatively effective when used in recommended amounts for the indication(s) noted in the "Will It Work for You?" section. See the "Will It Harm You?" section for warnings, however.

What Is Kava?

Kava (or kava-kava) is a drink prepared by steeping the knotty underground roots of a large, hardy flowering shrub indigenous to the South Pacific called *Piper methysticum.* More than twenty varieties of this pepper family member have been recognized so far.

What It Is Used For:

South Pacific islanders prepare a relaxing "cocktail" with kava root that plays an important part in their social and ceremonial life, much as wine does in other parts of the world. Ailments traditionally treated with the decoction include migraine headache, venereal disease, gout, rheumatic conditions, colds and respiratory tract problems, wounds, and menstrual problems. Many sources recommend—and manufacturers tout—kava as a relaxant, antistress agent, remedy for nervous anxiety, sedative and insomnia cure, diuretic ("water pill"), aphrodisiac, sexual stimulant, antidepressant, and antidote to muscle spasm and cramping (including menstrual cramps). Several of these uses reflect folk traditions.

Forms Available Include:

Capsule, decoction, liquid extract, powder, root. Kava appears in numerous "herb drinks."

Varying degrees of composition and concentration of the active ingredients can be found in the many kava varieties. Preparations standardized for active ingredients may be available.

Dosage Commonly Reported:

A bowl of traditionally prepared kava drink contains about 250 milligrams kavalactones, and several bowls are often consumed at one sitting. Follow package instructions on commercial preparations. One or two 250-milligram capsules each of the extract, representing 75 milligrams of kavalactones each, are taken once or twice a day. A common dosage for a calming effect is 24 to 70 milligrams kavalactones three times per day; for a sedative effect, some sources recommend 180 to 210 milligrams kavalactones one hour before bedtime.

Will It Work for You? What the Studies Say:

After decades of analysis, many scientists now contend that the sensation of sleepiness and tranquillity that many people describe after drinking kava preparations can be largely explained by the presence of pharmacologically active compounds that depress (slow down) the central nervous system. These compounds, referred to as kavalactones (or kava alphapyrones), are found in the root. Other substances may be involved as well; their combined effects pose considerable risks if abused (see "Will It Harm You?" below). As long as various precautions are taken, German health authorities approve of kava for treating conditions of nervous anxiety, stress, and restlessness.[1] Certain kava compounds are marketed in Europe as mild sedatives for the elderly.

Kava drinkers report feeling more sociable, tranquil, articulate, sensitive to sound, and generally happy.[2] In a double-blind, placebo-controlled, four-week study, kava was shown to minimize anxiety symptoms such as nervousness, palpitations, headache, dizziness, and stomach upset in humans.[3] No side effects were reported. One clinical trial demonstrated benefits of kava in treating menopause-related symptoms.[4] Certain substances in kava apparently act directly on muscle contractility to produce a muscle-relaxing effect.[5]

Animal studies indicate that kava has sedative and antispasmodic properties. It apparently promotes sleep in the absence of sedation.[6] Full consciousness is maintained with even fatal doses.[7] It slows hyperactivity (in mice), although not nearly as much as standard antipsychotic drugs.[8]

Kava also boasts local pain-relieving properties. When chewed, the root produces numbness in the mouth similar to what one would experience with cocaine and longer-lasting than what one would experience with benzocaine.[9]

Will It Harm You? What the Studies Say:

Serious toxic reactions can develop when kava is not used with care. High doses can cause visual and skin problems, muscle weakness, and sleepiness. Kava appears in herb drinks that have caused serious health problems related to central nervous system depression, such as breathing problems, in people who apparently took doses higher than recommended. This prompted the FDA in 1997 to issue a warning on the drinks.[10] If kava is used over extended periods of time, a syndrome referred to as "kawaism" or "kawa dermopathy" may develop, with such symptoms as reddened eyes, scaly skin eruptions, and yellowish discoloration of skin, hair, and nails.[11] This discoloration has been attributed to the presence of two yellow pigments in the plant.[12]

Heavy users are also more likely to experience such general health problems as rashes, puffiness in the face, weight loss, blood in the urine, and blood abnormalities, among other problems.[13] These have been attributed to the kava, although heavy alcohol and cigarette use may also play a role.[14]

Even typically recommended doses may impair motor reflexes, judgment, and other factors necessary for driving and working heavy machinery safely.[15] Avoid mixing kava with other substances that act on the central nervous system, such as alcohol, barbiturates, and psychopharmacologic substances.[16] Drinking alcohol at the same time, for example, appears to increase the potential toxicity of kava.[17]

Allergic skin reactions to kava are possible.[18] German health authorities warn that it should not be taken in cases of depression or by women who are pregnant or nursing.[19]

Kava is not hallucinogenic, addictive, or dependency-causing.[20]

GENERAL SOURCES:

Review of Natural Products. St. Louis: Facts and Comparisons, November 1996.

Leung, A.Y., and S. Foster. *Encyclopedia of Common Natural Ingredients Used in Food, Drugs, and Cosmetics.* 2nd ed. New York: John Wiley & Sons, 1996.

Mindell, E. *Earl Mindell's Herb Bible.* New York: Simon & Schuster/Fireside, 1992.

Murray, M.T. *The Healing Power of Herbs: The Enlightened Person's Guide to the Wonders of Medicinal Plants.* Revised and expanded 2nd ed. Rocklin, CA: Prima Publishing, 1995.

Weiner, M.A., and J.A. Weiner. *Herbs That Heal: Prescription for Herbal Healing.* Mill Valley, CA: Quantum Books, 1994.

Weiss, R.F. *Herbal Medicine,* trans. A.R. Meuss, from the 6th German edition. Beaconsfield, England: Beaconsfield Publishers, Ltd., 1988.

TEXT CITATIONS:

1. M. Blumenthal, J. Gruenwald, T. Hall, and R. S. Rister, eds., *The Complete German Commission E Monographs: Therapeutic Guide to Herbal Medicine* (Boston: Integrative Medicine Communications, 1998).

2. *Review of Natural Products* (St. Louis: Facts and Comparisons, November 1996).

3. E. Kinzler et al., *Arzneimittel-Forschung,* 116(4) (1991): 469–74.

4. G. Warnecke, *Fortschritte der Medizine,* 109 (1991): 120–22.

5. Y. Lebot et al., *Kava, the Pacific Drug* (New Haven, CT: Yale University Press, 1992).

6. E. Holm et al., *Arzneimittel-Forschung,* 41(7) (1991): 673–83.

7. R.F. Weiss, *Herbal Medicine,* trans. A.R. Meuss, from the 6th German edition. (Beaconsfield, England: Beaconsfield Publishers, Ltd., 1988).

8. D.D. Jamieson and P.H. Duffield, *Clinical and Experimental Pharmacology and Physiology,* 17(7) (1990): 495–507.

9. *Review of Natural Products,* op. cit.

10. "FDA Warns That Herb Drink May Cause Health Problems," *New York Times,* January 3 (1997).

11. *Review of Natural Products,* op. cit.

12. A.T. Shulgin, *Bulletin on Narcotics,* 25 (1973): 59.

13. J.D. Matthews et al., *Medical Journal of Australia,* 148(11) (1988): 548–55.

14. M.T. Murray, *The Healing Power of Herbs: The Enlightened Person's Guide to the Wonders of Medicinal Plants,* revised and expanded 2nd ed. (Rocklin, CA: Prima Publishing, 1995).

15. Blumenthal et al., op. cit.

16. Ibid.

17. *Review of Natural Products,* op. cit. D.D. Jamieson and P.H. Duffield, *Clinical and Experimental Pharmacology and Physiology,* 17(7) (1990): 509–14.

18. Blumenthal et al., op. cit.

19. Ibid.

20. A.Y. Leung and S. Foster, *Encyclopedia of Common Natural Ingredients Used in Food, Drugs, and Cosmetics,* 2nd ed. (New York: John Wiley & Sons, 1996).

K

Kava

PRIMARY NAME:
KELP

SCIENTIFIC NAME:

Fucus vesiculosus, Ascophyllum nodosum, and various *Laminaria* (e.g., *Laminaria digitata* and *Laminaria japonica*), *Macrocystis,* and *Nereocystis* species. Family: Fucaceae

COMMON NAMES:

Bladder fucus, bladderwrack (*Fucus vesiculosus*), brown algae, cutweed, fucales, fucus, horsetail, kun bu, laminaria, rockweed, sea girdles, seawrack, sea vegetables, wakame

RATING:

4 = Research indicates that this substance will not fulfill the claims made for it. Its safety appears to depend on careful use; see the "Will It Harm You?" section.

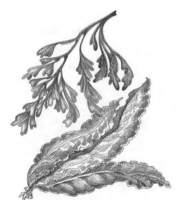

Bladderwrack (above)
Fucus vesiculosus
Kelp (below)
Laminaria saccharina

What Is Kelp?

The definition of kelp is steeped in confusion. All of the seaweeds noted under "Scientific Name" can be found in products marketed as kelp, as may others. For the most part, these flat, ribbonlike organisms grow attached to rocks by means of holdfasts, and have a salty and fishy taste and a mucilaginous consistency. They are found primarily in the cold waters of the Atlantic and Pacific oceans. The brown alga known as bladderwrack (*Fucus vesiculosus*) is a particularly common source of kelp. The entire plant body is used medicinally and for other purposes.

What It Is Used For:

Kelp has long served as a standard part of the Japanese diet and appears on any basic sushi menu. For decades in early America, iodide-rich kelp was valued highly for preventing goiter, an often unsightly enlargement of the thyroid gland caused by a deficiency in iodine. It was also popular as an antiseptic for wounds. A tincture was billed as a treatment for ailments ranging from syphilis to vaginal discharge, menstrual cramps, liver disorders, ovarian tumors, gallstones, bronchitis and asthma, ulcers, and testicle enlargement. Today, kelp tablets containing dried seaweed are still sold as sources of iodide as well as energy boosters, antiobesity agents, and weight loss ("slimming") aids. Some sources claim they can protect the consumer from arteriosclerosis and heart disease and from the harmful effects of exposure to radiation and toxic heavy metals.

Forms Available Include:

Capsule, infused oil, infusion, liquid extract, powder, raw (including granulated or powdered), tablet, tea (instant, often in herbal blends), tincture.

The mineral concentrations (including iodine) of various seaweeds used to make kelp preparations vary depending on such factors as the species used, the time it was harvested, and the age of the plant. Select a preparation with a standardized amount of the mineral desired. To avoid ingesting contaminants, do not collect your own kelp; buy it from a commercial source.

Dosage Commonly Reported:

An infusion is made using 2 to 3 teaspoons of dried powdered frond per cup of water and is drunk up to three times a day. Follow package instructions for dosage of commercial preparations.

Will It Work for You? What the Studies Say:

At one time, kelp may well have played an important role in providing critical minerals such as iodine. But in the age of iodized salt, few people living in developed countries are deficient in this mineral, which the adult body requires in small amounts (150 micrograms a day). Higher daily intake of iodine not only is worthless but may pose significant health hazards over time.

Iodine activates the thyroid gland. The argument that iodine-rich kelp will fight obesity applies only to situations in which a person is suffering from iodine deficiency and associated thyroid problems, an unlikely scenario given the plentiful stores of iodized salt in the American diet.[1] Critics contend that the iodine in kelp offers nothing superior to iodine from other, often cheaper and more standardized sources.[2] There is no evidence that the iodine in kelp will speed up your metabolism and help you lose weight if your thyroid function is normal.

German health authorities declined to approve of bladderwrack as a source of iodine for thyroid deficiency—they called this application obsolete—or for use in "slimming remedies" or to treat digestive disorders.[3] Claims that the iodine in kelp can benefit atherosclerosis by "cleansing" and "toning" blood vessels are unfounded,[4] and the German health authorities have not approved of it for these purposes either.

Some sources argue that the sodium alginate in kelp can help prevent absorption of heavy metals such as barium, plutonium, cesium, and radioactive strontium 90, a by-product of nuclear power and weapons plants and nuclear explosions.[5] Strontium 90 builds up in the body and has been linked to the development of leukemia, Hodgkin's disease, and other cancers. Studies have shown that sodium alginate can reduce the absorption of radioactive strontium in both animals and humans.[6] But several sources have questioned the need for this type of routine prevention in a society not experiencing major radioactive leaks or explosions.[7] They also point out that the recommended dosage could induce or worsen excess thyroid levels in the body.

Investigators are examining a possible role for laminaria in explaining the relatively low breast cancer rates in Japan[8] and have looked at potential anti-tumor-promoting properties in various models.[9] They have also examined anti-HIV components in bladderwrack.[10]

Will It Harm You? What the Studies Say:

The thyroid gland has only a limited capability for processing iodine. If taken in doses of more than 150 micrograms a day, the mineral poses the risk of inducing[11] or aggravating hyperthyroidism, possibly signaled by symptoms such as palpitations, sleeplessness, and restlessness. Or it may actually decrease thyroid function through a negative feedback mechanism.[12]

Do not take kelp if you suffer from hyperthyroidism, have heart problems, or are pregnant or nursing.[13] Kelp contains concentrations of sodium high enough to pose problems for people who have been told to reduce their sodium intake.[14]

The blood disorders autoimmune thrombocytopenia and dyserythropoiesis were linked to the ingestion of kelp supplements in one case.[15] Kelp has even been associated with cases of acnelike skin eruptions[16] and elevated urinary arsenic levels.[17]

GENERAL SOURCES:

American Pharmaceutical Association. *Handbook of Nonprescription Drugs.* 11th ed. Washington, D.C.: American Pharmaceutical Association, 1996.

Balch, J.F., and P.A. Balch. *Prescription for Nutritional Healing: A Practical A to Z Reference to Drug-Free Remedies Using Vitamins, Minerals, Herbs & Food Supplements.* 2nd ed. Garden City Park, NY: Avery Publishing Group, 1997.

Barrett, S., and V. Herbert. *The Vitamin Pushers: How the "Health Food" Industry Is Selling America a Bill of Goods.* Amherst, NY: Prometheus Books, 1994.

Bisset, N.G., ed. *Herbal Drugs and Phytopharmaceuticals.* Stuttgart: medpharm GmbH Scientific Publishers, 1994.

Blumenthal, M., J. Gruenwald, T. Hall, and R.S. Rister, eds., *The Complete German Commission E Monographs: Therapeutic Guide to Herbal Medicine.* Boston: Integrative Medicine Communications, 1998.

Bradley, P.C., ed. *British Herbal Compendium: A Handbook of Scientific Information on Widely Used Plant Drugs*, vol. 1. Bournemouth (Dorset), England: British Herbal Medicine Association, 1992.

Castleman, M. *The Healing Herbs: The Ultimate Guide to the Curative Power of Nature's Medicines.* New York: Bantam Books, 1995.

Lawrence Review of Natural Products. St. Louis: Facts and Comparisons, May 1992.

Tyler, V.E. *The Honest Herbal.* Binghamton, NY: Haworth Press/Pharmaceutical Products Press, 1993.

Tyler, V.E., L.R. Brady, and J.E. Robbers, eds. *Pharmacognosy.* Philadelphia: Lea & Febiger, 1988.

Weiss, R.F. *Herbal Medicine*, trans. A.R. Meuss, from the 6th German edition. Beaconsfield, England: Beaconsfield Publishers, Ltd., 1988.

TEXT CITATIONS:

1. V.E. Tyler, L.R. Brady, and J.E. Robbers, eds., *Pharmacognosy* (Philadelphia: Lea & Febiger, 1988).
2. R.F. Weiss, *Herbal Medicine*, trans. A.R. Meuss, from the 6th German edition (Beaconsfield, England: Beaconsfield Publishers, Ltd., 1988).
3. M. Blumenthal, J. Gruenwald, T. Hall, and R. S. Rister, eds., *The Complete German Commission E Monographs: Therapeutic Guide to Herbal Medicine* (Boston: Integrative Medicine Communications, 1998).
4. *Lawrence Review of Natural Products* (St. Louis: Facts and Comparisons, May 1992).
5. M. Castleman, *The Healing Herbs: The Ultimate Guide to the Curative Power of Nature's Medicines* (New York: Bantam Books, 1995).
6. Y.F. Gong et al., *Biomedical & Environmental Sciences*, 4(3) (1991): 273–82.
7. V.E. Tyler, *The Honest Herbal* (Binghamton, NY: Haworth Press/Pharmaceutical Products Press, 1993).
8. J. Teas, *Nutrition & Cancer*, 4(3) (1983): 217–22.
9. H. Ohigashi et al., *Bioscience, Biotechnology & Biochemistry*, 56(5) (1992): 994–95.
10. A. Beress et al., *Journal of Natural Products*, 56(4) (1993): 478–88.
11. P.A. de Smet et al., *Nederland Tijdschrift voor Geneeskunde*, 134(21) (1990): 1058–59.
12. American Pharmaceutical Association, *Handbook of Nonprescription Drugs*, 11th ed. (Washington, D.C.: American Pharmaceutical Association, 1996).
13. P.C. Bradley, ed., *British Herbal Compendium: A Handbook of Scientific Information on Widely Used Plant Drugs*, vol. 1 (Bournemouth [Dorset], England: British Herbal Medicine Association, 1992).
14. Tyler, Brady, and Robbers, op. cit.

15. K.G. Pye et al., *The Lancet*, 339 (1992): 8808.
16. B.L. Harrell and A.H. Rudolf, *Archives of Dermatology*, 112(4) (1976): 560.
17. O. Walkin and D.E. Douglas, *Canadian Medical Association Journal*, 111(12) (1974): 1301–2.

PRIMARY NAME:

KOLA (COLA)

SCIENTIFIC NAME:
Cola acuminata (Beauv.) Schott et Endl., and *Cola nitida* (Vent.) Schott et Endl. Family: Sterculiaceae

COMMON NAMES:
Guru nut, kola (cola) nut, kola (cola) seed

RATING:
2 = According to a number of well-designed studies and common use, this substance appears to be relatively effective and safe when used in recommended amounts for the indication(s) noted in the "Will It Work for You?" section.

What Is Kola?

The evergreen kola tree has long leathery leaves and bears purple-spotted yellow flowers. It produces fruits with seed-containing pods. For medicinal and other purposes, the dried seed, commonly called the "nut," is used. The seed coat is removed and the nut is ground to a powder. The more than one hundred *Kola* species are all indigenous to tropical West Africa. Both *Cola acuminata* and *Cola nitida*, which is cultivated in the tropics of Brazil, Jamaica, Sri Lanka, and other countries, are used commercially.

What It Is Used For:

West Africans have been chewing on the kola nut for its stimulant effect since time immemorial. They also consider kola valuable for reducing fevers. Sold to slave owners in Brazil and the Caribbean, the West Africans introduced the kola nut into these places, where they earned a reputation for treating fluid retention (as a diuretic, or "water pill"), fatigue, diarrhea, neuralgia (nerve pain), and digestive system problems, and for sexual stimulation. Kola nuts were also considered tonic and astringent.

Kola nut and coca leaf extracts (coca being the plant that produces cocaine) appear in the original Coca-Cola recipe introduced to Americans and the world in the late 1800s. Only minute amounts of kola nut purportedly remain in the "secret formula," as does decocainized coca leaf extract.[1] But contemporary herbalists continue to extol the kola nut for its stimulant effect and its purported ability to help treat asthma, enhance the effects of aspirin, and aid depression, diarrhea, migraine headache, and appetite loss. Kola commonly appears in diet and "energy" formulas.

Forms Available Include:

Concentrated drops, decoction (made with powder), extract, powder, tincture. Small amounts appear in cola beverages.

Dosage Commonly Reported:

A decoction is made using 1 to 2 teaspoons powdered nuts per cup of water and is drunk up to three times per day. A common dosage of tincture, extract, or concentrated drops is ½ to 1 dropperful.

Will It Work for You? What the Studies Say:

The primary active ingredient in kola nut is caffeine, although contrary to popular belief there is not as much as in a cup of coffee. A 12-ounce can of cola gives you about 40 milligrams of caffeine, compared with about 100 milligrams in a cup of brewed coffee and 60 milligrams in a cup of instant coffee. Some of the caffeine in the cola has probably been added by the manufacturer, however.

Presumably because of this caffeine content, German health authorities approve of kola nut for battling mental and physical fatigue.[2] Caffeine has also been recommended as an asthma treatment because it dilates (opens up) the bronchial tubes (airways), which swell and start to close during a typical attack. Kola also contains small amounts of theobromine, which likewise dilates the bronchial tubes. One source recommends cola drinks to help manage asthma in children, who may well prefer its taste to standard asthma medicines.[3] Whether cola drinks consistently contain enough caffeine or theobromine to help control asthma is unclear, however, and cola should never be relied upon to treat an asthma attack that is under way or be substituted for standard medicines unless a doctor recommends it. Caffeine's side effects, such as the jitters and hyperactivity, will probably become obvious and bothersome long before any significant antiasthma actions of the cola are seen.[4]

Migraine sufferers sometimes rely on cola drinks as a source of caffeine for preventing or controlling the headache, but quite a bit (equivalent to 100 to 200 milligrams) is generally needed to produce any benefit. Many combine the kola with aspirin.[5] Caffeine-containing substances such as kola and coffee are also mildly diuretic, but they are not commonly used for this purpose because unwanted side effects develop before adequate levels can accumulate.

Will It Harm You? What the Studies Say:

The risks associated with kola are the same as those seen with other caffeine-containing substances, such as tea (see **Tea, Black**) and **Maté**. The FDA categorizes kola nut as "Generally Recognized As Safe" (GRAS) for food consumption.

GENERAL SOURCES:

Blumenthal, M., J. Gruenwald, T. Hall, and R.S. Rister, eds. *The Complete German Commission E Monographs: Therapeutic Guide to Herbal Medicine.* Boston: Integrative Medicine Communications, 1998.

Castleman, M. *The Healing Herbs: The Ultimate Guide to the Curative Power of Nature's Medicines.* New York: Bantam Books, 1995.

Dobelis, I.N., ed. *The Magic and Medicine of Plants: A Practical Guide to the Science, History, Folklore, and Everyday Uses of Medicinal Plants.* Pleasantville, NY: Reader's Digest Association, 1986.

Leung, A.Y., and S. Foster. *Encyclopedia of Common Natural Ingredients Used in Food, Drugs, and Cosmetics.* 2nd ed. New York: John Wiley & Sons, 1996.

Mayell, M. *Off-the-Shelf Natural Health: How to Use Herbs and Nutrients to Stay Well.* New York: Bantam Books, 1995.

Tierra, M. *The Way of Herbs.* New York: Pocket Books, 1990.

Tyler, V.E. *Herbs of Choice: The Therapeutic Use of Phytomedicinals.* Binghamton, NY: Haworth Press/Pharmaceutical Products Press, 1994.

TEXT CITATIONS:

1. I.N. Dobelis, ed., *The Magic and Medicine of Plants: A Practical Guide to the Science, History, Folklore, and Everyday Uses of Medicinal Plants* (Pleasantville, NY: Reader's Digest Association, 1986).

2. M. Blumenthal, J. Gruenwald, T. Hall, and R. S. Rister, eds., *The Complete German Commission E Monographs: Therapeutic Guide to Herbal Medicine* (Boston: Integrative Medicine Communications, 1998).

3. C.C. Yarbrough, *Journal of the American Medical Association*, 230 (1974): 701.

4. V.E. Tyler, *Herbs of Choice: The Therapeutic Use of Phytomedicinals* (Binghamton, NY: Haworth Press/Pharmaceutical Products Press, 1994).

5. Ibid.

PRIMARY NAME:
KOMBUCHA (MANCHURIAN MUSHROOM)

SCIENTIFIC NAME:
N/A

COMMON NAMES:
Champagne of life, combucha tea, Dr. Sklenar's kombucha mushroom infusion, fungus Japonicus, kardasok tea, kombucha tea, kwassan, Manchurian tea, spumonto, t'chai from the sea, teekwass, tschambucco

RATING:
4 = Research indicates that this substance will not fulfill the claims made for it. Safety is a concern; see the "Will It Harm You?" section.

What Is Kombucha?

Kombucha is *not* a mushroom or a fungus, but rather a patty of gray material composed of various living organisms—usually yeast, bacteria, and lichen—that is used to ferment a tea in a mixture of water, black tea, sugar, or other prescribed elements. This fermented liquid or "brew" is subsequently drunk for its purported healing actions and has become quite a popular health beverage. As the patty grows, it is divided to create "daughter" "mushrooms" that are similarly used. The "mushrooms" are not themselves eaten at any point.

What It Is Used For:

Many enthusiasts claim that kombucha has been handed down through the centuries from Asian and Russian users. The practice of drinking fermented teas of various types certainly dates back some time in Eastern nations.[1] Introduced into North American in the mid-1990s, kombucha has been hailed by importers as a nutrient-rich, energizing brew and systemwide detoxifier and a preventive and therapeutic tool for slowing or reversing the course of aging and countless diseases ranging from intestinal disorders to cancer, rheumatism, multiple sclerosis, and AIDS. In Japan, the brew is concocted in seaweed (kombu) tea rather than black tea as is the custom in Western countries; hence the name "kombucha."[2]

Forms Available Include:

Capsule (as an ingredient in multiformulas), fluid extract, "mushroom," prepared tea.

Dosage Commonly Reported:

To use commercial kombucha preparations, follow the package instructions.

Will It Work for You? What the Studies Say:

No sound scientific evidence can be found to substantiate any of the numerous claims made for kombucha. According to various analyses, the fermented tea may contain sugar, alcohol, gluconic and lactic acids, yeasts, and possibly antibiotic substances.[3] Given that bacteria are involved in the fermenting process, the resulting tea may contain bacteria that alter the bacterial state of the gut.[4] In the 1960s, Dr. R. Sklenar developed his own system for diagnosing and treating cancer with kombucha as the featured ingredient. The handful of cases he reported to justify the value of his cancer regimen are devoid of sound medical data.[5] No human trials on kombucha can be found in the recent medical literature.

Will It Harm You? What the Studies Say:

Kombucha tea occasionally causes nausea and allergic reactions,[6] and several cases of severe illness and one fatality have been linked to it.[7] Homemade brews concocted in unsterile environments pose unique dangers because of the distinct risk of contamination with potentially harmful organisms. After analyzing the chemical constituents of several homemade brews in Germany, investigators recommended that while most are safe for normally healthy individuals, anyone whose immune system is suppressed should consume only kombucha beverages that are commercially prepared and controlled.[8]

GENERAL SOURCES:

Balch, J.F., and P.A. Balch. *Prescription for Nutritional Healing: A Practical A to Z Reference to Drug-Free Remedies Using Vitamins, Minerals, Herbs & Food Supplements.* 2nd ed. Garden City Park, NY: Avery Publishing Group, 1997.
Lawrence Review of Natural Products. St. Louis: Facts and Comparisons, August 1995.

TEXT CITATIONS:

1. *Lawrence Review of Natural Products* (St. Louis: Facts and Comparisons, August 1995).
2. R. Marin and N.A. Biddle, *Newsweek* (January 9, 1995): 64.
3. P. Mayser et al., *Mycoses,* 38(7–8) (1995): 289–95.
4. *Lawrence Review of Natural Products,* op. cit.
5. S.P. Hauser, *Schweizerische Rundschau für Medizin Praxis,* 79(9) (1990): 243–46.
6. *Lawrence Review of Natural Products,* op. cit.
7. A.D. Perron et al., *Annals of Emergency Medicine,* 26(5) (1995): 660–61. *Journal of the American Medical Association,* 275(2) (January 10, 1996): 96–98. W. Hearn, *American Medical News,* 38(17) (1995): 16.
8. Mayser, op. cit.

PRIMARY NAME:
KUDZU

SCIENTIFIC NAME:
Pueraria lobata (Willd.) Ohwi, *Pueraria thunbergiana* (Sieb. et Zucc.) Benth, and various other *Pueraria* species. Family: Leguminosae (Fabaceae)

COMMON NAMES:
Ge gen, Japanese arrowroot, ko ken, ku zu (Japan)

What Is Kudzu?

Introduced into the United States from eastern Asia a century ago, this hardy, hairy vine, a popular ground cover and fodder plant, now runs wild in the southeastern part of the country. Its tuberous roots and occasionally its flowers are used medicinally.

What It Is Used For:

Asian-Americans and certain other Asian communities enjoy kudzu root in soups and other foods. In traditional Asian medicine—Chinese, Japanese, Fijian—it has been used for centuries to treat ailments ranging from the common cold to allergies, flu, headache, neck stiffness, and diarrhea. Most intriguing to contemporary Western herbalists are reports that extracts of the plant can be used to treat alcoholism[1] and related alcohol toxicity, such as hangovers.[2] The flower is sometimes enlisted for this purpose as well. In recent times, kudzu

RATING:
3 = Studies on the effectiveness and safety of this substance are conflicting, or there are not enough studies to draw a conclusion.

has also been used to treat a host of other ailments including hives, psoriasis, high blood pressure, sudden deafness, and diabetes.

Forms Available Include:

Capsule, extract, flower, kudzu starch, root (dried slices or chopped pieces). Products may be standardized to the contained compound daidzin.

Dosage Commonly Reported:

Three 100-milligram capsules of the root extract, representing 1 milligram of daidzin, are taken daily. A standard daily dose of the root slices or pieces is 4.5 to 9 grams. Take commercial extracts according to package directions.

Will It Work for You? What the Studies Say:

Various parts of this twining vine—the root, starch, and flower—have shown promise in rapidly and dramatically curbing the desire for alcohol in small animals.[3] This was demonstrated in a classic animal model for testing alcohol-control substances.[4] In the model, alcohol-hungry Syrian golden hamsters are administered a substance and their drive to consume alcohol is then measured. Not only did a crude extract of kudzu injected into the hamsters significantly suppress their desire to consume the alcohol, but so did two major chemical compounds in the plant: daidzen and daidzin. These compounds are both powerful (and reversible) inhibitors of enzymes involved in the body's ability to metabolize alcohol (human alcohol dehydrogenase; ADH).[5] So far, however, no clinical trials appear to have been conducted to verify kudzu's effectiveness or safety in treating alcoholism in humans.

Another isoflavone compound, puerarin, represents the major active principle in the root.[6] Its actions help explain a number of traditional uses. For example, it and other isoflavones have been shown, through rat studies primarily, to lower blood pressure, block chemically induced irregular heart rhythms, lower blood sugar, and increase coronary and cerebral blood flow (by dilating coronary and cerebral vessels).[7] Human trials to verify that these actions occur in humans have yet to be done.

Will It Harm You? What the Studies Say:

Kudzu's long history of use as a food and medicinal herb in Asia testifies at least to some extent to its relative safety. No adverse reactions were noted in humans taking daily oral doses of 50 to 100 grams (of the root).[8] Overall, however, much remains to be learned about the chemical components of kudzu and their relative safety.

GENERAL SOURCES:
Lawrence Review of Natural Products. St. Louis: Facts and Comparisons, June 1994.
Leung, A.Y., and S. Foster. *Encyclopedia of Common Natural Ingredients Used in Food, Drugs, and Cosmetics.* 2nd ed. New York: John Wiley & Sons, 1996.
Mayell, M. *Off-the-Shelf Natural Health: How to Use Herbs and Nutrients to Stay Well.* New York: Bantam Books, 1995.
Tierra, M. *The Way of Herbs.* New York: Pocket Books, 1990.

K

Kudzu

TEXT CITATIONS:

1. *American Journal of Hospital Pharmacy*, 51 (1994): 750.
2. A.Y. Leung and S. Foster, *Encyclopedia of Common Natural Ingredients Used in Food, Drugs, and Cosmetics*, 2nd ed. (New York: John Wiley & Sons, 1996).
3. *American Journal of Hospital Pharmacy*, op. cit.
4. W.M. Keung and B.L. Vallee, *Proceedings of the National Academy of Sciences of the United States of America*, 90(21) (1993): 10008–12.
5. W.M. Keung, *Alcoholism, Clinical & Experimental Research*, 17(6) (1993): 1254–60.
6. Leung and Foster, op. cit.
7. Ibid.
8. Ibid.

PRIMARY NAME:
LABRADOR TEA

SCIENTIFIC NAME:
Ledum groenlandicum L.,
Ledum palustre L., *Ledum
latifolium* Jacq., and other
Ledum species. Family:
Ericaceae

COMMON NAMES:
Continental tea, James tea,
marsh tea, wild rosemary

RATING:
3 = Studies on the effectiveness
of this substance are
conflicting. Safety is a concern,
however; see the "Will It Harm
You?" section.

What Is Labrador Tea?

Labrador tea is made from the dried leaves of *Ledum* species, aromatic ever-green shrubs found in Greenland and throughout North America, including Labrador. They have bright green, dull-tipped leaves and bear seed-filled fruit capsules and white, bell-shaped flowers. The plant threatens to become endan-gered in parts of the United States.[1]

What It Is Used For:

This flavorful tea filled the bellies of early Americans engaged in the American Revolution who were unable to get their preferred commercial tea.[2] Through the decades it has also been taken to treat upper respiratory ailments such as coughs, colds, and bronchial infections. Many people have turned to it to treat headaches, rheumatism, kidney problems, diarrhea, and cancers. Strong decoc-tions are applied to itchy, red, or otherwise irritated skin. Other skin conditions such as acne and insect stings have also been treated with external formula-tions. Homeopaths recommend minute amounts for asthma and various other ailments. (See page 2 for a discussion of homeopathy.)

Forms Available Include:

Decoction, dried leaves, infusion.

Dosage Commonly Reported:

Given safety concerns with strong infusions, use only 1 teaspoon of dried leaves per cup of hot water,[3] and steep for a brief period of time. A stronger decoction is reserved for external use.

Will It Work for You? What the Studies Say:

Certain *Ledum* species such as *Ledum latifolium* and *Ledum groenlandicum* con-tain astringent tannins that are known to help constrict tissue and reduce ooz-ing and bleeding. Strong decoctions of the plant placed on inflamed, itchy, or oozing skin conditions or wounds may therefore help in healing. No studies have been done to verify this effect, however. Likewise, the volatile oil in the leaves contains camphor (ledol)[4] that may contribute to the tea's apparent ben-efit for symptoms related to colds and other upper respiratory tract conditions, but no research on the subject can be found to confirm this.

Will It Harm You? What the Studies Say:

While external formulations of this tea are probably relatively safe to use, be sure to stick to small doses and weak concentrations of the tea internally or you may risk serious adverse reactions. The plant has narcotic properties that can cause delirium and poisoning followed by paralysis and even death.[5] The toxic element is grayanotoxin, which can slow the pulse, lower blood pressure, and cause convulsions and more grave reactions such as paralysis.[6] Serious respira-tory conditions such as pulmonary infections or even persistent cough should be examined by a qualified health care professional.

GENERAL SOURCES:
Duke, J.A. *CRC Handbook of Medicinal Herbs*. Boca Raton, FL: CRC Press, 1985.
Review of Natural Products. St. Louis: Facts and Comparisons, November 1996.

TEXT CITATIONS:
1. *Review of Natural Products* (St. Louis: Facts and Comparisons, November 1996).
2. Ibid.
3. Ibid.
4. J.A. Duke, *CRC Handbook of Medicinal Herbs* (Boca Raton, FL: CRC Press, 1985).
5. *Review of Natural Products*, op. cit.
6. W.H. Lewis et al., *Medical Botany: Plants Affecting Man's Health* (New York: John Wiley & Sons, Inc., 1977).

L

Lady's Mantle

LADY'S MANTLE

SCIENTIFIC NAME:
Alchemilla xanthochlora
Rothm., also referred to as
Alchemilla vulgaris auct. non L.
Family: Rosaceae

COMMON NAMES:
Alchemilla, alchemille, heavenly dew

RATING:
3 = Studies on the effectiveness and safety of this substance are conflicting. Safety appears to depend on judicious use; see the "Will It Harm You" section.

What Is Lady's Mantle?

This light-green perennial bears rosettes of fan-shaped leaves that close into a funnel shape at night, efficiently collecting droplets of rainwater or dew by early morning. Although it is a member of the rose family, the plant's tiny yellow-green flowers grow in tight clusters and are nondescript. Lady's mantle grows in North America, Europe, and Asia. The flowering stems and basal leaves—and occasionally the entire aboveground part of the plant—are used medicinally.

What It Is Used For:

The Latin name *Alchemilla* reflects this plant's long association with alchemy, a medieval form of chemistry. Alchemists attributed magical and medicinal powers to the drops of liquid they found nestled in the leaf center in the morning. They called it "heavenly dew." Lady's mantle has been used externally to promote healing in wounds and bruises and to control vaginal discharge. Many folk healers considered it astringent and anti-inflammatory.

Contemporary herbalists recommend the herb for many of the same disorders it was valued for in the past: to lessen excessive menstrual bleeding, promote menstrual regularity, control diarrhea, counter muscle spasms, boost the appetite, promote urine production (as a diuretic, or "water pill"), and treat wounds and stop bleeding in the form of a poultice or wash. Baths and cosmetics containing lady's mantle have also been popular. The herb appears in European gynecological remedies as well as oral hygiene products.

Forms Available Include:

- *For internal use:* Dried herb, infusion, tincture.
- *For external use:* Decoction and diluted extracts for washes, douches, gargles, bath preparations, and poultices.

Dosage Commonly Reported:

A common daily dosage of tincture is 5 to 10 grams. An infusion is made using 1 to 2 teaspoons (1 to 2 grams) herb per cup of water.

Will It Work for You? What the Studies Say:

Intensive scientific investigations conducted years ago failed to uncover any notable healing properties in lady's mantle, although using it internally for diarrhea and externally for wounds and bleeding is somewhat justified by the presence of astringent tannins (6 to 8 percent). Tannins are believed to control or stop diarrhea by reducing inflammation in the intestines and to help wounds heal by constricting (tightening) tissue and reducing oozing and bleeding. German health authorities approve of lady's mantle in internal form for mild diarrhea not due to underlying disease.[1]

In one of the few studies done in humans so far, an extract of the herb reduced both the blood flow and the length of the menstrual cycle in 341 Romanian teenagers suffering from irregular or excessive menstrual bleeding (including bleeding between periods).[2] The girls, aged eleven to seventeen, took the extract by mouth. The herb demonstrated antibleeding properties within three to five days, and appeared to have a protective effect overall when taken ten to fifteen days before the periods were due. The quality of this study and its implications are relatively unclear because the report is accessible only in abbreviated abstract form.

Test-tube studies of this herb have yielded mixed results in terms of the herb's potentially beneficial or harmful effects. On the positive side, extracts may help fight fungi, according to one investigation, although they do so inconsistently.[3] The herb may also have antioxidant properties and inhibit enzymes that can damage connective and elastic tissue.[4] (Antioxidants control the formation of dangerous substances in the body called free radicals, which may contribute to cancer cell formation.) On the other hand, some investigators have found that the herb may have mutagenic properties,[5] meaning that it may promote the development of potentially cancerous cell changes. Other studies indicate that a fraction of the herb may be cytostatic, meaning that it stops the normal functioning of some normal cells.[6]

Will It Harm You? What the Studies Say:

Neither internal nor external use of this traditional healing herb has been associated with serious adverse reactions, although specific toxicity studies have yet to be done. Stick to recommended doses. Ingestion of any tannin-rich substance for long periods should be avoided, given indications that tannins may raise the risk of cancer. German health authorities cite no known side effects or situations in which the herb should not be used, but do advise that any diarrhea lasting more than three to four days be examined by a doctor.[7] Some experts consider the risk of possible liver damage cited by the German Standard License; some other plant experts consider this caution exaggerated.[8]

Although it has never been shown to induce miscarriage, pregnant women may want to avoid the herb given its long-standing use for menstrual irregularities.

GENERAL SOURCES:

Bisset, N.G., ed. *Herbal Drugs and Phytopharmaceuticals.* Stuttgart: medpharm GmbH Scientific Publishers, 1994.

Blumenthal, M., J. Gruenwald, T. Hall, and R.S. Rister, eds. *The Complete German Commission E Monographs: Therapeutic Guide to Herbal Medicine.* Boston: Integrative Medicine Communications, 1998.

Dobelis, I.N., ed. *The Magic and Medicine of Plants: A Practical Guide to the Science, History, Folklore, and Everyday Uses of Medicinal Plants.* Pleasantville, NY: Reader's Digest Association, 1986.

Lawrence Review of Natural Products. St. Louis: Facts and Comparisons, August 1996.

Mindell, E. *Earl Mindell's Herb Bible.* New York: Simon & Schuster/Fireside, 1992.

Stary, F. *The Natural Guide to Medicinal Herbs and Plants.* Prague: Barnes & Noble, Inc., in arrangement with Aventinum Publishers, 1996.

Tierra, M. *The Way of Herbs.* New York: Pocket Books, 1990.

Weiss, R.F. *Herbal Medicine*, trans. A.R. Meuss, from the 6th German edition. Beaconsfield, England: Beaconsfield Publishers, Ltd., 1988.

TEXT CITATIONS:

1. M. Blumenthal, J. Gruenwald, T. Hall, and R. S. Rister, eds., *The Complete German Commission E Monographs: Therapeutic Guide to Herbal Medicine* (Boston: Integrative Medicine Communications, 1998).

2. P. Petcu et al., *Clujul Medica*, 52 (1979): 266–70.

3. J.C. Guerin and H.P. Reveillere, *Annales Pharmaceutiques Françaises*, 42(6) (1984): 553–59.

4. M. Jonadet et al., *Journal de Pharmacologie*, 17(1) (1986): 21. *Lawrence Review of Natural Products* (St. Louis: Facts and Comparisons, August 1996).

5. O. Schimmer et al., *Mutation Research*, 206(2) (1988): 201–8.

6. *Lawrence Review of Natural Products*, op. cit.

7. Blumenthal et al., op. cit.

8. N.G. Bisset, ed., *Herbal Drugs and Phytopharmaceuticals* (Stuttgart: medpharm GmbH Scientific Publishers, 1994).

PRIMARY NAME:
LADY'S SLIPPER

SCIENTIFIC NAME:

Cypripedium pubescens Wills. and related species, including *Cypripedium calceolus* L. var *pubescens* and *Cypripedium acaule*. Family: Orchidaceae

COMMON NAMES:

American valerian, cypripedium, moccasin flower, nerveroot, whippoorwill's shoe, yellow Indian shoe

What Is Lady's Slipper?

The various perennial orchids referred to as lady's slipper all have broad, lance-shaped leaves and strong stems upon which appear complex and remarkable flowers ranging in color from golden yellow to pink. One of the petals forms a pouchlike structure reminiscent of a slipper, hence the name "lady's slipper." The rhizomes (underground stems) and roots have been used medicinally. *Cypripedium pubescens* is native to eastern North America and once populated the woods and pastures until overharvesting depleted it. It is now endangered in many states and officially protected in some.

What It Is Used For:

In nineteenth-century America, this Native American herb was recommended by many folk healers as a sedative for nervous headache, anxiety states, hysteria, depression, headache, menstrual and labor pains, epilepsy, neuralgia, and emo-

RATING:

4 = Research indicates that this subtance will not fulfill the claims made for it, but that it is also unlikely to cause any harm.

tional tension. Native Americans valued it highly as an antispasmodic and insomnia remedy, especially for anxiety-related insomnia. The nickname "American valerian" does not point to any resemblance to true valerian (*Valeriana officinalis*), a widely recognized sedative herb (see **Valerian**), although lady's slipper does have a reputation as a mild hypnotic and sedative. Few contemporary herbalists recommend the herb.

Forms Available Include:

Dried root, infusion, liquid extract. However, the herb is rarely available.

Dosage Commonly Reported:

In times past, an infusion was made with 2 to 4 grams of the dried rhizome or root and taken three times a day; 2 to 4 milliliters of the liquid extract was taken three times a day.

Will It Work for You? What the Studies Say:

Lady's slipper is a poorly researched herb, and none of its purported healing properties have been scientifically proved. More importantly, *the ethics of using this now rare plant are questionable.*

Will It Harm You? What the Studies Say:

Science has revealed even less about the potential toxicity of this herb than about its potential effectiveness. Ingesting the herb can cause allergic reactions in sensitized individuals, and handling it can cause contact dermatitis.[1] The sensitizing substance may be a chemical called a quinone, according to one of the few research papers on the herb.[2] Lady's slipper can cause psychedelic reactions, according to one source, and large doses may result in restlessness, giddiness, visual hallucinations, and mental excitement.[3]

GENERAL SOURCES:

Chevallier, A. *The Encyclopedia of Medicinal Plants: A Practical Reference Guide to More Than 550 Key Medicinal Plants & Their Uses.* 1st American ed. New York: Dorling Kindersley Publications, 1996.

Dobelis, I.N., ed. *The Magic and Medicine of Plants: A Practical Guide to the Science, History, Folklore, and Everyday Uses of Medicinal Plants.* Pleasantville, NY: Reader's Digest Association, 1986.

Newall, C.A., et al. *Herbal Medicines: A Guide for Health-Care Professionals.* London: The Pharmaceutical Press, 1996.

TEXT CITATIONS:

1. C.A. Newall et al., *Herbal Medicines: A Guide for Health-Care Professionals* (London: The Pharmaceutical Press, 1996).
2. H. Schmalle and B.M. Hausen, *Naturwissenschaften,* 66 (1979): 527–28.
3. Newall, op. cit.

L

Lady's Slipper

PRIMARY NAME:
LAVENDER

SCIENTIFIC NAME:
Lavendula angustifolia Mill., sometimes referred to as *Lavendula spica* L., *Lavendula officinalis* Chaix., or *Lavendula vera* DC. Other Lavendula species have been used medicinally as well, including *Lavendula latifolia* Medic. or Vill. and *Lavendula pubescens* Decne. Family: Labiatae (Lamiaceae)

COMMON NAMES:
Lavendula angustifolia: garden lavender, true lavender; *Lavendula latifolia:* aspic, broad-leafed lavender, spike lavender; lavandin (a hybrid)

RATING:
3 = Studies on the effectiveness and safety of this herb are conflicting, or there are not enough studies to draw a conclusion.

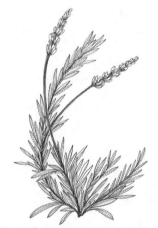

Lavender
Lavendula angustifolia

What Is Lavender?

This aromatic, evergreen half-shrub features spikes of small white, blue, or purple flowers. The flowers are collected and specially treated to extract a fragrant essential oil. Both the flowers and the oil are used medicinally. Lavender is indigenous to the Mediterranean region.

What It Is Used For:

Lavender is a heady-smelling herb that can claim centuries of renown as a perfume component as well as a general tonic, sedative, antispasmodic, diuretic ("water pill"), digestive aid, and gas remedy. In parts of the world including Europe, the herb is still added to "sleep pillows" and appears in sleep aids and sedatives and formulas for nervousness, depression, emotional upset, stress, headache, psoriasis and other skin problems, delayed menstruation, cancer, diabetes,[1] and digestive system upset due to bile or gallbladder problems. Steamed flowers have been used to treat colds. Special tonics and nerve pain baths and rubs contain lavender.

The essential oil features prominently in aromatherapy for sleep problems, fatigue, depresed mood, anxiety, and poor mental functioning.[2] Many still treasure it in perfumes, potpourris, and sachets; on linens; and in herbal formulas that might otherwise smell unpleasant. Extracts of spike lavender in particular are used in European insect and moth repellents.[3] Very small amounts of the herb and its oil are used to flavor teas and foods. Lavender is also cultivated for its beauty.

Forms Available Include:

Decoction, dried flowers, infusion, oil, tincture. Extracts—usually of the cheaper spike lavender—appear in many commercial products, including soaps and other bath products.

Dosage Commonly Reported:

A tea is made using 1 to 2 teaspoons lavender flowers per cup of water and is drunk several times per day, especially before bedtime. One to four drops of the oil on a sugar cube are taken internally. For external use, one to five drops oil are added to bathwater.

Will It Work for You? What the Studies Say:

Depending on the species, lavender flowers contain from 0.5 to 1.5 percent or more of a complex, highly aromatic volatile oil. Most of the therapeutic qualities ascribed to the herb can be attributed to this oil. Preliminary evidence indicates that it functions as a sedative and antispasmodic (calming agent) in humans, although much more research is needed to make any firm conclusions.[4] German health authorities endorse the use of lavender tea (or oil on a sugar cube) for restlessness and difficulty sleeping.[5] Extracts appear in prepared sedatives and tonics. In mouse experiments, the oil depresses (slows down) the central nervous system, inhibits spontaneous movement (motor activity), counters convulsions, and enhances the narcotic effects of another medicine (chloral hydrate).[6] Studies also show that spike lavender oil has antispasmodic actions in smooth muscles of various laboratory animals.[7]

In one of the few human trials done with lavender so far, investigators reported in *The Lancet*, a distinguished peer-reviewed British medical journal, that the oil may benefit insomniacs when used in the form of an aromatherapy.[8] The investigators in a six-week study involving only four geriatric nursing home patients with insomnia found that when they perfumed the sleeping ward with lavender and lavender oil for two weeks, patients slept as long as they did during a separate two-week interval in which they took their regularly prescribed powerful hypnotics. They were also less restless while sleeping. In contrast, sleep time diminished notably in a two-week interval in which the drug-free patients were exposed to no lavender at all.

The herb's value in soothing stomach upset, reducing excess gas, or encouraging bile flow remains unclear. Conceding a dearth of pharmacological information, German health authorities nonetheless decided to endorse the use of lavender tea (or oil on a sugar cube) for functional disturbances of the upper abdomen such as nervous irritable stomach.[9] Many volatile oils help with such discomforts, but direct evidence to support lavender's value cannot be found.[10] One German medicinal textbook considers lavender secondary to other herbs for gallbladder or bile duct disorders that influence the digestive process; its ability to promote the production, flow, or discharge of bile (choleretic or cholagogic effects) and thus aid the digestive process appears to be relatively weak.[11] German health authorities note that in combination with other herbs lavender may be particularly beneficial as both a sedative and a gas remedy.[12]

In Germany, lavender baths are considered valuable for stimulating the skin and body as a whole, treating wounds, and soothing and strengthening the nervous system.[13] German health authorities officially approve of lavender as a bath additive to treat functional circulation disorders.[14] Evidence to prove its effectiveness for these conditions cannot be found, although some sources cite the ability of lavender to irritate the olfactory nerves and hence influence the "autonomic centers in the midbrain."[15] The astringent tannins and demonstrated antimicrobial actions of the oil help explain its value for treating wounds.[16] A 1994 study described success in relieving postchildbirth perianal discomfort; the women reported less discomfort on the third, fourth, and fifth days when they added true lavender oil to their bath rather than a placebo or synthetic oil.[17]

Studies have found that lavender oil from certain species (*Lavendula stoechas*, *Lavendula latifolia*, *Lavendula dentata*) lowers blood sugar levels in rats with normal blood sugar levels (but not necessarily in those with chemically induced diabetes).[18] The implications for manipulating blood sugar levels—and diabetes—in humans are still far from clear, however.

Although spike lavender oil and lavandin oil contain many of the same chemicals that true lavender oil does, they are considered of lower quality because they contain relatively fewer active ingredients.

Will It Harm You? What the Studies Say:

Most research indicates that lavender and its oil are not likely to sensitize or irritate human skin, although allergic skin reactions have been reported recently.[19] Teas and other internal formulations have not been associated with serious adverse reactions. However, avoid ingesting or applying large doses of the oil, given the risk of contact dermatitis or even reactions similar to narcotic poisoning.[20]

GENERAL SOURCES:

Balch, J.F., and P.A. Balch. *Prescription for Nutritional Healing: A Practical A to Z Reference to Drug-Free Remedies Using Vitamins, Minerals, Herbs & Food Supplements.* 2nd ed. Garden City Park, NY: Avery Publishing Group, 1997.

Bisset, N.G., ed. *Herbal Drugs and Phytopharmaceuticals.* Stuttgart: medpharm GmbH Scientific Publishers, 1994.

Blumenthal, M., J. Gruenwald, T. Hall, and R.S. Rister, eds. *The Complete German Commission E Monographs: Therapeutic Guide to Herbal Medicine.* Boston: Integrative Medicine Communications, 1998.

Review of Natural Products. St. Louis: Facts and Comparisons, December 1996.

Leung, A.Y., and S. Foster. *Encyclopedia of Common Natural Ingredients Used in Food, Drugs, and Cosmetics.* 2nd ed. New York: John Wiley & Sons, 1996.

Stary, F. *The Natural Guide to Medicinal Herbs and Plants.* Prague: Barnes & Noble, Inc., in arrangement with Aventinum Publishers, 1996.

Tierra, M. *The Way of Herbs.* New York: Pocket Books, 1990.

Weiss, R.F. *Herbal Medicine,* trans. A.R. Meuss, from the 6th German edition. Beaconsfield, England: Beaconsfield Publishers, Ltd., 1988.

TEXT CITATIONS:

1. *Review of Natural Products* (St. Louis: Facts and Comparisons, December 1996).
2. I. Leshchinkskaia et al., *Kosmicheskaia Biologiia i Meditsina,* 17(2) (1983): 80–83. C. Dunn et al., *Journal of Advanced Nursing,* 21(1) (1995): 34–40.
3. D.M. Secoy and A.E. Smith, *Economic Botany,* 37 (1983): 28.
4. N.G. Bisset, ed., *Herbal Drugs and Phytopharmaceuticals* (Stuttgart: medpharm GmbH Scientific Publishers, 1994).
5. M. Blumenthal, J. Gruenwald, T. Hall, and R.S. Rister, eds., *The Complete German Commission E Monographs: Therapeutic Guide to Herbal Medicine* (Boston: Integrative Medicine Communications, 1998).
6. A.Y. Leung and S. Foster, *Encyclopedia of Common Natural Ingredients Used in Food, Drugs, and Cosmetics,* 2nd ed. (New York: John Wiley & Sons, 1996).
7. Ibid.
8. M. Hardy et al., *The Lancet,* 346 (September 9, 1995): 701.
9. Blumenthal et al., op. cit. Bisset, op. cit.
10. *Review of Natural Products,* op. cit.
11. R.F. Weiss, *Herbal Medicine,* trans. A.R. Meuss, from the 6th German edition (Beaconsfield, England: Beaconsfield Publishers, Ltd., 1988).
12. Bisset, op. cit.
13. Weiss, op. cit.
14. Blumenthal et al., op. cit.
15. Weiss, op. cit.
16. Leung and Foster, op. cit.
17. A. Dale et al., *Journal of Advanced Nursing,* 19(1) (1994): 89–96.
18. M.J. Gamez et al., *Pharmazie,* 43 (1988): 441.
19. M. Rademaker, *Contact Dermatitis,* 31(1) (1994): 58–59. M. Schaller et al., *Clinical & Experimental Dermatology,* 20(2) (1995): 143–45.
20. M. De Vincenzi and M.R. Dessi, *Fitoterapia,* 62(1) (1991): 39.

PRIMARY NAME:
LECITHIN

SCIENTIFIC NAME:
N/A

COMMON NAME:
N/A

RATING:
3 = Studies on the effectiveness and safety of this substance are conflicting, or there are not enough studies to draw a conclusion.

What Is Lecithin?

Lecithin is a natural compound found in all living organisms. It is a lipid (fat) manufactured by the liver and also present in brain and other tissues, as well as in many foods (such as egg yolks, soybeans, whole grains). It is the common name for a group of compounds called phosphatidylcholines (PPCs) and is the major source of the chemical nutrient choline. (Popular sources often make little distinction between the benefits of lecithin and choline.)

A distinction must be made between natural and commercially produced lecithin. Lecithin that is manufactured commercially, usually from soybeans or egg yolks, and that is now being sold as a dietary supplement, contains variable amounts of PPCs (30 to 90 percent) combined with other substances. It is unlikely that choline in PPCs or in any other form can be classified as a vitamin, as some proponents have claimed, given that the body can make choline on its own.

What It Is Used For:

The cells of all living organisms contain lecithin, which must be present for the body to function normally. Large concentrations in particular are found in the human nervous system and brain. The food industry has long used commercial lecithin in processed foods such as margarine and ice cream to act as a thickener, emulsifier, or stabilizer. The pharmaceutical and cosmetic industries use it similarly. Lecithin is partly soluble in water.

Recently some sources have started to recommend taking lecithin supplements to help remedy a host of ailments including gallstones, skin and nerve disorders, and liver damage caused by alcohol consumption. Some say lecithin will help strengthen weak muscles, boost brain function and memory, and improve balance. A few even argue that lecithin causes cholesterol and other fats to be dissolved in water and flushed out of the body, thus protecting against artery-clogging fatty buildup and aiding in the prevention of heart disease. Individuals taking niacin or nicotinic acid for high serum cholesterol and triglycerides are advised to integrate lecithin supplements into their diets. Finally, some contend that lecithin's value as an emulsifying agent can help boost digestion of fats, especially if taken before a meal, and may in this and other ways encourage weight loss. Recently, lecithin derived from egg yolks rather than soybeans has been promoted for use by people suffering from herpes, AIDS, chronic fatigue syndrome, or age-related immune disorders.[1]

Forms Available Include:

Capsule, granules, liquid.

Dosage Commonly Reported:

A common dosage is 5 to 10 grams in capsule form (or 1 to 2 tablespoons granules) of lecithin that is 20 percent phosphatidylcholine.

Will It Work for You? What the Studies Say:

The choline in lecithin is biologically necessary for the synthesis of a neurotransmitter called acetylcholine. Research indicates that in many neurologic disorders, acetylcholine activity is abnormal. On the basis of this observation, attempts have been made to recalibrate the level of this important neurotransmitter by flooding the system with its chemical precursors such as lecithin and its contained substance, choline. Very pure lecithin (90 percent PPC) improved the condition of manic individuals in one small but well-designed study.[2] Evidence also indicates that lecithin may prove beneficial in controlling certain neurologic disorders such as Tourette's syndrome[3] and Parkinson's disease,[4] although much more research is needed. A 1986 study of eighteen adults with tardive dyskinesia found no clinically important improvements in the disease compared with a placebo when the subjects took lecithin along with their lithium.[5]

Researchers have found that individuals with Alzheimer's disease have significantly depleted stores of acetylcholine in certain parts of the brain. Trials attempting to restore these levels and thus improve memory have been inconclusive. In one double-blind study, daily supplements for up to six weeks helped improve memory deficits in individuals with senile dementia (Alzheimer's, for example),[6] but later studies failed to replicate these positive findings.[7] Lecithin's role in preventing memory problems in individuals at risk for senile dementia is likewise unclear, as is the value of long-term supplementation with lecithin (or choline) to stabilize the course of Alzheimer's disease.[8] The capacity of lecithin (or choline) supplements to improve memory in normal, healthy adults is even hazier. A well-designed but small 1983 study in normal adults found that taking 20 grams of lecithin five hours before a memory test did not improve performance in any significant way.[9]

Limited evidence indicates that lecithin supplements reduce gallstone pain; in a small trial of individuals who had a tendency to develop cholesterol gallstones, lecithin supplements lessened the frequency of visceral pain. The subjects took the supplement for up to a year. The existing gallstones did not get smaller, however.[10] Interestingly, the gallbladder rests just under the liver. German health authorities have approved of soybean lecithin for improving subjective complaints such as appetite loss and sensations of pressure around the liver in cases of liver disease and chronic hepatitis.[11]

Relatively little sound clinical data can be found to support the claim that lecithin supplements will consistently reduce high cholesterol levels and decrease the incidence or progression of atherosclerosis and attendant coronary heart disease.[12] German health authorities, however, have approved of lecithin from soybeans to treat less severe forms of high cholesterol in which diet and other medical interventions have shown no results.[13] Evidence for any brain-boosting, mood-elevating, weight-reducing, or sexual stimulant properties is weak and has not been put to the test of clinical trials.

Will It Harm You? What the Studies Say:

Lecithin supplements taken in recommended amounts have not been associated with significant adverse reactions, although large doses have caused stomach and intestinal upset, vomiting, loose stools, and sweating in some individuals.[14] Most adults can tolerate doses up to 20 grams per day, and in some cases 30 grams per day, with no noticeable side effects. On the basis of studies in which the pups of rats who had been fed a diet containing 5 percent crude lecithin developed various abnormalities, pregnant women should probably avoid lecithin supplements.[15]

GENERAL SOURCES:

American Pharmaceutical Association. *Handbook of Nonprescription Drugs.* 11th ed. Washington, D.C.: American Pharmaceutical Association, 1996.

Balch, J.F., and P.A. Balch. *Prescription for Nutritional Healing: A Practical A to Z Reference to Drug-Free Remedies Using Vitamins, Minerals, Herbs & Food Supplements.* 2nd ed. Garden City Park, NY: Avery Publishing Group, 1997.

Barrett, S., and V. Herbert. *The Vitamin Pushers: How the "Health Food" Industry Is Selling America a Bill of Goods.* Amherst, NY: Prometheus Books, 1994.

Blumenthal, M., J. Gruenwald, T. Hall, and R.S. Rister, eds. *The Complete German Commission E Monographs: Therapeutic Guide to Herbal Medicine.* Boston: Integrative Medicine Communications, 1998.

Der Marderosian, A., and L. Liberti. *Natural Product Medicine. A Scientific Guide to Foods, Drugs, Cosmetics.* Philadelphia: George F. Stickley, 1988.

Griffith, H.W. *Complete Guide to Vitamins, Minerals, Nutrients & Supplements.* Tucson: Fisher Books, 1988.

Levy, R. *The Lancet.* 2(8299) (1982): 671–72.

Mayell, M. *Off-the-Shelf Natural Health: How to Use Herbs and Nutrients to Stay Well.* New York: Bantam Books, 1995.

Tyler, V.E., L.R. Brady, and J.E. Robbers, eds. *Pharmacognosy.* Philadelphia: Lea & Febiger, 1988.

TEXT CITATIONS:

1. J.F. Balch and P.A. Balch, *Prescription for Nutritional Healing: A Practical A to Z Reference to Drug-Free Remedies Using Vitamins, Minerals, Herbs & Food Supplements,* 2nd ed. (Garden City Park, NY: Avery Publishing Group, 1997).
2. B.M. Cohen et al., *American Journal of Psychiatry,* 137 (1980): 242.
3. A. Barbeau, *New England Journal of Medicine,* 302 (1980): 1310.
4. A. Der Marderosian and L. Liberti, *Natural Product Medicine. A Scientific Guide to Foods, Drugs, Cosmetics* (Philadelphia: George F. Stickley, 1988). J.R. Tweedy and C.A. Garcia, *European Journal of Clinical Investigation,* 12 (1982): 87.
5. J. Volavka et al., *Psychiatry Research,* 19(2) (1986): 101–4.
6. G.S. Rosenberg and K.L. Davis, *American Journal of Clinical Nutrition,* 36 (1982): 709.
7. Der Marderosian and Liberti, op. cit. L.J. Fitten et al., *American Journal of Psychiatry,* 147(2) (1990): 239–42. A. Little et al., *Journal of Neurology, Neurosurgery & Psychiatry,* 48(8) (1985): 736–42.
8. S. Gauthier et al., *Canadian Journal of Neurological Sciences,* 16(4 Suppl.) (1989): 543–46.
9. C.M. Harris et al., *American Journal of Psychiatry,* 140(8) (1983): 1010–2.
10. S. Tuzhilin et al., *American Journal of Gastroenterology,* 65(3) (1976): 231–35.
11. M. Blumenthal, J. Greenwald, T. Hall, and R. S. Rister, eds., *The Complete German Commission E Monographs: Therapeutic Guide to Herbal Medicine* (Boston: Integrative Medicine Communications, 1998).
12. Der Marderosian and Liberti, op. cit.
13. Blumenthal et al., op. cit.
14. American Pharmaceutical Association, *Handbook of Nonprescription Drugs,* 11th ed. (Washington, D.C.: American Pharmaceutical Association, 1996).
15. *Hospital Practice,* 19 (1984): 29. Der Marderosian and Liberti, op. cit.

PRIMARY NAME:
LEMONGRASS

SCIENTIFIC NAME:

Cymbopogon citratus (DC.) Stapf., sometimes referred to as *Andropogon citratus* DC. *Cymbopogon flexuosus* W. Wats. is a related plant that is also used medicinally. Family: Gramineae

COMMON NAMES:

Andropogon citratus: Guatemala lemongrass, Madagascar lemongrass; *Cymbopogon citratus:* capim-cidrao.

RATING:

4 = Research indicates that this substance will not fulfill the claims made for it, but that it is also unlikely to cause any harm.

What Is Lemongrass?

This sweetly scented flowering perennial grass grows in bushy clumps in its native India and Sri Lanka. It is cultivated in tropical regions worldwide, including Central and South America. As it grows, bulbous stems develop into narrow leaf blades. These are partially dried for medicinal use. An essential oil derived from the leaves is also used medicinally.

What It Is Used For:

The traditional cuisines of Thailand and various other countries feature lemongrass prominently. Traditional South American medicine has relied heavily on this herb. Herbalists today recommend a leaf tea for many of the uses common in that part of the world: as an antiseptic and to treat nervous and digestive problems (including diarrhea, stomach cramps, and gas), cough, fever, high blood pressure, and flu. External formulations are recommended for reducing rheumatic pain. Traditional Indian (Ayurvedic) healers apply a paste made with the leaves to ringworm infections.

The essential oil appears in foods and cosmetics, and aromatherapists recommend it for boosting muscle tone and circulation. Some herbalists also ascribe antiseptic properties to the oil.

Forms Available Include:

Herb, infusion, oil. The herb is now available as a food in many United States grocery stores.

Dosage Commonly Reported:

Approximately 2 to 3 teaspoons of the chopped herb are infused in a cup of water; two to three cups are drunk daily.

Will It Work for You? What the Studies Say:

While lemongrass pleases the palette and yields an important flavoring and scent oil (citral), it appears to be devoid of medicinal properties when taken as a tea or in any other oral form.[1] This is the conclusion of extensive research in both animals and humans. High oral doses administered to rats and mice failed to show fever-reducing or painkilling properties in one extensive round of testing.[2] They did not alter EEG (brain wave) activity, show anticonvulsive or anxiolytic (anxiety-reducing) properties, or induce changes in spontaneous motor activity, any of which may have indicated a calming and soothing effect for lemongrass. The high doses similarly failed to affect the time it takes for a certain type of food to pass through the intestines, which would have indicated potential for treating intestinal ailments.

Human trials have proved no more hopeful in inducing any type of medicinal actions. For example, no significant sedative properties—sleep quality, time to fall asleep, dream recall, reawakening—were noted in a double-blind study that involved fifty subjects sipping lemongrass tea or a placebo drink over three nights.[3] Volunteers who took a single oral dose of lemongrass or drank lemongrass tea every day for two weeks developed no notable changes in tests of their urine, blood, or brain wave or cardiac activity.[4]

Administration by injection has proved a different story, however. Injection of lemongrass reduced blood pressure in rats in one study, for example,[5] though apparently very high doses—doses twenty times greater than what would be typically given to humans—were needed to produce these blood pressure changes.

Will It Harm You? What the Studies Say:

All indicators suggest that lemongrass is very safe to take orally even in medicinal amounts. In human trials, subjects report no side effects and various laboratory tests show no deviations from normal parameters.[6] Rats fed high doses over long periods of time showed no adverse reactions.[7]

GENERAL SOURCES:

Bremness, L. *Herbs.* 1st American ed. Eyewitness Handbooks. New York: Dorling Kindersley Publications, 1994.

Chevallier, A. *The Encyclopedia of Medicinal Plants: A Practical Reference Guide to More Than 550 Key Medicinal Plants & Their Uses.* 1st American ed. New York: Dorling Kindersley Publications, 1996.

Lawrence Review of Natural Products. St. Louis: Facts and Comparisons, October 1989.

TEXT CITATIONS:

1. *Lawrence Review of Natural Products* (St. Louis: Facts and Comparisons, October 1989).
2. D. Carbajal et al., *Journal of Ethnopharmacology,* 25 (1989): 103.
3. J.R. Leite et al., *Journal of Ethnopharmacology,* 17 (1986): 75.
4. *Lawrence Review of Natural Products,* op. cit.
5. Ibid.
6. Carbajal et al., op. cit.
7. M.L.O.S. Formigoni et al., *Journal of Ethnopharmacology,* 17 (1986): 65.

PRIMARY NAME:
LETTUCE OPIUM

SCIENTIFIC NAME:

Derived from *Lactucosa virosa* L. and related species including *Lactucosa sativa* var. *capitata* L. (garden lettuce). Family: Asteraceae (Compositae)

COMMON NAMES:

The following refer to the plants that produce lettuce opium: acrid lettuce, garden lettuce, German lactucarium, greater

What Is Lettuce Opium?

Lettuce opium refers to the milky-white juice that oozes from the stems of various flowering *Lactucosa* plants when snapped or cut. This juice, or latex, collected when the large-leafed plants flower from July to September, is dried (at which point it turns brown) and sold as a medicinal substance called lactucarium.

What It Is Used For:

In ancient times the similarity in appearance, taste, and odor of the milky-white juice from wild lettuce to that of the opium poppy was noted and gave rise to the belief that the lettuce juice might have soporific (sleep-inducing) properties.[1] Its popularity as a mild sedative for restlessness and nervous excitability (particularly in children), sleep problems, and rheumatic and other pains endured over the centuries. It was reportedly used as a substitute for opium in European remedies for irritable cough.[2] The *U.S. Pharmacopoeia* officially listed prickly lettuce, green endive, lactucarium, strong-scented lettuce, wild lettuce

RATING:

4 = Research indicates that this substance will not fulfill the claims made for it, but that it is also unlikely to cause any harm.

lactucarium for nearly a century, until 1926. North Americans had virtually forgotten about it until the 1970s, when enthusiasts revived interest in smoking lettuce opium preparations as a means of getting high. Some sources touted it as a hallucinogen, and others recommended smoking it with marijuana to boost flavor and strength.[3]

Forms Available Include:

Latex (often referred to as juice or sap, sometimes dried), tincture.

Dosage Commonly Reported:

The dried latex extract is taken in doses of 0.3 to 1 gram three times a day.

Will It Work for You? What the Studies Say:

The purported sedative properties of the juice of wild lettuce have been attributed to the presence of two bitter principles: sesquiterpene lactones, called lactucopicrin, and lactucin. Both have been shown to depress (slow down) the central nervous system in small animals, counteracting the stimulant effects of coffee and tea.[4] A 1992 study in mice found that crude preparations from *Lactuca virosa* and lactucin have sedative and painkilling properties.[5] However, these compounds not only are chemically unstable but tend to appear in extremely small concentrations—if at all—in commercial lactucarium.[6] Reports from the early 1900s that the fresh herb contains trace amounts of hyoscyamine, a poisonous alkaloid with antispasmodic and sedative effects, have since been refuted.[7] No researcher since has reported detecting hyoscyamine in the dried herb or lactucarium. Claims that lettuce opium is in any way hallucinogenic are likewise poorly substantiated, although anticipation of and desire for an effect may help produce one.[8]

Lactucarium continues to appear in cough teas and other cough preparations in Europe particularly, although there have apparently been no studies to justify its use in this way and German plant specialists consider its use somewhat obsolete, particularly for severe acute coughs.[9]

The implications for human health of other scattered research findings over the years—that extracts of *Lactuca sativa* can lower blood pressure in dogs, for example, as well as inhibit the growth of the *Candida albicans* fungus in a test tube[11]—remain unclear.

Will It Harm You? What the Studies Say:

No reports of significant adverse reactions survive centuries of use, although the safety of smoking the herb—a relatively recent approach—remains unclear. Also, allergic reactions to this member of the daisy family, including contact dermatitis, have been reported.[12]

GENERAL SOURCES:

Bradley, P.C., ed. *British Herbal Compendium: A Handbook of Scientific Information on Widely Used Plant Drugs*, vol. 1. Bournemouth (Dorset), England: British Herbal Medicine Association, 1992.

Der Marderosian, A., and L. Liberti. *Natural Product Medicine. A Scientific Guide to Foods, Drugs, Cosmetics.* Philadelphia: George F. Stickley, 1988.

Lampe, K.E., and M.A. McCann. *AMA Handbook of Poisonous and Injurious Plants.* Chicago: American Medical Association, 1985.

Lawrence Review of Natural Products. St. Louis: Facts and Comparisons, November 1991.

Mayell, M. *Off-the-Shelf Natural Health: How to Use Herbs and Nutrients to Stay Well.* New York: Bantam Books, 1995.

Tyler, V.E., L.R. Brady, and J.E. Robbers, eds. *Pharmacognosy.* Philadelphia: Lea & Febiger, 1988.

Weiner, M.A., and J.A. Weiner. *Herbs That Heal: Prescription for Herbal Healing.* Mill Valley, CA: Quantum Books, 1994.

Weiss, R.F. *Herbal Medicine,* trans. A.R. Meuss, from the 6th German edition. Beaconsfield, England: Beaconsfield Publishers, Ltd., 1988.

TEXT CITATIONS:

1. V.E. Tyler, L.R. Brady, and J.E. Robbers, eds., *Pharmacognosy* (Philadelphia: Lea & Febiger, 1988).
2. P.C. Bradley, ed., *British Herbal Compendium: A Handbook of Scientific Information on Widely Used Plant Drugs*, vol. 1 (Bournemouth [Dorset], England: British Herbal Medicine Association, 1992).
3. Z.J. Huang et al., *Journal of Pharmaceutical Sciences*, 71(2) (1982): 270.
4. A.W. Forst, *Archiv für Experimentelle Pathologie und Pharmakologie*, 195 (1940): 1–25.
5. D. Gromek et al., *Phytotherapy Research*, 6(5) (1992): 285–87.
6. *Lawrence Review of Natural Products* (St. Louis: Facts and Comparisons, November 1991).
7. Bradley, op. cit.
8. A. Der Marderosian and L. Liberti, *Natural Product Medicine. A Scientific Guide to Foods, Drugs, Cosmetics* (Philadelphia: George F. Stickley, 1988).
9. R.F. Weiss, *Herbal Medicine,* trans. A.R. Meuss, from the 6th German edition (Beaconsfield, England: Beaconsfield Publishers, Ltd., 1988).
10. J. Moulin-Traffort et al., *Mycoses*, 33(7–8) (1990): 383.
11. *Lawrence Review of Natural Products*, op. cit.
12. H.S. Bernton, *Journal of the American Medical Association*, 230(4) (1974): 613. K.E. Lampe and M.A. McCann, *AMA Handbook of Poisonous and Injurious Plants* (Chicago: American Medical Association, 1985).

PRIMARY NAME:

LICORICE

SCIENTIFIC NAME:

Glycyrrhiza glabra L. and occasionally other Glycyrrhiza species. Family: Leguminosae (Fabaceae)

What Is Licorice?

Licorice consists of an extract prepared from the sweet-tasting dried roots and rhizomes (underground stems) of varieties of *Glycyrrhiza glabra*, a shrub that grows in subtropical climates. Greece, Turkey, and Asia Minor commonly export licorice to the United States.

What It Is Used For:

The most commonly recognized use for licorice in the United States is as a flavoring in candies, chewing tobacco, and pharmaceutical preparations such as throat lozenges. Contrary to common belief, very little candy sold as licorice in

COMMON NAMES:
Gan cao, glycyrrhiza, Italian licorice, licorice root, Russian licorice, Spanish licorice, sweet wood, Turkish licorice

RATING:
2 = According to a number of well-designed studies and common use, this substance appears to be relatively effective and safe when used in recommended amounts for the indication(s) noted in the "Will It Work for You?" section. However, see safety warnings in the "Will It Harm You?" section.

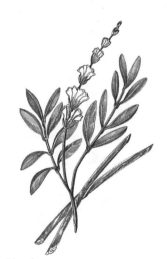

Licorice
Glycyrrhiza glabra

the United States actually contains licorice; most is flavored with anise oil. True licorice candy is far more common in Europe.

In some parts of the world, licorice has been used for more than three thousand years to treat coughs, colds, congestion, rashes, arthritis, constipation, cancer, and hepatitis, and to promote healing of stomach and mouth ulcers. Many people use it to mask the bitter taste of other herbs. Native Americans drank a tea brewed from licorice as a laxative and to treat coughs and earaches. Licorice is extremely popular and highly regarded as a healing herb in China.

In the United States, herbalists long recommended licorice for menstrual complaints, but it was used primarily as a flavoring agent until the 1950s, when interest mounted in its ability to treat peptic (gastric or duodenal) ulcers. Enthusiasm for this use faded, however, when certain adverse reactions were observed. Herbalists today recommend licorice to remedy indigestion, clear congestion (as an expectorant), and treat various genitourinary, gastrointestinal, and respiratory problems.

Forms Available Include:

Capsule, decoction, extract, fluid infusion, root and rhizome, solid extract (chopped, powered), tea, tincture. Found in many candy, tobacco, and pharmaceutical products, including cough drops, syrups, antismoking lozenges, and shampoos.

Dosage Commonly Reported:

A common—albeit conservative—dosage is 1 to 2 grams powdered root (Chinese sources commonly cite 2 to 12 grams, and European sources cite 5 to 15 grams), 2 to 4 milliliters fluid extract, or 250 to 500 milligrams solid extract, three times per day. For premenstrual syndrome, licorice is taken two weeks prior to menstruation in the preceeding amounts. Licorice should not be taken for longer than four to six weeks. As an expectorant, a pinch of licorice is added to herbal teas. Take commercially prepared capsules according to package directions.

Will It Work for You? What the Studies Say:

Licorice is a powerful drug that studies suggest is probably useful in treating a number of conditions. In terms of one of its oldest uses—as a cough remedy—laboratory findings indicate that licorice has merit; it contains a chemical called glycyrrhetinic acid, which has cough-suppressant elements. It stimulates mucosal secretions in the trachea, helping to loosen sticky phlegm so it is easier to cough up.[1] These expectorant properties have been seen in test rabbits.[2] Many European cough formulations contain licorice. German health authorities approve of licorice preparations for treating upper respiratory tract congestion (bronchitis).[3] Adding licorice to tea to soothe a sore throat is also likely to work; it contains soothing demulcent ingredients.

Test-tube studies also indicate that licorice extracts fight disease-causing bacteria such as *Staphylococci* and *Streptococci*, the *Herpes simplex* virus (responsible for cold sores and genital herpes), and *Candida albicans*, the fungus responsible for vaginal yeast infections and oral thrush.[4] Studies show that extracts have weak antiviral activity in laboratory animals as well as in the test tube.[5]

Licorice apparently helps to heal ulcers by encouraging a local concentration of prostaglandins, hormone-like chemicals that promote the secretion of stomach mucus,[6] and promoting an increase in certain stomach cells. In the West, interest in the medicinal properties of licorice was sparked by a 1946 study that showed that a paste prepared from an extract of the *Glycyrrhiza glabra* plant could alleviate abdominal symptoms in individuals with gastric ulcers. Imaging studies also indicated a healing effect, and studies in animals showed that it helped prevent the formation of gastric ulcers. In controlled clinical trials, the active substances in licorice were shown to speed the healing of gastric ulcers. German health authorities approve of licorice for helping to treat peptic ulcers.[7]

Researchers have also found that licorice has anti-inflammatory properties due to the presence of a steroid-like action from glycyrrhizin and liquiritin,[8] and animal studies have indicated an anti-inflammatory and antiarthritic effect.[9] This may explain its traditional use for inflammatory conditions such as arthritis. But there are also risks associated with glychrrhizin and liquiritin (see "Will It Harm You?" section).

Finally, according to an intriguing 1996 study in mice, licorice may beneficially lower levels of complexes formed in autoimmune diseases such as systemic lupus erythematosus.[10] More research is needed to determine whether licorice may one day prove valuable in treating this disease.

Will It Harm You? What the Studies Say:

Licorice in candies and other foods poses no risk of harm at typical levels. German health authorities consider maximum doses of up to 100 milligrams of glycyrrhizin a day acceptable and safe.[11] But there are real hazards to be aware of in taking licorice in higher (medicinal) amounts, or even in 100-milligram doses daily over the long term. Although licorice appears to help heal peptic ulcers, for example, it is limited for this purpose by substantial toxic effects, with one in five individuals developing swelling of the face and other body parts. In a number of cases, headache, stiffness, shortness of breath, and upper abdominal pain became apparent.

Research indicates that licorice, when consumed over time in large amounts in everything from tea to candies, appears to act like powerful steroid hormones (glucocorticoid and mineralocorticoid). This can result in a hypermineralocorticoid syndrome known as pseudoaldosteronism,[12] which is characterized by arterial hypertension (high blood pressure), edema (swelling), hypernatremia (abnormally high blood levels of sodium), and hypokalemia (abnormally low blood concentrations of potassium). Pseudoaldosteronism can be so severe that it leads to muscular disease and even death. The medical literature is littered with cases of pseudoaldosteronism caused by eating enormous amounts of licorice candy or by constantly swallowing the saliva produced by licorice-flavored chewing tobacco.

Just how much licorice has to be consumed for toxic effects to appear is not clear, in part because many studies have used confectionery products containing licorice in varying amounts rather than pure licorice. One study indicates that consumption of products containing licorice in amounts up to 100 grams a day for several years is dangerous.[13] Another suggests that life-threatening hypokalemia has resulted from consumption of the equivalent of less than 50 grams of licorice a day.[14] One otherwise healthy individual had to be hospitalized for four days after eating 700 grams (about 1.5 pounds) of licorice candy in nine days.

If you wish to use licorice medicinally, discuss it with your doctor. German health authorities warn that you should not take licorice for more than four to six weeks without medical advice. Certain individuals need to be particularly careful: pregnant and nursing women; individuals with high blood pressure, glaucoma, diabetes, kidney, or liver disease; or those who are taking hormonal therapy (because the licorice may interfere with it).[15] Anyone taking digitalis (sensitivity to it may be increased if your system suffers from potassium loss) or who has had a stroke or heart disease should take licorice only under the direction of a doctor. Individuals with eating disorders who may already be predisposed to hypokalemia for other reasons may be at heightened risk for pseudoaldosteronism.[16] Some sources recommend that anyone who has a cardiovascular-related disorder not consume licorice at all.[17] Keep in mind that you may be getting licorice from other sources as well, such as candies and drinks.

GENERAL SOURCES:

American Pharmaceutical Association. *Handbook of Nonprescription Drugs.* 11th ed. Washington, D.C.: American Pharmaceutical Association, 1996.

Baker, M.E. *Steroids.* 59 (1994): 136–41.

Bernardi, M., et al. *Life Sciences.* 55(11) (1994): 863–72.

Bradley, P.C., ed. *British Herbal Compendium: A Handbook of Scientific Information on Widely Used Plant Drugs,* vol. 1. Bournemouth (Dorset), England: British Herbal Medicine Association, 1992.

Castleman, M. *The Healing Herbs: The Ultimate Guide to the Curative Power of Nature's Medicines.* New York: Bantam Books, 1995.

Lawrence Review of Natural Products. St. Louis: Facts and Comparisons, June 1989.

Leung, A.Y., and S. Foster. *Encyclopedia of Common Natural Ingredients Used in Food, Drugs, and Cosmetics.* 2nd ed. New York: John Wiley & Sons, 1996.

Newall, C.A., et al. *Herbal Medicines: A Guide for Health-Care Professionals.* London: The Pharmaceutical Press, 1996.

Schambelan, M. *Steroids.* 59 (1994): 127–30.

Tyler, V.E. *The Honest Herbal.* Binghamton, NY: Haworth Press/Pharmaceutical Products Press, 1993.

TEXT CITATIONS:

1. C.A. Newall et al., *Herbal Medicines: A Guide for Health-Care Professionals* (London: The Pharmaceutical Press, 1996).
2. M. Blumenthal, J. Gruenwald, T. Hall, and R. S. Rister, eds., *The Complete German Commission E Monographs: Therapeutic Guide to Herbal Medicine* (Boston: Integrative Medicine Communications, 1998).
3. Ibid.
4. R.F. Chandler, *Canadian Pharmaceutical Journal,* 118 (1985): 420–24.
5. *Lawrence Review of Natural Products.* St. Louis: Facts and Comparisons, June 1989.
6. H. Wagner et al., eds., *Economic and Medicinal Plant Research,* vol. 1 (London: Academic Press, 1985).

7. Blumenthal et al., op. cit.
8. H. Hikino and Y. Kiso, "Natural Products for Liver Disease," *Economic and Medicinal Plant Research*, vol. 2 (New York: Academic Press, 1988, 39–72).
9. *Lawrence Review of Natural Products*, op. cit.
10. T. Matsumoto et al., *Journal of Ethnopharmacology*, 53 (1996): 1–4.
11. Blumenthal et al., op. cit.
12. M.T. Epstein et al., *British Medical Journal*, 1 (1977): 488–90. P.M. Stewart et al., *The Lancet*, II (1987): 821–24.
13. R.V. Farese et al., *New England Journal of Medicine*, 325 (1991): 1223–27.
14. J.M. Cereda et al., *The Lancet*, 1 (1983): 1442.
15. Newall, op. cit.
16. J. Brayley and J. Jones, *American Journal of Psychiatry*, 151(4) (1994): 617–18.
17. Newall, op. cit.

PRIMARY NAME:
LIFE ROOT

SCIENTIFIC NAME:
Senecio aureus L. Family: Asteraceae (Compositae)

COMMON NAMES:
Cocashweed, coughweed, false valerian, female regulator, golden groundsel, golden senecio, ragwort, senecio, squaw weed

RATING:
5 = Studies indicate that there is a definite health hazard to using this substance, even in recommended amounts.

What Is Life Root?

This perennial flourishes in swamps and other moist environments in the eastern and central parts of the United States and is cultivated in Europe. Bunches of delicate, bright yellow flowers crown the primary stem. All parts of the plant, once dried, have been used medicinally.

What It Is Used For:

Native American women sipped life root tea to speed up labor and relieve labor pains, induce menstruation, and remedy various reproductive tract disorders. Enthusiasm for the herb's reported ability to promote menstruation persisted for decades after the settlers arrived; hence the common name, "female regulator." Life root counted among the principal ingredients in Lydia Pinkham's Vegetable Compound, a famous nineteenth-century proprietary cure-all for "female weaknesses." Certain tribes also used it to control bleeding and encourage wound healing. Other uses have been encouraged as well, including controlling worms and calming colic.

Forms Available:

Dried herb or root, infusion, liquid extract.

Dosage Commonly Reported:

The dry herb or root is taken in doses of 2 to 4 grams, and the liquid extract in doses of 2 to 4 milliliters.

Will It Work for You? What the Studies Say:

Many scientists agree that although life root has an impact on female reproductive organs, the presence of toxic pyrrolizidine alkaloids (PAs) puts it out of the running as a practical herb for managing or alleviating related problems (see "Will It Harm You?"). There is scant information to indicate that life root can alter hormone levels in women or in any way soothe or restore health to the uterus.[1] The English-language literature contains little information about this herb.

Will It Harm You? What the Studies Say:

Life root contains toxic pyrrolizidine alkaloids (PAs), such as senecionine and senecine. Scientists believe these alkaloids play a role in liver diseases, including primary liver cancer, and can increase resistance to blood flow through the lungs (hypertensive pulmonary vascular disease).[2] Given such findings, most experts have concluded that the potential hazards involved in taking life root are far too high, even though the level of PAs is relatively low.[3] Some manufacturers remain unimpressed with this information and continue to add life root to menstrual and gynecologic remedies.

GENERAL SOURCES:

Bisset, N.G., ed. *Herbal Drugs and Phytopharmaceuticals.* Stuttgart: medpharm GmbH Scientific Publishers, 1994.
Duke, J.A. *CRC Handbook of Medicinal Herbs.* Boca Raton, FL: CRC Press, 1985.
Lawrence Review of Natural Products. St. Louis: Facts and Comparisons, July 1992.
Tyler, V.E. *The Honest Herbal.* Binghamton, NY: Haworth Press/Pharmaceutical Products Press, 1993.
Tyler, V.E., L.R. Brady, and J.E. Robbers, eds. *Pharmacognosy.* Philadelphia: Lea & Febiger, 1988.

TEXT CITATIONS:

1. *Lawrence Review of Natural Products* (St. Louis: Facts and Comparisons, July 1992).
2. Ibid.
3. R.H.F. Manske and H.L. Holmes, *The Alkaloids*, vol 1. (New York: Academic Press, 1950).

PRIMARY NAME:
LINDEN FLOWER

SCIENTIFIC NAME:
Tilia species, for medicinal purposes especially *Tilia cordata* Mill. and *T. platyphyllos* Scop. Family: Tiliaceae

COMMON NAMES:
Basswood, European linden, lime tree flower

What Is Linden Flower?

The yellowish-white flowers of the shade-giving *Tilia* species are picked in late spring and quickly dried to retain their honeylike scent and medicinal properties. The tree, which can grow close to an imposing one hundred feet high and boasts numerous drooping clusters of these flowers, is native to Europe and now grows in North America. The flowers make an excellent honey; an aromatic, pleasant-tasting drinking tea; and a medicinal tea.

What It Is Used For:

The practice of sipping hot (or very warm) linden flower tea to promote sweating began in medieval Europe. Feverish colds, flu, and other conditions associated with chilling were treated this way. Use of linden teas for these purposes as well as to alleviate congestion-associated cough and throat irritation can be found in the United States, Europe, and other parts of the world.

Linden flowers have also enjoyed popularity as a folk remedy for such broad-ranging ailments as headache, diarrhea, and indigestion. Especially in Latin American countries the flowers have been used to treat nervousness and other conditions believed to benefit from a sedative or tranquilizer. Home-

RATING:

2 = According to a number of well-designed studies and common use, this substance appears to be relatively effective and safe when used in recommended amounts for the indication(s) noted in the "Will It Work for You?" section.

opaths recommend minute amounts of linden for various illnesses. (See page 2 for a discussion of homeopathy.)

Forms Available Include:

Dried flowers, infusion, liquid flower extract, tea bag. The flower and its extracts can be found in herbal blends. To keep linden flowers fresh and fragrant, store them in an airtight, light-resistant container.

Dosage Commonly Reported:

An infusion is made using 1 to 2 teaspoons (2 to 4 grams) flowers and is drunk once or twice per day. The liquid flower extract is taken in doses of 2 to 4 milliliters.

Will It Work for You? What the Studies Say:

Linden flower tea will make a person start to sweat, but probably only after the person has drunk quite a bit. To get enough of the sweat-producing ingredient into the body, select a more flavorful tea from a *Tilia* species, one that boasts a relatively high concentration of substances called tannins. Examples include *Tilia cordata* and *Tilia platyphyllos*. Choosing teas with the flowers from these trees may prove difficult, however, because commercial brands do not always list their sources.[1] Advocates assert that particular ingredients in the herb—quercitin, kaempferol, and p-coumaric acid—are responsible for causing sweating. But plant scientists question whether the sweating does not result simply from drinking a hot liquid. German health authorities approve of the remedy for treating chills, colds, and associated coughs.[2] A gooey substance called mucilage is presumed to soothe cough-related throat irritation.

Several studies indicate that in addition to stimulating sweating, linden flowers may enhance a person's resistance to certain kinds of infection. A team of French investigators reported that an extract of linden flowers could fight the kind of bacteria commonly associated with mouth infections, at least in the test tube.[3] In another study, investigators reported that children with flulike symptoms who were treated with linden flowers, bed rest, and in some cases an antibiotic or a few aspirin (although aspirin is no longer recommended for children with flu symptoms because of the risk of Reyes syndrome) developed fewer middle ear infections and other complications than children with flulike symptoms given only an antibiotic.[4] They also recovered more quickly. More research on this subject is needed.

The ability of linden flowers to induce sedation (drowsiness) has not been extensively studied, although investigators have found that the flowers of at least one species—*Tilia tomentosa*—contain a compound that has an anxiety-relieving effect on mice when injected.[5] No one has demonstrated that this translates into a similar reaction in humans, particularly when they drink rather than inject the herb. This apparent anxiety-relieving property is intriguing, given that the herb was once used to treat hysteria, convulsions, and premenstrual tension, a practice that may persist in some parts of Germany.

L

Linden Flower

Will It Harm You? What the Studies Say:

Science has relatively little to say about the potential toxicity of linden flowers, but on the basis of centuries of use, the herb appears to be safe to use in moderation. German health authorities cite no known side effects, situations in which the herb should not be taken, or dangerous interactions with other remedies.[6] If drunk excessively, however, the herb may cause heart damage. For this reason, people with heart problems may want to avoid drinking linden tea.[7] The warning that tea made from very old linden flowers could cause symptoms of narcotic intoxication appears to be unsubstantiated.[8]

GENERAL SOURCES:

Bisset, N.G., ed. *Herbal Drugs and Phytopharmaceuticals.* Stuttgart: medpharm GmbH Scientific Publishers, 1994.

Blumenthal, M., J. Gruenwald, T. Hall, and R.S. Rister, eds. *The Complete German Commission E Monographs: Therapeutic Guide to Herbal Medicine.* Boston: Integrative Medicine Communications, 1998.

Duke, J.A. *CRC Handbook of Medicinal Herbs.* Boca Raton, FL: CRC Press, 1985.

Hallowell, M. *Herbal Healing: A Practical Introduction to Medicinal Herbs.* Garden City Park, NY: 1994.

Lawrence Review of Natural Products. St. Louis: Facts and Comparisons, December 1990.

Tyler, V.E. *The Honest Herbal.* Binghamton, NY: Haworth Press/Pharmaceutical Products Press, 1993.

Tyler, V.E., L.R. Brady, and J.E. Robbers, eds. *Pharmacognosy.* Philadelphia: Lea & Febiger, 1988.

Weiss, R.F. *Herbal Medicine*, trans. A.R. Meuss, from the 6th German edition. Beaconsfield, England: Beaconsfield Publishers, Ltd., 1988.

TEXT CITATIONS:

1. V.E. Tyler, *The Honest Herbal* (Binghamton, NY: Haworth Press/Pharmaceutical Products Press, 1993).
2. M. Blumenthal, J. Gruenwald, T. Hall, and R. S. Rister, eds., *The Complete German Commission E Monographs: Therapeutic Guide to Herbal Medicine* (Boston: Integrative Medicine Communications, 1998).
3. G. Sucie et al., *Revue de Chirurgie, Oncologie, Radiologie,* 35 (1988): 191.
4. R.F. Weiss, *Herbal Medicine*, trans. A.R. Meuss, from the 6th German edition (Beaconsfield, England: Beaconsfield Publishers, Ltd., 1988).
5. H. Viola et al., *Journal of Ethnopharmacology,* 44(1) (1994): 47–53.
6. Blumenthal et al., op. cit.
7. Tyler, op. cit.
8. Ibid.

PRIMARY NAME:
LOBELIA

SCIENTIFIC NAME:
Lobelia inflata L. Family: Campanulaceae

What Is Lobelia?

This hairy, erect flowering plant, indigenous to open woods and meadows of eastern North America, now grows wild across the continent. It is also widely cultivated. The aboveground herb—from the dainty, two-lipped blue flowers to the ovate or oblong leaves—is used medicinally once dried. In autumn, the flowers are replaced by many-seeded fruit.

COMMON NAMES:
Asthma weed, emetic herb, gagroot, Indian tobacco, pukeweed, vomit wort, wild tobacco

RATING:
5 = Studies indicate that there is a definite health hazard to using this substance internally, even in recommended amounts.

What It Is Used For:

Controversy over the use of lobelia is not new. Native Americans familiar with the plant reportedly smoked its leaves to relieve asthma and other upper respiratory complaints. With the encouragement of a nineteenth-century herbal medicine movement led by Samuel Thompson, lobelia's popularity as an antiasthmatic, expectorant, antispasmodic (for convulsive disorders), and agent for numerous other ailments persisted, despite documented poisonings. In fact, practitioners of this movement became known as "lobelia doctors," a derogatory term. Samuel Thompson fatally poisoned one of his patients with lobelia and was accused of murder; but the judge released him, declaring that "no one should have been dumb enough to take him seriously."[1]

Large doses of lobelia cause vomiting, a quality once considered valuable for treating food poisoning. In recent times the plant has also been used as an antismoking agent; enthusiasts claim it can alleviate the symptoms of nicotine poisoning as well as ease withdrawal symptoms. Some sources tout the herb's expectorant properties and recommend it for asthma, chronic bronchitis, pneumonia, whooping cough, colds and flu, viral infections, and cardiovascular disease. Others promote smoking lobelia leaves, concocting a tea, or taking the herb in capsule form to get "high." Tragic consequences such as fast heartbeat followed by coma and death have resulted from this practice as well as other misuses of lobelia. Some herbalists recommend external formulations for sprains, bruises, insect bites, ringworm, poison ivy symptoms, and other topical irritations. However, apparently little research has been done on its external uses.

Forms Available Include:

- *For internal use:* Capsule, decoction, dried herb, infusion, liquid extract, lozenge, powder, tablet.
- *For external use:* Tincture.

Dosage Commonly Reported:

The lack of standardized preparations for internal use, among other things, makes this herb hazardous to use. An infusion or decoction for internal or external use was typically made using 50 to 200 milligrams of dried herb per cup of water and drunk up to three times a day. Antismoking chewing gum, tablets, and other preparations sold outside the United States (or formerly sold in the United States) typically contain 2 to 4 milligrams of lobeline.

Will It Work for You? What the Studies Say:

Lobelia contains several alkaloids, but the most important one by far is lobeline. This substance affects the body much the way nicotine does, although less powerfully.[2] Scientists cite lobeline as the ingredient responsible for the herb's expectorant properties;[3] an expectorant typically helps clear congestion by loosening sticky secretions (phlegm), making them easier to cough up. Its traditional use for upper respiratory tract congestion is probably justified. The herb's long-standing use for spastic muscle conditions may be attributed to lobeline's ability to relax the smooth muscles of the body.[4]

Lobeline causes changes in the body similar to what occurs when a person smokes a cigarette, giving rise to the theory that the herb might help mask withdrawal symptoms from nicotine. It has been used as a nicotine-free tobacco substitute and may precondition the taste buds to be nonresponsive to nicotine. Clinical trials to test the herb's effectiveness for this purpose have proved disappointing overall, however.[5] Antismoking preparations sold in the United States are no longer allowed to contain lobeline.[6]

Will It Harm You? What the Studies Say:

Lobelia poses serious health risks, and the FDA has declared it a poisonous plant. Even in recommended doses, it can cause side effects similar to those experienced with nicotine: nausea, vomiting, diarrhea, tremors, coughing, and dizziness. As long ago as the 1920s, studies reported that after initially exciting the central nervous system, the herb then slows it down. As a result, even recommended doses can at first lead to dilation of the bronchial tubes and increased breathing, properties valuable in treating asthma. But if too much is taken, unpleasant reactions such as profuse sweating and fast heartbeat may develop, possibly followed by depression of the central nervous system with attendant hypothermia, convulsions, low blood pressure, suppressed and irregular breathing, coma, and death due to respiratory failure (paralysis of the respiratory system) in some cases.[7] Few, if any, studies have been done on the effectiveness or safety of external uses.

GENERAL SOURCES:

Bradley, P.C., ed. *British Herbal Compendium: A Handbook of Scientific Information on Widely Used Plant Drugs.* Vol. 1. Bournemouth (Dorset), England: British Herbal Medicine Association, 1992.

Dobelis, I.N., ed. *The Magic and Medicine of Plants: A Practical Guide to the Science, History, Folklore, and Everyday Uses of Medicinal Plants.* Pleasantville, NY: Reader's Digest Association, 1986.

Duke, J.A. *CRC Handbook of Medicinal Herbs.* Boca Raton, FL: CRC Press, 1985.

Leung, A.Y. *Encyclopedia of Common Natural Ingredients Used in Food, Drugs, and Cosmetics.* New York: John Wiley & Sons, 1980.

Murray, M.T. *The Healing Power of Herbs: The Enlightened Person's Guide to the Wonders of Medicinal Plants.* Rev. Rocklin, CA: Prima Publishing, 1995.

Newall, C.A., et al. *Herbal Medicines: A Guide for Health-Care Professionals.* London: The Pharmaceutical Press, 1996.

Tierra, M. *The Way of Herbs.* New York: Pocket Books, 1990.

Tyler, V.E. *Herbs of Choice: The Therapeutic Use of Phytomedicinals.* Binghamton, NY: Haworth Press/Pharmaceutical Products Press, 1994.

———. *The Honest Herbal.* Binghamton, NY: Haworth Press/Pharmaceutical Products Press, 1993.

Weiner, M.A., and J.A. Weiner. *Herbs That Heal: Prescription for Herbal Healing.* Mill Valley, CA: Quantum Books, 1994.

TEXT CITATIONS:

1. J.A. Duke, *CRC Handbook of Medicinal Herbs* (Boca Raton, FL: CRC Press, 1985).
2. W. Martindale, *Martindale: The Extra Pharmacopoeia,* 29th ed. (London: The Pharmaceutical Press, 1989).
3. A.Y. Leung, *Encyclopedia of Common Natural Ingredients Used in Food, Drugs, and Cosmetics* (New York: John Wiley & Sons, 1980).
4. Ibid.

5. Ibid.
6. Ibid.
7. Martindale, op. cit.

LOVAGE

SCIENTIFIC NAME:
Levisticum officinale Koch. Also referred to as *Angelica levisticum* Baillon and *Hipposelinum levisticum* Britt. and Rose. Family: Umbelliferae (Apiaceae)

COMMON NAMES:
Maggi plant, smellage

RATING:
2 = According to a number of well-designed studies and common use, this substance appears to be relatively effective and safe when used in recommended amounts for the indication(s) noted in the "Will It Work for You?" section.

What Is Lovage?

The underground parts (the rhizome and roots) of this highly fragrant perennial are used in medicinal teas. The plant, long cultivated in North America, bears yellow-brown fruits and clusters of small yellow flowers.

Take care not to confuse lovage with the toxic plants *Oenanthe aquatica* L. Lam (water fennel) or *Oenanthe cocata* L. (water lovage), also of the Umbelliferae Family.

What It Is Used For:

Lovage has held an esteemed position in folk medicine for several centuries, being highly valued for increasing urine flow in the form of a diuretic ("water pill"), calming stomach upset, and reducing excess gas. It has also been used to treat sore throat, malaria, kidney stones, bladder problems, and boils. Europeans still turn to lovage for these and a number of other ailments, including congestion, rheumatism, and migraine headache. Its suggestive name— "lovage"—has inspired many to add it to love potions (in vain).

Forms Available Include:

Capsule, decoction, dried root, liquid extract, tablet, tea. Appears in numerous herbal blends.

Dosage Commonly Reported:

A common daily dosage is 4 to 8 grams. A decoction is made using 1 to 2 teaspoons (2 to 4 grams) dried root per cup of water. As a stomach soother, it is drunk between meals. As a diuretic, it is drunk two or three times per day. The liquid extract is taken in doses of 0.3 to 2 milliliters. Commercially prepared tablets and capsules should be used per package directions.

Will It Work for You? What the Studies Say:

The few laboratory studies done so far indicate that lovage contains several active ingredients, with the volatile oil (at concentrations of about 2 percent) ranking as the most important. For relieving stomach upset, gas, bloating, and heartburn, lovage tea may work in several ways: the volatile oil may lessen the amount of gas within the stomach and intestines or one of the oil's ingredients (ligustilide) may reduce intestinal spasms.[1] Alternatively, the slightly spicy and bitter taste of the tea may alleviate these discomforts simply by boosting the secretion of saliva and gastric juices.[2] Whatever the mechanism, and although Western medical literature contains little scientific evidence to confirm or disprove lovage tea's effectiveness, thousands continue to sip it expectantly.

Studies indicate that lovage has promise as a diuretic; when injected with

L

Lovage

lovage extracts or oil, mice and rabbits urinate more than they did before.[3] The herb probably promotes urination by irritating the kidneys. Unfortunately, studies demonstrating this effect in humans, and in oral rather than injectable form, do not appear to have been done. Many herbalists and health authorities seem to feel confident of lovage's diuretic properties, however. German health authorities approve of lovage for irrigating (flushing out) an inflamed urinary tract and helping to prevent kidney stones.[4] The herb's diuretic action is also put to work reducing water retention and swelling in parts of the body such as the feet.[5]

Will It Harm You? What the Studies Say:

Despite the dearth of information on lovage, it is by all indications safe for most people to use. Exceptions include people with inflamed kidneys or impaired kidney function.[6] Given the herb's diuretic action, one should take care to consume adequate amounts of fluid with it. Earlier concerns that lovage could make susceptible individuals develop a rash or other adverse skin reaction to the sun appear to have abated; the risk appears to be greatest among people who have handled the plant.[7] The FDA places lovage on its list of foods that are "Generally Recognized As Safe" (GRAS).

GENERAL SOURCES:

Bisset, N.G., ed. *Herbal Drugs and Phytopharmaceuticals.* Stuttgart: medpharm GmbH Scientific Publishers, 1994.

Blumenthal, M., J. Gruenwald, T. Hall, and R.S. Rister, eds. *The Complete German Commission E Monographs: Therapeutic Guide to Herbal Medicine.* Boston: Integrative Medicine Communications, 1998.

Review of Natural Products. St. Louis: Facts and Comparisons, April 1997.

Leung, A.Y. *Encyclopedia of Common Natural Ingredients Used in Food, Drugs, and Cosmetics.* New York: John Wiley & Sons, 1980.

Opdyke, D.L.J. *Food & Cosmetics Toxicology.* 16 (Suppl. 1) (1978): 813.

Tyler, V.E. *Herbs of Choice: The Therapeutic Use of Phytomedicinals.* Binghamton, NY: Haworth Press/Pharmaceutical Products Press, 1994.

———. *The Honest Herbal.* Binghamton, NY: Haworth Press/Pharmaceutical Products Press, 1993.

Weiss, R.F. *Herbal Medicine,* trans. A.R. Meuss, from the 6th German edition. Beaconsfield, England: Beaconsfield Publishers, Ltd., 1988.

TEXT CITA\TIONS:

1. V.E. Tyler, *Herbs of Choice: The Therapeutic Use of Phytomedicinals* (Binghamton, NY: Haworth Press/Pharmaceutical Products Press, 1994).
2. C. Vollmann, *Zeitschrift für Phytotherapie,* 9 (1988): 128.
3. Ibid.
4. M. Blumenthal, J. Gruenwald, T. Hall, and R. S. Rister, eds., *The Complete German Commission E Monographs: Therapeutic Guide to Herbal Medicine* (Boston: Integrative Medicine Communications, 1998).
5. N.G. Bisset, ed., *Herbal Drugs and Phytopharmaceuticals* (Stuttgart: medpharm GmbH Scientific Publishers, 1994).
6. Ibid.
7. A.Y. Leung, *Encyclopedia of Common Natural Ingredients Used in Food, Drugs, and Cosmetics* (New York: John Wiley & Sons, 1980). M.G. Ashwood-Smith, *Contact Dermatitis,* 26(5) (1992): 356–57.

PRIMARY NAME:
L-LYSINE

SCIENTIFIC NAME:

N/A

COMMON NAME:

Lysine

RATING:

4 = Research indicates that this substance will not fulfill the claims made for it, but that it is also unlikely to cause any harm.

What Is L-Lysine?

L-lysine is an essential amino acid. "Essential" means that your body cannot manufacture it on its own and must get it through the foods you eat.

What It Is Used For:

The body uses this amino acid to promote growth and tissue repair and to encourage the production of hormones, antibodies, and enzymes. Advocates assert that taking lysine supplements will help during recovery from surgery and injuries, fight or even prevent herpes outbreaks (when taken with vitamin C and bioflavonoids), and lower high triglyceride levels.

Forms Available Include:

Capsule, tablet. This amino acid appears in many multivitamin and multimineral preparations.

Dosage Commonly Reported:

A common dosage for treating herpes is 1,000 milligrams L-lysine with each meal.

Will It Work for You? What the Studies Say:

There is no conclusive evidence to indicate that L-lysine will help treat cold sores.[1] A balanced diet including such L-lysine-rich foods as cheese, eggs, milk, lima beans, fish, potatoes, red meat, yeast, and soy products will fulfill the average body's need for this amino acid. See **L-Tyrosine** for information on the use of single amino acids such as this as supplements.

Will It Harm You? What the Studies Say:

There are no known side effects or adverse reactions associated with this amino acid or risks of overdose from it. At the same time, the safety of taking it in high doses or over long periods of time has not been closely examined. Avoid taking it if you are allergic to food proteins such as milk, wheat, or eggs; suffer from diabetes; or follow a nutrition-poor diet.[2] Concerns have also been raised about the wisdom of supplementing the diet with any single amino acid; see **L-Tyrosine** for more information.

GENERAL SOURCES:

American Pharmaceutical Association. *Handbook of Nonprescription Drugs*. 11th ed. Washington, D.C.: American Pharmaceutical Association, 1996.

Balch, J.F., and P.A. Balch. *Prescription for Nutritional Healing: A Practical A to Z Reference to Drug-Free Remedies Using Vitamins, Minerals, Herbs & Food Supplements*. 2nd ed. Garden City Park, NY: Avery Publishing Group, 1997.

Barrett, S., and V. Herbert. *The Vitamin Pushers: How the "Health Food" Industry Is Selling America a Bill of Goods*. Amherst, NY: Prometheus Books, 1994.

Griffith, H.W. *Complete Guide to Vitamins, Minerals, Nutrients & Supplements*. Tucson: Fisher Books, 1988.

TEXT CITATIONS:

1. American Pharmaceutical Association, *Handbook of Nonprescription Drugs*, 11th ed. (Washington, D.C.: American Pharmaceutical Association, 1996).

2. H.W. Griffith, *Complete Guide to Vitamins, Minerals, Nutrients & Supplements* (Tucson: Fisher Books, 1988).

L

L-Lysine

PRIMARY NAME:
MARIJUANA

SCIENTIFIC NAME:
Cannabis sativa L. Family:
Cannabinaceae

COMMON NAMES:
Bhang, ganja, grass, hashish,
hemp, huo ma ren, Mary Jane,
pot, reefer

RATING:
2 = According to a number of
well-designed studies, this herb
appears to be relatively effective
when used in recommended
amounts for the indication(s)
noted in the "Will It Work for
You?" section. Safety is a major
concern, however; see the "Will
It Harm You?" section.

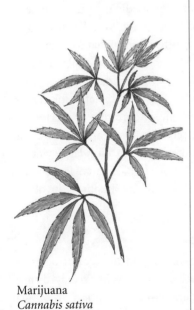

Marijuana
Cannabis sativa

What Is Marijuana?

This famous leafy annual is now cultivated worldwide for both legal (in the case
of fiber and seeds) and illegal (recreational drug use) purposes. It is an erect,
branching plant with long-toothed leaflets and small greenish flowers. There
are more than one hundred species of *Cannabis,* many of which grow as common weeds in parts of North America.

What It Is Used For:

Ancient Egyptian, Chinese, and other cultures recognized marijuana as an
important source of fiber (hemp) and oilseed, and as a valuable medicinal remedy. They and the traditional healers who followed recommended the leaves
and seeds for ailments ranging from congestion to pain, sleeplessness, nervous
disorders, fever, appetite loss, obesity, asthma, dandruff, hemorrhoids, inflammatory disorders, and leprosy. People going into surgery in the third century
reportedly sipped an infusion of the leaves to brace themselves for the pain, and
Queen Victoria relied on the herb as a painkiller, as did many nineteenth-
century women who took marijuana for menstrual cramps.[1]

Today, many people smoke or ingest marijuana as an intoxicant or psychoactive drug, a socially acceptable practice in some parts of Africa and Asia.
In the United States, scientists are investigating the herb as a treatment for nausea due to radiation therapy and cancer chemotherapy, asthma symptoms, the
physical wasting associated with AIDS, the muscle spasms associated with multiple sclerosis, seizures caused by epilepsy, and certain types of glaucoma. Marijuana hemp was the original material used for making blue jeans.[2] Hemp seeds
are a popular component of birdseed.

Forms Available Include:

Except for allowances in some states for treating such ailments as cancer, glaucoma, AIDS, and intractable pain, it is illegal to grow, possess, or use marijuana
in the United States. A pill containing the plant's primary active ingredient,
THC (see the "Will It Work for You" section), is available by prescription.

Dosage Commonly Reported:

To use THC capsules or other preparations, follow prescription instructions.

Will It Work for You? What the Studies Say:

A vast body of research supports the painkilling, anti-inflammatory, and sedative properties of marijuana. Its ability to induce feelings of exhilaration and
euphoria is well documented. Scientists have identified more than four hundred compounds and sixty types of cannabinoids (organic compounds
believed responsible for some, if not all, of the herb's pharmacologic action).
The principal cannabinoid—and the one apparently unique to marijuana—is
delta 9-tetrahydrocannabinol (THC). Its concentration varies depending on
the species and plant part it is derived from. Marijuana also contains steroidal
compounds, alkaloids, and volatile components.[3]

THC is largely responsible for the psychoactive effects of marijuana experienced when inhaling or ingesting the plant. In capsule form, THC has proved effective in treating otherwise intractable nausea caused by cancer treatments such as methotrexate and radiotherapy.[4] There are even data to indicate that it is as effective as the conventional drug, prochlorperazine, in reducing chemotherapy-related nausea and vomiting.[5] Some benefit has also been documented for treating spasticity associated with strokes, multiple sclerosis, and other neurologic disorders.[6]

There is evidence that marijuana may help control epileptic seizures,[7] although one team of investigators reports that it can also worsen grand mal convulsions.[8] The increased eye pressure associated with glaucoma may respond to marijuana and THC, according to research collected so far, but more data are needed to determine whether this actually preserves visual function.[9]

The value of marijuana as a medicinal plant is difficult to separate from political maneuvering in the United States and many other countries, where powerful lobbies both for and against its use have developed and a public health debate has ensued. Most recently, the tide has started to shift in favor of carefully controlled and limited use of the plant for such disorders as AIDS (to boost the appetite and counter physical wasting), glaucoma, chemotherapy-related nausea, and intractable pain. In early 1997, a panel of experts convened by the National Institutes of Health (NIH) recommended that researchers more fully explore the medicinal potential of the plant for certain ailments.

Many people interested in taking marijuana for medicinal purposes heatedly assert that no other substance offers the same quality of relief from pain and other symptoms. Opponents argue, among other things, that users are simply attempting to legally acquire an intoxicating substance not available to the rest of the population. The NIH commission recommended that scientists determine whether marijuana can offer equal or superior benefits for certain diseases and whether it can be designed so that no intoxicating properties are felt.[10] THC is already available in prescription pill form for treating various ailments, and pharmacology experts assert that there is more abundant evidence for the pill's effectiveness than there is for smoked marijuana. Proponents counter that the smoked form is superior, especially in situations involving digestive system upset.[11]

Will It Harm You? What The Studies Say:

Marijuana is a mind-altering substance. Smoking it can induce various psychomotor reactions that the user may experience positively or may dislike. These include changes in motor coordination and visual perception, emotional disturbances such as panic reactions, and even visual and auditory hallucinations. Marijuana can impair judgment and coordination in potentially dangerous situations such as driving a car or operating heavy machinery.

Nausea, vomiting, and dryness in the mouth have been associated with the use of marijuana, and allergic reactions have been documented in small animals.[12] Adverse reactions to THC treatment for cancer-related nausea in more than 1,500 patients have included fast heartbeat, seizure, and agitation.[13]

Smoking marijuana irritates the lungs and bronchial tubes. There is evidence that long-term use may impair the function of the lungs and may even cause constrictive lung disease.[14] Smoking the plant in many cases also exposes the user's lungs to contaminants such as molds and may increase the risk of lung cancer.[15] The potential for these types of complications severely limits its value as an asthma treatment, despite the fact that the user experiences a brief initial period of reduced bronchospasm and increased dilation of the bronchial tubes, which makes it easier to breathe.

Inhaling or ingesting marijuana often causes increased heart rate[16] but does not appear to adversely affect the cardiovascular system in any way. When used over the long term, marijuana can cause menstrual irregularities including missed cycles in women. Animal studies indicate that it can damage a fetus, a finding that apparently also applies to humans.[17]

GENERAL SOURCES:

Bremness, L. *Herbs*. 1st American ed. Eyewitness Handbooks. NY: Dorling Kindersley Publications, 1994.

Chevallier, A. *The Encyclopedia of Medicinal Plants: A Practical Reference Guide to More Than 550 Key Medicinal Plants & Their Uses*. 1st American ed. New York: Dorling Kindersley Publications, 1996.

Dobelis, I.N., ed. *The Magic and Medicine of Plants: A Practical Guide to the Science, History, Folklore, and Everyday Uses of Medicinal Plants*. Pleasantville, NY: Reader's Digest Association, 1986.

Duke, J.A. *CRC Handbook of Medicinal Herbs*. Boca Raton, FL: CRC Press, 1985.

Lawrence Review of Natural Products. St. Louis: Facts and Comparisons, August 1990.

Scigliano, J.A. *Journal of Clinical Pharmacology*. 21(8–9 Suppl.) (1981): 113S-121S.

Weiner, M.A., and J.A. Weiner. *Herbs That Heal: Prescription for Herbal Healing*. Mill Valley, CA: Quantum Books, 1994.

TEXT CITATIONS:

1. A. Chevallier, *The Encyclopedia of Medicinal Plants: A Practical Reference Guide to More than 550 Key Medicinal Plants & Their Uses*, 1st American ed. (New York: Dorling Kindersley Publications, 1996).
2. L. Bremness, *Herbs*, 1st American ed. Eyewitness Handbooks (New York: Dorling Kindersley Publications, 1994).
3. A.P. Mason et al., *Journal of Forensic Science*, 30 (1985): 615.
4. *Lawrence Review of Natural Products* (St. Louis: Facts and Comparisons, August 1990).
5. J.T. Ungerleider et al., *Cancer*, 50(4) (1982): 636–45.
6. D.J. Petro and C. Ellenberger, Jr., *Journal of Clinical Pharmacology*, 21(8–9 Suppl.) (1981): 413S-416S.
7. P.F. Consroe et al., *Journal of the American Medical Association*, 234 (1975): 306.
8. M.H. Keeler and C.F. Reifler, *Diseases of the Nervous System*. 28 (1967): 474. *Lawrence Review of Natural Products*, op. cit.
9. *Journal of the American Medical Association*, 242 (1979): 1962.
10. *Lawrence Review of Natural Products*, op. cit. W. Leary, *New York Times* (February 21, 1997): A27.
11. Leary, op. cit.
12. E.S. Watson et al., *Journal of Pharmaceutical Sciences*, 72 (1983): 954, 1983.
13. *Lawrence Review of Natural Products*, op. cit.
14. Ibid.
15. S.L. Kagen, *New England Journal of Medicine*, 304 (1981): 483.

16. Council on Scientific Affairs, *Journal of the American Medical Association*, 246 (1981): 1823.

17. *Lawrence Review of Natural Products*, op. cit.

MARJORAM, SWEET

SCIENTIFIC NAME:
Origanum majorana L. Also known as *Majorana hortensis* Moench. Family: Labiatae (Lamiaceae)

COMMON NAMES:
Knotted marjoram, marjoram

M

Marjoram, sweet

RATING:
4 = Research indicates that this substance will not fulfill the claims made for it, but that it is also unlikely to cause any harm when properly used.

What Is Sweet Marjoram?

This bushy but tender native Mediterranean perennial has small oval leaves and white, lavender, or pink flowers that grow together in knotlike clusters. The dried leaves and flowers are used for cooking and healing. Steam distillation produces sweet marjoram oil.

Do not confuse this plant with oregano (*Origanum vulgare*), commonly called wild marjoram (see **Oregano**).

What It Is Used For:

Sweet marjoram is widely used as a kitchen herb. As a folk remedy, it is said to have many of the same qualities as its similar-tasting cousin, oregano: digestive aid and stomach soother, reducer of excess gas, expectorant to clear coughs and other respiratory ailments, tranquilizer, perspiration-inducer, and antispasmodic for such discomforts as menstrual cramps. Healers in times past used it to treat cancers.[1] Some contemporary herbalists also recommend marjoram as a diuretic ("water pill"), headache treatment, tool to prevent motion sickness, and antiviral agent. Sweet marjoram and its oil are commonly used as fragrance components and flavoring ingredients in many foods.

Forms Available Include:

Dried herb, infusion, tincture.

Dosage Commonly Reported:

An infusion is made using 1 to 2 teaspoons dried leaves and flowers per cup of water and is drunk up to three times per day. The tincture is taken in dosages of ½ to 1 teaspoon up to three times per day.

Will It Work for You? What the Studies Say:

Sweet marjoram may have a mild stomach-settling effect, probably due to the presence of a volatile oil (about 1 percent) and reported antispasmodic properties[2] that may soothe the digestive tract muscles. Overall, however, there is limited substantiation for this. German health authorities, citing a lack of evidence, declined to approve of sweet marjoram herb or oil as a medicinal remedy.[3]

In the test tube, at least, liquid extracts of sweet marjoram inhibit the growth of *Herpes simplex*, the virus responsible for cold sores and genital herpes.[4] Follow-up studies are needed to determine whether this antiviral action occurs in living tissue and has any role to play in preventing or treating herpes outbreaks.

Sweet marjoram extracts have demonstrated antioxidative properties on lard, which means that they may help remove toxic by-products that may contribute to the formation of cancer cells.[5] Much more research is needed to determine if this effect occurs in humans and whether it is strong enough to have any practical value in preventing cancer.

Will It Harm You? What the Studies Say:

No significant adverse reactions have been associated with the use of sweet marjoram in culinary or medicinal concentrations. The FDA has placed sweet marjoram on its list of substances "Generally Recognized As Safe" (GRAS) for food consumption. However, although the oil will not irritate or sensitize the skin, the fresh herb may cause skin or eye inflammation, and cases of contact dermatitis have been reported.[6]

GENERAL SOURCES:

Blumenthal, M., J. Gruenwald, T. Hall, and R.S. Rister, eds. *The Complete German Commission E Monographs: Therapeutic Guide to Herbal Medicine.* Boston: Integrative Medicine Communications, 1998.

Castleman, M. *The Healing Herbs: The Ultimate Guide to the Curative Power of Nature's Medicines.* New York: Bantam Books, 1995.

Leung, A.Y., and S. Foster. *Encyclopedia of Common Natural Ingredients Used in Food, Drugs, and Cosmetics.* 2nd ed. New York: John Wiley & Sons, 1996.

Stary, F. *The Natural Guide to Medicinal Herbs and Plants.* Prague: Barnes & Noble, Inc., in arrangement with Aventinum Publishers, 1996.

TEXT CITATIONS:

1. J.L. Hartwell, *Lloydia*, 32 (1969): 247.
2. A.Y. Leung and S. Foster, *Encyclopedia of Common Natural Ingredients Used in Food, Drugs, and Cosmetics*, 2nd ed. (New York: John Wiley & Sons, 1996).
3. M. Blumenthal, J. Gruenwald, T. Hall, and R. S. Rister, eds., *The Complete German Commission E Monographs: Therapeutic Guide to Herbal Medicine* (Boston: Integrative Medicine Communications, 1998).
4. E.C. Herrmann and L.S. Kucera, *Proceedings of the Society for Experimental Biology and Medicine*, 124 (1967): 874.
5. Leung and Foster, op. cit.
6. D.L.J. Opdyke, *Food and Cosmetics Toxicology*, 14 (1976): 469. Leung and Foster, op. cit. J. Farkas, *Contact Dermatitis*, 7(2) (1981): 121.

PRIMARY NAME:

MARSHMALLOW

SCIENTIFIC NAME:
Althaea officinalis L. Family: Malvaceae

COMMON NAMES:
Althea, kitmi, mallards, malvavisco

What Is Marshmallow?

True to its name, marshmallow grows in marshes. It also flourishes in meadows, bogs, and other moist places across the United States, its native Europe, and other parts of the world. Primarily the tall root of this perennial is used for medicinal purposes, although the velvety-hairy leaves and even the large pale pink or white flowers, which bloom in summer, are occasionally used as well.

What It Is Used For:

Historians believe that people ate marshmallow during famines long ago. The herb's popularity as a folk remedy reaches far back into time as well. Consider

MARSHMALLOW (Continued)

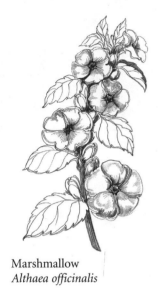

Marshmallow
Althaea officinalis

that the root of its botanical name, *Althea,* is *altho,* the Greek word for healing. Several years ago, investigators searching a Neanderthal grave found flowers of this plant type (*Althea*) that they believed were used medicinally.[1] Hippocrates, the father of Western medicine, recommended the herb, as did folk healers in medieval Europe and colonial America. Internal preparations such as decoctions were put to work treating colds, stomach troubles, vomiting, diarrhea, and kidney and bladder ailments. Some considered it an antidote for poison.

In topical forms, marshmallow is revered as an emollient and wound healer. Burns, bites, scalds, and bruises have been treated with it through the ages, as have toothaches and tissue irritations. Marshmallow ointments have been used to soothe chapped hands and cold-induced swellings or sores called chilblains. In the nineteenth century, doctors regularly whipped up a foamy meringue with the root juices, egg whites, and sugar; waited for the concoction to harden; and gave it to children with sore throats to suck on. However, the magical gooey mass toasted over campfires today no longer contains the actual herb.

Marshmallow held official drug status in the United States for a number of years. Although this is no longer true, most contemporary herbalists still place it high on their lists of winning medicinal herbs. Today it may be most popular as a cough remedy and soothing agent for throat irritation caused by coughs, colds, and bronchitis. Many herbalists recommend marshmallow tea for relieving stomach upset and controlling urinary bladder inflammation (cystitis) and other urinary complaints. Some herbal manufacturers sell it as a diuretic ("water pill"). Topical forms of marshmallow, from gels to ointments and pastes, are enlisted to encourage healing in minor cuts, scrapes, abrasions, and burns, including sunburns.

Marshmallow extracts occasionally appear as a flavoring agent in beverages (alcoholic included), candies, breads, and other foods.

Forms Available Include:

- *For internal use:* Capsule, decoction, dried leaves, infusion (of dried leaf), root (powdered), syrup, tea bag, tincture. Teas should be made with cold water to retain important active ingredients, and then gently warmed before drinking.
- *For external use:* Gargle, gel, ointment, poultice or paste (made from powdered or chopped root mixed with a little water), root (powdered), tincture.

Dosage Commonly Reported:

Marshmallow leaf tea is made using 1 heaping teaspoon leaves per cup of water. A decoction is made using 1 to 2 teaspoons root per cup of water. The syrup is taken in doses of 10 grams. A preparation for external use is made by applying enough water to the chopped root to form a paste.

Will It Work for You? What the Studies Say:

Marshmallow largely deserves the praise heaped upon it. The root contains up to 5 to 10 percent mucilage, a critical substance that becomes gooey when combined with liquid and has a sound reputation for softening, protecting, and soothing irritated mucous membranes or skin. German health authorities approve of marshmallow root tea for calming inflammation in the mouth, throat, upper respiratory tract, stomach, and intestines.[2] By soothing the throat, the herb also helps to suppress coughing, cutting short the vicious circle of irritation-cough-irritation. A study involving cats demonstrated this property; those fed marshmallow root extracts coughed much less than those that were not.[3] The subject does not appear to have been put to the test of clinical trials, but the mere presence of mucilage seems to satisfy most experts. The mucilage has also shown notable blood-sugar-lowering actions in healthy mice; the implication for individuals with associated problems such as diabetes is unclear.[4]

In addition to soothing irritated body tissues, marshmallow fights certain types of disease-causing bacteria[5] and may also give the immune system a kick. A team of investigators reported that in their experiments the herb enhanced the power of white blood cells to engulf and disarm certain kinds of germs.[6] Herbalists point to such findings when recommending marshmallow root for wounds, burns, and other skin irritations. No human trials have been done to confirm that it works, however.

As for the other proposed uses for this herb, scientific justification is weak or nonexistent. This includes popular claims that it will clear chest congestion (as an expectorant), promote diuresis, control diarrhea, or cure cystitis.

Will It Harm You? What the Studies Say:

Marshmallow root is a safe bet according to all sources. German health authorities cite no known side effects. The only precaution to consider is that the herb may delay the absorption of other drugs taken at the same time.[7] It may also interfere with treatments for lowering blood sugar.[8]

GENERAL SOURCES:

Bisset, N.G., ed. *Herbal Drugs and Phytopharmaceuticals.* Stuttgart: medpharm GmbH Scientific Publishers, 1994.

Blumenthal, M., J. Gruenwald, T. Hall, and R.S. Rister, eds. *The Complete German Commission E Monographs: Therapeutic Guide to Herbal Medicine.* Boston: Integrative Medicine Communications, 1998.

Castleman, M. *The Healing Herbs: The Ultimate Guide to the Curative Power of Nature's Medicines.* New York, NY: Bantam Books, 1995.

Hallowell, M. *Herbal Healing: A Practical Introduction to Medicinal Herbs.* Garden City Park, NY: 1994.

Heinerman, J. *Heinerman's Encyclopedia of Healing Herbs and Spices.* West Nyack, NY: Parker Publishing Co., 1996.

Huriez, C., and C. Fagez. *Lille Medical.* 13 (2 Suppl.) (1968): 121–23.

Leung, A.Y. *Encyclopedia of Common Natural Ingredients Used in Food, Drugs, and Cosmetics.* New York: John Wiley & Sons, 1980.

Mindell, E. *Earl Mindell's Herb Bible.* New York: Simon & Schuster/Fireside, 1992.

Newall, C.A., et al. *Herbal Medicines: A Guide for Health-Care Professionals.* London: The Pharmaceutical Press, 1996.

Ody, P. *The Herb Society's Complete Medicinal Herbal.* London: Dorling Kindersley Limited, 1993.

Weiss, R.F. *Herbal Medicine,* trans. A.R. Meuss, from the 6th German edition. Beaconsfield, England: Beaconsfield Publishers, Ltd., 1988.

TEXT CITATIONS:

1. J. Lietava, *Journal of Ethnopharmacology*, 35(3) (1992): 263–66.
2. M. Blumenthal, J. Gruenwald, T. Hall, and R. S. Rister, eds., *The Complete German Commission E Monographs: Therapeutic Guide to Herbal Medicine* (Boston: Integrative Medicine Communications, 1998).
3. G. Nosal'ova et al., *Pharmazie*, 47(3) (1992): 224–26.
4. M. Tomoda, *Planta Medica*, 53 (1987): 8–12.
5. M.C. Recio et al., *Phytotherapy Research*, 3 (1989): 77–80.
6. M. Tomoda et al., *Chemical and Pharmaceutical Bulletin*, 28 (1980): 824.
7. Blumenthal et al., op. cit.
8. C.A. Newall et al., *Herbal Medicines: A Guide for Health-Care Professionals* (London: The Pharmaceutical Press, 1996).

PRIMARY NAME:
MATÉ

SCIENTIFIC NAME:
Ilex paraguariensis St. Hill. Also referred to as *Ilex paraguensis* and *Ilex paraguayensis*. Family: Aquifoliaceae

COMMON NAMES:
Jesuit tea, Paraguay tea, St. Bartholomew's tea, yerba maté

RATING:
2 = According to a number of well-designed studies and common use, this substance appears to be relatively effective and safe when used in recommended amounts for the indication(s) noted in the "Will It Work for You?" section.

What Is Maté?

Maté is a caffeine-containing beverage made from an infusion of the dried, leathery leaves of *Ilex paraguariensis*, a small perennial holly shrub or tree that grows wild in Central and South America. It is also cultivated extensively, although not in the United States. The small red, black, or yellow fruit (berries) are not used in the beverage, which is pronounced MAH-tay.

What It Is Used For:

Many Argentineans, Brazilians, and other South and Central Americans prefer maté tea to coffee or black tea. It is traditionally drunk through a tube from a small gourd. With its 2 percent of caffeine, it gives some of the same kick that tea and coffee do and also promotes urine flow. It is drunk both hot and cold, and appears in sodas as a flavoring agent. Some sources consider it a digestive aid, appetite suppressant, "slimming" agent, and body cleanser. Centuries ago, Jesuit missionaries started to cultivate the plant when they realized that South American Indians on an otherwise all-meat diet often escaped the scourge of scurvy and other vitamin deficiency ailments when they drank maté.[1] The average Argentinean reportedly consumes eleven pounds of maté every year.[2]

Forms Available Include:

Infusion (with hot or cold water), liquid extract, tea (including instant). Also an ingredient in certain sodas.

Dosage Commonly Reported:

An infusion is made using 1 teaspoon of maté per cup of water and is steeped only briefly. The liquid leaf extract is taken in doses of 2.5 to 5 milliliters.

Will It Work for You? What the Studies Say:

Maté's caffeine content—there are about 25 to 50 milligrams of caffeine in a 6-ounce cup—explains its effectiveness as a mild stimulant. The same amount of brewed coffee contains as much as three to four times that amount of caffeine (about 100 milligrams), while a cup of breakfast cocoa contains about half (about 13 milligrams).[3] German health authorities approve of maté for mental and physical fatigue, presumably because of this caffeine content.[4] Some sources also cite the caffeine content as reason to promote maté as a slimming aid, claiming that it raises body heat and promotes the burning of fat when taken regularly. There is little good evidence for this, although one team of investigators did find that maté reduced appetite.

Caffeinated drinks such as maté, tea, and coffee are widely recognized mild diuretics. Responsible herbalists do not recommend caffeine-containing products for weight reduction because lost weight represents transitory fluid loss. Sources who promote maté as a cold and flu remedy cite its vitamin C content, which is high but can easily be obtained from other sources as well.

Maté also contains theophylline and theobromine, substances that have been used at much higher levels than are present in this herb to treat asthma.

Will It Harm You? What the Studies Say:

South Americans have been drinking maté beverages for centuries to no apparent ill effect. Considerable concern was raised by a study that found a significantly increased risk of esophageal cancer among very heavy maté drinkers in Uruguay.[5] Investigators compared the maté-drinking habits of 226 esophageal cancer patients with those of 469 controls who did not have the cancer. Analysis revealed that the cancer risk was higher the more maté the person drank on average. The risk was particularly high in women. The authors speculate that the heat of the drink, the high level of tannins—7 to 14 percent—or the presence of other ingredients may have played a role in causing the cancer.[6] A 1995 study of maté-associated esophageal cancer risk in Paraguay isolated the temperature of the maté drink as a key risk factor for developing esophageal cancer in the general population, with very hot maté significantly increasing risk.[7] However, the risk of developing esophageal cancer if you simply drink the brew in moderate amounts at something other than very high temperatures appears to be minimal. German health authorities cite no known side effects or adverse interactions with other medicines.[8] The FDA includes maté among several other caffeine-containing plants on its "Generally Recognized As Safe" (GRAS) list for use as a food additive.

GENERAL SOURCES:

Bisset, N.G., ed. *Herbal Drugs and Phytopharmaceuticals.* Stuttgart: medpharm GmbH Scientific Publishers, 1994.

Blumenthal, M., J. Gruenwald, T. Hall, and R.S. Rister, eds. *The Complete German Commission E Monographs: Therapeutic Guide to Herbal Medicine.* Boston: Integrative Medicine Communications, 1998.

Castleman, M. *The Healing Herbs: The Ultimate Guide to the Curative Power of Nature's Medicines.* New York: Bantam Books, 1995.

Lawrence Review of Natural Products. St. Louis: Facts and Comparisons, April 1988.

Mindell, E. *Earl Mindell's Herb Bible.* New York: Simon & Schuster/Fireside, 1992.

Tyler, V.E. *Herbs of Choice: The Therapeutic Use of Phytomedicinals.* Binghamton, NY: Haworth Press/Pharmaceutical Products Press, 1994.

———. *The Honest Herbal.* Binghamton, NY: Haworth Press/Pharmaceutical Products Press, 1993.

Tyler, V.E., L.R. Brady, and J.E. Robbers, eds. *Pharmacognosy.* Philadelphia: Lea & Febiger, 1988.

Weiner, M.A., and J.A. Weiner. *Herbs That Heal: Prescription for Herbal Healing.* Mill Valley, CA: Quantum Books, 1994.

TEXT CITATIONS:

1. F. Alikaridis, *Journal of Ethnopharmacology*, 20 (1987): 121. A. Meyer, *Suddeutcher Apotheker-Zeitung*, 77 (1937): 1001–2.
2. *Lawrence Review of Natural Products* (St. Louis: Facts and Comparisons, April 1988).
3. V.E. Tyler, *The Honest Herbal* (Binghamton, NY: Haworth Press/Pharmaceutical Products Press, 1993).
4. M. Blumenthal, J. Gruenwald, T. Hall, and R. S. Rister, eds., *The Complete German Commission E Monographs: Therapeutic Guide to Herbal Medicine* (Boston: Integrative Medicine Communications, 1998).
5. A. Vassalo et al., *Journal of the National Cancer Institute*, 75 (1985): 1005.
6. *Lawrence Review of Natural Products*, op. cit.
7. P.A. Rolon et al., *Cancer Epidemiology, Biomarkers & Prevention*, 4(6) (1995): 595–605.
8. Blumenthal et al., op. cit.

PRIMARY NAME:

MAYAPPLE, AMERICAN

SCIENTIFIC NAME:

Podophyllum peltatum L.
Family: Poedophiliac
(Berberidaceae)

COMMON NAMES:

American mandrake, American podophyllum, devil's apple, duck's foot, mandrake, podophyllin, vegetable mercury, wild lemon, wild mandrake

RATING:

- *For external use:* 1 = Years of use and extensive, high-quality studies indicate that this substance is very effective when used in recommended amounts for the indications noted in the "Will It Work for You?" section. The safety of this potentially very damaging herb depends on proper use, however; see the "Will It Harm You?" section.

- *For internal use:* 5 = Studies indicate that there is a definite health hazard to using this herb.

What Is American Mayapple?

This common perennial, a native of eastern North America that favors shady wet environments, bears one or two large shieldlike lobed leaves between which a solitary white, waxy flower grows. Mayapple also produces an edible fruit. The dried rhizomes (underground stems) and roots are used medicinally, as is a resinous extract from these parts of the plant called podophyllin. The related and similarly used *Podophyllum hexandrum* Royle is referred to as Indian podophyllum. It grows wild and is cultivated in India and Pakistan and is now considered an endangered species.[1]

Do not confuse *Podophyllum peltatum* with the European mandrake (*Mandragora officinarum* L.), as it exerts other types of pharmacologic influence.

What It Is Used For:

Various Native American tribes and settlers used the root as a cathartic (a very strong laxative), a liver treatment for such ailments as hepatitis and jaundice, a poisoning antidote, a cure for worms and syphilis, and a cancer-fighter. Today, although some herbalists still recommend ingesting it—in small and carefully controlled doses—for constipation and bile and digestive obstructions, most consider it too toxic for any internal purpose. The extract known as podophyllin finds widespread use in conventional medicine for topically treating certain benign skin tumors, especially venereal warts. Other cancers are occasionally treated with semisynthetic derivatives of the plant.

Forms Available Include:

For external use only: Powder, tincture, various prescription formulations.

Dosage Commonly Reported:

When using prescription formulations, powders, and tinctures, follow instructions very carefully.

Will It Work for You? What the Studies Say:

Most herbalists and plant experts agree that mayapple preparations pose too great a risk of toxicity to be taken internally for any ailment. Although it is a proven cathartic, U.S. health authorities no longer allow it to be used in over-the-counter laxative preparations.[2] The plant's resin—podophyllin, present in concentrations of about 5 percent, and even higher in *Podophyllum hexandrum*—is believed to cause bowel evacuation by irritating the colon.

If used with care, however, topically applied tinctures have proved relatively effective in melting away warts, particularly genital warts. They most likely accomplish this by inflicting cell damage on the rapidly dividing tumor cells. Prescription formulations are available. German health authorities endorse the use of topical formulations for condyloma acuminatum (genital warts).[3]

Inspired in part by the traditional use of this plant for treating internal cancers as well, components of podophyllin resin are used to produce semisynthetic agents such as etoposide and teniposide, which have shown promise when administered intravenously for treating stubborn testicular tumors, ovarian cancers, small-cell lung cancers, lymphomas, certain kinds of leukemias, and various other neoplastic diseases.[4]

Interestingly, some European doctors are using semisynthetic derivatives of podophyllum to treat rheumatoid arthritis. They cite studies showing superiority over placebos in improving the way patients feel, as well as improvements in various clinical and immunological measurements.[5] Semisynthetic derivatives have also been used to treat psoriasis.[6]

Will It Harm You? What the Studies Say:

Except for the fully ripe fruit, the entire American mayapple plant and its extracts (e.g., podophyllin) are poisonous. Severe multisystem toxicity with lingering neurologic problems and even death have occurred in people who take it internally as a laxative (chronically) or who have overdosed on it. Native Americans once ate the young shoots to commit suicide.[7]

Topical formulations must be used with extreme care, as they can cause severe irritation to mucous membranes. If improperly applied—placed on large areas of tissue, left on too long, not correctly removed—the substance can be absorbed into the body and cause systemwide toxicity as severe as if it had been ingested.[8] Follow prescription instructions precisely.

Pregnant women should never be treated with podophyllin, either internally or externally; it has caused limb deformities, heart defects, and other congenital abnormalities in the fetus, and even fetal death in some cases.[9] It should never be given to children.

GENERAL SOURCES:

Blumenthal, M., J. Gruenwald, T. Hall, and R.S. Rister, eds. *The Complete German Commission E Monographs: Therapeutic Guide to Herbal Medicine.* Boston: Integrative Medicine Communications, 1998.

Duke, J.A. *CRC Handbook of Medicinal Herbs.* Boca Raton, FL: CRC Press, 1985.

Lawrence Review of Natural Products. St. Louis: Facts and Comparisons, January 1992.

Leung, A.Y., and S. Foster. *Encyclopedia of Common Natural Ingredients Used in Food, Drugs, and Cosmetics.* 2nd ed. New York: John Wiley & Sons, 1996.

Tierra, M. *The Way of Herbs.* New York: Pocket Books, 1990.

Tyler, V.E. *Herbs of Choice: The Therapeutic Use of Phytomedicinals.* Binghamton, NY: Haworth Press/Pharmaceutical Products Press, 1994.

Weiss, R.F. *Herbal Medicine,* trans. A.R. Meuss, from the 6th German edition. Beaconsfield, England: Beaconsfield Publishers, Ltd., 1988.

TEXT CITATIONS:

1. A.Y. Leung and S. Foster, *Encyclopedia of Common Natural Ingredients Used in Food, Drugs, and Cosmetics,* 2nd ed. (New York: John Wiley & Sons, 1996).
2. *Lawrence Review of Natural Products* (St. Louis: Facts and Comparisons, January 1992). G. Rosenstein et al., *Pediatrics,* 57 (1976): 419.
3. Leung and Foster, op. cit.
4. J.A. Sinkule, *Pharmacotherapy,* 4(2) (1984): 61–73. R. Canetta et al., *Cancer Chemotherapy and Pharmacology,* 7 (1982): 9. Leung and Foster, op. cit. M. Rozencweig et al., *Cancer,* 40 (1977): 334.
5. A. Larsen et al., *British Journal of Rheumatology,* 28(2) (1989): 124.
6. Leung and Foster, op. cit.
7. J.A. Duke, *CRC Handbook of Medicinal Herbs* (Boca Raton, FL: CRC Press, 1985).
8. G. White and A. McFarlane, *Australian Prescriber,* 13(2) (1990): 36.
9. M.D. Karol et al. *Clinical Toxicology,* 16(3) (1980): 283. J.E. Cullis, *The Lancet,* 2 (1962): 511. *Lawrence Review of Natural Products,* op. cit.

PRIMARY NAME:
MEADOWSWEET

SCIENTIFIC NAME:
Filipendula ulmaria L. Maxim., formerly referred to as *Spiraea ulmaria* L. Family: Rosaceae

COMMON NAMES:
Bridewort, queen-of-the-meadow, spirea

RATING:
2 = According to a number of well-designed studies and common use, this substance appears to be relatively effective and safe when used in recommended amounts for the indication(s) noted in the "Will It Work for You?" section.

What Is Meadowsweet?

This tall, sweet-smelling herb bears large drooping clusters of creamy white blossoms. Both these flowering tops and the plant's leaves—but not its fruits—are used medicinally. Meadowsweet can be found in meadows, along streambanks, and in other damp environments in Europe and North America. It is also commonly grown in gardens.

What It Is Used For:

Treasured as an air freshener and bridal bouquet in medieval Europe, this delicately scented herb gradually developed a reputation for remedying arthritis, lowering fever, aiding respiratory ailments, controlling diarrhea (in children especially), blunting menstrual cramp pain, resolving indigestion and heartburn, preventing and helping to heal peptic ulcers, and promoting urination (as a diuretic, or "water pill"). In the mid-1800s a German chemist found the same ingredient in the plant's flower buds that had recently been discovered in white willow bark: salicin, a potent painkiller, anti-inflammatory, and fever-reducer. Nearly fifty years later, the Bayer pharmaceutical company introduced acetylsalicylic acid, a far more potent compound synthesized from meadowsweet's salicin, under the brand name Aspirin, which is now a generic term.

Herbalists today highlight the value of meadowsweet as a diuretic and diaphoretic (sweat-inducer) for feverish chills and colds and as a treatment for digestive system upset, diarrhea, low-grade fever, and pain caused by muscle aches, arthritis and other rheumatic complaints, headaches, and toothaches.

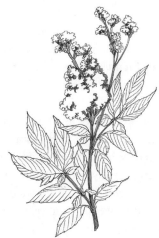

Meadowsweet
Filipendula ulmaria

Forms Available Include:

Dried flowers and leaves, infusion, liquid extract, tincture. Appears as an ingredient in herbal blends.

Dosage Commonly Reported:

An infusion is made using 1 to 2 teaspoons flower and is drunk very hot several times per day. The liquid extract is taken in doses of 2 to 4 milliliters.

Will It Work for You? What the Studies Say:

Meadowsweet preparations are no match for the painkilling or anti-inflammatory potency of aspirin, not even when taken as strong infusions or tinctures. Whether you actually experience any pain relief or reduction in inflammation is unclear; while the herb contains the substances known to exert these effects, no studies to test the herb's practical value in humans have been done. Do not count on the herb to lower a fever, either, especially if it is high. The only condition for which German health authorities approve of meadowsweet is the common cold, and then only as a supportive (secondary) treatment.[1] The standard license there notes that taking the herb in the form of a hot infusion may help increase sweating and urine output. Substances in meadowsweet (salicylate aglycones) have anti-inflammatory and diuretic actions.[2]

Meadowsweet also contains a considerable amount of astringent tannins (10 to 15 percent), which may explain its traditional use for digestive disorders such as acid indigestion and diarrhea.[3] (Tannins are believed to control or stop diarrhea by reducing inflammation in the intestines.) According to a 1960s study, the tannins in meadowsweet may also kill certain bacteria, some of which are commonly held responsible for infectious diarrhea (e.g., *Shigella dysenteriae*).[4] Flower extracts have been shown to fight bacteria commonly involved in urinary tract infections, such as *Staphylococcus aureus* and *Escherichia coli*.[5] Studies to confirm meadowsweet's practical value in treating such infections have apparently not been done.

Meadowsweet may help prevent stomach ulcers caused by certain irritants or medical procedures, according to studies in rats and mice.[6] Liquid extracts of the flowers appear to be most promising in this regard.[7] No human trials can be found in the recent medical literature, however.

Russian scientists have discovered a substance in the flowers and seeds that inhibits blood clotting (specifically, it is anticoagulant and fibrinolytic) in laboratory animals and is very similar in structure to one of the standard drugs prescribed for this purpose, heparin.[8] Aspirin (and heparin for more serious cases) is now commonly given to help prevent blood clots and associated complications, such as stroke. Despite these intriguing findings, do not rely on meadowsweet to prevent such potentially deadly clots because the herb's consistency in this regard has not been verified in human trials.

Also unclear are the implications of Russian research indicating that meadowsweet administered to rats can suppress certain kinds of tumors, including laboratory-induced brain and spinal cord tumors, and help to inhibit cervical and vaginal cancer in both mice and humans when systematically inserted into the vagina.[9]

Will It Harm You? What the Studies Say:

Use meadowsweet in moderation, given its high tannin content,[10] as the role of tannins in suppressing or promoting cancers remains poorly defined. German health authorities cite no known side effects or harmful interactions with other remedies.[11] The FDA placed meadowsweet on its formerly maintained list of "Herbs of Undefined Safety."

Because it is far less potent than aspirin, meadowsweet poses much less risk of the type of side effects—mainly stomach upset—that annoy many aspirin users. But precisely because of their chemical similarity, avoid the herb if you have had any type of an allergic reaction to aspirin or any other salicylate-containing substance. Although no direct link has ever been demonstrated, pregnant women may likewise want to avoid meadowsweet, given evidence linking aspirin use to birth defects and other complications, and studies indicating that the herb increases uterine tone in rabbits.[12]

Do not give meadowsweet to children under sixteen with flu or chicken pox symptoms, given the risk of a rare but serious ailment called Reye's syndrome that has been associated with aspirin in this age group. If you have asthma, use meadowsweet with caution; it has stimulated bronchial spasms in some people.[13]

GENERAL SOURCES:

Bisset, N.G., ed. *Herbal Drugs and Phytopharmaceuticals.* Stuttgart: medpharm GmbH Scientific Publishers, 1994.

Blumenthal, M., J. Gruenwald, T. Hall, and R.S. Rister, eds. *The Complete German Commission E Monographs: Therapeutic Guide To Herbal Medicine.* Boston: Integrative Medicine Communications, 1998.

Bradley, P.C., ed. *British Herbal Compendium: A Handbook of Scientific Information on Widely Used Plant Drugs*, vol. 1. Bournemouth (Dorset), England: British Herbal Medicine Association, 1992.

Castleman, M. *The Healing Herbs: The Ultimate Guide to the Curative Power of Nature's Medicines.* New York: Bantam Books, 1995.

Mayell, M. *Off-the-Shelf Natural Health: How to Use Herbs and Nutrients to Stay Well.* New York: Bantam Books, 1995.

Mindell, E. *Earl Mindell's Herb Bible.* New York: Simon & Schuster/Fireside, 1992.

Newall, C.A., et al. *Herbal Medicines: A Guide for Health-Care Professionals.* London: The Pharmaceutical Press, 1996.

TEXT CITATIONS:

1. M. Blumenthal, J. Gruenwald, T. Hall, and R. S. Rister, eds., *The Complete German Commission E Monographs: Therapeutic Guide to Herbal Medicine* (Boston: Integrative Medicine Communications, 1998).
2. P.C. Bradley, ed., *British Herbal Compendium: A Handbook of Scientific Information on Widely Used Plant Drugs*, vol. 1 (Bournemouth [Dorset], England: British Herbal Medicine Association, 1992).
3. E. Haslam et al., *Planta Medica*, 55 (1989): 1–8. Bradley, op. cit.
4. L.S. Kazarnosvskii et al., *Trudy Khar'kovskogo Gosudazt vennogo Farmatsevticheskogo Instituta*, 2 (1962): 23–26.
5. I. Catanicin-Hintz et al., *Clujul-Medica*, 56 (1983): 381–84.
6. O.D. Barnaulov and P.P. Denisenko, *Farmakologiia I Toksikologia* (Moscow), 43 (1980): 700–5. C.A. Newall et al., *Herbal Medicines: A Guide for Health-Care Professionals* (London: The Pharmaceutical Press, 1996).

7. A.Y. Yanutsh et al., *Farmatsevtichnii Zhurnal* (Kiev), 37 (1982): 53–56.
8. B.A. Kudriashov et al., *Vestnik Moskovskogo Universiteta Seriya 16: Biologiya*, 3 (1994): 15–16. B.A. Kudrifashov, *Izvestiia Akademii Nauk SSR. Serria Biologicheskaia*, 6 (1991): 939–42. L.A. Liapina and G.A. Koval'chuk, *Izvestiia Akademii Serria Biologischeskaia*, 4 (1993): 625–28.
9. V.G. Bespalov et al., *Khimico-Farmatsevticheskii Zhurnal*, 26(1) (1992): 59–61. A.P. Paresun'ko et al., *Voprosy Onkologii*, 39(12) (1993): 291–95.
10. Newall, op. cit.
11. Blumenthal et al., op. cit.
12. O.D. Barnaulov et al., *Rastitel'nye Resursy*, 14 (1978): 573–79.
13. Newall, op. cit.

PRIMARY NAME:

MELATONIN

SCIENTIFIC NAME:
N/A

COMMON NAME:
N/A

RATING:
2 = According to a number of well-designed studies and common use, this substance appears to be relatively effective and safe when used in recommended amounts for the indication(s) noted in the "Will It Work for You?" section.

What Is Melatonin?

Melatonin is a hormone secreted by the tiny pineal gland at the base of the brain. The pineal gland starts to excrete melatonin at the fall of darkness around 9 P.M., with peak output occurring between 2 A.M. and 4 A.M. At the appearance of light in the morning, melatonin excretion drops off. Dietary supplements containing both synthetic melatonin and melatonin extracted from animal pineal glands are available.

What It Is Used For:

Melatonin is integrally involved in setting your internal "clock" and is responsible for the sleepiness you feel at night and your wakefulness during the day. With age, natural levels of melatonin decline.

As a hot-selling dietary supplement, melatonin is most famous for its purported ability to fight jet lag and insomnia. Many sources also claim that it can slow the aging process, elevate mood and fight certain types of depression, protect the body against toxins, function as an antioxidant, reduce the release of estrogen, boost immune system function, and relax the body, among other things.

Forms Available Include:

Capsule, cream (for external use), liquid, spray, tablet. To avoid the risk of contamination, select synthetic versions rather than those made from animal tissue. Some sources recommend storing melatonin in the refrigerator.[1]

Dosage Commonly Reported:

Melatonin is commonly taken in doses of 0.5 to 6 milligrams, depending on the desired effect. People are often advised to begin with a low dose and increase the dose if necessary. Use the commercially prepared creams and sprays according to package instructions.

Will It Work for You? What the Studies Say:

By far the strongest scientific evidence for use of melatonin is for its ability to hasten sleep and to minimize jet lag. Lower-than-normal levels of circulating melatonin have been documented in insomniacs both young and old.[2]

Although there have been no large or long-term controlled trials on the subject, the data collected so far indicate that taking a very small amount of melatonin—a fraction of a milligram in some cases—can hasten sleep in insomniacs as well as people who do not normally have trouble sleeping. Low doses of melatonin efficiently promote falling asleep, the data indicate, although higher doses may be needed to help individuals who have trouble staying asleep.[3]

One double-blind crossover trial reported that when six healthy volunteers took 0.3 or 1 milligram of melatonin one to two hours before they usually went to sleep, it took them less time to fall asleep, to initiate a deeper sleep (stage 2 sleep), and to experience rapid eye movement (REM) sleep.[4] The subjects did not report drowsiness the following day. In another study that involved twelve elderly insomniacs, melatonin supplements reduced by fourteen minutes the average time it took to fall asleep.[5] The subjects also experienced improved sleep efficiency and reduced by twenty-four minutes the time spent awake after initially falling asleep.

These sleep-regulating properties may be of particular benefit for blind people whose melatonin production is not set to a twenty-four-hour cycle because light and dark do not affect them the same way they do sighted people. Many blind people suffer from chronic daytime drowsiness and fatigue as a result. In one study, nighttime insomnia and daytime drowsiness receded in blind men who took 5 milligrams of melatonin supplements at bedtime for three weeks.[6]

The goal of taking melatonin for jet lag is to help your twenty-four-hour cycle readjust to the new time zone more quickly. Studies on the hormone's ability to prevent jet lag have produced mixed results, although recent studies seem to support the practice if carried out properly.[7] Most subjects say they are less fatigued the next day, their mood is improved, their subsequent sleep cycles are less disturbed, and they are able to recover from time-zone switches more quickly.[8] Various regimens have been investigated, but the ideal one has yet to be elucidated. There is good evidence that taking melatonin at the wrong time could worsen jet lag.

Several experts recommend taking a small dose (such as 0.5 milligram) in the middle of the afternoon the day before flying from west to east, so that your body can prepare for an earlier fall of darkness.[9] Take it again on the day of departure, they advise, but two hours earlier. Take it again on the first full day spent at the eastern location and the day after that, but an hour or two earlier. Get out into the sun as early as possible upon arriving at your eastern destination. When traveling in the opposite direction, take a similarly small dose in the morning on the day before traveling, as well as the morning you leave and your first few days at the western location, so that your body experiences a delayed dawn.[10] The day you arrive, spend time outside without sunglasses for at least thirty minutes late in the day.[11]

In one placebo-controlled trial, less fatigue was noted among the fifteen volunteers flying from North America to France who took 8 milligrams of melatonin at about 10 P.M. French time on the day of the flight and around the same hour for the next three days in France.[12] The severity and duration of jet lag symptoms, such as days needed to recover a normal sleep pattern and an absence of fatigue during the day, were also less pronounced with melatonin than with a placebo in a trial involving twenty volunteers flying a great distance—from New Zealand to London and back.[13] The volunteers took 5 milligrams of melatonin once a day starting three days before the flight and continuing for three days after their arrival.

Evidence that melatonin can alter female hormone levels involved in menstruation—it can actually inhibit ovulation, according to a study of thirty-two women who took it along with synthetic progestin for four months—has inspired some researchers to examine its potential as a contraceptive.[14]

Some sources blame a malfunction in melatonin secretion for the melancholy and other symptoms that people suffering from seasonal affective disorder (SAD) experience during the long winter months of sunlight deprivation. Melatonin supplements have been recommended for such cases. Human trials on the subject do not appear in the recent medical literature, however.

Although more well-designed trials are needed before any conclusions can be made, melatonin has shown promise in fighting cancer. It appears to stimulate natural killer cells within the body as well as to exert antioxidant activity[15]; antioxidants help to remove toxic by-products that may contribute to the formation of cancer cells. One-year survival rates improved in individuals with metastatic lung cancer who took a daily supplement of 10 milligrams of melatonin in a 1995 study.[16] The hormone is being tested in individuals with various types of tumors that are either unresponsive to other types of therapy or have metastasized.[17]

Will It Harm You? What the Studies Say:

Most studies in humans report no major adverse reactions to melatonin and no side effects with small doses (i.e., 3 milligrams or less). Only minor side effects were seen with doses up to 8 milligrams, such as headache, transient depression, a sensation of heaviness in the head,[18] and worsening of depression in already depressed psychiatric patients.[19] Common recommended dosages are lower—1.5 to 3 milligrams of melatonin.

Despite these promising data, much still remains unknown about the potential for adverse reactions to melatonin, especially with long-term use, and the FDA has not yet conducted standard safety tests. Much also remains to be learned about proper dosages and potential interactions with other medicines. Critics say that such a potent hormone poses unknown risks, particularly when taken chronically or in high doses. The purity of melatonin products also raises some concern; one survey found that four of six melatonin products purchased at health food stores contained unidentifiable impurities.[20]

Many sources recommend that pregnant or nursing women avoid this hormone, as should anyone with kidney disease, depression, epilepsy, diabetes, or autoimmune disease. Women trying to conceive may want to avoid melatonin, given that it can function as a contraceptive at high doses. Children (under twenty years old) should not take it; they produce it in abundance.

Exercise care in driving or operating heavy machinery—or avoid it altogether—after taking melatonin because it may make you drowsy within thirty minutes for about one hour.[21] Also keep in mind that a number of the conditions for which melatonin is being taken, including seasonal affective disorders (SAD) and emotional disturbances, should be evaluated by a qualified medical professional.

GENERAL SOURCES:

Brody, J.E. *New York Times.* (April 30, 1997): C10.

Lawrence Review of Natural Products. St. Louis: Facts and Comparisons, January 1996.

Mayell, M. *Off-the-Shelf Natural Health: How to Use Herbs and Nutrients to Stay Well.* New York: Bantam Books, 1995.

TEXT CITATIONS:

1. M. Mayell, *Off-the-Shelf Natural Health: How to Use Herbs and Nutrients to Stay Well* (New York: Bantam Books, 1995).
2. S.M. Webb and M. Puig-Domingo, *Clinical Endocrinology,* 42(3) (1995): 221. *Lawrence Review of Natural Products* (St. Louis: Facts and Comparisons, January 1996).
3. *Lawrence Review of Natural Products,* op. cit.
4. I.V. Zhdanova et al., *Clinical Pharmacology and Therapeutics,* 57 (1995): 552.
5. D. Garfinkel et al., *The Lancet,* 346 (1995): 541.
6. R.L. Sack et al., *Journal of Biological Rhythms,* 6 (1991): 249.
7. R.J. Croughs and T.W. de Bruin, *Netherlands Journal of Medicine,* 49(4) (1996): 164–66.
8. *Lawrence Review of Natural Products,* op. cit.
9. J.E. Brody, *New York Times,* (April 30, 1997): C10.
10. Ibid. G. Cowley, "Melatonin Mania," *Newsweek,* (November 6, 1995): 60–63.
11. Brody, op. cit.
12. B. Claustrat et al., *Biological Psychiatry,* 32 (1992): 705.
13. K. Petrie et al., *British Medical Journal,* 298 (1989): 705–7.
14. B.C.G. Voordouw et al., *Journal of Clinical Endocrinology,* 74 (1992): 108. *Lawrence Review of Natural Products,* op. cit.
15. *Lawrence Review of Natural Products,* op. cit.
16. Webb and Puig-Domingo, op. cit.
17. P. Lissoni et al., *Oncology,* 52 (1995): 163. P. Lissoni et al., *Oncology,* 48 (1991): 448. S. Barni et al., *Oncology,* 52 (1995): 243.
18. J.E. Jan et al., *Developmental Medicine and Child Neurology,* 36 (1994): 97. *Lawrence Review of Natural Products,* op. cit.
19. J.S. Carman et al., *American Journal of Psychiatry,* 133(10) (1976): 1181–86.
20. *Medical Letter,* 37(962) (1995): 111–12.
21. *Lawrence Review of Natural Products,* op. cit.

PRIMARY NAME:
MENTHOL

What Is Menthol?

Menthol is an alcohol found in peppermint (*Mentha x piperta*) and other mint oils. It can also be synthetically produced.

SCIENTIFIC NAME:
N/A

COMMON NAME:
N/A

RATING:
1 = Years of use and extensive, high-quality studies indicate that this substance is very effective and safe when used in recommended amounts for the indication(s) noted in the "Will It Work for You?" section. However, see the "Will It Harm You?" section for warnings about pure menthol.

What It Is Used For:

Several valuable healing properties have been ascribed to menthol, including an ability to numb pain, stop itching, and produce a distracting and cooling sensation when applied to the skin. It is used to relieve indigestion and gas when taken in the form of peppermint preparations, help clear sinuses when inhaled in the form of a vapor, and quiet coughs and minor throat irritations when applied to the chest in the form of a rub. See **Peppermint** for more information.

Forms Available Include:

Multiple; see **Peppermint**.

Dosage Commonly Reported:

See **Peppermint**.

Will It Work for You? What the Studies Say:

Menthol is widely accepted by conventional and alternative medical traditions as an effective agent for numerous ailments, including indigestion and gas, clogged sinuses, coughs, and sore throats. See **Peppermint** for more information.

Will It Harm You? What the Studies Say:

Menthol qualifies as a safe substance to use in recommended amounts. Take special precautions in treating infants and small children with menthol- or peppermint-containing substances, however. *Never ingest pure menthol;* it is poisonous and as little as a teaspoonful (1 gram per kilogram of body weight) can be fatal.

GENERAL SOURCES:
Castleman, M. *The Healing Herbs: The Ultimate Guide to the Curative Power of Nature's Medicines.* New York: Bantam Books, 1995.
Leber, M.R., et al. *Handbook of Over-the-Counter Drugs and Pharmacy Products.* Berkeley: Celestial Arts Publishing, 1994.
Tyler, V.E. *Herbs of Choice: The Therapeutic Use of Phytomedicinals.* Binghamton, NY: Haworth Press/Pharmaceutical Products Press, 1994.

PRIMARY NAME:
MILK THISTLE

SCIENTIFIC NAME:
Silybum marianum L. Gaertn.
Family: Asteraceae
(Compositae)

What Is Milk Thistle?

Milk thistle is native to the Mediterranean region but now grows in many parts of Europe and the Americas, including California and the eastern seaboard of the United States. Milk thistle has been cultivated as a vegetable and ornamental. The tall, weedlike plants have large prickly leaves and the stems contain a milky sap that oozes out when cracked open. Small fruits ("seeds") nestle in the feathery reddish-purple flowers and are used to make the medicinal extract known as silymarin. Most commercial preparations are standardized to contain

M

Milk Thistle

COMMON NAMES:
Marian, Mary thistle, Our Lady's thistle, St. Mary's, silybum

RATING:
1 = Years of use and extensive, high-quality studies indicate that this substance is very effective and safe when used in recommended amounts for the indication(s) noted in the "Will It Work for You?" section.

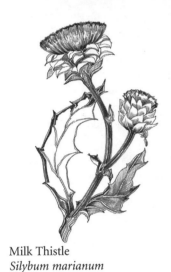

Milk Thistle
Silybum marianum

at least 70 percent of this substance. Other parts of the plant have occasionally been used for medicinal purposes as well.

Do not confuse milk thistle (*Silybum marianum*) with the similarly named **Blessed Thistle** or holy thistle (*Cnicus benedictus*), which is used differently.

What It Is Used For:

For more than two thousand years, Europeans considered milk thistle a remedy for liver ailments, digestive system upset, excessive menstrual flow, and various other ills. Ancient Greek and Roman texts mention the herb. But by the early part of the twentieth century, most people had lost interest in it. Then German investigators identified chemicals in the fruit important to liver function, lending scientific weight to the nearly forgotten folk practice of taking the herb as a liver tonic. Today, milk thistle preparations are considered an all-around cure for this major organ so critical to proper digestion, waste processing, and other body functions. Extracts are taken to protect the liver from exposure to biologic and chemical toxins, as well as to treat the organ after damage has been done. The herb's renown for regenerating wounded liver cells and boosting the organ's overall function has inspired many to treat chronic liver diseases with it, including inflammatory conditions such as hepatitis and alcohol-induced cirrhosis. Thousands if not millions of people—especially Europeans—have expectantly taken milk thistle preparations for these ailments.

Milk thistle fruit also has a reputation, although far less formidable, for alleviating mild digestive disorders, stimulating the production of mother's milk, and treating functional gallbladder disease. In Europe, prepared gastrointestinal, biliary, and phlebitis (vein inflammation) remedies containing milk thistle extracts are available. Homeopaths prescribe minute amounts of the herb for various ailments. (See page 2 for a discussion of homeopathy.)

Forms Available Include:

Capsule, concentrated drops, decoction, fruit (to be crushed for making tea), injection, powder solution, tablet, tea bag, tincture.

Dosage Commonly Reported:

An extract standardized to 70 percent silymarin is typically used in various forms. The usual daily dose is 12 to 15 grams fruit (whole or powdered) or about 200 to 420 milligrams silymarin. A decoction is made using 1 heaping teaspoon (about 3 to 5 grams) crushed fruit and is drunk three or four times per day thirty minutes before meals.

Will It Work for You? What the Studies Say:

German scientists made a breakthrough in the late 1960s when they isolated liver-protectant principles in the fruit.[1] They called these silymarin. Extensive studies in test tubes, small animals, and humans have demonstrated just how good to the liver this complex mixture of flavonoid compounds is.

Of the many compliments paid to silymarin, one of the greatest is that it actually protects the liver. Research indicates that it does this by altering the outer structure of liver cell membranes in such a way that certain toxic substances are blocked from entering. Studies in small animals have illustrated this protective action for a number of liver toxins, including carbon tetrachloride, radiation, and certain foods such as the highly poisonous amanita (deathcap) mushroom.[2] Studies involving individuals suffering from amanita poisoning have shown that the death rate drops significantly below previously known levels among those treated with an intravenous formulation of the herb called silibinin.[3] Silymarin also helps cleanse the liver of dangerous toxins by scavenging for substances called free radicals that can damage the organ.[4]

Silymarin boasts another remarkable property: by encouraging the regeneration of liver cells it can actually reverse damage and help cure the liver. In technical terms, it does this by stimulating protein synthesis (RNA polymerase A), thus activating the liver's ability to regenerate itself through increased formation of new liver cells called hepatocytes.[5] In a series of experiments, liver cells were regenerated in rats who had parts of their livers cut out and were then fed silymarin. More importantly, numerous clinical trials in humans confirm that silymarin can effectively treat liver ailments such as chronic cirrhosis and toxic liver.[6]

In one well-designed, randomized trial that included a control group given a dummy drug for comparison, silymarin taken in 140-milligram doses three times a day significantly reduced the death rate among individuals with alcohol-induced liver cirrhosis.[7] Other trials have shown that individuals suffering from alcohol- and drug-induced liver complaints who are treated with silymarin fare much better than those given a placebo.[8] German health authorities have officially approved of milk thistle fruit for toxic liver damage and as a supportive treatment for chronic inflammatory liver conditions and liver cirrhosis.[9]

Milk thistle also helps control mild digestive disorders, according to various plant experts. German health authorities have endorsed it for this purpose (in infusion form).[10] A recent study in rats indicated that silymarin may even battle stomach ulcers, but more research on the subject is needed.[11]

When considering taking milk thistle, keep in mind that various formulations work differently. For example, although some herbalists recommend them, milk thistle teas probably do not contain enough active ingredients to be medicinally effective.[12] The critical ingredient—silymarin—does not dissolve well in water, so the tea ends up containing only trace amounts of it. The stomach and intestines do not absorb silymarin well, which means that very little if any would make it into the body's circulation. For these reasons, concentrated forms of the herb, such as drops, are a wise selection. Injection solutions may be optimal. In Germany, milk thistle teas are recommended only for functional gallbladder disorders.[13]

Will It Harm You? What the Studies Say:

According to extensive studies done over the past few decades, milk thistle (and silymarin) are very safe in typically recommended amounts. Mild but transient diarrhea appears to be the only risk. Not even large doses seem to be toxic, possibly because excess amounts are simply flushed out of the body in the urine.[14] German health authorities do not cite any situations in which the herb or its extracts should be avoided or any harmful interactions with other remedies.[15] German texts indicate the herb is even safe for pregnant women, although you should probably discuss this with an obstetrician.[16] However, liver diseases are serious ailments; talk to your doctor about taking this or any other medicine for them.

GENERAL SOURCES:

American Pharmaceutical Association. *Handbook of Nonprescription Drugs.* 11th ed. Washington, D.C.: American Pharmaceutical Association, 1996.

Bisset, N.G., ed. *Herbal Drugs and Phytopharmaceuticals.* Stuttgart: medpharm GmbH Scientific Publishers, 1994.

Blumenthal, M., J. Gruenwald, T. Hall, and R.S. Rister, eds. *The Complete German Commission E Monographs: Therapeutic Guide to Herbal Medicine.* Boston: Integrative Medicine Communications, 1998.

Foster, S. *Milk Thistle: Botanical Series.* American Botanical Council. Number 305, 1991.

Review of Natural Products. St. Louis: Facts and Comparisons, January 1997.

Lorenz, D., et al. *Planta Medica.* 45 (1982): 216.

Mayell, M. *Off-the-Shelf Natural Health: How to Use Herbs and Nutrients to Stay Well.* New York: Bantam Books, 1995.

Mindell, E. *Earl Mindell's Herb Bible.* New York: Simon & Schuster/Fireside, 1992.

Tyler, V.E. *Herbs of Choice: The Therapeutic Use of Phytomedicinals.* Binghamton, NY: Haworth Press/Pharmaceutical Products Press, 1994.

———. *The Honest Herbal.* Binghamton, NY: Haworth Press/Pharmaceutical Products Press, 1993.

Valenzuela, V., et al. *Planta Medica.* 52 (1986): 438.

Wagner, H., et al. *Arzneimittel-Forschung.* 18 (1968): 688–96.

Weiss, R.F. *Herbal Medicine,* trans. A.R. Meuss, from the 6th German edition. Beaconsfield, England: Beaconsfield Publishers, Ltd., 1988.

TEXT CITATIONS:

1. H. Wagner et al., *Plant Drug Analysis* (New York: Springer-Verlag, 1984).
2. G. Vogel and I. Temme, *Arzneimittel-Forschung,* 19 (1969): 613–15.
3. C. Hruby, *Forum,* 6 (1984): 23–26.
4. H. Hikino and Y. Kiso, "Natural Products for Liver Disease," *Economic and Medicinal Plant Research,* vol. 2 (New York: Academic Press, 1988), 39–72.
5. V.E. Tyler, *Herbs of Choice: The Therapeutic Use of Phytomedicinals* (Binghamton, NY: Haworth Press/Pharmaceutical Products Press, 1994). N.G. Bisset, ed., *Herbal Drugs and Phytopharmaceuticals* (Stuttgart: medpharm GmbH Scientific Publishers, 1994). S. Foster, *Milk Thistle: Botanical Series,* American Botanical Council, Number 305, 1991.
6. Bisset, op. cit.
7. P. Ferenci et al., *Journal of Hepatology,* 9 (1989): 105–13.
8. Foster, op. cit.
9. M. Blumenthal, J. Gruenwald, T. Hall, and R. S. Rister, eds., *The Complete German Commission E Monographs: Therapeutic Guide to Herbal Medicine* (Boston: Integrative Medicine Communications, 1998).
10. Ibid. V. Fintelmann, *Planta Medica,* 57(7) (1991): S48–52.
11. A.C. Alarcon de la Lastra et al., *Planta Medica,* 61(2) (1995): 116–19.
12. V.E. Tyler, *The Honest Herbal* (Binghamton, NY: Haworth Press/Pharmaceutical Products Press, 1993).
13. Bisset, op. cit.
14. Ibid.
15. Blumenthal et al., op. cit.
16. R.F. Weiss, *Herbal Medicine,* trans. A.R. Meuss, from the 6th German edition (Beaconsfield, England: Beaconsfield Publishers, Ltd., 1988).

MISTLETOE

SCIENTIFIC NAME:

In North America, species of the *Phoradendron* genus, most commonly *Phoradendron flavescens* (Pursh) Nuttal, *Phoradendron serotinum* (Raf.) M.C. Johnston, and *Phoradendron tomentosum* (DC) Englem. In Europe: *Viscum album* L. and related species. Family: Loranthaceae

COMMON NAMES:

All heal, birdlime, devil's fuge, golden bough, herb de la croix, lignum crucis, viscum

RATING:

5 = Studies indicate that there is a definite health hazard to using this herb.

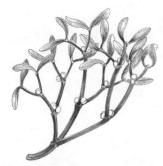

Mistletoe
Phoradendron flavescens

What Is Mistletoe?

Mistletoes are branching, semiparasitic evergreen shrubs that root into the bark of oak, apple, and other deciduous trees. Their sticky white berries, leathery leaves, and young twigs have been used medicinally.

What It Is Used For:

Holiday revelers kissing under the mistletoe may not know that the plant has a history of medicinal use stretching back to antiquity. Leaf preparations in particular have been used to treat nervous disorders and blood pressure ailments, and to fight certain cancers. Many ancient herbalists quickly recognized the herb's toxic effects and confined their recommendations to external formulations for skin problems such as sores and abscesses.

For years, herbalists have made a distinction between the effects of European and American mistletoe; the former has a reputation as a calming agent, antispasmodic, and blood pressure reducer, while the latter is considered good for increasing blood pressure and stimulating the uterus and intestines. Interest in European mistletoe's anticancer potential (in injection form) is mounting.[1]

Forms Available Include:

Infusion (made with leaves). The following commercial forms are hard to obtain in the United States: capsule, injection, liquid extract, tincture.

Dosage Commonly Reported:

An infusion is made using 1 teaspoon of chopped leaves per cup of water and is drunk once or twice per day.

Will It Work for You? What the Studies Say:

Although folk wisdom has it that American and European mistletoe (stems and leaves) affect the body in opposite ways, laboratory findings indicate that they in fact share active ingredients—the toxic proteins phoratoxins and viscotoxins—and produce similar reactions. In laboratory animals, these substances cause dose-dependent drops or increases in blood pressure, stimulate uterine and gastrointestinal contractions, and slow and weaken the heartbeat.[2]

Whether any of these actions occur in humans has yet to be proved. For example, evidence that mistletoe—particularly in oral form such as a tea—can benefit high blood pressure is vague at best. Experts believe that the active ingredients break down and are not fully absorbed in the gastrointestinal tract.[3] Citing the need for sounder evidence, German health authorities declined to endorse the use of mistletoe to treat high blood pressure.[4]

Mistletoe's reputation as a cancer cure persists, although misinformation abounds and more research is needed before firm conclusions can be made about its value and safety in treating human cancers. Experiments indicate that mistletoe extracts (phoratoxins, viscotoxins, other lectins) can inhibit the growth of tumor cells, both in test tubes and in laboratory animals.[5] A proprietary crude plant juice formulation called Iscador™ was used for many of these studies. German health authorities endorse the use of mistletoe leaves in specially prepared, commercially sterile injection form to treat malignant tumors, although such uses are not approved in the United States.[6] This is done only by injecting the extract intravenously or into the tumor itself, not by drinking mistletoe tea or taking it in any other oral form. No convincing data from large clinical trials can be found, although Iscador™ given to groups of people suffering from breast, stomach, colon, cervix, and other cancers has been reported to slightly improve the disease course compared with controls, especially in the case of colon cancer.[7] In a 1979 study, a mistletoe formulation statistically increased survival among women with ovarian cancer.[8] Immune-system stimulating properties have also been identified in Iscador™ and are believed to contribute to its anticancer activity.[9]

German health authorities also endorse the use of specially prepared, commercially sterile injection solutions for degenerative joint inflammation.[10] They do not, however, endorse the use of mistletoe *fruit* for any ailment, owing, in part, to a lack of proven efficacy.

Will It Harm You? What the Studies Say:

Until more definitive information becomes available and controversy on the subject is settled, the safest approach is to presume that all parts of the European and American mistletoe plant are toxic.[11] In any case, take the herb only under supervision of a qualified practitioner. Some sources contend that parts of the mistletoe are in fact not very toxic, including the berries of the European mistletoe and the leaves of the American mistletoe. A review of three hundred cases of accidental ingestion of European mistletoe (berries for the most part) among adults indicated that there were no fatalities; the majority did not even develop symptoms of poisoning.[12] Yet children have died after eating just a berry or two. Hepatitis developed in a woman taking an herbal blend containing mistletoe; experts attributed the disease to the mistletoe specifically.[13]

Citing safety concerns, the FDA has withheld the sale of mistletoe capsules.[14] The herb may interfere with medications you are taking for high or low blood pressure, depression, heart disease, and certain other ailments.[15] Signs and symptoms of berry or leaf poisoning include nausea, diarrhea and vomiting with possible dehydration, slowed heartbeat, stomach upset, delirium, high blood pressure, and heart attack. Potential side effects following injection of mistletoe extracts include death of the tissue around the injection sight, shivering, high fever, headache, chest pain complications, and allergic reactions.[16]

GENERAL SOURCES:

Bisset, N.G., ed. *Herbal Drugs and Phytopharmaceuticals*. Stuttgart: medpharm GmbH Scientific Publishers, 1994.

Blumenthal, M., J. Gruenwald, T. Hall, and R.S. Rister, eds. *The Complete German Commission E Monographs: Therapeutic Guide to Herbal Medicine*. Boston: Integrative Medicine Communications, 1998.

Castleman, M. *The Healing Herbs: The Ultimate Guide to the Curative Power of Nature's Medicines*. New York: Bantam Books, 1995.

Lampe, K.E., and M.A. McCann. *AMA Handbook of Poisonous and Injurious Plants*. Chicago: American Medical Association, 1985.

Lawrence Review of Natural Products. St. Louis: Facts and Comparisons, December 1992.

Leung, A.Y., and S. Foster. *Encyclopedia of Common Natural Ingredients Used in Food, Drugs, and Cosmetics.* 2nd ed. New York: John Wiley & Sons, 1996.

Newall, C.A., et al. *Herbal Medicines: A Guide for Health-Care Professionals.* London: The Pharmaceutical Press, 1996.

Tyler, V.E. *Herbs of Choice: The Therapeutic Use of Phytomedicinals.* Binghamton, NY: Haworth Press/Pharmaceutical Products Press, 1994.

———. *The Honest Herbal.* Binghamton, NY: Haworth Press/Pharmaceutical Products Press, 1993.

Weiner, M.A., and J.A. Weiner. *Herbs That Heal: Prescription for Herbal Healing.* Mill Valley, CA: Quantum Books, 1994.

TEXT CITATIONS:

1. V.E. Tyler, *Herbs of Choice: The Therapeutic Use of Phytomedicinals* (Binghamton, NY: Haworth Press/Pharmaceutical Products Press, 1994).

2. *Lawrence Review of Natural Products* (St. Louis: Facts and Comparisons, December 1992). V.E. Tyler, *The Honest Herbal* (Binghamton, NY: Haworth Press/Pharmaceutical Products Press, 1993). T. Fukunaga et al., *Journal of the Pharmaceutical Society of Japan*, 109 (1989): 600. S. Rosell and G. Samuelsson, *Toxicon*, 4 (1966): 107.

3. N.G. Bisset, ed., *Herbal Drugs and Phytopharmaceuticals* (Stuttgart: medpharm GmbH Scientific Publishers, 1994).

4. M. Blumenthal, J. Gruenwald, T. Hall, and R. S. Rister, eds., *The Complete German Commission E Monographs: Therapeutic Guide to Herbal Medicine* (Boston: Integrative Medicine Communications, 1998).

5. M.L. Jung et al., *Cancer Letters* (1990) 51:103. *Lawrence Review of Natural Products*, op. cit. C.A. Newall et al., *Herbal Medicines: A Guide for Health-Care Professionals* (London: The Pharmaceutical Press, 1996).

6. V.E. Tyler, *The Honest Herbal* (Binghamton, NY: Haworth Press/Pharmaceutical Products Press, 1993). Blumenthal et al., op. cit.

7. Newall, op. cit.

8. W. Hassauer et al., *Onkologie*, 2(1) (1979): 28.

9. Newall, op. cit. H. Franz, *Oncology*, 43(S1) (1984): 23.

10. Blumenthal et al., op. cit.

11. Tyler, *The Honest Herbal*, op. cit.

12. H.A. Hall et al., *Annals of Emergency Medicine*, 15 (1986): 1320.

13. J. Harvey and D.G. Colin-Jones, *British Medical Journal*, 282 (1981): 186–87.

14. *Lawrence Review of Natural Products*, op. cit.

15. Newall, op. cit.

16. Blumenthal et al., op. cit.

PRIMARY NAME:

MORMON TEA

SCIENTIFIC NAME:

Ephedra nevadensis Wats.
Family: Ephedraceae

What Is Mormon Tea?

Mormon tea is brewed from the fresh or dried stems and branches of *Ephedra nevadensis*, a small, many-branched shrub native to the dry, rocky soils of the American Southwest and Mexico. Yellow-green flowers bloom on the weather-beaten shrub in spring, followed by small dark seeds. *Ephedra nevadensis* is often referred to as an American species of ephedra (see **Ephedra** for more information), but it actually contains none of that herb's active ingredients, such as alkaloids.

COMMON NAMES:

Brigham tea, desert tea, joint fir, Mexican tea, Nevada jointfir, popotillo, squaw tea, teamster's tea, whorehouse tea

RATING:

4 = Research indicates that this substance will not fulfill the claims made for it, but that it is also unlikely to cause any harm.

What It Is Used For:

Before European settlers arrived, Native Americans reportedly enjoyed a refreshing tea made from the stems of this indigenous plant. Mexicans and numerous early frontiersmen are said to have sipped what they referred to as Mormon tea—so-called because it was caffeine-free—to "purify the blood" or as a "spring tonic," both euphemisms for treating venereal diseases such as syphilis and gonorrhea. The tea is said to have mild diuretic properties, which may account for this and other traditional uses, such as for kidney disorders. Other folk uses include the treatment of headaches and colds. The dried, powdered twigs were once used to make poultices and ointments to place on burns and sores.

Forms Available Include:

Infusion (of dried whole or powdered stems).

Dosage Commonly Reported:

None commonly reported.

Will It Work for You? What the Studies Say:

Although it is related to the Chinese plant *Ephedra sinica*, this herb contains none of the ephedrine that has earned that plant its renown as a decongestant, central nervous system stimulant, and bronchodilator. In fact, other than astringent substances called tannins, a resin, and a volatile oil, Mormon tea appears to contain no active principles, according to the limited data collected over the years.[1] The astringent tannins endow it with a distinct flavor and thirst-quenching quality that many people enjoy, and appear to contribute to a slight constipating action.[2] Plant experts also report that infusions and fluid extracts increase urine output,[3] but no studies on the subject can be found in the recent medical literature.

Will It Harm You? What the Studies Say:

After decades of use, there are no reports of serious adverse reactions to Mormon tea. Given its relatively high concentration of tannins, however, avoid very large doses or long-term use, as tannins may irritate the stomach or even increase the risk of cancer if taken in these ways.[4]

GENERAL SOURCES:

Duke, J.A. *CRC Handbook of Medicinal Herbs.* Boca Raton, FL: CRC Press, 1985.

Hylton, W.H. ed. *The Rodale Herb Book. How to Use, Grow, and Buy Nature's Miracle Plants.* Emmaus, PA: Rodale Press, Inc., 1974.

Tyler, V.E. *Herbs of Choice: The Therapeutic Use of Phytomedicinals.* Binghamton, NY: Haworth Press/Pharmaceutical Products Press, 1994.

————. *The Honest Herbal.* Binghamton, NY: Haworth Press/Pharmaceutical Products Press, 1993.

Tyler, V.E., L.R. Brady, and J.E. Robbers, eds. *Pharmacognosy.* Philadelphia: Lea & Febiger, 1988.

TEXT CITATIONS:

1. V.E. Tyler, *The Honest Herbal* (Binghamton, NY: Haworth Press/Pharmaceutical Products Press, 1993).
2. V.E. Tyler, L.R. Brady, and J.E. Robbers, eds., *Pharmacognosy* (Philadelphia: Lea & Febiger, 1988).
3. J.A. Duke, *CRC Handbook of Medicinal Herbs* (Boca Raton, FL: CRC Press, 1985). Tyler, op. cit.
4. Tyler, op. cit.

PRIMARY NAME:

MOTHERWORT

SCIENTIFIC NAME:
Leonurus cardiaca L. Family: Labiatae (Lamiaceae)

COMMON NAMES:
Heartwort, lion's tail

RATING:
3 = Studies on the effectiveness and safety of this herb are conflicting, or there are not enough studies to draw a conclusion.

What Is Motherwort?

This large perennial's palm-shaped leaves and whorls of small pink or white flowers are used medicinally once they have been dried. Motherwort is native to Asia but now grows in parts of Europe and North America.

What It Is Used For:

Motherwort has a long history of folk use in China, Europe, North America, and other parts of the world as a "heart tonic" for nervousness-related heart complaints, such as palpitations and fast heartbeat. It has also been used as a general calmative, sedative, nerve tonic, epilepsy treatment, and agent for stimulating delayed or suppressed menstruation, encouraging labor, and relaxing the uterus after childbirth. Contemporary herbalists recommend many of these same applications today. Germans have taken it as an adjuvant treatment for symptoms of hyperthyroidism (an overactive thyroid gland). Chinese healers have tested indigenous *Leonurus* species such as *Leonurus artemisia* for numerous ailments, including prostate enlargement[1] (in an herbal blend) and stroke.[2]

Forms Available Include:

Dried herb, infusion, liquid extract, tincture. Given its bitter taste, you may want to add honey, lemon, or another favorite flavoring to improve the flavor.

Dosage Commonly Reported:

An infusion is made using 1 to 2 teaspoons dried herb per cup of water and is drunk once or twice per day. The tincture is taken is dosages of 10 to 15 drops up to three times per day. The liquid herb extract is taken in doses of 2 to 4 milligrams.

Will It Work for You? What the Studies Say:

Studies indicate that motherwort may have a justifiable role to play in treating nervous heart conditions. Controlled clinical trials in humans appear to be lacking, but several European health authorities, including those in Germany, consider the evidence strong enough to approve of motherwort for such conditions as long as the heart is essentially healthy.[3] Alkaloids in the herb such as leonurine and possibly stachydrine have been reported to lower blood pressure and depress (slow down) the central nervous system in laboratory animals; this was shown first in the test tube, then in animal hearts isolated in chemical baths, and then in the animals themselves.[4] This kind of action may also explain the herb's long-standing reputation as a mild sedative and antispasmodic, although animal studies done some time ago reported mixed results regarding the sedative action of motherwort.[5] Overall, research on the subject has been somewhat limited.

One German physician notes personal success in treating problems arising from poor regulation of the electrical system of the heart, but says that long-term treatment is required and the results are usually mild.[6] Chinese researchers have reported success in preventing stroke in animals and treating coronary heart disease with motherwort-hawthorn mixtures (see **Hawthorn**).[7] Reports that motherwort can prevent blood clots are based on studies in a related plant, *Leonurus heterophyllus*, and have apparently not been tested in *Leonurus cardiaca*.[8]

German health authorities also approve of motherwort as an adjuvant treatment for hyperthyroidism, which can cause such unpleasant symptoms as excessive sweating, palpitations, fatigue, and anxiety.[9]

Motherwort's impact on the uterus—and thus its value for treating menstrual irregularities or labor—remains unclear.[10] An alkaloid with oxytocic (birth-hastening) activity called stachydrine has been identified in the herb through test-tube studies.[11]

Will It Harm You? What the Studies Say:

After centuries of use, there are no reports of serious adverse reactions to motherwort, and the herb causes no known side effects or harmful interactions with other medications.[12] But use it in moderation. If you suffer from a heart disorder or take any medicine for a heart condition, consult your doctor before taking this herb. Bear in mind that high blood pressure, palpitations, other heart ailments, and hyperthyroidism are often serious conditions that require professional care. Pregnant women should avoid motherwort, given how little is known about its action on the uterus.

GENERAL SOURCES:

Blumenthal, M., J. Gruenwald, T. Hall, and R.S. Rister, eds. *The Complete German Commission E Monographs: Therapeutic Guide to Herbal Medicine.* Boston: Integrative Medicine Communications, 1998.

Bradley, P.C., ed. *British Herbal Compendium: A Handbook of Scientific Information on Widely Used Plant Drugs*, vol. 1. Bournemouth (Dorset), England: British Herbal Medicine Association, 1992.

Bremness, L. *Herbs.* 1st American ed. Eyewitness Handbooks. New York: Dorling Kindersley Publications, 1994.

Castleman, M. *The Healing Herbs: The Ultimate Guide to the Curative Power of Nature's Medicines.* New York: Bantam Books, 1995.

Chevallier, A. *The Encyclopedia of Medicinal Plants: A Practical Reference Guide to More Than 550 Key Medicinal Plants & Their Uses.* 1st American ed. New York: Dorling Kindersley Publications, 1996.

Mindell, E. *Earl Mindell's Herb Bible.* New York: Simon & Schuster/Fireside, 1992.

Newall, C.A., et al. *Herbal Medicines: A Guide for Health-Care Professionals.* London: The Pharmaceutical Press, 1996.

Stary, F. *The Natural Guide to Medicinal Herbs and Plants.* Prague: Barnes & Noble, Inc., in arrangement with Aventinum Publishers, 1996.

Tierra, M. *The Way of Herbs.* New York: Pocket Books, 1990.

Weiner, M.A., and J.A. Weiner. *Herbs That Heal: Prescription for Herbal Healing.* Mill Valley, CA: Quantum Books, 1994.

Weiss, R.F. *Herbal Medicine*, trans. A.R. Meuss, from the 6th German edition. Beaconsfield, England: Beaconsfield Publishers, Ltd., 1988.

TEXT CITATIONS:

1. S.Q. Zhang et al., *Journal of Traditional Chinese Medicine*, 8(4) (1988): 254–56.
2. P.G. Kuang et al., *Journal of Traditional Chinese Medicine*, 8(1) (1988): 37–40.
3. P.C. Bradley, ed., *British Herbal Compendium: A Handbook of Scientific Information on Widely Used Plant Drugs*, vol. 1. (Bournemouth [Dorset], England: British Herbal Medicine Association, 1992).
4. Ibid. P.G. Kuang et al., *Journal of Traditional Chinese Medicine*, 8 (1988): 37–40.
5. D.D. Yablokov, *Soviet Medicine*, 4 (1943): 23–25.
6. R.F. Weiss, *Herbal Medicine*, trans. A.R. Meuss, from the 6th German edition (Beaconsfield, England: Beaconsfield Publishers, Ltd., 1988).
7. Kuang, op. cit. Bradley, op. cit.
8. C.A. Newall et al., *Herbal Medicines: A Guide for Health-Care Professionals* (London: The Pharmaceutical Press, 1996).
9. M. Blumenthal, J. Gruenwald, T. Hall, and R. S. Rister, eds., *The Complete German Commission E Monographs: Therapeutic Guide to Herbal Medicine* (Boston: Integrative Medicine Communications, 1998).
10. Newall, op. cit.
11. Ibid.
12. Blumenthal et al., op. cit.

PRIMARY NAME:

MUGWORT

SCIENTIFIC NAME:
Artemisia vulgaris L. Family: Asteraceae (Compositae)

COMMON NAMES:
Ai ye, Carline thistle

RATING:
4 = Research indicates that this substance will not fulfill the claims made for it, but that it is also unlikely to cause any harm when used as commonly recommended.

What Is Mugwort?

The leaves, small yellow or reddish flowering tops, and root of the tall *Artemisia vulgaris* plant are used medicinally. Mugwort grows throughout North America, Europe, and Asia, and has a pleasant odor and somewhat spicy, bitter taste.

What It Is Used For:

This herb is awash in legend and superstition. It may well be named after its use as a substitute for hops to flavor beer (consider: *mug*wort),[1] and it continues to be used as a food seasoning in some parts of the world. Folk healers from China to Europe and North America (including Native Americans) have recommended it through the centuries to relieve painful menstrual cramps, to induce menstruation, and to treat other gynecological problems.[2] It has also been used to combat intestinal worms, improve poor liver performance, and function as a bitter aromatic to aid digestion, lessen stomach upset, stimulate a flagging appetite, and reduce gas and bloating. Many consider it useful for calming nervousness and associated shaking and insomnia—years ago epilepsy was treated with it—in some cases by smoking the herb. A number of contemporary herbalists recommend mugwort for these and other ailments.

Many South Asian cultures, including Japan, also use mugwort leaves to make moxas; these ancient herbal preparations are placed on the skin, ignited, and allowed to burn down to the skin and form a scar. In various Eastern traditions, moxas are believed to stimulate the immune system in a positive way and help reduce pain and cold spasms, revive sensation in deadened limbs, and stop hemorrhage, among other things.

Forms Available Include:

Decoction, dried herb, infusion, root extract, smoking formulation, tincture.

Dosage Commonly Reported:

To stimulate the appetite, a tea made using 1 teaspoon (1.2 grams) of herb in 1 cup of water is drunk two or three times per day before meals. The liquid root extract is taken in doses of 0.5 to 5 milliliters.

Will It Work for You? What the Studies Say:

The medical literature contains no scientific studies that justify the use of mugwort for any of its traditional uses. The herb contains a volatile oil, a bitter principle, tannins, and a number of other relatively common plant constituents. The volatile oil and bitter-tasting substances in the herb may explain its long-standing use for soothing stomach upset and stimulating the appetite. The volatile oil also has antibacterial and antifungal properties, as well as considerable insecticidal and larvicidal properties, according to research in some cases reported decades ago.[3] Unfortunately, the concentration and quality of the volatile oil vary widely.[4]

Some samples also contain ingredients found in mugwort's botanical cousin, **Wormwood**, such as camphor and thujone. Wormwood has traditionally been used in similar ways but is considered far more effective.[5] Citing a lack of substantiation, German health authorities declined to endorse mugwort as a healing herb.[6]

The ability of moxas to affect human health can be judged only through a full understanding of traditional Eastern healing.

Will It Harm You? What the Studies Say:

Commonly recommended doses of mugwort are unlikely to cause harm.[7] Given the meager data on how it affects the human body, however, not to mention the presence (although variable) of certain potentially toxic substances such as thujone, stick to commonly recommended amounts. Allergic reactions including contact dermatitis may occur in previously sensitized individuals,[8] although a well-designed clinical trial reported in 1995 found that hay fever reactions to the herb could be significantly minimized through herbal immunotherapy.[9]

Avoid internal forms of mugwort during pregnancy, given lingering questions about its ability to stimulate the uterus and possibly cause miscarriage; pregnancy loss has apparently never been documented, however.

GENERAL SOURCES:

Bisset, N.G., ed. *Herbal Drugs and Phytopharmaceuticals.* Stuttgart: medpharm GmbH Scientific Publishers, 1994.

Blumenthal, M., J. Gruenwald, T. Hall, and R.S. Rister, eds. *The Complete German Commission E Monographs: Therapeutic Guide to Herbal Medicine.* Boston: Integrative Medicine Communications, 1998.

Chevallier, A. *The Encyclopedia of Medicinal Plants: A Practical Reference Guide to More Than 550 Key Medicinal Plants & Their Uses.* 1st American ed. New York: Dorling Kindersley Publications, 1996.

Duke, J.A. *CRC Handbook of Medicinal Herbs.* Boca Raton, FL: CRC Press, 1985.

Ody, P. *The Herb Society's Complete Medicinal Herbal.* London, England: Dorling Kindersley Limited, 1993.

Tierra, M. *The Way of Herbs.* New York: Pocket Books, 1990.

Weiner, M.A., and J.A. Weiner. *Herbs That Heal: Prescription for Herbal Healing.* Mill Valley, CA: Quantum Books, 1994.

Weiss, R.F. *Herbal Medicine,* trans. A.R. Meuss, from the 6th German edition. Beaconsfield, England: Beaconsfield Publishers, Ltd., 1988.

TEXT CITATIONS:

1. J.A. Duke, *CRC Handbook of Medicinal Herbs* (Boca Raton, FL: CRC Press, 1985).
2. V.J. Broendgarrd, *Svensk Farmaceutisk Tidskrift,* 69(23) (1965): 669–79.
3. V.K. Kaul et al., *Indian Journal of Pharmacology,* 38 (1976): 21. Y.S. Hwang et al., *Journal of Chemical Ecology,* 11(9) (1985): 1297–306. R.N. Chopra et al., *Journal of the Malaria Institute of India,* 3 (1940): 495–98.
4. N.G. Bisset, ed., *Herbal Drugs and Phytopharmaceuticals* (Stuttgart: medpharm GmbH Scientific Publishers, 1994).
5. R.F. Weiss, *Herbal Medicine,* trans. A.R. Meuss, from the 6th German edition (Beaconsfield, England: Beaconsfield Publishers, Ltd., 1988).
6. M. Blumenthal, J. Gruenwald, T. Hall, and R. S. Rister, eds., *The Complete German Commission E Monographs: Therapeutic Guide to Herbal Medicine* (Boston: Integrative Medicine Communications, 1998).
7. Bisset, op. cit.
8. G. Kurz and M.J. Rapaport, *Contact Dermatitis,* 5 (1979): 407.
9. O.T. Olsen et al., *Allergologia et Immunopathologia,* 23(2) (1995): 73–78.

PRIMARY NAME:
MUIRA PUAMA

SCIENTIFIC NAME:
Ptychopetalum olacoides Benth. and *Ptychopetalum uncinatum* Anselmino. Family: Olacaceae. At one time incorrectly referred to as *Liriosma ovata* Miers and possibly *Acanthea virilis.*[1]

COMMON NAME:
Potency wood

What Is Muira Puama?

The root and stem wood of these two species of Brazilian shrubs (*Ptychopetalum olacoides* and *Ptychopetalum uncinatum*) have been used medicinally.

What It Is Used For:

Muira puama has a long history in Brazilian folk medicine, most notably among native tribes, as an aphrodisiac and as a remedy for sexual impotence and frigidity. The "cure" sometimes involved bathing the genitals with a strong decoction.[2] The plant has also been used as a central nervous system tonic; to treat hookworm, infectious diarrhea, acute poliomyelitis, chronic rheumatism, and menstrual irregularities; and to stimulate the appetite and ease indigestion.[3] Topical formulations are applied to rheumatic joints and paralyzed muscles. Contemporary American and European herbalists occasionally recommend muira puama as an aphrodisiac, nerve tonic, stimulant, and astringent.

RATING:

4 = Research indicates that this substance will not fulfill the claims made for it, and very little is known about its potential toxicity.

Forms Available Include:

- *For internal use:* Concentrated drops, decoction, liquid extract, powder, tincture.
- *For external use:* Concentrated drops, decoction.

Dosage Commonly Reported:

As an aphrodisiac, muira puama is taken in daily doses of 2 to 4 milligrams liquid root extract; alternatively, a dropperful of tincture is taken prior to sexual intercourse. The concentrated drops are sometimes applied to the genitals and are also used topically to treat rheumatic pains. Use commercial preparations according to package directions.

Will It Work for You? What the Studies Say:

Plant experts do not consider any of the chemical constituents identified in muira puama—from lupeol to a resin to relatively common plant ingredients such as tannins and a volatile oil—particularly notable, and none scientifically justifies the folk uses for this herb, including its reported aphrodisiac effects.[4] Evidence to support claims that the resin has central-nervous-system-stimulating activity cannot be found in the recent medical literature; no animal or human clinical trials have apparently been done. Because of this lack of proven efficacy, German health authorities have declined to approve of muira puama as an aphrodisiac or for preventing any sexual disorder.[5]

Will It Harm You? What the Studies Say:

No reports of serious adverse reactions to muira puama appear in the recent medical literature, and none of the compounds identified so far raises major concerns. Unfortunately, this does not rule out the possibility that muira puama can cause harm, even given its long-term use in Brazilian folk medicine.

GENERAL SOURCES:

Blumenthal, M., J. Gruenwald, T. Hall, and R.S. Rister, eds. *The Complete German Commission E Monographs: Therapeutic Guide To Herbal Medicine.* Boston: Integrative Medicine Communications, 1998.

Duke, J.A. *CRC Handbook of Medicinal Herbs.* Boca Raton, FL: CRC Press, 1985.

Mayell, M. *Off-the-Shelf Natural Health: How to Use Herbs and Nutrients to Stay Well.* New York: Bantam Books, 1995.

Mindell, E. *Earl Mindell's Herb Bible.* New York: Simon & Schuster/Fireside, 1992.

Steinmetz, E.F. *Quarterly Journal of Crude Drug Research.* 11(3) (1971): 1787–89.

Tierra, M. *The Way of Herbs.* New York: Pocket Books, 1990.

Tyler, V.E. *The Honest Herbal.* Binghamton, NY: Haworth Press/Pharmaceutical Products Press, 1993.

Tyler, V.E., L.R. Brady, and J.E. Robbers, eds. *Pharmacognosy.* Philadelphia: Lea & Febiger, 1988.

TEXT CITATIONS:

1. J.A. Duke, *CRC Handbook of Medicinal Herbs* (Boca Raton, FL: CRC Press, 1985).
2. H. Gaebler, *Deutsche Apotheker,* 22(3) (1970): 94–96. A. Toyota et al., *Shoyakugaku Zasshi,* 33(2) (1979): 57–64.
3. V.E. Tyler, *The Honest Herbal* (Binghamton, NY: Haworth Press/Pharmaceutical Products Press, 1993).

4. V.E. Tyler, L.R. Brady, and J.E. Robbers, eds., *Pharmacognosy* (Philadelphia: Lea & Febiger, 1988).
5. M. Blumenthal, J. Gruenwald, T. Hall, and R. S. Rister, eds., *The Complete German Commission E Monographs: Therapeutic Guide to Herbal Medicine* (Boston: Integrative Medicine Communications, 1998).

PRIMARY NAME:
MULLEIN

SCIENTIFIC NAME:
Verbascum thapsus L. and occasionally other *Verbascum* species such as *Verbascum thapsiforme* Schrad. Family: Scrophulariaceae

COMMON NAMES:
Aaron's rod, candleflower, candlewick, feltwort, flannel plant, hightaper, longwort, shepherd's staff, torches, velvet dock. *Verbascum thapsiforme:* European or orange mullein

RATING:
2 = This substance appears to be relatively effective and safe when used in recommended amounts for the indication(s) noted in the "Will It Work for You?" section.

What Is Mullein?

This hardy biennial first produces large elliptical gray-green woolly leaves that form a basal rosette, and in the second year sends up a stiff stem reaching four feet or more that is crowned by a grand cylindrical spike of medium-sized yellow flowers. Primarily the flowers and leaves are used medicinally. Mullein grows worldwide in temperate climates.

What It Is Used For:

Traditional healers from many parts of the globe have long used this herb. Both now and in times past it was popular as a remedy for respiratory problems such as cough, bronchitis, and asthma. Some people even smoked the leaves for these troubles. It was also considered a tuberculosis remedy. Many Native Americans reportedly adopted these practices when settlers introduced the plant to North America. The plant also has an enduring reputation for soothing throat irritation and clearing congestion, controlling diarrhea, and increasing urine production (as a diuretic, or "water pill"), and externally for treating wounds, calming hemorrhoidal pain and inflammation, and generally softening and protecting the skin. Contemporary herbalists recommend mullein for similar ailments, but for the most part emphasize its value for cough and sore throat. The yellow flowers were once used as a blond hair dye, and the stems and leaves were combined to create candlewicks.

Forms Available Include:

- *For internal use:* Flowers, infusion (typically sweetened to make it palatable), leaves.
- *For external use:* Compress (made with cooled infusion), tincture.

Dosage Commonly Reported:

An infusion is made using 3 to 4 teaspoons (1.5 to 2 grams) of the flowers per cup of water and is drunk once or twice per day or used in a compress.

Will It Work for You? What the Studies Say:

Mullein contains a substance called mucilage that swells upon contact with liquid, rendering it slippery and hence soothing and softening to irritated skin and mucous membranes. These properties would be expected to make mullein potentially effective in treating sore throat and coughs. However, the amount of mucilage is relatively small—about 3 percent—so do not expect dramatic effects.

Mullein also contains tannins, astringent substances that constrict (tighten)

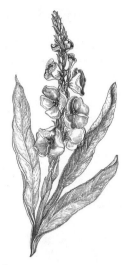

Mullein
Verbascum thapsus

tissue and reduce oozing and bleeding. Wounds and hemorrhoids may be expected to respond favorably when these tannins are used externally. The presence of tannins also helps explain the herb's traditional use for diarrhea; they are believed to control diarrhea by reducing inflammation in the intestines. Saponins may have an anti-inflammatory action. As far as can be determined, however, none of these external or internal healing properties has been tested in humans.

Other ingredients, including a volatile oil and saponins, may explain the herb's reputation for clearing congestion in coughs and colds. As an expectorant, it is believed to loosen sticky phlegm (mucus) so that it is easier to cough up. The saponins probably contribute even more to the herb's expectorant action than mucilage, in fact.[1] German health authorities approve of mullein for treating respiratory congestion.[2] One German doctor considers it particularly useful for chronic rather than acute bronchitis.[3]

Will It Harm You? What the Studies Say:

Avoid the seeds of this plant; they are toxic. There have been no reports of significant adverse reactions linked to medicinal preparations made from the leaves, flowers, or roots, however. The FDA lists mullein as "Generally Recognized As Safe" (GRAS) for food use. Prolonged use of any tannin-containing plant is unwise, however, given lingering questions about its cancer-causing potential.

GENERAL SOURCES:

Bisset, N.G., ed. *Herbal Drugs and Phytopharmaceuticals.* Stuttgart: medpharm GmbH Scientific Publishers, 1994.

Blumenthal, M., J. Gruenwald, T. Hall, and R.S. Rister, eds. *The Complete German Commission E Monographs: Therapeutic Guide to Herbal Medicine.* Boston: Integrative Medicine Communications, 1998.

Castleman, M. *The Healing Herbs: The Ultimate Guide to the Curative Power of Nature's Medicines.* New York: Bantam Books, 1995.

Lawrence Review of Natural Products. St. Louis: Facts and Comparisons, September 1989.

Mindell, E. *Earl Mindell's Herb Bible.* New York: Simon & Schuster/Fireside, 1992.

Stary, F. *The Natural Guide to Medicinal Herbs and Plants.* Prague: Barnes & Noble, Inc., in arrangement with Aventinum Publishers, 1996.

Tyler, V.E. *Herbs of Choice: The Therapeutic Use of Phytomedicinals.* Binghamton, NY: Haworth Press/Pharmaceutical Products Press, 1994.

———. *The Honest Herbal.* Binghamton, NY: Haworth Press/Pharmaceutical Products Press, 1993.

Weiner, M.A., and J.A. Weiner. *Herbs That Heal: Prescription for Herbal Healing.* Mill Valley, CA: Quantum Books, 1994.

Weiss, R.F. *Herbal Medicine,* trans. A.R. Meuss, from the 6th German edition. Beaconsfield, England: Beaconsfield Publishers, Ltd., 1988.

TEXT CITATIONS:

1. J. Kraus and G. Franz, *Deutsche Apotheker Zeitung,* 127 (1987): 665–669.
2. V.E. Tyler, *The Honest Herbal* (Binghamton, NY: Haworth Press/Pharmaceutical Products Press, 1993). M. Blumenthal, J. Gruenwald, T. Hall, and R. S. Rister, eds., *The Complete German Commission E Monographs: Therapeutic Guide to Herbal Medicine* (Boston: Integrative Medicine Communications, 1998).
3. R.F. Weiss, *Herbal Medicine,* trans. A.R. Meuss, from the 6th German edition (Beaconsfield, England: Beaconsfield Publishers, Ltd., 1988).

SCIENTIFIC NAME:

Black mustard: *Brassica nigra* L. Koch. Brown mustard: *Brassica juncea* L. Czern. et Coss., sometimes referred to as *Sinapis juncea* L. White mustard: *Brassica alba* L. Rabenh, sometimes referred to as *Sinapis alba* L. Family: Cruciferae

COMMON NAMES:

Brassica alba: bai jie zi, yellow mustard; *Brassica juncea:* Indian mustard

RATING:

1 = Years of use and extensive, high-quality studies indicate that this substance is very effective and safe when used in recommended amounts for the indication(s) noted in the "Will It Work for You?" section. Saftey is a concern, however; see the warnings in the "Will It Harm You?" section.

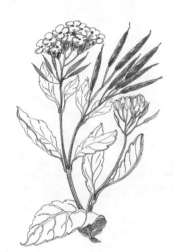

Mustard
Black: Brassica nigra
Brown: Brassica juncea
White: Sinapis alba

What Is Mustard?

Mustard plants yield seeds that after ripening and drying are highly valued for culinary and drug purposes. Brown mustard is native to Asia. White and black mustards are native to Eurasia. All three flowering plants are now cultivated worldwide. The fixed oil from brown and black mustard yields, after special processing, what is known as volatile mustard oil, which contains high concentrations of an important ingredient called allyl isothiocyanate.

What It Is Used For:

The pungent-tasting mustard seed qualifies as a popular condiment in most parts of the globe. It can also claim a long and distinguished history as a traditional medicine. Both the seeds and the oil have long been used in poultice, plaster, and other external formulations for upper respiratory tract congestion, joint pain, inflammation, and pain in the lower back or lumbar region. Internal formulations have been popular for improving digestion and stimulating the appetite, as well as for use as diuretics ("water pills"), as emetics (vomiting agents), and to aid fat metabolism.

Some dog and cat repellents contain mustard oil, as do certain lubricants and other commercial preparations. Mustard seeds are the flavoring in table mustard, and mustard greens are eaten as a salad ingredient. Mustard oil serves as a flavoring in many beverages and foods.

Forms Available Include:

- *For internal use:* Seed (ground and whole). Also available as a condiment (table, or prepared, mustard).
- *For external use:* Liniment, oil, ointment, paste, plaster (typically made by mixing prepared mustard with flour and water to create a paste), poultice.

Dosage Commonly Reported:

To relieve chest congestion, two handfuls ground mustard seed are mixed with lukewarm water to make a paste (some recipes call for equal parts powdered seeds and flour). This paste is spread on a cloth and placed on the chest; the cloth is removed when a strong burning sensation is felt. Alternatively, mustard oil is applied externally in concentrations of 0.5 to 5 percent up to three or four times per day.

Will It Work for You? What the Studies Say:

The ingredient critical to volatile mustard oil, allyl isothiocyanate, irritates, reddens, and can even blister the skin when left on for long enough. This irritating substance explains mustard's medicinal value. Plant experts classify the oil as a counterirritant and rubefacient. A counterirritant induces surface skin irritation so that deeper, underlying pain is masked; and a rubefacient dilates surface blood vessels, increasing the blood supply to the area, reddening it, helping it to heal, and helping the muscles to relax.

The oil must be properly diluted (such as 1 part oil to 50 parts diluent[1]) for these purposes. The FDA considers volatile mustard oil a safe and effective counterirritant in concentrations of 0.5 to 5 percent.[2] German health authorities approve of white mustard seed in the form of a poultice for helping to allay symptoms related to joint and soft tissue diseases.[3] Footbaths for aching feet may well work, although no studies on the subject appear in the recent medical literature.

German physicians report that mustard oil can help relieve congestion in the lungs when applied externally in the form of an ointment or liniment. The theory is that the oil, once absorbed through the skin, is eliminated through the lungs.[4] Health authorities in Germany endorse its use for upper respiratory tract congestion. No studies to verify the effectiveness and safety of this practice can be found in other recent medical literature, however.

The oil fights bacteria and fungi,[5] although the practical value of these properties remains unclear, given its irritating properties. The same is true for evidence that mustard seeds ingested whole can ease constipation and reduce stomach upset caused by acid indigestion.[6]

Will It Harm You? What the Studies Say:

Mustard seed preparations can cause excessive skin irritation; use them sparingly, in diluted form only, and for short periods of time (typically less than ten or fifteen minutes). Blistering, pain, ulceration, and tissue damage may develop if the preparation is left on too long. Never taste or inhale the undiluted oil; it qualifies as one of the most toxic essential oils known.[7]

Mustard seed and its oil are so pungent that they may well make you tear. In large doses the mustard-oil glycosides will cause vomiting; they were once commonly used for this purpose. Toxic mustard gases used in warfare contain derivatives of allyl isothiocyanate,[8] as do certain antitumor agents.

People with severe circulation disorders, varicose veins, or other venous disorders should not use mustard-oil preparations.[9] Cases of hyperthyroidism with goiter (enlarged thyroid gland) in both humans[10] and animals[11] have been traced to the use of the isothiocyanates in mustard.

GENERAL SOURCES:

Balch, J.F., and P.A. Balch. *Prescription for Nutritional Healing: A Practical A to Z Reference to Drug-Free Remedies Using Vitamins, Minerals, Herbs & Food Supplements.* 2nd ed. Garden City Park, NY: Avery Publishing Group, 1997.

Bisset, N.G., ed. *Herbal Drugs and Phytopharmaceuticals.* Stuttgart: medpharm GmbH Scientific Publishers, 1994.

Blumenthal, M., J. Gruenwald, T. Hall, and R.S. Rister, eds. *The Complete German Commission E Monographs: Therapeutic Guide to Herbal Medicine.* Boston: Integrative Medicine Communications, 1998.

Dobelis, I.N., ed. *The Magic and Medicine of Plants: A Practical Guide to the Science, History, Folklore, and Everyday Uses of Medicinal Plants.* Pleasantville, NY: Reader's Digest Association, 1986.

Lawrence Review of Natural Products. St. Louis: Facts and Comparisons, February 1992.

Leung, A.Y., and S. Foster. *Encyclopedia of Common Natural Ingredients Used in Food, Drugs, and Cosmetics.* 2nd ed. New York: John Wiley & Sons, 1996.

Tyler, V.E. *Herbs of Choice: The Therapeutic Use of Phytomedicinals.* Binghamton, NY: Haworth Press/Pharmaceutical Products Press, 1994.

Weiner, M.A., and J. Weiner. *Weiner's Herbal: A Guide to Herb Medicine.* Mill Valley, CA: Quantum Books, 1991.

Weiss, R.F. *Herbal Medicine.*, trans. A.R. Meuss, from the 6th German edition. Beaconsfield, England: Beaconsfield Publishers, Ltd., 1988.

TEXT CITATIONS:

1. A.Y. Leung and S. Foster, *Encyclopedia of Common Natural Ingredients Used in Food, Drugs, and Cosmetics*, 2nd ed. (New York: John Wiley & Sons, 1996).
2. V.E. Tyler, *Herbs of Choice: The Therapeutic Use of Phytomedicinals* (Binghamton, NY: Haworth Press/Pharmaceutical Products Press, 1994).
3. M. Blumenthal, J. Gruenwald, T. Hall, and R. S. Rister, eds., *The Complete German Commission E Monographs: Therapeutic Guide to Herbal Medicine* (Boston: Integrative Medicine Communications, 1998).
4. R.F. Weiss, *Herbal Medicine*, trans. A.R. Meuss, from the 6th German edition (Beaconsfield, England: Beaconsfield Publishers, Ltd., 1988).
5. Leung and Foster, op. cit.
6. Tyler, op. cit.
7. Leung and Foster, op. cit.
8. *Lawrence Review of Natural Products.* St. Louis: Facts and Comparisons, February 1992.
9. N.G. Bisset, ed., *Herbal Drugs and Phytopharmaceuticals* (Stuttgart: medpharm GmbH Scientific Publishers, 1994).
10. Leung and Foster, op. cit.
11. P. Ahmad and A.J. Muztar, *Pakistani Journal of Biochemistry*, 4 (1971): 72.

PRIMARY NAME:

MYRRH

SCIENTIFIC NAME:
Commiphora molmol Engl. and other *Commiphora* species.
Family: Burseraceae

COMMON NAMES:
Bal, bol, bola, heerabol, gum myrrh, mo yao, myrrha.
Commiphora molmol: African myrrh, Somali myrrh;
Commiphora abyssinica: Arabian and Yemen myrrh

RATING:
2 = According to a number of well-designed studies and common use, this substance appears to be relatively effective and safe when used in recommended amounts for the indication(s) noted in the "Will It Work for You?" section.

What Is Myrrh?

Myrrh is a fragrant pale yellow-white liquid (an oleo gum resin) that oozes from cracks or incisions made in the whitish-gray bark of certain *Commiphora* tree species. The liquid hardens into tear-shaped globules. The trees (or shrubs in some cases) grow in northeastern Africa and the Arabian peninsula.

For information on the oleo gum resin referred to as guggul from the related *Commiphora* species *Commiphora mukul* Hook, see **Guggul**.

What It Is Used For:

Even cursory students of history will recognize myrrh as an important component of religious ceremonies in ancient times. As an incense and perfume, it has a pedigree that few substances can match. Less well known is that this aromatic resin was also considered an important healing agent, having been used for centuries in Western cultures as an antiseptic for sores and gingivitis, and as a stimulant, an expectorant for congestion caused by cough or asthma, an antispasmodic, a stomach soother, a menstruation promoter, and a remedy for loose teeth, leprosy, and cancer. Traditional Chinese healers valued it for treating bleeding, pain, swelling, and wounds.

Contemporary herbalists value myrrh in many of the same ways, but rate it particularly highly as a topical antiseptic for wounds, hemorrhoids, bedsores, and the like. Its astringent properties are put to work in oral formulations such as gargles and rinses for mild mucous membrane inflammations such as sore throat, hoarseness, and gingivitis. Internal formulations, although less commonly recommended, are said to relieve gas, indigestion, ulcers, and nasal and bronchial congestion, and to stimulate menstrual flow. Myrrh was formerly listed in the *U.S. Pharmacopoeia* and in the *National Formulary*. It is sometimes used as a flavoring in foods.

Forms Available Include:
- *For external use:* Gargle, mouth rinse, powder, tincture. Also an ingredient in lip balm, tooth powder and toothpaste.
- *For internal use:* Capsule, extract, infusion, powder, tincture.

Dosage Commonly Reported:
A gargle or rinse is made using 5 to 10 drops tincture per glass of water. The undiluted tincture is applied to canker sores or sore gums. An infusion is made with 1 teaspoon of powdered myrrh per cup of water and is drunk once or twice per day. Two to three capsules containing 657 milligrams of myrrh gum are taken two to three times a day. Eight to 10 drops of myrrh extract are taken up to four times a day.

Will It Work for You? What the Studies Say:
Myrrh contains a complex mixture of chemicals, the actions of which are only partially understood. It contains about 8 percent of a volatile oil, 25 to 40 percent resin, and 50 to 60 percent gum. Most plant experts agree that, partly because of its resin content, myrrh is mildly astringent[1] and antiseptic (according to test-tube studies).[2] It is included in various commercial mouthwashes and gargles as an astringent, and in toothpastes in some parts of the world.

Studies with rodents indicate that myrrh also has anti-inflammatory,[3] fever-lowering,[4] immune-system-stimulating,[5] analgesic (painkilling),[6] and possibly blood-sugar-reducing properties.[7] Myrrh's aromatic, stimulating odor may help in clearing congestion. Future research may conclude that these actions explain or even justify some of the traditional uses for myrrh, but as yet it is still very unclear whether they occur in humans at all. No studies of humans appear in the recent medical literature.

The German health authorities endorse the use of myrrh for mild inflammations of the mouth and throat mucosa, such as gingivitis and stomatitis.[8] British health authorities recognize its value as a gargle for soothing sore throat and tonsillitis pain, as a mouthwash for gingivitis and canker sores in the mouth, and as a tincture for minor skin inflammations and sinusitis (used topically).[9]

Will It Harm You? What the Studies Say:
People have been using myrrh for centuries to no apparent ill effect. Commenting on external uses for myrrh, German health authorities cite no known side effects, potentially negative interactions with other remedies, or situations in which the herb should not be used. Research indicates that it is not irritating, sensitizing, or sun-sensitizing to human or animal skin.[10] Dermatitis and allergic reactions have been reported, however.[11] Always dilute the tincture, as undiluted forms may irritate the mouth or cause a burning sensation.[12]

Much less is known about the potential for adverse reactions to internal formulations of myrrh. Limit your intake to typically recommended amounts.

GENERAL SOURCES:

Bisset, N.G., ed. *Herbal Drugs and Phytopharmaceuticals.* Stuttgart: medpharm GmbH Scientific Publishers, 1994.

Blumenthal, M., J. Gruenwald, T. Hall, and R.S. Rister, eds. *The Complete German Commission E Monographs: Therapeutic Guide to Herbal Medicine.* Boston: Integrative Medicine Communications, 1998.

Bradley, P.C., ed. *British Herbal Compendium: A Handbook of Scientific Information on Widely Used Plant Drugs*, vol. 1. Bournemouth (Dorset), England: British Herbal Medicine Association, 1992.

Castleman, M. *The Healing Herbs: The Ultimate Guide to the Curative Power of Nature's Medicines.* New York: Bantam Books, 1995.

Lawrence Review of Natural Products. St. Louis: Facts and Comparisons, February 1994.

Leung, A.Y., and S. Foster. *Encyclopedia of Common Natural Ingredients Used in Food, Drugs, and Cosmetics.* 2nd ed. New York: John Wiley & Sons, 1996.

Michie, C.A., and E. Cooper. *Journal of the Royal Society of Medicine.* 84(10) (1991): 602–5.

Murray, M.T. *The Healing Power of Herbs: The Enlightened Person's Guide to the Wonders of Medicinal Plants.* Rev. 2nd ed. Rocklin, CA: Prima Publishing, 1995.

Newall, C.A., et al. *Herbal Medicines: A Guide for Health-Care Professionals.* London: The Pharmaceutical Press, 1996.

Tierra, M. *The Way of Herbs.* New York: Pocket Books, 1990.

Tyler, V.E. *Herbs of Choice: The Therapeutic Use of Phytomedicinals.* Binghamton, NY: Haworth Press/Pharmaceutical Products Press, 1994.

———. *The Honest Herbal.* Binghamton, NY: Haworth Press/Pharmaceutical Products Press, 1993.

Weiner, M.A., and J.A. Weiner. *Herbs That Heal: Prescription for Herbal Healing.* Mill Valley, CA: Quantum Books, 1994.

TEXT CITATIONS:

1. V.E. Tyler, *The Honest Herbal* (Binghamton, NY: Haworth Press/Pharmaceutical Products Press, 1993).

2. A.Y. Leung and S. Foster, *Encyclopedia of Common Natural Ingredients Used in Food, Drugs, and Cosmetics.* 2nd ed. (New York: John Wiley & Sons, 1996). G.E. Trease and W.C. Evans, *Trease and Evans' Pharmacognosy*, 13th ed. (Philadelphia: Bailliere Tindall, 1989).

3. M. Tariq et al., *Agents & Actions*, 17 (1986): 381–82.

4. A. Mohsin et al., *Fitoterapia*, 60 (1989): 174–77.

5. P. Deleveau et al., *Planta Medica*, 40 (1980): 49–54.

6. P. Dolara et al., *Nature*, 379(6560) (1996): 29.

7. F.M. Al-Awadi and K.A. Gumaa, *Acta Diabetologica Latina*, 24 (1987): 37–41. C.A. Newall et al., *Herbal Medicines: A Guide for Health-Care Professionals* (London: The Pharmaceutical Press, 1996).

8. M. Blumenthal, J. Gruenwald, T. Hall, and R.S. Rister, eds., *The Complete German Commission E Monographs: Therapeutic Guide to Herbal Medicine* (Boston: Integrative Medicine Communications, 1998).

9. P.C. Bradley, ed., *British Herbal Compendium: A Handbook of Scientific Information on Widely Used Plant Drugs*, vol. 1 (Bournemouth [Dorset], England: British Herbal Medicine Association, 1992).

10. Leung and Foster, op. cit.

11. T.Y. Lee and T.H. Lam, *Contact Dermatitis*, 28 (1993): 89; 29(5) (1993): 279.

12. N.G. Bisset, ed., *Herbal Drugs and Phytopharmaceuticals* (Stuttgart: medpharm GmbH Scientific Publishers, 1994).

PRIMARY NAME:

NEEM

SCIENTIFIC NAME:
Azadirachta indica A. Juss.
Formerly known as *Melia
azadirachta* L. Family:
Meliaceae

COMMON NAMES:
Margosa, margosa oil, nim,
nimba

RATING:
3 = Studies on the effectiveness
of this substance are
conflicting, or there are not
enough studies to draw a
conclusion. Its safety appears
to depend on judicious use: see
the "Will It Harm You?"
section.

What Is Neem?

Nearly every part of this tall, shade-giving East Indian evergreen tree has been
used medicinally. It has compound leaves and bears small white flowers and
olive-shaped fruit. Neem is widely cultivated in tropical regions of Asia and
other parts of the world for its aromatic seed oil, gum, and bitter-tasting bark.
It is also valued for its wood.

What It Is Used For:

In India and neighboring countries, the neem tree has long been valued as providing a traditional tonic and astringent, and its oil has been regarded as a virtual panacea through the centuries. Various plant parts have been used to treat
skin diseases, hemorrhoids, scabies, inflammations, worm infections, diabetes,
peptic ulcers, fevers, heart disease, and other ailments.[1] The leaves are rubbed
against the teeth to treat gum disease and inhibit the formation of sticky plaque,
and the twigs are used as toothpicks. Some commercial toothpastes currently
marketed in India and Pakistan contain neem.[2] The seed oil is used as a hair-
dressing and a base for other remedies. Neem has also been heavily used for its
pesticide and insect-repellent properties (especially its antimosquito powers).

Forms Available Include:

Capsule (of powder or leaves), decoction (of leaves or bark), seed oil, tincture.

Dosage Commonly Reported:

Two to four 500-milligram powder capsules are taken with meals, or two to
three 505-milligram leaf capsules are taken two times a day.

Will It Work for You? What the Studies Say:

Preliminary research supports the traditional use of neem and certain extracts
to clean teeth, inhibit plaque formation, and help prevent gum inflammation.[3]
Test-tube studies reveal anti-inflammatory and antimicrobial properties, and
limited clinical studies in humans indicate that it is an effective dentifrice,
although more study is needed.[4]

These anti-inflammatory and antimicrobial actions also support neem's traditional use for skin diseases. One group of investigators found evidence that the
oil can fight as many as two hundred types of bacteria.[5] Neem's astringent tannins
also probably contribute to its long-standing use for skin wounds, as they help to
promote healing by constricting (tightening) tissue and controlling oozing and
bleeding. A paste made of neem and turmeric proved effective in treating chronic
ulcers and scabies in more than eight hundred rural villagers in India.[6]

Neem may also have promise as a pain reliever; in a 1994 experiment, leaf
extracts not only controlled inflammation but significantly limited pain in rats,
both at apparently nontoxic doses.[7] Although relatively higher doses were
needed to be effective, neem leaf extracts also reduced fever in these test rats,
suggesting that its traditional use as a fever-controller may have merit.[8]

The yellow oil drawn from the seed kernels in concentrations of about 10
percent smells something like garlic. It contains glycerides and important bitter

principles. Various studies indicate that this oil may be a safe, nonirritating, and effective contraceptive. In test-tube experiments it immobilizes human sperm within thirty seconds, and insertion of the oil into the vagina before intercourse prevented pregnancy in ten couples over four menstrual cycles without altering the timing of ovulation.[9] The contraceptive potential of neem oil in injection form is also being explored.[10]

Positive results from preliminary rat studies suggest that neem oil helps control blood glucose levels in diabetes, implying but not proving that its traditional use for this disease may be justified.[11] The tree holds promise as a weapon against malaria in developing countries: 2 percent neem oil mixed in coconut oil provided protection from mosquito bites for twelve hours in a group of volunteers[12] (mosquitoes often carry the disease). Neem extracts have also demonstrated antimalarial properties in test-tube studies.[13]

Neem extracts (azadirachtin in particular) have proved to be extremely effective agricultural pesticides and insect repellents. The Environmental Protection Agency has endorsed the limited use of a neem formulation as a pesticide for certain crops not destined for human consumption.[14] As a pesticide, neem apparently does not harm warm-blooded animals, fish, or birds.

Will It Harm You? What the Studies Say:

Although neem seeds are poisonous in large doses, the traditional ways of using this plant appear to be safe for most people. Stick to recommended doses, however, as excessive doses caused breathing problems, stupor, convulsions, and ultimately death in laboratory rats.[15] Although apparently safe for adults in recommended doses, neem oil (sometimes referred to as margosa oil) is potentially poisonous to infants and small children because of a still undefined toxin to which they appear to be particularly susceptible.[16] Signs of poisoning resembled Reye's syndrome, a rare but potentially fatal disease.[17] Characteristic reactions recorded in a group of thirteen infants included drowsiness, metabolic acidosis, seizures, loss of consciousness, coma, and in two cases death (due to encephalopathy).[18] Studies indicate that the oil does *not* cause cell changes that may make them prone to cancer.[19]

A 1995 study in mice and rabbits found neem oil safe to apply externally to wounds; it proved to have no adverse effects on the kidneys and liver and was nonirritating to the skin.[20]

GENERAL SOURCES:

Bremness, L. *Herbs.* 1st American ed. Eyewitness Handbooks. New York: Dorling Kindersley Publications, 1994.

Chevallier, A. *The Encyclopedia of Medicinal Plants: A Practical Reference Guide to More Than 550 Key Medicinal Plants & Their Uses.* 1st American ed. New York: Dorling Kindersley Publications, 1996.

Lawrence Review of Natural Products. St. Louis: Facts and Comparisons, April 1991.

Tierra, M. *The Way of Herbs.* New York: Pocket Books, 1990.

Tyler, V.E. *Herbs of Choice: The Therapeutic Use of Phytomedicinals.* Binghamton, NY: Haworth Press/Pharmaceutical Products Press, 1994.

Van der Nat, J.M., et al. *Journal of Ethnopharmacology.* 35(1) (19910): 1–24.

TEXT CITATIONS:

1. *Lawrence Review of Natural Products*. St. Louis: Facts and Comparisons, April 1991.
2. V.K. Patel and H. Venkatakrishna-Bhatt, *International Journal of Clinical Pharmacology, Therapy, and Toxicology*, 26 (1988): 176–84.
3. Ibid.
4. V.E. Tyler, *Herbs of Choice: The Therapeutic Use of Phytomedicinals* (Binghamton, NY: Haworth Press/Pharmaceutical Products Press, 1994).
5. D.V.K. Rao et al., *Indian Journal of Medical Research*, 84 (1986): 314.
6. V. Charles and S.X. Charles, *Tropical & Geographical Medicine*, 44(1–2) (1992): 178–81.
7. K.M. Koley et al., *Fitoterapia*, 65(6) (1994): 524–28.
8. Ibid.
9. K.C. Sinha et al., *Indian Journal of Medical Research*, 79 (1984): 131.
10. *Lawrence Review of Natural Products*, op. cit. R.K. Tewari et al., *Journal of Ethnopharmacology*, 25 (1989): 281.
11. V.P. Dixit et al., *Journal of Ethnopharmacology*, 17 (1986): 95.
12. V.P. Sharma et al., *Journal of the American Mosquito Control Association*, 9(3) (1993): 359–60.
13. S.A. Khalid et al., *Journal of Natural Products*, 52 (1989): 922.
14. *Lawrence Review of Natural Products*, op. cit.
15. M. Gandhi et al., *Journal of Ethnopharmacology*, 23 (1988): 39.
16. R. Sinniah et al., *Journal of Pathology*, 159 (1989): 255.
17. D. Sinniah and G. Baskaran, *The Lancet*, 1 (1981): 487.
18. S.M. Lai et al., *Singapore Medical Journal*, 31(5) (1990): 463–65.
19. K. Polasa and C. Rukmini, *Food and Chemical Toxicology*, 25 (1987): 763.
20. S.K. Tandan et al., *Fitoterapia*, 66(1) (1995): 69–72.

PRIMARY NAME:

NETTLE

SCIENTIFIC NAME:
Urtica dioica L. Family: Urticaceae

COMMON NAMES:
Common nettle, greater nettle, stinging nettle

RATING:

• *For internal use:* 3 = Studies on the effectiveness and safety of this substance are conflicting, or there are not enough studies to draw a conclusion.

What Is Nettle?

This flowering perennial populates wastelands in the United States, Canada, and Europe. Upon contact with skin or other surfaces, bristles on the dark green leaves spring into action something like tiny hypodermic needles and cause quite a sting. Medicinal preparations made from the leaves, stems, and roots of nettle are used both internally and externally. Some of the information for nettle also applies to the small stinging nettle *Urtica urens*, and hybrids thereof.

What It Is Used For:

Nettle has been valued since ancient times for reducing congestion, controlling coughs, and relieving asthma symptoms. Less commonly it has been used to promote urine flow (as a diuretic, or "water pill"), encourage menstruation, control diabetes, and stimulate and soothe the body in the form of a general tonic. Various Native American tribes made nettle formulations to facilitate delivery and stanch uterine bleeding.

Today's Western herbalists have scaled down the recommendations list, although not dramatically. Some tout nettles for controlling female discomforts such as heavy menstrual periods and vaginal infections and boosting milk out-

- *For external use:* 4 = Research indicates that this substance will not fulfill the claims made for it, but that it is also unlikely to cause any harm.

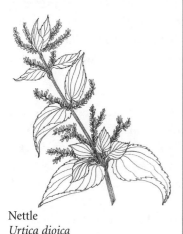

Nettle
Urtica dioica

put in nursing mothers. Others recommend the plant as a hay fever remedy, diuretic, and potential treatment for benign prostatic hyperplasia (BPH). Topical nettle lotions and teas are said to stop bleeding, help wounds heal, encourage hair growth, and lessen nerve pains and rheumatic aches. Through the ages, the herb's nutritious, tender young shoots have been eaten as a vegetable and added to beer and other drinks and foods. The vitamin C–rich shoots were once enlisted to treat scurvy. Nettle has served as fodder for crops, as fiber for textiles, and as a source for dye in the form of chlorophyll.

Forms Available Include:

- *For internal use:* Capsule, decoction, extract, infusion, juice, leaves and stems, powdered root, tea.
- *For external use:* Skin lotion, tea, tincture. Extracts appear in topical formulations.

Dosage Commonly Reported:

As a diuretic, nettle is taken in an infusion made by steeping 3 to 4 teaspoons (about 4 to 6 grams) leaves and stems in 150 milliliters of boiling water; this is drunk three to four times a day along with additional water. One to two 480-milligram leaf capsules are taken two to three times a day (or one to two 250-milligram leaf extract capsules). A common dose of the root is 4 to 6 grams per day in the form of a decoction (1 teaspoon powdered root equals about 1.3 grams).

Will It Work for You? What the Studies Say:

Studies confirm the mild diuretic effect of nettle; consuming the dried leaves will slightly increase urine output.[1] This has led some manufacturers and herbalists to recommend nettles as a diet aid and remedy for premenstrual bloating and venous insufficiency (chronic poor drainage of leg veins). But experts remain unclear about which constituents cause the diuretic effect and many feel the supporting data are weak.[2] German health authorities, however, approve of nettle for increasing urination to treat inflammatory conditions of the lower urinary tract, and to help prevent and treat kidney stones; they do not recommend nettle if a person has edema (swelling) due to impaired kidney or heart function, however.[3] Responsible herbalists do not recommend diuretic diet aids, because any lost weight is likely to return.

Although no definitive studies of humans have been done so far, mounting scientific evidence supports the use of nettle for early symptoms of BPH, a noncancerous prostate enlargement that plagues millions of men around the world and can cause difficulties starting the urine flow, sensations of incomplete emptying, and other annoying complications. Investigators report that nettle extracts may suppress growth of prostate cells (involved in BPH) as well as certain vital functions within them.[4] In a mid-1980s randomized study, men who took an extract of nettles experienced improvements in certain symptoms, but so did those who took a dummy drug.[5] German health authorities endorse the use of nettle for treating BPH; but they warn that although the herb could be expected to possibly reduce symptoms, it would not shrink the prostate itself. **Saw Palmetto** is another medicinal plant popularly used to treat BPH in the United States and abroad.

Research indicates that nettles may reduce hay fever symptoms including sneezing and itching. In the sole clinical trial on the subject, half of the sixty-nine hay fever sufferers who took nettle capsules declared the herb equivalent or superior to medications they had taken in the past.[6] A week into the study, 58 percent of those taking nettles said they felt moderate to excellent relief, compared with only 37 percent of those taking a placebo; 42 percent rated the herb ineffective. Two of the study subjects taking nettles, however, withdrew from the study because of an intensification of their allergy symptoms. The study was done at the National College of Naturopathic Medicine in Oregon. Confirmatory studies are needed.

Recent investigations indicate that drinking nettle tea to lower blood sugar levels and help control diabetes may actually be counterproductive. Upon analyzing the sugar-lowering (hypoglycemic) effect of plants used in Mexico as antidiabetic drugs, researchers detected slightly *increased* blood sugar levels in rabbits fed nettle.[7] In a separate study the herb aggravated the diabetic condition in experimental mice.[8] German authorities have issued warnings about the safety of using nettles for diabetes.[9]

Although there are indications that nettle may help stanch bleeding, scientific evidence to support the use of nettles in juice, infusion, or other topical forms to reduce pain caused by gout, sprains, tendinitis, or rheumatisms such as arthritis is shaky at best. German health authorities endorse the use of nettle both externally and internally for rheumatic conditions, however.[10] Some German physicians continue to recommend it for asthma as well. No one has ever proved that the herb can grow hair on a bald head, as some promoters claim.

Will It Harm You? What the Studies Say:

Nettle appears to be relatively safe to use for most ailments. Stick to typically recommended dosages, however. Sometimes nettle tea or other oral preparations—especially in large amounts—can cause stomach upset, urine suppression, burning sensations on the skin, and other uncomfortable reactions. Be sure to drink plenty of fluids if you are taking nettle preparations as a diuretic. Given reports that the herb can cause uterine contractions in rabbits, pregnant women may want to avoid oral formulations altogether, just to be safe, although no cases of miscarriage or other pregnancy-related complications can be found in the literature. In rare cases, nettle causes allergic reactions. The FDA placed it on their formerly maintained list of "Herbs of Undefined Safety."

GENERAL SOURCES:

Bisset, N.G., ed. *Herbal Drugs and Phytopharmaceuticals.* Stuttgart: medpharm GmbH Scientific Publishers, 1994.

Blumenthal, M., J. Gruenwald, T. Hall, and R.S. Rister, eds. *The Complete German Commission E Monographs: Therapeutic Guide to Herbal Medicine.* Boston: Integrative Medicine Communications, 1998.

Bradley, P.C., ed. *British Herbal Compendium: A Handbook of Scientific Information on Widely Used Plant Drugs*, vol. 1. Bournemouth (Dorset), England: British Herbal Medicine Association, 1992.

Castleman, M. *The Healing Herbs: The Ultimate Guide to the Curative Power of Nature's Medicines*. New York: Bantam Books, 1995.

Dreikorn, K., and P.S. Schonhofer. *Urologie*. Ausgabe, A. 34(2) (1995): 119–29.

Duke, J. *HerbalGram* 1(4) (1984): 10.

Edwards, E.K., Jr., and E.K. Edwards, Sr. *Contact Dermatitis*. 27(4) (1992): 264–65.

Heinerman, J. *Heinerman's Encyclopedia of Healing Herbs and Spices*. West Nyack, NY: Parker Publishing Co., 1996.

Review of Natural Products (St. Louis: Facts and Comparisons, April 1997).

Tyler, V.E. *Herbs of Choice: The Therapeutic Use of Phytomedicinals*. Binghamton, NY: Haworth Press/Pharmaceutical Products Press, 1994.

Weiss, R.F. *Herbal Medicine*, trans. A.R. Meuss, from the 6th German edition. Beaconsfield, England: Beaconsfield Publishers, Ltd., 1988.

TEXT CITATIONS:

1. P.C. Bradley, ed., *British Herbal Compendium: A Handbook of Scientific Information on Widely Used Plant Drugs*, vol. 1 (Bournemouth [Dorset], England: British Herbal Medicine Association, 1992).
2. *Review of Natural Products* (St. Louis: Facts and Comparisons, April 1997).
3. M. Blumenthal, J. Gruenwald, T. Hall, and R.S. Rister, eds., *The Complete German Commission E Monographs: Therapeutic Guide to Herbal Medicine* (Boston: Integrative Medicine Communications, 1998).
4. T. Hirano et al., *Planta Medica*, 60(1) (1994): 30–33. Z. Dunzendorfer, *Phytotherapie*, 5 (1984): 800.
5. G. Schonefeld et al., *Klinische und Experimentelle Urologie*, 4 (1982): 179. Stahl, *Zeitschrift Allgemein Medizin*, 60 (1984): 128. 1984
6. P. Mittman, *Planta Medica*, 56 (1990): 44–47.
7. R.R. Roman et al., *Archives of Medical Research*, 23(1) (1992): 59–64.
8. S.K. Swanston-Flatt et al., *Diabetes Research*, 10(2) (1989): 69–73.
9. R.F. Weiss, *Herbal Medicine*, trans. A.R. Meuss, from the 6th German edition (Beaconsfield, England: Beaconsfield Publishers, Ltd., 1988).
10. Blumenthal et al., op. cit.

PRIMARY NAME:

NEW ZEALAND GREEN-LIPPED MUSSEL

SCIENTIFIC NAME:
Perna canaliculus. Family: *Mytilidae*

COMMON NAMES:
NZGLM, sea mussel

What Is New Zealand Green-Lipped Mussel?

This marine bivalve mollusk is commonly recognized by its dark, elongated shell. Special marine farms (most, if not all, of them abroad) harvest and freeze-dry this mussel, then sell it in capsule form.

What It Is Used For:

Manufacturers of New Zealand green-lipped mussel (NZGLM) market it as a risk-free remedy for pain, restriction of movement, joint distortion, and other signs and symptoms of rheumatoid and osteoarthritis.

Forms Available Include:

Capsule.

RATING:

4 = Research indicates that this substance will not fulfill the claims made for it, but that it is also unlikely to cause any harm.

Dosage Commonly Reported:

New Zealand green-lipped mussel is commonly sold in 625-milligram capsules and is taken for periods ranging from three to eighteen weeks; follow the package instructions.

Will It Work for You? What the Studies Say:

Scientists know very little about the chemicals contained in NZGLM. Controversy persists over its value as an anti-inflammatory agent for arthritis or osteoarthritis. Results of rat studies have been conflicting,[1] with no anti-inflammatory activity noted when the substance was fed to the rodents rather than injected into them.[2] Advocates of NZGLM point to findings of a 1980 study that reported relief from various symptoms of rheumatoid arthritis and osteoarthritis.[3] In that double-blind study, which involved sixty-six subjects split between those assigned to take the NZGLM or a placebo, 39 percent of those taking the medicine and only 18 percent of those taking the placebo showed improvement at the end of the first three months. But a follow-up study in rheumatoid arthritis patients reported in 1981 found no significant differences between NZGLM and a placebo in improvement of the disease.

The FDA and the National Institute for Arthritis, Metabolism, and Digestive Diseases criticized the first study as being small and poorly analyzed.[4] The authors of the first study then objected to findings of the second study, contending that the length of that trial (one month) was far too short to observe a benefit.[5] The Arthritis Foundation expressed concerns that the product would raise false hopes among arthritis sufferers and possibly steer them away from proven treatment regimens.[6] In a further blow to enthusiasts, another 1981 study found that NZGLM could not carry through its promise as a pain reliever for rheumatoid arthritis and osteoarthritis.[7] In that study NZGLM and a placebo were added to a regimen of naproxen, a conventional anti-inflammatory and painkiller; when naproxen was stopped after the sixth week, nearly as many subjects on NZGLM as on a placebo withdrew from the study because of inadequate pain relief.

Despite the fact that the FDA issued an "Import Alert" on NZGLM in 1980, it can still be found in the marketplace.

Will It Harm You? What the Studies Say:

Few adverse reactions have been noted in the clinical trials done so far. The most common ones were diarrhea, nausea, and flatulence.[8] Laboratory tests likewise found no signs of significant adverse changes.[9] However, a recent report describing hepatitis, jaundice, colicky stomach pains, anorexia, and malaise in a sixty-four-year-old woman taking NZGLM suggests that she had a drug reaction to the substance.[10] Pregnant women should probably not take it, given evidence of slowed fetal development and delayed birth in rats.[11] Obviously, avoid NZGLM if you are allergic to shellfish.

GENERAL SOURCES:

Der Marderosian, A., and L. Liberti. *Natural Product Medicine: A Scientific Guide to Foods, Drugs, Cosmetics.* Philadelphia: George F. Stickley, 1988.

Review of Natural Products. St. Louis: Facts and Comparisons, April 1997.

Tyler, V.E. *The Honest Herbal.* Binghamton, NY: Haworth Press/Pharmaceutical Products Press, 1993.

TEXT CITATIONS:

1. K.D. Rainsford and M.W.N. Whitehouse, *Arzneimittel-Forschung,* 30 (1980): 2128. A. Der Marderosian and L. Liberti, *Natural Product Medicine: A Scientific Guide to Foods, Drugs, Cosmetics* (Philadelphia: George F. Stickley, 1988).
2. V.E. Tyler, *The Honest Herbal* (Binghamton, NY: Haworth Press/Pharmaceutical Products Press, 1993).
3. R.G. Gibson et al., *Practitioner,* 224 (1980): 955.
4. *Review of Natural Products* (St. Louis: Facts and Comparisons, April 1997).
5. Ibid.
6. *Drug Intelligence & Clinical Pharmacy,* 15 (1981): 157.
7. Anonymous, *The Lancet,* 1 (1981): 85.
8. Ibid.
9. M. Ahern et al., *Medical Journal of Australia,* 2(August 9, 1980): 151–52.
10. *Review of Natural Products,* op. cit.
11. T. Miller et al., *New Zealand Medical Journal,* 97(757) (1984): 355–57.

PRIMARY NAME:
NUTMEG (and MACE)

SCIENTIFIC NAME:

Myristica fragrans Houtt., sometimes referred to as *Myristica officinalis* L.f. Family: Myristicaceae

COMMON NAMES:

Nutmeg: myristica, nux moschata, rou dou kou; Mace: macis, muscade

RATING:

4 = Research indicates that this substance will not fulfill the claims made for it. Safety appears to depend on cautious and conservative use; see the "Will It Harm You?" section.

What Is Nutmeg?

Myristica fragrans is a tall, slow-growing, and densely foliated evergreen tree that bears small fleshy fruit. When ripe, this fruit splits open, revealing a single seed kernel contained in a bright red, netlike encasement called the aril. The kernel is dried to produce nutmeg and the aril is dried to produce mace. Steam distillation of both yields an essential oil. The tree grows in India, Ceylon, Malaysia, and Granada.

What It Is Used For:

Both nutmeg and mace are treasured as strong but warm, sweet spices for baking and cooking. For centuries, traditional healers around the world also recommended them as remedies for stomach discomforts ranging from indigestion to excess gas, nausea, vomiting, and diarrhea. Some also suggested the herbs for kidney problems, insomnia, and cancers. Nutmeg in particular has earned respect as a soothing remedy for stomach disorders and rheumatic problems, as an aphrodisiac, and, in the past century particularly, as an agent for stimulating menstruation. (This use is now obsolete.) People can still be found using it for diarrhea, mouth sores, and insomnia. Nutmeg's purported hallucinogenic and sedative properties, recognized for centuries now, have recently been examined.[1]

Nutmeg oil has a reputation as a topical tonic and pain reliever for such ailments as mouth sores and toothaches. It serves as a flavoring and fragrance in many commercial products. Some herbalists recommend mace or mace oil in ointment form for rheumatic pains.[2]

Forms Available Include:

- *Nutmeg:* Capsule, decoction, extract, kernel (raw; whole or ground), oil.
- *Mace:* Ground (raw), oil, ointment.

Dosage Commonly Reported:

Powdered nutmeg or mace is taken in doses of 0.3 to 1 gram, and the essential oil in doses of 0.05 to 0.2 gram. Follow package directions for commercial preparations of mace and nutmeg.

Will It Work for You? What the Studies Say:

Research has revealed a number of intriguing properties in nutmeg and mace, but so far no clinical studies have been done to prove their effectiveness or safety in humans. Citing a lack of substantiating data, German health authorities have declined to approve of nutmeg or mace for any of the health claims made for them.[3] Their essential oils are chemically similar. Both contain myristicin (methoxysafrole; about 4 percent), a toxic substance that can cause psychotropic reactions in adequate doses (see the "Will It Harm You?" section). Experts attribute much of the pharmacologic activity of these spices to myristicin.

Alcoholic mace extracts have shown anti-inflammatory activity in the classic animal model for testing this, the swollen rat paw,[4] but the implications for treating inflammatory conditions in humans are far from clear.[5] The same is true for findings indicating that extracts fight certain fungi and bacteria, including several commonly found in the mouth.[6] Oils from both nutmeg and mace have larvicidal properties.[7]

Investigators identified strong antioxidant components in both nutmeg and mace and their extracts as long ago as the 1960s. High concentrations of antioxidants are believed to help scavenge toxic by-products that may contribute to cancer cell formation. More recent animal studies indicate that mace in particular has promise as an anticancer agent.[8] Topical application of mace to the skin of experimental mice reduced the incidence of skin tumors in one study, for example.[9]

Nutmeg has been used successfully to treat diarrhea in calves[10] and diarrhea caused by thyroid cancer in humans.[11] A 1995 study indicated that high cholesterol levels in rabbits were lowered by feeding them nutmeg extracts[12]; the subject requires considerably more investigation to assess its importance for humans.

Will It Harm You? What the Studies Say:

Experts consider both of these spices harmless when used in culinary amounts or even typically recommended medicinal concentrations. Be aware, however, that a dose of about 5 to 20 grams of nutmeg (equivalent to one to three whole nuts or two grated nuts, or about 2 tablespoons of commercial ground nutmeg) has been reported to produce such psychoactive reactions as hallucinations, euphoria, delusions, and feelings of unreality.[13] High doses are also likely to cause very unpleasant toxic reactions such as nausea and vomiting, flushing, a fast heartbeat, delirium, stupor, and a sense of impending doom.[14] Very large amounts can be fatal.[15] Experts attribute these reactions to the oil's myristicin.

Considerable variation in the level of myristicin explains why these reactions occur in some cases and not in others.[16] Some sources have questioned whether nutmeg has hallucinogenic or other psychoactive properties, conceding only that it may have a mild sedative action.[17]

Nutmeg oil also contains very small amounts of a safrole that research indicates can promote liver cancers in mice.[18] Some people may develop mild skin irritation or an allergic reaction when consuming nutmeg as a spice.[19]

Comparatively little is known about the specifics of mace intoxication,[20] but caution is recommended. Allergic reactions have been reported.

GENERAL SOURCES:

Blumenthal, M., J. Gruenwald, T. Hall, and R.S. Rister, eds. *The Complete German Commission E Monographs: Therapeutic Guide to Herbal Medicine.* Boston: Integrative Medicine Communications, 1998.

Der Marderosian, A., and L. Liberti. *Natural Product Medicine: A Scientific Guide to Foods, Drugs, Cosmetics.* Philadelphia: George F. Stickley, 1988.

Duke, J.A. *CRC Handbook of Medicinal Herbs.* Boca Raton, FL: CRC Press, 1985.

Lawrence Review of Natural Products. St. Louis: Facts and Comparisons, September 1987 (nutmeg), September 1995 (mace).

Leung, A.Y., and S. Foster. *Encyclopedia of Common Natural Ingredients Used in Food, Drugs, and Cosmetics.* 2nd ed. New York: John Wiley & Sons, 1996.

Ody, P. *The Herb Society's Complete Medicinal Herbal.* London, England: Dorling Kindersley Limited, 1993.

Weiss, R.F. *Herbal Medicine,* trans. A.R. Meuss, from the 6th German edition. Beaconsfield, England: Beaconsfield Publishers, Ltd., 1988.

TEXT CITATIONS:

1. R.A. Faguet and K.F. Rowland, *American Journal of Psychiatry,* 135 (1978): 860.
2. S.S. Handa et al., *Fitoterapia,* 63(1) (1992): 3.
3. M. Blumenthal, J. Gruenwald, T. Hall, and R.S. Rister, eds., *The Complete German Commission E Monographs: Therapeutic Guide to Herbal Medicine* (Boston: Integrative Medicine Communications, 1998).
4. A.Y. Leung and S. Foster, *Encyclopedia of Common Natural Ingredients Used in Food, Drugs, and Cosmetics,* 2nd ed. (New York: John Wiley & Sons, 1996).
5. Y. Ozaki et al., *Japanese Journal of Pharmacology,* 49(2) (1989): 155–63.
6. K.Y. Orabi et al., *Journal of Natural Products,* 54(3) (1991): 856–59. Y. Saeki et al., *Bulletin of Tokyo Dental College,* 30(3) (1989): 129.
7. N. Nakumura et al., *Chemical & Pharmaceutical Bulletin,* 36(7) (1988): 2685.
8. *Lawrence Review of Natural Products* (St. Louis: Facts and Comparisons, September 1987 [nutmeg], September 1995 [mace]).
9. L.N. Jannu et al., *Cancer Letters,* 56(1) (1991): 59–63.
10. *Lawrence Review of Natural Products,* op. cit. J.F. Stamford and A. Bennett, *Veterinary Record,* 106 (1980): 389.
11. J.A. Barrowman, *British Medical Journal,* 3 (1975): 11.
12. A. Sharma et al., *Indian Journal of Physiology & Pharmacology,* 39(4) (1995): 407–10.
13. Leung and Foster, op. cit. R.B. Mack, *North Carolina Medical Journal* (June 1982): 439.
14. M.K. Abernethy and L.B. Becker, *American Journal of Emergency Medicine,* 10(5) (1992): 429. Leung and Foster, op. cit. *Lawrence Review of Natural Products,* op. cit.
15. D.L.T. Opdyke, *Food & Cosmetics Toxicology,* 14 (1976): 631.
16. *Lawrence Review of Natural Products,* op. cit.

17. C. Van Gils and P.A. Cox, *Journal of Ethnopharmacology*, 42(2) (1994): 117–24.
18. E.C. Miller et al., *Cancer Research*, 43 (1983): 1124. *Lawrence Review of Natural Products*, op. cit.
19. A. Dooms-Goossens et al., *Dermatology Clinics*, 8(1) (1990): 89.
20. *Lawrence Review of Natural Products*, op. cit.

PRIMARY NAME:

NUX VOMICA

SCIENTIFIC NAME:
Strychnos nux-vomica L. Family: Loganiaceae

COMMON NAMES:
Ma qianz, poison nut plant

RATING:

- *In homeopathic concentrations:* 4 = Research indicates that this substance will not fulfill the claims made for it, but that it is also unlikely to cause any harm.
- *All other forms:* 5 = Studies indicate that there is a definite health hazard to using this substance; see toxicity warnings in the "Will It Harm You?" section.

What Is Nux Vomica?

Nux vomica is a highly diluted homeopathic remedy derived from the toxic, strychnine-rich seeds of the poison nut plant (*Strychnos nux-vomica*). This small Asian evergreen tree has oval leaves, yellowish-white tubular flowers, and yellow fruits; the seeds nestle inside the fruits. Strychnine, a lethal alkaloid, is extracted as a white crystalline material from these grayish seeds.

What It Is Used For:

Traditional Chinese healers have used external formulations of this plant to reduce pain, treat paralysis, and fight various tumors. Europeans started importing seeds from the East in the Middle Ages to poison rodents and game animals. They reportedly first used it medicinally—as a stimulant in the mid-1600s—but soon appreciated its toxicity.[1] Today, some European plant experts consider the plant a powerful bitter tonic that in carefully controlled doses can serve as an important nervous system stimulant.[2] In Europe, this remedy is often prescribed for children and the elderly. Other herbalists view it as an effective heart stimulant and agent to increase alertness.

By far the most widespread contemporary use of nux vomica is in extremely dilute concentrations as a homeopathic remedy. Homeopaths recommend nux vomica for boosting energy (including sexual drive); alleviating digestive problems such as gas; and treating nausea and vomiting (especially from motion sickness or overeating or drinking), constipation, certain types of coughs, fevers, backaches, headaches, cold sensations, and irritability. (See page 2 for more information on homeopathy.)

Forms Available Include:

Homeopathic formulations: Pellet, tablet.

Dosage Commonly Reported:

A common dose of the commercial homeopathic preparation is two to four tablets of 12X to 30X strength up to four times per day.

Will It Work for You? What the Studies Say:

The value of nux vomica in homeopathic formulations is highly questionable given the inconsistent manner in which they are prepared.

The author of a standard German textbook on plant medicines considers nux vomica an indispensable nerve tonic for such conditions as nervous exhaustion.[3] The text recommends controlled, small doses of nux vomica tincture, which is available in that country, as a tonic bitter taken in a large glass of water to mask its extremely bitter taste. Clinical studies to demonstrate the value of nux vomica for these purposes cannot be found in the recent medical literature, however. The numerous alkaloids in the seeds, including strychnine, are presumably involved in the reported actions, but this is difficult to confirm. German health authorities do not approve of nux vomica for any of its proposed uses, including appetite stimulation or the treatment of nervous system conditions, depression, migraine, gastrointestinal disorders, or circulatory system diseases such as Raynaud's disease.[4]

In a 1996 study, Chinese researchers reported that crude alkaloids from the dried seeds reduced pain in test mice.[5] Investigators there also reported identifying alkaloids active against certain tumor cells in the test tube, suggesting possible treatment strategies for cancer in traditional Chinese medicine.[6] The implications of these findings for treating pain or cancer in humans remain far from clear, however. Popular claims that Chinese researchers have successfully treated Bell's palsy symptoms with a paste made from the seeds[7] could not be confirmed.

Will It Harm You? What the Studies Say:

All parts of this plant contain a lethal poison, strychnine. Many countries have imposed legal restrictions on the herb's use. Poisoning can cause restlessness, anxiety, and intense intestinal spasms. Severe cases may involve bodywide muscle spasms, hyperthermia, anoxia, dangerous increases in blood acidity, and death.[8] Despite its toxicity, herbalists and physicians in some countries such as Germany continue to recommend nux vomica in doses greater than the ones seen in homeopathic preparations, which are generally considered safe because the herb has been so diluted. Homeopathic formulations of this herb are essentially the only ones available in North America. It should be noted, however, that German health authorities do not approve of nux vomica in any form for medicinal use, given the risks of central nervous system stimulation.[9] They note that the risks are particularly high for individuals with liver damage because strychnine accumulates in that organ.

GENERAL SOURCES:

Blumenthal, M., J. Gruenwald, T. Hall, and R.S. Rister, eds. *The Complete German Commission E Monographs: Therapeutic Guide to Herbal Medicine.* Boston: Integrative Medicine Communications, 1998.

Chevallier, A. *The Encylopedia of Medicinal Plants: A Practical Reference Guide to More Than 550 Key Medicinal Plants & Their Uses.* 1st American ed. New York: Dorling Kindersley Publications, 1996.

Duke, J.A. *CRC Handbook of Medicinal Herbs.* Boca Raton, FL: CRC Press, 1985.

Lampe, K.E., and M.A. McCann. *AMA Handbook of Poisonous and Injurious Plants.* Chicago: American Medical Association, 1985.

Mayell, M. *Off-the-Shelf Natural Health: How to Use Herbs and Nutrients to Stay Well.* New York: Bantam Books, 1995.

Weiss, R.F. *Herbal Medicine*, trans. A.R. Meuss, from the 6th German edition. Beaconsfield, England: Beaconsfield Publishers, Ltd., 1988.

TEXT CITATIONS:

1. A. Chevallier, *The Encyclopedia of Medicinal Plants: A Practical Reference Guide to More Than 550 Key Medicinal Plants & Their Uses*, 1st American ed. (New York: Dorling Kindersley Publications, 1996).

2. R.F. Weiss, *Herbal Medicine*, trans. A.R. Meuss, from the 6th German edition (Beaconsfield, England: Beaconsfield Publishers, Ltd., 1988).

3. Ibid.

4. M. Blumenthal, J. Gruenwald, T. Hall, and R.S. Rister, eds., *The Complete German Commission E Monographs: Therapeutic Guide to Herbal Medicine* (Boston: Integrative Medicine Communications, 1998).

5. B. Cai et al., *Biological & Pharmaceutical Bulletin*, 19(1) (1996): 127–31.

6. B. Cai et al., *National Medicine*, 1995; 49(1): 39–42.

7. Chevallier, op. cit.

8. K.E. Lampe and M.A. McCann, *AMA Handbook of Poisonous and Injurious Plants* (Chicago: American Medical Association, 1985).

9. Blumenthal et al., op. cit.

OAK BARK

SCIENTIFIC NAME:
Quercus alba, L. Family:
Fagaceae. *Quercus robur* and
Quercus petraea are also used.

COMMON NAMES:
Stave oak, stone oak, tanner's
oak

RATING:
- *For external use:* 2 =
According to a number of
well-designed studies and
common use, this substance
appears to be relatively
effective and safe when used
in recommended amounts
for the indication(s) noted in
the "Will It Work for You"
section.
- *For internal use:* 4 = Research
indicates that this substance
will not fulfill the claims
made for it, but that it is also
unlikely to cause any harm.

What Is Oak Bark?

The smooth bark and occasionally the acorn of hundreds of species of the ancient oak genus *Quercus* found in the northern hemisphere have been used medicinally, including that of *Quercus petraea* (Matt.) Liebl. (winter oak) and *Quercus robur* L. (British oak). Of the seventy or so species native to North America, *Quercus alba* probably ranks as the most important for medicinal purposes. Deciduous forms bear lobed leaves.

What It Is Used For:

Through countless generations, people have relied on this majestic tree for everything from timber to food to shade. The acorns served as a food staple for many Native American tribes. The tree's high-grade wood made it a favorite among early American furniture, whisky-barrel, and ship builders. As a healing agent its primary value has been as an astringent wash for inflammatory skin conditions, oozing wounds, weeping eczema, bleeding hemorrhoids, bruises, varicose leg ulcers, chilblains, eye ailments, and sweaty feet. Gargles and mouth-washes have been taken for inflamed gums and sore throats, and decoctions sipped for diarrhea and other stomach and intestinal ailments. Some contemporary herbalists limit their recommendations to use in animals only.

Forms Available Include:

- *For external use:* Bark (chopped and powdered), bath formulation (sometimes available in commercial preparations), compress, decoction (of chopped or powdered bark), extract, gargle, lotion, mouthwash, oral paint, poultice.
- *For internal use:* Capsule, decoction, liquid extract.

Dosage Commonly Reported:

A gargle or rinse is made with 2 tablespoons of oak bark per 500 milliliters (1 pint) of water and is used several times per day. The decoction is also used at room temperature as a compress or lotion, or is added to bathwater. Internally, a common daily dose is 3 grams (about 1 teaspoon) in decoction form. Three capsules of 434 milligrams each are taken three times a day.

Will It Work for You? What the Studies Say:

Although no clinical studies appear to have been done and few other important ingredients have been identified, scientists have confirmed that *Quercus alba* contains large amounts (6 to 11 percent) of an astringent tannin, quercitannic acid. Experts regard tannin highly for its astringent and mild antiseptic qualities. It constricts (tightens) tissue, reduces oozing, and shields injured tissue by forming a protective coating. Many consider it effective, when present at adequate levels (as is the case with oak bark), for controlling minor bleeding and accelerating healing in skin ulcers, inflamed hemorrhoids, itchy rashes and eczema, inflammatory eye conditions, bleeding or infected mouth sores, and similar conditions. German health authorities approve of using the closely related *Quercus robur* and *Quercus petraea* bark in poultices or lotions—even in baths—for inflammatory skin complaints, including those affecting the genital

O

Oak Bark

and anal regions.[1] Gargles (typically, undiluted decoctions) are approved for mild inflammation of the gums and mucous membranes of the throat. Certain European oak species are also marketed in Germany for excessive sweating of the feet and as a supplementary treatment of chilblains and anal fissures.

German health authorities also approve of internal formulations of *Quercus robur* and *Quercus petraea* bark for acute cases of diarrhea not due to underlying disease[2]; when taken internally, tannins are believed to control or stop diarrhea by reducing inflammation in the intestines.

Will It Harm You? What the Studies Say:

On the basis of years of use and what scientists have learned so far, oak bark apparently does not irritate the skin or mucous membranes[3] or induce allergic reactions. Take care, however, not to place oak bark preparations on large swaths of damaged skin. Along the same lines, German health authorities recommend not using oak baths if you have large areas of damaged skin, a fever or infectious disease, weeping eczema, hypertonia, or moderately serious cardiac insufficiency.[4]

German health authorities cite no known side effects with internal use, and no situations in which the herb should not be used, although they do note that it may reduce or inhibit the absorption of other drugs.[5] Avoid ingesting any tannin-rich herb for prolonged periods, given the still poorly understood cancer risks. Oak bark pollen is a common allergen.[6]

GENERAL SOURCES:

Bisset, N.G., ed. *Herbal Drugs and Phytopharmaceuticals.* Stuttgart: medpharm GmbH Scientific Publishers, 1994.

Blumenthal, M., J. Gruenwald, T. Hall, and R.S. Rister, eds. *The Complete German Commission E Monographs: Therapeutic Guide to Herbal Medicine.* Boston: Integrative Medicine Communications, 1998.

Dobelis, I.N., ed. *The Magic and Medicine of Plants: A Practical Guide to the Science, History, Folklore, and Everyday Uses of Medicinal Plants.* Pleasantville, NY: Reader's Digest Association, 1986.

Foster, S. *Forest Pharmacy: Medicinal Plants in American Forests.* Durham, NC: Forest History Society, 1995.

Heinerman, J. *Heinerman's Encyclopedia of Healing Herbs and Spices.* West Nyack, NY: Parker Publishing Co., 1996.

Tierra, M. *The Way of Herbs.* New York: Pocket Books, 1990.

Weiner, M.A., and J.A. Weiner. *Herbs That Heal: Prescription for Herbal Healing.* Mill Valley, CA: Quantum Books, 1994.

―――. *Weiner's Herbal: A Guide to Herb Medicine.* Mill Valley, CA: Quantum Books, 1991.

Stary, F. *The Natural Guide to Medicinal Herbs and Plants.* Prague: Barnes & Noble, Inc., in arrangement with Aventinum Publishers, 1996.

Tyler, V.E. *Herbs of Choice: The Therapeutic Use of Phytomedicinals.* Binghamton, NY: Haworth Press/Pharmaceutical Products Press, 1994.

Weiss, R.F. *Herbal Medicine,* trans. A.R. Meuss, from the 6th German edition. Beaconsfield, England: Beaconsfield Publishers, Ltd., 1988.

TEXT CITATIONS:

1. M. Blumenthal, J. Gruenwald, T. Hall, and R.S. Rister, eds., *The Complete German Commission E Monographs: Therapeutic Guide to Herbal Medicine* (Boston: Integrative Medicine Communications, 1998).

2. Ibid.
3. R.F. Weiss, *Herbal Medicine*, trans. A.R. Meuss, from the 6th German edition (Beaconsfield, England: Beaconsfield Publishers, Ltd., 1988).
4. Blumenthal et al., op. cit.
5. Ibid.
6. R.C. Loria et al., *Journal of Allergy & Clinical Immunology*, 84(1) (1989): 9–18.

PRIMARY NAME:
OATS

SCIENTIFIC NAME:
Avena sativa L. Family:
Gramineae

COMMON NAME:
Wild oats

Rating:

- *Oat extracts for external use:*
  2 = According to a number of well-designed studies and common use, this substance appears to be relatively effective and safe when used in recommended amounts for the indication(s) noted in the "Will It Work for You?" section.

- *Oat bran to reduce cholesterol:* 2 = According to a number of well-designed studies and common use, this substance appears to be relatively effective and safe when used in recommended amounts for the indication(s) noted in the "Will It Work for You?" section.

- *Oat straw for internal use:* 4 = Research indicates that this substance will not fulfill the claims made for it, but that it is also unlikely to cause any harm.

What Are Oats?

Hearty foods such as oatmeal are made from the grains (seeds) of this familiar, erect annual grass, of which there are many varieties. Oat bran is made from the ground inner husks of the grains, while oatmeal consists of the ground whole grains. The young, whole plant (known as oat straw) and unripe grain are also used medicinally in a variety of ways.

What They Are Used For:

Oats have been cultivated for centuries as a nutritious food staple as well as a feed for livestock. Many contemporary herbalists carry on the tradition of their predecessors in recommending oat straw tea and other formulations as antidepressants, sedatives for sleeplessness, restorative tonics for nervous exhaustion or a "weakened" nervous system, and diuretics ("water pills") for fluid retention, and to help treat degenerative diseases and rheumatic illnesses. Some even recommend oat straw as a mild aphrodisiac, impotence remedy, and agent to lower uric-acid levels in the blood. It appears in many herbal blends. Traditional Indian healers have treated opium and cigarette addiction with oat extracts. Homeopaths recommend minute doses of oat extracts as sedatives and occasionally for other purposes. (For more information on homeopathy, see page 2.)

Oat extracts have long been valued as soothing topical emollients. A powdered form of oatmeal for baths called colloidal oatmeal turns into a gooey mass when mixed with liquid, coating the skin and sealing in moisture, thereby relieving itching due to such conditions as poison ivy dermatitis. Europeans in particular are known to take oat baths for rheumatism, bladder problems, and kidney ailments. Oatmeal is included in many soaps and moisturizers for its reported soothing and exfoliating actions. Many sources hail oat bran's high soluble fiber content as a mechanism for lowering cholesterol levels and combating a number of other ailments.

Forms Available Include:

Bran, capsule, concentrated drops, extract, grain (in various forms for use in foods), powder (colloidal oatmeal for use in baths), tea, tincture. Also available in herbal blends, and in bath preparation, soaps, and moisturizers.

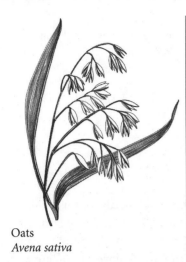

Oats
Avena sativa

Dosage Commonly Reported:

Consumption of 3 grams of oat bran (soluble fiber) daily is recommended for reducing cholesterol levels. The tincture or concentrated drops are taken in doses of ½ to 1 dropperful two or three times per day. To use bath preparations containing colloidal oatmeal or herbal blends containing oat straw, follow the package instructions.

Will They Work for You? What the Studies Say:

Oat bran contains considerable amounts of soluble fiber (meaning that the fiber dissolves in water). Most vegetables and fruits contain soluble fiber as well. Several controlled clinical trials have shown that ingesting large amounts of soluble fiber (40 grams a day) such as that found in oat bran may significantly reduce blood cholesterol levels within two to three weeks.[1] Such conclusions remain a subject of heated debate among experts, however.

Studies published in various respected journals indicate that consumption of 3 grams of oat soluble fiber a day can reduce cholesterol levels by about 5 percent, and that this holds true especially for individuals with cholesterol levels above 240.[2] In 1997, the FDA gave permission to the Quaker Oats company and other manufacturers to make the following claim on their products as long as each serving contains 0.75 gram of soluble fiber: "Soluble fiber from oatmeal, as part of a low-saturated-fat, low-cholesterol diet, may reduce the risk of heart disease."[3] A 1-ounce serving of Quaker Oat Bran High Fiber Oat Cereal, for example, offers 19 grams of oat bran, of which 7.6 grams is soluble. A serving of regular Quaker Oat Bran Hot Cereal contains 4.1 grams of total dietary fiber, of which 1.9 grams is soluble.

Despite a long-standing reputation, no sound evidence can be found to support the use of oat straw internally as a nerve tonic, sedative, stress- and anxiety-reducer, antidepressant, or booster of sexual desire or performance. No sedative properties of any oat formulation have been proven. Citing a lack of demonstrated efficacy, German health authorities declined to approve of oat formulations for proposed medicinal uses, including the treatment of diabetes and gastrointestinal complaints.[4]

Although no studies can be found to confirm the value of oat straw baths for such conditions as paralysis, arthritis, rheumatism, liver disorders, or hypertonia, derivatives of the grain in baths and other formulations have proved successful in treating itchy and irritated skin and other skin disorders. This soothing and moisturizing property is attributed to the plant's gluten content.[5]

The findings of a 1971 placebo-controlled trial indicate that an alcoholic extract of the fresh oat plant can curtail the desire to smoke cigarettes in heavy users, but researchers failed to reproduce these findings in follow-up studies.[6]

Will They Harm You? What the Studies Say:

No reports of significant adverse reactions to oats in any form, including as a medicinal herb in recommended doses, appear in the medical literature. Any high-fiber food such as oat bran should be consumed with plenty of liquids, and some people find the increase in the bulk of their stool, and the associated gas, quite troublesome.[7] People with celiac disease should avoid oats because they contain gluten. Some people have allergic skin reactions to oat flour.

GENERAL SOURCES:

Bisset, N.G., ed. *Herbal Drugs and Phytopharmaceuticals*. Stuttgart: medpharm GmbH Scientific Publishers, 1994.

Blumenthal, M., J. Gruenwald, T. Hall, and R.S. Rister, eds. *The Complete German Commission E Monographs: Therapeutic Guide to Herbal Medicine*. Boston: Integrative Medicine Communications, 1998.

Der Marderosian, A., and L. Liberti. *Natural Product Medicine: A Scientific Guide to Foods, Drugs, Cosmetics*. Philadelphia: George F. Stickley, 1988.

Lawrence Review of Natural Products. St. Louis: Facts and Comparisons, January 1991.

Mayell, M. *Off-the-Shelf Natural Health: How to Use Herbs and Nutrients to Stay Well*. New York: Bantam Books, 1995.

Mindell, E. *Earl Mindell's Herb Bible*. New York: Simon & Schuster/Fireside, 1992.

Murray, M.T. *The Healing Power of Herbs: The Enlightened Person's Guide to the Wonders of Medicinal Plants*. Revised and expanded 2nd ed. Rocklin, CA: Prima Publishing, 1995.

Ody, P. *The Herb Society's Complete Medicinal Herbal*. London, England: Dorling Kindersley Limited, 1993.

Tierra, M. *The Way of Herbs*. New York: Pocket Books, 1990.

Tyler, V.E. *The Honest Herbal*. Binghamton, NY: Haworth Press/Pharmaceutical Products Press, 1993.

Weiner, M.A., and J.A. Weiner. *Herbs That Heal: Prescription for Herbal Healing*. Mill Valley, CA: Quantum Books, 1994.

Weiss, R.F. *Herbal Medicine*, trans. A.R. Meuss, from the 6th German edition. Beaconsfield, England: Beaconsfield Publishers, Ltd., 1988.

TEXT CITATIONS:

1. *Lawrence Review of Natural Products* (St. Louis: Facts and Comparisons, January 1991). *Medical Letter*, 30 (1988): 111.
2. M. Burros, *New York Times* (February 26, 1997): C5.
3. Ibid.
4. M. Blumenthal, J. Gruenwald, T. Hall, and R.S. Rister, eds., *The Complete German Commission E Monographs: Therapeutic Guide to Herbal Medicine* (Boston: Integrative Medicine Communications, 1998).
5. A. Der Marderosian and L. Liberti, *Natural Product Medicine: A Scientific Guide to Foods, Drugs, Cosmetics* (Philadelphia: George F. Stickley, 1988).
6. C.L. Anand, *Nature*, 233 (1971): 496. C. Bye et al., *Nature*, 252 (1974): 580.
7. *Lawrence Review of Natural Products*, op. cit.

PRIMARY NAME:

OLIVE LEAF

SCIENTIFIC NAME:

Olea europa var. *europaea.*
Family: Oleaceae

COMMON NAME:

Lucca

What Is Olive Leaf?

The leathery leaf of this ancient olive tree, an evergreen, is used medicinally. For information on the oil, see **Olive Oil**.

What It Is Used For:

The olive branch has symbolized peace and prosperity since biblical times, and the meaty olive has served as a source of culinary pleasure and precious oil for centuries. Medicinally, olive leaf formulations have been recommended as

RATING:

3 = Studies on the effectiveness and safety of this substance are conflicting, or there are not enough studies to draw a conclusion.

diuretics ("water pills") and antihypertensives. Recent interest has focused on their purported ability to reduce blood sugar levels to help manage diabetes. The leaves have long been used externally to treat wounds.

Forms Available Include:

Decoction, fluid extract, tincture.

Dosage Commonly Reported:

To use commercial olive leaf preparations, follow the package instructions.

Will It Work for You? What the Studies Say:

Animal studies dating back to the 1930s indicate that extracts (decoctions or tinctures) of olive leaves can help reduce high blood pressure. One of the active ingredients has been identified as the glycoside oleuropeoside ("oleuropein").[1] This blood-pressure-lowering action has been demonstrated in rats, dogs, and other animals, but apparently no human clinical trials have been conducted.[2] A German textbook recommends that this treatment be reserved for labile (easily changeable) and medium to severe high blood pressure.[3] German health authorities, however, do not approve of the extracts for this use, citing a lack of documented effectiveness.[4]

The implications for treating diabetes in humans remain far from clear, but studies have shown that olive leaf extracts can reduce blood sugar levels in animals with chemically induced diabetes.[5] Leaf extracts have also shown diuretic ("water pill") properties in various studies. German health authorities did not find evidence of the effectiveness of olive leaves as a diuretic convincing and do not approve of them for this purpose.[6]

Scientists have studied the effect of leaf extracts on heart function in dogs, but no conclusions have been made.[7] In a 1941 investigation, olive leaf extracts failed to reduce fever in guinea pigs, suggesting that this folk use may be invalid.[8] Antioxidant properties have been identified in both olive leaves and olive oil.[9] Antioxidants control the formation of dangerous substances in the body called free radicals. These substances damage cells through oxidation, which may contribute to cancer cell formation. What role these antioxidants may play in preventing or treating cancer in humans is still unclear.

Will It Harm You? What the Studies Say:

Significant adverse reactions have not been associated with the use of olive leaf preparations. Because leaf preparations may irritate the stomach lining, they should always be taken after meals. If you have diabetes, keep in mind that this is a serious condition, and a medical professional should oversee its management.

GENERAL SOURCES:

American Pharmaceutical Association. *Handbook of Nonprescription Drugs.* 11th ed. Washington, D.C.: American Pharmaceutical Association, 1996.

Blumenthal, M., J. Gruenwald, T. Hall, and R.S. Rister, eds. *The Complete German Commission E Monographs: Therapeutic Guide to Herbal Medicine.* Boston: Integrative Medicine Communications, 1998.

Bremness, L. *Herbs.* 1st American ed. Eyewitness Handbooks. New York: Dorling Kindersley Publications, 1994.

Chevallier, A. *The Encyclopedia of Medicinal Plants: A Practical Reference Guide to More Than 550 Key Medicinal Plants & Their Uses.* 1st American ed. New York: Dorling Kindersley Publications, 1996.

Hallowell, M. *Herbal Healing: A Practical Introduction to Medicinal Herbs.* Garden City Park, NY, 1994.

Mindell, E. *Earl Mindell's Herb Bible.* New York: Simon & Schuster/Fireside, 1992.

Weiss, R.F. *Herbal Medicine,* trans. A.R. Meuss, from the 6th German edition. Beaconsfield, England: Beaconsfield Publishers, Ltd., 1988.

TEXT CITATIONS:
1. M. Gonzalez et al., *Planta Medica* 58(6) (1992): 513–15.
2. A. Trovato et al., *Plantes Medicinales et Phytotherapie,* 26(4) (1993): 300–8.
3. R.F. Weiss, *Herbal Medicine,* trans. A.R. Meuss, from the 6th German edition (Beaconsfield, England: Beaconsfield Publishers, Ltd., 1988).
4. M. Blumenthal, J. Gruenwald, T. Hall, and R.S. Rister, eds., *The Complete German Commission E Monographs: Therapeutic Guide to Herbal Medicine* (Boston: Integrative Medicine Communications, 1998).
5. Gonzalez, op. cit. Trovato, op. cit.
6. Blumenthal et al., op. cit.
7. F. Occhiuto et al., *Phytotherapy Research,* 4(4) (1990): 140–43.
8. J. Delphaut et al., *Comptes Rendus Sociologique Biologique,* 135 (1941): 1458–60.
9. I. Susnik-Rybarski et al., *Hrana Ishrana,* 24(1–2) (1983): 11–15. B. Berra et al., *Riv Ital Sostanze Grasse,* 72(7) (1995): 285–88.

PRIMARY NAME:
OLIVE OIL

SCIENTIFIC NAME:
Olea europa var. *europaea.*
Family: Oleaceae

COMMON NAME:
Lucca

RATING:
- *For external use:* 2 = According to a number of well-designed studies and common use, this substance appears to be relatively effective and safe when used in recommended amounts for the indication(s) noted in the "Will It Work for You?" section.
- *For internal use:* 3= Studies on the effectiveness of this substance are conflicting, or there are not enough studies to draw a conclusion.

What Is Olive Oil?

The graceful olive tree, an evergreen, is one of the longest-surviving species in the plant kingdom. Its bark is gnarled and deeply grooved. Both the familiar oil from the green to blue-black fruits and the leathery leaves have been used medicinally. The medicinal uses of olive oil are discussed here; see **Olive Leaf** for information on olive leaf preparations.

What It Is Used For:

The olive branch has symbolized peace and prosperity since biblical times, and the meaty olive has served as a source of culinary pleasure and precious oil for centuries. Medicinally, olive oil has long been valued as an emollient and topical lubricant. Some contemporary herbalists recommend it as a wound dressing for minor burns and psoriasis, insect bites, scalds, eczema (small patches), and other skin irritations, and, when warmed, to condition dry hair and an itchy scalp. In combination formulations it has been used to prevent and treat pregnancy-related stretch marks, to firm breasts, to function as nose drops, to soften hardened earwax, to relieve burning and itching in the ear, and to smother insects invading the ear.

The oil has been recommended internally for bowel diseases, intestinal colic, gallstones, and constipation (as a laxative). Recent interest has focused on its purported ability to reduce cholesterol levels, control high blood pressure, reduce blood sugar levels to help manage diabetes, and inhibit platelet aggregations (which has implications for preventing blood clots).

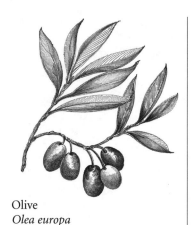

Olive
Olea europa

Forms Available Include:

Oil.

Dosage Commonly Reported:

Olive oil is consumed in moderation as part of the diet. As a laxative, it is commonly taken in dosages of 1 to 2 ounces. For a protective effect on the gastrointestinal tract, 1 tablespoon of the oil is taken in the morning. Externally, the undiluted oil is rubbed onto the affected areas.

Will It Work for You? What the Studies Say:

Olive oil will soothe and soften the skin.[1] Placing it in the ear canal will help soften earwax, as well as alleviate any itching or burning. It is safe for smothering an insect that gets trapped in the ear canal.[2] Olive oil is given internally to treat chronic stomach conditions in some parts of Europe. A German medical textbook recommends a tablespoon of olive oil in the morning on an empty stomach to protect the stomach lining;[3] no scientific studies that verify the effectiveness of this appear in the recent medical literature, however. Its purported laxative properties are also hard to confirm. German health authorities do not approve of olive oil for these or any other conditions, and recommend against its use for gallstones because of the risk of triggering gallbladder colic.[4]

The implications for treating diabetes in humans remain far from clear, but studies have shown that olive oil extracts can reduce blood sugar levels in animals with a chemically induced version of diabetes.[5]

Olive oil is high in monounsaturated fats, a type of fat many experts now consider beneficial in reducing the level of low-density-lipoprotein cholesterol (the "bad" cholesterol) and, in association, reducing the risk of heart disease. Future studies may clarify this still debatable issue.

Researchers are finding increasing amounts of information indicating that olive oil extracts may prove useful in preventing blood clots. In various test-tube experiments, components in olive oil have been shown not only to inhibit the aggregation of platelets but also to affect other blood components in positive ways.[6] Anti-blood-clotting actions are being compared to those of vitamin E and aspirin.

Will It Harm You? What the Studies Say:

No significant adverse reactions have been associated with the use of olive oil preparations.

GENERAL SOURCES:

American Pharmaceutical Association. *Handbook of Nonprescription Drugs.* 11th ed. Washington, D.C.: American Pharmaceutical Association, 1996.

Blumenthal, M., J. Gruenwald, T. Hall, and R.S. Rister, eds. *The Complete German Commission E Monographs: Therapeutic Guide to Herbal Medicine.* Boston: Integrative Medicine Communications, 1998.

Bremness, L. *Herbs.* 1st American ed. Eyewitness Handbooks. New York: Dorling Kindersley Publications, 1994.

Chevallier, A. *The Encyclopedia of Medicinal Plants: A Practical Reference Guide to More Than 550 Key Medicinal Plants & Their Uses.* 1st American ed. New York: Dorling Kindersley Publications, 1996.

Hallowell, M. *Herbal Healing: A Practical Introduction to Medicinal Herbs.* Garden City Park, NY, 1994.

Mindell, E. *Earl Mindell's Herb Bible.* New York: Simon & Schuster/Fireside, 1992.

Weiss, R.F. *Herbal Medicine*, trans. A.R. Meuss, from the 6th German edition. Beaconsfield, England: Beaconsfield Publishers, Ltd., 1988.

TEXT CITATIONS:

1. American Pharmaceutical Association, *Handbook of Nonprescription Drugs*, 11th ed. (Washington, D.C.: American Pharmaceutical Association, 1996).

2. Ibid.

3. R.F. Weiss, *Herbal Medicine*, trans. A.R. Meuss, from the 6th German edition (Beaconsfield, England: Beaconsfield Publishers, Ltd., 1988).

4. M. Blumenthal, J. Gruenwald, T. Hall, and R.S. Rister, eds., *The Complete German Commission E Monographs: Therapeutic Guide to Herbal Medicine* (Boston: Integrative Medicine Communications, 1998).

5. M. Gonzalez et al., *Planta Medica*, 58(6) (1992): 513–15. A. Trovato et al., *Plantes Medicinales et Phytotherapie*, 26(4) (1993): 300–8.

6. A. Petroni et al., *Thrombosis Research*, 78(2) (1995): 151–60. M. Salami et al., "Fatty Acids and Lipids: Biological Aspects," *World Review Nutrition and Dietetics*, 75 (1994): 169–72.

PRIMARY NAME:

ONION

SCIENTIFIC NAME:

Allium cepa L. Family: Liliaceae

COMMON NAME:

N/A

RATING:

2 = According to a number of well-designed studies and common use, this substance appears to be relatively effective and safe when used in recommended amounts for the indication(s) noted in the "Will It Work for You?" section.

What Is Onion?

The common onion is cultivated worldwide. There are many forms and varieties of this aromatic vegetable, a member of the lily family, although the most common are the white, yellow, and red globe onions. Greenish-white flowers grow at the end of a long, cylindrical hollow stem that emerges from the bulb. The meaty bulb is used medicinally.

What It Is Used For:

Like its close relative, garlic, the onion is considered a healing agent and as a food, a seasoning, and even a religious ointment. Over the centuries, it has been used to relieve gas, eliminate worms, reduce swelling (as a diuretic, or "water pill"), counter stubborn coughs and colds by loosening sticky secretions associated with congestion, control asthma, fight infections, and soothe stomach upset. External preparations are considered antiseptic and valuable for fighting fungal infections, warts, and unwanted blemishes; for reducing pain from sprains and bruises; and for lessening earaches. With the weight of increasing scientific research behind them, contemporary herbalists also highlight the onion's potential for reducing high cholesterol, preventing blood clots, controlling high blood pressure, and lowering blood sugar in diabetes.

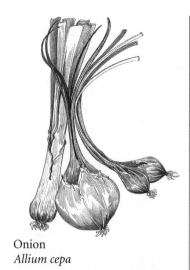

Onion
Allium cepa

Forms Available Include:

- *For internal use:* Capsule and tablet containing dehydrated onion, extracts, fresh onion (eaten raw, juiced).
- *For external use:* Fresh juice.

Dosage Commonly Reported:

Two to 5 ounces of fresh onion (about ¼ to 1 cup chopped onion) or its equivalent is ingested daily for its cardiovascular benefits. Onion juice is taken in dosages of 1 teaspoon three to four times per day. A cough syrup is made by mixing the juice with honey. The fresh juice is also applied to minor cuts and to athlete's foot.

Will It Work for You? What the Studies Say:

Several studies—a number of them with humans—report that both fresh onions and commercial onion extracts may reduce the risk of cardiovascular disease by lowering blood lipid levels (e.g., cholesterol), reducing blood pressure, and preventing the formation of blood clots.[1] Investigators have challenged the design (some were not randomized or blinded) and size (many were quite small) of many of these studies.[2] Some of the proposed properties have support from test-tube and animal studies, however. For example, animal studies indicate that consumption of onions can counteract high cholesterol levels.[3] Test-tube studies and studies with small animals indicate that liquid onion extracts in relatively large doses inhibit the formation of blood clots in various ways,[4] although it is not clear whether the same will occur in humans.[5] German health authorities officially recognize the ability of onion to lower lipid and blood pressure levels, as well as its anticlotting properties.[6] They endorse its use for helping to prevent atherosclerosis.

Research indicates that onions contain sulphur compounds that can lower blood sugar levels, a property considered valuable in treating diabetes.[7] Whether it makes sense for a diabetic to try to control his or her blood sugar levels with onion is a different matter altogether, however, given the serious need for consistent results.

Test-tube and rodent studies support the notion that onion oil and other extracts stop tumor growth in rats.[8] A 1989 Chinese study found that eating relatively large amounts of *Allium* vegetables such as onions and garlic was associated with a significantly reduced risk of stomach cancer.[9] The results were based on interviews with more than 560 patients with stomach cancer and 1,130 controls. This appears to be the first such study in humans.

Onion's reputation for treating asthma got something of a boost in 1990 when scientists reported identifying a chemical in onion with moderate ability to prevent the chemical and biological steps that lead to the inflammatory reactions seen with the disease.[10] Much remains to be learned about this property in humans, however.

Liquid extracts of onion fight various bacteria and fungi; this helps explain onion's traditional use as an external anti-infective.[11] German health authorities endorse its use as an antibacterial agent. Garlic may be more potent, however, and onion's practicality for fighting infections is far from clear.

Will It Harm You? What the Studies Say:

Other than the tears you are likely to shed when chopping fresh onions, and the memorable onion odor left on your breath after consuming them, the herb is not associated with any adverse reactions. Contact allergy can occur after handling the plant, however.[12] German health authorities cite no known adverse side effects or situations in which the herb should not be used.[13]

GENERAL SOURCES:

Dobelis, I.N., ed. *The Magic and Medicine of Plants: A Practical Guide to the Science, History, Folklore, and Everyday Uses of Medicinal Plants.* Pleasantville, NY: Reader's Digest Association, 1986.

Fenwick, G.R., and A.B. Hanley. *Critical Review in Food Science & Nutrition.* 23(1) (1985): 1–73.

Leung, A.Y., and S. Foster. *Encyclopedia of Common Natural Ingredients Used in Food, Drugs, and Cosmetics.* 2nd ed. New York: John Wiley & Sons, 1996.

Mindell, E. *Earl Mindell's Herb Bible.* New York: Simon & Schuster/Fireside, 1992.

Murray, M.T. *The Healing Power of Herbs: The Enlightened Person's Guide to the Wonders of Medicinal Plants.* Revised and expanded 2nd ed. Rocklin, CA: Prima Publishing, 1995.

Tyler, V.E. *Herbs of Choice: The Therapeutic Use of Phytomedicinals.* Binghamton, NY: Haworth Press/Pharmaceutical Products Press, 1994.

Weiner, M.A., and J. Weiner. *Weiner's Herbal: A Guide to Herb Medicine.* Mill Valley, CA: Quantum Books, 1991.

Weiss, R.F. *Herbal Medicine,* trans. A.R. Meuss, from the 6th German edition. Beaconsfield, England: Beaconsfield Publishers, Ltd., 1988.

TEXT CITATIONS:

1. M.M. Mittal et al., *Indian Journal of Medical Sciences,* 28(3) (1974): 144–48. G.S. Sainani et al., *Indian Journal of Medical Research,* 69 (1979): 776–780. K.K. Sharma et al., *Indian Journal of Medical Research,* 65 (1977): 422–29.

2. J. Kleijnen et al., *British Journal of Clinical Pharmacology,* 28(5) (1989): 535–44.

3. A.Y. Leung and S. Foster, *Encyclopedia of Common Natural Ingredients Used in Food, Drugs, and Cosmetics,* 2nd ed. (New York: John Wiley & Sons, 1996).

4. G.S. Sainani et al., *Japanese Heart Journal,* 20(3) (1979): 351–57. K.C. Srivastava, *Biomedica Biochimica Acta,* 43(8–9) (1984): S335–46. K.C. Srivas, *Prostaglandins, Leukotrienes & Medicine,* 13(2) (1984): 227–35. A.N. Makheja et al., *Prostaglandins & Medicine,* 2(6) (1979): 413–24.

5. Leung and Foster, op. cit.

6. M. Blumenthal, J. Gruenwald, T. Hall, and R.S. Rister, eds., *The Complete German Commission E Monographs: Therapeutic Guide to Herbal Medicine* (Boston: Integrative Medicine Communications, 1998).

7. R.F. Weiss, *Herbal Medicine,* trans. A.R. Meuss, from the 6th German edition (Beaconsfield, England: Beaconsfield Publishers, Ltd., 1988). B.O. Bever and G.R. Zahnd, *Quarterly Journal of Crude Drug Research,* 17 (1979): 139–96.

8. S. Belman, *Carcinogenesis,* 4(8) (1983): 1063–65. D.P. Nepkar et al., *Indian Journal of Experimental Biology,* 19 (1981): 598–600.

9. W.C. You et al., *Journal of the National Cancer Institute,* 81(2) (1989): 162–64.

10. *Science News* (June 16, 1990).

11. E.I. Elnima et al., *Pharmazie,* 38(11) (1983): 747–48.

12. R. Lautier and V. Wendt, *Occupational & Environmental Dermatoses,* 33(6) (1985): 213–15.

13. Blumenthal et al., op. cit.

O

Onion

PRIMARY NAME:
OREGANO

SCIENTIFIC NAME:
Origanum vulgare L. Family:
Labiatae (Lamiaceae). Also
Lippia graveolens H.B.K., *Lippia palmeri* S. Wats., and other
Lippia species. Family:
Verbenaceae

COMMON NAMES:
Origanum vulgare: European
oregano, origanum, wild
marjoram; *Lippia* species:
Mexican marjoram, Mexican
oregano, wild sage

RATING:
4 = Research indicates that this
substance will not fulfill the
claims made for it, but that it is
also unlikely to cause any harm.

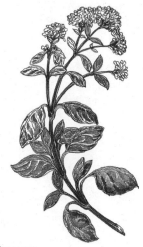

Oregano
Origanum vulgare

What Is Oregano?

The name "oregano" refers to more than two dozen species whose flowering tops or leaves bring to mind the characteristic oregano flavor.[1] The dried leaves of the aromatic, flowering *Origanum vulgare*, a hardy perennial with purplish-red flowers native to Europe, are used, as are the leaves and dried herb of Mexican *Lippia graveolens* and *Lippia palmeri* shrubs or trees.

What It Is Used For:

Few Americans fail to recognize the distinctive spicy, slightly minty flavor of this basic pizza topping, particularly of the somewhat milder and more commonly used Eurasian type. In addition to its long-standing tradition as a culinary spice, many healing properties have been attributed to the herb over the centuries. Today's herbalists typically highlight its ability to make a warm, spicy infusion for clearing congestion in coughs and other respiratory ailments, as well as to relieve stomach upset and aid digestion, bring about relaxation and drowsiness, and promote menstruation. In years past, oregano was also used to stimulate the appetite, alleviate toothaches and oral inflammations, induce sweating (typically to bring down a fever), resolve nervous headaches, and relieve aching in arthritic joints. Traditional Chinese healers have recommended oregano for a number of these and other conditions including diarrhea, jaundice, and itchy skin.

Forms Available Include:

Dried herb, infusion (for drinking, gargling, or adding to baths), oil.

Dosage Commonly Reported:

An infusion made using 1 to 2 teaspoons of dried herb per cup of water is drunk up to three times per day. The diluted oil is applied externally to ease toothache and rheumatism. Dilute according to package directions.

Will It Work for You? What the Studies Say:

The essential oil in most *Origanum* species (up to 1 percent in *Origanum vulgare*) contains the phenols carvacrol and thymol, both recognized for various healing properties such as expectoration (loosening sticky phlegm so that it is easier to cough up) and an ability to kill fungi and worms. Other herb oils such as thyme contain these ingredients as well. With oregano oil, however, the relative proportion of these and other active ingredients varies widely, from 0 to 90 percent in some cases.[2]

Origanum vulgare is reported to have antispasmodic and choleretic (bile-stimulating) properties, possibly explaining its reputation as a digestive aid in terms of soothing the digestive tract muscles and settling indigestion symptoms such as pain and bloating, for example; but none of these properties has been proved to work in human trials. German health authorities, citing a lack of confirmed efficacy, declined to endorse the medicinal use of *Origanum vulgare*.[3]

According to at least one source, a recently identified substance called lapachenole in *Lippia graveolens* may have both carcinogenic (cancer-causing) and antifertility properties.[4] What this means for people taking oregano medicinally remains to be determined.

Will It Harm You? What the Studies Say:

No significant adverse reactions have been associated with the use of oregano in culinary or medicinal concentrations. The FDA has placed oregano on its list of substances "Generally Recognized As Safe" (GRAS) for food consumption. Some sources recommend that pregnant women avoid consuming medicinal concentrations of oregano, given its traditional use for promoting menstruation. There is no evidence that it has ever been effective for this purpose.

GENERAL SOURCES:

Blumenthal, M., J. Gruenwald, T. Hall, and R.S. Rister, eds. *The Complete German Commission E Monographs: Therapeutic Guide to Herbal Medicine.* Boston: Integrative Medicine Communications, 1998.

Castleman, M. *The Healing Herbs: The Ultimate Guide to the Curative Power of Nature's Medicines.* New York: Bantam Books, 1995.

Dobelis, I.N., ed. *The Magic and Medicine of Plants: A Practical Guide to the Science, History, Folklore, and Everyday Uses of Medicinal Plants.* Pleasantville, NY: Reader's Digest Association, 1986.

Dominquez, X.A., et al. *Planta Medica.* 55 (1989): 208.

Leung, A.Y., and S. Foster. *Encyclopedia of Common Natural Ingredients Used in Food, Drugs, and Cosmetics.* 2nd ed. New York: John Wiley & Sons, 1996.

Stary, F. *The Natural Guide to Medicinal Herbs and Plants.* Prague: Barnes & Noble, Inc., in arrangement with Aventinum Publishers, 1996.

Tyler, V.E., L.R. Brady, and J.E. Robbers, eds. *Pharmacognosy.* Philadelphia: Lea & Febiger, 1988.

Weiss, R.F. *Herbal Medicine*, trans. A.R. Meuss, from the 6th German edition. Beaconsfield, England: Beaconsfield Publishers, Ltd., 1988.

TEXT CITATIONS:

1. A.Y. Leung and S. Foster, *Encyclopedia of Common Natural Ingredients Used in Food, Drugs, and Cosmetics*, 2nd ed. (New York: John Wiley & Sons, 1996).
2. Ibid.
3. M. Blumenthal, J. Gruenwald, T. Hall, and R.S. Rister, eds., *The Complete German Commission E Monographs: Therapeutic Guide to Herbal Medicine* (Boston: Integrative Medicine Communications, 1998).
4. X.A. Dominquez et al., *Planta Medica*, 55 (1989): 208.

PANGAMIC ACID

SCIENTIFIC NAME:
N/A

COMMON NAMES:
Calcium pangamate, dimethylglycine (DMG), Pangamate, Russian formula, Vitamin B_{15}, various proprietary names

RATING:
3 = Studies on the effectiveness and safety of this substance are conflicting, or there are not enough studies to draw a conclusion.

What Is Pangamic Acid?

In 1949, Ernst T. Krebs and his son Ernst Jr. received a patent for a product said to be derived from apricot kernels (*Prunus armeniaca* L.), rice, and barley. They called it pangamic acid and the trade name became "Vitamin B_{15}." Products subsequently labeled as Vitamin B_{15} or one of the names noted under "Common Names", consist of various ingredients that vary according to brand. In years past, many brands contained calcium gluconate and N,N-dimethylglycine (DMG), an amino acid. There is no official standard for identifying pangamic acid. It is not a vitamin, despite the fact that it is often referred to as one. The FDA has seized stores of these "pangamic acid" products because they fail to meet the widely accepted standards of classification as a vitamin; absence of the "vitamin" could not be associated with any deficiency state. Many sources now market DMG alone as pangamic acid.

What It Is Used For:

Many claims have been made for products sold as Vitamin B_{15} or one of the other names noted above, including that they offer protection against toxins as well as various diseases, and that they will relieve symptoms associated with heart disease, arthritis, asthma, eczema, nerve pain, and a host of other ailments.[1] Manufacturers suggest that DMG in supplement form is able to help maintain high energy levels, enhance the immune system, possibly control epileptic seizures, and increase mental alertness.

Forms Available Include:

Liquid, lozenge, tablet (including sublingual).

Dosage Commonly Reported:

To use commercial formulations, follow the package instructions.

Will It Work for You? What the Studies Say:

No sound scientific study has ever substantiated the value of pangamic acid in treating any medical disorder. It is not a vitamin and has no nutritional or therapeutic value.[2] The original patent application offered no scientific or clinical evidence to support the claims that it could detoxify body products or effectively treat any disease.[3]

Pangamic acid has not been shown to increase athletic performance or stamina. A 1982 treadmill study that examined its effect on the performance of sixteen male track athletes found that it conferred no benefit over a placebo.[4] The investigators tested, among other things, maximal heart rate, blood sugars, and short-term maximal treadmill performance.

There is, however, some supporting evidence for taking DMG alone for certain purposes, although more research is definitely needed. For example, the substance may enhance the body's immune system, according to a double-blind clinical trial.[5] The authors based this conclusion on an analysis of immune system factors in the blood of twenty subjects given either DMG (orally) or a placebo after receiving a pneumococcal vaccine. No other studies on the subject appear in the recent medical literature.

There have been contradictory reports regarding the ability of DMG to affect epileptic seizures. A 1982 study reported a dramatic improvement in seizure control,[6] but there were weaknesses in the study, including the fact that it involved only one individual.[7] A 1989 study of nineteen subjects found no difference in seizure frequency between subjects taking a placebo or DMG, or any improvement of the condition of the subjects, since the beginning of the study.[8]

Will It Harm You? What the Studies Say:

The potential of a product sold as pangamic acid or its "equivalents" depends largely on the ingredients in the particular product you purchase. Many of the common ingredients are not toxic. Still, pangamic acid products present something of a wild card. The DMG in many of them has shown mutation-causing (and thus potentially cancer-causing) properties.[10] Yet in 1978 an FDA Vitamin and Mineral Panel concluded, from tests on mice fed DMG, that the substance was "not terribly toxic" and a person would have to ingest large amounts (i.e., 22 pounds according to one source) before dying from it.[11]

GENERAL SOURCES:
American Pharmaceutical Association. *Handbook of Nonprescription Drugs*. 11th ed. Washington, D.C.: American Pharmaceutical Association, 1996.
Barrett, S., and V. Herbert. *The Vitamin Pushers: How the "Health Food" Industry Is Selling America a Bill of Goods.* Amherst, NY: Prometheus Books, 1994.
Der Marderosian, A., and L. Liberti. *Natural Product Medicine: A Scientific Guide to Foods, Drugs, Cosmetics.* Philadelphia: George F. Stickley, 1988.
Drug Topics. 125(5) (1981): 20.
Jukes, T.H. *Journal of the American Medical Association.* 242 (1979): 719–20.
Tyler, V.E. *The Honest Herbal.* Binghamton, NY: Haworth Press/Pharmaceutical Products Press, 1993.
Tyler, V.E., L.R. Brady, and J.E. Robbers, eds. *Pharmacognosy.* Philadelphia: Lea & Febiger, 1988.

TEXT CITATIONS:
1. American Pharmaceutical Association, *Handbook of Nonprescription Drugs*, 11th ed. (Washington, D.C.: American Pharmaceutical Association, 1996).
2. Ibid.
3. V.E. Tyler, *The Honest Herbal* (Binghamton, NY: Haworth Press/Pharmaceutical Products Press, 1993).
4. M.E. Gray and L.W. Titlow, *Medicine & Science in Sports & Exercise*, 14(6) (1982): 424–27.
5. C.D. Graber et al., *Journal of Infectious Diseases*, 143(1) (1981): 101–5.
6. E.S. Roach and L. Carlin, *New England Journal of Medicine*, 307 (1982): 1081.
7. V. Herbert, *New England Journal of Medicine*, 308(9) (1983): 527–28.
8. G. Gascon et al., *Epilepsia*, 30(1) (1989): 90–93.
9. A. Der Marderosian and L. Liberti, *Natural Product Medicine: A Scientific Guide to Foods, Drugs, Cosmetics* (Philadelphia: George F. Stickley, 1988). F.N. Marshall et al.,

International Proceedings of the Society of Experimental Biology and Medicine, 107 (1961): 420.

10. N. Colman et al., *Proceedings of the Society for Experimental Biology & Medicine*, 164(1) (1980): 9–12. R.V. Kendall, *Annals of Pharmacotherapy*, 28(7–8) (1994): 973. Tyler, op. cit.

11. Der Marderosian and Liberti, op. cit. E. Hettich, *Science Digest* (July 1982): 38.

PANSY

SCIENTIFIC NAME:
Viola tricolor, Viola tricolor hortensis (cultivated variety), L. Family: Violaceae

COMMON NAMES:
Field pansy, heartsease, Johnny-jump-up, ladies'-delight

RATING:
3 = Studies on the effectiveness and safety of this substance are conflicting, or there are not enough studies to draw a conclusion.

P

Pansy

What Is Pansy?

Pansy is easily recognized by its handsome, delicate flowers, which range in color from deep blue and bright yellow to pale violet and white. These flowers bloom from May to September and can be seen growing wild across temperate regions of North America and their native Europe, Asia, and North Africa. The plant is also widely cultivated. The aboveground parts, including the flowers and the lobed oval leaves, are used medicinally.

What It Is Used For:

In years past, pansy had a reputation in folk medicine as an expectorant to help clear upper respiratory tract congestion, bronchitis, and whooping cough. It was also used to treat feverish chills and increase urination in the form of a diuretic ("water pill"). A gargle was used for throat inflammation. Some prepared herbal remedies for these conditions still contain pansy or its extracts.

Contemporary herbalists for the most part recommend pansy in topical form for skin disorders such as eczema, mild seborrhea (including "cradle cap"), acne, itching, and impetigo. It also has a reputation as an internal "blood purifier" that can purportedly abolish toxins responsible for such skin disorders. The colorful blossoms are sometimes added as decorations to cakes, candies, and other foods.

Forms Available Include:

- *For external use:* Flowers, gargle, leaves, lotion, wet dressing made with an infusion.
- *For internal use:* Flowers, infusion. The herb and its extracts appear in herbal blends.

Dosage Commonly Reported:

An infusion is made using 1 to 2 teaspoons of flowers per cup of water and is taken internally or used in a wet dressing.

Will It Work for You? What the Studies Say:

Scientists continue to hunt for the ingredients responsible for pansy's healing properties. So far they have considered salicylic acid (present in concentrations up to about 0.3 percent), saponins, and mucilage (which has softening and soothing actions). Salicylic acid, which belongs to the same class of medicines as aspirin, is used in commercial over-the-counter formulations at higher concentrations—1.8 to 3 percent—to treat seborrhea, dandruff, acne, and other skin disorders. It promotes skin healing by generating a more rapid turnover of new skin cells. Apparently on the basis of this and positive findings in rat experiments, German health authorities endorse the use of a pansy infusion applied externally to mild seborrhoeic skin complaints, including seborrhea of the scalp in nursing infants.[1]

What contributions, if any, the other ingredients (or as yet unidentified ones) offer for ailments traditionally treated with pansy, such as mucilage for soothing the respiratory tract, remains speculative and unclear.[2] The medical literature contains no references to human studies testing pansy directly for any ailment. Apparently the herb in the form of a diuretic does not increase urination, although it may alter the composition of the urine in some ways.[3]

Will It Harm You? What the Studies Say:

A dearth of data on the medicinal properties of this herb makes it very difficult to determine whether it is potentially harmful in any way. Topical formulations, at least, cause no known side effects, according to German health authorities, and no known interactions with other remedies.[4] The recent medical literature contains no references to adverse reactions. However, logic dictates that, given the presence of salicylic acid (albeit in very low concentrations), you should watch for any extra irritation, dryness, peeling, or other reactions on the skin after using it externally, and stop using it if any occur. Do not leave it on large parts of the body or apply it to open wounds.

GENERAL SOURCES:

Bisset, N.G., ed. *Herbal Drugs and Phytopharmaceuticals.* Stuttgart: medpharm GmbH Scientific Publishers, 1994.

Blumenthal, M., J. Gruenwald, T. Hall, and R.S. Rister, eds. *The Complete German Commission E Monographs: Therapeutic Guide to Herbal Medicine.* Boston: Integrative Medicine Communications, 1998.

Chevallier, A. *The Encyclopedia of Medicinal Plants: A Practical Reference Guide to More Than 550 Key Medicinal Plants & Their Uses.* 1st American ed. New York: Dorling Kindersley Publications, 1996.

Dobelis, I.N., ed. *The Magic and Medicine of Plants: A Practical Guide to the Science, History, Folklore, and Everyday Uses of Medicinal Plants.* Pleasantville, NY: Reader's Digest Association, 1986.

TEXT CITATIONS:

1. M. Blumenthal, J. Gruenwald, T. Hall, and R.S. Rister, eds., *The Complete German Commission E Monographs: Therapeutic Guide to Herbal Medicine* (Boston: Integrative Medicine Communications, 1998). N.G. Bisset, ed., *Herbal Drugs and Phytopharmaceuticals* (Stuttgart: medpharm GmbH Scientific Publishers, 1994).
2. Bisset, op. cit.
3. H. Vollmer and R. Weidlich, *Archives of Experimental Pathology and Pharmacology*, 186 (1936): 574.
4. Blumenthal et al., op. cit.

P

Pansy

PRIMARY NAME:

PAPAYA

SCIENTIFIC NAME:
Carica papaya L. Family:
Caricaceae

COMMON NAMES:
Melon tree, pawpaw

RATING:
2 = According to a number of
well-designed studies and
common use, this substance
appears to be relatively
effective and safe when used in
recommended amounts for the
indication(s) noted in the "Will
It Work for You?" section.

What Is Papaya?

The small papaya tree, found throughout the tropics, has large, hand-shaped leaves and yellowish-green, pear-shaped melons (or fruit) valued for their edible orange-yellow pulp. These fruits can weigh several pounds. Scoring the fully grown unripe melon produces a milky juice (sap, or latex) that contains a mixture of plant protein-degrading enzymes termed papain (or vegetable pepsin). The juice is collected and dried. Smaller concentrations of papain appear in the leaves as well. Papain is also used commercially. This latex and the papaya fruit, leaves, and seeds are all used medicinally.

What It Is Used For:

In regions where the papaya grows naturally, the fruit and its derivative, papain, have long been treasured as digestive aids and remedies for stomach upset, especially following heavy, protein-rich meals. The seeds in particular have traditionally been used to fight intestinal worms. Papain tablets and leaf infusions to take during the meal are sold in parts of Europe for chronic gastritis and other stomach upset.

While North Americans increasingly recognize papaya as a healing herb, most still come into contact with the plant through papain and its use in commercial meat tenderizers, where it is used to break down proteins in the meat, softening it. Papain is also added as a purported softening agent to facial and other skin creams and cleansers, and some manufacturers even tout its ability to "digest freckles and other sun blemishes."[1] Poorly healing wounds, psoriasis, ringworm, wound infections, and other skin disorders have all been treated with papain as well as the leaves. Papain appears in some commercial douche products to "break down" excess vaginal discharge,[2] as well as in substances to control surgical or trauma-related swelling and inflammation,[3] and in preparations to chill-proof beer.

Forms Available Include:

- *For internal use:* Fruit (fresh and dried), infusion, juice, leaf, tablet (papain).
- *For external use:* Latex, leaves, powder (of dried papain).

Dosage Commonly Reported:

An infusion is made using 1 to 2 teaspoons dried, or, preferably, fermented, leaves per cup of water. Avoid boiling, which deactivates papain. Fermented leaves may yield a richer mixture of proteolytic enzymes.[4] This is drunk during or after meals to aid digestion. The fruit juice is taken in doses of 1 to 3 teaspoons as needed. Tablets containing 10 to 50 milligrams papain are available as a digestive aid. The latex is applied externally to wounds and warts.

Will It Work for You? What the Studies Say:

Papaya's popularity as a digestive aid and meat tenderizer can be attributed to the presence of several important digestive enzymes, the most notable being papain. Papain encourages the breakdown of proteins as well as carbohydrates and fats,[5] much the way natural human digestive enzymes do. It tenderizes meat by essentially predigesting it. Something similar occurs when humans take it orally, although several plant experts contend that its performance is rather unpredictable in the digestive juices of the human gastrointestinal tract.[6] Studies in the test tube indicate that papain can destroy worms by dissolving their protective outer cuticle.[7] But the same destabilizing action of the body's digestive juices may compromise papain's ability to destroy worms in humans, a property once valued by traditional healing cultures. German health authorities, citing a lack of substantiating evidence, declined to approve of papaya or its extracts for easing digestion or as a vermifuge (to fight intestinal worms).[8]

Investigators have reported that a natural Japanese health food prepared with fermented papaya can inhibit the production of potentially damaging free radicals in blood components taken from rats and humans,[9] raising hopes that it may qualify as an antioxidant capable of helping to prevent or fight certain cancers and counter immune system deficiency. More studies are needed before any conclusions can be made about this property, however.

Although it is doubtful that papain can "digest" skin blemishes such as freckles, studies do support the notion that papaya and its extract may benefit certain skin disorders. Extracts have shown bacteria-fighting actions, for example, which means that they may be of value in treating wound infections.[10] Test-tube studies indicate that the latex inhibits the growth of *Candida albicans*, a fungus responsible for such disorders as ringworm.[11]

Papaya seeds can reverse sterility without affecting libido or causing other adverse reactions, according to several studies in male rats and mice fed liquid extracts.[12] Whether this holds true for humans has not been examined. Follow-up studies have failed to confirm research findings that papaya latex may help protect against ulcers in rats.[13]

The FDA has approved of the use of injectable forms of chymopapain, a papaya enzyme less potent than papain, to treat herniated ("slipped") vertebral disks. The treatment is considered only in cases in which conservative treatment fails. Although apparently effective, it has proved controversial, with persistent safety concerns.[14] The latest findings indicate that severe allergic reactions such as anaphylaxis occur in fewer than 0.5 percent of patients—a much lower figure than initially reported—and that other adverse reactions are rare.[15] Other investigators have proposed ways of removing potentially allergy-causing substances in chymopapain to reduce the risk.[16]

Will It Harm You? What the Studies Say:

When eaten in moderation, ripe papaya fruit is unlikely to cause any harm, although in sensitive individuals severe allergic reactions to both the fruit and the latex have occurred.[17] There have also been reports of perforated esophagus in people who ate large amounts of the fruit or latex.[18] Papain has the potential to cause severe stomach inflammation (gastritis) when taken internally,[19] and to induce dermatitis and other skin irritation when applied externally.

Concerns raised by 1960s and 1970s rat studies indicating that papaya taken in various stages of pregnancy can cause birth defects and poison embryos have not been reinforced by further research. A 1995 study that examined the effect of papain on different phases of prenatal development in rats found that oral papain in doses up to 800 milligrams per kilogram does not disturb prenatal development or cause toxicity in the mother rat.[20] However, pregnant women may want to play it safe and confine their consumption to moderate amounts of the ripe fruit.

GENERAL SOURCES:

American Pharmaceutical Association. *Handbook of Nonprescription Drugs.* 11th ed. Washington, D.C.: American Pharmaceutical Association, 1996.

Blumenthal, M., J. Gruenwald, T. Hall, and R.S. Rister, eds. *The Complete German Commission E Monographs: Therapeutic Guide to Herbal Medicine.* Boston: Integrative Medicine Communications, 1998.

Castleman, M. *The Healing Herbs: The Ultimate Guide to the Curative Power of Nature's Medicines.* New York: Bantam Books, 1995.

Duke, J.A. *CRC Handbook of Medicinal Herbs.* Boca Raton, FL: CRC Press, 1985.

Lawrence Review of Natural Products. St. Louis: Facts and Comparisons, August 1991.

Mindell, E. *Earl Mindell's Herb Bible.* New York: Simon & Schuster/Fireside, 1992.

Tierra, M. *The Way of Herbs.* New York: Pocket Books, 1990.

Tyler, V.E. *The Honest Herbal.* Binghamton, NY: Haworth Press/Pharmaceutical Products Press, 1993.

Weiner, M.A., and J.A. Weiner. *Herbs That Heal: Prescription for Herbal Healing.* Mill Valley, CA: Quantum Books, 1994.

Weiss, R.F. *Herbal Medicine,* trans. A.R. Meuss, from the 6th German edition. Beaconsfield, England: Beaconsfield Publishers, Ltd., 1988.

TEXT CITATIONS:

1. V.E. Tyler, *The Honest Herbal* (Binghamton, NY: Haworth Press/Pharmaceutical Products Press, 1993).
2. American Pharmaceutical Association, *Handbook of Nonprescription Drugs,* 11th ed. (Washington, D.C.: American Pharmaceutical Association, 1996).
3. *Lawrence Review of Natural Products* (St. Louis: Facts and Comparisons, August 1991).
4. Tyler, op. cit.
5. *Lawrence Review of Natural Products,* op. cit.
6. Tyler, op. cit.
7. R. Giordan et al., *Mycoses,* 34(11–12) (1991): 469–77. F. Satrija et al., *Journal of Ethnopharmacology,* 48(3) (1995): 161–64. Tyler, op. cit.
8. M. Blumenthal, J. Gruenwald, T. Hall, and R.S. Rister, eds., *The Complete German Commission E Monographs: Therapeutic Guide to Herbal Medicine* (Boston: Integrative Medicine Communications, 1998).
9. J.A. Osato et al., *Nutrition,* 11(5 Suppl.) (1995): 568–72.
10. A.C. Emeruwa, *Journal of Natural Products,* 45(2) (1982): 123–27.
11. R. Giordan et al., *Mycoses,* 39(3–4) (1996): 103–10.
12. N.K. Lohiya et al., *Planta Medica.* 60(5) (1994): 400–4. N.J. Chinou et al., *Reproductive Toxicology,* 8(1) (1994): 75–79.
13. C.R. Chen et al., *American Journal of Chinese Medicine,* 9(3) (1981): 205–12.
14. *Lawrence Review of Natural Products,* op. cit.
15. Ibid. P.H. Wright, *Journal of the American Medical Association,* 263(7) (1990): 948.
16. P.M. Dando et al., *Spine,* 20(9) (1995): 981–85.

17. A.Y. Leung and S. Foster, *Encyclopedia of Common Natural Ingredients Used in Food, Drugs, and Cosmetics*, 2nd ed. (New York: John Wiley & Sons, 1996).
18. *Lawrence Review of Natural Products*, op. cit.
19. J.A. Duke, *CRC Handbook of Medicinal Herbs* (Boca Raton, FL: CRC Press, 1985).
20. H. Schmidt, *Reproductive Toxicology*, 9(1) (1995): 49–55.

PARSLEY

SCIENTIFIC NAME:
Petroselinum crispum (Mill.)
Nym., *Petroselinum sativum*
Hoffm., *Petroselinum hortense*
Hoffm. Family: Umbelliferae
(Apiaceae)

COMMON NAMES:
Common parsley, fairy feathers, flat-leaf parsley, garden parsley, Italian parsley, rock parsley, rock selinon

RATING:
3 = Studies on the effectiveness and safety of this substance are conflicting, or there are not enough studies to draw a conclusion.

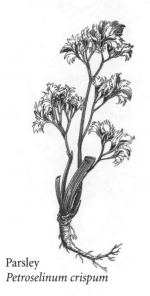

Parsley
Petroselinum crispum

What Is Parsley?

Many varieties of this bright green aromatic herb are cultivated worldwide. They are distinguished largely by whether the leaves are divided, featherlike, curly, or flat. The characteristically spicy tiny fruits ("seeds") are gray to grayish-brown. Small yellowish flowers grow in clusters. The leaves, seeds, juicy stems, and roots are used in cooking and medicine, as is an oil extracted separately through steam distillation of the herb and seed.

For information on Chinese parsley (cilantro), which looks a lot like flat-leaf parsley but actually bears no relation to the parsley varieties discussed here, see **Coriander**.

What It Is Used For:

Few herbs rival parsley as a universally recognized condiment and garnish. It makes its appearance before most other herbs in spring and is celebrated as a symbol of new beginnings in the ritual Jewish Passover meal, seder. For centuries, folk healers have recommended parsley to freshen the breath, soothe indigestion, and generally settle the stomach after a meal; help expel excess gas; reduce colicky stomach upset; encourage urine production in the form of a diuretic ("water pill"); stimulate the menstrual flow; and increase breast milk production. Arthritis, cough- and cold-related congestion, liver and spleen disorders, and other ailments have been treated with various parts of the herb. Parsley juice has been sipped to treat kidney ailments, and the oil taken to regulate menstrual flow.

Bruised leaves are applied externally to bruises, tumors, insect bites, lice and other parasitic infestations, and skin infections. Rubbing the leaves into the scalp will purportedly stimulate hair growth. The essential oil of the seeds serves as food flavoring.

Forms Available Include:

Decoction, infusion, liquid extract (of the rootstock), leaf and sprig (fresh or dried), root, seed, tea (made from seeds), tincture.

Dosage Commonly Reported:

To freshen the breath, chew a few sprigs of fresh parsley. A decoction is made using 1 to 2 teaspoons dried leaves or root or 1 teaspoon (about 1.4 grams) bruised seeds per cup of water. When making parsley seed tea, do not let the water boil because the all-important volatile oil will quickly dissipate.[1] To encourage urination, the leaves or roots are often taken in doses of 6 grams per day (1 teaspoon chopped root equals about 2 grams).

Will It Work for You? What the Studies Say:

Parsley's nutritional value is beyond dispute: it is packed with vitamins and minerals from carotene (a precursor of vitamin A) to B vitamins and vitamin C, iron, and calcium. But beyond this, experts dispute the validity of most claims made for the herb's healing properties. Several factors make it hard to resoundingly endorse the herb: the amount of volatile oil among parsley varieties differs notably, as does the concentration of and perceived safety of two particularly important active ingredients within the oils—apiole and the chemically related myristicin.

What little data are available clearly indicate that these two substances, as well as flavonoids, promote urine production, so the herb can be designated a diuretic. It probably works by irritating kidney tissue and thus increasing the blood flow and the rate at which the kidneys filter out toxins (the kidney glomerular filtration rate).[2] Diuretics are traditionally used to treat urinary tract infections and such potentially grave conditions as high blood pressure and fluid retention from congestive heart failure. German health authorities endorse the use of parsley leaves and roots as diuretics to subdue urinary tract inflammation and help prevent and treat kidney stones.[3] But citing health risks and a lack of proven efficacy, they declined to approve of parsley seed formulations for these purposes. Actually, the seeds tend to contain more of the active essential oil than the leaves (2 to 7 percent versus 0.3 to 0.5 percent, respectively), which is why many sources recommend infusions of crushed seeds for diuresis.[4] The ability of leaf and stem preparations to aid digestion or increase urine flow remains unclear.

Research indicates that apiole and myristicin can stimulate the uterus, which helps explain why women once used parsley to promote menstruation.[5] A Russian product containing parsley juice (85 percent) is used to stimulate uterine contractions during labor.[6]

The relatively high level of volatile oil in parsley seeds may also explain their effectiveness in settling the stomach and relieving gas, although the overall effect is probably mild.[7] In part because of the volatile oil's variability, do not count on the proven fever-reducing properties in the oil's apiole to control a fever.[8] Parsley's high chlorophyll content accounts for its ancient use as a breath freshener. Various other properties have been attributed to the herb and its constituents as well, but none has been properly studied in humans or even in animals.

In the 1960s, people reportedly smoked parsley in an attempt to get a "high"; the myristicin in the herb, also present in nutmeg seeds, has hallucinogenic properties.[9] But it is not at all clear that smoking parsley produces any type of desired reaction, and the practice did not endure despite high hopes. The myristicin concentration is in any case much lower than that for nutmeg seed.[10]

Mild antibacterial and antifungal properties have been observed in test-tube studies, possibly explaining a slight antiseptic action.[11] Apparently no studies have been done to show that these properties persist in the human body, however. Researchers are exploring parsley's ability to inhibit the mutagenic (mutation-causing) elements in the urine of cigarette smokers, possibly helping to protect them against dangerous cell changes.[12]

Will It Harm You? What the Studies Say:

Parsley is safe to use in culinary amounts, but avoid very high doses or extended use. German health sources advise against using parsley seed preparations because the seeds contain relatively higher amounts of the volatile oil, and thus myristicin and apiole, than other parts of the plant. Large amounts of this oil may irritate the stomach, intestines, or kidneys, and possibly cause headaches, loss of balance, convulsions, nerve damage, and other complications.[13] Also, the contained myristicin, it is believed, may cause giddiness, low blood pressure, and paralysis, and even stimulate and then induce a narcotic state.[14] Parsley oil also contains substances called psoralens (and related compounds) that can cause skin sensitivity reactions to sunlight.[15]

Both myristicin and apiole may stimulate the muscles in the uterus and could therefore cause serious complications and possibly even miscarriage in pregnant women, so many herbalists and plant medicine experts recommend that women who are hoping to conceive or who are pregnant should avoid taking large amounts of parsley as a food, or parsley oil, juice, or seeds.

People with kidney problems may want to use parsley judiciously, given the ability of the volatile oil to increase urine production by irritating the kidneys. Avoid parsley if you are allergic to other members of the same plant family, such as carrots or celery.

GENERAL SOURCES:
Bradley, P.C., ed. *British Herbal Compendium: A Handbook of Scientific Information on Widely Used Plant Drugs*, vol. 1. Bournemouth (Dorset), England: British Herbal Medicine Association, 1992.
Castleman, M. *The Healing Herbs: The Ultimate Guide to the Curative Power of Nature's Medicines.* New York: Bantam Books, 1995.
Hallowell, M. *Herbal Healing: A Practical Introduction to Medicinal Herbs.* Garden City Park, NY, 1994.
Lawrence Review of Natural Products. St. Louis: Facts and Comparisons, February 1991.
Leung, A.Y., and S. Foster. *Encyclopedia of Common Natural Ingredients Used in Food, Drugs, and Cosmetics.* 2nd ed. New York: John Wiley & Sons, 1996.
Mayell, M. *Off-the-Shelf Natural Health: How to Use Herbs and Nutrients to Stay Well.* New York: Bantam Books, 1995.
Middleton, E., and G. Drzewiecki. *Biochemical Pharmacology.* 33 (1984): 333.
Mindell, E. *Earl Mindell's Herb Bible.* New York: Simon & Schuster/Fireside, 1992.
Newall, C.A., et al. *Herbal Medicines: A Guide for Health-Care Professionals.* London: The Pharmaceutical Press, 1996.
Petkov, V. *American Journal of Chinese Medicine.* 7 (1979): 197.
Smith, D.A. *Practitioner.* 229 (1985): 673.
Stary, F. *The Natural Guide to Medicinal Herbs and Plants.* Prague: Barnes & Noble, Inc., in arrangement with Aventinum Publishers, 1996.

P

Parsley

Tyler, V.E. *Herbs of Choice: The Therapeutic Use of Phytomedicinals.* Binghamton, NY: Haworth Press/Pharmaceutical Products Press, 1994.

———. *The Honest Herbal.* Binghamton, NY: Haworth Press/Pharmaceutical Products Press, 1993.

Tyler, V.E., L.R. Brady, and J.E. Robbers, eds. *Pharmacognosy.* Philadelphia: Lea & Febiger, 1988.

Wickelgren, I. *Science News.* 6 (July 13, 1989): 5.

Weiss, R.F. *Herbal Medicine,* trans. A.R. Meuss, from the 6th German edition. Beaconsfield, England: Beaconsfield Publishers, Ltd., 1988.

TEXT CITATIONS:

1. R.F. Weiss, *Herbal Medicine,* trans. A.R. Meuss, from the 6th German edition (Beaconsfield, England: Beaconsfield Publishers, Ltd., 1988).

2. G. Marczal et al., *Acta Agron Acad Sci Hung,* 26 (1977): 7. P.C Bradley, ed., *British Herbal Compendium: A Handbook of Scientific Information on Widely Used Plant Drugs,* vol. 1 (Bournemouth [Dorset], England: British Herbal Medicine Association, 1992). V.E. Tyler, *Herbs of Choice: The Therapeutic Use of Phytomedicinals* (Binghamton, NY: Haworth Press/Pharmaceutical Products Press, 1994).

3. Bradley, op. cit.

4. A.Y. Leung and S. Foster, *Encyclopedia of Common Natural Ingredients Used in Food, Drugs, and Cosmetics,* 2nd ed. (New York: John Wiley & Sons, 1996). F. Stary, *The Natural Guide to Medicinal Herbs and Plants* (Prague: Barnes & Noble, Inc., in arrangement with Aventinum Publishers, 1996). Weiss, op. cit.

5. V.E. Tyler, *The Honest Herbal* (Binghamton, NY: Haworth Press/Pharmaceutical Products Press, 1993).

6. N.G. Bisset, ed., *Herbal Drugs and Phytopharmaceuticals* (Stuttgart: medpharm GmbH Scientific Publishers, 1994).

7. *Lawrence Review of Natural Products* (St. Louis: Facts and Comparisons, February 1991).

8. Leung and Foster, op. cit.

9. C.A. Newall et al., *Herbal Medicines: A Guide for Health-Care Professionals* (London: The Pharmaceutical Press, 1996). *Lawrence Review of Natural Products,* op. cit.

10. Newall, op. cit.

11. Marczal, op. cit.

12. S. Ohyama et al., *Mutation Research,* 192(1) (1987): 7–10.

13. *Lawrence Review of Natural Products,* op. cit.

14. Bisset, op. cit. Newall, op. cit.

15. K. Lagey et al., *Burns,* 21(7) (1995): 542–43. C.L. Egan and G. Sterling, *Cutis,* 51(1) (1993): 41–42.

PRIMARY NAME:
PASSIONFLOWER

SCIENTIFIC NAME:
Passiflora incarnata L. Family: Passifloraceae

What Is Passionflower?

Of the hundreds of species of passionflower, the one most commonly used for medicinal purposes is *Passiflora incarnata,* an American native generally found in the southeastern part of the country. The dried flowers and oval pulpy fruit from this perennial climbing vine are used medicinally. Unlike other *Passiflora* species, *Passiflora incarnata* does not produce the edible, succulent fruit referred to as passion fruit. Passionflower does not contain the poison cyanide, as some sources incorrectly suggest; they may have mistaken *Passiflora incarnata* for *Passiflora caerulea,* the ornamental blue passionflower that does contain this toxin.

COMMON NAMES:

Apricot vine, maypop, passiflora, water lemon, wild passionflower

RATING:

2 = According to a number of well-designed studies and common use, this substance appears to be relatively effective and safe when used in recommended amounts for the indications noted in the "Will It Work for You?" section.

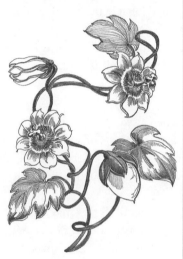

Passionflower
Passiflora incarnata

What It Is Used For:

Sixteenth-century Spanish explorers who came across the showy, oddly attractive passionflower in Peru concluded that the flowers were symbolic of the Passion of Christ, and thus a sign of Christ's approval of their endeavors. Other notions followed, including the idea, based on its name, that the flower could inspire emotional or physical passion.

Passionflower has a long history as a sedative (calming agent) and tranquilizer. In the early part of the twentieth century, the *National Formulary* even listed it for this purpose. Belief in passionflower's sedating capacity never waned in Europe, where commercial preparations still sell very well, often in herbal mixtures. A 1986 survey found that in Britain passionflower ranks as the most popular herbal sedative. Some American herbalists contend that passionflower is one of nature's best tranquilizers. Many recommend it for promoting a good night's sleep (especially in cases of anxiety-related insomnia), soothing jangled nerves, relaxing the body, calming emotional upset, controlling anxiety-related muscle spasms, treating headaches and pain, and aiding digestion. It has also been used traditionally to reduce exaggerated awareness of heart palpitations. Homeopaths suggest taking it in minute amounts for numerous disorders, including insomnia and nervous exhaustion. (See page 2 for a discussion of homeopathic medicine.) Passionflower adorns many gardens around the world and is also a popular houseplant.

Forms Available Include:

Concentrated drops, extracts, flowers, fruit, infusion (made from dried flowers), poultice, tincture.

Dosage Commonly Reported:

An infusion is made using 1 teaspoon dried flowers per cup of water. As a sleep aid it is drunk before bedtime; in other cases it is drunk up to three times per day. The tincture is used in doses of ½ to 1 teaspoon up to three times per day. The solid extract is taken in doses of 150 to 300 milligrams per day.

Will It Work for You? What the Studies Say:

Modern research indicates that passionflower's long-standing reputation as a sedative and tranquilizer has some merit, although exactly why remains unclear. While scientists have found low concentrations of chemicals that can depress (slow down) the central nervous system, they have also discovered chemicals that can stimulate it, causing confusion about the true nature of this so-called sedative. Recent investigations offer a partial explanation; according to a 1974 study, the chemicals that depress the central nervous system may overwhelm or sufficiently counter the ones that stimulate it, resulting in an overall sedating and tranquilizing effect.[1] Animal studies illustrate this complex stimulant and depressant activity, likewise indicating that the latter wins out. In a 1988 study, rats injected with passionflower extract slept longer and slowed down physically compared with those not given passionflower.[2] An investigation a few years later found that rats given passionflower extract to eat over a long period of time became less physically active.[3] Other studies have shown that passionflower increases the rate of respiration and causes a temporary drop in blood pressure, and that it can dampen the stimulant effect of drugs like methamphetamine in mice.

Apparently on the basis of such findings, German health authorities endorse the use of passionflower for nervous unrest.[4] But other sources assert that passionflower's sedating and tranquilizing effects have yet to be proved in well-designed human trials.[5] In 1978, unconvinced of its effectiveness or safety, the FDA banned the herb from over-the-counter sleep aids.

Animal studies indicate that passionflower may work as a digestive aid and soothing agent for menstrual discomfort. The herb's harmala alkaloids appear to relax certain smooth muscles such as those lining the digestive tract and uterus. Researchers have yet to examine whether passionflower will work these ways in humans.

Native Americans used to place poultices of crushed passionflower leaves on cuts and bruises to help them heal. Years later, experiments show that passionflower in fact kills many different kinds of bacteria, yeasts, and fungi in the test tube.[6] This germ-fighting quality dissipates quite quickly, however. Passionflower has also been reported to have painkilling properties, although relatively little is known about this. Despite the alluring name, the flower can claim no aphrodisiac properties.

Will It Harm You? What the Studies Say:

Passionflower probably poses no health risk when used in typically recommended amounts. After centuries of use, there are no reports of serious harm. Mice injected with extracts develop no adverse reactions.[7] German health authorities cite no known side effects, interactions with other medicines, or situations in which the herb should not be used.[8]

Avoid large doses, however, as the plant contains chemicals that may depress (slow down) the central nervous system. Pregnant women should not take it, given that it contains components (harman and harmaline) that affect the uterus,[9] although no reports of miscarriage associated with passionflower can be found in the medical literature. Unlike many drugs used for their sedative or tranquilizing effects, passionflower is not a narcotic. Thus it poses no risk of addiction, and in European countries where it is sold, the consumer needs no prescription.

GENERAL SOURCES:

Blumenthal, M., J. Gruenwald, T. Hall, and R.S. Rister, eds. *The Complete German Commission E Monographs: Therapeutic Guide to Herbal Medicine.* Boston: Integrative Medicine Communications, 1998.

Bradley, P.C., ed. *British Herbal Compendium: A Handbook of Scientific Information on Widely Used Plant Drugs*, vol. 1. Bournemouth (Dorset), England: British Herbal Medicine Association, 1992.

Castleman, M. *The Healing Herbs: The Ultimate Guide to the Curative Power of Nature's Medicines.* New York: Bantam Books, 1995.

Duke, J.A. *CRC Handbook of Medicinal Herbs.* Boca Raton, FL: CRC Press, 1985.

Della Loggia, R., et al. *Rivista di Neurologia,* 51(5) (1981): 297–310.

Lawrence Review of Natural Products. St. Louis: Facts and Comparisons, May 1989.

Leung, A.Y. *Encyclopedia of Common Natural Ingredients Used in Food, Drugs, and Cosmetics.* New York: John Wiley & Sons, 1980.

Mindell, E. *Earl Mindell's Herb Bible.* New York: Simon & Schuster/Fireside, 1992.

Newall, C.A., et al. *Herbal Medicines: A Guide for Health-Care Professionals.* London: The Pharmaceutical Press, 1996.

Tyler, V.E. *Herbs of Choice: The Therapeutic Use of Phytomedicinals.* Binghamton, NY: Haworth Press/Pharmaceutical Products Press, 1994.

Tyler, V.E., L.R. Brady, and J.E. Robbers, eds. *Pharmacognosy.* Philadelphia: Lea & Febiger, 1988.

TEXT CITATIONS:
1. N. Aoyagi et al., *Chemical and Pharmaceutical Bulletin,* 22 (1974): 1008.
2. E. Speroni and A. Minghetti, *Planta Medica,* 54 (1988): 488.
3. N. Sopranzi et al., *Clinical Therapeutics,* 132(5) (1990): 329–33.
4. M. Blumenthal, J. Gruenwald, T. Hall, and R.S. Rister, eds., *The Complete German Commission E Monographs: Therapeutic Guide to Herbal Medicine* (Boston: Integrative Medicine Communications, 1998).
5. *Lawrence Review of Natural Products* (St. Louis: May 1989).
6. J.M. Nicholls et al., *Antimicrobial Agents & Chemotherapy,* 3 (1973): 110–117.
7. Ibid.
8. Blumenthal et al., op. cit.
9. C.A. Newall et al., *Herbal Medicines: A Guide for Health-Care Professionals* (London: The Pharmaceutical Press, 1996).

PRIMARY NAME:
PAU D'ARCO

SCIENTIFIC NAME:
Tabebuia impetiginosa. Family: Bignoniaceae

COMMON NAMES:
Ipe roxo, lapacho, taheebo

RATING:
5 = Studies indicate that there is a definite health hazard to using this substance, even in recommended amounts.

What Is Pau d'Arco?

Pau d'arco is derived from the inner bark of various *Tabebuia* species, enormous, flowering trees found in South and Central America.

What It Is Used For:

In terms of popularity, this bark may lead the pack of recent herbal cancer "cures." It appears in remedies for leukemia, Hodgkin's disease, and cancers of the esophagus, head, intestines, tongue, and lungs. Herbalists also recommend taking the bark to promote overall health, lower blood sugar, and aid digestion. Some suggest dabbing topical formulations onto fungal infections such as athlete's foot. The list of older folk uses is quite extensive. Central and South Americans reportedly still rely on the bark for many ailments.

Forms Available Include:

Bark, capsule, decoction, extracts, tea bag.

Dosage Commonly Reported:

Three 505-milligram bark capsules are taken three times a day. The daily dosage for a decoction is 15 to 20 grams of the inner bark boiled in a pint of water.

Will It Work for You? What the Studies Say:

Many claims have been made for pau d'arco, but none stand up to scientific scrutiny or common safety standards. Scientists were optimistic at first; they found that the bark of the *Tabebuia* tree contains an active ingredient—lapachol—that can help fight various cancers in animals, including Yoshida sarcoma and Murphy-Sturm lymphosarcoma. But when studies in humans were initiated in the mid-1970s, such severe side effects developed that the subjects had to withdraw. So even if lapachol does help fight cancer in humans—and this has yet to be conclusively shown—it appears to be too toxic to use.[1] The National Cancer Institute, once very interested in lapachol, stopped studying the substance because it could document no "therapeutic effects."[2]

Apparently because of this toxicity risk, studies to explore whether ingredients in the bark also fight bacteria and parasites in humans have not been done; previous test-tube and animal experiments indicate that they may.[3]

Some herbal teas labeled as pau d'arco may contain little of the real thing. A related tree bark may be used instead, or inadequate amounts of the all-critical lapachol may be present. Investigators who put a dozen "pau d'arco" teas from Canadian health food stores into the test tube discovered that all but two had no active ingredient into any notable amounts.[4]

Will It Harm You? What the Studies Say:

At the point that pau d'arco reaches adequate concentrations in the bloodstream, highly unpleasant reactions develop, such as nausea, vomiting, a tendency to bleed, and anemia.[5] In a 1993 medical journal article, investigators reviewing seven "nutritional" anticancer therapies including pau d'arco tea came to the same conclusions about toxicity as earlier studies.[6] They also warned that herbal cancer "cures" pose the distinct risk that patients will abandon effective treatment.

GENERAL SOURCES:

Duke, J.A. *CRC Handbook of Medicinal Herbs.* Boca Raton, FL: CRC Press, 1985.

Heinerman, J. *Heinerman's Encyclopedia of Healing Herbs and Spices.* West Nyack, NY: Parker Publishing Co., 1996.

Lawrence Review of Natural Products. St. Louis: Facts and Comparisons, July 1990.

Mindell, E. *Earl Mindell's Herb Bible.* New York: Simon & Schuster/Fireside, 1992.

Tyler, V.E. *The Honest Herbal.* Binghamton, NY: Haworth Press/Pharmaceutical Products Press, 1993.

TEXT CITATIONS:

1. M. Girard et al., *Journal of Natural Products,* 51 (1988): 1023–24.
2. J.A. Duke, *CRC Handbook of Medicinal Herbs* (Boca Raton, FL: CRC Press, 1985).
3. O.A. Binutu and B.A. Lajubutu, *African Journal of Medicine & Medicinal Sciences,* 23(3) (1994): 269–73. C. Anesini and C. Perez, *Journal of Ethnopharmacology,* 39(2) (1993): 119–28. V.E. Tyler, *The Honest Herbal* (Binghamton, NY: Haworth Press/ Pharmaceutical Products Press, 1993).
4. *Journal of Herbs, Spices & Medicinal Plants,* 2(4) (1994): 37.

5. J.B. Block et al., *Cancer Chemotherapy Reports (Part 2)*, 4(4) (1974): 27–28. Duke, op. cit.
6. *CA: A Cancer Journal for Clinicians*, 43(5) (1993): 309–19.

PRIMARY NAME:
PENNYROYAL

SCIENTIFIC NAME:
American pennyroyal: *Hedeoma pulegioides* L. European pennyroyal: *Mentha pulegium* (L.) Persoom. Family: Labiatae (Lamiaceae)

COMMON NAMES:
Hedeoma, mosquito plant, squawmint, tickweed

RATING:
5 = Studies indicate that there is a definate health hazard to using this substance, even in recommended amounts.

What Is Pennyroyal?

Although American and European pennyroyal look different and have distinct Latin names, both belong to the mint family and share chemical similarities, uses, and risks. American pennyroyal grows in North American woods; European pennyroyal is native to Europe and western Asia but now also grows in parts of North America. The leaves and flowering tops have been used medicinally, as has an essential oil distilled from both.

What It Is Used For:

Centuries ago in Europe, pennyroyal earned the nickname "mosquito plant" because it repelled mosquitoes. Herbalists over the years recommended pennyroyal tea as a stimulating digestive tonic and for alleviating gassy indigestion, inducing perspiration (this was thought to break fevers and help eradicate colds and flus), and stimulating the menstrual flow. When European settlers arrived, Native Americans were using American pennyroyal for many of these same purposes. Like the Europeans, they valued it for repelling insects. But they also relied on the tea as a decongestant for colds, cough, and flu; for treating headaches; and externally for dressing wounds and various inflammatory skin disorders such as eczema.

Some contemporary herbalists recommend pennyroyal externally for such skin disorders and internally as a tea for colds, encouraging a productive cough, alleviating upset stomach and gas, and promoting menstruation. A number of modern users have attempted to use pennyroyal for inducing menstruation, often with tragic consequences. Many herbalists have apparently crossed the herb off their lists, deeming the risk of adverse reactions too high.

Forms Available Include:

- *For internal use:* Decoction (drunk hot or warm), dried herb extract, infusion, oil, tincture.
- *For external use:* Crushed fresh plant, essential oil, tincture.

Dosage Commonly Reported:

WARNING: *Pennyroyal should never be used medicinally.*

Will It Work for You? What the Studies Say:

No studies in the recent medical literature can be found to justify the use of pennyroyal for any ailment or condition, although, given its toxicity, it clearly contains active substances. Pennyroyal has a strong odor that may repel insects.

Will It Harm You? What the Studies Say:

An active but highly toxic substance called pulegone appears in high concentrations (up to 92 percent) in the volatile oil of American and European pennyroyal. Ingesting the oil either directly or through other preparations of the herb can cause nausea, abdominal pain, vomiting, diarrhea, fever, lethargy and agitation, rash, increased blood pressure and heart rate, gastrointestinal bleeding, inhibited clotting, liver damage, shock, and death.[1] There is no antidote for this poisoning.

Pregnant women in particular should not take pennyroyal in any form. There is no way to predict how the oil will affect you: one pregnant woman recovered fully after taking 7.5 milliliters of the oil,[2] while another woman died after ingesting just 1 ounce, and another died after ingesting 30 milliliters.[3] The oil can damage the central nervous system; one woman developed seizures and hallucinations after taking 5 milliliters of the oil, although she ultimately recovered.[4] Do not use the oil externally, either.

Pennyroyal tea and other extracts probably contain little of the toxic oil (and hence the toxin, pugelone) and should theoretically pose no risk of harm. But the risks may simply be too high for most, especially given the fact that none of the herb's purported healing properties has been proved. Large doses of pennyroyal in forms other than the pure essential oil may also cause nausea, vomiting, and other adverse reactions. Canadian health authorities have banned the sale of pennyroyal.[5]

GENERAL SOURCES:

Castleman, M. *The Healing Herbs: The Ultimate Guide to the Curative Power of Nature's Medicines.* New York: Bantam Books, 1995.

Chevallier, A. *The Encyclopedia of Medicinal Plants: A Practical Reference Guide to More Than 550 Key Medicinal Plants & Their Uses.* 1st American ed. New York: Dorling Kindersley Publications, 1996.

Der Marderosian, A., and L. Liberti. *Natural Product Medicine: A Scientific Guide to Foods, Drugs, Cosmetics.* Philadelphia: George F. Stickley, 1988.

Duke, J.A. *CRC Handbook of Medicinal Herbs.* Boca Raton, FL: CRC Press, 1985.

Lawrence Review of Natural Products. St. Louis: Facts and Comparisons, January 1992.

Mindell, E. *Earl Mindell's Herb Bible.* New York: Simon & Schuster/Fireside, 1992.

Newall, C.A., et al. *Herbal Medicines: A Guide for Health-Care Professionals.* London: The Pharmaceutical Press, 1996.

Tierra, M. *The Way of Herbs.* New York: Pocket Books, 1990.

Tyler, V.E. *The Honest Herbal.* Binghamton, NY: Haworth Press/Pharmaceutical Products Press, 1993.

Tyler, V.E., L.R. Brady, and J.E. Robbers, eds. *Pharmacognosy.* Philadelphia: Lea & Febiger, 1988.

Weiner, M.A., and J.A. Weiner. *Herbs That Heal: Prescription for Herbal Healing.* Mill Valley, CA: Quantum Books, 1994.

TEXT CITATIONS:

1. C.A. Newall et al., *Herbal Medicines: A Guide for Health-Care Professionals* (London: The Pharmaceutical Press, 1996).
2. Gunby, P., *Journal of the American Medical Association* 241 (1979): 2246–47. Sullivan, J. B. et al., *Journal of the American Medical Association* 242 (1979): 2873.
3. Vallance, W. B., *The Lancet* ii (1955): 850–51.

4. E.F. Early, *The Lancet*, 2 (1961): 580–81.
5. S. Waxman, *Washington Post*, (March 24, 1996): A22.

PEONY

SCIENTIFIC NAME:
Paeonia officinalis L. emend.
Willd., or *Paeonia mascula* (L.)
Miller *s.l.* L. Family:
Paeoniaceae

COMMON NAME:
King of flowers

RATING:
4 = Research indicates that this substance will not fulfill the claims made for it. Lack of data makes it difficult to determine whether it is safe to use.

What Is Peony?

The fragrant and sumptuous peony flower, named after the physician of the Greek gods (Paeon), bursts into bloom in early summer, with pink, purple-red, and white blossoms. It has been valued since ancient times as a decorative and medicinal plant. It is actually a double flower. A native of southern Europe and the Mediterranean region, peony can be found in mountain woodlands and cultivated as a garden plant. The flowers, roots, and seeds are used medicinally.

For information on white or Chinese peony—*Paeonia lactiflora*—see **Peony, White**.

What It Is Used For:

Traditional European healers once considered peony root antispasmodic and sedative, recommending it highly for epilepsy and nervous conditions, as well as for intestinal upset, whooping cough, and arthritis. The flowers have been used for skin and mucous membrane disorders including anal fissures, and for heart trouble, stomach upset, respiratory tract ailments, and nervous disorders, often in combination with other herbs. The seeds were used as a kitchen spice and (presumably in larger doses) to induce vomiting and stimulate menstrual flow. Today, peony is not widely used, and little research has been done on it. It is most commonly found in herbal blends to perk up their color. Homeopaths recommend minute amounts for phlebitis (vein inflammation), hemorrhoids, varicose veins, and a number of other conditions. (See page 2 for more information on homeopathy.) Dried petals are added to potpourris. The Chinese variety is much more heavily used and has been intensively studied.

Forms Available Include:

Flowers, infusion.

Dosage Commonly Reported:

An infusion is made by pouring boiling water over 1 teaspoon (about 1 gram) of the flowers, letting it steep for five to ten mintues, then straining it.

Will It Work for You? What the Studies Say:

The medical literature contains no data to support the use of peony flower and root for any of their traditional uses. Citing a lack of substantiating information, German health authorities declined to approve of peony as a medicinal herb.[1] The roots and flowers both contain astringent tannins, according to dated research, which may explain why they were once used to treat skin eruptions; tannins constrict tissue and reduce oozing and bleeding. Many other herbs contain more reliable and tested amounts of this substance, however.

Will It Harm You? What the Studies Say:

Exercise caution in taking this herb, as excessive amounts of the flowers, roots, or seeds can cause vomiting, colic, diarrhea, and other complications.[2] Except for these potential reactions, scientists have learned little about the safety of peony. According to German health authorities, it probably poses no risks when added to teas to make them more colorful.[3] Most herbalists recommend taking it only under professional supervision. Pregnant women may want to take extra care in avoiding peony, given its traditional use for stimulating menstruation.

GENERAL SOURCES:

Bisset, N.G., ed. *Herbal Drugs and Phytopharmaceuticals.* Stuttgart: medpharm GmbH Scientific Publishers, 1994.

Blumenthal, M., J. Gruenwald, T. Hall, and R.S. Rister, eds. *The Complete German Commission E Monographs: Therapeutic Guide to Herbal Medicine.* Boston: Integrative Medicine Communications, 1998.

Chevallier, A. *The Encyclopedia of Medicinal Plants: A Practical Reference Guide to More Than 550 Key Medicinal Plants & Their Uses.* 1st American ed. New York: Dorling Kindersley Publications, 1996.

Ody, P. *The Herb Society's Complete Medicinal Herbal.* London, England: Dorling Kindersley Publications, 1993.

TEXT CITATIONS:

1. M. Blumenthal, J. Gruenwald, T. Hall, and R.S. Rister, eds., *The Complete German Commission E Monographs: Therapeutic Guide to Herbal Medicine* (Boston: Integrative Medicine Communications, 1998).
2. N.G. Bisset, ed., *Herbal Drugs and Phytopharmaceuticals* (Stuttgart: medpharm GmbH Scientific Publishers, 1994).
3. Blumenthal et al., op. cit.

PRIMARY NAME:
PEONY, WHITE

SCIENTIFIC NAME:
Paeonia lactiflora, sometimes referred to as *Paeonia albiflora.* Family: Paeoniaceae

COMMON NAMES:
Bai shao yao, Chinese peony

RATING:
3 = Studies on the effectiveness and safety of this substance are conflicting, or there are not enough studies to draw a conclusion.

What Is White Peony?

The thick, tuberous white roots of this bushy perennial found growing throughout northeastern China and Inner Mongolia are used medicinally. Its large and bountiful white, red, or pink summer flowers have also qualified it as an ornamental in many parts of the world. For information on this plant's close European relative, *Paeonia officinalis,* see **Peony**.

What It Is Used For:

In addition to being cultivated for its dramatic and fragrant flowers, white peony has been a mainstay of Chinese medicine. Traditional Chinese healers have relied on its root for centuries as a tonic and pain reliever, particularly for such gynecologic discomforts as menstrual pain and breakthrough bleeding. They reportedly value it as well for nourishing the blood and liver, remedying anemia, and treating ailments ranging from headache to stiff joints, night sweats, and dizziness. A tonic known as "four things soup" contains the herb, along with **Rehmannia**, **Angelica**, and chuan xiong (Ligusticum wallichi). White peony is also used in numerous Asian skin care products.

Forms Available Include:

Decoction. Extracts appear in skin care products. Root.

Dosage Commonly Reported:

For menstrual pain, heavy bleeding, and hot flashes, a decoction made using 20 grams root to 750 milliliters of water is sipped throughout the day.

Will It Work for You? What the Studies Say:

Intensive research on the part of primarily Chinese investigators has revealed a number of interesting properties in this plant, several of which lend support to traditional uses. Investigators have identified glycosides as the root's critical compounds, with paeonol and paeoniflorin playing leading roles.

Anti-inflammatory, sedative, antibacterial, antifungal, and antiviral properties in paeoniflorin and other glycosides have been demonstrated, mostly through animal studies.[1] The bitter and sour-tasting root can also fight tumors, improve the memory, fight cell mutations, prolong survival, and possibly help prevent blood clots by reducing platelet stickiness, according to research findings.[2]

While the recent medical literature—at least that available in the West—fails to verify the root's effectiveness in treating menstrual or other gynecologic discomforts such as menstrual cramps and related disorders, analgesic and antispasmodic actions seen in animal studies may indirectly explain its value for these purposes. Clearly, more research on the subject is needed.

A substance called TBM—the total glucosides of the peony cortex—has shown promise in preventing liver injury in laboratory mice,[3] positively affecting immune system function in arthritic rats,[4] encouraging anticonvulsant actions in mice,[5] and inducing antistress properties in rats.[6] Extracts have also shown analgesic properties in mice,[7] immune-system-modulating effects in mice,[8] heart-protectant actions (against damage from blood flow after lack of oxygen) in rats,[9] and anti-inflammatory actions in the classic rat-paw edema test.[10]

Whether the root's anti-inflammatory, antimicrobial, and astringent effects actually improve the quality of skin care products to which it is added has apparently not been tested in humans, although these products are popular, especially in Asian parts of the globe.[11]

Will It Harm You? What the Studies Say:

The medical literature contains no reports of serious adverse reactions to this classic Chinese herb. Rat studies indicate that the toxicity of both the root and its extracts, such as paeoniflorin, is low.

P

Peony, White

GENERAL SOURCES:

Bremness, L. *Herbs.* 1st American ed. Eyewitness Handbooks. New York: Dorling Kindersley Publications, 1994.

Chevallier, A. *The Encyclopedia of Medicinal Plants: A Practical Reference Guide to More Than 550 Key Medicinal Plants & Their Uses.* 1st American ed. New York: Dorling Kindersley Publications, 1996.

Leung, A.Y., and S. Foster. *Encyclopedia of Common Natural Ingredients Used in Food, Drugs, and Cosmetics.* 2nd ed. New York: John Wiley & Sons, 1996.

TEXT CITATIONS:

1. A.Y. Leung and S. Foster, *Encyclopedia of Common Natural Ingredients Used in Food, Drugs, and Cosmetics,* 2nd ed. (New York: John Wiley & Sons, 1996). Y. Liu and Y. Ma, *Zhongcaoyao,* 26(8) (1995): 437–40.
2. Leung and Foster, op. cit.
3. L. Dai et al., *Zhongguo Yaolixue Tongbao,* 10(1) (1994): 58–60.
4. Z. Ge et al., *Zhongguo Yaolixue Tongbao,* 11(4) (1995): 303–5.
5. Yan Zhang et al., *Zhongguo Yaolixue Tongbao,* 10(5) (1994): 372–74.
6. H. Zhou et al., *Zhongguo Yaolixue Tongbao,* 10(6) (1994): 429–32.
7. X. Liu et al., *Zhongguo Yaolixue Tongbao,* 9(6) (1993): 464–67.
8. X. Wang et al., *Zhongguo Yaolixue Tongbao,* 6(6) (1990): 363–66.
9. W.G. Zhang and Z.S. Zhang, *Yaoxue Xuebao,* 29(2) (1994): 145–48. J. Tang et al., *Zhongcaoyao,* 21(12) (1990): 547–49.
10. G. Wu et al., *Zhongguo Yaoke Daxue Xuebao,* 20(3) (1989): 147–50.
11. Leung and Foster, op. cit.

P

Peppermint

PRIMARY NAME:
PEPPERMINT

SCIENTIFIC NAME:
Mentha x piperta L. Family: Labiatae (Lamiaceae)

COMMON NAMES:
Varieties include those commonly known as black mint (*M. piperta* var. *vulgaris Sole*) and white mint (*M. piperta* var. *officinalis Sole*).

What Is Peppermint?

This esteemed mint-family member was born in an English field of spearmint in the 1700s; it represents a natural hybrid between spearmint (*Mentha spicata*) and water mint (*Mentha aquatica*). Peppermint sports the classic square stems of the mint family, oblong to oval leaves, and dense spikes of lilac-pink flowers that bloom in summer. Various types of peppermint are cultivated around the world. The leaves (dried and fresh) and flowering tops have been used medicinally for centuries.

An intensely spicy, cooling, and aromatic oil is extracted from the leaves and the fresh or partially dried aboveground and flowering part of the herb. In the late 1800s, chemists distilled the all-important component, menthol, from this oil (see **Menthol** for more information).

What It Is Used For:

In the kingdom of mints, peppermint and spearmint reign as king and queen. Both Western and Eastern cultures have long brewed teas with the peppermint leaf to treat indigestion, sore throat, nausea, colds, cancers, gas, and cramplike stomach and intestinal discomforts. (Although spearmint contains a volatile oil that is responsible for its distinctive aroma and taste, as well as its medicinal properties, it does not contain the all-important menthol found in peppermint oil and is therefore not considered as diverse or potent an herbal remedy.) The

RATING:

1 = Years of use and extensive, high-quality studies indicate that this substance is very effective and safe when used in recommended amounts for the indication(s) noted in the "Will It Work for You?" section. However, see the warnings in the "Will It Harm You?" section.

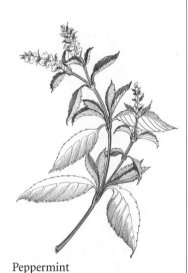

Peppermint
Mentha x piperta

English started to use peppermint medicinally and cultivate it commercially in the mid-1700s. The Americans followed close behind. The United States now grows more peppermint than any other country in the world.

Herbalists today recommend the herb internally for many of the same ailments their predecessors did. Some tout its ability to counter motion sickness, congestion, headache, heartburn, fever, and sleeplessness. It is considered a valuable antispasmodic. The leaf and extracts appear in numerous European laxatives, bile-duct remedies, and bile-stimulating formulations. For tension and weariness, many sources recommend a peppermint-scented bath. Topical formulations are suggested for inflammation and itching.

In addition to being popular as a flavoring, peppermint oil contains the medicinally active substance known as menthol and is therefore widely used as a digestion regulator, gas remedy, and antiseptic and local anesthetic agent in everything from cold and cough preparations (lozenges and syrups) to formulas for insect bites, hemorrhoids, toothaches, and musculoskeletal pain. It is being investigated as a treatment for irritable bowel syndrome. Peppermint oil also commonly appears in lotions, aromatic mists, and aromatherapy formulations.

Forms Available Include:

- *For internal use:* A flavoring agent in candy, capsule, infusion (of dried leaves), leaves (fresh and dried), lozenge, oil, syrup, tincture. A tea made from dried peppermint leaves will not necessarily yield medicinal concentrations.
- *For external use:* Oil, ointment, tincture. The oil appears in many commercial formulations; it usually contains substantial amounts of menthol. Sometimes formulations contain extracted menthol only.

Dosage Commonly Reported:

The dried leaf is typically taken in doses of 1.5 to 3 grams, or an infusion is made with that amount. The strength of tinctures varies considerably, and so do recommended dosages. A tincture taken in doses of 2 to 3 milliliters is typical when the ratio of peppermint to liquid is 1 to 5, and contains 45 percent ethanol. For gastrointestinal complaints and as a cholagogue (to stimulate bile production), 3 to 6 grams of the leaves is taken daily. A tea is made using 1 tablespoon (1.5 grams) leaves per cup of water and is drunk three to four times per day between meals. The essential oil is taken in doses of 0.05 to 0.2 milliliter. Enteric-coated capsules of peppermint oil are taken in doses of 0.2 to 0.4 milliliter or up to 0.6 to 1.2 milliliters a day (the enteric coating probably allows for a higher dosage than would be seen with the essential oil taken directly). For gallstones or irritable bowel syndrome, a common dosage is one to two enteric-coated peppermint oil capsules (0.2 milliliters per capsule) three times a day between meals. The undiluted oil is applied externally as a counterirritant. A few drops of the oil are used in steam inhalations.

WARNING: *Never ingest pure menthol;* it is poisonous and as little as a teaspoonful (1 gram per kilogram of body weight) can be fatal.

Will It Work for You? What the Studies Say:

The primary healing component in peppermint is its volatile oil, which contains rich stores (50 percent or more) of menthol, a crystalline alcohol with notable medicinal properties. The menthol is probably responsible for peppermint's renown as a stomach-soother and gas-reducer; studies show that it calms the smooth muscles of the digestive tract (antispasmodic) and facilitates belching.[1] Menthol and other components (probably flavonoids[2]) also stimulate the liver's production of bile, a body fluid that helps break down fats, and thus helps promote digestion.[3] German health authorities approve of peppermint and its volatile oil as an antispasmodic, especially for upper digestive tract conditions, and consider it effective in promoting stomach secretions.[4] The FDA, on the other hand, has declared peppermint oil ineffective as a digestive aid and no longer allows it to be used for this purpose in nonprescription remedies.[5] This decision was reportedly based on a lack of convincing evidence presented to the agency.

The FDA does, however, approve of peppermint oil as a common cold remedy, and both peppermint oil and menthol alone appear in numerous cough and throat lozenges, topical nasal decongestants, inhalants, ointments, and other formulations. Most users report a clearing of congestion in the nose and sinuses.

German health authorities endorse the use of peppermint oil for reducing the symptoms of irritable bowel syndrome, a condition characterized by colicky abdominal pain, bloating, and disturbed bowel habits.[6] Talk to your doctor if you are interested in using peppermint oil for this purpose.

Peppermint has proved itself as an infection fighter in various studies, possibly justifying its traditional use as a wound-healer. It demonstrates antibacterial and antiviral properties in test-tube studies. The oil not only kills numerous bacteria but fights various viruses, including the herpes simplex viruses (types 1 and 2) responsible for cold sores and genital herpes.[7] It has apparently not been well studied for practical treatment of these kinds of infections, however.

Menthol's analgesic and counterirritant properties are widely accepted by the medical establishment, and both menthol and peppermint oil in many cases can be expected to effectively numb pain or produce a cooling sensation on the skin that helps relieve inflammatory pain such as that caused by arthritis and tendinitis.

Will It Harm You? What the Studies Say:

Most adults can drink peppermint tea regularly without worrying about an adverse reaction; the relative concentration of menthol in peppermint tea is actually quite low. Most peppermint-related complaints occur when there are high concentrations of menthol or menthone in the preparation, or when products made with high concentrations of the oil, such as menthol cigarettes, are used.

Take care in giving infants or small children peppermint tea or any preparations of peppermint oil. They may be startled or even gag or choke because of the intense fragrance and the menthol. There have been reports of instant collapse in infants who have had a menthol-containing ointment applied to their nostrils to treat cold symptoms.[8] Talk to a doctor before using peppermint if you suffer from a hiatal hernia, as the oil may exacerbate your symptoms.[9]

If you ingest peppermint oil directly in more than the typically recommended amount, you may be at risk for heartburn and acid reflux. Internal overdosage of the oil has caused dose-dependent brain lesions in rats.[10] If applied undiluted or in high doses, peppermint oil may irritate the skin or mucous membranes, although even recommended doses of peppermint oil or menthol can cause a rash or contact dermatitis in sensitive individuals.

Avoid all peppermint products if you are allergic to menthol, to avoid such reactions as headache, rash, and flushing.[11] Several sources recommend that people with gallstones either consult a doctor before taking peppermint-containing preparations or avoid them altogether.[12]

GENERAL SOURCES:

American Pharmaceutical Association. *Handbook of Nonprescription Drugs.* 11th ed. Washington, D.C.: American Pharmaceutical Association, 1996.

Bisset, N.G., ed. *Herbal Drugs and Phytopharmaceuticals.* Stuttgart: medpharm GmbH Scientific Publishers, 1994.

Blumenthal, M., J. Gruenwald, T. Hall, and R.S. Rister, eds. *The Complete German Commission E Monographs: Therapeutic Guide to Herbal Medicine.* Boston: Integrative Medicine Communications, 1998.

Bradley, P.C., ed. *British Herbal Compendium: A Handbook of Scientific Information on Widely Used Plant Drugs*, vol. 1. Bournemouth (Dorset), England: British Herbal Medicine Association, 1992.

Castleman, M. *The Healing Herbs: The Ultimate Guide to the Curative Power of Nature's Medicines.* New York: Bantam Books, 1995.

Dobelis, I.N., ed. *The Magic and Medicine of Plants: A Practical Guide to the Science, History, Folklore, and Everyday Uses of Medicinal Plants.* Pleasantville, NY: Reader's Digest Association, 1986.

Foster, S. *Peppermint: Mentha x piperta.* American Botanical Council, Botanical Series No. 306. 1991.

Hallowell, M. *Herbal Healing: A Practical Introduction to Medicinal Herbs.* Garden City Park, NY, 1994.

Lawrence Review of Natural Products. St. Louis: Facts and Comparisons, July 1990.

Leung, A.Y., and S. Foster. *Encyclopedia of Common Natural Ingredients Used in Food, Drugs, and Cosmetics.* 2nd ed. New York: John Wiley & Sons, 1996.

Mayell, M. *Off-the-Shelf Natural Health: How to Use Herbs and Nutrients to Stay Well.* New York: Bantam Books, 1995.

Tyler, V.E. *Herbs of Choice: The Therapeutic Use of Phytomedicinals.* Binghamton, NY: Haworth Press/Pharmaceutical Products Press, 1994.

———. *The Honest Herbal.* Binghamton, NY: Haworth Press/Pharmaceutical Products Press, 1993.

TEXT CITATIONS:

1. American Pharmaceutical Association, *Handbook of Nonprescription Drugs*, 11th ed. (Washington, D.C.: American Pharmaceutical Association, 1996).
2. V.E. Tyler, *The Honest Herbal* (Binghamton, NY: Haworth Press/Pharmaceutical Products Press, 1993).
3. G.D. Bell and J. Doran, *British Medical Journal*, 278 (1979): 24. W.R. Ellis and G.D. Bell, *British Medical Journal*, 282 (1981): 611.

4. M. Blumenthal, J. Gruenwald, T. Hall, and R.S. Rister, eds., *The Complete German Commission E Monographs: Therapeutic Guide to Herbal Medicine* (Boston: Integrative Medicine Communications, 1998).
5. Tyler, op. cit.
6. American Pharmaceutical Association, op. cit.
7. A.Y. Leung and S. Foster, *Encyclopedia of Common Natural Ingredients Used in Food, Drugs, and Cosmetics*, 2nd ed. (New York: John Wiley & Sons, 1996).
8. Ibid.
9. *Lawrence Review of Natural Products* (St. Louis: Facts and Comparisons, July 1990).
10. P. Olsen and I. Thorup, *Archives of Toxicology* (Suppl. 7) (1984): 408.
11. *Lawrence Review of Natural Products* (St. Louis: Facts and Comparisons, July 1990).
12. V.E. Tyler, *Herbs of Choice: The Therapeutic Use of Phytomedicinals* (Binghamton, NY: Haworth Press/Pharmaceutical Products Press, 1994).

PRIMARY NAME:

PERIWINKLE, LESSER

SCIENTIFIC NAME:

Vinca minor L. Family: Apocynaceae

COMMON NAMES:

Common periwinkle, myrtle, running myrtle, sorcerer's violet

RATING:

5 = Studies indicate that there is a definite health hazard to using this substance, even in recommended amounts.

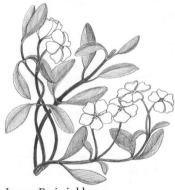

Lesser Periwinkle
Vinca minor

What Is Lesser Periwinkle?

Vinca minor is a hardly evergreen undershrub, the blue-violet flowers, bright green oval leaves, and other aboveground parts of which are used medicinally. The plant is a common ground cover in its native Europe and now grows wild in parts of North America, having escaped the gardens and other enclosed areas in which it was planted.

Although they are related, do not confuse *Vinca minor* with *Vinca major* (greater periwinkle), a somewhat larger plant; or with *Vinca rosea* (formerly *Catharanthus roseus*), a plant with considerably different pharmacologic properties.

What It Is Used For:

The modern applications of this herb differ notably from the recommendations of medieval herbalists, especially in France, where it was referred to as "violette des sorciers" (violet of the sorcerers) in recognition of its perceived ability to ward off evil spirits. Then, it was used to treat such conditions as dizziness and headaches. Today, traditional healers suggest taking periwinkle as a hemostatic (for stopping bleeding) for such conditions as excessive menstrual flow, and to treat circulation disorders (especially for increasing oxygen supply to the brain), protect against aging of brain cells, prevent memory and concentration problems, increase mental productivity, lower blood pressure, alleviate nervous disorders, boost immune function, alleviate sore throat and intestinal inflammation, and remedy a host of other ailments. They recommend it externally as an astringent and hemostatic in wounds. Homeopaths prescribe minute amounts for various ailments. (See page 2 for a discussion of homeopathy.)

Forms Available Include:

Tincture.

Dosage Commonly Reported:

No dosage information available.

Will It Work for You? What the Studies Say:

Lesser periwinkle contains an alkaloid called vincamine, which has been intensively studied since its discovery in the early 1950s and found to have a notable ability to lower blood pressure and counteract cerebral blood flow problems, including strokes and related complications such as memory problems.[2] Many of these studies were apparently well designed, but they all relied on standardized concentrations of purified vincamine, not the herb itself, which contains notoriously low and inconsistent amounts of the alkaloid.[3] For these reasons, and given the fact that the herb's effectiveness for most of the claimed applications is weak, German health authorities declined to approve of periwinkle as a medicinal agent.[4] They also cited health risks.

Will It Harm You? What the Studies Say:

A number of sources have cited concerns about the safety of this herb. The FDA placed lesser periwinkle on its formerly maintained list of "unsafe" herbs. German health authorities cite findings from animal experiments in which the herb lowered levels of critical immune system cells such as lymphocytes and other white blood cells.[5]

GENERAL SOURCES:

Blumenthal, M., J. Gruenwald, T. Hall, and R.S. Rister, eds. *The Complete German Commission E Monographs: Therapeutic Guide to Herbal Medicine.* Boston: Integrative Medicine Communications, 1998.

Dobelis, I.N., ed. *The Magic and Medicine of Plants: A Practical Guide to the Science, History, Folklore, and Everyday Uses of Medicinal Plants.* Pleasantville, NY: Reader's Digest Association, 1986.

Hylton, W.H. ed. *The Rodale Herb Book: How to Use, Grow, and Buy Nature's Miracle Plants.* Emmaus, PA: Rodale Press, Inc., 1974.

Mayell, M. *Off-the-Shelf Natural Health: How to Use Herbs and Nutrients to Stay Well.* New York: Bantam Books, 1995.

Weiner, M.A., and J.A. Weiner. *Herbs That Heal: Prescription for Herbal Healing.* Mill Valley, CA: Quantum Books, 1994.

Weiss, R.F. *Herbal Medicine*, trans. A.R. Meuss, from the 6th German edition. Beaconsfield, England: Beaconsfield Publishers, Ltd., 1988.

TEXT CITATIONS:

1. Dobelis, I.N., ed. *The Magic and Medicine of Plants: A Practical Guide to the Science, History, Folklore, and Everyday Uses of Medicinal Plants* (Pleasantville, NY: Reader's Digest Association, 1986).

2. Weiss, R.F. *Herbal Medicine*, trans. A.R. Meuss, from the 6th German edition (Beaconsfield, England: Beaconsfield Publishers, Ltd., 1988).

3. Ibid.

4. M. Blumenthal, J. Gruenwald, T. Hall, and R.S. Rister, eds., *The Complete German Commission E Monographs: Therapeutic Guide to Herbal Medicine* (Boston: Integrative Medicine Communications, 1998).

5. Ibid.

PRIMARY NAME:
L-PHENYLALANINE

SCIENTIFIC NAME:
N/A

COMMON NAME:
Phenylalanine

RATING:
4 = Research indicates that this substance will not fulfill the claims made for it, but that it is also unlikely to cause any harm.

What Is L-Phenylalanine?

L-phenylalanine is an essential amino acid. "Essential" means that your body cannot manufacture it on its own and must get it through the foods you eat.

What It Is Used For:

The body uses this essential amino acid in many ways. One of the most important is to convert it into another amino acid, L-tyrosine, endowed with its own task of producing the important neurotransmitters dopamine, norepinephrine, and epinephrine (see **L-Tyrosine**). Advocates assert that taking L-phenylalanine supplements will boost alertness, memory, and learning, increase energy, suppress the appetite, diminish pain, reverse mental depression and generally elevate mood, and stimulate the libido. Conditions it is recommended for include obesity, migraine headache, arthritis, depression, schizophrenia, and Parkinson's disease.

Forms Available Include:

Capsule, powder. So-called "smart drinks" (combinations of fruit, juice, and nutritional supplements) often contain L-phenylalanine. Good dietary sources of this amino acid include bananas, almonds, cottage cheese, peanuts, nonfat dried milk, and sesame seeds.

Dosage Commonly Reported:

Capsules or powders are commonly taken in dosages of 375 to 500 milligrams once or twice daily thirty minutes before a meal. DL-phenylalanine (a mixed form of L-phenylalanine and d-phenylalanine, also called DLPA) is typically taken in doses of 500 to 1,000 milligrams.

Will It Work for You? What the Studies Say:

Despite numerous claims made for the benefit of supplementing the diet with single amino acids like L-phenylalanine, there is little information in the recent medical literature to support them. See **L-Tyrosine** for more information.

Will It Harm You? What the Studies Say:

Concerns have been raised about the wisdom of supplementing the diet with any single amino acid; see **L-Tyrosine** for more information. Several sources warn that pregnant and nursing women as well as individuals who are afflicted with high blood pressure, taking a monoamine oxidase (MAO) inhibitor, or suffering from the disorder known as phenylketonuria should not take L-phenylalanine supplements.

GENERAL SOURCES:

Balch, J.F., and P.A. Balch. *Prescription for Nutritional Healing: A Practical A to Z Reference to Drug-Free Remedies Using Vitamins, Minerals, Herbs & Food Supplements.* 2nd ed. Garden City Park, NY: Avery Publishing Group, 1997.

Griffith, H.W. *Complete Guide to Vitamins, Minerals, Nutrients & Supplements.* Tucson: Fisher Books, 1988.

Mayell, M. *Off-the-Shelf Natural Health: How to Use Herbs and Nutrients to Stay Well.* New York: Bantam Books, 1995.

Weiner, M.A., and J.A. Weiner. *Herbs That Heal: Prescription for Herbal Healing*. Mill Valley, CA: Quantum Books, 1994.

PRIMARY NAME:
PICRORHIZA

SCIENTIFIC NAME:
Picrorhiza kurroa Royle ex Benth. Family: Scrophulariaceae

COMMON NAME:
Hu huang lian

RATING:
3 = Studies on the effectiveness and safety of this substance are conflicting, or there are not enough studies to draw a conclusion.

What Is Picrorhiza?

The roots and rhizomes (underground stems) of this flowering perennial are used medicinally. It is native to mountainous regions of India, Tibet, and Nepal.

What It Is Used For:

Traditional Indian (Ayurvedic) healers have relied on this plant for centuries to treat lung and liver disorders including hepatitis and poor bile production, constipation, digestive upset, and snakebites, among other ailments. Traditional Chinese healers have treated infectious and chronic diarrhea with it, reportedly using the species known as *Picrorhiza scrophylariaeflora* interchangeably with *Picrorhiza kurroa*. Picrorhiza is increasingly available in the United States.

Forms Available Include:

Capsule (containing picroliv in standardized form).

Dosage Commonly Reported:

Take this herb only under professional supervision.

Will It Work for You? What the Studies Say:

Researchers in India particularly have focused on this herb and its medicinal potential. Their studies, most of them on rodents or small animals, indicate that the herb and standardized extracts of it, such as picroliv, may help protect the liver, control asthma, reduce inflammation, stimulate the immune system, fight viruses, positively affect bile output, and even help control potentially dangerous cell changes that sometimes develop into cancers. The studies reported did not involve human beings, but this may now be changing. Picroliv in particular is reportedly now being tested in humans (in phase II clinical trials) in India.[1]

Indian investigators have hailed picroliv as a powerful liver-protectant. The compound and a mixture of glycosides from the rhizomes and roots called kutkin have proved effective in protecting rats from chemically induced liver damage in various studies.[2] Several experiments have displayed the power of this component to help stimulate liver growth in rats who have had part of this organ removed,[3] and a few experiments have found picroliv more potent than silymarin, a widely reported liver-protectant from milk thistle (see **Milk Thistle**), in protecting rat liver cells placed in a test tube.[4] Another group of researchers found the protectant properties of kutkin comparable if not superior to silibinin—an intravenous formulation made from the milk thistle herb—in mice exposed to toxic substances from the highly poisonous amanita

505

(deathcap) mushroom (*Amanita phalloides*).[5] Unlike these milk thistle components, however, the liver-protectant properties of *Picrorhiza kurroa* have reportedly never been studied in humans.

Antiasthmatic properties have also been observed in small-animal studies.[6] In a 1991 investigation involving guinea pigs, the glycoside androsin helped prevent the bronchial obstruction caused by certain components of the inflammatory cascade.[7] The same investigators found in test-tube studies that other substances in the herb helped inhibit inflammatory white cells involved in the release of histamine and generalized asthmatic responses. In another investigation, researchers identified anti-inflammatory properties and possibly even anticlotting properties in apocynin, another compound isolated from *Picrorhiza kurroa*.[8]

Although it is still far from clear that kutkin and other substances in the herb will have the same effect in humans, they have showed promise as generalized anti-inflammatory substances when injected into rats and mice subjected to a variety of standard inflammation models.[9] Lipid-lowering properties have also been found in rats administered picroliv.[10] Hamster studies have shown that picroliv increases immune system activity after the animals are infected with the parasite that causes the tropical disease leishmaniasis.[11]

Will It Harm You? What the Studies Say:

Little is known about the potential of this plant to cause harm. However, although no reports of serious adverse reactions appear in the recent medical literature, it is clear from test-tube and animal studies that it has active components that may well affect the human body. For this reason, it should probably be taken only under professional supervision, at least until sound toxicity studies in humans have been conducted. Pregnant women should definitely avoid it until more data are available.

GENERAL SOURCES:

Chevallier, A. *The Encyclopedia of Medicinal Plants: A Practical Reference Guide to More Than 550 Key Medicinal Plants & Their Uses.* 1st American ed. New York: Dorling Kindersley Publications, 1996.

TEXT CITATIONS:

1. B.N. Dhawan, *Med Chem Res.* 5(8) (1995): 595–605.
2. R.A. Ansari et al., *Indian Journal of Medical Research.* 87(April 1988): 401–4. Y. Dwivedi et al., *Pharmacology and Toxicology,* 71(5) (1992): 383–87.
3. S. Saksena et al., *Phytotherapy Research,* 9(7) (1995): 518–21.
4. P.K.S. Visen et al., *Phythotherapy Research,* 5(5) (1991): 224–27.
5. G.L. Floersheim et al., *Agents and Actions,* 29(3–4) (1990): 386–87.
6. W. Dorsch and H. Wagner, *International Archives of Allergy and Applied Immunology,* 94(1–4) (1991): 262–65.
7. W. Dorsch et al., *International Archives of Allergy and Applied Immunology,* 95(2–3) (1991): 128–33.
8. F. Engels et al., *FEBS Letters for the Rapid Publication of Short Reports in Biochemistry, Biophysics and Molecular Biology,* 305(3) (1992): 254–56.
9. G. Singh et al., *Phytotherapy Research,* 7(6) (1993): 402–7.

10. A.K. Khanna et al., *Phytotherapy Research*, 8(7) (1994): 403–7.
11. A. Puri et al., *Planta Medica*, 58(6) (1992): 528–32.

PINEAPPLE

SCIENTIFIC NAME:
Ananas comosus L. Merr., sometimes referred to as *Ananas sativus* Schult. f. Family: Bromeliaceae

COMMON NAME:
N/A

RATING:
3 = Studies on the effectiveness of this substance are conflicting, or there are not enough studies to draw a conclusion. Its safety depends on judicious use, however; see the "Will It Harm You?" section.

What Is Pineapple?

Most North Americans have no trouble identifying this large, distinctively shaped, succulent reddish-yellow fruit. The tropical perennial has lance-shaped leaves with spiny edges and a short, sturdy stem. It has no seeds. The fruit, juice, leaves, and extracted enzymes called bromelains are used medicinally. Pineapple also contains at least three other proteolytic (protein-digesting) enzymes, but they have not been as thoroughly studied as the bromelains.[1]

What It Is Used For:

In addition to its fame as a juicy treat, the ripe pineapple fruit has long been valued as a folk remedy for settling gas, soothing other digestive upsets, reducing constipation (it is high in fiber), controlling nervous exhaustion, and destroying intestinal worms. Herbalists classify pineapple juice as a digestive tonic and diuretic ("water pill"). The sour, unripe fruit is also said to improve the appetite, encourage good digestion, and relieve indigestion. Traditional Indian healers consider it a uterine tonic. The leaves have traditionally been used to stimulate menstrual periods and ease painful menstruation. The fresh fruit has been made into facial masks.

Commercial manufacturers extract bromelain, one of the plant's enzymes, for use as a meat tenderizer. It has also been promoted as relieving a number of ailments (and as improving digestion) by helping to break down food more completely. Some sources recommend bromelain for removing dead tissue from skin burns; for treating inflammation and edema (fluid retention or swelling) caused by surgery, trauma, allergies, arthritis, and infections; and for easing diarrhea due to digestive enzyme deficiency. Others promote it for respiratory tract infections, painful menses, vein inflammation (thrombophlebitis) and varicose veins, wound-healing, pain and swelling in sports injuries, and ulcer prevention, and as an adjunct to cancer therapy. Bromelain appears in cosmetics such as facial cleansers and bath preparations and in food as an agent to chill-proof beer and modify dough. It is often used as a substitute for the more costly proteolytic enzyme called papain, derived from the unripe papaya fruit (see **Papaya**).

There are two types of bromelain: that taken from the fruit, called fruit bromelain; and that taken from the stem, called stem bromelain. Commercial bromelain is typically made with stem bromelain.[2]

Forms Available Include:

- *Pineapple:* Candied, canned, fresh fruit, juice, syrup.
- *Bromelain:* Tablet (usually with indication of potency based on enzyme units established by the supplier). The extract also appears in vitamin and herbal blends.

P

Pineapple

Dosage Commonly Reported:

Bromelain is taken three times a day in doses of 250 to 500 milligrams. As a digestive aid it is taken after meals; otherwise it is taken on an empty stomach.

Will It Work for You? What the Studies Say:

Pineapple juice has been reported to be diuretic, meaning that it increases urine output. This may explain its popularity in folk medicine for bladder ailments, kidney stones, venereal diseases, and certain other disorders. Apparently its effectiveness for these illnesses has not been properly tested in humans, although animal studies indicate that topical formulations of enzymes from pineapple may indeed help burn wounds heal.[3]

As many as two hundred or more scientific papers have been published on bromelain since it was first introduced as a medicinal agent in the late 1950s.[4] Overall they indicate a broad spectrum of actions, from the ability to reduce inflammation to an ability to relax smooth muscles, prevent ulcers, relieve sinus inflammation, enhance the absorption of antibiotics, inhibit the appetite, shorten labor, treat urinary tract infections, reduce pain, interfere with the growth of malignant cells, break up blood clots (fibrinolytic), and inhibit blood platelet aggregation (thus decreasing the risk of clotting).[5]

However, the American medical community no longer prescribes bromelain as it once did because clinical trials failed to prove that it was actually effective for most of these ailments when given to human beings.[6] Today, bromelain is widely sold as a dietary supplement in health food and other outlets and is still used in conventional medicine to treat inflammation and swelling caused by surgery, injuries, allergies, and infections, and to remove dead skin tissue associated with burns. Still, the wisdom of these uses has been challenged, given a lack of supporting data from clinical trials.[7]

For information on bromelain's success in aiding digestion, see **Papaya**, which contains a discussion of a similarly used enzyme, papain.

Will It Harm You? What the Studies Say:

Ripe pineapple is considered harmless in moderate doses, but stay away from the unripe fruit; it is poisonous and can cause violent vomiting.[8] Large doses of the ripe fruit juice have reportedly caused uterine contractions, so pregnant women may want to take extra care to limit themselves to moderate amounts.[9] Eating large amounts of the fruit can also cause mouth sores involving a breakdown of the lip tissue.[10] Nausea, vomiting, diarrhea, skin rash, and excessive menstrual flow have been reported in individuals taking medicinal doses of bromelain.[11] Bromelain can cause allergic reactions if you have been sensitized to the substance or are exposed to it over long periods of time in your job.[12] An odd reaction among pineapple cutters has been noted: repeated exposure to the bromelain destroys their fingerprints.[13]

GENERAL SOURCES:

Duke, J.A. *CRC Handbook of Medicinal Herbs.* Boca Raton, FL: CRC Press, 1985.
Lawrence Review of Natural Products. St. Louis: Facts and Comparisons, July 1993.

Leung, A.Y., and S. Foster. *Encyclopedia of Common Natural Ingredients Used in Food, Drugs, and Cosmetics.* 2nd ed. New York: John Wiley & Sons, 1996.

Mayell, M. *Off-the-Shelf Natural Health: How to Use Herbs and Nutrients to Stay Well.* New York: Bantam Books, 1995.

Murray, M.T. *The Healing Power of Herbs: The Enlightened Person's Guide to the Wonders of Medicinal Plants.* Rev. 2nd ed. Rocklin, CA: Prima Publishing, 1995.

Weiss, R.F. *Herbal Medicine*, trans. A.R. Meuss, from the 6th German edition. Beaconsfield, England: Beaconsfield Publishers, Ltd., 1988.

TEXT CITATIONS:

1. *Lawrence Review of Natural Products* (St. Louis: Facts and Comparisons, July 1993).
2. A.Y. Leung and S. Foster, *Encyclopedia of Common Natural Ingredients Used in Food, Drugs, and Cosmetics*, 2nd ed. (New York: John Wiley & Sons, 1996).
3. A.D. Rowan et al., *Burns*, 16(4) (1990): 243.
4. M.T. Murray, *The Healing Power of Herbs: The Enlightened Person's Guide to the Wonders of Medicinal Plants*, rev. 2nd ed. (Rocklin, CA: Prima Publishing, 1995).
5. Leung and Foster, op. cit. S.J. Taussig and S. Batkin, *Journal of Ethnopharmacology*, 22(2) (1988): 191–203.
6. *Lawrence Review of Natural Products*, op. cit.
7. Leung and Foster, op. cit. S. Kumakura et al., *European Journal of Pharmacology*, 150 (1988): 295.
8. J.A. Duke, *CRC Handbook of Medicinal Herbs* (Boca Raton, FL: CRC Press, 1985).
9. Leung and Foster, op. cit.
10. Duke, op cit.
11. Leung and Foster, op. cit.
12. Murray, op. cit.
13. Duke, op. cit.

PRIMARY NAME:

PLEURISY ROOT

SCIENTIFIC NAME:

Asclepias tuberosa L. Family: Asclepiadaceae

COMMON NAMES:

Asclepias, butterfly weed, pipple root, silkweed, swallow wort, tuber root, wind root

RATING:

5 = Studies indicate that there is a definite health hazard to using this substance in many cases, even in recommended amounts.

What Is Pleurisy Root?

Asclepias tuberosa is a hardy perennial shrub that grows in dry soils across the Americas. Its stiff stems send off loose spirals of long, pointed leaves, and clusters of showy, nectar-rich orange flowers that bloom from May through September. Seed-filled pods open in autumn. The root is used medicinally.

What It Is Used For:

Considering the primary name, it comes as no surprise that this plant was traditionally used to treat pleurisy, a painful inflammation of the lung lining. The *U.S. Pharmacopoeia* listed it for this purpose for seventy years, up until 1890. Native Americans and settlers reportedly turned to it for other respiratory conditions as well, such as asthma, colds, flu, bronchitis, and even pneumonia, and as an expectorant to clear lung and nasal congestion. Large doses were used to induce vomiting. A root poultice was placed on rheumatic pains, bruises, and other external ailments.

A number of contemporary herbalists consider pleurisy root effective for pleurisy, chest congestion, and other respiratory disorders, and some encourage

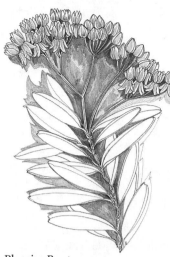

Pleurisy Root
Asclepias tuberosa

its use for easing digestion, soothing stomach upset, and reducing a fever by inducing perspiration.

Forms Available Include:
Decoction, liquid extract, powder (of dried root), tincture.

Dosage Commonly Reported:
1 tablespoon of powdered root is mixed in 8 ounces of warm liquid and drunk once a day. The liquid root extract is taken in doses of 2.5 to 5 milliliters.

Will It Work for You? What the Studies Say:
Researchers have largely ignored this herb, and consequently very little is known about its potential for healing. Concerns about toxicity preclude its widespread use in any case (see "Will It Harm You?" section). Some states have declared *Asclepias tuberosa* a protected plant.[1]

Will It Harm You? What the Studies Say:
Research has revealed enough about this herb to determine that it can be harmful. People with heart problems in particular may want to proceed with caution; pleurisy root contains toxic cardiac glycosides,[2] a class of medications with important effects on the muscle and electrical conduction system of the heart. Digitalis is a cardiac glycoside, for example. A simple tea made from pleurisy root was found to have digoxinlike activity (increasing the heart's ability to contract forcefully with a regular rhythm).[3] The herb may interfere with certain heart medicines.[4]

The few experiments that have been done on this herb indicate that it has estrogenlike effects (estrogen is a female hormone) and can cause uterine contractions in animals.[5] Given these findings, pregnant women may want to avoid the herb. Very large doses of the root may also interfere with hormonal therapy and medicines that alter amine concentrations in the brain, such as antidepressants.[6]

GENERAL SOURCES:
Bradley, P.C., ed. *British Herbal Compendium: A Handbook of Scientific Information on Widely Used Plant Drugs*, vol. 1. Bournemouth (Dorset), England: British Herbal Medicine Association, 1992.
Dobelis, I.N., ed. *The Magic and Medicine of Plants: A Practical Guide to the Science, History, Folklore, and Everyday Uses of Medicinal Plants.* Pleasantville, NY: Reader's Digest Association, 1986.
Mindell, E. *Earl Mindell's Herb Bible.* New York: Simon & Schuster/Fireside, 1992.
Newall, C.A., et al. *Herbal Medicines: A Guide for Health-Care Professionals.* London: The Pharmaceutical Press, 1996.
Tierra, M. *The Way of Herbs.* New York: Pocket Books, 1990.
Tyler, V.E. *The Honest Herbal.* Binghamton, NY: Haworth Press/Pharmaceutical Products Press, 1993.
Weiner, M.A., and J.A. Weiner. *Herbs That Heal: Prescription for Herbal Healing.* Mill Valley, CA: Quantum Books, 1994.

TEXT CITATIONS:

1. I.N. Dobelis, ed., *The Magic and Medicine of Plants: A Practical Guide to the Science, History, Folklore, and Everyday Uses of Medicinal Plants* (Pleasantville, NY: Reader's Digest Association, 1986).
2. J.N. Seiber et al., *Plant Toxicology. Proceedings of the Australia/USA Poisonous Plants Symposium* (1985): 427–37.
3. L. Longerich et al., *Clinical & Investigative Medicine*, 16(3) (1993): 210–18.
4. C.A. Newall et al., *Herbal Medicines: A Guide for Health-Care Professionals* (London: The Pharmaceutical Press, 1996).
5. P.C. Bradley, ed., *British Herbal Compendium: A Handbook of Scientific Information on Widely Used Plant Drugs*, vol. 1 (Bournemouth [Dorset], England: British Herbal Medicine Association, 1992). C.H. Costello and C.L. Butler, *Journal of the American Pharmaceutical Association. Scientific Edition*, 39 (1949): 233–37. W.E. Hassan and H.L. Reed, *Journal of the American Pharmaceutical Association. Scientific Edition*, 41 (1952): 298–300.
6. Newall, op. cit.

PRIMARY NAME:
POKEWEED

SCIENTIFIC NAME:
Phytolacca americana L. and various other *Phytolacca* species. Family: Phytolaccaceae

COMMON NAMES:
Cancer jalap, cancer root, chongras, coakum, crowberry, garget, inkberry, pigeonberry, poke, pokeberry, pokeroot, red ink plant, scoke, shang lu

RATING:
5 = Studies indicate that there is a definite health hazard to using this substance, even in recommended amounts.

What Is Pokeweed?

This hardy, shrublike perennial, something of a wayside weed, sprouts a profusion of small greenish-white flowers on its many branches. Over time, these blossoms turn into clusters of dark purple, nearly black juicy berries. Pokeweed grows abundantly in North America, to which it is indigenous, as well as in southern Europe and northern Africa. The roots and leaves have been used medicinally.

What It Is Used For:

Herbalists have recommended pokeweed for a dizzying spectrum of ailments, from indigestion to rheumatism and painful menstrual periods. Its slow-acting but proven ability to induce vomiting and clear the bowels has long been noted. Various Native American tribes reportedly drank pokeweed berry tea for rheumatism and treated cancer with the powdered root. The berry juice and the root in ointment or decoction form, sometimes as a poultice, were traditionally used to treat skin infections, ulcers, tumors, cancers, inflamed joints, and hemorrhoids. In Europe, pokeweed has a reputation as a lymph system cleanser. Well-cooked young shoots have been used as greens and potherbs, and properly treated berries have been enjoyed as fruits. Scientists occasionally use pokeweed extracts in laboratory studies.

Forms Available Include:

Capsule, poultice, root (dried or powdered), tincture.

Dosage Commonly Reported:

Pokeweed should not be used medicinally.

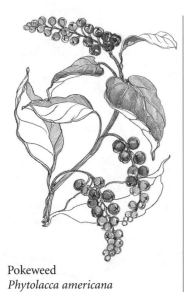

Pokeweed
Phytolacca americana

Will It Work for You? What the Studies Say:

Pokeweed is not a practical healing herb; vomiting and catharsis (bowel evacuation) can be expected, owing to its contained toxins. The implications of various study findings are hard to determine, for this and other reasons. Researchers have isolated a protein that fights many plant and human viruses quite vigorously, including the virus that causes AIDS (HIV).[1] In test-tube studies, extracts effectively destroy leukemia cells.[2] Anti-inflammatory substances called triterpenoid saponins have been identified in the roots.[3]

Will It Harm You? What the Studies Say:

Except for properly treated young (still green) leaves and well-cooked berries, all parts of the mature pokeweed plant can cause toxic reactions. The rootstock is the most poisonous. Fatalities in children and serious adverse reactions requiring hospitalization in adults have been reported. Poisonings occurred frequently in nineteenth-century America, often because people mistook pokeweed for the similar-appearing Jerusalem artichoke, horseradish, or parsnip.[4] Pokeweed teas also caused poisonings.[5]

Toxicity is due to a saponin mixture called phytolaccatoxin, as well as a protein called pokeweed mitogen, which can cause blood cell abnormalities. Signs and symptoms of poisoning, which are usually self-limited (ceasing without intervention), include severe stomach cramping, nausea, frothy diarrhea, intense vomiting, weakness, dizziness, headache, slow and labored breathing, spasms, low blood pressure, and convulsions. One middle-aged male developed heart block after eating raw or possibly cooked pokeweed leaves.[6] Mild poisonings can last for twenty-four hours. The toxic elements in the plant can enter the circulation through cuts on the skin, so protective gloves should be worn when handling it.[7] The FDA placed pokeweed on its formerly maintained list of "Herbs of Undefined Safety," citing narcotic effects.

In 1979, the Herb Trade Association issued a policy statement saying that the plant should not be sold as a food or herbal beverage and that any products containing it should be labeled with toxicity warnings regarding internal use.[8]

GENERAL SOURCES:

Duke, J.A. *CRC Handbook of Medicinal Herbs.* Boca Raton, FL: CRC Press, 1985.

Lawrence Review of Natural Products. St. Louis: Facts and Comparisons, April 1991.

Newall, C.A., et al. *Herbal Medicines: A Guide for Health-Care Professionals.* London: The Pharmaceutical Press, 1996.

Ody, P. *The Herb Society's Complete Medicinal Herbal.* London: Dorling Kindersley Limited, 1993.

Tyler, V.E. *The Honest Herbal.* Binghamton, NY: Haworth Press/Pharmaceutical Products Press, 1993.

Tyler, V.E., L.R. Brady, and J.E. Robbers, eds. *Pharmacognosy.* Philadelphia: Lea & Febiger, 1988.

TEXT CITATIONS:

1. Y. Hur et al., *Proceedings of the National Academy of Sciences of the United States of America,* 92(18) (1995): 8448–52.
2. J.Y. Chu et al., *Journal of Tongji Medical University,* 10(1) (1990): 15–18.

3. W.S. Woo et al., *Planta Medica*, 34 (1978): 87.
4. W.H. Lewis and P.R. Smith, *Journal of the American Medical Association* (letter), 242 (1975): 2759.
5. Ibid.
6. R.J. Hamilton et al., *Veterinary & Human Toxicology*, 37(1) (1995): 66–67.
7. V.E. Tyler, L.R. Brady, and J.E. Robbers, eds., *Pharmacognosy* (Philadelphia: Lea & Febiger, 1988).
8. Ibid.

POPPY

SCIENTIFIC NAME:
Papaver somniferum L. Family: Papaveraceae

COMMON NAMES:
Opium poppy, poppyseed poppy

RATING:
1 = Years of use and extensive, high-quality studies indicate that this substance is very effective when used in recommended amounts for the indication(s) noted in the "Will It Work for You?" section. Its safety depends on judicious use, however; see the "Will It Harm You?" section.

What Is Poppy?

The large, showy flowers of this erect annual have white, pink, red, or purple petals with dark basal spots. The flowers bloom in May across cultivated fields in Asia and the Mideast. The leaves are dark green and have serrated edges. The unripe seed capsules contain a thick white latex known as opium. The seeds themselves range in color from off-white to blue-black.

What It Is Used For:

The Sumerians living in Mesopotamia in 3000 B.C. called the opium poppy the "joy plant." The Greeks, Arabs, and Romans valued it as a medicinal herb capable of inducing sedation and sleepiness, although they also recognized its addictive potential. Few major cultures around the world have not come into contact with the poppy over the centuries or failed to recognize its double-edged gift of pain relief and smothering addiction. When smoked, opium is an addictive intoxicant. A German pharmacist isolated the first plant alkaloid ever—morphine—in 1803. Just over seventy years later, heroin was created through the mixture of morphine and acetic anhydride. Codeine is also derived from opium alkaloids, as are narcotine, papaverine, and laudenine. These alkaloids are variously used for their narcotic, analgesic (painkilling), sedative, hypnotic, antispasmodic, and cough-suppressant properties.

Today, opium derivatives still figure prominently in cough medicines, painkillers, and diarrhea medicines. Efforts to control the illegal use of morphine, codeine, and heroin—all addictive narcotics—have had limited success.

Poppy seeds, which contain no opium, are popular for use in breads and sweets and as a base for an industrial drying oil.

Forms Available Include:

Derivatives such as codeine are added to many prescription medications. Seeds (for use in cooking).

Dosage Commonly Reported:

Follow the doctor's instructions for prescription medications containing opium derivatives.

Will It Work for You? What the Studies Say:

Few if any other plants outrank the opium poppy in their power to control pain and induce other medicinal actions or in their potential for harm. Researchers have learned a lot about the chemical structure of the plant, carefully studying the more than thirty alkaloids in the milky latex from the unripe seed capsules. Interestingly, the ripened and opened seed capsules contain none of the active (or potentially harmful) alkaloids.

The poppy plant continues to represent a major source of morphine and codeine. Morphine is considered one of the most effective analgesics. It controls pain by blocking the nerve impulses that transmit pain messages to the brain. Addicts take it for its associated ability to melt away anxiety, inhibition, fear, and other unwanted feelings, inducing a state of euphoria and stimulation. Codeine is, like morphine, sedative and analgesic, and appears in prescriptions for minor pain. Both alkaloids also relax smooth muscles and can therefore reduce cramping and control diarrhea. Codeine's capacity to suppress the cough reflex explains why it is added to prescription cough medicines. Another alkaloid, papaverine, is prescribed for asthma-related respiratory spasms, intestinal and stomach spasms, and other muscular contractions because it effectively relaxes involuntary smooth muscles. It also increases blood flow to the brain.

Investigators are searching for other *Papaver* species that contain the critical morphine derivatives capable of being synthesized into codeine.[1]

Will It Harm You? What the Studies Say:

Even a cursory student of history learns about the devastating impact this herb has had on the health of millions who have abused it. An overdose will typically cause cold, clammy skin; a fast, weak pulse; fluid in the lungs; cyanosis; constriction of the pupils; and subsequent death from circulatory and respiratory failure unless emergency treatment is given promptly. Opium addicts can reportedly tolerate as much as 2,000 milligrams over four hours, but most people will probably die after taking as little as 300 milligrams.[2]

Poppy seeds contain none of the medicinal properties of opium. They do not pose any risk of adverse reactions; they contain none of the narcotic alkaloids. However, testing for illegal drugs has brought to light that eating foods containing these seeds can increase codeine and morphine in the urine to suspicious levels. These opiates have been detected in the urine of people who had consumed poppy-seed-containing foods, such as poppy-seed bagels, as much as forty-eight hours earlier.[3]

GENERAL SOURCES:

Bremness, L. *Herbs.* 1st American ed. Eyewitness Handbooks. New York: Dorling Kindersley Publications, 1994.

Dobelis, I.N., ed. *The Magic and Medicine of Plants: A Practical Guide to the Science, History, Folklore, and Everyday Uses of Medicinal Plants.* Pleasantville, NY: Reader's Digest Association, 1986.

Duke, J.A. *CRC Handbook of Medicinal Herbs.* Boca Raton, FL: CRC Press, 1985.

Lawrence Review of Natural Products. St. Louis: Facts and Comparisons, December 1990.

Weiss, R.F. *Herbal Medicine*, trans. A.R. Meuss, from the 6th German edition. Beaconsfield, England: Beaconsfield Publishers, Ltd., 1988.

TEXT CITATIONS:
1. *Lawrence Review of Natural Products* (St. Louis: Facts and Comparisons, December 1990).
2. J.A. Duke, *CRC Handbook of Medicinal Herbs* (Boca Raton, FL: CRC Press, 1985).
3. L.W. Hayes et al., *Clinical Chemistry*, 33 (1987): 806.

PRICKLY ASH (NORTHERN and SOUTHERN)

SCIENTIFIC NAME:
Zanthoxylum clava-herculis L. (southern) and *Zanthoxylum americanum* Mill. (northern), with *Zanthoxylum* sometimes spelled *Xanthoxylum*. Family: Rutaceae

COMMON NAMES:
Northern prickly ash: Angelica tree, suterberry, toothache tree; Southern prickly ash: Hercules' club

RATING:
3 = Studies on the effectiveness and safety of this substance are conflicting, or there are not enough studies to draw a conclusion.

What Is Prickly Ash?

The northern prickly ash, native to the northern, central, and western regions of the United States, is a deciduous, flowering shrub with thorny branches and compound leaves that smell lemony when crushed. Lemon-scented dots can also be found on the round, reddish berries. As the name suggests, the closely related southern prickly ash grows in central and southern regions of the country. It is larger than its northern cousin, and has knotty, rough bark. The bark and berries of both varieties are used medicinally.

What It Is Used For:

Northern and southern prickly ash have traditionally been used in similar ways. Native American tribes used to chew dried bark pieces and pack the moist mass around a painful toothache, hence the popular name, toothache tree.[1] They reportedly also chewed the bark for rheumatism and to stimulate the circulation, although the berries may have been more heavily used or even preferred for these purposes.[2] In any case, many settlers picked up the practice, sometimes using pulverized root or bark. Prickly ash was also commonly used as a diaphoretic (to stimulate perspiration) and antispasmodic, and folk healers counted on it to treat venereal disease, flatulence (gas), typhoid pneumonia, and diarrhea. It was included in Harry Hoxey's renowned (and ultimately debunked) cancer cure.

Many contemporary herbalists place prickly ash high on their lists of remedies for alleviating toothache and gum pain, and a number cite it for treating rheumatic conditions, inducing sweating, and reversing sluggish circulation due to such ailments as Raynaud's disease and intermittent claudication (narrowing of arteries). Poultices made with the bark are said to encourage healing of stubborn wounds.

Forms Available Include:

Bark (to chew and place around aching teeth), berries, decoction (of bark), liquid extract from bark, lotion, tablet, tincture.

Dosage Commonly Reported:

A small amount of the bark is chewed and the moist mass packed around an aching tooth. A decoction made with 1 to 2 grams of the dried bark is taken three times a day. The liquid bark extract is taken in doses of 1 to 3 milliliters three times a day, and the liquid fruit extract is taken in doses of 0.5 to 1.5 milliliters.

Will It Work for You? What the Studies Say:

Scant scientific information has been collected on the healing properties of prickly ash, particularly the northern type.[3] The chemical makeup of the southern type has been relatively well documented,[4] although how the constituents will affect human health is not altogether clear. The herb may have anti-inflammatory and painkilling properties, at least according to studies that involved feeding rats chelerythrine, an alkaloid extract found in the plants.[5] Research has also demonstrated that the contained alkaloid nitidine lowers blood pressure in mice.[6] Whether humans who take prickly ash preparations will experience these effects is unknown.

According to widespread experience in humans, chewing the bark of either northern or southern prickly ash will cause tingling sensations in the mouth and help relieve toothache pain,[7] although scientists are still not sure to which constituent to ascribe this local anesthetic and anti-inflammatory action. Some experts suspect that an aromatic substance called fagaramide found in a related species indigenous to West Africa, *Zanthoxylum zanthoxyloides* (Lam.) Watson, may be responsible.[8] Scientists still have to determine whether the North American prickly ash species contain fagaramide. Prickly ash bark apparently induces copious salivation, which may further reduce pain.[9]

Zanthoxylum species native to other parts of the world have been much more intensively studied than the North American types, and antibacterial, cardiovascular, and anthelmintic (antiworm) properties documented in them. Interestingly, studies have found extensive antibacterial and antifungal (against *Candida*) microbial properties in a common Nigerian "chewing stick" made from the root of the *Zanthoxylum zanthoxyloides*.[10]

As for the other traditional uses for prickly ash, even less substantiating information can be found. The recent medical literature contains no references to test-tube, animal, or human tests of prickly ash. The *U.S. Pharmacopoeia* listed the dried bark as a treatment for chronic rheumatism from 1820 to 1926, and the *National Formulary* included the berries from 1916 to 1947 for reported stimulant, antirheumatic, and antispasmodic properties. But whether the plant lives up to the reputation suggested by these former listings is hard to determine.

Will It Harm You? What the Studies Say:

There are no reports of harm linked to short-term and moderate use of this herb in humans, but given what little is known about it, it would be best to stick to moderate dosages. There are reports of cattle, chicken, and fish dying as a result of ingesting southern prickly ash, probably owing to the bark's neuromuscular blocking properties.[11] Northern prickly ash contains coumarins that could, theoretically, interfere with anticoagulant (anticlotting) medicines.[12] Pregnant and nursing women should definitely avoid medicinal concentrations, given the lack of data on the herb.[13] The FDA includes prickly ash bark on its list of substances "Generally Recognized As Safe" (GRAS) for food use as a flavoring.

GENERAL SOURCES:

Bradley, P.C., ed. *British Herbal Compendium: A Handbook of Scientific Information on Widely Used Plant Drugs*, vol. 1. Bournemouth (Dorset), England: British Herbal Medicine Association, 1992.

Chevallier, A. *The Encyclopedia of Medicinal Plants: A Practical Reference Guide to More Than 550 Key Medicinal Plants & Their Uses.* 1st American ed. New York: Dorling Kindersley Publications, 1996.

Foster, S., and J.A. Duke. *The Peterson Field Guide Series: A Field Guide to Medicinal Plants. Eastern and Central North America.* Boston: Houghton Mifflin Company, 1990.

Hallowell, M. *Herbal Healing: A Practical Introduction to Medicinal Herbs.* Garden City Park, NY, 1994.

Hylton, W.H., ed. *The Rodale Herb Book: How to Use, Grow, and Buy Nature's Miracle Plants.* Emmaus, PA: Rodale Press, Inc., 1974.

Mowrey, D.B. *Proven Herbal Blends: A Rational Approach to Prevention and Remedy.* (Condensed from *The Scientific Validation of Herbal Medicine.*) New Canaan, CT: Keats Publishing, Inc: 1986.

Newall, C.A., et al. *Herbal Medicines: A Guide for Health-Care Professionals.* London: The Pharmaceutical Press, 1996.

Tierra, M. *The Way of Herbs.* New York: Pocket Books, 1990.

Tyler, V.E. *Herbs of Choice: The Therapeutic Use of Phytomedicinals.* Binghamton, NY: Haworth Press/Pharmaceutical Products Press, 1994.

Weiner, M.A., and J.A. Weiner. *Herbs That Heal: Prescription for Herbal Healing.* Mill Valley, CA: Quantum Books, 1994.

TEXT CITATIONS:

1. V.E. Tyler, *Herbs of Choice: The Therapeutic Use of Phytomedicinals* (Binghamton, NY: Haworth Press/Pharmaceutical Products Press, 1994).

2. A. Chevallier, *The Encyclopedia of Medicinal Plants: A Practical Reference Guide to More Than 550 Key Medicinal Plants & Their Uses*, 1st American ed. (New York: Dorling Kindersley Publications, 1996).

3. F. Fish et al., *Lloydia*, 38 (1975): 268–70.

4. C.A. Newall et al., *Herbal Medicines: A Guide for Health-Care Professionals* (London: The Pharmaceutical Press, 1996).

5. J. Lenfield et al., *Planta Medica*, 43 (1981): 161–65. Newall, op. cit.

6. I. Addae-Mensah et al., *Planta Medica*, 52(Suppl.) (1986): 58.

7. Tyler, op. cit.

8. Ibid.

9. S. Foster and J.A. Duke, *The Peterson Field Guide Series: A Field Guide to Medicinal Plants: Eastern and Central North America* (Boston: Houghton Mifflin Company, 1990).

10. Newall, op. cit.

11. J.M. Bowen and R.J. Cole, *Federal Proceedings*, 40 (1981): 696. Newall, op. cit.

12. Newall, op. cit.

13. P.C. Bradley, ed., *British Herbal Compendium: A Handbook of Scientific Information on Widely Used Plant Drugs*, vol. 1. (Bournemouth [Dorset] England: British Herbal Medicine Association, 1992).

PRIMARY NAME:

PROPOLIS

SCIENTIFIC NAME:
N/A

COMMON NAMES:
Bee glue, bee rue, hive dross, propolis balsam, propolis resin, propolis wax

RATING:
3 = Studies on the effectiveness and safety of this substance are conflicting, or there are not enough studies to draw a conclusion.

What Is Propolis?

Propolis is a reddish-brown, resinous substance produced by honeybees from the buds of poplar and conifer trees. It is an extremely complicated mixture of natural substances. The bees use it inside their hives as a form of glue.

What It Is Used For:

The antiseptic and local anesthetic properties of this pleasant-smelling resin were reportedly recognized in prehistoric times and enlisted for the earliest of surgical procedures.[1] Over the centuries, propolis has been used as a dressing for leg ulcers and battle wounds (reportedly used heavily in the Boer War[2]), as a crucial element in throat lozenges, and in numerous soaps and cosmetics. Propolis may have reached its zenith of popularity as a healing agent several centuries ago in Europe—most major pharmacies in seventeenth-century England carried it—before falling out of favor until a recent revival in interest on the part of laypersons and scientists alike.[3]

A variety of medicinal properties have been ascribed to propolis in recent years, including an ability to fight bacteria, viruses, and protozoa involved in various infectious diseases, such as tuberculosis, certain kinds of dermatitis, and giardiasis. Some sources recommend it for treating herpes simplex virus type 1 (oral herpes), the influenza virus, hepatitis B virus, and avian herpes viruses. Proposed anti-inflammatory, antitumoral, tissue-regenerative, fever-reducing, and antioxidant capabilities have made propolis a popular agent for treating common colds, duodenal ulcers, stomach problems, and various inflammatory processes including arthritis. Recent claims that propolis boasts immune-system-stimulating properties have also met with great interest. The resin has attracted interest from dentists for treating a variety of oral and dental complications, including fungal infections (moniliasis), and for encouraging postsurgical healing.[4]

Propolis can also be found in some soaps and cosmetics and serves as a varnish for high-quality violins.

Forms Available Include:

Capsule (sometimes in combination with pollen), chips (like chewing gum), cream, powder, throat lozenges, tincture.

Dosage Commonly Reported:

To use commercial propolis formulations, follow the package instructions.

Will It Work for You? What the Studies Say:

Most scientific evidence for propolis is based on test-tube or small-animal studies. Its mechanism of action appears to be very complex and is still not fully understood. Recent test-tube research confirms the presence of modest antibacterial, antifungal, and antiviral properties, although the value of these in the modern era of standard anti-infectives is questionable. For example, test-tube research has demonstrated that propolis effectively fights certain types of bacteria and fungi.[5] Because propolis is so complex—some twenty-five compounds have been tested—simple analogies to the mode of action of classic antibiotics cannot be made.[6] Clinical trials reported by Central European researchers indicate that it may help wounds heal and fight fungal and bacterial infections.[7] Flavonoids appear to be the most active ingredients.

Scientists conducting test-tube studies also report detecting action against herpes simplex virus type 1, the influenza virus, hepatitis B virus, and avian herpes viruses, polio virus, and other viruses.[8] Proponents say that propolis stimulates the immune system by elevating the body's natural resistance to infection, but solid evidence for this cannot be found in the medical literature.

Studies have ascribed anti-inflammatory, antitumor, and antioxidant effects to propolis. Preparations fared well in tests of anti-inflammatory activity and certain types of chemically induced arthritis in rats, for example.[9] Several investigators have reported intriguing antitumor properties in test-tube studies that they attribute to a component called caffeic acid pheneythyl ester.[10] Alcoholic extracts have demonstrated slight antioxidant properties, which means the extracts are believed to help scavenge toxic by-products that may contribute to cancer cell formation.[11] In a possible demonstration of this property, mice given propolis and then exposed to high doses of radiation have been shown to live longer than those not given the extract.[12] Overall, however, more studies are needed to verify that any of these properties translate into meaningful healing actions in humans.

A team of investigators found that propolis failed to demonstrate any fever-reducing or antiamebic properties.[13]

Will It Harm You? What the Studies Say:

Since no sophisticated clinical trials have been conducted in human beings, it is impossible to determine exactly what adverse effects propolis might cause. The resin has caused dermatitis, according to reports from people who have used propolis-containing skin cosmetics[14] and others who work with the substance.[15] Allergic mouth reactions, characterized by inflammation and ulceration, have also been reported following the use of lozenges that contain the resin.[16] Overall, however, side effects are likely to be minimal. The subject clearly demands further study.

GENERAL SOURCES:

Castleman, M. *Healing Herbs: The Ultimate Guide to the Curative Power of Nature's Medicines.* New York: Bantam Books, 1995.

Lawrence Review of Natural Products. St. Louis: Facts and Comparisons, February 1996.

Tyler, V.E. *The Honest Herbal.* Binghamton, NY: Haworth Press/Pharmaceutical Products Press, 1993.

TEXT CITATIONS:

1. W.M. Thomson, *Medical Journal of Australia*, 153(11–12) (1990): 654.
2. Ibid.
3. V.E. Tyler, *The Honest Herbal* (Binghamton, NY: Haworth Press/Pharmaceutical Products Press, 1993).
4. O. Magro-Fiho and A.C. Perri de Carvalho, *Journal of the Nihon University School of Dentistry*, 36(2) (1994): 102–11.
5. J.W. Dobrowski et al., *Journal of Ethnopharmacology*, 35 (1991): 77–82.

6. N.B. Takaisi-Kikuni and H. Schilcher, *Planta Medica*, 60 (1994): 222–27.
7. *Lawrence Review of Natural Products* (St. Louis: Facts and Comparisons, February 1996).
8. M. Amoros et al., *Journal of Natural Products*, 57(5) (1994): 644–47.
9. Dobrowski, op. cit.
10. *Lawrence Review of Natural Products*, op. cit.
11. S. Scheller et al., *International Journal of Radiation Biology*, 57(3) (1990): 461. *Lawrence Review of Natural Products*, op. cit.
12. S. Scheller et al., *Zeitschrift für Naturforschung*, 44(11–12) (1989): 1049.
13. Dobrowski, op. cit.
14. C. Pincelli et al., *Contact Dermatitis*, 11(1) (1984): 49.
15. *Lawrence Review of Natural Products*, op. cit.
16. K.D. Hay and D.E. Greig, *Oral Surgery Oral Medicine Oral Pathology*, 70(5) (1990): 584.

PRIMARY NAME:
PSYLLIUM

SCIENTIFIC NAME:
Plantago psyllium L., *Plantago lanceolata* L., *Plantago arenaria* Waldst. and Kit., *Plantago indica* L. (Spanish or French psyllium), and *Plantago ovata* Forsk. (blonde psyllium or Indian plantago). Family: Plantaginaceae

COMMON NAME:
fleawort seed

RATING:
1 = Years of use and extensive, high-quality studies indicate that this substance is very effective and safe when used in recommended amounts for the indication(s) noted in the "Will It Work for You?" section.

What Is Psyllium?

There are about 250 species of plantain (or psyllium), typically hardy perennial herbs or shrubby plants found throughout the globe, growing wild in fields along roads and in lawns, for instance. Most have basal or narrow linear leaves and small flowers that grow in dense round spikes. After this summer bloom, the flowers turn into seed pods. The wind spreads the seeds, as do birds and other animals who consume them and then leave the seeds in yet another location in their feces.[1] The dried, cleaned, ripened psyllium seeds, which are small and dark red or brown, as well as the seed husks, are used medicinally.

Do not confuse the species of *Plantago* plantain discussed here with the tree (*Musa paradisiaca*) that produces the small cooking banana by the same name.

What It Is Used For:

Psyllium seeds and husks are a proven bulk-producing laxative widely used to treat chronic constipation and other situations in which a soft stool is desired, including hemorrhoids, operations on the anal or rectal area, and anal fissures. The seeds and husks have also been used to treat overly loose stools, as in diarrhea, because they endow the stool with bulk and shape. Traditional Chinese, Indian (Ayurvedic), and European healers have long recognized the value of psyllium seeds or husks for treating these kinds of discomfort, as well as other intestinal upsets, urinary problems, and high blood pressure. Although it took until the twentieth century to reach North American shores, psyllium now qualifies as one of the nation's most widely used laxatives. Think of Metamucil, Fiberall, and Naturacil; these and many other common laxatives contain psyllium.

Forms Available Include:

Fresh leaves, powdered husk, seeds. Both seeds and husks can be found in many commercial laxatives.

Dosage Commonly Reported:

As a laxative, a common dosage of psyllium is 2 heaping teaspoons (7.5 grams) seeds or 1 teaspoon of husks taken in a glass of liquid. Follow with extra liquids to avoid complications. Follow the package directions on commercial psyllium-containing laxatives, and be sure to take them with plenty of water.

Will It Work for You? What the Studies Say:

Psyllium seeds are covered with a substance called mucilage that swells into a gummy, gelatinous mass when it absorbs fluid in the intestines, thus lubricating the gut wall. The increased bulk also stimulates the gut wall, encouraging peristalsis (the wavelike movement we experience as the "urge") and defecation; the result is a softened and better-formed stool. The mucilage also helps reduce diarrhea by adsorbing excess fluid. It is important to drink plenty of liquid to enable the mucilage to work properly.

This softening and forming of the stool help lessen the itching, bleeding, pain, and other symptoms of hemorrhoids, according to a handful of reports. A double-blind study of more than fifty individuals suffering from hemorrhoid-associated bleeding and pain found that nearly 85 percent reported an elimination of or improvement in these symptoms when they supplemented their diet with a psyllium-containing preparation, compared with only 52 percent of those taking a placebo.[3] Itching, secretions, and prolapse of the rectum were also significantly reduced at three weeks, but insignificantly so at six weeks. Anal fissures likewise respond well to such treatment, according to a 1978 report involving nearly 395 patients.[4]

German health authorities approve of psyllium seed for constipation, hemorrhoids, and pregnancy, and in other situations in which a soft stool is desired. They also approve of the seed as a supportive (secondary) treatment for irritable bowel syndrome (IBS), a condition characterized by alternating constipation and diarrhea and frequently accompanied by crampy abdominal pain. Study results on this subject have been somewhat mixed. People with this syndrome who are not already on a high-fiber diet may benefit the most, according to 1983 findings.[5]

High cholesterol is a significant risk factor for coronary artery diseases. A number of studies show that integrating a high-fiber food such as psyllium seeds into the diet (they contain up to 80 percent soluble fiber) effectively lowers total cholesterol and the "harmful" cholesterol known as low-density-lipoprotein (LDL) cholesterol.[6] In an eight-week study involving twenty-six individuals with high cholesterol, supplementing the diet with psyllium three times a day (3.4 grams) significantly lowered total serum cholesterol levels, LDL levels, and the ratio of LDL to the "good" cholesterol known as high-density lipoprotein (HDL), compared with placebo treatment and initial readings of these parameters.[7] Similarly, a twelve-week study conducted in 1989 documented a 5 percent cholesterol drop in subjects who supplemented their diets with psyllium.[8] Although German health authorities approve of using both the seeds and the husks for this purpose, United States authorities do not.[9] Efforts to add psyllium seed to breakfast cereals have forced regulators to grapple with the issue of whether it is a food or drug.[10]

Preliminary findings indicate that psyllium may also have a justified role to play in diabetes management. When it was taken before breakfast and dinner, the typical rise in glucose and insulin concentrations seen in people with non-insulin-dependent diabetes was notably reduced in one study.[11] This crossover study involved eighteen subjects. More research is needed.

Several herbalists note that psyllium may help reduce the risk of colon cancer indirectly by bulking up the stool and thus allowing toxic chemicals to have less direct contact with intestinal tissue.[12] However, no well-designed studies have been done to verify that this translates into protection from colon or any other cancer.

Will It Harm You? What the Studies Say:

Experts consider psyllium one of the safest laxatives known, partly because it works like many high-fiber foods. But German health authorities point out that the herb should not be used by people who suffer intestinal tract blockage or stenosis (hardening) of the esophagus or the gastrointestinal tract. Diabetes sufferers also should not take it.[14] The powdered and liquid forms of plantain remedies in particular have caused allergic reactions in rare cases; the reactions were severe in a few. The risk appears to be particularly high in people who are constantly exposed to the plant, such as pharmaceutical workers.[15]

Pregnant women should not take this or any other laxative without talking to their doctors first. A regimen of other high-fiber foods such as fruits and vegetables, plenty of liquids, and exercise may well reduce constipation and eliminate the need for a laxative.

GENERAL SOURCES:

American Pharmaceutical Association. *Handbook of Nonprescription Drugs.* 11th ed. Washington, D.C.: American Pharmaceutical Association, 1996.

Bisset, N.G., ed. *Herbal Drugs and Phytopharmaceuticals.* Stuttgart: medpharm GmbH Scientific Publishers, 1994.

Castleman, M. *The Healing Herbs: The Ultimate Guide to the Curative Power of Nature's Medicines.* New York: Bantam Books, 1995.

Lawrence Review of Natural Products. St. Louis: Facts and Comparisons, August 1988.

Leung, A.Y., and S. Foster. *Encyclopedia of Common Natural Ingredients Used in Food, Drugs, and Cosmetics.* 2nd ed. New York: John Wiley & Sons, 1996.

Tierra, M. *The Way of Herbs.* New York: Pocket Books, 1990.

Tyler, V.E. *Herbs of Choice: The Therapeutic Use of Phytomedicinals.* Binghamton, NY: Haworth Press/Pharmaceutical Products Press, 1994.

Weiner, M.A., and J.A. Weiner. *Herbs That Heal: Prescription for Herbal Healing.* Mill Valley, CA: Quantum Books, 1994.

Weiss, R.F. *Herbal Medicine,* trans. A.R. Meuss, from the 6th German edition. Beaconsfield, England: Beaconsfield Publishers, Ltd., 1988.

TEXT CITATIONS:

1. *Lawrence Review of Natural Products* (St. Louis: Facts and Comparisons, August 1988).
2. A.Y. Leung and S. Foster, *Encyclopedia of Common Natural Ingredients Used in Food, Drugs, and Cosmetics,* 2nd ed. (New York: John Wiley & Sons, 1996).

3. F. Moesgaard et al., *Diseases of the Colon and Rectum*, 25 (1982): 454. *Lawrence Review of Natural Products*, op. cit.
4. H.A. Shub et al., *Diseases of the Colon and Rectum*, 21 (1978): 582.
5. Y. Arthurs and J.F. Fielding, *Irish Medical Journal*, 76 (1983): 253. *Lawrence Review of Natural Products*, op. cit.
6. American Pharmaceutical Association, *Handbook of Nonprescription Drugs*, 11th ed. (Washington, D.C.: American Pharmaceutical Association, 1996). D.L. Sprecher et al., *Annals of Internal Medicine*, 119 (1993): 545–54.
7. J.W. Anderson et al., *Archives of Internal Medicine*, 148 (1988): 292.
8. L.P. Bell et al., *Journal of the American Medical Association*, 261 (1989): 1195.
9. V.E. Tyler, *Herbs of Choice: The Therapeutic Use of Phytomedicinals* (Binghamton, NY: Haworth Press/Pharmaceutical Products Press, 1994).
10. Ibid.
11. J.G. Pastors et al., *American Journal of Clinical Nutrition*, 33(6) (1991): 1431-35.
12. M. Castleman, *The Healing Herbs: The Ultimate Guide to the Curative Power of Nature's Medicines* (New York: Bantam Books, 1995).
13. S. Duckett, *New England Journal of Medicine*, 303 (1980): 383.
14. American Pharmaceutical Association, op. cit.
15. Ibid. R. Suhonen et al., *Allergy*, 38 (1983): 363.

PRIMARY NAME:
PULSATILLA

SCIENTIFIC NAME:
Pulsatilla vulgaris Miller (syn. with *Anemone pulsatilla* L.) and *Pulsatilla pratensis* L. Family: Ranunculaceae

COMMON NAME:
Pasqueflower

RATING:
3 = Studies on the effectiveness of this substance are conflicting, or there are not enough studies to draw a conclusion. Safety is a major concern, however; see the "Will It Harm You?" section.

What Is Pulsatilla?

The lovely and quite poisonous pulsatilla bears purple-blue, bell-shaped flowers with bright yellow centers that become seed heads over time. The herb's leaves are finely divided, with a feathery appearance. This European native blooms at Easter (hence the common name, "pasqueflower"). The dried aboveground parts are used medicinally.

What It Is Used For:

Although less popular than in past times, when it was recommended for coughs, asthma, headaches, and warts, and as a sedative for sleep problems, pulsatilla still finds use as an herbal remedy for painful menstrual cramps and other cramp- or spasm-related pain in the male or female reproductive tract. It is poisonous when fresh, but not when properly dried. In some parts of Europe it maintains a reputation for remedying cough, sleeping problems, migraine headache, eye disorders (including cataracts and glaucoma), lung disease, and skin eruptions complicated by inflammation and bacterial infections. Homeopaths are quick to recommend this popular remedy in minute dosages for, among other things, painful or absent menstruation, indigestion, runny nose, earache, certain eye disorders, nerve pain, depression, toothache, and urticaria (allergic itch).[1] (See page 2 for a discussion of homeopathy.)

Forms Available Include:

Decoction, infusion, liquid extract, tincture. Pulsatilla is commonly found in herbal blends.

Dosage Commonly Reported:

To use commercial herbal blends, homeopathic remedies, or other formulations containing pulsatilla, follow the package instructions. See page 2 for information on interpreting homeopathic dosages.

Will It Work for You? What the Studies Say:

Very little research has been done on pulsatilla, and almost none of it in recent years. According to animal studies done in the 1910s, the herb does indeed have an impact on the uterus; it apparently both stimulates and depresses the muscle.[2] But many European physicians consider the herb obsolete for treating painful menstrual cramps or other genital conditions.[3] No hormonal effect has ever been documented. Citing a lack of scientific confirmation, German health authorities declined to approve of pulsatilla for reproductive tract problems, restlessness, migraine, infections or inflammations of the skin or mucous membranes, neuralgia (nerve pain), or urinary or gastrointestinal tract ailments.[4]

Rodent studies indicate that certain components in pulsatilla—anemonin and protoanemonin—have sedative and fever-reducing properties.[5] Protoanemonin also fights bacteria.[6] Unfortunately, these are the highly toxic substances in the fresh herb that should be avoided.

The herb's value as a homeopathic remedy depends on your perspective regarding these agents in general.

Will It Harm You? What the Studies Say:

Never ingest or topically apply fresh pulsatilla, which is poisonous. The toxic component in its volatile oil, protoanemonin, reportedly loses its toxicity quite quickly as drying degrades it.[7] Avoid handling the plant. Protoanemonin from the fresh plant can cause severe skin and mucous membrane irritation with reddening, itching, and blistering.[8] When inhaled, pulsatilla's volatile oil may irritate the eyes and mucous membranes in the nose.[9] High internal doses can cause kidney and urinary tract irritation.[10] Animal tests indicate that anemonin is toxic to cells; this has implications for causing cancer, although it has not been documented in humans.[11]

As for dried pulsatilla, it is not considered toxic in any way, but stick to moderate doses, as excessive ones can cause violent stomach upset. Allergic reactions have been reported as well.[12] Pregnant women should never take pulsatilla, particularly given evidence that it can affect the menstrual cycle[13] and has caused pregnancy losses and birth defects in animals grazing on the plant.[14]

GENERAL SOURCES:

Blumenthal, M., J. Gruenwald, T. Hall, and R.S. Rister, eds. *The Complete German Commission E Monographs: Therapeutic Guide to Herbal Medicine.* Boston: Integrative Medicine Communications, 1998.

Bradley, P.C., ed. *British Herbal Compendium: A Handbook of Scientific Information on Widely Used Plant Drugs,* vol. 1. Bournemouth (Dorset), England: British Herbal Medicine Association, 1992.

Bremness, L. *Herbs.* 1st American ed. Eyewitness Handbooks. New York: Dorling Kindersley Publications, 1994.

Chevallier, A. *The Encyclopedia of Medicinal Plants: A Practical Reference Guide to More Than 550 Key Medicinal Plants & Their Uses.* 1st American ed. New York: Dorling Kindersley Publications,1996.

Duke, J.A. *CRC Handbook of Medicinal Herbs.* Boca Raton, FL: CRC Press, 1985.

Mayell, M. *Off-the-Shelf Natural Health: How to Use Herbs and Nutrients to Stay Well.* New York: Bantam Books, 1995.

Newall, C.A., et al. *Herbal Medicines: A Guide for Health-Care Professionals.* London: The Pharmaceutical Press, 1996.

Weiss, R.F. *Herbal Medicine,* trans. A.R. Meuss, from the 6th German edition. Beaconsfield, England: Beaconsfield Publishers, Ltd., 1988.

TEXT CITATIONS:

1. J.A. Duke, *CRC Handbook of Medicinal Herbs* (Boca Raton, FL: CRC Press, 1985).
2. J.M. Pilcher et al., *Surgery, Gynecology and Obstetrics,* 18 (1918): 97–99. J.M. Pilcher et al., *Archives of Internal Medicine* 18 (1916): 557–83.
3. R.F. Weiss, *Herbal Medicine,* trans. A.R. Meuss, from the 6th German edition (Beaconsfield, England: Beaconsfield Publishers, Ltd., 1988).
4. M. Blumenthal, J. Gruenwald, T. Hall, and R.S. Rister, eds., *The Complete German Commission E Monographs: Therapeutic Guide to Herbal Medicine (Boston:* Integrative Medicine Communications, 1998).
5. M.L. Martin et al., *Journal of Ethnopharmacology,* 24 (1988): 185–91.
6. S.A. Hifny, *Planta Medica,* 16 (1968): 231–38.
7. C.A. Newall et al., *Herbal Medicines: A Guide for Health-Care Professionals* (London: The Pharmaceutical Press, 1996).
8. Blumenthal et al., op. cit. Weiss, op. cit.
9. Newall, op. cit.
10. Blumenthal et al., op. cit.
11. Newall, op. cit.
12. Ibid.
13. Ibid.
14. Blumenthal et al., op. cit.

PRIMARY NAME:

PYCNOGENOL

SCIENTIFIC NAME:
N/A

COMMON NAME:
Pine bark extract

RATING:
3 = Studies on the effectiveness and safety of this substance are conflicting, or there are not enough studies to draw a conclusion.

What Is Pycnogenol?

In the health food industry the term "pycnogenol" refers to an extract of certain pine trees, most commonly the European coastal pine, *Pinus maritima,* sometimes referred to as *Pinus nigra* var. *maritima.* It is billed as an antioxidant and consists of a proprietary blend of biologically active substances called flavonoids. Technically, the term also refers to the group of flavonoids known as flavan-3-ol derivatives.[1]

What It Is Used For:

Dietary supplement manufacturers bill pycnogenol as a powerful antioxidant. Taken orally as a dietary supplement for its contained procyanidolic oligomers (PCOs), pycnogenol can be used interchangeably with **Grape Seed Extract**. Pycnogenol is said to protect against tumor formation, help fight aging, improve circulation to the benefit of peripheral vascular diseases, reduce inflammation, control diabetes, aid wound healing, treat retinopathy, and fight the breakdown of collagen, which can occur with aging and a number of inflammatory collagen diseases. A U.S. patent claims that its pycnogenol compound can help rectify the impact of oxygen deprivation associated with strokes, heart attacks, atherosclerosis (hardening of the arteries), inflammation, and certain connective tissue diseases.[2]

Pycnogenol is also used externally. Many European "antiaging" creams and "wrinkle therapies" contain pycnogenol and can now be purchased in the United States. The cream is marketed as a substance that can nourish the collagen fibers that endow skin with firmness and elasticity.

Forms Available Include:

- *For internal use:* Capsule, liquid extract, tablet.
- *For external use:* Creams and other formulations.

Dosage Commonly Reported:

Tablets or capsules are initially taken in daily doses of 75 to 300 milligrams for up to three weeks; then the daily dosage is lowered to 40 to 80 milligrams.

Will It Work for You? What the Studies Say:

Preliminary data from human trials, most of them carried out in Europe, indicate that pycnogenol has some benefit for various illnesses. It appears to function as an antioxidant, although there is some disagreement as to the true benefits of these substances. (See **Beta-Carotene** for a full discussion of antioxidants.) Antioxidants are believed to control the formation of dangerous substances in the body called free radicals. These substances damage cells through oxidation; some may contribute to cancer cell formation. According to preliminary trials conducted in Europe, pycnogenol may also aid disorders involving hypoxia (lack of oxygen), such as inflammatory collagen disease, peripheral vascular disease, atherosclerosis, heart attack, and stroke.[3] A 1981 study of individuals suffering from peripheral circulation disorders reported that the subjects experienced a decrease in limb heaviness, pain, and swelling after taking oral doses of pycnogenol for thirty days.[4]

No studies appear in the recent medical literature to verify that pycnogenol will absorb efficiently into the skin and be of any value in "antiaging" creams.

Will It Harm You? What the Studies Say:

No reports of serious adverse reactions to pycnogenol have been reported in human trials. Its toxicity does not appear to have been specifically examined, however. Much about this subject remains unknown.

GENERAL SOURCES:

American Pharmaceutical Association. *Handbook of Nonprescription Drugs.* 11th ed. Washington, D.C.: American Pharmaceutical Association, 1996.

Lawrence Review of Natural Products. St. Louis: Facts and Comparisons, February 1991.

Leung, A.Y., and S. Foster. *Encyclopedia of Common Natural Ingredients Used in Food, Drugs, and Cosmetics.* 2nd ed. New York: John Wiley & Sons, 1996.

TEXT CITATIONS:

1. J. Masquelier et al., *International Journal of Vitamin and Nutrition Research*, 49 (1979): 307. *Lawrence Review of Natural Products* (St. Louis: Facts and Comparisons, February 1991).
2. *Lawrence Review of Natural Products*, op. cit.
3. American Pharmaceutical Association, *Handbook of Nonprescription Drugs*, 11th ed. (Washington, D.C.: American Pharmaceutical Association, 1996). H. Mollmann and P. Rohdewald, *Therapiewoche*, 33 (1983): 4967.
4. L. Sarrat, *Bordeaux Medical*, 14 (1981): 685.

QUASSIA

SCIENTIFIC NAME:
Picrasma excelsa (Sw.) Planch.
Family: Simaraoubaceae. Also
Quassia amara L.

COMMON NAMES:
Bitterwood, Jamaican quassia,
picrasma

RATING:
3 = Studies on the effectiveness
and safety of this substance are
conflicting, or there are not
enough studies to draw a
conclusion. See warnings in the
"Will It Harm You?" section.

What Is Quassia?

The pale yellow, intensely bitter-tasting wood of the West Indian quassia tree is granulated to prepare a medicinal remedy. Clusters of small, rose-colored flowers and long pinnate leaves grow on this tall tree. The wood of the Surinam quassia, *Quassia amara* L., a smaller tree that grows in Colombia, Argentina, Guyana, and Panama, is also used.

What It Is Used For:

West Indian natives familiar with this tree reportedly carved "quassia cups" out of the wood, added hot water, and let these stand long enough that the extremely bitter resin in the wood would be drawn into the water. They then sipped the mixture when indigestion or other stomach upsets developed or the appetite needed a boost. Quassia became a common European bitter tonic for similar conditions once it was imported to the continent in the 1700s. Although it is little used for these purposes today, quassia does appear in a number of prepared stomach-soothing and bile-stimulating herbal formulas.[1] The extract, quassin, has been similarly used, and a number of contemporary herbalists recommend it for stimulating liver, gallbladder, kidney, and other internal "juices." Homeopaths prescribe minute dosages of quassia for a variety of ailments. (See page 2 for more information on homeopathy.)

The use of oral and rectal (enema) formulations for intestinal worms, once quite popular, has become dated. Topical quassia formulations such as lotions are sometimes applied to combat body lice. Many aperitifs, liqueurs, and tonic wines contain this bitter wood. It also serves as a flavoring in foods and beverages. Gardeners regard it as an effective insect repellent and pesticide.

Forms Available Include:

Decoction, dried stem wood for infusions, enema, fluid extract, infusion (including concentrated form), lotion, tea bag, tincture.

Dosage Commonly Reported:

A decoction is made using a scant ¼ teaspoon (0.5 gram) powdered wood per cup of water and is drunk about thirty minutes before meals. The tincture is taken in doses of 2.5 to 5 milliliters, the concentrated wood tea in doses of 2.5 to 5 milliliters. Oral formulations such as infusions are drunk cold.

Will It Work for You? What the Studies Say:

The wood contains substances called quassinoids that are reportedly fifty times more bitter than the widely recognized bitter, quinine. Quassin is the primary quassinoid. Scientists believe that bitters such as this stimulate the appetite and settle the stomach by promoting salivation and the excretion of stomach juices. Although there are no studies to verify this property with quassia specifically, years of use with this and other bitters should certainly be taken into account. Although the data are limited, one team of investigators reported success in combating head lice in 454 individuals with a quassia tincture scalp lotion.[2] Investigators have reported conflicting results in fighting parasitic (amebic) infections with quassia, but limited data indicate success in treating thread-worms with an enema made with quassia.[3]

Although the implications for human cancers remain unclear, it should be noted that researchers report positive test-tube activity for quassin in cancers affecting the throat and nasal passages, and have identified significant antitumor actions (against a type of lymphatic leukemia) in mice experiments.[4] In test-tube studies, alkaloids called beta-carbolines[5] have shown antibacterial and antifungal actions, as well as a potential ability to increase the squeezing force of the heart muscle.[6] Whether these properties translate into anything meaningful for humans requires further examination.

Will It Harm You? What the Studies Say:

Avoid higher-than-recommended doses of quassia, as they may cause stomach irritation and vomiting. High doses may also complicate heart or blood-thinning treatments.[7] Also, given the risk of vomiting, do not take quassia during pregnancy or while nursing.[8] The FDA has placed quassia on its list of foods "Generally Regarded As Safe" (GRAS).

GENERAL SOURCES:

Bisset, N.G., ed., *Herbal Drugs and Phytopharmaceuticals* Stuttgart: medpharm GmbH Scientific Publishers, 1994.

Dobelis, I.N., ed. *The Magic and Medicine of Plants: A Practical Guide to the Science, History, Folklore, and Everyday Uses of Medicinal Plants.* Pleasantville, NY: Reader's Digest Association, 1986.

Newall, C.A., et al. *Herbal Medicines: A Guide for Health-Care Professionals.* London: The Pharmaceutical Press, 1996.

Weiner, M.A., and J.A. Weiner. *Herbs That Heal: Prescription for Herbal Healing.* Mill Valley, CA: Quantum Books, 1994.

TEXT CITATIONS:

1. N.G. Bisset, ed., *Herbal Drugs and Phytopharmaceuticals* (Stuttgart: medpharm GmbH Scientific Publishers, 1994).
2. C.A. Newall et al., *Herbal Medicines: A Guide for Health-Care Professionals* (London: The Pharmaceutical Press, 1996).
3. Ibid.
4. Ibid.
5. P. Barbetti et al., *Planta Medica*, 53 (1987): 289.
6. Newall, op. cit.
7. Ibid.
8. Bisset, op. cit.

PRIMARY NAME:
RASPBERRY

SCIENTIFIC NAME:
Rubus idaeus L. and occasionally other *Rubus* varieties. Family: Rosaceae

COMMON NAMES:
Bramble, hindberry, red raspberry

RATING:
3 = Studies on the effectiveness and safety of this substance are conflicting, or there are not enough studies to draw a conclusion.

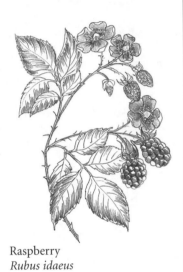

Raspberry
Rubus idaeus

What Is Raspberry?

The tall, thorny-stemmed raspberry shrub bears the sweet red berries so deeply admired in many parts of the world including North America, where it grows widely and is also heavily cultivated. Small white flowers appear in summer. Primarily the plant's lance-shaped leaves are used for medicinal purposes.

What It Is Used For:

Ancient Greeks, Native Americans, and many other peoples have treasured the delectable flavor of the raspberry. Through the years, the berries have been added to medicines to improve their flavor and concocted in vinegars for coughs and sore throats. Today, however, it is the medicinal value of the leaves that endures. Leaf preparations were once—and still are in some places—highly esteemed for treating diarrhea, stomach upset (especially with cold tea), wounds, ulcers, fever blisters, hemorrhoids, and other skin inflammations. Warm raspberry leaf tea has a reputation for soothing mouth sores (including canker sores), sore throats, and other mouth and throat inflammations, and is sometimes prepared as an astringent gargle for this purpose. An eyewash made with the tea has been used to calm and clear the eyes. It appears in a number of blood- and skin-"purifying" teas. In France it is regarded as a tonic for the prostate gland.

But perhaps the most enduring reputation for raspberry leaf preparations is as a pregnancy aid and remedy for "female troubles." The practice got a big boost in the 1940s with scientific reports that the leaves contain a principle that relaxes the uterus in animals.[1] Since then, raspberry leaf tea has been widely touted as the ideal drink for expectant mothers. Some herbalists recommend sipping it regularly through the last month or two of pregnancy to prepare the uterus for childbirth. Others suggest battling morning sickness with it. Women in various parts of the world sip the tea to combat a threatened miscarriage or treat labor pains. Other "female troubles" treated with raspberry leaf tea include menstrual cramping and profuse menstrual flow.

Raspberry leaves can also be found in various herbal remedies for diabetes, fever, respiratory problems, heart ailments, and other conditions.

Forms Available Include:

- *For internal use:* Capsule, extract, infusion (made with fresh and dried leaves, sometimes as a cold maceration), leaves, tea bag, tincture. Raspberry leaf frequently appears as an ingredient in herbal blends. When buying prepared tea, check the label carefully to make sure the leaves are the main ingredient.[2]
- *For external use:* Eyewash, poultice, tea for mouthwash or gargle.

Dosage Commonly Reported:

An infusion is made by pouring a cup of water over 1 to 2 teaspoons of crushed leaves, allowing it to steep, and straining. Alternatively, the leaves are allowed to sit in cold water for a period of time, and then strained; this is called a cold maceration. As a treatment for menstrual cramps or diarrhea, either drink is taken up to six times a day. For capsules, one to three 384-milligram capsules are taken three times a day.

Will It Work for You? What the Studies Say:

Raspberry leaves live up to a few, but not all, of the traditional claims made for them. Infusions and other drinks made with the leaves may well calm intestinal inflammation and help stop diarrhea because they contain rich stores of tannins, substances that are believed to help control diarrhea by reducing inflammation in the intestines. They probably also help hinder further absorption of toxic material.[3] These astringent properties may also justify to some extent the use of raspberry leaf tea mouthwashes and gargles for mouth or throat inflammations, including sore throats. (Tannins constrict tissues and reduce bleeding.)

The capacity of raspberry leaf tea to aid pregnancy and treat "female disorders" appears to be overblown. Confusion and disagreement on the subject persist. Some herbalists point to a 1941 report in the British medical journal *Lancet* and later reports that the herb contains principles that can help relax the uterus as well as the intestines.[4] Interestingly, no chemical has actually been found in the herb that explains this supposed reaction. No clinical studies have ever been done to demonstrate that some as yet unidentified constituent affects the uterus in any way.[5] In the 1950s a team of investigators reported that leaf extracts administered to tissue taken from guinea pigs and frogs definitely exerted some type of effect, but that the overall reaction was unclear[6]; in somewhat contradictory fashion, the extracts stopped spasms and stimulated smooth muscle at the same time. A 1970 study further complicated the scenario; it reported that raspberry leaf promoted contraction of normal uterine tissue taken from women in early pregnancy (at ten to sixteen weeks), but that it had no impact on uterine tissue taken from women who were not pregnant.[7] Citing a lack of substantiating scientific evidence, German health authorities conclude that raspberry leaves cannot be recommended for "female troubles," or any other disorder for that matter.[8]

Researchers have also reported that leaves from a closely related species, *Rubus fructicosus*,[9] help reduce blood sugar (glucose) levels in diabetic rats. What this may mean for treating diabetes in humans remains unclear. The leaves of this plant contain plentiful stores of vitamin C, although the concentration varies depending on how they are dried and stored.

Will It Harm You? What the Studies Say:

Raspberry leaf preparations appear to be relatively harmless when taken in typically recommended amounts, although the true risks involved, especially when taken over long periods, are unknown. This is particularly relevant for pregnancy. No long-term studies have been done to prove that the fetus is not adversely affected in any way. Herbalists offer mixed advice. One cautions against using high doses during early pregnancy because of the risk of stimulating the uterus,[10] while another advises not taking it until the seventh month.[11] German health authorities say the risks are "unknown."

Eyewashes made with raspberry leaves are not appropriate for treating conjunctivitis or other eye infections or inflammation.[12] Consider the fundamentals of hygiene whenever you put foreign material in your eye; if it is not sterile, it could irritate your eye even more. Homemade solutions are particularly risky.

GENERAL SOURCES:

Bisset, N.G., ed. *Herbal Drugs and Phytopharmaceuticals*. Stuttgart: medpharm GmbH Scientific Publishers, 1994.

Castleman, M. *The Healing Herbs: The Ultimate Guide to the Curative Power of Nature's Medicines*. New York, NY: Bantam Books, 1995.

Dobelis, I.N., ed. *The Magic and Medicine of Plants: A Practical Guide to the Science, History, Folklore, and Everyday Uses of Medicinal Plants*. Pleasantville, NY: Reader's Digest Association, 1986.

Mindell E. *Earl Mindell's Herb Bible*. New York: Simon & Schuster/Fireside, 1992.

Newall, C.A., et al. *Herbal Medicines: A Guide for Health-Care Professionals*. London: The Pharmaceutical Press, 1996.

Ody, P. *The Herb Society's Complete Medicinal Herbal*. London: Dorling Kindersley Limited, 1993.

Tierra, M. *The Way of Herbs*. New York: Pocket Books, 1990.

Tyler, V.E. *Herbs of Choice: The Therapeutic Use of Phytomedicinals*. Binghamton, NY: Haworth Press/Pharmaceutical Products Press, 1994.

———. *The Honest Herbal*. Binghamton, NY: Haworth Press/Pharmaceutical Products Press, 1993.

Weiner, M.A., and J.A. Weiner. *Herbs That Heal: Prescription for Herbal Healing*. Mill Valley, CA: Quantum Books, 1994.

TEXT CITATIONS:

1. J.H. Burn and E.R. Withell, *The Lancet*, II (6149) (1941): 1.
2. V.E. Tyler, *The Honest Herbal* (Binghamton, NY: Haworth Press/Pharmaceutical Products Press, 1993).
3. V.E. Tyler, *Herbs of Choice: The Therapeutic Use of Phytomedicinals* (Binghamton, NY: Haworth Press/Pharmaceutical Products Press, 1994).
4. Burn and Withell, op. cit.
5. V.E. Tyler, *The Honest Herbal*, op. cit.
6. A.H. Beckett et al., *Journal of Pharmacy and Pharmacology*, 6 (1954): 785–96.
7. D.S. Bamford et al., *British Journal of Pharmacology*, 40(1) (1970): 161P–162P. V.E. Tyler, *Herbs of Choice*, op. cit.
8. M. Blumenthal, J. Gruenwald, T. Hall, and R.S. Rister, eds., *The Complete German Commission E Monographs: Therapeutic Guide to Herbal Medicine* (Boston: Integrative Medicine Communications, 1998).
9. R. Alonso et al., *Planta Medica*, 40(Suppl.) (1980): 102–6.
10. P. Ody, *The Herb Society's Complete Medicinal Herbal* (London: Dorling Kindersley Limited, 1993).
11. E. Mindell, *Earl Mindell's Herb Bible* (New York: Simon & Schuster/Fireside, 1992).
12. C.A. Newall et al., *Herbal Medicines: A Guide for Health-Care Professionals* (London: The Pharmaceutical Press, 1996).

SCIENTIFIC NAME:

Aspalathus linearis (Burm. f.) R. Dahlgr. Sometimes referred to as *Borbonia pinifolia* Marloth or *Aspalathus contaminata* (Thunb.) Druce. Family: Leguminosae

COMMON NAME:

N/A

RATING:

3 = Studies on the effectiveness of this herb are conflicting, or there are not enough studies to draw a conclusion. Safety is not a major concern.

What Is Red Bush?

Red bush is a low-lying bush native to the mountainous regions of South Africa. A tea, called red bush or Rooibos tea, is made from its dried flowering twigs and leaves. The long, needlelike leaves turn red when bruised, endowing the brew with a distinctive red color.

What It Is Used For:

Red bush tea is one of the most popular commercial teas in South Africa, and the plant is extensively cultivated there.[1] One of its great appeals is that, unlike so many other tasty hot beverages, it contains no stimulants such as caffeine or significant amounts of any active compounds that might cause unwanted reactions. Many people find that this refreshing drink settles the stomach. Some herbalists contend that it reduces allergies.

Forms Available Include:

Dried flowering twigs and leaves (to make an infusion), tea bag.

Dosage Commonly Reported:

An infusion is made by pouring a cup of boiling water over 1 to 4 teaspoons of dried leaves. This is taken three times a day. It is commonly mixed with sugar and milk.

Will It Work for You? What the Studies Say:

Any stomach-settling sensation you feel may be accounted for by a low level of astringent tannins, but the tea contains so little (less than 5 percent) that the settling effect may be more imagined than real. The tea contains some vitamin C and no caffeine.[2] As a nonstimulating, refreshing drink, it appears to be a good selection.

Although the implications for preventing or treating human cancers are still very unclear, investigators in the mid-1990s started issuing reports that red bush tea contains substances (flavonoids) that appear to help scavenge potentially damaging and cancer-causing free radicals.[3] In other words, it may be antioxidant. Most of these studies were done on mice. One found a protective effect against gamma-ray irradiation in mice fed an infusion of the tea.[4] Another reported that cancerous cell changes due to X-ray exposure were suppressed in mouse cells exposed to red bush tea in the test tube.[5] The greater the red bush tea concentration, the researchers found, the greater the protective effect.

This antioxidant may have implications for the aging process, according to some sources. With aging, substances called lipid peroxides appear to accumulate in the brain; rats continuously given red bush tea in a 1995 study did not experience this accumulation, although the rats treated with plain water instead of the tea did.[6] Although this is intriguing, much more research is needed to determine whether it happens in human beings and whether it makes any difference in the aging process.

Will It Harm You? What the Studies Say:

Despite decades of use, no reports of significant adverse reactions to this plant or the tea made from it appear in the medical literature. A 1979 study of ten healthy men confirmed that red bush tea did not affect the absorption of iron, as some experts had feared.[7]

GENERAL SOURCES:

Bremness, L. *Herbs.* 1st American ed. Eyewitness Handbooks. New York: Dorling Kindersley Publications, 1994.

Lawrence Review of Natural Products. St. Louis: Facts and Comparisons, August 1990.

Tyler, V.E. *The Honest Herbal.* Binghamton, NY: Haworth Press/Pharmaceutical Products Press, 1993.

Tyler, V.E., L.R. Brady, and J.E. Robbers, eds. *Pharmacognosy.* Philadelphia: Lea & Febiger, 1988.

TEXT CITATIONS:

1. *Lawrence Review of Natural Products* (St. Louis: Facts and Comparisons, August 1990).
2. V.E. Tyler, *The Honest Herbal* (Binghamton, NY: Haworth Press/Pharmaceutical Products Press, 1993). *Lawrence Review of Natural Products,* op. cit.
3. Y.F. Sasaki et al., *Mutation Research,* 286(2) (1993): 221–32.
4. K. Shimoi et al., *Mutation Research,* 350(1) (1996): 153–61.
5. K. Komatsu et al., *Cancer Letters,* 77(1) (1994): 33–38.
6. O. Inanami et al., *Neuroscience Letters,* 196(1–2) (1995): 85–88.
7. P.B. Hesseling et al., *South African Medical Journal,* 55(16) (1979): 631–32.

PRIMARY NAME:
RED CLOVER

SCIENTIFIC NAME:
Trifolium pratense L. Family: Leguminosae

COMMON NAMES:
Cow clover, meadow clover, pink clover, purple clover, sweet clover, trefoil

RATING:
4 = Research indicates that this substance will not fulfill the claims made for it, but that it is also unlikely to cause any harm.

What Is Red Clover?

The distinctive, fragrant round flower heads of this perennial are used medicinally after drying. The rose-to-pink flower heads are composed of miniature florets that develop on hairy upright stems along with oval leaflets that grow in groups of three and bear a pale crescent marking. Red clover grows in North America and many other parts of the world and is widely cultivated as silage and forage, and as a cover crop.

What It Is Used For:

This ancient agricultural crop is rich in historical and religious symbolism; its likeness even appears on the clubs suit in playing cards. The plant's significance as a healing agent extends far back into history; red clover has been used over the years as a tumor and cancer remedy (for breast cancer particularly), a treatment for skin disorders, and an expectorant to clear chest congestion caused by coughs, colds, and bronchitis. Around the turn of the twentieth century, Americans could get a dose of red clover in "Trifolium compound" preparations, herbal mixtures touted for venereal diseases such as syphilis, skin diseases, and tuberculosis of the lymph nodes.[1] In the 1940s, red clover blossoms appeared in Harry Hoxey's highly controversial herbal anticancer formula.

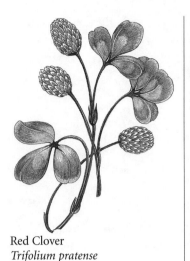

Red Clover
Trifolium pratense

Herbalists still recommend infusions and other internal preparations for calming coughs and clearing chest congestion, reducing uncomfortable menopausal symptoms, and improving overall health as a generalized tonic. Red clover continues to appear in some herbal blends for cancer. External preparations are used for rashes, psoriasis, eczema, and other skin disorders. The *National Formulary* listed it as a skin-disease remedy until the mid-1900s.

Forms Available Include:
- *For internal use:* Capsule, dried flowers, infusion, liquid extract.
- *For external use:* Infusion, liquid extract, ointment.

Dosage Commonly Reported:
An infusion is made using 1 to 3 teaspoons dried flower tops per cup of water. This is drunk up to three times per day, or 2.5 to 10 milliliters of the liquid flower extract is taken.

Will It Work for You? What the Studies Say:
Red clover has not been carefully examined as a healing agent. It contains compounds that function something like the female hormone estrogen: isoflavones as well as trace amounts of an estrogenic coumarin, coumestrol. Some herbalists have suggested putting these estrogenlike compounds to work in treating menopausal symptoms. A small 1994 study found increases in teat size and certain measurements of the uterus, along with other suggestive estrogen-like reactions, in three heifers fed large amounts of red clover silage for fourteen days.[2] No study has ever been done to demonstrate that any type of estrogen-like reactions occur in humans or that the active compounds are present at the safe, consistent levels that would be needed to treat an hormonal imbalance.

Red clover contains compounds that may have anticancer potential, such as daidzein and genisten, but the herb's cancer-fighting powers remain unclear. Preliminary test-tube studies indicate some potential.[3] Other constituents are mildly antispasmodic and expectorant, which means that the herb may help in treating congestion for spasmodic coughs.[4] There is no evidence to support the use of red clover for venereal disease.

Although herbalists continue to tout red clover as a healing agent for psoriasis, eczema, and rashes, scant information on the herb's powers to heal these types of skin disorders can be found. At most, a complex volatile oil containing methyl salicylate and benzyl alcohol may explain mild antiseptic or anti-inflammatory properties.

Will It Harm You? What the Studies Say:
There is little evidence to suggest that red clover poses any risk of serious adverse reactions in humans, although the subject has not been well studied. The FDA places red clover on its list of herbs "Generally Recognized As Safe" (GRAS) for food use. Given the herb's still poorly understood estrogen-like effects, common sense would dictate caution if you are taking birth control pills or hormone replacement therapy, have heart disease, are at risk for blood clots,

or suffer from an estrogen-dependent cancer.[5] Also avoid this herb if you are pregnant or are taking blood-thinning medicines. All tumors or possible symptoms of cancer should be examined and treated by a qualified physician before you consider using this or any other herb.

GENERAL SOURCES:
Bradley, P.C., ed. *British Herbal Compendium: A Handbook of Scientific Information on Widely Used Plant Drugs*, vol. 1. Bournemouth (Dorset), England: British Herbal Medicine Association, 1992.
Bremness, L. *Herbs*. 1st American ed. Eyewitness Handbooks. New York: Dorling Kindersley Publications, 1994.
Castleman, M. *The Healing Herbs: The Ultimate Guide to the Curative Power of Nature's Medicines*. New York: Bantam Books, 1995.
Chevallier, A. *The Encyclopedia of Medicinal Plants: A Practical Reference Guide to More Than 550 Key Medicinal Plants & Their Uses*. 1st American ed. New York: Dorling Kindersley Publications, 1996.
Dobelis, I.N., ed. *The Magic and Medicine of Plants: A Practical Guide to the Science, History, Folklore, and Everyday Uses of Medicinal Plants*. Pleasantville, NY: Reader's Digest Association, 1986.
Mindell, E. *Earl Mindell's Herb Bible*. New York: Simon & Schuster/Fireside, 1992.
Tierra, M. *The Way of Herbs*. New York: Pocket Books, 1990.
Tyler, V.E. *The Honest Herbal*. Binghamton, NY: Haworth Press/Pharmaceutical Products Press, 1993.

TEXT CITATIONS:
1. V.E. Tyler, *The Honest Herbal* (Binghamton, NY: Haworth Press/Pharmaceutical Products Press, 1993). M. Castleman, *The Healing Herbs: The Ultimate Guide to the Curative Power of Nature's Medicines* (New York: Bantam Books, 1995).
2. A.I. Nwannenna et al., *Acta Veterinaria Scandinavica*, 35(2) (1994): 173–83.
3. J.M. Cassady et al., *Cancer Research*, 48(22) (1988): 6257–61.
4. P.C. Bradley, ed., *British Herbal Compendium: A Handbook of Scientific Information on Widely Used Plant Drugs*, vol. 1. (Bournemouth [Dorset], England: British Herbal Medicine Association, 1992).
5. Castleman, op. cit.

PRIMARY NAME:
RED PEPPER

SCIENTIFIC NAME:
Capsicum annum L., *Capsicum frutescens* L., and other *Capsicum* varieties and hybrids. Family: Solanaceae

COMMON NAMES:
African chilis, bird pepper, capsicum, cayenne, chili pepper, Guinea pepper, hot pepper,

What Is Red Pepper?

Plant experts estimate that hot peppers derive from about five different species and their hybrids.[1] The shape, size, color, and pungency of the pepper can differ markedly. For medicinal purposes, the dried, ripe fruit is used. The source of the leathery, shiny red pepper is the shrubby perennial *Capsicum annum* native to tropical America and now cultivated worldwide. *Capsicum frutescens* yields a piquant, oblong fruit also referred to as red pepper. It is a small spreading annual native to tropical Africa.

Do not confuse red peppers with the black and white pepper spices found on most kitchen tables in America. These represent the unripened fruit of *Piper nigrum*. Also, do not confuse them with sweet bell peppers.

Louisiana long (and short) pepper, Mexican chili, paprika, tabasco pepper

RATING:
1 = Years of use and extensive, high-quality studies indicate that this substance is very effective when used properly and in recommended amounts for the indication(s) noted in the "Will It Work for You?" section. Safety depends on judicious use; see the "Will It Harm You?" section.

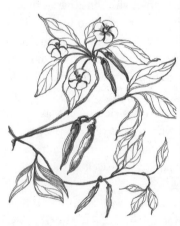

Red Pepper
Capsicum frutescens

What It Is Used For:

Few cultures around the world are unfamiliar with peppers as a spice—think of Tabasco® sauce in America—and many use their local varieties for myriad medicinal purposes as well. Contemporary Western herbalists recommend red pepper in the form of a tea for soothing indigestion and excess gas, stimulating the appetite, and controlling bowel problems. Many advise taking the herb to lessen severe and chronic pain, reduce milder pain such as that caused by headaches, control chills and other cold symptoms, reduce inflammation related to such disorders as psoriasis and arthritis, lower blood cholesterol, and mildly stimulate the body in the form of a tonic.

People suffering from stiffness and pain due to muscle soreness or arthritis and rheumatism may benefit from a red pepper formulation applied to the skin for its rubefacient and counterirritant properties. Commercial preparations containing the active ingredient capsaicin are used to control severe pain caused by neuritis syndromes such as shingles. Red pepper's irritating effect on mucous membranes is also put to use in self-defense sprays. More than a few folk healers have advised frustrated parents to sprinkle red pepper powder onto the thumbs of children who cannot seem to stop thumb-sucking.

Forms Available Include:

- *For internal use:* Capsule, concentrated drops, dried fruit, infusion, powder, tea, tincture.
- *For external use:* Cream, gel liniment, plaster. Many external formulations are standardized to contain specific concentrations of capsaicin, a critical active ingredient. The FDA has approved the use of a cream containing 0.075 percent capsaicin for over-the-counter sale.

Dosage Commonly Reported:

As a digestive aid and appetite stimulant, an infusion is made using ¼ to ½ teaspoon ground spice per cup of water; this is drunk after meals. The tincture is taken in doses of ¼ to ½ dropperful. Creams containing 0.025 to 0.075 percent capsaicin are sold over the counter. Follow package instructions carefully on how to apply capsaicin; sometimes a special applicator comes with it. The medicine must be applied several times daily—and in the dose prescribed—to be effective. If applied less than three to four times a day (or as directed), it will not be nearly as able to reduce pain and may actually lengthen the time that you feel common side effects such as warmth, burning, and stinging.

Will It Work for You? What the Studies Say:

The ingredient responsible for the piquancy of red peppers—a phenolic chemical called capsaicin—is also the one responsible for its medicinal properties. In fact, the more piquant the pepper, the more likely it is to offer healing benefits.

Red pepper has proven itself as a rubefacient and counterirritant, which means that it reddens and slightly irritates the skin, flooding the area with a sensation of warmth and helping to mask deeper pain. A burning sensation develops if concentrations are high. When applied repeatedly, capsaicin eventually causes the nerve cells to run out of a chemical they need to send pain signals to the brain. Capsaicin is now available in the form of an over-the-counter cream or gel to help alleviate a type of severe pain known as neuralgia, which can occur as a result of infection with the herpes zoster virus (responsible for chicken pox and shingles), diabetes, lumbago, and other disorders. It has also been used to control the pain of mastectomies and amputations, cluster headaches, arthritis, and psoriasis, and to manage minor pain from sprains, strains, and backaches.

Capsaicin has been tested as an inhalation solution for dulling the nasal nerves involved in causing such symptoms as sneezing and congestion. This kind of desensitization was observed in eight volunteers treated with capsaicin nose sprays.[2] According to another study, capsaicin can eliminate constriction of the bronchial tubes and airway swelling caused by irritants such as cigarette smoke, but only if it is given before exposure to the irritant.[3]

By jogging the flow of saliva and stomach secretions, the piquancy of red pepper aids digestion in many people, although those with sensitive stomachs may experience only irritation. Mixed results have been reported for the effect of red pepper on the secretion of stomach acids and the healing of ulcers. Several sources have suggested that ingesting red peppers will desensitize areas of ulcer pain, but no study has conclusively shown this.[4] Overall, red peppers do not appear either to help ulcers heal or to aggravate them.[5] In a 1972 report, no significant change in acid or pepsin secretion or gastric mucus was noted in individuals suffering from duodenal ulcers who were given red peppers to eat.[6] Ingesting capsaicin directly, however, has been shown to increase stomach acid concentrations in individuals with duodenal ulcers as well as those without ulcers.[7]

Claims that red pepper reduces cholesterol levels are weak. A 1987 study in rats fed a high-fat diet reported a significant reduction in blood triglyceride levels, but serum cholesterol levels overall were not altered.[8] No human trials on the subject appear to have been done so far.

Red peppers are a good source of vitamin C.

Will It Harm You? What the Studies Say:

Anyone who has accidentally touched his or her eyes—or any other mucous membrane—after handling red peppers is not likely to have forgotten the experience. Red peppers are famous for their irritating qualities. The responsible components—the capsaicinoids—can remain on the body for several hours, especially under fingernails. If you do develop eye irritation, try flushing out the eye with water and flushing any other affected part of the body with warm (not hot) soapy water; milk may help, according to anecdotal reports.[9] Vinegar reportedly works well, although it can itself be irritating. Another strategy is preventive: handle red peppers only with rubber gloves on. In any case, wash your hands well in warm soapy water every time you handle red peppers. The same holds true after applying capsaicin in over-the-counter formulations. Capsaicin will not blister skin.

Some people develop stomach upset with small doses of red peppers, while others find the plant soothing to the stomach. If you have never tried red pepper before, start slowly to see how you react. To lower the risk of a burning sensation, remove the seeds first[10] or eat a banana along with the pepper.[11] If taken in high doses over long periods of time, red peppers may cause kidney or liver damage or gastroenteritis.[12] If you are interested in taking red pepper internally and also take a prescription medicine, talk to a doctor first, as the red pepper may increase the liver's metabolism of other medicines and even interfere with high blood pressure medicines or monoamine oxidase (MAO) inhibitors.[13]

Many people develop skin irritation in reaction to the commercial creams. Sometimes the burning sensation is intolerable and the person stops using the product. For most people the capsaicin will cause feelings of warmth, burning, or stinging for the first few days. Sometimes this sensation lasts as long as two to four weeks or more, although it almost always lessens as treatment continues. Do not stop applying the capsaicin or reduce the dose because of these sensations, as this could make the symptoms worse. Keep cool, as heat, humidity, and sweat can heighten these side effects.

Never place red pepper or commercial products containing it on wounds or broken or irritated skin.

Pepper sprays can immediately blind an attacker and cause irritation for up to thirty minutes without causing permanent vision damage.

GENERAL SOURCES:

Castleman, M. *The Healing Herbs: The Ultimate Guide to the Curative Power of Nature's Medicines.* New York: Bantam Books, 1995.

Der Marderosian, A., and L. Liberti. *Natural Product Medicine: A Scientific Guide to Foods, Drugs, Cosmetics.* Philadelphia: George F. Stickley, 1988.

Lampe, K.E., and M.A. McCann. *AMA Handbook of Poisonous and Injurious Plants.* Chicago: American Medical Association, 1985.

Lawrence Review of Natural Products. St. Louis: Facts and Comparisons, July 1993.

Leung, A.Y., and S. Foster. *Encyclopedia of Common Natural Ingredients Used in Food, Drugs, and Cosmetics.* 2nd ed. New York: John Wiley & Sons, 1996.

Mayell, M. *Off-the-Shelf Natural Health: How to Use Herbs and Nutrients to Stay Well.* New York: Bantam Books, 1995.

Mindell, E. *Earl Mindell's Herb Bible.* New York: Simon & Schuster/Fireside, 1992.

Murray, M.T. *The Healing Power of Herbs: The Enlightened Person's Guide to the Wonders of Medicinal Plants.* Rev. 2nd ed. Rocklin, CA: Prima Publishing, 1995.

Newall, C.A., et al. *Herbal Medicines: A Guide for Health-Care Professionals.* London: The Pharmaceutical Press, 1996.

Ody, P. *The Herb Society's Complete Medicinal Herbal.* London: Dorling Kindersley Limited, 1993.

Tyler, V.E. *Herbs of Choice: The Therapeutic Use of Phytomedicinals.* Binghamton, NY: Haworth Press/Pharmaceutical Products Press, 1994.

———. *The Honest Herbal.* Binghamton, NY: Haworth Press/Pharmaceutical Products Press, 1993.

Weiner, M.A., and J.A. Weiner. *Herbs That Heal: Prescription for Herbal Healing.* Mill Valley, CA: Quantum Books, 1994.

TEXT CITATIONS:

1. *Lawrence Review of Natural Products* (St. Louis: Facts and Comparisons, July 1993).

2. M. Snyder, *USA Today*, (March 18, 1992).
3. S.H. Buck and T.F. Burks, *Tips*, 4 (1983): 84. *Lawrence Review of Natural Products*, op. cit.
4. C.A. Newall et al., *Herbal Medicines: A Guide for Health-Care Professionals* (London: The Pharmaceutical Press, 1996).
5. N. Kumar et al., *British Medical Journal*, 288 (1984): 1803.
6. B.N.D. Pimparker et al., *Journal of the Association of Physicians in India*, 20 (1972): 901–10.
7. R.A. Locock, *Canadian Pharmaceutical Journal*, 118 (1985): 517–19.
8. T. Kawada et al., *Journal of Nutrition*, 116 (1986): 1272–78. V.E. Tyler, *The Honest Herbal* (Binghamton, NY: Haworth Press/Pharmaceutical Products Press, 1993).
9. *Lawrence Review of Natural Products*, op. cit.
10. R.J. Prevost, *The Lancet*, 8277(l) (1982): 917.
11. *Lawrence Review of Natural Products*, op. cit. R.M. Roberts, *The Lancet*, 8270(l) (1982): 519.
12. Newall, op. cit.
13. Ibid.

PRIMARY NAME:
REHMANNIA

SCIENTIFIC NAME:
Rehmannia glutinosa (Gaertn.). Family: Scrophulariaceae

COMMON NAMES:
Chinese foxglove, di huang, earth yellow, gan dihuang (dried rehmannia), sheng dihuang (raw rehmannia), shu dihuang (cured rehmannia), sok-day-sang-day. The Japanese name for rehmannia is jio.

RATING:
3 = Studies on the effectiveness and safety of this substance are conflicting, or there are not enough studies to draw a conclusion.

What Is Rehmannia?

This flowering Chinese perennial is a hardy plant with large oval leaves and purple flowers. The thick, fleshy root is used medicinally.

What It Is Used For:

Rehmannia has been used for a millennium or more in traditional Chinese medicine as a nourishing *yin* tonic; it is found in many important herbal formulas and ranks among the most commonly used Chinese herbs.[1] Experts draw an important distinction between dried and cured rehmannia; the former is considered a cooling agent to treat what are considered "febrile" ailments, such as skin eruptions, restlessness, and nosebleeds, while the latter is normally used as a warming agent to nourish the "vital essence" and "tone" the blood,[2] properties considered useful in Chinese medicinal tradition for treating conditions such as heavy menstrual bleeding, dizziness, and premature hair graying.

Contemporary Western herbalists do not make a distinction between dried and cured rehmannia, characterizing it as one herb for a wide range of ills such as anemia and related fatigue, injured bones and tendons, and liver disease. In China, both forms are also consumed in soups and other foods to promote longevity and prevent disease. Extracts, valued for their anti-inflammatory and antimicrobial actions, appear in various Chinese hair-care and skin products.

Forms Available Include:

Decoction, extract, root (dried or cured; processed or unprocessed).

Dosage Commonly Reported:

To aid the liver and boost metabolism, 5 grams of root is chewed one to three times per day. Alternatively, a decoction is made using 5 grams of root per cup of water and drunk one to three times a day.[3] For blood loss and anemia, 15 grams of root is simmered in 500 milliliters of red wine. For heavy menstrual bleeding the root is taken as a decoction or as part of an herbal mixture known as "four things soup."[4]

Will It Work for You? What the Studies Say:

China and Japan have been the foci of research into this ancient medicinal root. Most studies have been conducted in the test tube or on laboratory animals; human trials do not appear in the medical literature accessible in the West. On the basis of research findings, rehmannia may indeed "nourish" the blood; in one study, for example, dried and prepared rehmannia helped promote the regeneration of red blood cells, helping laboratory mice to recover from anemia.[5] Whether this translates into similar reactions in humans has not been determined. Preliminary studies in hyperthyroid rats indicate that rehmannia may also help normalize certain cellular blood changes associated with hyperthyroidism.[6]

In one of several studies with potential implications for treating rheumatoid arthritis, an alcoholic extract from steamed and dried rehmannia demonstrated positive effects in the condition of the blood of arthritic and thrombotic (blood-clot-prone) rats, such as inhibiting deformations and drops in red blood cell counts, although it did nothing to prevent the development of edema (swelling) or inflammation.[7] Rehmannia's reputation as an antidiabetic agent was explored in various animal studies done in the 1930s, most of which found the root effective in decreasing high blood sugar levels in healthy rabbits.

Although the implications for manipulating the human immune system or treating cancers remain unclear, investigators have published intriguing findings based on rodent studies. One team reported in 1995 that a new component isolated from the herb—a polysaccharide fraction, Rehmannia glutinosa polysaccharide b—could inhibit the growth of various transplanted tumors when injected into laboratory mice, most likely through its impact on the immune system.[8] Dried rehmannia has demonstrated intriguing immune system–enhancing actions as well; in one study the root (type not specified) helped improve the immune-system defenses (specifically, cell-mediated and nonspecific immunity) in experimental mice.[9] Other studies have reported tranquilizing, diuretic, and liver-protectant actions.[10]

Will It Harm You? What the Studies Say:

According to mouse studies and long-term human use, often as a food, the toxicity of rehmannia is low. Properly controlled trials to confirm this have not been done, however, so moderation is advised.

GENERAL SOURCES:

Bremness, L. *Herbs.* 1st American ed. Eyewitness Handbooks. New York: Dorling Kindersley Publications, 1994.

Chevallier, A. *The Encyclopedia of Medicinal Plants: A Practical Reference Guide to More Than 550 Key Medicinal Plants & Their Uses.* 1st American ed. New York: Dorling Kindersley Publications, 1996.

Leung, A.Y., and S. Foster. *Encyclopedia of Common Natural Ingredients Used in Food, Drugs, and Cosmetics.* 2nd ed. New York: John Wiley & Sons, 1996.

Mindell, E. *Earl Mindell's Herb Bible*. New York: Simon & Schuster/Fireside, 1992.

Tierra, M. *The Way of Herbs*. New York: Pocket Books, 1990.

TEXT CITATIONS:

1. A.Y. Leung and S. Foster, *Encyclopedia of Common Natural Ingredients Used in Food, Drugs, and Cosmetics*, 2nd ed. (New York: John Wiley & Sons, 1996).
2. Ibid.
3. A. Chevallier, *The Encylopedia of Medicinal Plants: A Practical Reference Guide to More Than 550 Key Medicinal Plants & Their Uses*, 1st American ed. (New York: Dorling Kindersley Publications, 1996).
4. Ibid.
5. Y. Yuan et al., *Chung-Kuo Chung Yao Tsa Chih—China Journal of Chinese Materia Medica*, 17(6) (1992): 388–98.
6. J.C. Shan, *Chung-Kuo Chung Hsi I Chieh Ho Tsa Chih*, 14(2) (1994): 69–70, 96–98.
7. M. Kubo et al., *Biological & Pharmaceutical Bulletin*, 17(9) (1994): 1282–86.
8. L.Z. Chen et al., *Chung-Kuo Yao Li Hsueh Pao—Acta Pharmacologica Sinica*, 16(4) (1995): 337–40. L.Z. Chen et al., *Zhongguo Yaolixue Yu Dulixue Zazhi* (1993): 7(2)153–56.
9. Z.H. Luo, *Chinese Journal of Plastic Surgery & Burns*, 9(1) (1993): 56–58, 80.
10. Leung and Foster, op. cit.

PRIMARY NAME:

REISHI MUSHROOM

SCIENTIFIC NAME:

Ganoderma lucidum (Leyss. ex Fr.) Karst. and *Ganoderma japonicum* (Fr.) Lloyd. Family: Polyporaceae

COMMON NAMES:

Holy mushroom, ling chi, ling zhi cao, mannentake. *Ganoderma japonicum:* purple lingzhi; *Ganoderma lucidum:* red lingzhi

RATING:

3 = Studies on the effectiveness and safety of this substance are conflicting, or there are not enough studies to draw a conclusion.

What Is Reishi Mushroom?

Reishi is a fleshy fungus with a shiny, hard-crusted, off-center cap that changes from yellow to chestnut brown, or from dull purple to black in the case of *Ganoderma japonicum*. The mushrooms are collected in autumn, and the cap and stem are used medicinally. The Japanese prefer *Ganoderma lucidum*, a species that grows in the United States and is also the type primarily imported into this country. Both fungi grow throughout China.

What It Is Used For:

Oriental cuisines hold this flavorful mushroom in high esteem. The fungus, considered the "elixir of life,"[1] commands a venerable status in traditional Chinese healing. Stores were once reserved for Chinese emperors. Reishi still ranks as one of the premier Chinese tonics and in addition to reportedly benefiting vital *qi* energy and boosting energy and resistance to disease and stress, not to mention promoting longevity, it is traditionally used to treat a myriad of ailments ranging from general weakness to cough, indigestion, appetite loss, and high blood pressure. Extracts can be found in moisturizing complexion creams and other skin care products. Reishi mushroom's aroma can be detected in Chinese soups and herbal drinks.

Contemporary Western herbalists recommend reishi mushroom to stimulate the immune system, prevent or slow cancerous growths, control allergies, lower cholesterol, help prevent blood clots, and balance the system overall. Along with the shiitake (see **Shiitake Mushroom**), reishi is one of America's most popular medicinal mushrooms.

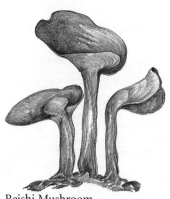

Reishi Mushroom
Ganoderma lucidum

Forms Available Include:

Capsule, concentrated drops, liquid extract, mushroom (fresh and dried), standardized extracts, tablet, tea (bags and granules), tincture.

Dosage Commonly Reported:

Three to six 606-milligram capsules are taken daily.

Will It Work for You? What the Studies Say:

Most of the research on reishi mushroom has been done on *Ganoderma lucidum.* Studies of animals and in a few cases of humans indicate that it has a broad range of activity. According to a number of them, it affects the central nervous system with possible painkilling, sedative, and anticonvulsive properties[2] and may help inhibit some of the chemical steps involved in allergic reactions (including antihistamine effects),[3] reduce inflammation,[4] jog the immune system (in the case of a particular immunomodulator in the mushroom, ling zhi-8),[5] lower blood sugar levels,[6] inhibit the aggregation of platelets and therefore possibly have a role to play in preventing blood clots and treating atherosclerotic disease,[7] protect against radiation damage,[8] lower blood cholesterol levels,[9] shield the user from environmentally induced liver damage[10] (in some cases through an antioxidant activity),[11] increase coronary blood flow as well as increase and decrease blood pressure,[12] and fight certain types of tumors or tumor cells (in most cases).[13] Future studies may or may not conclude that some of these actions occur in human beings taking reishi.

Will It Harm You? What the Studies Say:

Studies indicate that reishi mushrooms are very safe to take, causing no toxic reactions in mice at high doses, and only rarely producing adverse reactions in humans after long-term (three to six months) and continuous use. These reactions may include dizziness, itching, stomach upset, bloody stools, nosebleeds, and dryness in the mouth, nose, and throat.[14] Allergic reactions are also possible.

GENERAL SOURCES:

Bremness, L. *Herbs.* 1st American ed. Eyewitness Handbooks. New York: Dorling Kindersley Publications, 1994.

Leung, A.Y., and S. Foster. *Encyclopedia of Common Natural Ingredients Used in Food, Drugs, and Cosmetics.* 2nd ed. New York: John Wiley & Sons, 1996.

Mayell, M. *Off-the-Shelf Natural Health: How to Use Herbs and Nutrients to Stay Well.* New York: Bantam Books, 1995.

Weiner, M.A., and J.A. Weiner. *Herbs That Heal: Prescription for Herbal Healing.* Mill Valley, CA: Quantum Books, 1994.

TEXT CITATIONS:

1. A.Y. Leung and S. Foster, *Encyclopedia of Common Natural Ingredients Used in Food, Drugs, and Cosmetics,* 2nd ed. (New York: John Wiley & Sons, 1996).
2. Ibid. Y. Kasahara and H. Hikino, *Phytotherapy Research,* 1(1) (1987): 17. Y. Kasahara and H. Hikino, *Phytotherapy Research.* 1(4) (1987): 173.
3. K. Tasaka et al., *Agents & Actions,* 23(3–4) (1988): 153–56. H. Kohda et al., *Chemical & Pharmaceutical Bulletin,* 33 (1985): 1367. M. Nogami et al., *Yakugaku Zasshi,* 106 (1986): 594.

4. J.M. Lin et al., *American Journal of Chinese Medicine*, 21(1) (1993): 59-69.
5. K. Kino et al., *International Journal of Immunopharmacology*, 13(8) (1991): 1109–15.
6. H. Hikino et al., *Planta Medica*, 4 (1985): 339. H. Hikino and T. Mizuno, *Planta Medica*, 55 (1989): 385.
7. J. Tao and K.Y. Feng, *Journal of Tongji Medical University*, 10(4) (1990): 240–43. A. Shimizu et al., *Chemical & Pharmaceutical Bulletin*, 33 (1985): 3012. M. Kubo et al., *Yakugaku Zasshi*, 103 (1983): 871.
8. H.Y. Hsu et al., *American Journal of Chinese Medicine*, 18(1–2) (1990): 61–69.
9. M.J. Lee and M.H. Chung, *Korean Journal of Pharmacognosy*, 18 (1987): 254.
10. Ibid. G.T. Liu et al., *Chinese Medical Journal*, 92 (1979): 496.
11. J.M. Lin et al., *Journal of Ethnopharmacology*, 47(1) (1995): 33–41.
12. A. Morigiwa et al., *Chemical & Pharmaceutical Bulletin*, 34 (1986): 3052.
13. H. Maruyama et al., *Journal of Pharmacobio-Dynamics*, 12(2) (1989): 118–23. Y. Sone et al., *Agricultural and Biological Chemistry*, 49 (1985): 2641. T. Miyazaki and M. Nishijima, *Chemical & Pharmaceutical Bulletin*, 29 (1981): 3611. T.K. Yun et al., *Anticancer Research*, 15(3) (1995): 839–45. C.W. Lieu et al., *Anticancer Research*, 12(4) (1992): 1211–15. T.W. Chen et al., *Chung Hua I Hsueh Tsa Chih— Chinese Medical Journal*, 48(1) (1991): 54–58.
14. Leung and Foster, op. cit.

PRIMARY NAME:
RHATANY

SCIENTIFIC NAME:
Krameria triandra Ruiz & Pav. Also referred to as *Krameria argentea* Mart. Family: Krameriaceae

COMMON NAMES:
Krameria root, Peruvian rhatany, rhatany root

RATING:
2 = According to a number of well-designed studies and common use, this substance appears to be relatively effective and safe when used in recommended amounts for the indication(s) noted in the "Will It Work for You?" section.

What Is Rhatany?

Rhatany is the reddish-brown, bitter-tasting root of *Krameria triandra*, an undershrub native to the Andean region of South America that bears large red flowers, and the related species *Krameria ayentea*. The root is dried for medicinal use.

What It Is Used For:

This traditional South American healing herb was highly valued for its astringent properties. Gargles, tinctures, and oral paints were typically used to treat inflamed or bleeding gums, other oral inflammations such as canker sores (noninfectious kinds), gingivitis, sore throat, and tongue fissures. Internally it was taken for diarrhea (including dysentery) and other gastrointestinal tract problems. Modern Western herbalists recommend many of these uses, emphasizing the root's astringent and anti-infective properties.

Forms Available Include:

- *For mouth and throat ailments:* Decoction to make gargles and mouthwashes, extract, tincture (undiluted or mixed with another herb as an oral paint, or diluted with water as a mouthwash), root.
- *For hemorrhoids:* Ointment, suppository.

Dosage Commonly Reported:

As a mouthwash or gargle, rhatany is used in a decoction made from 1 teaspoon chopped root per glass of water; this is taken two or three times a day. Alternatively, 1 to 2 teaspoons tincture is added to a glass of water. The undiluted tincture is applied to canker sores. The root extract is taken in doses of 0.3 to 1 gram.

Will It Work for You? What the Studies Say:

Rhatany contains high levels of tannins[1] (10 percent or more, often more than 20 percent), astringent substances that tighten tissue and inhibit blood and other fluid secretions. German health authorities approve of using rhatany externally for mild mouth and throat inflammations[2] such as canker sores and sore throat. Gargles and mouthwashes made from a root decoction are common formulations.

Root preparations may also help fight infections, according to studies that have attributed antimicrobial properties to some of the tannins (procyanidins)[3] and other substances (benzofuran compounds of the ratanhiaphernol type) in the plant.[4] These astringent and anti-infective properties may explain why the root has traditionally been used to treat hemorrhoids and bleeding wounds. No animal or human studies to prove these treatments effective have apparently been done.

Taken internally, tannins are believed to control or stop diarrhea by reducing inflammation in the intestines. Because of this known property, rhatany root taken internally may well control diarrhea. Very high tannin concentrations (taken internally) pose their own risks, however. German health authorities make no comment on the effectiveness of rhatany for diarrhea.

Will It Harm You? What the Studies Say:

Evidence indicates that topical rhatany formulations pose no risk of harm, although German health authorities recommend seeking medical advice before using them for more than two weeks. The only potential negative reaction to topical forms of the herb is an allergic reaction in the mucous membranes, such as swelling in the mouth.

Avoid long-term use of any tannin-rich drug, given the still poorly understood health hazards, such as stomach irritations and cancer. The FDA approves rhatany as a food ingredient in the form of a flavoring; it appears on the list of items "Generally Recognized As Safe" (GRAS).

GENERAL SOURCES:

Bisset, N.G., ed. *Herbal Drugs and Phytopharmaceuticals*. Stuttgart: medpharm GmbH Scientific Publishers, 1994.

Blumenthal, M., J. Gruenwald, T. Hall, and R.S. Rister, eds. *The Complete German Commission E Monographs: Therapeutic Guide to Herbal Medicine*. Boston: Integrative Medicine Communications, 1998.

Bradley, P.C., ed. *British Herbal Compendium: A Handbook of Scientific Information on Widely Used Plant Drugs*, vol. 1. Bournemouth (Dorset), England: British Herbal Medicine Association, 1992.

Chevallier, A. *The Encyclopedia of Medicinal Plants: A Practical Reference Guide to More Than 550 Key Medicinal Plants & Their Uses*. 1st American ed. New York: Dorling Kindersley Publications, 1996.

Tyler, V.E. *Herbs of Choice: The Therapeutic Use of Phytomedicinals*. Binghamton, NY: Haworth Press/Pharmaceutical Products Press, 1994.

TEXT CITATIONS:
1. E. Scholz and H. Rimpler, *Planta Medica*, 55 (1989): 379–84.
2. M. Blumenthal, J. Gruenwald, T. Hall, and R.S. Rister, eds., *The Complete German Commission E Monographs: Therapeutic Guide to Herbal Medicine* (Boston: Integrative Medicine Communications, 1998).
3. Scholz and Rimpler, op. cit.
4. A. Arnone et al., *Gazzetta Chimica Italiana*, 118 (1988): 675–82. P.C. Bradley, ed., *British Herbal Compendium: A Handbook of Scientific Information on Widely Used Plant Drugs*, vol. 1 (Bournemouth [Dorset], England: British Herbal Medicine Association, 1992).

PRIMARY NAME:

RHUBARB, CHINESE

SCIENTIFIC NAME:

Rheum palmatum L. or *Rheum officinale* Baill., or hybrids or mixtures of these two species. Family: Polygonaceae

COMMON NAMES:

Canton rhubarb, medicinal rhubarb, shensi rhubarb

RATING:

2 = According to a number of well-designed studies and common use, this substance appears to be relatively effective and safe when used in recommended amounts for the indication(s) noted in the "Will It Work for You?" section. However, see warnings in the "Will It Harm You?" section.

What Is Chinese Rhubarb?

This tall, sturdy perennial has conspicuous palm-shaped leaves, winged fruits, and purplish-red to white flowers. The dried and peeled rhizomes (underground stems) and roots, which yield a bright yellowish to brown powder, are used medicinally. The highest-quality herb grows at high altitudes in Asia, either in the wild or cultivated.[1]

Do not confuse this type of rhubarb with the common garden rhubarb, *Rheum rhaponticum*, typically used as a food or vegetable.

What It Is Used For:

Over the centuries, traditional Chinese healers have honored the two notable and somewhat contradictory properties of this herb—laxative and astringent (hence antidiarrheal)—by prescribing carefully calculated amounts to achieve the desired action. At higher doses, the herb is said to ease constipation, while at lower doses it is said to control diarrhea. A valued medicine in Europe as early as the first century after Christ, Chinese rhubarb (henceforth referred to as "rhubarb") came to play an important role in commercial trade with China.[2]

Traditional Chinese healers also prescribe rhubarb for cancer, fever, headache, sores, toothache, and assorted other ills. In Western countries, it has a reputation as a stomach-soothing agent as well. European plant medicines for "blood cleansing," "slimming," and stimulating bile flow or easing stomach upset sometimes contain rhubarb, as do the famous Swedish herbal bitters.

Forms Available Include:

Decoction, infusion, root (powdered or chopped), tincture. Both the decoction and the infusion are made with finely chopped or powdered roots or powdered extracts of the roots. Rhubarb is also added to herbal blends.

Dosage Commonly Reported:

As a laxative, the root is taken in daily doses of 1.2 to 4.8 grams; as a stomachic, 0.12 to 0.36 gram. A decoction is made using ½ to 1 teaspoon powdered or finely chopped root per cup of water. For constipation, a cup of the decoction is drunk once or twice per day, in the morning and/or at night. As a stomachic, the decoction is made with 0.1 to 0.2 gram powdered root (1 teaspoon equals

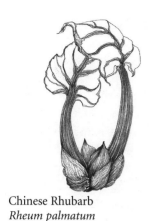

Chinese Rhubarb
Rheum palmatum

2.5 grams) and is drunk once or twice per day. (In China, daily doses of the root range from 3 to 12 grams.) The tincture is taken in daily dosages up to 15 milliliters.

Will It Work for You? What the Studies Say:

This chemically complex herb contains two ingredients of particular note: anthraquinones and considerable concentrations of astringent tannins. Anthraquinones are powerful laxative chemicals that were long believed to work by irritating the large intestine. They inhibit the uptake of water and electrolytes (salts) in the large intestine and also influence movement through the intestines.[3] Other constituents may contribute to the herb's laxative effect as well, or may play an even more significant role than these properties.[4]

German health authorities endorse the use of rhubarb for constipation and various ailments for which a soft stool is desired, such as hemorrhoids and anal fissures.[5] As intestinal irritants, anthraquinones, which are also found in such powerful laxative herbs as aloe juice (see **Aloe Vera**), can cause severe intestinal cramping and colic. For this reason, anthraquinone-containing herbs are often mixed with other agents. Rhubarb also serves as a component in European cholagogues (to increase bile flow to the intestines).[6]

Rhubarb's astringent tannins are also believed to control or stop diarrhea by reducing inflammation in the intestines. Traditional Chinese and European healers, among others, have been using the herb for this purpose for centuries, and German health authorities officially approve of small doses of rhubarb as an astringent to counter diarrhea.[7] Interestingly, rhubarb extracts have also been used in China to treat upper digestive tract bleeding, reportedly with notable success.[8]

The presence of astringent tannins, which are known to constrict (tighten) tissue and reduce oozing and bleeding, probably also inspired the herb's traditional application for external wounds and ulcers. Research indicates that one of the constituent tannins also has analgesic and anti-inflammatory properties,[9] which would obviously help wounds heal as well.

Rhubarb's bitter taste is also put to use in herbal digestive "tonics" such as Swedish bitters to increase salivation, get digestive juices flowing, and thereby help soothe stomach upset. Studies have also shown that components in the tannins contain notable painkilling and anti-inflammatory properties.[10]

Rhubarb has also been studied, primarily by Chinese investigators, as a treatment for chronic renal failure[11] and endometriosis,[12] and for preventing pregnancy-induced high blood pressure.[13]

Will It Harm You? What the Studies Say:

When used properly, rhubarb has not generally been linked to any side effects. The exception to this is griping (sharp stomach pain) associated with its use as a laxative. For this reason, some sources consider the herb inappropriate for laxative use; the amount of active substance in the herb varies enough that it is difficult to know if you are getting too much or too little. Also, taking rhubarb habitually, very frequently (for more than a few days), or in excessive amounts can also lead to loss of important bodily fluids and salts such as potassium, and loss of pigmentation of intestinal mucosa. Whenever considering taking a laxative, keep in mind the gentler approaches to reducing constipation, including increasing your fluid and fiber intake and exercising.

There are several situations in which taking rhubarb would probably be unwise. German health authorities warn that the herb should not be used if the intestines are obstructed in any way, or taken during pregnancy or lactation because of the risk of reflex stimulation of the uterus or substances in the rhubarb passing to the infant.[14] Some European authorities advise against taking rhubarb preparations if you suffer from a kidney disorder[15] or are taking a cardiotonic glycoside such as digitalis, because rhubarb may enhance the effect of the medicine. Rhubarb may temporarily (and harmlessly) discolor urine to a deep yellowish to reddish brown.

To avoid absorption and possible toxic reactions to the contained tannins, do not apply topical formulations to burned skin or large areas of skin. The plant's leaf blades are poisonous and can cause severe vomiting and liver and kidney damage if accidentally ingested.[16]

GENERAL SOURCES:

Bisset, N.G., ed. *Herbal Drugs and Phytopharmaceuticals.* Stuttgart: medpharm GmbH Scientific Publishers, 1994.

Blumenthal, M., J. Gruenwald, T. Hall, and R.S. Rister, eds. *The Complete German Commission E Monographs: Therapeutic Guide to Herbal Medicine.* Boston: Integrative Medicine Communications, 1998.

Bradley, P.C., ed. *British Herbal Compendium: A Handbook of Scientific Information on Widely Used Plant Drugs,* vol. 1. Bournemouth (Dorset), England: British Herbal Medicine Association, 1992.

Dobelis, I.N., ed. *The Magic and Medicine of Plants: A Practical Guide to the Science, History, Folklore, and Everyday Uses of Medicinal Plants.* Pleasantville, NY: Reader's Digest Association, 1986.

Duke, J.A. *CRC Handbook of Medicinal Herbs.* Boca Raton, FL: CRC Press, 1985.

Leung, A.Y., and S. Foster. *Encyclopedia of Common Natural Ingredients Used in Food, Drugs, and Cosmetics.* 2nd ed. New York: John Wiley & Sons, 1996.

Mayell, M. *Off-the-Shelf Natural Health: How to Use Herbs and Nutrients to Stay Well.* New York: Bantam Books, 1995.

Newall, C.A., et al. *Herbal Medicines: A Guide for Health-Care Professionals.* London: The Pharmaceutical Press, 1996.

Tierra, M. *The Way of Herbs.* New York: Pocket Books, 1990.

Tyler, V.E. *Herbs of Choice: The Therapeutic Use of Phytomedicinals.* Binghamton, NY: Haworth Press/Pharmaceutical Products Press, 1994.

Weiner, M.A., and J.A. Weiner. *Herbs That Heal: Prescription for Herbal Healing.* Mill Valley, CA: Quantum Books, 1994.

Weiss, R.F. *Herbal Medicine,* trans. A.R. Meuss, from the 6th German edition. Beaconsfield, England: Beaconsfield Publishers, Ltd., 1988.

TEXT CITATIONS:

1. P.C. Bradley, ed., *British Herbal Compendium: A Handbook of Scientific Information on Widely Used Plant Drugs,* vol. 1 (Bournemouth [Dorset], England: British Herbal Medicine Association, 1992).

2. J.A. Duke, *CRC Handbook of Medicinal Herbs* (Boca Raton, FL: CRC Press, 1985).

3. A.Y. Leung and S. Foster, *Encyclopedia of Common Natural Ingredients Used in Food, Drugs, and Cosmetics,* 2nd ed. (New York: John Wiley & Sons, 1996).

4. T. Yamagishi et al., *Chemical & Pharmaceutical Bulletin*, 35 (1987): 3132.
5. M. Blumenthal, J. Gruenwald, T. Hall, and R.S. Rister, eds., *The Complete German Commission E Monographs: Therapeutic Guide to Herbal Medicine* (Boston: Integrative Medicine Communications, 1998).
6. N.G. Bisset ed. *Herbal Drugs and Phytopharmaceuticals* (Stuttgart: medpharm GmbH Scientific Publishers, 1994).
7. Blumenthal et al., op. cit.
8. D.H. Jiao et al., *Pharmacology*, 20(Suppl. 1) (1980): 128. D.A. Sun et al., *Chinese Journal of Integrative Medicine*, 6 (1986): 4589. Leung and Foster, op. cit.
9. Bisset, op. cit.
10. G.I. Nonaka et al., *Chemical & Pharmaceutical Bulletin*, 29 (1981): 2862.
11. Z. Kang et al., *Journal of Traditional Chinese Medicine*, 13(4) (1993): 249–52. G. Zhang and A.M. el Nahas, *Nephrology, Dialysis, Transplantation*, 11(1) (1996): 186–90.
12. D.Z. Wang et al., *Chung Hsi I Chieh Ho Tsa Chih—Chinese Journal of Modern Developments in Traditional Medicine*, 11(9) (1991): 515, 524–26.
13. Z.J. Zhang et al., *Chinese Journal of Obstetrics & Gynecology*, 29(8) (1994): 463–64, 509.
14. Bisset, op. cit.
15. Bradley, op. cit.
16. Leung and Foster, op. cit.

PRIMARY NAME:
ROSE HIP

SCIENTIFIC NAME:
Rosa canina L., *Rosa gallica* L., *Rosa rugosa* Thunb., *Rosa villosa* L., and other *Rosa* species. Family: Rosaceae

COMMON NAMES:
Heps, hipberries

RATING:
3 = Studies on the effectiveness and safety of this substance are conflicting, or there are not enough studies to draw a conclusion.

What is Rose Hip?

The rosebush, a native of Europe and Asia, is now extensively cultivated around the world for its graceful, fragrant flowers. Rose hip is marble-sized, brilliantly red fruit that forms on the prickly branch after the petals of the blossom fall away. The major commercial source of rose hip is *Rosa canina* (dog rose).

What It Is Used For:

The discovery of vitamin C (ascorbic acid) in the 1930s and the realization that rose hips contained large amounts revived enthusiasm for this herb among herbalists.[1] In the past, rose hips had been recommended as a laxative, diuretic, and skin astringent and as a treatment for headache, mouth sores, and numerous other ills. As a natural source of vitamin C, rose hips became popular as ingredients in "natural" vitamin supplements such as teas, capsules, tablets, extracts, and even foods that could then boast a nutritional content. Many sources tout rose hip formulations as the key to preventing and treating the common cold and flu; this accepts the controversial premise that saturating the body with vitamin C will enhance the body's resistance. Many herbalists also note the thirst-quenching, laxative, and diuretic ("water pill") properties of rose hips.

Forms Available Include:

Capsule, hips (fresh and dried), infusion, tablet, tea bag, tincture.

Dosage Commonly Reported:

An infusion is made using a scant ¾ teaspoon of dried, chopped hips per cup of water and is taken as needed. The tea is drunk cold for fever. Take commercially prepared capsules, tablets, and tinctures according to package directions.

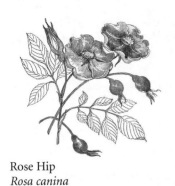

Rose Hip
Rosa canina

Will It Work for You? What the Studies Say:

The pleasant taste of rose hips appeals to many palates, but the herb constitutes an unreliable and expensive source of vitamin C. The concentration of the vitamin varies widely, depending on a number of factors, including the species the rose hips were taken from, the climate they were grown in, and the ripeness of the hips when picked.[2] By the time they make it onto the drugstore shelf, much of the vitamin originally present—concentrations range from 0.24 to 1.25 percent—has been eliminated during extraction or ordinary drying. Some commercial samples contain no detectable amount of vitamin C.[3]

To ensure an acceptable vitamin C content, many manufacturers fortify their "natural" rose hip products with synthetic ascorbic acid. There is often no way for the consumer to discern the source of the vitamin C.[4] In any case, your body will not know the difference, although at the steep prices for the "natural" label, your pocketbook might.

Given these variables, it may not be wise to rely on commercial rose hip products as a source of vitamin C. Also keep in mind that an infusion will extract only a part of the vitamin C. Rose hips certainly do not represent the only food source for this vitamin. If they are of the highest quality and still fresh, rose hips contain about 1,250 milligrams of vitamin C per 100 grams; other excellent sources include citrus fruits (about 50 milligrams), kiwi fruit and uncooked broccoli (about 100 milligrams), and Barbados cherry (about 1,000 to 2,330 milligrams).[5] Lemon juice is the best source of vitamin C.[6]

Taking rose hips to prevent or shorten cold or flu symptoms assumes that saturating the body with vitamin C will help, a controversial theory. German health authorities, normally open to the potential benefits of herbs and other unconventional methods of medicine, do not consider the evidence for vitamin C as a cold- or flu-preventor sufficient to endorse it.[7] On the other hand, drinking a lot of rose hip tea will help ensure that your fluid intake is high, which is widely considered beneficial for keeping secretions fluid. When drunk hot, the tea may well relieve sensations of soreness in the throat.

In addition to vitamin C, rose hips contain chemicals—malic and citric acid in particular—that explain their traditional use as a mild laxative and diuretic. The medical literature contains no references to clinical trials on this subject.

Will It Harm You? What the Studies Say:

Rose hips do not pose a risk of serious adverse reactions, at least according to common experience and data collected so far. Vitamin C is a water-soluble vitamin, so the body generally flushes out any excess amount. High doses of vitamin C are hard to get from rose hips anyway. Megadose vitamin C supplements that may or may not contain rose hips have, however, been associated with cases in which the kidneys are strained and complications such as kidney and bladder (oxalate) stones develop. There have also been reports that the dust from the hips can cause severe respiratory allergies in people repeatedly exposed to them, such as production workers.[8]

GENERAL SOURCES:

Balch, J.F., and P.A. Balch. *Prescription for Nutritional Healing: A Practical A to Z Reference to Drug-Free Remedies Using Vitamins, Minerals, Herbs & Food Supplements.* 2nd ed. Garden City Park, NY: Avery Publishing Group, 1997.

Castleman, M. *The Healing Herbs: The Ultimate Guide to the Curative Power of Nature's Medicines.* New York: Bantam Books, 1995.

Lawrence Review of Natural Products. St. Louis: Facts and Comparisons, September 1991.

Leung, A.Y., and S. Foster. *Encyclopedia of Common Natural Ingredients Used in Food, Drugs, and Cosmetics.* 2nd ed. New York: John Wiley & Sons, 1996.

Mayell, M. *Off-the-Shelf Natural Health: How to Use Herbs and Nutrients to Stay Well.* New York: Bantam Books, 1995.

Tyler, V.E. *The Honest Herbal.* Binghamton, NY: Haworth Press/Pharmaceutical Products Press, 1993.

Tyler, V.E., L.R. Brady, and J.E. Robbers, eds. *Pharmacognosy.* Philadelphia: Lea & Febiger, 1988.

Weiss, R.F. *Herbal Medicine,* trans. A.R. Meuss, from the 6th German edition. Beaconsfield, England: Beaconsfield Publishers, Ltd., 1988.

TEXT CITATIONS:

1. M. Castleman, *The Healing Herbs: The Ultimate Guide to the Curative Power of Nature's Medicines* (New York: Bantam Books, 1995).
2. A.Y. Leung and S. Foster, *Encyclopedia of Common Natural Ingredients Used in Food, Drugs, and Cosmetics,* 2nd ed. (New York: John Wiley & Sons, 1996).
3. V.E. Tyler, *The Honest Herbal* (Binghamton, NY: Haworth Press/Pharmaceutical Products Press, 1993).
4. V.E. Tyler, L.R. Brady, and J.E. Robbers, eds., *Pharmacognosy* (Philadelphia: Lea & Febiger, 1988).
5. *Lawrence Review of Natural Products* (St. Louis: Facts and Comparisons, September 1991).
6. R.F. Weiss, *Herbal Medicine,* trans. A.R. Meuss, from the 6th German edition (Beaconsfield, England: Beaconsfield Publishers, Ltd., 1988).
7. M. Blumenthal, J. Gruenwald, T. Hall, and R.S. Rister, eds., *The Complete German Commission E Monographs: Therapeutic Guide to Herbal Medicine* (Boston: Integrative Medicine Communications, 1998).
8. A. Kwaselow et al., *Journal of Allergy and Clinical Immunology,* 85(4) (1990): 704–8.

PRIMARY NAME:
ROSEMARY

SCIENTIFIC NAME:
Rosmarinus officinalis L.
Family: Labiatae (Lamiaceae)

COMMON NAMES:
Mi die xiang, old man, rosemarine

What Is Rosemary?

Rosemary is a small, camphor-scented evergreen shrub with thick, needlelike leaves that are dark on top and whitish underneath. It is native to the Mediterranean region but is now cultivated worldwide. The leaves are used medicinally and steam distillation of the fresh pale blue flowers produces an essential oil.

What It Is Used For:

Europeans have treasured this aromatic herb since ancient times as both a flavoring and a healing agent. Centuries ago, meats were wrapped in rosemary leaves to help preserve them. Superstition held that rosemary could ward off evil spirits, cure paralysis, and perform a number of other remarkable feats; it even earned a reputation for helping to sharpen and preserve memory.

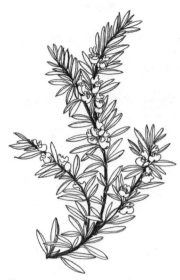

Rosemary
Rosmarinus officinalis

Many herbalists today contend that it can stimulate the digestive, circulatory, and nervous systems. Rosemary and its oil have been used for calming indigestion and stomach upset, relieving gas, promoting menstrual flow, encouraging hair growth (when applied externally), repelling insects, and treating headaches (including migraines). Head colds, muscle pain, joint inflammation, bad breath, nervous tension, mental fatigue, depression, poorly healing wounds, eczema, and cancers have all been treated with it. Rosemary baths are popular in parts of Europe for relaxing the body as well as stimulating blood circulation to the skin. German herbal textbooks recommend rosemary spirits externally for nerve pain, rheumatic complaints, and certain (functional) heart complaints.[1] Traditional Chinese healers have used the herb similarly over the centuries.

Rosemary extracts appear in foods as flavorings and in cosmetics; the oil is a popular fragrance component in soaps, perfumes, and other commercial products.

Forms Available Include:

- *For internal use:* Fresh and dried stems with leaves, infusion, powder, spirit, tincture.
- *For external use:* Essential oil, ointment. Also an ingredient in bath preparations.

Dosage Commonly Reported:

Four to 6 grams of rosemary are taken internally. An infusion is made using 1 teaspoon (2 grams) of chopped leaves per cup of water. Rosemary spirit is taken internally in doses of 0.3 to 1.2 milliliters, or applied externally for rheumatic pains. The essential oil is used externally in combined preparations and also in aromatherapy. For a bath additive, an aqueous extract is made using 50 grams leaves per liter of water.

Will It Work for You? What the Studies Say:

Researchers have uncovered a number of intriguing properties in rosemary, a few of which give some credence to long-standing folk uses. But so far, no properly conducted clinical trials have conclusively verified that any of these properties works in humans. The volatile oil (1 to 2.5 percent) in the leaves is probably responsible for the herb's medicinal properties; it contains such ingredients as camphor, monoterpene hydrocarbons, borneol, and cineol. The oil fights certain bacteria as well as fungi; this may explain its reputation as an infection-fighter.

The volatile oil contained in the leaves offers some carminative properties valuable for relieving gas in the stomach and intestines, as well as for calming indigestion, stimulating the appetite, and reducing bloating sensations.[2] Extracts show spasm-reducing properties in the small intestine and bile duct, a type of stomach-soothing property often seen in culinary herbs.[3] German health authorities endorse the use of rosemary leaves internally for indigestion.[4]

Rosemary also contains camphor, a skin irritant that increases blood supply to the skin. Because of this property, rosemary oil or ointment is used, often in the form of a bath, to reduce pain in rheumatic muscles and joints. German physicians recommend rosemary baths (made with infusions or oil) as tonics to improve chronic circulatory weaknesses such as low blood pressure, varicose veins, rheumatic pain, bruises, and sprains.[5] Some plant experts question whether this strategy actually improves deeper circulation,[6] although it may feel as if it does. The essential oil has even been massaged into the skin around the heart to treat the symptoms of (functional) heart complaints such as chest pain; the effectiveness of this may have to do largely with the sufferer's feeling that he or she is doing something about the problem.[7] German health authorities endorse rosemary in external formulations for rheumatism of the muscles and joints.[8] Its value as an internal stimulant is still being debated.[9]

One of the most intriguing recent discoveries is that rosemary may help fight cancer, as the folk use suggests. Contemporary herbalists consider the herb a good source of antioxidants.[10] In humans, antioxidants are believed to control the formation of dangerous substances in the body called free radicals. These substances damage cells through oxidation, some of which may contribute to cancer cell formation. Plant experts contend that in some cases rosemary herb and its oil are comparable in their antioxidant activity to commercial food preservatives such as BHT and BHA.[11] Interestingly, rosemary has been used for centuries as a preservative to protect packaged foods from rotting. In 1995, Japanese investigators reported identifying two compounds (carnosol and carnosic acid) in the herb that may protect body tissue and cells against oxidative stresses that have been linked to such disorders as diabetes, aging, and coronary arteriosclerosis.[12] In one study, rosemary extract significantly inhibited (by nearly half) the development of laboratory-induced mammary (breast tissue) tumors in laboratory mice, compared with those not fed the extract.[13]

Will It Harm You? What the Studies Say:

Rosemary is safe to use as a kitchen herb. The oil does not usually cause irritation or allergic reactions when applied to the skin, although skin redness and dermatitis have been reported in people whose skin is sensitive to it.[14] But avoid ingesting the essential oil—as this can irritate the stomach and intestines and even cause kidney damage—or applying large amounts of it.[15] German health authorities advise pregnant women not to take medicinal rosemary preparations because of potential adverse effects from the essential oil.[16] The herb has reportedly never been shown to induce abortion.

GENERAL SOURCES:

Bisset, N.G., ed. *Herbal Drugs and Phytopharmaceuticals.* Stuttgart: medpharm GmbH Scientific Publishers, 1994.

Blumenthal, M., J. Gruenwald, T. Hall, and R.S. Rister, eds. *The Complete German Commission E Monographs: Therapeutic Guide to Herbal Medicine.* Boston: Integrative Medicine Communications, 1998.

Castleman, M. *The Healing Herbs: The Ultimate Guide to the Curative Power of Nature's Medicines.* New York: Bantam Books, 1995.

Lawrence Review of Natural Products. St. Louis: Facts and Comparisons, February 1992.

Leung, A.Y., and S. Foster. *Encyclopedia of Common Natural Ingredients Used in Food, Drugs, and Cosmetics.* 2nd ed. New York: John Wiley & Sons, 1996.

Mayell, M. *Off-the-Shelf Natural Health: How to Use Herbs and Nutrients to Stay Well.* New York: Bantam Books, 1995.

Mindell E. *Earl Mindell's Herb Bible.* New York: Simon & Schuster/Fireside, 1992.

Newall, C.A., et al. *Herbal Medicines: A Guide for Health-Care Professionals.* London: The Pharmaceutical Press, 1996.

Tierra, M. *The Way of Herbs.* New York: Pocket Books, 1990.

Tyler, V.E. *Herbs of Choice: The Therapeutic Use of Phytomedicinals.* Binghamton, NY: Haworth Press/Pharmaceutical Products Press, 1994.

————. *The Honest Herbal.* Binghamton, NY: Haworth Press/Pharmaceutical Products Press, 1993.

Weiner, M.A., and J.A. Weiner. *Herbs That Heal: Prescription for Herbal Healing.* Mill Valley, CA: Quantum Books, 1994.

Weiss, R.F. *Herbal Medicine,* trans. A.R. Meuss, from the 6th German edition. Beaconsfield, England: Beaconsfield Publishers, Ltd., 1988.

TEXT CITATIONS:

1. R.F. Weiss, *Herbal Medicine,* trans. A.R. Meuss, from the 6th German edition (Beaconsfield, England: Beaconsfield Publishers, Ltd., 1988).
2. N.G. Bisset, ed., *Herbal Drugs and Phytopharmaceuticals* (Stuttgart: medpharm GmbH Scientific Publishers, 1994).
3. Ibid.
4. M. Blumenthal, J. Gruenwald, T. Hall, and R.S. Rister, eds., *The Complete German Commission E Monographs: Therapeutic Guide to Herbal Medicine* (Boston: Integrative Medicine Communications, 1998).
5. Weiss, op. cit.
6. V.E. Tyler, *Herbs of Choice: The Therapeutic Use of Phytomedicinals* (Binghamton, NY: Haworth Press/Pharmaceutical Products Press, 1994).
7. Weiss, op. cit.
8. Blumenthal et al., op. cit.
9. Weiss, op. cit.
10. S.S. Chang et al., *Journal of Food Sciences,* 42 (1977): 1102.
11. A.Y. Leung and S. Foster, *Encyclopedia of Common Natural Ingredients Used in Food, Drugs, and Cosmetics,* 2nd ed. (New York: John Wiley & Sons, 1996). Bisset, op. cit.
12. H. Haraguchi et al., *Planta Medica,* 61 (1995): 333–36.
13. K.W. Singletary and J.M. Nelshoppen, *Cancer Letters,* 60(2) (1991): 169.
14. D.L.J. Opdyke, *Food and Cosmetics Toxicology,* 12 (Suppl.) (1974): 977.
15. Bisset, op. cit.
16. Blumenthal et al., op. cit.

PRIMARY NAME:

ROSE OIL (and ROSE WATER)

SCIENTIFIC NAME:
Rosa gallica L., *Rosa alba* L., *Rosa centifolia* L., and *Rosa damascena* Mill. Family: Rosaceae

COMMON NAME:
N/A

What Is Rose Oil?

The fresh flowers of the prickly rose bush are typically harvested early in the morning when their essential oil content is the highest,[1] and then subjected to steam distillation to produce a yellow-green oil. Rose water refers to the watery portion left over. Only selected cultivars of this old plant, of which there are now thousands of species, are used to make rose oil.

What It Is Used For:

The ancients reveled in the powerful aroma of rose oil, attributing various powers to it, and treasured it as a cosmetic. Some herbalists still recommend the oil and the water as healing astringents, and they are even included as astringents in some cold creams and other pharmaceutical preparations. Not unlike the healers of another time who trumpeted the oil's powers to allay nervous system disorders, aromatherapists today hail rose oil for calming nervous anxiety, rejuvenating the body and spirit, instilling a feeling of well-being and lifting a depressive mood, stimulating sexual desire, and treating appetite loss, headache, and circulation problems. Rose water is used in a compress for sore eyes.

Rose oil and rose water are widely used as fragrance components in perfumes, medicines, tobacco (only the oil), and various cosmetics. Very low levels of oil can even be found as a "fruity" flavor component in foods and drinks.

Forms Available Include:

Essential oil, rose water.

Common Dosage:

Rose oil is used in aromatherapy.

Will It Work for You? What the Studies Say:

The power of rose oil to lift a depressive mood, stimulate sexual desire, or inspire any other emotion depends largely on your personal reaction to the aroma and your belief in the powers of aromatherapy. True rose oil is expensive because it takes so many rose petals (a few hundred) to produce just a small vial of high-quality product.

Astringent substances such as tannins and certain alcohols in rose oil and stronger rose water may explain why they had such a reputation in cosmetics centuries ago and are still used for this purpose today; astringents help heal skin by tightening it. German health authorities endorse the use of *Rosa gallica* flower extracts for treating mild mouth and throat inflammation.[2] Rose oil is listed in the *National Formulary*.

Will It Harm You? What the Studies Say:

Rose oil has not been linked to any reports of serious adverse reactions, although data are relatively scant overall. Tests of rose oil from Morocco, Bulgaria, and Turkey on human skin found that it was not irritating, sensitizing, or sun-sensitizing, although undiluted oil did irritate rabbit skin.[3]

GENERAL SOURCES:
Lawrence, B.M. *Perfumes and Flavorings,* 1991; 16(6): 43.
Leung, A.Y., and S. Foster. *Encyclopedia of Common Natural Ingredients Used in Food, Drugs, and Cosmetics.* 2nd ed. New York. John Wiley & Sons, 1996.
Weiner, J.A. *Weiner's Herbal: A Guide to Herb Medicine.* Mill Valley, CA: Quantum Books, 1991.
Weiss, R.F. *Herbal Medicine,* trans. A.R. Meuss, from the 6th German edition. Beaconsfield, England: Beaconsfield Publishers, Ltd., 1988.

TEXT CITATIONS:
1. A.Y. Leung and S. Foster, *Encyclopedia of Common Natural Ingredients Used in Food, Drugs, and Cosmetics,* 2nd ed. (New York: John Wiley & Sons, 1998).
2. Leung and Foster, op. cit.
3. Leung and Foster, op. cit.

PRIMARY NAME:
ROYAL JELLY

SCIENTIFIC NAME:
N/A

COMMON NAMES:
Apilak, feng wang jiang, gelée royale, queen bee jelly

RATING:
4 = Research indicates that this substance will not fulfill the claims made for it, but that it is also unlikely to cause any harm.

What Is Royal Jelly?

Young worker bees of the species *Apis mellifers* L.—minions in the palace of the queen bee—spend their days feeding the queen a milky-white substance secreted by their pharyngeal (salivary) glands. This nutritious nectar accounts for the dramatic differences in size, fertility, and life span of the queen bees, who, compared with worker bees, grow to about twice the size, lay some 2,000–3,000 eggs a day more than the infertile worker bees, and live five to eight years.[1] Worker bees live, on average, four to six weeks. Harvesters scrape "royal jelly" from bee hives by means of suction or manual scraping, remove impurities, and then process it for further purification and packaging.

What It Is Used For:

Folk healers contend that benefits similar to those experienced by queen bees, from increased growth to improved fertility, will accrue to humans who take royal jelly. Various traditional medicine cultures have also treated malnutrition in children, debility in the elderly, and ailments such as diabetes, arthritis, high blood pressure, and hepatitis with the substance. Traditional Chinese healers attribute invigorating, anti-aging, strengthening, and nourishing properties to it. Western sources have promoted it as a key to longevity, improving sexual performance, and controlling menopausal symptoms, among other things. Many claim it will boost energy levels and combat fatigue.

Royal jelly is added to many external formulations, including skin tonics, creams, lotions, soaps, and toothpastes, for its purported nourishing, skin clearing, and antiwrinkle properties. Even hair growth stimulants on occasion contain royal jelly.

Forms Available Include:

- *For internal use:* Capsule, liquid, tablet. Appears in combination with Asian ginseng in "energizing" herbal blends.
- *For external use:* Appears as an ingredient in creams, ointments, and other topical formulations.

Common Dosage:

For commercial royal jelly formulations, follow the package instructions.

Will It Work for You? What the Studies Say:

Intensive laboratory analysis of royal jelly reveals that it is a complex and nutritious substance, rich in proteins, lipids, carbohydrates, and B vitamins in particular. Claims that it represents a good "energizing" supplement are far-fetched, however, given that many foods and a balanced diet offer the same nutritional complex, often at much lower prices.

According to test-tube and rat studies, royal jelly is antiseptic, fighting a number of infectious organisms including *Staphylococcus aureus, Escherichia coli, Streptococcus hemolyticus,* and *Bacillus subtilis.*[2] Whether these antibacterial properties occur in humans and are of any benefit for preventing or treating infections remains unclear. A mouse test also showed antitumor activity for royal jelly, with an ability to inhibit the growth of tumors and leukemia.[3] More research on this subject is needed before any conclusions about treating human cancers can be drawn.

An investigator reporting a critical evaluation of royal jelly determined that the substance does not influence growth, fertility, or longevity in animals, and that it has no estrogenlike properties.[4] A set of investigators report that royal jelly does not qualify as a sound diet therapy for individuals with chronic fatigue syndrome, despite promotional material indicating that it does.[5] Royal jelly also failed to show any notable skin-rejuvenating properties in a three-month trial of twenty-four women with dry skin, with ten women reporting improvement but ten experiencing no changes at all and four developing skin irritation.[6]

Studies also indicate that royal jelly can affect the adrenal cortex and produce hyperglycemia.[7]

Will It Harm You? What the Studies Say:

Royal jelly may irritate the skin in sensitive individuals. Allergic reactions have also been reported but are generally rare,[8] although there has been at least one case of fatal royal-jelly-induced asthma.[9] Obviously, if you have an allergy to bees, avoid royal jelly. The recent medical literature contains no references to serious adverse reactions from taking royal jelly internally, however.

GENERAL SOURCES:
Der Marderosian, A., and L. Liberti. *Natural Product Medicine: A Scientific Guide to Foods, Drugs, Cosmetics.* Philadelphia: George F. Stickley, 1988.
Lawrence Review of Natural Products. St. Louis,: Facts and Comparisons, March 1992.
Leung, A.Y., and S. Foster. *Encyclopedia of Common Natural Ingredients Used in Food, Drugs, and Cosmetics.* 2nd ed. New York: John Wiley & Sons, 1996.
Mayell M. *Off-the-Shelf Natural Health: How to Use Herbs and Nutrients to Stay Well.* New York: Bantam Books, 1995.
Tyler, V.E. *The Honest Herbal.* Binghamton, NY: Haworth Press/Pharmaceutical Products Press, 1993.
Worthinton-Roberts, B., and M.A. Breskin. *American Pharmacy,* 23(8) (1983): 30.

TEXT CITATIONS:
1. A. Der Marderosian and L. Liberti, *Natural Product Medicine: A Scientific Guide to Foods, Drugs, Cosmetics* (Philadelphia: George F. Stickley, 1988).
2. M.S. Blum et al., *Science,* 130 (1959): 452. Y.D. Xu, *Zhongguo Yangfeng,* 6 (1989) 28. A.Y. Leung and S. Foster, *Encyclopedia of Common Natural Ingredients Used in Food, Drugs, and Cosmetics,* 2nd ed. (New York: John Wiley & Sons, 1996).

3. G.F. Townsend et al., *Nature*, 183 (1959): 1270. Leung and Foster, op. cit.
4. A.D. Dayan, *Journal of Pharmacy and Pharmacology*, 12 (1960): 377–83.
5. D.H. Morris and F.S. Stare, *Archives of Family Medicine*, 2(2) (1993): 181–85.
6. V.E. Tyler, *The Honest Herbal* (Binghamton, NY: Haworth Press/Pharmaceutical Products Press, 1993).
7. *Lawrence Review of Natural Products* (St. Louis: Facts and Comparisons, March 1992).
8. Leung and Foster, op. cit.
9. F.C. Thien et al., *Medical Journal of Australia*, 159(9) (1993): 639. R.J. Bullock et al., *Medical Journal of Australia*, 160(1) (1994): 44.

PRIMARY NAME:

RUE

SCIENTIFIC NAME:

Ruta graveolens L. Family: Rutaceae

COMMON NAMES:

Common rue, countryman's-treacle, garden rue, German rue, herb-of-grace

RATING:

5 = Studies indicate that there is a definite health hazard to using this substance, even in recommended amounts.

R

Rue

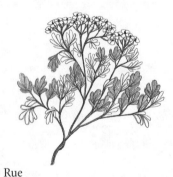

Rue
Ruta gravelones

What Is Rue?

Rue, a native of Europe, is cultivated worldwide, including in North America. The fresh leaves and occasionally other parts of this evergreen shrub have been used medicinally. Its bright yellow flowers have a distinctively disagreeable odor. Steam distillation of the fresh flowering plant yields an essential oil.

What It Is Used For:

Rue has been used as a healing herb since ancient times. Of the numerous purposes for which it has been used, perhaps the most prominent include stimulating menstruation, relieving intestinal and menstrual cramps, killing intestinal worms, inducing sedation, and suppressing coughs. Both rue tea and the essential oil have been used to induce miscarriage, an extremely dangerous practice. Rue also has a reputation for repelling insects; bouquets were placed in law courts of the Middle Ages to repel the vermin and germs of filthy prisoners.[1] Some contemporary herbalists continue to recommend the herb for various disorders, although the majority discourage its use altogether because of health risks.

Forms Available Include:

Herb (dried), infusion, leaf, oil, tincture (for external use).

Dosage Commonly Reported:

Rue should not be used medicinally.

Will It Work for You? What the Studies Say:

Rue has proved itself both an active herb and a hazardous one. It is packed with active constituents, including a volatile oil, bitters, rutin, and an astringent tannin. Intensive investigation has revealed the presence of chemicals (alkaloids such as arborinine and coumarins) with reversible antispasmodic properties on smooth muscles, explaining the herb's traditional use for menstrual cramps and digestive upset of some types. Animal studies have demonstrated this antispasmodic action in smooth muscle tissue such as the heart, stomach, and intestines. Rue's complex chemistry also contains potent antibacterial, antifungal, and worm-fighting properties[2] that explain some of its traditional uses.

Given both the health hazards in taking rue and the lack of proven effectiveness in humans, German health authorities have declined to endorse the herb for any ailment.[3]

Will It Harm You? What the Studies Say:

Rue is a toxic herb. When taken internally, the fresh plant can cause stomach upset and other complications. This is due to the volatile oil, which can cause severe stomach pain, vomiting, convulsive twitching, life-threatening miscarriage, and other serious complications, including fatal ones if taken in large doses.[4] Drying decreases the volatile oil content, but the risk of a toxic reaction is still present, particularly if large doses of the dried leaves are ingested.[5] No scientific evidence supports the claim made by some sources that administering **Goldenseal** will counteract adverse reactions from an overdose of rue.[6]

Women of childbearing age—and pregnant women in particular—should completely avoid all forms of this herb because it can cause miscarriage or interfere with a normal menstrual cycle.

Handling the fresh leaves exposes you to rue oil, which can cause redness, blisters, swelling, and burning sensations. Substances called psoralens make the skin extremely sensitive to the sun. Several cases of severe skin reaction appear in the medical literature, including one in which a woman and her two small children developed hives and massive blisters after rubbing the fresh leaves onto their skin; they had read that it could repel insects.[7]

GENERAL SOURCES:

Blumenthal, M., J. Gruenwald, T. Hall, and R.S. Rister, eds. *The Complete German Commission E Monographs: Therapeutic Guide to Herbal Medicine.* Boston: Integrative Medicine Communications, 1998.

Dobelis, I.N., ed. *The Magic and Medicine of Plants: A Practical Guide to the Science, History, Folklore, and Everyday Uses of Medicinal Plants.* Pleasantville, NY: Reader's Digest Association, 1986.

Lawrence Review of Natural Products. St. Louis: Facts and Comparisons, July 1989.

Leung, A.Y., and S. Foster. *Encyclopedia of Common Natural Ingredients Used in Food, Drugs, and Cosmetics.* 2nd ed. New York: John Wiley & Sons, 1996.

Mayell, M. *Off-the-Shelf Natural Health: How to Use Herbs and Nutrients to Stay Well.* New York: Bantam Books, 1995.

Tierra, M. *The Way of Herbs.* New York: Pocket Books, 1990.

Tyler, V.E. *The Honest Herbal.* Binghamton, NY: Haworth Press/Pharmaceutical Products Press, 1993.

Weiner, M.A., and J.A. Weiner. *Herbs That Heal: Prescription for Herbal Healing.* Mill Valley, CA: Quantum Books, 1994.

Weiss, R.F. *Herbal Medicine,* trans. A.R. Meuss, from the 6th German edition. Beaconsfield, England: Beaconsfield Publishers, Ltd., 1988.

TEXT CITATIONS:

1. I.N. Dobelis, ed., *The Magic and Medicine of Plants: A Practical Guide to the Science, History, Folklore, and Everyday Uses of Medicinal Plants* (Pleasantville, NY: Reader's Digest Association, 1986).

2. A.Y. Leung and S. Foster, *Encyclopedia of Common Natural Ingredients Used in Food, Drugs, and Cosmetics,* 2nd ed. (New York: John Wiley & Sons, 1996). B. Wolters and U. Eilert, *Planta Medica,* 43 (1981): 166.

R

Rue

3. M. Blumenthal, J. Gruenwald, T. Hall, and R.S. Rister, eds., *The Complete German Commission E Monographs: Therapeutic Guide to Herbal Medicine* (Boston: Integrative Medicine Communications, 1998).

4. Leung and Foster, op. cit.

5. V.E. Tyler, *The Honest Herbal* (Binghamton, NY: Haworth Press/Pharmaceutical Products Press, 1993).

6. Ibid.

7. N.S. Heskel et al., *Contact Dermatitis*, 9(4) (1983): 278–80.

SAFFRON

SCIENTIFIC NAME:
Crocus sativus L. Family: Iridaceae

COMMON NAMES:
Hay saffron, saffron crocus, Spanish saffron

RATING:
- *For internal use:* 3 = Studies on the effectiveness and safety of this substance are conflicting, or there are not enough studies to draw a conclusion. See "Will It Harm You?" section for important warnings.

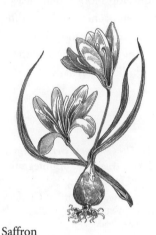

Saffron
Crocus sativus

What Is Saffron?

The yellow-red stigmata of the violet, lilylike flowers of *Crocus sativus* are dried to make the highly valued spice known as saffron. Saffron is one of the most expensive spices in the world; it takes about 75,000 flowers to yield 1 pound of saffron. Some manufacturers try to pass off the less expensive American saffron (safflower) as the more costly genuine variety.

What It Is Used For:

The ancients treasured saffron as a spice, a dye, an aphrodisiac, and a perfume. They also valued it as a medicinal agent. Some contemporary herbalists recommend it as a sedative, expectorant, sexual stimulant, antispasmodic (to relieve smooth muscle spasms), digestive aid, diaphoretic (sweat inducer), pain reliever, and dry skin balm. Traditional Indian and Chinese doctors prescribe it for these and other uses.

Forms Available Include:

- *For internal use:* Tea, threads, tincture.
- *For external use:* Paste.

Dosage Commonly Reported:

Saffron is used primarily in cooking. As a medicine it is taken in doses of 0.5 to 1.5 grams. A tea is made with 10 to 15 saffron threads (stigmata), and tastes mildly like honey.

Will It Work for You? What the Studies Say:

As a medicine for daily ills, this ancient spice no longer commands much respect, but research has sparked interest in its potential to help prevent and cure such complex conditions as heart disease and cancer. Patents have been awarded to crocetin, the most active component in saffron, for the treatment of spinal cord injuries, benign skin tumors, high blood pressure, and cerebral edema (swelling) in cats.[1] Whether this glycoside can aid human beings in these ways has yet to be shown, however.

Some scientists suggest that the incidence of cardiovascular disease in parts of Spain is low because the locals consume so much saffron,[2] although others attribute their healthy hearts to the liberal use of olive oil. Interestingly, significant reduction of cholesterol was noted in a number of studies that involved injecting animals with saffron; high cholesterol is believed to increase the risk for heart disease. Whether this translates into a cholesterol drop in humans who consume saffron (rather than injecting it) is still unclear.

Saffron may reduce the risk of heart disease in another way as well: by increasing the oxygen supply to the bloodstream. Research indicates that extra oxygen in the bloodstream may help prevent situations in which vessel walls are hungry for oxygen and artery-clogging plaque begins to deposit along crucial vessels feeding the heart, causing atherosclerosis.[3] Scientists still have a lot to learn about these connections, but they appear optimistic. In any case, more studies on the potential of saffron to protect against heart disease are clearly needed.

Saffron may also help fight cancer, according to research being done around the world. No studies involving humans have been reported so far, but in a number of experiments, mice with various kinds of cancers who were fed saffron extracts lived longer than mice not fed saffron extracts.[4] Test-tube studies found that extracts killed certain tumor cells, including human leukemia cells, and that they inhibited the synthesis of nucleic acids in tumor cells.[5] Saffron is rich in carotenoids (antioxidants), substances that research indicates may help fight cancer, prevent cell mutations, and contribute to the control of the immune system.

There is no scientific evidence that saffron's long-standing reputation as a menstruation promoter has any merit.[6] German health authorities could find no evidence that the herb calms jangled nerves, relieves muscle cramps, or alleviates asthma symptoms.[7] Medicinal mixtures that include saffron have been used abroad for restoring hair growth and preventing premature ejaculation, but it is not at all clear whether saffron plays the active role.

Will It Harm You? What the Studies Say:

Keep your consumption of saffron below a hefty 1.5 grams a day—that comes to many cups of saffron tea or dozens of saffron-spiced curries—and you run no apparent risk of a toxic reaction. With much more than this, however, past experience indicates that a person may vomit or develop bloody diarrhea or urine, vertigo, yellowing of the skin and mucous membranes, and bleeding from the nose, lips, and eyelids. Large doses can also cause sedation.[8] A dose of 10 grams reportedly can cause uterine bleeding, and doses of 20 grams or more can be lethal. Saffron appears to pose no risk when applied externally.

GENERAL SOURCES:

Bisset, N.G., ed. *Herbal Drugs and Phytopharmaceuticals.* Stuttgart: medpharm GmbH Scientific Publishers, 1994.

Blumenthal, M., J. Gruenwald, T. Hall, and R.S. Rister, eds. *The Complete German Commission E Monographs: Therapeutic Guide to Herbal Medicine.* Boston: Integrative Medicine Communications, 1998.

Der Marderosian, A., and L. Liberti. *Natural Product Medicine. A Scientific Guide to Foods, Drugs, Cosmetics.* Philadelphia: George F. Stickley, 1988.

Gainer, J.L., and G.M. Chisolm. *Atherosclerosis.* 19 (1974): 135.

Lawrence Review of Natural Products. St. Louis: Facts and Comparisons, April 1993.

Mindell, E. *Earl Mindell's Herb Bible.* New York: Simon & Schuster/Fireside, 1992.

Salomi, M.J., et al. *Nutrition and Cancer.* 16(1) (1991): 67–72.

Weiss, R.F. *Herbal Medicine,* trans. A.R. Meuss, from the 6th German edition. Beaconsfield, England: Beaconsfield Publishers, Ltd., 1988.

TEXT CITATIONS:

1. A. Der Marderosian and L. Liberti, *Natural Product Medicine. A Scientific Guide to Foods, Drugs, Cosmetics* (Philadelphia: George F. Stickley, 1988).
2. S. Grisolia, *The Lancet* , 7871 (1974): 41.
3. *Lawrence Review of Natural Products* (St. Louis: Facts and Comparisons, April 1993).
4. S.C. Nair et al., *Cancer Letters,* 57(2) (1991): 109–14. M.J. Salomi et al., *Nutrition and Cancer,* 16(1) (1991): 67–72.
5. S.C. Nair et al., *Cancer Biotherapy,* 10(4) (1995): 257–64. F.L. Abdullaev and G.D. Frenkel, *Biofactors,* 3 (1992): 201.

6. *Lawrence Review of Natural Products*, op. cit.

7. M. Blumenthal, J. Gruenwald, T. Hall, and R.S. Rister, eds., *The Complete German Commission E Monographs: Therapeutic Guide to Herbal Medicine* (Boston: Integrative Medicine Communications, 1998).

8. M. Bricklin and A. Der Marderosian, *The Encyclopedia of Natural Healing* (Emmaus, PA: Rodale Press, 1976).

SAGE

SCIENTIFIC NAME:
Dalmation sage: *Salvia officinalis* L. Spanish sage: *Salvia lavandulaefolia* Vahl.

COMMON NAMES:
Garden sage, meadow sage, red sage, scarlet sage, true sage

RATING:
- *For internal use:* 3 = Studies on the effectiveness and safety of this substance are conflicting, or there are not enough studies to draw a conclusion. However, see "Will It Work for You?" and "Will It Harm You" for important warnings.

- *For external use:* 2 = According to a number of well-designed studies and common use, this substance appears to be relatively effective and safe when used in recommended amounts for the indication(s) noted in the "Will It Work for You?" section.

What Is Sage?

Numerous species of this small, shrubby evergreen perennial are cultivated around the world, but *Salvia officinalis* L. (Dalmation sage) and *Salvia lavandulaefolia* Vahl. (Spanish sage) rank as the most commercially important. The grayish-green leaves (fresh and dried) are used medicinally, as is the volatile oil produced through steam distillation. Do not confuse sage with the similarly named **Salvia** (*Salvia miltiorrhiza*).

What It Is Used For:

Sage is a common kitchen herb, an aromatic member of the mint family. It appears in everything from foods to perfumes, deodorants, and insecticides. The early Greeks and generations since have used it to preserve meat. The plant's botanical name stems from the Latin word *salvus*, meaning healthy, which is apt, considering the number of conditions herbalists from Europe to China, India, and North America have recommended it for through the ages. Principal among them are excessive perspiration and salivation, and digestive system upsets such as stomach cramps and gas. Not long ago, people racked with tuberculosis-induced night sweats were urged to sip sage tea to slow or stop the sweating. Sage ranks as something of a natural antiperspirant; The German sage product Salysat is marketed this way. Some say sage will help dry up a mother's milk when she decides to stop nursing. Since antiquity, women in certain cultures have taken the herb to induce and increase the menstrual flow, as well as to alleviate menstrual pains.

Antiseptic, anti-inflammatory, and astringent properties have long been attributed to sage, and nervous conditions, depression, diarrhea, rheumatic pains, sprains, and insect bites have all been treated with it at some point. Herbalists commonly recommend sage tea as a mouthwash or hot gargle to calm mouth or throat inflammations including sore throat, bleeding gums, and canker sores. Sage tea is also recommended for dry cough or swallowing problems. Sage has been promoted as a toothpaste and toothache balm. Plasters made from the powdered leaf and other topical sage preparations were once used to treat cancers.[1] Some German physicians recommend sage (combined with chamomile especially) as an anti-inflammatory douche.[2] Numerous moisturizers contain the herb for its reported soothing and healing effects.

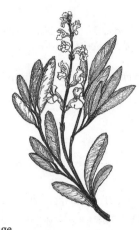

Sage
Salvia officinalis

Forms Available Include:

- *For internal use:* Infusion, leaf (fresh and dried), liquid extract, tincture.
- *For external use:* Extracts, gargle, mouthwash, paste, plaster.

Dosage Commonly Reported:

An infusion made using about 2 teaspoons (5 grams) finely cut herb per cup of water is used as a mouthwash or gargle. Take commercial preparations according to package directions.

Will It Work for You? What the Studies Say:

Research indicates that several of the traditional uses for sage make sense. On the downside, medicinal concentrations of sage can pose health hazards if not used carefully. Conservatives recommend using only topical forms of medicinal-strength sage, such as mouthwashes or gargles for mouth and throat inflammations.

The volatile oil and tannins play a critical role, performing as astringents and increasing blood flow to the area.[3] Other components (phenolic acids) in sage fight certain bacteria such as *Staphylococcus aureus*, possibly encouraging healing.[4] German health authorities approve of using sage in the form of a mouthwash or gargle made from an infusion. Sage extracts appear in a number of European mouth and throat remedies. Until the early years of the twentieth century, American medical textbooks recommended sage gargles for sore throats.

A number of trials with animals and humans, some conducted as early as 1896, indicate that sage fulfills the folk promise of reducing sweating, in some cases by 50 percent.[5] It is no surprise that people instinctively turned to it to control fevers. German health authorities approve of using sage to treat excessive sweating.[6] Not all sources indicate that it works this way, however. Reports from the 1940s indicated that sage failed to reduce perspiration in small laboratory animals.[7] (The investigator also found no antibacterial actions or efficacy in a number of other proposed properties.)

Sage is said to have mild estrogen-like effects, possibly explaining its traditional use as a menstruation-promoter, for example. Apparently no animal or human studies have been done to explore this subject. Similarly, little sound evidence can be found to justify the use of sage for lowering blood pressure, despite studies indicating that a liquid extract of the herb may have mild blood-pressure-lowering effects in humans, especially when taken on an empty stomach.[8]

According to animal studies, the volatile oil in sage helps alleviate excess gas and relax the smooth muscle lining of the digestive tract, both qualities considered useful for treating stomach and intestinal upset. German health authorities have officially approved of sage for treating indigestion.[9] Extracts of the plant appear in products for bile stimulation, although there is no scientific evidence to verify that the herb will work in this way.

Exciting new research indicates that sage extracts exert strong antioxidant activity.[10] (Antioxidants control the formation of dangerous substances in the body called free radicals, agents that damage cells through oxidation, some of which may contribute to cancer-cell formation.) Much more research is needed before conclusions can be made about the implications for human health. Antioxidants may also help prevent meat spoilage, explaining sage's reputation as a preservative.

Will It Harm You? What the Studies Say:

The volatile oil in sage contains relatively high concentrations of a toxic chemical called thujone. This does not pose a risk if you are cooking with the leaves, since the chemical probably dissipates with heat.[11] Herb-scented cooking oils are safe as well. But it puts into question the wisdom of using internal forms of sage medicinally. Certainly *do not ingest purified sage oil; it is toxic.* The medical literature contains reports of convulsions in both humans and animals consuming sage oil.[12] If consumed in small doses over long stretches of time the thujone in sage oil can cause numerous complications including physical and mental deterioration, and large doses can lead to convulsions and coma.[13] Thujone is the infamous ingredient in absinthe that many say made Vincent Van Gogh go mad. See **Wormwood** for more information on the toxic effects of thujone.

Several investigators have noted that unlike purified sage oil, which is definitely dangerous, most medicinal sage preparations contain very small amounts of the oil (and hence thujone) and are therefore unlikely to cause an adverse reaction.[14] German health authorities warn that prolonged consumption of sage tea could be hazardous to health and that extended use of the essential oil or tincture could result in convulsions.[15] There have been a few cases of people developing inflamed mucous tissues of the mouth and lips after drinking sage tea.[16] In contrast, using sage tea as a mouthwash or gargle does not pose these hazards and is considered harmless; always spit the material out, however. Undiluted forms of the oil placed on the skin in a series of tests did not result in irritation or allergic sensitization.[17] Until the experts know more about the herb's estrogen-like effects, pregnant women may want to avoid medicinal-strength dosages of sage in any form.

GENERAL SOURCES:

Bisset, N.G., ed. *Herbal Drugs and Phytopharmaceuticals.* Stuttgart: medpharm GmbH Scientific Publishers, 1994.

Blumenthal, M., J. Gruenwald, T. Hall, and R.S. Rister, eds. *The Complete German Commission E Monographs: Therapeutic Guide to Herbal Medicine.* Boston: Integrative Medicine Communications, 1998.

Castleman, M. *The Healing Herbs: The Ultimate Guide to the Curative Power of Nature's Medicines.* New York: Bantam Books, 1995.

Debelmas, A.M., and J. Rochat. *Plantes Medicinales et Phytotherapie,* 1 (1967): 23.

Duke, J.A. *CRC Handbook of Medicinal Herbs.* Boca Raton, FL: CRC Press, 1985.

Hartwell, J.L. *Lloydia.* 32 (1969): 247.

Lawrence Review of Natural Products. St. Louis: Facts and Comparisons, August 1992.

Leung, A.Y., and S. Foster. *Encyclopedia of Common Natural Ingredients Used in Food, Drugs, and Cosmetics.* 2nd ed. New York: John Wiley & Sons, 1996.

Mayell, M. *Off-the-Shelf Natural Health: How to Use Herbs and Nutrients to Stay Well.* New York: Bantam Books, 1995.

Mindell, E. *Earl Mindell's Herb Bible.* New York: Simon & Schuster/Fireside, 1992.

Mitchell, J.C., and A. Rook. *Botanical Dermatology.* Vancouver: Greenglass, 1979.

Newall, C.A., et al. *Herbal Medicines: A Guide for Health-Care Professionals.* London: The Pharmaceutical Press, 1996.

Tyler, V.E. *Herbs of Choice: The Therapeutic Use of Phytomedicinals.* Binghamton, NY: Haworth Press/Pharmaceutical Products Press, 1994.

———. *The Honest Herbal.* Binghamton, NY: Haworth Press/Pharmaceutical Products Press, 1993.

Weiss, R.F. *Herbal Medicine*, trans. A.R. Meuss, from the 6th German edition. Beaconsfield, England: Beaconsfield Publishers, Ltd., 1988.

TEXT CITATIONS:

1. J.L. Hartwell, *Lloydia*, 32 (1969): 247.
2. R.F. Weiss, *Herbal Medicine*, trans. A.R. Meuss, from the 6th German edition. Beaconsfield, England: Beaconsfield Publishers, Ltd., 1988.
3. V.E. Tyler, *Herbs of Choice: The Therapeutic Use of Phytomedicinals* (New York: Haworth Press/Pharmaceutical Products Press, 1994).
4. D.L.J. Opdyke, *Food & Cosmetics Toxicology*, 14 (Suppl.) (1976): 857.
5. V.E. Tyler, *The Honest Herbal* (Binghamton, NY: Haworth Press/Pharmaceutical Products Press, 1993). N.G. Bisset, ed., *Herbal Drugs and Phytopharmaceuticals* (Stuttgart: medpharm GmbH Scientific Publishers, 1994).
6. M. Blumenthal, J. Gruenwald, T. Hall, and R.S. Rister, eds., *The Complete German Commission E Monographs: Therapeutic Guide to Herbal Medicine* (Boston: Integrative Medicine Communications, 1998).
7. V.E. Tyler, *The Honest Herbal* (Binghamton, NY: Haworth Press/Pharmaceutical Products Press, 1993).
8. Ibid.
9. Blumenthal et al., op. cit.
10. H. Masaki et al., *Biological & Pharmaceutical Bulletin*, 18(1) (1995): 162–66. M. Takacsova et al., *Nahrung*, 39(3) (1995): 241–43.
11. V.E. Tyler, *The Honest Herbal* (Binghamton, NY: Haworth Press/Pharmaceutical Products Press, 1993).
12. C.A. Newall et al., *Herbal Medicines: A Guide for Health-Care Professionals* (London: The Pharmaceutical Press, 1996).
13. H.B.J. van Rijn, *Pharmaceutisch Weekblad*, 84 (1949): 337–43.
14. V.E. Tyler, *The Honest Herbal* (Binghamton, NY: Haworth Press/Pharmaceutical Products Press, 1993).
15. Blumenthal et al., op. cit.
16. J.C. Mitchell and A. Rook, *Botanical Dermatology* (Vancouver: Greenglass, 1979).
17. Opdyke, op. cit.

PRIMARY NAME:
ST. JOHN'S WORT

SCIENTIFIC NAME:
Hypericum perforatum L.
Family: Hypericaceae

COMMON NAMES:
Amber touch-and-heal, goatweed, John's wort, klamath weed, rosin rose

What Is St. John's Wort?

This shrubby perennial, indigenous to Europe and considered an aggressive weed in western North America and Australia,[1] bears striking, bright yellow star-shaped flowers. Spots on the small oblong leaves are glands that contain a volatile oil and resin. The fresh or dried flowering tops are used medicinally.

What It Is Used For:

St. John's wort, possibly named by early Christians in honor of John the Baptist, can claim a folk tradition centuries old. Up through the Middle Ages, it was believed to possess magical powers and a capacity to repel evil spirits. Folk heal-

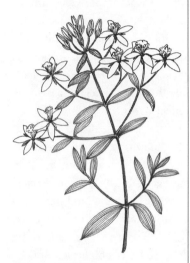

St. John's Wort
Hypericum perforatum

ers long used it to treat anxiety, depression, insomnia, diarrhea, stomach irritation, fluid retention (as a diuretic, or "water pill"), bladder ailments, kidney and lung disorders, and even cancer. A distinctively red tincture consisting of the chopped flowers steeped in oil was popular for placing on wounds, bruises, sores, and other skin disorders to fight infection and inflammation.

Contemporary herbalists recommend external formulations for promoting healing in wounds and hemorrhoids. But the internal use of St. John's wort had essentially disappeared until relatively recently, when fresh research sparked interest in its value as an antidepressant, a sedative for anxiety and nervous disturbances, a tranquilizer, a remedy for menstrual cramps, an expectorant for colds and chest congestion, and a potential tool in fighting viral infections, including HIV (the virus that causes AIDS). Homeopaths recommend minute amounts for numerous ailments. (See page 2 for a discussion of homeopathy.)

Forms Available Include:

- *For internal use:* Capsule, decoction, fluid extract, infusion, oil, tincture. Preparations standardized for the active ingredient, a pigment called hypericin, are available, although the quality of these formulations varies widely.[2]
- *For external use:* Oil, ointment.

Dosage Commonly Reported:

The herb is taken in daily doses of 2 to 4 grams, calculated to contain 0.2 to 1.0 milligram of hypericin. Capsules containing 300 milligrams of the extract (and 0.3 percent of the active ingredient hypericin) are typically taken three times a day. An infusion is made by pouring 1 cup of boiling water over 1 to 2 heaping teaspoons (2 to 4 grams) of flowers, allowing it to steep for ten minutes, and then straining the liquid. This is drunk once or twice a day over the course of four to six weeks.

Will It Work for You? What the Studies Say:

Several well-designed human studies indicate that a standardized extract of St. John's wort can help alleviate mild to moderate depression or temporary depressive moods. German health authorities endorse its use for mild depressive states, anxiety, or nervous unrest.[3] A dose of 2 to 4 grams of the herb (0.2 to 1.0 milligram of hypericin) is used for mild antidepressant action or nervous disturbances.[4]

Several clinical trials support the herb's reputation for these types of disorders. In a four-week trial involving 105 individuals with mild to moderate depression or a depressive mood, a large number (65 percent) of those given St. John's wort extract (standardized for hypericin) reported significant relief from feelings of sadness, hopelessness, uselessness, and fear, as well as disturbed sleep and other classic signs and symptoms of depression.[5] Only 28 percent of those given a placebo experienced this kind of improvement. During the study, neither the subjects nor the researchers knew who was taking the drug. These results reinforce the positive findings of earlier animal studies and human trials.[6]

In an analysis published in 1996 of twenty-three randomized clinical trials involving a total of 1,757 outpatients with primarily mild or moderately severe depression, investigators found that St. John's wort consistently offered more relief than a placebo.[7] It is particularly important to consider that no studies have been done to demonstrate that St. John's wort is as effective as—or more effective than—conventional antidepressants,[8] especially if you suffer from severe depression. The herb may cause fewer side effects, however.

Also keep in mind that subjects in this and other studies took an extract standardized for hypericin content, not a tea or another preparation of the herb that could contain variable amounts of this apparently critical ingredient. Research indicates that hypericin (or possibly even other parts of the plant) inhibits the activity of the enzyme monoamine oxidase (MAO), enabling the level of various nerve-impulse transmitters critical to mood and emotional stability in the brain to increase.[9] This mechanism of action places St. John's wort among other important antidepressants known as MAO inhibitors. Plant experts now consider the herb, long categorized as a sedative, an antidepressant.[10] It may take several weeks or more for users to notice the antidepressant effect. German textbooks note that neither true melancholia (nonsituational depression), nor severe and acute depression should be treated with this herb.[11] Talk to your physician or psychiatrist about taking St. John's wort, and about an effective dosage.

Research supports the use of the herb as a wound treatment and infection-fighter. Its rich stores of astringent substances called tannins would be expected to help constrict tissue and dry up oozing of secretions. The herb also contains substances active against common infection-causing agents such as *Staphylococcus aureus*.[12] According to test-tube and small-animal studies, hypericin (and pseudohypericin) fight certain viruses.[13] German health authorities approve of the oil externally for first-degree burns, injuries, and muscle pain. In Europe, skin abrasions and inflammations are also commonly treated with the herb.[14] German health authorities also approve of taking the oil internally for dyspeptic complaints.[15]

Researchers are currently investigating hypericin's powers to fight retroviruses such as HIV, which causes AIDS. The FDA now allows researchers to use hypericin in testing on humans[16]; studies are under way.

Will It Harm You? What the Studies Say:

St. John's wort is not generally associated with serious adverse reactions in controlled clinical trials. Be aware, however, that it poses a risk of sun-sensitivity reactions (photosensitivity) in light-skinned livestock.[17] The only time this kind of reaction has been seen in humans was when they were taking a synthetic form of the active ingredient, hypericin.[18] In any case, you should avoid direct sunlight after ingesting the herb in any form, especially if you are light-skinned or have had sun-sensitivity reactions before.[19] Given that scientists still have a lot to learn about how the herb works, avoid treating yourself with it for long-term periods. Talk to your doctor before combining it with another antidepressant.

Fifteen of the twenty-three trials in the analysis noted above were placebo-controlled. In those, 4.8 percent of the subjects given St. John's wort reported side effects, compared with 4.1 percent of the subjects given a placebo. This is a favorable comparison. Reported side effects have included restlessness, mild allergic reactions, and gastrointestinal upset.

Concerns about the risk of cell damage and possibly dangerous mutations caused by a substance called quercetin in the herb have been defused by the recognition that quercetin appears in many plants and that taking this herb medicinally will not significantly add to the overall intake for most people.[20]

GENERAL SOURCES:

American Pharmaceutical Association. *Handbook of Nonprescription Drugs.* 11th ed. Washington, D.C.: American Pharmaceutical Association, 1996.

Castleman, M. *The Healing Herbs: The Ultimate Guide to the Curative Power of Nature's Medicines.* New York: Bantam Books, 1995.

Blumenthal, M., J. Gruenwald, T. Hall, and R. S. Rister, eds. *The Complete German Commission E Monographs: Therapeutic Guide to Herbal Medicine.* Boston: Integrative Medicine Communications, 1998.

Lawrence Review of Natural Products. St. Louis: Facts and Comparisons, January 1995.

Leung, A.Y., and S. Foster. *Encyclopedia of Common Natural Ingredients Used in Food, Drugs, and Cosmetics.* 2nd ed. New York: John Wiley & Sons, 1996.

Mindell, E. *Earl Mindell's Herb Bible.* New York: Simon & Schuster/Fireside, 1992.

Murray, M.T. *The Healing Power of Herbs: The Enlightened Person's Guide to the Wonders of Medicinal Plants.* Rev. 2nd ed. Rocklin, CA: Prima Publishing, 1995.

Tierra, M. *The Way of Herbs.* New York: Pocket Books, 1990.

Tyler, V.E. *Herbs of Choice: The Therapeutic Use of Phytomedicinals.* Binghamton, NY: Haworth Press/Pharmaceutical Products Press, 1994.

Weiss, R.F. *Herbal Medicine*, trans. A. R. Meuss, from the 6th German edition. Beaconsfield, England: Beaconsfield Publishers, Ltd., 1988.

TEXT CITATIONS:

1. A.Y. Leung and S. Foster, *Encyclopedia of Common Natural Ingredients Used in Food, Drugs, and Cosmetics*, 2nd ed. (New York: John Wiley & Sons, 1996).
2. V.E. Tyler, *Herbs of Choice: The Therapeutic Use of Phytomedicinals* (Binghamton, NY: Haworth Press/Pharmaceutical Products Press, 1994).
3. M. Blumenthal, J. Gruenwald, T. Hall, and R. S. Ritter, eds., *The Complete German Commission E Monographs: Therapeutic Guide to Herbal Medicine* (Boston: Integrative Medicine Communications, 1998).
4. Leung and Foster, op. cit.
5. G. Harrer and H. Sommer, *Phytomedicine*, 1 (1994): 3–8.
6. S.N. Okpanyi, *Arzneimittel-Forschung*, 43 (1987): 10.
7. K. Linde et al. *British Medical Journal*, 313 (1996): 253–58.
8. Tyler, op. cit.
9. J. Holzl, *Deutsche Apotheker Zeitung*, 130 (1990): 367. Tyler, op. cit. R.F. Weiss, *Herbal Medicine*, trans. by A.R. Meuss, from the 6th German edition (Beaconsfield, England: Beaconsfield Publishers, Ltd., 1988).
10. American Pharmaceutical Association, *Handbook of Nonprescription Drugs*, 11th ed. (Washington, D.C.: American Pharmaceutical Association, 1996).
11. Weiss, op. cit.
12. Leung and Foster, op. cit. P. Maisenbacher and K.A. Kovar, *Planta Medica*, 58 (1992): 291.
13. D. Muruelo et al., *Proceedings of the National Academy of Science, U.S.A.*, 85 (1988): 5230–34.
14. Leung and Foster, op. cit.
15. Ibid.
16. *Lawrence Review of Natural Products* (St. Louis: Facts and Comparisons, January 1995).
17. Tyler, op. cit.

18. R. Gulick et al., *International Conference on AIDS*, 8 (1992): B90.
19. American Pharmaceutical Association, op. cit.
20. Tyler, op. cit.

SALVIA

SCIENTIFIC NAME:
Salvia miltiorrhiza. Family:
Labiatae (Lamiaceae)

COMMON NAMES:
Dang shen, red sage

RATING:
3 = Studies on the effectiveness
and safety of this substance are
conflicting, or there are not
enough studies to draw a
conclusion.

What Is Salvia?

The dried, reddish-colored root of this hardy perennial is used medicinally. The plant grows in China and Mongolia; has serrated, oval leaves; and bears spikes of purple-blue flowers.

Do not confuse salvia with the similarly named **Sage** (*Salvia officinalis*).

What It Is Used For:

This classic Chinese herb has long been used to treat a variety of ailments, including irregular menstruation, excessive uterine bleeding, and abdominal bloating. Traditional healers contend that it can "stimulate" or "invigorate" the blood, and thus combat circulation problems. It also has a reputation for improving heart function, encouraging recovery from heart attacks, and reducing chest pain (angina pectoris). Some herbalists attribute sedative actions to salvia as well.

Forms Available Include:

Decoction, dried root, injection formulations (for acupuncture points), liquid extract, tincture. Some of these formulations may be available only in China.

Dosage Commonly Reported:

Salvia is taken in daily doses of 6 to 15 grams of dried root.

Will It Work for You? What the Studies Say:

Nearly all of the published research on salvia has been reported by Chinese investigators. The herb contains substances called tanshinones that may help benefit heart ailments, according to their findings. Studies on its effectiveness in treating heart disease, including coronary artery stenosis,[1] and in improving circulation in individuals with coronary heart disease,[2] have been promising. A number of studies indicate that the root prevents the aggregation of platelets, meaning that it may help to prevent blood clots and associated complications such as heart attacks.[3] Other investigators have found that salvia may reduce chest pain by dilating coronary vessels, although whether this translates into a direct positive effect on high blood pressure, as the investigators theorized, remains unclear.[4] Animal studies indicate that the root encourages a drop in blood pressure.[5] Whether the clot-preventing property also helps ameliorate painful menstrual cramping remains speculative.

Chinese scientists also report promising results with salvia in treating lupus[6] (an autoimmune disorder) and cerebral infarction (stroke) in humans,[7] among other things. One team reports success in regenerating liver tissue.[8] Although intriguing, these and other findings require further exploration and confirmation with large and well-designed clinical trials.

Will It Harm You? What the Studies Say:

To some extent, time attests to the safety of salvia; traditional Chinese healers have reportedly prescribed it for thousands of years. No reports of significant adverse reactions can be found in the medical literature available in the West, but given the limited accessible data, it is probably wise to exercise moderation and caution.

GENERAL SOURCES:

Bisset, N.G., ed. *Herbal Drugs and Phytopharmaceuticals.* Stuttgart: medpharm GmbH Scientific Publishers, 1994.

Bremness, L. *Herbs.* 1st American ed. Eyewitness Handbooks. New York: Dorling Kindersley Publications, 1994.

Chevallier, A. *The Encyclopedia of Medicinal Plants: A Practical Reference Guide to More Than 550 Key Medicinal Plants & Their Uses.* 1st American ed. New York: Dorling Kindersley Publications, 1996.

Tierra, M. *The Way of Herbs.* New York: Pocket Books, 1990.

Mindell, E. *Earl Mindell's Herb Bible.* New York: Simon & Schuster/Fireside, 1992.

TEXT CITATIONS:

1. H.T. Xu et al., *Chung Hsi i Chieh Ho Tsa Chih—Chinese Journal of Modern Developments in Traditional Medicine,* 10(12) (1990): 710, 737–39.

2. G.R. Yu, *Chung Hsi i Chieh Ho Tsa Chih—Chinese Journal of Modern Developments in Traditional Medicine,* 8(10) (1988): 581, 596–98.

3. M. Onitsuka et al., *Chemical & Pharmaceutical Bulletin,* 31(5) (1983): 1670–75. N. Wang et al., *Planta Medica.* 55(4) (1989): 390–91.

4. X.L. Lei and G.C. Chiou., *American Journal of Chinese Medicine,* 14(3–4) (1986): 145–52.

5. C.P. Li et al., *American Journal of Chinese Medicine,* 18(3–4) (1990): 157–66.

6. X.L. Lei and G.C. Chiou, *American Journal of Chinese Medicine,* 14(1–2) (1986): 26–32. Z.Y. Wang, *Chung Hsi i Chieh Ho Tsa Chih—Chinese Journal of Modern Developments in Traditional Medicine,* 9(8) (1989): 452, 465–68.

7. B.Q. Wu, *Chung Hsi i Chieh Ho Tsa Chih—Chinese Journal of Modern Developments in Traditional Medicine,* 9(11) (1989): 644, 656–57.

8. X.H. Ma, *Chung Hsi i Chieh Ho Tsa Chih—Chinese Journal of Modern Developments in Traditional Medicine,* 3(3) (1983): 180–81.

PRIMARY NAME:
SARSAPARILLA

SCIENTIFIC NAME:

Smilax officinalis and related species, including *Smilax regelii* Killip et Morton (from Honduras), *Smilax aristolochiaefolia* Mill. (from Mexico), and *Smilax fibrifuga* Kunth (from Ecuador). Family: Smilacaceae

What Is Sarsaparilla?

Sarsaparilla is a perennial vine native to tropical America and the West Indies. There are several related species. The long, tuberous rootstock emerges aboveground as a climbing vine with prickly stems and greenish flowers. Medicinal preparations are made from the dried rhizome (underground stem) and roots.

What It Is Used For:

Around the turn of the century, Americans regularly imbibed sarsaparilla-flavored root beer and soda pop. For many, it was not only the taste that attracted them; the drink had a widespread reputation as a "blood purifier," a euphemism for syphilis remedy. This ill-founded fame persisted into the early

COMMON NAMES:

American sarsaparilla, Ecuadoran sarsaparilla, Honduran sarsaparilla, Jamaican sarsaparilla, Mexican sarsaparilla, Vera Cruz sarsaparilla

RATING:

4 = Research indicates that this substance will not fulfill claims made for it, but that it is also unlikely to cause any harm.

part of the twentieth century. The *U.S. Pharmacopeia* and the *National Formulary* listed sarsaparilla as a (secondary) syphilis remedy for nearly 150 years. The pharmaceutical industry flavored medicines with it.

Sarsaparilla found favor for other ailments as well. Central American Indians treated rheumatism, skin diseases, stomach upset and digestive disorders, fevers, and venereal diseases such as gonorrhea with the plant. Modern Mexicans and Hondurans, among others, turn to it for many of these same ailments. Traditional Chinese healers use *Smilax* species native to their country in similar ways, as well as to treat skin disorders. Over the years, certain species have been used to fight cancer.

Few contemporary herbalists in the United States recommend sarsaparilla for syphilis or other sexually transmitted diseases anymore, although some continue to suggest taking it to control urinary tract disorders or battle a cough, cold, or fever. Many Americans, Europeans, and other peoples take it to reduce arthritic swelling and pain and to treat psoriasis. Sarsaparilla's reputation as a strengthening and rejuvenating tonic, especially for males interested in boosting their sexual potency, endures in some circles. Take this herb (alone or in combination with other herbs), some promoters say, and your performance and endurance will skyrocket and muscle mass will accumulate. Some sources even claim that the herb's steroid-like compounds (saponin glycosides) include male hormones such as testosterone and that these will function like anabolic steroids once in the body.

Forms Available Include:

Capsule, decoction, liquid extract, powdered root, tincture.

Dosage Commonly Reported:

A decoction is made using 1 to 2 teaspoons powdered root per cup of water and is drunk up to three times per day. The tincture is taken in doses of ¼ to ½ teaspoon up to three times per day.

Will It Work for You? What the Studies Say:

Although a number of findings and theories regarding sarsaparilla are intriguing, the scientific evidence does not weigh in positively for this herb. Those looking to sarsaparilla for a syphilis cure are likely to be sorely disappointed. A contingent of physicians challenged the claim that the herb could eliminate the infection more than a century ago, but it took decades for others to start listening. No Western studies have ever shown that sarsaparilla or any of its ingredients can fight syphilis.

The latest sarsaparilla "bodybuilding" rage has likewise proved unfounded. Simply put, these promoters are advertising sarsaparilla as a legal alternative to illegal steroidal drugs,[1] but facts are not on their side.[2] Intensive chemical analyses have yet to reveal any testosterone in sarsaparilla (or any other higher plant, for that matter), and the plant contains no substance that will raise testosterone levels. Sarsaparilla does contain steroids—including sarsapogenin and smilagenin and their glycosides (saponins)—but these do not function as anabolic steroids.[3]

This is not to say that sarsaparilla is inert. Rigorous laboratory analysis of the herb over the years has actually led to the identification of important properties such as saponins. Some herbalists say these chemicals, which have laxative and expectorant properties, may prove quite valuable. Saponins are also known to promote sweating and exert a significant diuretic ("water pill") effect[4]; perhaps early syphilis sufferers noticed that they urinated more frequently while taking sarsaparilla "cures," and thought that this would help "clear" the illness from their systems. The body would also have cooled down through increased sweating. The unanswered question is whether any of these actions are potent enough to make a difference to human health.

One of the few human trials of sarsaparilla reported promising findings in the treatment of psoriasis. Unfortunately the study, published in 1942, was not particularly well designed; the subjects and the researchers knew who was getting the sarsaparilla compound and who was getting a placebo, allowing potential bias to enter into the results.[5] Unimpressed with the data, German health authorities have declined to approve of sarsaparilla for psoriasis or any other skin disease.[6]

Intriguing evidence has also been collected in animal studies. Saudi Arabian investigators have demonstrated that sarsaparilla significantly inhibits inflammation in rats; this has led the researchers to speculate that the herb's traditional use in treating arthritis, rheumatism, and other inflammatory diseases may be justified if further studies confirm the findings.[7] So far, apparently none has. In the test tube, extracts of certain *Smilax* species have been shown to fight fungi responsible for certain kinds of skin infections[8] and bacteria responsible for gastrointestinal disorders.[9] Some researchers speculate that the steroidal elements in sarsaparilla may some day prove valuable as a source for the semisynthetic production of anti-inflammatory steroidal drugs like cortisone.[10] German health authorities, after reviewing the literature collected so far, declined to approve of sarsaparilla for treating rheumatic complaints or kidney disorders.[11]

Will It Harm You? What the Studies Say:

Decades of uneventful use suggest that sarsaparilla is safe to use. Stick to typically recommended amounts, however, as high doses can reportedly cause stomach and intestinal upset and unpleasant burning sensations in the mouth and throat.[12] Be wary of sarsaparilla-containing diet programs; any lost weight will consist of important body fluids quick to return. The chemicals in sarsaparilla called saponins may intensify the absorption of other drugs.

Carefully read the ingredients listed on any sarsaparilla product you buy. Analysts in 1988 found that instead of *Smilax* species from tropical America, a number of products contained another plant altogether: *Hemidesimus indicus* L. Shult, sometimes called Indian sarsaparilla or false sarsaparilla.[13] Although not hazardous, it contains none of sarsaparilla's active ingredients, and the two plants share only a name. They resemble each other neither in effects nor in appearance.

GENERAL SOURCES:

Blumenthal, M., J. Gruenwald, T. Hall, and R.S. Rister, eds. *The Complete German Commission E Monographs: Therapeutic Guide to Herbal Medicine.* Boston: Integrative Medicine Communications, 1998.

Bradley, P.C., ed. *British Herbal Compendium: A Handbook of Scientific Information on Widely Used Plant Drugs*, vol. 1. Bournemouth (Dorset), England: British Herbal Medicine Association, 1992.

Castleman, M. *The Healing Herbs: The Ultimate Guide to the Curative Power of Nature's Medicines.* New York: Bantam Books, 1995.

Fitzpatrick, F.K. *Antibiotics and Chemotherapy.* 4(5) (1954): 528.

Heinerman, J. *Heinerman's Encyclopedia of Healing Herbs and Spices.* West Nyack, NY: Parker Publishing Co., 1996.

Hobbs, C. *HerbalGram.* 17 (1988): 10.

Leung, A.Y., and S. Foster. *Encyclopedia of Common Natural Ingredients Used in Food, Drugs, and Cosmetics.* 2nd ed. New York: John Wiley & Sons, 1996.

Mindell, E. *Earl Mindell's Herb Bible.* New York: Simon & Schuster/Fireside, 1992.

Newall, C.A., et al. *Herbal Medicines: A Guide for Health-Care Professionals.* London: The Pharmaceutical Press, 1996.

Thurmon, F.M. *New England Journal of Medicine.* 227 (1942): 128.

Tyler, V.E. *Herbs of Choice: The Therapeutic Use of Phytomedicinals.* Binghamton, NY: Haworth Press/Pharmaceutical Products Press, 1994.

———. *The Honest Herbal.* Binghamton, NY: Haworth Press/Pharmaceutical Products Press, 1993.

Tyler, V.E. *Nutrition Forum.* 5 (1988): 23.

Tyler, V.E., L.R. Brady, and J.E. Robbers, eds. *Pharmacognosy.* Philadelphia: Lea & Febiger, 1988.

TEXT CITATIONS:

1. V.E. Tyler, *Nutrition Forum,* 5 (1988): 23.
2. K.K. Grunewald and R.S. Bailey, *Sports Medicine*, 15(2) (1993): 90–103.
3. V.E. Tyler, *Herbs of Choice: The Therapeutic Use of Phytomedicinals* (Binghamton, NY: Haworth Press/Pharmaceutical Products Press, 1994).
4. M. Blumenthal, J. Gruenwald, T. Hall, and R.S. Rister, eds., *The Complete German Commission E Monographs: Therapeutic Guide to Herbal Medicine* (Boston: Integrative Medicine Communications, 1998).
5. F.M. Thurmon, *New England Journal of Medicine*, 227 (1942): 128–33.
6. Blumenthal et al., op. cit.
7. A.M. Ageel et al., *Drugs Under Experimental & Clinical Research*, 15(8) (1989): 369–72.
8. A. Caceres et al., *Journal of Ethnopharmacology*, 31(3) (1991): 263–76.
9. A. Caceres et al., *Journal of Ethnopharmacology*, 30(1) (1990): 55–73.
10. V.E. Tyler, L.R. Brady, and J.E. Robbers, eds., *Pharmacognosy* (Philadelphia: Lea & Febiger, 1988).
11. Blumenthal et al., op. cit.
12. M. Castleman, *The Healing Herbs: The Ultimate Guide to the Curative Power of Nature's Medicines* (New York: Bantam Books, 1995).
13. M. Blumenthal, *Health Foods Business*, 34(4) (1988): 58.

SASSAFRAS

SCIENTIFIC NAME:
Sassafras albidum (Nuttal)
Nees., sometimes referred to as
Sassafras officinale Nees et
Eberm or *Sassafras variifolium*
(Salisb.) Kuntzel. Family:
Lauracea

COMMON NAMES:
Ague tree, cinnamon wood,
common sassafras, saloop

RATING:
5 = Studies indicate that there
is a definite health hazard to
using this substance, even in
recommended amounts.

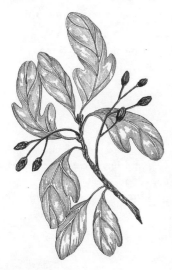

Sassafras
Sassafras albidum

What Is Sassafras?

This small deciduous tree is native to eastern regions of North America. All parts, from the variably shaped leaves to the miniature yellowish flowers and bark, emit a strong spicy odor. The dried root bark is used medicinally.

What It Is Used For:

This formerly popular scent and flavoring—it once flavored root beer—was traditionally used in North American and Europe as a "spring tonic," or syphilis cure. Its purported ability to increase urination probably prolonged this traditional application. Native Americans introduced it to settlers as a remedy for numerous ailments, and its use reportedly persists in parts of the South such as Appalachia. It has been used both internally and externally for rheumatic pains, colds and flus, high blood pressure in elderly individuals, gout, bronchitis, kidney problems, cancers, and skin eruptions (including acne, measles, and poison ivy rash), and to induce sweating and reduce excess gas. Despite concerns about toxicity, a number of sources recommend sassafras tea for these and other ailments, including a very recent report recommending it for breast inflammation following childbirth.[1]

Forms Available Include:

Infusion, safrole-free extract, tea bag, tincture.

Dosage Commonly Reported:

Sassafras should not be used medicinally.

Will It Work for You? What the Studies Say:

No study has ever shown that taking sassafras or its volatile oil internally cures syphilis, enhances performance, or significantly remedies any ailment. Interest in and enthusiasm about the herb dissipated in the 1960s when researchers reported that a toxic substance called safrole (a phenolic ether) in the aromatic root bark oil at concentrations of 80 to 90 percent caused liver tumors in laboratory rats and mice. This prompted the FDA in 1960 to ban both sassafras volatile oil and safrole for use as food additives or flavors and in 1976 to prohibit the interstate marketing of sassafras bark for making tea.[2] A safrole-free extract is now produced and allowed for use in food.[3] There are concerns that other substances in the herb may be cancer-causing as well, however.

Sassafras tea has reportedly been effectively used to produce sweating (diaphoresis),[4] which may help explain why it was once believed to "sweat out" toxins.[5] Other constituents in sassafras include tannins, alkaloids, and resins. Along with safrole, the volatile oil (present in concentrations of 5 to 9 percent) contains small amounts of eugenol, camphor, thujone, and other components. Some of these substances may explain certain folk uses, but their value in sassafras has not been explored, presumably because of the health risks posed by the safrole.

Sassafras oil reportedly has anti-infective and lice-destroying properties,[6] and may still be used externally for these purposes.

Will It Harm You? What the Studies Say:

The volatile oil in sassafras consists of large amounts (80 to 90 percent) of the toxic substance safrole. Signs of poisoning may include vomiting, stupor, collapse, and paralysis. Reportedly, as little as one teaspoonful of the oil can kill an adult, and only a few drops can kill a toddler.[7] Numerous studies have shown that safrole causes liver tumors in animals; these tumors are benign or malignant depending on the dose given. Other cancers have also been observed in laboratory animals, such as esophageal cancer.[8] Safrole-free products are available, but studies indicate that even these pose an increased risk of tumors.[9]

Depending on how long it was allowed to steep and other factors, drinking one cup of tea made with 2.5 grams of sassafras could put as much as 200 milligrams of safrole into your system (equivalent to 3 milligrams per kilogram); compare this with the potentially hazardous dose for human beings, which has been placed at 0.66 milligram per kilogram.[10] A 1994 report found that safrole levels greater than 10,000 milligrams per kilogram (1 percent) were commonly found in unbrewed sassafras tea mixtures easily obtainable in health food outlets.[11] It is important to consider such findings in context, however. A 1977 study posed the possibility that human beings metabolize the cancer-causing element in safrole differently from animals, which could mean that humans would not be at the same risk for developing cancer as experimental animals would be.[12] More research on this subject is needed.

The risks involved in using the herb or its oil in topical formulations are not clear, although contact dermatitis can occur in sensitized people who have contact with sassafras oil.[13]

GENERAL SOURCES:

Duke, J.A. *CRC Handbook of Medicinal Herbs.* Boca Raton, FL: CRC Press, 1985.

Lawrence Review of Natural Products. St. Louis: Facts and Comparisons, January 1988.

Leung, A.Y., and S. Foster. *Encyclopedia of Common Natural Ingredients Used in Food, Drugs, and Cosmetics.* 2nd ed. New York: John Wiley & Sons, 1996.

Newall, C.A., et al. *Herbal Medicines: A Guide for Health-Care Professionals.* London: The Pharmaceutical Press, 1996.

Tierra, M. *The Way of Herbs.* New York: Pocket Books, 1990.

Tyler, V.E. *Herbs of Choice: The Therapeutic Use of Phytomedicinals.* Binghamton, NY: Haworth Press/Pharmaceutical Products Press, 1994.

——. *The Honest Herbal.* Binghamton, NY: Haworth Press/Pharmaceutical Products Press, 1993.

Tyler, V.E., L.R. Brady, and J.E. Robbers, eds. *Pharmacognosy.* Philadelphia: Lea & Febiger, 1988.

Weiner, M.A., and J.A. Weiner. *Herbs That Heal: Prescription for Herbal Healing.* Mill Valley, CA: Quantum Books, 1994.

Weiss, R.F. *Herbal Medicine*, trans. A.R. Meuss, from the 6th German edition. Beaconsfield, England: Beaconsfield Publishers, Ltd., 1988.

TEXT CITATIONS:

1. L. Lieberman, *Midwifery Today & Childbirth Education*, 26 (1993): 9.
2. V.E. Tyler, *Herbs of Choice: The Therapeutic Use of Phytomedicinals* (Binghamton, NY: Haworth Press/Pharmaceutical Products Press, 1994).

3. A.Y. Leung and S. Foster, *Encyclopedia of Common Natural Ingredients Used in Food, Drugs, and Cosmetics*, 2nd ed. (New York: John Wiley & Sons, 1996).

4. J.D. Haines, Jr., *Postgraduate Medicine*, 90(4) (1991): 75–76. Leung and Foster, op. cit.

5. *Merck Index*, 10th ed. (Rahway, NJ: Merck & Co., 1983).

6. Leung and Foster, op. cit.

7. C.A. Newall et al., *Herbal Medicines: A Guide for Health-Care Professionals* (London: The Pharmaceutical Press, 1996).

8. G.J. Kapadia et al., *Journal of the National Cancer Institute*, 60(3) (1978): 683–86.

9. V.E. Tyler, *The Honest Herbal* (Binghamton, NY: Haworth Press/Pharmaceutical Products Press, 1993).

10. Ibid.

11. D.L. Heikes, *Journal of Chromatographic Science*, 32(7) (1994): 253–88.

12. M.S. Benedetti et al., *Toxicology*, 7 (1977): 69.

13. J.A. Duke, *CRC Handbook of Medicinal Herbs* (Boca Raton, FL: CRC Press, 1985).

PRIMARY NAME:
SAVORY

SCIENTIFIC NAME:
Summer savory: *Satureja hortensis* L. Winter savory: *Satureja montana.*

COMMON NAMES:
Bean herb, white thyme

RATING:
3 = Studies on the effectivess and safety of this herb are conflicting, or there are not enough studies to draw a conclusion.

What Is Savory?

Summer and winter savory are extensively cultivated aromatic herbs that grow to about two feet and have narrow oblong leaves and lavender or pink-white flowers. Americans commonly use summer savory, which is native to Europe but can be found in many parts of North America. Winter savory is also grown in North America. The dried leaves and tender stems of this annual are used medicinally, as is an oil made through steam distillation of the entire dried herb. The same parts of winter savory, a perennial, are used.

What It Is Used For:

Cooks have been using these mint-family members for centuries. Both types exude a spicy aroma and flavor reminiscent of thyme and oregano, although summer savory is somewhat sweeter and often favored as a cooking herb. Along the way, summer savory also acquired a reputation for boosting sexual drive, while winter savory became known for damping it. Both savories were used in folk medicine, typically in tea form, as tonics and treatments for cough and congestion, sore throat, diarrhea, appetite loss, and gastrointestinal upsets such as cramps, gas, and indigestion. Contemporary herbalists recommend the savories for a number of these purposes, but especially for stomach upset, coughs, and colds in children; they reputedly have mild effects.

Forms Available Include:

Herb (fresh and dried), infusion, oil, tincture.

Dosage Commonly Reported:

An infusion made using 4 teaspoons herb (1 to 2 teaspoons for children) per cup of water is drunk up to three times per day. The tincture is taken in doses of 1 teaspoon (½ teaspoon for children) up to three times per day.

S

Savory

Will It Work for You? What the Studies Say:

On the basis of what researchers have learned about the herb's chemical constituents, the traditional use of summer savory as an infusion for simple diarrhea and mild digestive system upset may be justified. The herb has yet to be properly studied in humans, however.

Dried summer savory contains about 1 percent of a volatile oil that features mild antibacterial and antifungal properties, as well as an astringent tannin (4 to 8.5 percent). This tannin and substances in the oil (phenolic compounds, specifically) explain the herb's popularity for treating mild diarrhea.[1] (Tannins are believed to control or stop diarrhea by reducing inflammation in the intestines.) Research indicates that savory oil also has antispasmodic effects on isolated smooth muscles[2]; it may calm the digestive tract in this way. A German medical textbook attributes summer savory's value for treating acute enterocolitis to a carminative (gas-relieving) action.[3]

The volatile oil and astringent tannins in summer savory may also be expected to soothe minor coughs and throat irritations, albeit mildly.[4] Both it and winter savory feature an expectorant called cineole, which is valuable for treating congestion.

Winter savory contains about 1.6 percent of a volatile oil. It has demonstrated diuretic ("water pill") activity in laboratory rats, but the property has yet to be properly examined in humans.[5]

Science fails to support the reputation of either summer or winter savory for arousing or damping sexual desire.

Will It Harm You? What the Studies Say:

After years of use with no reports of harm, both types of savory appear to be safe to use as culinary herbs and herbal remedies. No clinical study has carefully addressed the toxicity risk for humans of medicinal concentrations, however. Diluted summer savory oil tested on human skin proved to be nonirritating and nonsensitizing, although the skin of rabbits and guinea pigs subjected to undiluted oil became very irritated.[6] Undiluted oil applied to the backs of hairless mice proved fatal to 50 percent within forty-eight hours.[7] The FDA places savory on its list of foods "Generally Recognized As Safe" (GRAS).

GENERAL SOURCES:

Castleman, M. *The Healing Herbs: The Ultimate Guide to the Curative Power of Nature's Medicines.* New York: Bantam Books, 1995.

Duke, J.A. *CRC Handbook of Medicinal Herbs.* Boca Raton, FL: CRC Press, 1985.

Lawrence Review of Natural Products. St. Louis: Facts and Comparisons, March 1992.

Leung, A.Y., and S. Foster. *Encyclopedia of Common Natural Ingredients Used in Food, Drugs, and Cosmetics.* 2nd ed. New York: John Wiley & Sons, 1996.

Tyler, V.E. *The Honest Herbal.* Binghamton, NY: Haworth Press/Pharmaceutical Products Press, 1993.

Weiss, R.F. *Herbal Medicine*, trans. A.R. Meuss, from the 6th German edition. Beaconsfield, England: Beaconsfield Publishers, Ltd., 1988.

TEXT CITATIONS:

1. V.E. Tyler, *The Honest Herbal* (Binghamton, NY: Haworth Press/Pharmaceutical Products Press, 1993).

2. A.Y. Leung and S. Foster., *Encyclopedia of Common Natural Ingredients Used in Food, Drugs, and Cosmetics*, 2nd ed. (New York: John Wiley & Sons, 1996).

3. R.F. Weiss, *Herbal Medicine*, trans. A.R. Meuss, from the 6th German edition (Beaconsfield, England: Beaconsfield Publishers, Ltd., 1988).

4. Tyler, op. cit.

5. G. Stanic and I. Samarzija, *Phytotherapy Research*, 7(5) (1993): 363.

6. D.L.J. Opdyke, *Food & Cosmetics Toxicology*, 14(Suppl.) (1976): 859.

7. Leung and Foster, op. cit.

PRIMARY NAME:

SAW PALMETTO

SCIENTIFIC NAME:
Serenoa repens (Bart.) Small, sometimes referred to as *Serenoa serrulata* Hook., F, *Sabal serrulata* Schult., or *Serenoa serrulata* (Michx.) Nichols. Family: Palmaceae (Arecaceae)

COMMON NAMES:
American dwarf palm tree, cabbage palm, serenoa

RATING:
1 = Years of use and high-quality studies indicate that this substance is very effective when used in recommended amounts for the indication(s) noted in the "Will It Work for You?" section. It appears to be safe when judiciously used; see the "Will It Harm You" section, however.

What Is Saw Palmetto?

This shrubby palm can be found in sandy soils throughout the southeastern United States and parts of the Mediterranean region. It grows to about ten feet and is distinguished by clusters of long, double-pointed, swordlike leaf blades. The dark, olive-sized fruit ("berry") is picked when ripe, then partially dried and used medicinally.

What It Is Used For:

In the early part of the twentieth century, conventional medicine in America and Europe began to investigate the potential of saw palmetto, which Native Americans had apparently relied on as a food, to fulfill its claimed value as a remedy for such ailments as chronic cystitis (bladder inflammation), urinary tract infections, sex hormone disorders, impotence and frigidity, and respiratory tract diseases. It also had a reputation as an aphrodisiac, sperm booster, and breast-enhancer. For many years people took it to increase urine output in the form of a diuretic, or "water pill."

But saw palmetto's most widely held reputation through the years has been as a remedy for excessive need to urinate, especially at night, and other symptoms associated with prostate enlargement and inflammation. (The prostate is a glandular organ in men positioned between the bladder and urethra, so its enlargement can interfere with urinating.) Ultimately unconvinced of its effectiveness, conventional American medicine became disenchanted with the remedy in the 1940s and 1950s, and the *National Formulary* stopped listing it in 1950.[1] But modern herbalists extol this and other long-time uses for saw palmetto, and medical authorities in Germany, France, and Italy continue to recognize it officially as a treatment for symptoms of what is now commonly called benign (nonmalignant) prostatic hyperplasia (BPH).

Forms Available Include:

Capsule, concentrated drops, decoction (of dried, ground berries), extract (liquid or oil-based), fruit, tablet, tincture.

Dosage Commonly Reported:

A typical daily dose is 1 to 2 grams of the ground, dried fruit. Alternatively, 320 milligrams of an alcohol or hexane extract, standardized to 90 percent fatty acids/sterols, may be taken. Two to three 600-milligram fruit capsules are taken three times a day.

Will It Work for You? What the Studies Say:

Results from well-designed although generally small human trials indicate that certain extracts from saw palmetto berries help reduce the symptoms of early prostatic enlargement (specifically, BPH). Compared with a placebo, treatment strengthened (increased) the flow of urine, decreased the number of times needed to urinate (including at night), reduced residual (leftover) urine, and made it easier to start urinating.[2] According to animal studies, it apparently does this not by shrinking the gland, but by inhibiting the actions of male hormones (androgens) in various ways[3] and exerting anti-inflammatory and antiswelling effects.[4] Recent findings from a human trial indicate that the prostate itself might shrink somewhat.[5] Earlier thinking held that the substance worked by promoting the activity of the female hormone, estrogen, but this has since been dismissed.[6]

Experts have yet to identify the responsible ingredients. They do know, however, that a liquid extract of the fruit, such as a tea, will probably not work because the critical ingredients do not dissolve in water; it has to be extracted with a fat-soluble substance such as alcohol or hexane.[7]

Saw palmetto fruit and extracts do not cause changes in testosterone or other hormone levels,[8] and claims that they can boost sperm production or increase sexual vigor or interest are not only unsubstantiated but the opposite of what one would expect from an antiandrogen.[9] The fruit and extracts also have antiallergic and immune-system-stimulating properties, according to evidence from small-animal studies,[10] but the implications of these findings for human disorders remain unclear.

Will It Harm You? What the Studies Say:

On the basis of years of use, experience in clinical trials, and data on the ingredients in saw palmetto, the herb appears to be safe for medicinal use. Cases of headache have been reported but are uncommon, and only one subject withdrew from a particular clinical trial because of an adverse reaction—stomach upset.[11] Large doses may cause diarrhea.[12] Well-designed, long-term studies still need to be done to fully assess the risks posed by this herb, however. The FDA placed saw palmetto on its formerly maintained list of "Herbs of Undefined Safety."

If you suspect that you have prostate problems, a urinary tract infection, or any other type of genitourinary disorder, see a doctor before using this or any other herb, as all these problems have the potential to cause serious complications. Given its documented hormonal actions, also keep in mind that the herb may interact negatively with prostate medicines or hormonal treatments (including hormone replacement therapy), possibly canceling out their effectiveness or causing unwanted side effects, and may be unwise to take if you suffer from a hormone-dependent illness such as breast cancer.[13] Pregnant and nursing women should not take it, for the same reasons.

GENERAL SOURCES:

American Pharmaceutical Association. *Handbook of Nonprescription Drugs.* 11th ed. Washington, D.C.: American Pharmaceutical Association, 1996.

Lawrence Review of Natural Products. St. Louis: Facts and Comparisons, March 1994.

Leung, A.Y., and S. Foster. *Encyclopedia of Common Natural Ingredients Used in Food, Drugs, and Cosmetics.* 2nd ed. New York: John Wiley & Sons, 1996.

Mayell, M. *Off-the-Shelf Natural Health: How to Use Herbs and Nutrients to Stay Well.* New York: Bantam Books, 1995.

Murray, M.T. *The Healing Power of Herbs: The Enlightened Person's Guide to the Wonders of Medicinal Plants.* Rev. 2nd ed. Rocklin, CA: Prima Publishing, 1995.

Newall, C.A., et al. *Herbal Medicines: A Guide for Health-Care Professionals.* London: The Pharmaceutical Press, 1996.

Tierra, M. *The Way of Herbs.* New York: Pocket Books, 1990.

Tyler, V.E. *Herbs of Choice: The Therapeutic Use of Phytomedicinals.* Binghamton, NY: Haworth Press/Pharmaceutical Products Press, 1994.

———. *The Honest Herbal.* Binghamton, NY: Haworth Press/Pharmaceutical Products Press, 1993.

Weiner, M.A., and J.A. Weiner. *Herbs That Heal: Prescription for Herbal Healing.* Mill Valley, CA: Quantum Books, 1994.

TEXT CITATIONS:

1. V.E. Tyler, *The Honest Herbal* (Binghamton, NY: Haworth Press/Pharmaceutical Products Press, 1993).
2. G. Champault et al., *British Journal of Clinical Pharmacology,* 18 (1984): 461–62. A. Tasca et al., *Minerva Urologica e Nefrologica,* 37 (1985): 87–91. F. DiSilverio et al., *European Urology,* 21 (1992): 309. V.E. Tyler, *Herbs of Choice: The Therapeutic Use of Phytomedicinals* (Binghamton, NY: Haworth Press/Pharmaceutical Products Press, 1994).
3. C.A. Newall et al., *Herbal Medicines: A Guide for Health-Care Professionals* (London: The Pharmaceutical Press, 1996).
4. DiSilverio, op. cit. J.O. Carreras, *Archivos Espanoles de Urologia,* 40 (1987): 310–13.
5. J. Braeckman, *Current Therapeutic Research,* 55 (1994): 776–85.
6. M.I. Elghamry and R. Hansel, *Experientia,* 25 (1969): 828–29.
7. V.E. Tyler, *Herbs of Choice: The Therapeutic Use of Phytomedicinals* (Binghamton, NY: Haworth Press/Pharmaceutical Products Press, 1994). V.L. Begg, *Herb Quarterly,* 50 (1991): 33–35.
8. C. Casarosa et al., *Clinical Therapeutics,* 10 (1988): 558–85.
9. Tyler, op. cit.
10. *Lawrence Review of Natural Products* (St. Louis: Facts and Comparisons, March 1994). J.P. Tarayre et al., *Annales Pharmaceutiques Françaises,* 41 (1983): 559.
11. *Lawrence Review of Natural Products,* op. cit. Carreras, op. cit.
12. *Lawrence Review of Natural Products,* op. cit.
13. Ibid.

PRIMARY NAME:
SCHISANDRA

SCIENTIFIC NAME:
Schisandra chinensis (Turcz.) Bail., *Schisandra sphenanthera*

What Is Schisandra?

Schisandra is an aromatic, flowering woody vine native to eastern Asia. Its juicy, seed-bearing red berries (fruit), once fully ripened in autumn, are collected and dried to a shriveled brownish black for medicinal purposes. These have a sour and salty taste.

Reid et Wils., and other *Schisandra* species. Family: Schisandraceae

COMMON NAMES:

Five-flavor seed, gomishi, kita-gomishi (Japanese), wu wei zi

RATING:

3 = Studies on the effectiveness and safety of this substance are conflicting, or there are not enough studies to draw a conclusion.

What It Is Used For:

Chinese and other Asian healing traditions integrated schisandra into their repertoires many centuries ago. They value it for its purported tonic, antiseptic, and astringent properties, and have traditionally used it to treat cough, asthma and various other respiratory diseases, chronic diarrhea, insomnia, physical exhaustion, neurasthenia, thirst, and impotence.[1] It has a reputation as a kidney remedy and male tonic. Russian folk medicine relies on it heavily.

Schisandra has recently been promoted in the United States as a remedy for numerous disorders, but most consistently perhaps as a system-strengthening herb to increase stamina and fight fatigue and as an "adaptogen" to boost the body's resistance to "stressors" such as illness. Recently, researchers have focused much of their attention on the herb's potential liver-protectant properties.

Forms Available Include:

Capsule, concentrated drops, decoction (of crushed berries), extracts, herb (dried), powder, tablet, tincture.

Dosage Commonly Reported:

The dried herb is taken in doses of 1.5 to 9 grams. A decoction is made using 5 grams crushed berries per 100 milliliters water and is drunk in divided doses three times per day. In China, a chronic cough is typically treated with 1.5 to 3 grams of the dried herb, and for tonic purposes 6 to 9 grams are taken.

Will It Work for You? What the Studies Say:

Chinese, Japanese, and Russian investigators in particular have taken an interest in this herb. Their research reveals a myriad of actions in humans and laboratory animals. Although many findings are intriguing, none so far is based on well-designed human trials. The fruit contains a volatile oil (1 to 3 percent), and the enclosed seeds contain more than forty different lignans, including wu wei zi C, deoxygomisin A, shisantherin D, and gomisins A, C, and N. These lignans are believed to be the major active constituents in the herb,[2] and investigators have focused on them as substances that may protect the liver from toxins such as carbon tetrachloride. The medical literature features dozens of reports on schisandra's liver-protectant properties, including many in laboratory animals and some in humans, indicating that it may improve symptoms in individuals suffering from chronic hepatitis.

Adaptogens purportedly help the body to adapt to stress.[3] Schisandra has displayed adaptogenic properties similar to, although weaker (and potentially less toxic) than, those of common tonics such as ginseng and Siberian ginseng. In one experiment, racehorses given schisandra markedly improved their performance and endurance.[4] Many studies have shown that schisandra or its extracts can heighten reflexes and endurance in healthy humans,[5] exert antidepressant actions in mice, induce anticonvulsant and tranquilizing properties in rodents, encourage breathing in various laboratory animals, fight bacteria in the test tube, stimulate the uterus of rabbits in the test tube and in the animal, normalize blood pressure, exert antioxidant actions (antioxidants help prevent damage from free radicals, agents that damage cells through oxidation, which may be related to cancer cell formation),[6] and initiate antitussive (anticough) and muscle-relaxant actions in mice.[7] The implications of these findings are bright with potential yet untested by well-designed human trials.

Will It Harm You? What the Studies Say:

The medical literature contains no reports of serious adverse reactions to schisandra, although reportedly in rare cases it can cause stomach upset, hives, and decreased appetite.[8] It also has the potential to depress (slow down) the central nervous system, so use it with care.[9] Given its unclear impact on the liver, individuals with liver problems or those at risk for them may want to avoid the herb altogether. It may also affect how other medicines metabolized in the liver are processed.[10]

GENERAL SOURCES:

Chevallier, A. *The Encyclopedia of Medicinal Plants: A Practical Reference Guide to More Than 550 Key Medicinal Plants & Their Uses.* 1st American ed. New York: Dorling Kindersley Publications, 1996.

Lawrence Review of Natural Products. St. Louis: Facts and Comparisons, June 1988.

Leung, A.Y., and S. Foster. *Encyclopedia of Common Natural Ingredients Used in Food, Drugs, and Cosmetics.* 2nd ed. New York: John Wiley & Sons, 1996.

Mayell, M. *Off-the-Shelf Natural Health: How to Use Herbs and Nutrients to Stay Well.* New York: Bantam Books, 1995.

Tyler, V.E. *Herbs of Choice: The Therapeutic Use of Phytomedicinals.* Binghamton, NY: Haworth Press/Pharmaceutical Products Press, 1994.

———. *The Honest Herbal.* Binghamton, NY: Haworth Press/Pharmaceutical Products Press, 1993.

Tyler, V.E., L.R. Brady, and J.E. Robbers, eds. *Pharmacognosy.* Philadelphia: Lea & Febiger, 1988.

Weiner, M.A., and J.A. Weiner. *Herbs That Heal: Prescription for Herbal Healing.* Mill Valley, CA: Quantum Books, 1994.

TEXT CITATIONS:

1. A.Y. Leung and S. Foster, *Encyclopedia of Common Natural Ingredients Used in Food, Drugs, and Cosmetics,* 2nd ed. (New York: John Wiley & Sons, 1996).
2. Ibid.
3. I.I. Brekhman and I.V. Dardymov, *Annual Review of Pharmacology,* (1969): 419.
4. F. Ahumada et al., *Phytotherapy Research,* 3 (1989): 175.
5. B.X. Wang, *Tianjin Yiyao Zazhi,* 7 (1965): 338.
6. Leung and Foster, op. cit.
7. S. Maeda et al., *Yakugaky Zasshi,* 101 (1981): 1030.
8. Leung and Foster, op. cit.
9. *Lawrence Review of Natural Products* (St. Louis: Facts and Comparisons, June 1988).
10. Ibid.

PRIMARY NAME:
SCULLCAP

SCIENTIFIC NAME:
Scutellaria laterifolia L. and occasionally other *Scutellaria* species; in Europe and Asia, *Scutellaria baicalensis* Georgii is commonly used. Family: Labiatae (Lamiaceae)

COMMON NAMES:
Helmetflower, hoodwort, maddog weed, Quaker bonnet, skullcap, Virginia skullcap

RATING:
4 = Research indicates that this substance will not fulfill the claims made for it, but that it is also unlikely to cause any harm. However, see warnings in the "Will It Harm You?" section.

What Is Scullcap?

This erect perennial, a mint-family member, has branching square stems that support serrated oval leaves and small, tubular, bluish flowers in summer. It is a slender but hardy plant and favors moist woods and other damp environments in its native North America. The aboveground parts are used medicinally. As many as one hundred or more related species that grow in Europe and China have been used medicinally as well.

What It Is Used For:

As a folk medicine, scullcap was used to treat convulsions, hysteria, nervous tension, and epilepsy (grand mal seizures in particular). Traditional healers in Europe considered it valuable for these disorders as a sedative and anticonvulsant. Introduced into American medicine in the 1770s as a remedy for hydrophobia (fear of water) associated with rabies,[1] the herb eventually gained a reputation as a tonic, tranquilizer, antispasmodic, and remedy for various female ills. Many of these uses are recommended by herbalists today. The herb was officially recognized as a tranquilizer in the *U.S. Pharmacopoeia* for nearly fifty-five years, until 1916. Some contemporary sources also cite it as a cure for drug and alcohol withdrawal. Herbal blends for insomnia, anxiety, and women in particular often feature scullcap.

Forms Available Include:

Capsule, concentrated drops, infusion, liquid extract, tablet, teas, tincture. Appears as an ingredient in numerous herbal tea blends. Many people sweeten scullcap tea with honey or sugar.

Dosage Commonly Reported:

An infusion made using 1 to 2 teaspoons dried herb per cup of water is drunk up to three times per day. The tincture is taken in doses of 1 to 2 droppersful. Two to three 429-milligram capsules of the herb are taken three times a day. The liquid herb extract is taken in doses of 2 to 4 milliliters.

Will It Work for You? What the Studies Say:

Scant supporting evidence can be found to justify the use of scullcap (*Scutellaria laterifolia*, specifically) as a cure for rabies or as a tranquilizer, tonic, or antispasmodic. One has to hunt back into research reports from the early part of the twentieth century to find scientific material on this herb. In the 1910s, researchers reported that scullcap extracts added to a guinea pig uterus in a chemical bath slightly inhibited the ability of the uterine tissue to contract. More importantly, perhaps, tolerable ("normal") doses had no effect at all when given to the animal directly.[2] Follow-up experiments on frogs and small animals confirmed this apparent lack of antispasmodic or tranquilizing action on the central nervous system and circulation. Several experts have questioned a study indicating that a tincture of the related Asian species *Scutellaria baicalensis* can generate long-lasting drops in blood pressure.[3] Substances called flavonoids in certain *Scutellaria* species might be expected to exert some antispasmodic effect (and hence a possible calming action), but results of mouse experiments have not been promising.[4]

Numerous intriguing properties have been identified in *Scutellaria baicalensis*, including potential anti-HIV properties,[5] tumor-fighting actions,[6] and the presence of antiviral[7] and antifungal substances.[8] Japanese researchers report anti-inflammatory activity in laboratory animals that may be explained by inhibition of the enzyme sialidase, which has been implicated in certain inflammatory diseases.[9]

Will It Harm You? What the Studies Say:

Typically recommended doses of scullcap are unlikely to cause any harm, although large amounts of the tincture can cause giddiness, confusion, limb twitching, and signs of an epileptic seizure.[10] The FDA placed scullcap on its formerly maintained list of "Herbs of Undefined Safety." Liver damage from hepatitis developed in a forty-nine-year-old woman who had been drinking an herbal remedy containing scullcap, motherwort, kelp, and mistletoe; the authors identified mistletoe as the causative agent, however.

GENERAL SOURCES:

Bremness, L. *Herbs*. 1st American ed. Eyewitness Handbooks. New York: Dorling Kindersley Publications, 1994.

Castleman, M. *The Healing Herbs: The Ultimate Guide to the Curative Power of Nature's Medicines*. New York: Bantam Books, 1995.

Chevallier, A. *The Encyclopedia of Medicinal Plants: A Practical Reference Guide to More Than 550 Key Medicinal Plants & Their Uses*. 1st American ed. New York: Dorling Kindersley Publications, 1996.

Duke, J.A. *CRC Handbook of Medicinal Herbs*. Boca Raton, FL: CRC Press, 1985.

Lawrence Review of Natural Products. St. Louis: Facts and Comparisons, January 1993.

Mayell, M. *Off-the-Shelf Natural Health: How to Use Herbs and Nutrients to Stay Well*. New York: Bantam Books, 1995.

Newall, C.A., et al. *Herbal Medicines: A Guide for Health-Care Professionals*. London: The Pharmaceutical Press, 1996.

Tierra, M. *The Way of Herbs*. New York: Pocket Books, 1990.

Tyler, V.E. *The Honest Herbal*. Binghamton, NY: Haworth Press/Pharmaceutical Products Press, 1993.

Weiner, M.A., and J.A. Weiner. *Herbs That Heal: Prescription for Herbal Healing*. Mill Valley, CA: Quantum Books, 1994.

TEXT CITATIONS:

1. V.E. Tyler, *The Honest Herbal* (Binghamton, NY: Haworth Press/Pharmaceutical Products Press, 1993).
2. Ibid. T. Sollmann, *A Manual of Pharmacology*, 7th ed. (Philadelphia: W.B. Saunders, 1948).
3. Tyler, op. cit. B.A. Kumakov, *Farmakologiya I Toksikologiya* (Moscow), 206 (1957): 79–80.
4. S.G. Franzblau and C. Cross, *Journal of Ethnopharmacology*, 15 (1986): 279. *Lawrence Review of Natural Products* (St. Louis: Facts and Comparisons, January 1993).
5. B.Q. Li et al., *Cellular & Molecular Biology Research*, 39(2) (1993): 119–24.
6. T. Konoshima et al., *Chemical & Pharmaceutical Bulletin*, 40(2) (1992): 531–32.
7. T. Nagai et al., *Biological & Pharmaceutical Bulletin*, 18(2) (1995): 295–99.

8. D. Yang et al., *Annales Pharmaceutiques Françaises*, 53(3) (1995): 138–41.
9. T. Nagai et al., *Planta Medica*, 55 (1989): 27.
10. J.A. Duke, *CRC Handbook of Medicinal Herbs* (Boca Raton, FL: CRC Press, 1985).

PRIMARY NAME:
SELENIUM

SCIENTIFIC NAME:
N/A

COMMON NAME:
N/A

RATING:
3 = Studies on the effectiveness and safety of this substance are conflicting, or there are not enough studies to draw a conclusion. See the warnings in the "Will It Harm You?" section.

What Is Selenium?

Selenium is an essential trace element present in all body tissues.

What It Is Used For:

The human body needs selenium to function properly. The body relies on it as a cofactor in inhibiting the oxidation of lipids (fats), and as such it can be classified as an antioxidant. Deficiencies in the element are uncommon in industrialized countries. When they do occur, they are usually in individuals with alcoholic cirrhosis who may be getting an insufficient amount through a poor diet or who have an altered ability to metabolize the mineral because of their liver condition.[1] When the body is short of selenium, muscle pain, abnormal nail beds, and cardiomyopathy (a type of heart failure) may develop.

Various sources, including dietary supplement manufacturers, recommend taking selenium supplements for a myriad of purposes, including to prevent and treat heart disease and cancer. Increased rates of cancer and heart disease have been observed in regions of the world where levels of selenium in the soil are low. Several sources claim that selenium supplementation can reduce the risk of skin cancer and help to prevent cancers of the breast, lung, ovaries, large intestine, rectum, and prostate. Others assert that supplementing the diet with this element can improve mood, clear up skin conditions such as acne, forestall aging, boost the immune system, and even help prevent and counter immune-system-deficiency disorders such as AIDS. Various shampoos contain selenium for dandruff control.

Forms Available Include:

Capsule, tablet. Appears in many multivitamin and multimineral formulas.

Dosage Commonly Reported:

The Recommended Daily Allowance for selenium is 70 micrograms for adult men and 50 to 55 micrograms for adult women.[2] A commonly reported daily dosage is 50 to 100 micrograms. Selenium is often taken in combination with vitamin E.

Will It Work for You? What the Studies Say:

Although studies indicate that selenium may help prevent or treat a number of disorders, conclusive findings from well-designed, large-scale studies have yet to be made. Most Americans appear to get sufficient amounts through their diets. Particularly good sources of selenium include meat, fish, various cereal grains, mushrooms, poultry, egg yolks, wheat germ, garlic, cucumbers, asparagus, and Brazil nuts. The selenium content reflects the selenium-richness of the soil in which the plants grow.

Selenium qualifies as an antioxidant. These substances control the formation of dangerous substances in the body called free radicals, agents that damage cells through oxidation, some of which may contribute to cancer-cell formation. Dozens of studies in animals have shown that adding selenium to the diet helps protect the animals from various cancers.[3] In a study published in 1997, six hundred people taking daily selenium supplements of 200 micrograms a day for ten years developed many fewer cancers than those taking a placebo; there were 71 percent fewer prostate cancers, 67 percent fewer esophageal cancers, 62 percent fewer colorectal cancers, and 46 percent fewer lung cancers.[4] Whether the type of selenium available to the consumer will produce the same effects is not clear; the study subjects took special selenium-enriched yeast closely resembling the selenium that is normally consumed in the diet.[5] In any case, the body can probably use selenium from dietary sources better than it can from dietary supplements. Low dietary selenium levels may adversely affect mood, according to recently published research. A double-blind, placebo-controlled crossover study of twenty British subjects found that the lower the original level of selenium in the subjects' diet, the more they reported improvement in levels of depression and anxiety after taking 100 micrograms of selenium daily for five weeks.[6] However, none of the data collected in studies so far specifically indicate that supplementing the typical American diet with selenium pills will actually improve mood.[7]

Selenium has been shown to aid a potentially deadly heart disorder called Keshan disease. Keshan disease has been found at higher-than-normal rates in children living in regions of China where the concentrations of selenium in the soil are very low. Higher-than-normal rates of a joint disorder called Kaschin-Beck disease were also found in the children.

Will It Harm You? What the Studies Say:

A daily intake of between 50 micrograms and 200 micrograms of selenium is safe, according to the Food and Nutrition Board of the National Academy of Sciences. *But selenium is toxic if taken in more than the recommended concentrations,* causing nausea and vomiting, skin lesions, fatigue, hair and nail loss, tooth problems, and central nervous system effects in many cases.[8] Some of these reactions have been noted in people taking twenty-five times the recommended amount.[9] At least eleven people suffered selenium poisoning in the mid-1980s after taking supplements that accidentally contained 125 times the recommended amount.[10] Such serious conditions as muscular weakness, respiratory failure, infertility, growth retardation, swallowing difficulties, focal hepatic necrosis, and bronchopneumonia may signal selenium toxicity.[11]

No adverse reactions were noted in the study published in 1997 that involved six hundred subjects taking 200 micrograms of selenium daily for a decade.[12]

GENERAL SOURCES:

American Pharmaceutical Association. *Handbook of Nonprescription Drugs.* 11th ed. Washington, D.C.: American Pharmaceutical Association, 1996.

Balch, J.F., and P.A. Balch. *Prescription for Nutritional Healing: A Practical A to Z Reference to Drug-Free Remedies Using Vitamins, Minerals, Herbs & Food Supplements.* 2nd ed. Garden City Park, NY: Avery Publishing Group, 1997.

Brody, J.E. "Hopes Rising for Selenium." *New York Times.* (February 19, 1997): C8.

Mayell, M. *Off-the-Shelf Natural Health: How to Use Herbs and Nutrients to Stay Well.* New York: Bantam Books, 1995.

TEXT CITATIONS:

1. American Pharmaceutical Association, *Handbook of Nonprescription Drugs*, 11th ed. (Washington, D.C.: American Pharmaceutical Association, 1996).

2. Ibid.

3. J.E. Brody, "Hopes Rising for Selenium," *New York Times* (February 19, 1997): C8.

4. B.H. Patterson and O.A. Levander, *Cancer Causes and Control*, 6(1) (1997): 63–69. W.J. Blot, *Proceedings of the Society for Experimental Biology and Medicine*, 216(2) (1997): 291–96. R.E. Patterson et al., *Cancer Causes and Control*, 8(5) (1997): 786–802.

5. Brody, op. cit.

6. D. Benton and R. Cook. *Biological Psychiatry*, 29(11) (1991): 1092–98.

7. W.C. Hawkes and L. Hornbostel, *Biological Psychiatry*, 39(2) (1996): 121–28.

8. American Pharmaceutical Assocation, op. cit.

9. Brody, op. cit.

10. Ibid.

11. American Pharmaceutical Association, op. cit.

12. B. H. Patterson, op. cit. Blot, op. cit. R. E. Patterson, op. cit.

PRIMARY NAME:
SENEGA ROOT

SCIENTIFIC NAME:

Polygala senega L. and other closely related species cultivated in Japan and western Canada. Family: Polygalaceae. *Polygala senega* var. *latifolia* is a species commonly cultivated in Japan.

COMMON NAMES:

Milkwort, northern senega (Canada), rattlesnake root, seneca snakeroot, senega, senega snakeroot, snakeroot yuan zhi

What Is Senega Root?

This perennial is native to the woodlands of eastern North America. It has lance-shaped leaves and clusters of small whitish-green to pinkish flowers topping erect stems. The twisted roots and rootstock are used medicinally once dried.

What It Is Used For:

Seneca Indians and other North American tribes reportedly chewed the roots of this plant and then applied the pulp to rattlesnake bites—hence the name many people know it by: rattlesnake root. Early settlers apparently followed suit. Although the practice eventually faded, the herb's popularity as an expectorant for controlling respiratory tract congestion and for treating asthma, bronchitis, and pleurisy along with a number of other respiratory ills persisted for many decades in North America and was officially recognized in the *U.S. Pharmacopoeia*. Many healers considered it good for increasing salivation and promoting perspiration to reduce fever. Large doses were used to induce vomiting and diarrhea. Contemporary herbalists continue to extol its value for a number of these symptoms, but focus primarily on its use for coughs, colds, asthma, and bronchitis.

Forms Available Include:

Decoction, extract (in European cough and throat lozenges), infusion, liquid extract, syrup, tincture, tea.

Dosage Commonly Reported:

A decoction is made using 0.5 gram (about ⅕ teaspoon) of root per cup of water. Daily doses of more than 3 grams are not recommended.

Will It Work for You? What the Studies Say:

Senega root contains considerable amounts (up to 12 percent in some cases) of recognized expectorants called triterpenoid saponins. By irritating the stomach lining, they cause nausea and reflexively stimulate mucus production in the bronchial tubes and sweat glands.[1] This in turn loosens sticky secretions in the respiratory tract, making them easier to cough up. The official pharmacist's handbook—the *National Formulary*—listed it as an expectorant until 1960, but it is no longer officially recognized in the United States, presumably because safer and equally effective substances are available. German health authorities, however, approve of senega root for treating upper respiratory congestion.[2] The root's volatile oil contains small amounts of methyl salicylate, which imparts a wintergreen odor.

Not much else is known about *Polygala senega*, although animal studies have been done on other *Polygala* species. A patent awarded to a French company indicates that an acid extracted from the plant offers important anti-inflammatory properties.[3]

Will It Harm You? What the Studies Say:

Stick to recommended dosages (not more than 3 grams a day) or nausea, stomach upset, or diarrhea may develop.[4] The safety of long-term exposure to the active ingredient—the saponins—is unclear. It may eventually irritate the gastrointestinal tract in such a way as to allow toxins to enter the bloodstream.[5] If you already have an irritated stomach or stomach ulcer, avoid this herb.[6]

GENERAL SOURCES:

Blumenthal, M., J. Gruenwald, T. Hall, and R.S. Rister, eds. *The Complete German Commission E Monographs: Therapeutic Guide to Herbal Medicine.* Boston: Integrative Medicine Communications, 1998.

Bradley, P.C., ed. *British Herbal Compendium: A Handbook of Scientific Information on Widely Used Plant Drugs*, vol. 1. Bournemouth (Dorset), England: British Herbal Medicine Association, 1992.

Dobelis, I.N., ed. *The Magic and Medicine of Plants: A Practical Guide to the Science, History, Folklore, and Everyday Uses of Medicinal Plants.* Pleasantville, NY: Reader's Digest Association, 1986.

Newall, C.A., et al. *Herbal Medicines: A Guide for Health-Care Professionals.* London: The Pharmaceutical Press, 1996.

Tyler, V.E. *Herbs of Choice: The Therapeutic Use of Phytomedicinals.* Binghamton, NY: Haworth Press/Pharmaceutical Products Press, 1994.

———. *The Honest Herbal.* Binghamton, NY: Haworth Press/Pharmaceutical Products Press, 1993.

Weiner, M.A., and J.A. Weiner. *Herbs That Heal: Prescription for Herbal Healing.* Mill Valley, CA: Quantum Books, 1994.

TEXT CITATIONS:

1. V.E. Tyler, *The Honest Herbal* (Binghamton, NY: Haworth Press/Pharmaceutical Products Press, 1993).

S

Senega Root

2. M. Blumenthal, J. Gruenwald, T. Hall, and R.S. Rister, eds., *The Complete German Commission E Monographs: Therapeutic Guide to Herbal Medicine* (Boston: Integrative Medicine Communications, 1998).
3. P. Tuber, *France Demande Patent # 2,202,683.* C.A. Newall et al., *Herbal Medicines: A Guide for Health-Care Professionals* (London: The Pharmaceutical Press, 1996).
4. V.E. Tyler, *Herbs of Choice: The Therapeutic Use of Phytomedicinals* (Binghamton, NY: Haworth Press/Pharmaceutical Products Press, 1994).
5. Newall, op. cit.
6. P.C. Bradley, ed., *British Herbal Compendium: A Handbook of Scientific Information on Widely Used Plant Drugs*, vol. 1 (Bournemouth [Dorset], England: British Herbal Medicine Association, 1992).

PRIMARY NAME:

SENNA

SCIENTIFIC NAME:
Cassia senna L. (sometimes referred to as *Cassia acutifolia* Del. and *Senna alexandrina* Mill.), and *Cassia angustifolia* Vahl. (sometimes referred to as *Senna alexandrina* Mill.). Family: Leguminosae (Fabaceae)

COMMON NAMES:
Cassia. *Cassia senna:* Alexandrian senna, Khartoum senna; *Cassia angustifolia:* Fan xie ye, Indian senna, Tinnevelly senna

RATING:
1 = Years of use and extensive, high-quality studies indicate that this substance is very effective when used in recommended amounts for the indication(s) noted in the "Will It Work for You?" section. Safety depends on judicious use, however; see the "Will It Harm You" section.

What Is Senna?

Senna refers to the dried leaflets and leathery pods of two closely related herbaceous shrubs, *Cassia senna* and *Cassia angustifolia.* The first grows naturally along the Nile in northern Africa, and the second in parts of India and northeastern Africa. Both are cultivated in other parts of the world. So-called "wild sennas" can be found in eastern regions of North America.

What It Is Used For:

Arabs appear to have started using this plant medicinally before written records were kept, finally introducing it into European trade in the ninth or tenth century.[1] Senna's enduring fame is as a cathartic—a strong laxative. Cultures around the world have relied on cups of senna tea to dispel constipation. Although few modern herbalists fail to mention this ancient herb, most note the high risk of intestinal cramping and other side effects. The pods are said to have a gentler action. Native Americans reportedly used the herb to reduce fever.

Forms Available Include:

Capsule, infusion, powder, syrup, tincture. Aromatic herbs may be added to mask the herb's nauseating taste and smell. Senna is sold as a laxative in various over-the-counter forms, including liquids, powders, and tablets. Standardized commercial preparations are widely available.

Dosage Commonly Reported:

An infusion is made using ½ to 1 teaspoon (0.5 to 2 grams) herb per cup of water or by soaking the leaflets in cold water for ten to twelve hours. Two (one in the case of a child) of the 25-milligram senna extract capsules are taken once or twice a day.

Will It Work for You? What the Studies Say:

Senna is a potent, proven laxative. Anthraquinones, its key ingredients, were long believed to irritate or stimulate the bowel. The same substances appear in such herbs as **Aloe Vera** and Chinese rhubarb (see **Rhubarb, Chinese**). But

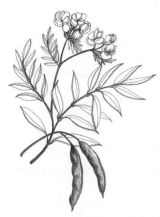

Senna
Cassia senna

experts now agree that another function may well account for the laxative activity, possibly including increased bowel activity due to the secretion of anthraquinones into the colon.[2]

Because side effects such as abdominal cramping and colic are largely unpredictable with a homemade remedy, most sources recommend taking a standardized commercial formulation that can be purchased over the counter. In any case, there are gentler approaches to reducing constipation, including increasing your fluid and fiber intake and exercising. Turn to a cathartic such as senna only if these measures or a gentler laxative cannot resolve the problem.

Will It Harm You? What the Studies Say:

Senna is a powerful medicine that can cause very uncomfortable and serious reactions if not taken properly. Even correct dosages may cause mild abdominal discomfort. Because the concentration of active ingredients in herbal formulations such as teas can vary so widely, some users may get doses that are too high and may experience diarrhea, nausea, severe cramps, dehydration, and related complications; other users may get no relief from the constipation at all.

Risks do not disappear with standardized commercial preparations, however. Take a stimulant laxative such as this only for short periods (a maximum of ten days); if taken for longer periods or abused, senna can cause chronic diarrhea and cramps, laxative dependence, pigment deposits (melanin) in the colon's mucous membranes, and the loss of critical fluids and salts (including potassium) that may lead to weakness and possibly other complications, including increased risks from heart medicines. One woman developed clubbing of the fingers after taking senna tablets for many years.[3] The leaves may cause a skin rash in sensitive individuals.

Do not take this herb if you suffer from any kind of intestinal obstruction or have appendicitis or abdominal pain of unknown cause, and take it only on the advice of a doctor if you suffer from inflammatory bowel disease.[4] If you are pregnant or nursing, do not use it or any other laxative except under the advice of a doctor; one source indicates that muscle contractions stimulated by the laxative may extend to the uterus and cause complications.[5] Senna may temporarily (and harmlessly) discolor urine.

GENERAL SOURCES:

Bradley, P.C., ed. *British Herbal Compendium: A Handbook of Scientific Information on Widely Used Plant Drugs*, vol. 1. Bournemouth (Dorset), England: British Herbal Medicine Association, 1992.

Castleman, M. *The Healing Herbs: The Ultimate Guide to the Curative Power of Nature's Medicines.* New York: Bantam Books, 1995.

Lawrence Review of Natural Products. St. Louis: Facts and Comparisons, January 1989.

Leung, A.Y., and S. Foster. *Encyclopedia of Common Natural Ingredients Used in Food, Drugs, and Cosmetics.* 2nd ed. New York: John Wiley & Sons, 1996.

Newall, C.A., et al. *Herbal Medicines: A Guide for Health-Care Professionals.* London: The Pharmaceutical Press, 1996.

Tyler, V.E. *Herbs of Choice: The Therapeutic Use of Phytomedicinals.* Binghamton, NY: Haworth Press/Pharmaceutical Products Press, 1994.

S

Senna

———. *The Honest Herbal*. Binghamton, NY: Haworth Press/Pharmaceutical Products Press, 1993.

Tyler, V.E., L.R. Brady, and J.E. Robbers, eds. *Pharmacognosy*. Philadelphia: Lea & Febiger, 1988.

Weiner, M.A., and J.A. Weiner. *Herbs That Heal: Prescription for Herbal Healing*. Mill Valley, CA: Quantum Books, 1994.

Weiss, R.F. *Herbal Medicine*, trans. A.R. Meuss, from the 6th German edition. Beaconsfield, England: Beaconsfield Publishers, Ltd., 1988.

TEXT CITATIONS:

1. V.E. Tyler, *The Honest Herbal* (Binghamton, NY: Haworth Press/Pharmaceutical Products Press, 1993).
2. A.Y. Leung, and S. Foster, *Encyclopedia of Common Natural Ingredients Used in Food, Drugs, and Cosmetics*. 2nd. ed. (New York, NY: John Wiley & Sons, 1996).
3. J. Prior and I. White, *The Lancet*, II (1978): 947.
4. C.A. Newall et al., *Herbal Medicines: A Guide for Health-Care Professionals* (London: The Pharmaceutical Press, 1996).
5. R.F. Weiss, *Herbal Medicine*, trans. A.R. Meuss, from the 6th German edition (Beaconsfield, England: Beaconsfield Publishers, Ltd., 1988).

PRIMARY NAME:

SHARK CARTILAGE (and SQUALAMINE)

SCIENTIFIC NAME:
N/A

COMMON NAME:
N/A

RATING:
4 = Research indicates that this substance will not fulfill the claims made for it. Its safety has not been determined.

What Is Shark Cartilage?

Shark cartilage and squalamine are derivatives of the predatory ocean sharks *Squalus acanthias* (spiny dogfish shark) and *Sphyrna lewini* (hammerhead shark) and other shark species. Shark cartilage supplements are prepared from the elastic but tough material called cartilage that makes up a shark's skeleton. The cartilage is cleaned, dried, pulverized, sterilized, and inserted into capsules. Pure shark cartilage is white.[1] Squalamine is a substance originally extracted from the stomach of the dogfish shark and now produced synthetically.

What It Is Used For:

Advocates assert that shark cartilage can cure cancer. It has also been promoted for the treatment of osteoarthritis, psoriasis, and eye disorders such as diabetic retinopathy.

Forms Available Include:

Capsule, powder, tablet.

Dosage Commonly Reported:

To use commercial shark cartilage formulations, follow the package instructions.

Will It Work for You? What the Studies Say:

There are no published studies of humans or animals that show that shark cartilage can cure cancer. Preliminary reports of a 1992 study conducted in Havana, Cuba, suggested that cancer sufferers treated with shark cartilage experienced some improvement in their condition. Details on the quality of the study and the exact type of improvement observed are hard to ascertain, given that the results are still not published. The National Cancer Institute did review the study, however, and on this basis apparently decided that the substance did not merit government-funded research.[2]

Backers cite several reasons for taking shark cartilage to fight cancer. They note that proteins in the cartilage inhibit the development of new blood vessels (angiogenesis) that can serve as "feeding networks" for tumors; without these networks, the argument goes, the tumors will not grow and existing ones will wither. The cartilage in sharks does not contain blood vessels, which may be why these animals so rarely get cancer. The theory concludes that ingesting the animal's cartilage may therefore inhibit the formation of tumor-forming new blood vessels in humans, and thus cure cancer.

The notion that inhibiting tumor angiogenesis may help control tumor growth has been around for a while.[3] A 1983 study reported that shark cartilage contains unidentified substances that inhibit tumor angiogenesis in rabbit corneas.[4] It is apparently on the basis of this line of thinking, the results of the rabbit study, anecdotal experience, unpublished studies of humans, and unreplicated findings in the Cuban trial that proponents claim shark cartilage supplements will cure cancer.[5]

But the bottom line is that no clinical trial has been published to show that shark cartilage can affect human cancer in any way. It is also important to note that the purported cancer-fighting protein is broken down by the body's digestive tract, which means that it never gets absorbed into the body intact, putting into question the value of taking the substance in oral form.[6] Moreover, sharks can and do get cancer in their cartilage, according to a Smithsonian Institution registry.[7]

Researchers examining other shark species have identified proteins that may have cancer-controlling properties,[8] and studies are under way to determine whether preliminary conclusions can be made about their ability to fight human cancers.

There is no good evidence that shark cartilage can benefit any other disorder. The FDA ordered a New York company to stop making unsubstantiated claims that its product could help reduce the symptoms of inflammatory disorders such as arthritis and psoriasis.[9] However, the same agency recently granted an application to investigate the potential of shark cartilage to treat prostate cancer and AIDS-associated Kaposi's sarcoma, a type of skin cancer.[10]

Interestingly, squalamine, a substance taken from the dogfish shark, has demonstrated notable antibacterial, antifungal, and antiprotozoal activity in the laboratory.[11] This steroidal antibiotic appears to offer broad-spectrum coverage that could prove useful in treating infectious diseases, although more research is needed.[12]

Will It Harm You? What the Studies Say:

There is little published research available to determine whether shark cartilage or squalamine is potentially harmful in any way, although a case of hepatitis caused by shark cartilage supplements was reported in 1996.[13] Some proponents warn that pregnant women, children, and people who have recently had a heart attack or undergone surgery should not take shark cartilage.[14]

GENERAL SOURCES:

Balch, J.F., and P.A. Balch. *Prescription for Nutritional Healing: A Practical A to Z Reference to Drug-Free Remedies Using Vitamins, Minerals, Herbs & Food Supplements.* 2nd ed. Garden City Park, NY: Avery Publishing Group, 1997.

Barrett, S., and V. Herbert. *The Vitamin Pushers: How the "Health Food" Industry Is Selling America a Bill of Goods.* Amherst, NY: Prometheus Books, 1994.

Hunt, T.J., and J.F. Connelly. *American Journal of Health-System Pharmacy.* 52 (1995): 1756.

Lawrence Review of Natural Products. St. Louis: Facts and Comparisons, September 1995.

Markman, M. *Cleveland Clinic Journal of Medicine.* 63(3) (1996): 179–80.

TEXT CITATIONS:

1. J.F. Balch and P.A. Balch, *Prescription for Nutritional Healing: A Practical A to Z Reference to Drug-Free Remedies Using Vitamins, Minerals, Herbs & Food Supplements,* 2nd ed. Garden City Park, NY: Avery Publishing Group, 1997).
2. J. Masslo Anderson, *MD Magazine,* 37 (1993): 43. *Lawrence Review of Natural Products* (St. Louis: Facts and Comparisons, September 1995).
3. J. Folkman, *Annals of Internal Medicine,* 82 (1975): 96–100.
4. A. Lee and R. Langer, *Science,* 221 (1983): 1185–87.
5. I.W. Lance, *Alternative & Complementary Therapies,* 1(4) (1995): 238–482.
6. S. Barrett and V. Herbert, *The Vitamin Pushers: How the "Health Food" Industry Is Selling America a Bill of Goods* (Amherst, NY: Prometheus Books, 1994).
7. Ibid.
8. *Lawrence Review of Natural Products,* op. cit.
9. Barrett and Herbert, op. cit.
10. T.J. Hunt and J.F. Connelly, *American Journal of Health-System Pharmacy,* 52 (1995): 1756.
11. K.S. Moore et al., *Proceedings of the National Academy of Sciences, USA,* 90(4) (1993): 1354.
12. *Lawrence Review of Natural Products,* op. cit.
13. B. Ashar and E. Vargo, *Annals of Internal Medicine,* 125(9) (1996): 780–81.
14. Balch and Balch, op. cit.

PRIMARY NAME:

SHEEP'S SORREL

SCIENTIFIC NAME:

Rumex acetosella. Family: Polygonacea

COMMON NAMES:

Common field sorrel, common sorrel, field sorrel, redtop sorrel, sourgrass

What Is Sheep's Sorrel?

Sheep's sorrel grows in temperate regions, including many parts of North America. The aboveground parts of this low-growing perennial are used medicinally. Its flowering spikes are topped with modest green flowers that turn red with the ripening of the seeds; the leaves are arrow-shaped.

What It Is Used For:

This herb, sometimes eaten as a salad green, has long been considered a mild laxative and "detoxifying" herb that promotes urination in the form of a diuretic ("water pill"). The closely related European native *Rumex acetosa,* which is commonly known as sorrel, once had a reputation as a "detoxifying" diuretic as well. Concerns about toxicity have put a stop to taking the herb for any of these purposes.

Sheep's sorrel also figured highly in a Native American cancer treatment called essiac, which also contained **Slippery Elm** and **Burdock Root**.

Forms Available Include:

Fresh juice, herb. The herb appears in various herbal blends sold in capsule form.

Dosage Commonly Reported:

To use commercial formulations containing sheep's sorrel, follow the package instructions.

Will It Work for You? What the Studies Say:

For a plant commonly included in modern herbal blends, remarkably little is known about this herb, and no test-tube, animal, or human trials appear in the recent medical literature. It is said to contain substances called oxalates, which may explain its bitter taste; and anthraquinones (emodin, chrysophanol), which are widely recognized as laxative and irritant. Anthraquinones stimulate a bowel movement either by increasing the volume of the bowel contents and initiating peristalsis, the wavelike contractions of the large intestine that we experience as the "urge," or by another, still poorly understood mechanism. Apparently no clinical trials have ever been done to test sheep's sorrel herb directly for these properties.

Will It Harm You? What the Studies Say:

There is scant information on the safety of this herb. Given its contained anthraquinones, however, long-term use should be avoided because of the potential loss of important salts (electrolytes), especially potassium. Laxative formulations in which the anthraquinones have not been standardized may be risky to take because their potency is unreliable. Overdoses may cause abdominal cramps, diarrhea, nausea, and excessive urination. See **Aloe Vera** or **Senna** for more information on the risks of anthraquinones. Given the way that sheep's sorrel encourages bowel movements, individuals with intestinal obstruction should not use it.

The oxalates in sheep's sorrel pose the risk of serious poisoning if large amounts are ingested. As with the related European plant *Rumex acetosa*, small children, old people, those in poor health, and those with kidney disorders (kidney stones in particular), gout, or rheumatism should avoid the herb because of these oxalates.[1] See **Yellow Dock** for more information on the potential toxicity of oxalates.

Sheep's sorrel can cause upper respiratory hypersensitivity reactions such as coughing and sneezing. Such reactions tend to occur in people who are similarly sensitive to grass, tree, or shrub pollens.[2]

GENERAL SOURCES:

Bremness, L. *Herbs.* 1st American ed. Eyewitness Handbooks. New York: Dorling Kindersley Publications, 1994.

Chevallier, A. *The Encyclopedia of Medicinal Plants: A Practical Reference Guide to More Than 550 Key Medicinal Plants & Their Uses.* 1st American ed. New York: Dorling Kindersley Publications, 1996.

Dobelis, I.N., ed. *The Magic and Medicine of Plants: A Practical Guide to the Science, History, Folklore, and Everyday Uses of Medicinal Plants.* Pleasantville, NY: Reader's Digest Association, 1986.

TEXT CITATIONS:

1. I.N. Dobelis, ed., *The Magic and Medicine of Plants: A Practical Guide to the Science, History, Folklore, and Everyday Uses of Medicinal Plants* (Pleasantville, NY: Reader's Digest Association, 1986).
2. B. Gniazdowska et al., *Pneumonologia I Alergologia Polska*, 61(7–8) (1993): 367–72.

PRIMARY NAME:

SHEPHERD'S PURSE

SCIENTIFIC NAME:

Capsella bursa-pastoris (L.) Medic., sometimes referred to as *Thlaspi bursa-pastoris.* Family: Cruciferae

COMMON NAMES:

Capsella, caseweed, lady's purse, mother's-heart, rattle pouches, rattle weed, shovelweed

RATING:

3 = Studies on the effectiveness and safety of this substance are conflicting, or there are not enough studies to draw a conclusion.

What Is Shepherd's Purse?

This foul-smelling annual can be found throughout temperate regions of the world. The pioneers introduced it to North America, and it promptly spread, weedlike, across the continent. The aboveground parts of this now common, hardy weed are used medicinally. Its name comes from the appearance of its delicate seedpods, which resemble small, heart-shaped purses (shepherd's *purse*) or small shovels (*shovel*weed). Thousands of yellow seeds reside in each pod. Small white flowers bloom year-round at the top of an erect stem that arises from a basal rosette of leaves.

What It Is Used For:

The seeds of this cabbage-family member were considered an effective laxative in ancient Greek and Roman times. But the plant's reputation as a healing herb began in earnest in medieval Europe, where it became known as an agent to stop bleeding. This reputation has persisted into modern times. In World War I, soldiers reportedly counted on it as an alternative to other antibleeding agents when those ran out. Herbalists today recommend the herb to stop or control various types of internal and external bleeding: profuse menstrual flow, bleeding due to endometriosis, postpartum bleeding, and blood in the urine, and blood in the vomit, and externally for wounds and hemorrhoids. Some also recommend it for triggering labor and treating cystitis (bladder infection), diarrhea, and gastrointestinal disorders. The seeds can serve as a substitute for mustard, and the young leaves can be eaten as a salad green.

Forms Available Include:

Concentrated drops, decoction, infusion, leaf, liquid extract, tincture. A sweetener is commonly added to the decoction or infusion to improve its taste.

Dosage Commonly Reported:

A tea is made using 1 teaspoon herb per cup of water and is drunk two to four times per day. The extract is taken in doses of 1 tablespoon two or three times per day, and the tincture is taken in doses of 20 to 30 drops two or three times per day.

Will It Work for You? What the Studies Say:

Study findings indicate that shepherd's purse has hemostatic properties, meaning that it can stop bleeding, but that these actions are inconsistent and relatively weak.[1] The critical ingredients may get destroyed in the stomach and intestines, or degrade with extended storage,[2] making it hard to know if a particular batch of the herb will work or not. Apparently no human studies have been done to test its hemostatic properties.

As for controlling excessive menstrual or other uterine bleeding specifically, implications of study results are likewise hazy. Components in the herb affect the uterus, according to researchers who have yet to pinpoint exactly which are responsible,[3] and test-tube studies of rat uteruses indicate that extracts can exert an action similar to oxytocin, the hormone critical to triggering labor.[4] Whether this qualifies the herb for managing uterine bleeding problems is far from clear.

Although investigators have initiated a number of animal studies on shepherd's purse, most of their findings reveal little or nothing about other traditional uses for this herb. They do, however, indicate that an alcoholic extract of the herb injected into rats enables them to recover from stress-induced ulcers much more quickly and to fight chemically induced inflammation more effectively than untreated rats.[5] Cats, dogs, rabbits, and rats injected with an herbal extract experienced a lowering of their blood pressure.[6] Extracts injected straight into the arteries of dogs slightly inhibited ventricular fibrillation of the heart.[7] Other studies indicate that shepherd's purse affects animal hearts in other ways as well.[8] A number of test-tube studies have shown that it stimulates smooth muscle tissues, including the small intestine of guinea pigs and the uterus of rats.[9] Mice injected or fed the herb experienced an increase in urination (diuresis).[10] Researchers have identified weak antibacterial activity in test-tube studies.[11] The conclusion that shepherd's purse taken orally in the form of an infusion will prevent ulcers, help control inflammatory diseases, fight urinary tract infections, or in other ways affect human health is quite a stretch. At most, these findings might be considered intriguing but in need of further investigation and human trials.

Will It Harm You? What the Studies Say:

Although people have been using shepherd's purse for centuries and there are no reports of serious adverse reactions to it in the recent medical literature, much remains to be learned about its relative safety. Moderation may be the best approach. Mouse studies suggest that its toxicity is low. Perhaps the greatest risk this herb poses is that people will rely on it to treat symptoms of potentially serious ailments that demand professional care. Excessive, persistent, or consistently unexpected menstrual or uterine bleeding should always be examined by a doctor, as should blood in the urine, stool, or vomit.

Always make cleaning and bandaging a wound a priority before applying this or any other herb, and keep in mind that you do not want to introduce other bacteria. Pregnant women should avoid shepherd's purse, given evidence that it may have oxytocinlike activity. Its still unproven reputation for inducing miscarriage and altering the menstrual cycle should also be taken into account.

GENERAL SOURCES:

Castleman, M. *The Healing Herbs: The Ultimate Guide to the Curative Power of Nature's Medicines.* New York: Bantam Books, 1995.

Chevallier, A. *The Encyclopedia of Medicinal Plants: A Practical Reference Guide to More Than 550 Key Medicinal Plants & Their Uses.* 1st American ed. New York: Dorling Kindersley Publications, 1996.

Dobelis, I.N., ed. *The Magic and Medicine of Plants: A Practical Guide to the Science, History, Folklore, and Everyday Uses of Medicinal Plants.* Pleasantville, NY: Reader's Digest Association, 1986.

Newall, C.A., et al. *Herbal Medicines: A Guide for Health-Care Professionals.* London: The Pharmaceutical Press, 1996.

Tierra, M. *The Way of Herbs.* New York: Pocket Books, 1990.

Weiner, M.A., and J.A. Weiner. *Herbs That Heal: Prescription for Herbal Healing.* Mill Valley, CA: Quantum Books, 1994.

Weiss, R.F. *Herbal Medicine,* translated by A.R. Meuss, from the 6th German edition. Beaconsfield, England: Beaconsfield Publishers, Ltd., 1988.

TEXT CITATIONS:

1. R.F. Weiss, *Herbal Medicine,* translated by A.R. Meuss, from the 6th German edition. (Beaconsfield, England: Beaconsfield Publishers, Ltd., 1988).
2. Ibid.
3. K. Kuroda and T. Kaku, *Life Sciences,* 8 (1969): 151–55.
4. K. Kuroda and K. Takagi, *Nature,* 220 (1968): 707–8.
5. K. Kuroda and K. Takagi, *Archives of International Pharmacodynamic Therapy,* 178 (1969): 392–99.
6. S. Jurrison, *Tartu Riiliku Ulikooli Toim,* 270 (1971): 71–79. Kuroda and Takagi, *Nature,* op. cit. C.A. Newall et al., *Herbal Medicines: A Guide for Health-Care Professionals* (London: The Pharmaceutical Press, 1996).
7. Jurrison, op. cit.
8. Newall, op. cit.
9. Kuroda and Takagi, *Nature,* op. cit.
10. Kuroda and Takagi, *Archives of International Pharmacodynamic Therapy,* op. cit.
11. S.A. Moskalenko, *Journal of Ethnopharmacology,* 15 (1986): 231–59.

PRIMARY NAME:

SHIITAKE MUSHROOM

SCIENTIFIC NAME:
Lentinula edodes (Berk.) Pegler, sometimes referred to as *Tricholomopsis edodes* Sing.

COMMON NAMES:
Black forest mushroom, hua gu, pasania fungus, snake butter

RATING:
3 = Studies on the effectiveness and safety of this substance are conflicting, or there are not enough studies to draw a conclusion.

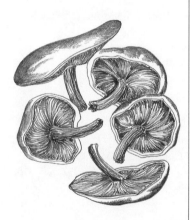

Shiitake Mushrooms
Lentinula edodes

What Is Shiitake Mushroom?

This flavorful brown fungus has a flat brown cap that develops cracks as it dries. Both the cap and the stem are used medicinally, as is lentinan, a complex polysaccharide first isolated from the mushroom in the 1970s.

What It Is Used For:

Shiitake mushroom has been cultivated in Asia for thousands of years as a food and medicine and has recently appeared in American supermarkets and health food outlets. Along with the **Reishi Mushroom**, it now qualifies as one of the country's most popular medicinal mushrooms. Manufacturers add lentinan to dietary supplement products said to enhance the ability of the immune system to fight infection and disease. It is reported to have antiviral, antimicrobial, and tumor-fighting properties. Some sources also recommend the mushroom and its extracts for lowering cholesterol.

Traditional Asian healers prescribe shiitake mushroom as a vitalizing tonic, blood-pressure reducer, cholesterol control agent, and treatment for anemia and diabetes. Traditional Japanese healers reportedly prescribe the mushroom to prevent and treat cancer, focusing particularly on lentinan for improving the outcome of cancer-related surgery of the breast and gastrointestinal tract.

Forms Available Include:

Capsule, decoction, mushroom (fresh and dried), tablet, tincture. Shiitake mushroom and its extracts are often added into herbal blends.

Dosage Commonly Reported:

One to three 606-milligram capsules are taken three times a day.

Will It Work for You? What the Studies Say:

This edible mushroom contains nutritious vitamins, carbohydrates, and protein. The extract, lentinan, may well fulfill a number of the claims made for it, according to mounting test-tube, animal, and human research. Laboratory research suggests that it enhances the effectiveness of the immune system in various ways, increasing the activity of such crucial infection-fighting cells as macrophages, T-helper cells, and other white blood cells, for example.[1] Whether these actions occur in human beings has apparently not been tested, however. Animal studies also suggest that lentinan increases resistance to bacterial infections[2] and protects against certain types of viral infections in mice, such as the virus that causes encephalitis (a potentially deadly inflammation of brain tissue).[3] Test-tube studies suggest that it may enhance the actions of a common AIDS drug, AZT (zidovudine).[4] Other research has shown that the mushroom may help treat the disease by increasing the activity of the immune system.

Although rat studies indicate that lentinan and other shiitake mushroom compounds can significantly lower cholesterol levels,[5] this has yet to be confirmed in human trials.

Lentinan also shows great promise as a cancer fighter, with early animal studies indicating that it inhibits cancerous tumors of various types when injected. Lentinan injections significantly increased the life span of rats with colon cancer in one study.[6] More important, positive results have been reported in human trials involving subjects with stomach cancer,[7] gastrointestinal tumors,[8] cervical cancer,[9] and breast cancer.[10]

Will It Harm You? What the Studies Say:

Shiitake mushrooms constitute a significant part of the diet in China and Japan. Studies indicate that both the mushrooms and lentinan are very safe to take, causing few if any toxic reactions in mice and other animals.[11] Few adverse reactions have been reported by people taking lentinan in clinical trials, with one study involving advanced cancer patients reporting only minor side effects in three of fifty subjects.[12] Allergic reactions are possible, however.[13]

GENERAL SOURCES:

Balch, J.F., and P.A. Balch. *Prescription for Nutritional Healing: A Practical A to Z Reference to Drug-Free Remedies Using Vitamins, Minerals, Herbs & Food Supplements.* 2nd ed. Garden City Park, NY: Avery Publishing Group, 1997.

Bremness, L. *Herbs.* 1st American ed. Eyewitness Handbooks. New York: Dorling Kindersley Publications, 1994.

Mayell, M. *Off-the-Shelf Natural Health: How to Use Herbs and Nutrients to Stay Well.* New York: Bantam Books, 1995.

Mindell, E. *Earl Mindell's Herb Bible.* New York: Simon & Schuster/Fireside, 1992.

Review of Natural Products. St. Louis: Facts and Comparisons, May 1997.

Weiner, M.A., and J.A. Weiner. *Herbs That Heal: Prescription for Herbal Healing.* Mill Valley, CA: Quantum Books, 1994.

TEXT CITATIONS:

1. J. Feher et al., *Immunopharmacology & Immunotoxicology*, 11(1) (1989): 55–62. *Review of Natural Products* (St. Louis: Facts and Comparisons, May 1997).
2. Y. Kaneko et al., *Advances in Experimental Medicines & Biology*, 319 (1992): 201–15.
3. K.S.S. Chang, *International Journal of Immunopharmacology*, 4 (1982): 267.
4. O. Yoshida et al., *Biochemical Pharmacology*, 37(15) (1988): 2887–91.
5. I. Chibata et al., *Experimentia*, 25 (1969): 1237.
6. J.F. Jeannin et al., *International Journal of Immunopharmacology*, 10 (1988): 855.
7. T. Tagachi, *Cancer Detection & Prevention*, 1(Suppl) (1987): 333–49.
8. S. Maekawa et al., *Gan To Kagaku Ryoho*, 17(1) (1990): 137–40.
9. Y. Shimizu et al., *Nippon Sanka Fujinka Gakkai Zasshi*, 42(1) (1990): 37–44.
10. A. Kosaka et al., *Gan To Kagaku Ryoho*, 14(2) (1987): 516–22.
11. G. Chihara et al., *Cancer Research*, 30 (1970): 2776. *Review of Natural Products*, op. cit.
12. J.F. Jeannin et al., *Journal of Immunopharmacology*, 10 (1988): 855.
13. K. Tarvainen et al., *Journal of the American Academy of Dermatology*, 24(1) (1991): 61–66.

SCIENTIFIC NAME:
Ulmus rubra Muhl., formerly referred to as *Ulmus fulva* Michx. Family: Ulmaceae

COMMON NAMES:
Indian elm, moose elm, red elm, soft elm

RATING:
1 = Years of use and extensive, high-quality studies indicate that this substance is very effective and safe when used in recommended amounts for the indication(s) noted in the "Will It Work for You?" section.

What Is Slippery Elm?

The inner bark of this stately tree, native to moist forests of eastern North America, is dried and used medicinally. The tree, recently ravaged by Dutch elm disease, has broad, toothed leaves. The slightly fragrant, gluelike, edible inner bark can be found beneath the deeply furrowed outer bark.

What It Is Used For:

Native Americans and early settlers found many uses for the slippery inner bark of this tree, from making canoes to soothing irritated and sore throats and controlling cough, diarrhea, digestive system upset, ulcers, and other external or internal mucous membrane inflammations. A soft and nourishing gruel concocted by grinding the bark and mixing it with water or milk was fed to ailing infants, children, and adults. A poultice was widely used for cold sores, boils, and other skin sores and wounds. For years, sore throat lozenges contained slippery elm. The *U.S. Pharmacopoeia* and the *National Formulary* listed this highly esteemed herb for several decades up to 1960.

Forms Available Include:

Capsule, decoction (of powdered bark), gruel (made with powdered bark), liquid extract, lozenge component, poultice (of powdered bark), powdered bark, tablet.

Dosage Commonly Reported:

Slippery elm is eaten as gruel by mixing 1 tablespoon powder with 1 tablespoon sugar and a cup of boiling water, or a simple decoction is made by using 1 to 3 teaspoons of powdered bark per cup of water and is drunk up to three times per day. A poultice is made by mixing the powdered bark with water to form a paste. Two 340-milligram capsules are taken as needed.

Will It Work for You? What the Studies Say:

Slippery elm's inner bark contains abundant amounts of mucilage, a substance that swells into a spongy "mass" when it then comes into contact with liquid. This material coats, protects, lubricates, and soothes inflamed and irritated mucous membranes in the mouth and throat, and in the digestive tract as well. Cough, esophagitis, gastritis, colitis, gastric and duodenal ulcers, and diarrhea may benefit from this kind of treatment.[1] The FDA has declared the inner bark a safe and effective demulcent (soothing agent) for treating sore throats, and it can be found in lozenges for this purpose. The mucilage is also nutritious and easy to digest and in many parts of the world is considered an excellent convalescent food.

These same soothing and protective properties serve well in poultice form for applying to minor wounds, burns, boils, and various other skin inflammations and sores. Be sure to clean any skin wound well before applying this or any other substance, however. The material will dry into an "herbal bandage."

Other than the mucilage and a small amount of astringent tannin, no other medically important ingredients have been identified in slippery elm.

S

Slippery Elm

Will It Harm You? What the Studies Say:

Severe and occasionally uncontrollable bleeding has developed in pregnant women attempting to induce an abortion by inserting strips of the bark into the cervix. Infection is also a risk. Trying this is unwise and very risky. In all other situations, slippery elm bark is considered quite safe to use in both internal and external forms; none of the ingredients poses a particular risk, and no reports of serious adverse reactions appear in the medical literature. Contact dermatitis after handling the plant is a possibility, however.[2]

GENERAL SOURCES:

American Pharmaceutical Association. *Handbook of Nonprescription Drugs.* 11th ed. Washington, D.C.: American Pharmaceutical Association, 1996.

Bradley, P.C., ed. *British Herbal Compendium: A Handbook of Scientific Information on Widely Used Plant Drugs.* Vol. 1. Bournemouth (Dorset), England: British Herbal Medicine Association, 1992.

Castleman, M. *The Healing Herbs: The Ultimate Guide to the Curative Power of Nature's Medicines.* New York: Bantam Books, 1995.

Duke, J.A. *CRC Handbook of Medicinal Herbs.* Boca Raton, FL: CRC Press, 1985.

Lawrence Review of Natural Products. St. Louis: Facts and Comparisons, March 1991.

Mayell, M. *Off-the-Shelf Natural Health: How to Use Herbs and Nutrients to Stay Well.* New York: Bantam Books, 1995.

Mindell, E. *Earl Mindell's Herb Bible.* New York: Simon & Schuster/Fireside, 1992.

Mowrey, D.B. *Proven Herbal Blends: A Rational Approach to Prevention and Remedy.* (Condensed from *The Scientific Validation of Herbal Medicine.*) New Canaan, CT: Keats Publishing, Inc: 1986.

Newall, C.A., et al. *Herbal Medicines: A Guide for Health-Care Professionals.* London: The Pharmaceutical Press, 1996.

Tierra, M. *The Way of Herbs.* New York: Pocket Books, 1990.

Tyler, V.E. *Herbs of Choice: The Therapeutic Use of Phytomedicinals.* Binghamton, NY: Haworth Press/Pharmaceutical Products Press, 1994.

Weiner, M.A., and J.A. Weiner. *Herbs That Heal: Prescription for Herbal Healing.* Mill Valley, CA: Quantum Books, 1994.

TEXT CITATIONS:

1. P.C. Bradley, ed., *British Herbal Compendium: A Handbook of Scientific Information on Widely Used Plant Drugs*, vol. 1 (Bournemouth [Dorset], England: British Herbal Medicine Association, 1992).
2. *Lawrence Review of Natural Products* (St. Louis: Facts and Comparisons, March 1991).

PRIMARY NAME:
SOAPWORT

SCIENTIFIC NAME:
Saponaria officinalis L. Family: Caryophyllaceae

What Is Soapwort?

The solitary stem of this tall perennial gives rise to lance-shaped leaves and fragrant clusters of white to light lavender flowers. But it is primarily the plant's round, reddish-brown roots that are used medicinally and commercially. Although native to Europe and regions of Asia, soapwort can now be found growing wild, often in pastures and roadsides, across the United States.

COMMON NAMES:
Bouncing bet, bruisewort, dog cloves, fuller's herb, lady's-washbowl, latherwort, old-maid's-ping, saponaria

RATING:
3 = Studies on the effectiveness and safety of this substance are conflicting, or there are not enough studies to draw a conclusion.

What It Is Used For:

Not wanting to be deprived of soapwort's key feature—an ability to lather up and clean like a true soap—European settlers introduced this herb into North America. Contemporary sources tout this feature in "natural" soaps and shampoos. The Pennsylvania Dutch concocted the foamy head on their beer with the saponins from this plant, a practice some brewers apparently still follow.[1]

Teas made from the root were once commonly used internally for constipation, upper respiratory tract congestion, rheumatic complaints, and fluid retention (as a diuretic, or "water pill"), as well as externally for acne, boils, psoriasis, and eczema.

Forms Available Include:

Infusion, root. Soapwort appears in some prepared European cough remedies.

Dosage Commonly Reported:

An infusion is made by pouring boiling water over 0.4 gram (roughly equivalent to ⅛ teaspoon) of the moderately finely chopped root, allowing it to steep, and straining the liquid. A daily dosage of 1.5 grams (about ⅓ teaspoon) of the herb is standard.

Will It Work for You? What the Studies Say:

Soapwort lives up to its name; all parts of the plant contain the saponins capable of foaming up into an impressive soapy lather.

German health authorities approve of the herb medicinally for treating upper respiratory tract congestion such as that which occurs with the common cold.[2] They cite the presence of components in the root that will irritate the stomach mucosa, indirectly causing mucus to clear from congested airways.

Interestingly, anti-inflammatory properties have also been demonstrated for the saponin extracts of soapwort,[3] and also painkilling properties.[4] Whether these actions explain certain traditional uses for the plant, such as treating skin eruptions or inflammatory diseases such as arthritis, remains to be determined.

Will It Harm You? What the Studies Say:

One popular source indicates that internal use of this plant may cause severe vomiting and diarrhea,[5] but the source of this information is not clear. In most cases, saponins are toxic only if injected.[6] German health authorities indicate that a majority of people tolerate soapwort preparations well, with notable stomach upset possible but rare.[7] They cite no known interactions with other medicines. People with ulcers or other gastrointestinal problems may do well to avoid using soapwort medicinally, however.[8]

GENERAL SOURCES:
Bisset, N.G., ed. *Herbal Drugs and Phytopharmaceuticals.* Stuttgart: medpharm GmbH Scientific Publishers, 1994.

Blumenthal, M., J. Gruenwald, T. Hall, and R.S. Rister, eds. *The Complete German Commission E Monographs: Therapeutic Guide to Herbal Medicine.* Boston: Integrative Medicine Communications, 1998.

Dobelis, I.N., ed. *The Magic and Medicine of Plants: A Practical Guide to the Science, History, Folklore, and Everyday Uses of Medicinal Plants.* Pleasantville, NY: Reader's Digest Association, 1986.

Lawrence Review of Natural Products. St. Louis: Facts and Comparisons, July 1993.

TEXT CITATIONS:

1. *Lawrence Review of Natural Products* (St. Louis: Facts and Comparisons, July 1993).
2. M. Blumenthal, J. Gruenwald, T. Hall, and R.S. Rister, eds., *The Complete German Commission E Monographs: Therapeutic Guide to Herbal Medicine* (Boston: Integrative Medicine Communications, 1998).
3. N.G. Bisset, ed., *Herbal Drugs and Phytopharmaceuticals* (Stuttgart: medpharm GmbH Scientific Publishers, 1994).
4. B. Cebo et al., *Herba Polonica*, 22 (1976): 154.
5. I.N. Dobelis, ed., *The Magic and Medicine of Plants: A Practical Guide to the Science, History, Folklore, and Everyday Uses of Medicinal Plants* (Pleasantville, NY: Reader's Digest Association, 1986).
6. *Lawrence Review of Natural Products*, op. cit.
7. Blumenthal et al., op. cit.
8. *Lawrence Review of Natural Products*, op. cit.

PRIMARY NAME:

SPEARMINT

SCIENTIFIC NAME:

Mentha spicata L. Family: Labiatae (Lamiaceae)

COMMON NAMES:

Garden mint, garden spearmint

RATING:

2 = According to a number of well-designed studies and common use, this substance appears to be relatively effective and safe when used in recommended amounts for the indication(s) noted in the "Will It Work for You?" section.

What Is Spearmint?

This fragrant perennial has the classic square stem of the mint family. Slender spikes of white-, pink-, or lilac-colored flower whorls bloom in midsummer. The wrinkly, lance-shaped leaves and flowering tops are dried and used medicinally. They also yield an important essential oil. Spearmint is cultivated and sometimes grows freely in temperate regions of North America. It looks a lot like peppermint except that it is shorter and has more wrinkled leaves; in fact, peppermint is a natural hybrid of spearmint and water mint (*Mentha aquatics*). See **Peppermint**.

What It Is Used For:

True to its botanical family, spearmint—a carminative—ranks high on the list of pleasant-tasting remedies for stomach and intestinal gas. Many meals of yore were concluded by chewing on a sprig of spearmint. Since ancient times, people have turned to what is fondly referred to as the "original" mint to control mild indigestion (especially after a large meal), relieve stomach and bowel spasms, and dispel nausea. Traditional Chinese and Indian (Ayurvedic) healers have treasured it through the ages as a digestive aid as well as a cough and cold treatment. Some even consider it good for controlling fever. Contemporary herbalists have embraced nearly all of these traditional uses, and a few have added the treatment of depression to the list. The essential oil is placed in vapor inhalations as a decongestant.

Spearmint is often added to other herbal blends and conventional medicines because its taste and aroma are so appealing. It can also be found in sauces, candies, liqueurs, baked goods, chewing gums, mint juleps, iced teas, and a myriad of other foods, not to mention as a flavoring or fragrance in a host of cosmetics, toothpastes, mouthwashes, deodorants and assorted toiletries. Most "mint"-flavored products contain an oil extracted from peppermint.

Forms Available Include:
Bath additive, fresh or dried herb, infusion, oil, tincture.

Dosage Commonly Reported:
An infusion made using 1 to 1.5 grams leaves (1 or 2 tablespoons) per cup of water is drunk several times a day. A cloth bag filled with a few handfuls of leaves is added to bathwater.

Will It Work for You? What the Studies Say:
Spearmint contains a volatile oil that is responsible for its distinctive aroma and taste, as well as its widely accepted ability to ease digestion and relieve stomach and intestinal gas.[1] However, it does not contain menthol, a critical ingredient in peppermint oil. For this reason, peppermint rightfully claims the reputation of being a more diverse and potent remedy for a host of discomforts, including indigestion and gas. As a decongestant, spearmint's essential oil is probably most effective in steam vapor formulations. Its role in other medicinal preparations is more as a pleasing flavoring and aroma than as anything else.[2]

Will It Harm You? What the Studies Say:
Generations have enjoyed spearmint to no apparent ill effect, and the medical literature contains no reports of serious harm as a result of ingesting spearmint as a food or medicine. On rare occasions, allergic reactions have occurred, probably to a component in the oil called carvone. People who are also allergic to members of the Asteraceae (Compositae) family of plants, such as ragweed and daisies, may be at increased risk of this type of reaction, although this theory requires confirmation.[3] Contact allergy to spearmint-flavored toothpastes, although rare, has also occurred.[4] The FDA places spearmint along with peppermint on its list of foods that are "Generally Recognized As Safe" (GRAS).

One important precaution, however: avoid giving infants and very young children any full-strength mint preparation because they may gag in response to the herb's pungency. This reaction is probably only to menthol, which is present in peppermint but not in spearmint, but play it safe. Stick to diluted spearmint preparations such as infusions for this age group.

GENERAL SOURCES:
Bisset, N.G., ed. *Herbal Drugs and Phytopharmaceuticals.* Stuttgart: medpharm GmbH Scientific Publishers, 1994.

S

Spearmint

Castleman, M. *The Healing Herbs: The Ultimate Guide to the Curative Power of Nature's Medicines.* New York: Bantam Books, 1995.

Dobelis, I.N., ed. *The Magic and Medicine of Plants: A Practical Guide to the Science, History, Folklore, and Everyday Uses of Medicinal Plants.* Pleasantville, NY: Reader's Digest Association, 1986.

Murray, M.T. *The Healing Power of Herbs: The Enlightened Person's Guide to the Wonders of Medicinal Plants.* Rev. 2nd ed. Rocklin, CA: Prima Publishing, 1995.

Tierra, M. *The Way of Herbs.* New York: Pocket Books, 1990.

Weiner, M.A., and J.A. Weiner. *Herbs That Heal: Prescription for Herbal Healing.* Mill Valley, CA: Quantum Books, 1994.

Weiss, R.F. *Herbal Medicine*, trans. A.R. Meuss, from the 6th German edition. Beaconsfield, England: Beaconsfield Publishers, Ltd., 1988.

TEXT CITATIONS:

1. N.G. Bisset, ed., *Herbal Drugs and Phytopharmaceuticals* (Stuttgart: medpharm GmbH Scientific Publishers, 1994).
2. Ibid.
3. E. Paulsen et al., *Contact Dermatitis*, 29(3) (1993): 138–43.
4. K.E. Andersen, *Contact Dermatitis*, 4(4) (1978): 195–98.

PRIMARY NAME:

SPIRULINA

SCIENTIFIC NAME:
Various *Spirulina* species, often including *Spirulina maxima* or *Spirulina platensis*. Family: Oscillatoriaceae

COMMON NAMES:
Dihe, tecuitiatl

RATING:
4 = Research indicates that this substance will not fulfill the claims made for it, but that it is also unlikely to cause any harm.

What Is Spirulina?

Spirulina is a blue-green alga. Harvesters collect it from freshwater lakes and ponds, allow it to dry, and then compress it into tablet, capsule, or powder form. It is also added to "health" or "green" drinks usually notable for their intensely green color.

What It Is Used For:

The Aztecs and natives of the Sahara desert reportedly harvested this blue-green alga centuries ago, the Azetcs from Lake Texcoco (now part of Mexico) in the form of "blue mud," and the Saharans from what moist ground there was in their desert environment,[1] and it may still qualify as a food staple in some parts of the world.[2] It tastes something like bean sprouts. North Americans have been buying it since the late 1970s, when it burst onto the scene as an "ideal" food and *the* way to lose weight. Marketers hail it is a "superior food" that offers a unique blend of nutrients, packed as it is with proteins, amino acids, minerals, and vitamins B, A, and E. Some highlight its purportedly high concentration of chlorophyll and carotenoids. Others claim that an amino acid in spirulina—phenylalanine—switches off hunger pangs rooted in the brain's appetite center,[3] aiding the dieter in his or her quest to lose weight. Some argue that eating spirulina suppresses hunger pangs by raising the body's blood sugar concentrations enough to influence the critical hunger center in the brain.[4] Spirulina has been promoted as an agent to boost immunity, increase energy and physical performance, lower cholesterol levels, help absorb minerals, and aid diabetes (by stabilizing blood sugar levels), anemia, stress, ulcers, and hair loss, among other disorders.[5]

Forms Available Include:

Capsules, powder, tablet. Spirulina often appears in herbal blends.

Dosage Commonly Reported:

To use commercial spirulina formulations, follow the package instructions.

Will It Work for You? What the Studies Say:

Spirulina is rich in protein and nutrients, including high levels of B-complex vitamins (although there is no B^{12} in a form the human body can use, as some sources claim[6]), iron, and all twenty-two amino acids.[7] Interestingly, soybeans offer about the same spread and concentration of nutrients[8] for a much lower price. In fact, spirulina is at least ten times as expensive as other protein sources such as milk, eggs, and beef.[9] It qualifies as a "body rejuvenator" because any nutrient gives the body energy.

There is absolutely no evidence that spirulina suppresses the appetite[10] and can in this or any other way help a person lose weight. An FDA advisory panel on over-the-counter drugs reported finding no reliable data to indicate that the substance is a safe and effective appetite suppressant.[11] The panel did not locate any evidence to support the theory that high levels of phenylalanine inhibit the appetite in any way.[12]

Will It Harm You? What the Studies Say:

Many cultures have used spirulina as a food, and it probably poses little risk to human health as long as it is taken in moderation and as long as mercury levels—which can be significant, according to some tests—are not too high.[13] Testing has established that it is not toxic to humans,[14] although some batches have been confiscated because of unacceptable levels of contaminants such as bird feathers, flies, and microbes (a risk when spirulina is grown on fermented animal waste).[15]

GENERAL SOURCES:

American Pharmaceutical Association. *Handbook of Nonprescription Drugs.* 11th ed. Washington, D.C.: American Pharmaceutical Association, 1996.

Balch, J.F., and P.A. Balch. *Prescription for Nutritional Healing: A Practical A to Z Reference to Drug-Free Remedies Using Vitamins, Minerals, Herbs & Food Supplements.* 2nd ed. Garden City Park, NY: Avery Publishing Group, 1997.

Barrett, S., and V. Herbert. *The Vitamin Pushers: How the "Health Food" Industry Is Selling America a Bill of Goods.* Amherst, NY: Prometheus Books, 1994.

Lawrence Review of Natural Products. St. Louis: Facts and Comparisons, February 1988.

Mayell, M. *Off-the-Shelf Natural Health: How to Use Herbs and Nutrients to Stay Well.* New York: Bantam Books, 1995.

Tyler, V.E. *The Honest Herbal.* Binghamton, NY: Haworth Press/Pharmaceutical Products Press, 1993.

Tyler, V.E., L.R. Brady, and J.E. Robbers, eds. *Pharmacognosy.* Philadelphia: Lea & Febiger, 1988.

TEXT CITATIONS:

1. *Lawrence Review of Natural Products* (St. Louis: Facts and Comparisons, February 1988).

2. S. Barrett and V. Herbert, *The Vitamin Pushers: How the "Health Food" Industry Is Selling America a Bill of Goods* (Amherst, NY: Prometheus Books, 1994).

3. American Pharmaceutical Association, *Handbook of Nonprescription Drugs*, 11th ed. (Washington, D.C.: American Pharmaceutical Association, 1996).

4. V.E. Tyler, *The Honest Herbal* (Binghamton, NY: Haworth Press/Pharmaceutical Products Press, 1993).

5. Ibid. C. Hills, ed., *The Secrets of Spirulina* (Boulder Creek, CA: University of the Trees, 1980).

6. V. Herbert and G. Drivas, *Journal of the American Medical Association*, 248 (1982): 3096.

7. *Lawrence Review of Natural Products* (St. Louis: Facts and Comparisons, February 1988).

8. Barrett and Herbert, op. cit.

9. V.E. Tyler, L.R. Brady, and J.E. Robbers, eds., *Pharmacognosy* (Philadelphia: Lea & Febiger, 1988).

10. American Pharmaceutical Association, op. cit.

11. *Pharmacy Practice*, 16 (1981): 82.

12. *FDA Consumer*, (September 1981): 3.

13. *Lawrence Review of Natural Products*, op. cit.

14. Ibid.

15. J.F. Wu and W.G. Pond, *Bulletin of Environmental Contamination and Toxicology*, 27 (1981): 151. Tyler et al., op. cit.

PRIMARY NAME:
SQUAW VINE

SCIENTIFIC NAME:
Mitchella repens L. Family: Rubiaceae

COMMON NAMES:
Deerberry, one-berry, partridgeberry, winter clover

RATING:
4 = Research indicates that this substance will not fulfill the claims made for it, but that it is also unlikely to cause any harm.

What Is Squaw Vine?

This creeping evergreen perennial is native to woodlands and dry areas of eastern and central North America. Its rounded shiny leaves have white markings. Long stems bear pairs of fragrant, fringed white flowers that merge to form a single bright red berry. The leaves and stems are used medicinally. Do not confuse this plant with *Gaultheria procumbens*, a plant with similar appearance and name (listed as wintergreen) but commonly known as partridgeberry.

What It Is Used For:

Women of various Native American tribes reportedly drank a tea made from the leaves of this plant during the final weeks of pregnancy to hasten and facilitate childbirth. The brew was believed to stimulate the uterus. Early settlers used it in much the same way. The *National Formulary* listed it for a little over two decades until 1947. Some modern herbalists recommend the herb for preparing a woman's womb for childbirth and for treating menstrual pain or irregularity at other times. Some consider it astringent and thus effective for diarrhea, as well as a diuretic ("water pill") and therefore useful for certain fluid retention and some urinary problems. The berry has reportedly been used for insomnia, rheumatic pains, poor milk flow in nursing women, and other disorders. Gardeners favor the plant as an ornamental ground cover.

Forms Available Include:

Infusion, liquid extract, tincture. Appears in herbal blends.

Dosage Commonly Reported:

The liquid extract is taken in doses of 4 milliliters. Take commercial preparations according to package directions.

Will It Work for You? What the Studies Say:

Scientists still know very little about the chemical makeup of squaw vine. Most contemporary sources cite the possible presence of glycosides, saponins, and tannins, although a 1931 report indicated that the herb contains neither of the first two ingredients.[1] The tannins, if present, may explain its use as an antidiarrheal; tannins are believed to control or stop diarrhea by reducing inflammation in the intestines. No research supports the herb's use for menstrual irregularities, hastening childbirth, or in any other way affecting the uterus. A 1916 study of numerous herbs reported that squaw vine failed to have any action on the guinea pig uterus in a laboratory dish.[2] Its reputation as a diuretic appears to be similarly unfounded.

Will It Harm You? What the Studies Say:

Scientists know very little about the safety profile of this herb. No reports of serious adverse reactions appear in the recent medical literature. To be safe, pregnant women may want to avoid squaw vine, given its reputation as a uterine stimulant, even though data to indicate that it affects the human uterus in any way cannot be found.

GENERAL SOURCES

Balch, J.F., and P.A. Balch. *Prescription for Nutritional Healing: A Practical A to Z Reference to Drug-Free Remedies Using Vitamins, Minerals, Herbs & Food Supplements.* 2nd ed. Garden City Park, NY: Avery Publishing Group, 1997.

Chevallier, A. *The Encyclopedia of Medicinal Plants: A Practical Reference Guide to More Than 550 Key Medicinal Plants & Their Uses.* 1st American ed. New York: Dorling Kindersley Publications, 1996.

Dobelis, I.N., ed. *The Magic and Medicine of Plants: A Practical Guide to the Science, History, Folklore, and Everyday Uses of Medicinal Plants.* Pleasantville, NY: Reader's Digest Association, 1986.

Duke, J.A. *CRC Handbook of Medicinal Herbs.* Boca Raton, FL: CRC Press, 1985.

Foster, S. *Forest Pharmacy: Medicinal Plants in American Forests.* Durham, NC: Forest History Society, 1995.

Griffith, H.W. *Complete Guide to Vitamins, Minerals, Nutrients Supplements.* Tucson: Fisher Books, 1988.

Tierra, M. *The Way of Herbs.* New York: Pocket Books, 1990.

Weiner, M.A., and J.A. *Herbs That Heal: Prescription for Herbal Healing.* Mill Valley, CA: Quantum Books, 1994.

TEXT CITATIONS:

1. W.P. Briggs, *Journal of the American Pharmaceutical Association*, 20 (1931): 224–26.
2. J.D. Pilcher, *Proceedings, Journal of Pharmacology*, 8 (1916): 110–11.

SQUILL

Urginea maritima L. Baker
(sometimes referred to as
Drimia maritima L. Stearn) and
Urginea indica (Roxb.) Kunth.
(sometimes referred to as *Scilla
indica* L. or *Drimia indica* L.
Stearn). Family: Liliaceae

COMMON NAMES:

Urginea maritima:
Mediterranean squill, red squill,
scilla, sea onion, sea squill,
white squill; *Urginea indica:*
Indian squill, white squill

RATING:

5 = According to a number of
well-designed studies and
common use, this substance
appears to be relatively
effective when used as
recommended in the "Will It
Work for You?" section.
However, studies also indicate
that there is a definite health
hazard to using this substance
in crude as well as in processed
forms when not properly
supervised by a qualified
medical practitioner. See the
"Will It Harm You?" section for
more information.

S

Squill

What Is Squill?

Squill consists of the dried fleshy inner layers of *Urginea maritima*, a scaly onion-like bulb native to the Mediterranean region. The color of the whitish or rose-hued flowers distinguishes the two basic varieties: white or red. Scientists have recently learned that *Urginea maritima* actually represents at least six chemically different species. Only a handful contain the necessary ingredients for fulfilling medicinal requirements as set forth by German health authorities, however. *Urginea indica* is considered a substitute for *Urginea maritima*. Today, the chemicals obtained from squill are harvested from the wild plants, although the herb is also cultivated.

What It Is Used For:

The white- and red-colored varieties of squill have traditionally been used differently. For centuries stretching back to the time of the ancient Greeks, European folk healers used white squill as a heart stimulant, diuretic ("water pill"), vomiting agent, and expectorant. Its heart-healing properties were particularly renowned. Some herbalists used it to treat cancer. Red squill, on the other hand, has a reputation as a rat (but not mouse) poison.

Forms Available Include:

Extract, tincture. Neither is commercially available in the United States.

Dosage Commonly Reported:

Not available for home use in the United States.

Will It Work for You? What the Studies Say:

Squill is a potent medicine. It contains powerful substances—cardiac glycosides—that can have a profound impact on heart function. In the proper dosage, these substances may stimulate the heart and help improve the condition of someone suffering from congestive heart failure, a condition in which the heart is so weak that it fails to pump blood efficiently to all parts of the body. The glycosides in squill are similar to those taken from the dried leaves of *Digitalis purpurea* L. and *Digitalis lanata*, drugs commonly known as digitoxin and digoxin. The squill glycosides work more quickly than these drugs, but they are not as strong, their effects do not last as long, and they are not as reliable.[1] Squill is not widely used because it offers no particular advantage over digitalis.[2] *Never take this herb without direct professional supervision.* Squill preparations are not used in the United States, although they are in parts of Europe, particularly when digitalis is not tolerated for some reason. German health authorities approve of squill for mild cardiac insufficiency.[3]

Scientists have identified other healing properties in white squill. It is an effective expectorant, irritating the stomach lining in such a way that it promotes the production of secretions in the respiratory tract and thus loosens sticky phlegm, making it easier to cough up. It will also induce vomiting at certain dosages.[4] These properties are somewhat irrelevant, however, given the herb's toxicity. Squill also increases urine production in the form of a diuretic, and German health authorities endorse its use for diminished kidney function.[5]

Will It Harm You? What the Studies Say:

Do not try to self-medicate with this herb. Side effects include nausea, vomiting, stomachache, diarrhea, and an irregular pulse. Overdose could be extremely serious and potentially fatal. German health authorities warn that the herb should not be used at the same time as digitalis or by individuals with a potassium deficiency (presumably because of its diuretic properties).[6] They also advise that squill not be taken at the same time as quinidine, calcium, laxatives, or saluretics, or in cases of long-term glucocorticoid treatment, because of the risk of interactions and side effects.

In the case of red squill, humans and animals start vomiting so quickly that they never have a chance to get enough of the herb into their systems to do any damage. Rats are not so lucky; they cannot vomit.

GENERAL SOURCES:

Blumenthal, M., J. Gruenwald, T. Hall, and R.S. Rister, eds. *The Complete German Commission E Monographs: Therapeutic Guide to Herbal Medicine.* Boston: Integrative Medicine Communications, 1998.

Bradley, P.C., ed. *British Herbal Compendium: A Handbook of Scientific Information on Widely Used Plant Drugs*, vol. 1. Bournemouth (Dorset), England: British Herbal Medicine Association, 1992.

Dobelis, I.N., ed. *The Magic and Medicine of Plants: A Practical Guide to the Science, History, Folklore, and Everyday Uses of Medicinal Plants.* Pleasantville, NY: Reader's Digest Association, 1986.

Leung, A.Y., and S. Foster. *Encyclopedia of Common Natural Ingredients Used in Food, Drugs, and Cosmetics.* 2nd ed. New York: John Wiley & Sons, 1996.

Tyler, V.E. *Herbs of Choice: The Therapeutic Use of Phytomedicinals.* Binghamton, NY: Haworth Press/Pharmaceutical Products Press, 1994.

Weiner, M.A., and J.A. Weiner. *Herbs That Heal: Prescription for Herbal Healing.* Mill Valley, CA: Quantum Books, 1994.

TEXT CITATIONS:

1. W.E. Court, *Pharmaceutical Journal*, 235 (1985): 194. P.C. Bradley, ed., *British Herbal Compendium: A Handbook of Scientific Information on Widely Used Plant Drugs*, vol. 1 (Bournemouth [Dorset], England: British Herbal Medicine Association, 1992).

2. V.E. Tyler, *Herbs of Choice: The Therapeutic Use of Phytomedicinals* (Binghamton, NY: Haworth Press/Pharmaceutical Products Press, 1994).

3. M. Blumenthal, J. Gruenwald, T. Hall, and R.S. Rister, eds., *The Complete German Commission E Monographs: Therapeutic Guide to Herbal Medicine* (Boston: Integrative Medicine Communications, 1998).

4. A.Y. Leung and S. Foster, *Encyclopedia of Common Natural Ingredients Used in Food, Drugs, and Cosmetics*, 2nd ed. (New York: John Wiley & Sons, 1996).

5. Blumenthal et al., op. cit.

6. Court, op. cit.

SCIENTIFIC NAME:
Stevia rebaudiana (Bertoni)
Bertoni, sometimes referred to
as *Eupatorium rebaudianum*
Bertoni. Family: Asteraceae
(Compositae)

COMMON NAMES:
Sweet herb, sweet leaf

RATING:
3 = Studies on the effectiveness
and safety of this herb for
medicinal purposes are
conflicting, or there are not
enough studies to draw a
conclusion. See the warnings in
the "Will It Harm You?" section.

What Is Stevia?

The dried leaves of this herbaceous perennial, a native of the highland regions of Paraguay and Brazil, are used as a sweetener and medicinal remedy. The lance-shaped, ridged leaves emerge off hairy stems. Clusters of white flower heads appear in season. Stevia is commercially produced in its native countries as well as Japan, China, Korea, and Thailand.

What It Is Used For:

Stevia's reputation rests on its sweetness; it is said to be three hundred times as sweet as granulated table sugar. Indian tribes in Paraguay have relied on it for centuries to sweeten what is now known as the national drink, maté (for more information, see **Maté**). Local inhabitants also used stevia to treat diabetes,[1] and other groups have apparently experimented with this as well.[2] Some say that the leaf can actively lower blood sugar levels and may fight infection.

Over the years there has been great interest in putting stevia to work as a sugar substitute, particularly for diabetics and people interested in noncaloric sweeteners. Japan is the biggest consumer, putting it in everything from soft drinks to pickles, although Paraguay and Brazil continue to use it heavily as well. The FDA banned stevia leaf in 1991 because of health concerns, but with the liberalization of standards associated with the Dietary Supplement Health and Education Act of 1994, the herb has returned to store shelves.

Forms Available Include:

Capsule, leaf (dried), liquid extract, powder, tea. Some herbal tea blends are sweetened with stevia.

Dosage Commonly Reported:

To use commercial stevia formulations, follow the package instructions.

Will It Work for You? What the Studies Say:

Few palates would deny that stevia is sweet. Researchers have calculated that a substance in the herb, a glycoside called stevioside, is about one hundred times sweeter than sucrose at a 10 percent concentration.[3] Its role in helping to manage diabetes is still unclear. In a small 1986 study, liquid extracts of the leaves significantly decreased plasma glucose levels after overnight fasting by sixteen healthy adult volunteers.[4] But according to studies in animals and most other data, stevia will not consistently lower blood sugar levels (i.e., it is not hypoglycemic).[5]

The herb fights microbes such as *Pseudomonas aeruginosa* and *Proteus vulgaris* weakly in test-tube studies.[6] Rat studies indicate that it dilates vessels,[7] causing lowered blood pressure and increased urine flow when given over long periods.[8] What this means for humans demands further examination.

Will It Harm You? What the Studies Say:

There has been some confusion regarding the safety of stevia, with the FDA at one point declaring it an "unsafe herb" but most recently asserting that it is safe to use in capsule form but not as a tea (unless labeled as a dietary supplement).[9] According to studies of rats, rabbits, guinea pigs, and fowl given very high concentrations of the sweetening element, the glycoside stevioside, stevia is not toxic.[10] Rats fed stevioside over a fifty-day period showed no signs of adverse reactions.[11]

Although various test-tube studies found no increased risk of mutations or gene abnormalities with stevioside,[12] one research study reported that a by-product of stevioside—the aglycone steviol—is mutagenic (can cause cell mutations) in the test tube.[13] Still to be determined is whether the human body metabolizes stevioside in such a way as to produce this dangerous substance; it may not. Given these unclear findings, moderation with stevia may be the wisest approach.

To play it safe, women who are pregnant or trying to become pregnant may want to avoid the herb, given limited data that it may help prevent conception[14]; Paraguayans reportedly used stevia as a contraceptive, and a report published in the late 1980s described reduced fertility in mice treated with the herb.[15] Other rodent studies, however, found no increased risk of birth defects or detrimental impact on mating performance or fertility.[16]

Unlike table sugar, stevia is not likely to cause cavities, at least according to studies of rats.[17]

GENERAL SOURCES:

Dobelis, I.N., ed. *The Magic and Medicine of Plants: A Practical Guide to the Science, History, Folklore, and Everyday Uses of Medicinal Plants.* Pleasantville, NY: Reader's Digest Association, 1986.

Leung, A.Y., and S. Foster. *Encyclopedia of Common Natural Ingredients Used in Food, Drugs, and Cosmetics.* 2nd ed. New York: John Wiley & Sons, 1996.

Mindell, E. *Earl Mindell's Herb Bible.* New York: Simon & Schuster/Fireside, 1992.

Weiss, R.F. *Herbal Medicine*, trans. A.R. Meuss, from the 6th German edition. Beaconsfield, England: Beaconsfield Publishers, Ltd., 1988.

TEXT CITATIONS:

1. A.Y. Leung and S. Foster, *Encyclopedia of Common Natural Ingredients Used in Food, Drugs, and Cosmetics,* 2nd ed. (New York: John Wiley & Sons, 1996). D.D. Soejarto et al., *Economic Botany*, 37(1) (1983): 71.
2. J.R. White, Jr., et al., *Diabetes Care,* 17(8) (1994): 940.
3. A.D. Kinghorn et al., eds., *Economic and Medicinal Plant Research,* vol. 1 (Orlando, FL: Academic Press, 1985).
4. R. Curi et al., *Brazilian Journal of Medical & Biological Research,* 19(6) (1986): 771–74.
5. Leung and Foster, op. cit.
6. Kinghorn, op. cit.
7. M.S. Melis, *Brazilian Journal of Medical & Biological Research,* 29(5) (1996): 669–75.
8. M.S. Melis, *Journal of Ethnopharmacology,* 47(3) (1995): 129–34.
9. R. McCaleb, *Controversial Products in the Natural Foods Market,* on-line article (Denver, Colorado: Herb Research Foundation).
10. Leung and Foster, op cit.
11. Kinghorn, op. cit.
12. M. Suttajit et al., *Environmental Health Perspectives,* 101, Suppl. 3 (1993): 53–56.
13. Kinghorn, op. cit. J.M. Pezzuto et al., *Proceedings of the National Academy of Sciences of the United States of America,* 82(8) (1985): 2478–82.

14. G. Mazzei Planas and J. Kuc, *Science*, 162(857) (1968): 1007.
15. Leung and Foster, op. cit. P. Nunes et al., *Brazilian Review of Pharmacy*, 69(1) (1988): 46.
16. Leung and Foster, op. cit.
17. S. Das et al., *Caries Research*, 26(5) (1992): 363–66.

SUMA

SCIENTIFIC NAME:
Pfaffia paniculata (Mart.) Kuntze. Also referred to as *Hebanthe paniculata* Mart. (may be more accurate). Family: Amaranthaceae

COMMON NAMES:
Brazilian ginseng, *para todo*

RATING:
4 = Research indicates that this substance will not fulfill the claims made for it, but that it is also unlikely to cause any harm.

S

Suma

What Is Suma?

The dried root of the tropical *Pfaffia paniculata*, a plant found in the rain forests of the Amazon, is used medicinally. Some sources indicate that the berries, leaves, and bark are used as well.

What It Is Used For:

Inhabitants of the Amazon reportedly consume suma as a food. In a nod to its enormous healing potential, many are said to refer to it as *para todo*, meaning "for all things." North American herbalists characterize the herb as an energizing adaptogen, a substance capable of boosting the immune system and hence the ability to contend with the stresses of everyday life. Some call it Brazilian ginseng. They say it helps fight fatigue and low energy, helps control diabetes, and may reduce menopausal symptoms and imbalances in the female hormone system. One herbalist describes using it to combat exhaustion from viral infections such as Epstein-Barr disease.[1] Suma has reportedly been used to help prevent cancer in humans, although details on this proved hard to get.

Forms Available Include:

Capsule, dried herb, tablet.

Dosage Commonly Reported:

Suma is commonly taken in dosages of 500 to 1,000 milligrams of dried herb two or three times per day. One to two 520-milligram root capsules are taken twice a day.

Will It Work for You? What the Studies Say:

Although suma is frequently likened to Asian ginseng, chemical studies indicate vast differences between the two.[2] Much remains to be learned about this plant and its potential healing qualities, if any. No sound scientific studies in humans appear in the medical literature. Not even claims that suma is an ancient Brazilian remedy could be confirmed.[3]

What little research has been done has focused on the plant's potential anticancer properties. In the late 1980s, Japanese researchers found that chemicals designated pfaffosides (saponins) in suma can inhibit the growth of tumor cell melanomas in the test tube[4] and display antitumor activity against ascites tumor in mice.[5] These interesting but preliminary findings say nothing conclusive about the ability of suma to inhibit certain cancers in humans, however. Researchers do not know how toxic suma can be to healthy cells.[6]

Will It Harm You? What the Studies Say:

Researchers know almost as little about the potential for adverse effects from suma as they do about its safety. It is not even clear that people have used it for generations, usually a rough guide to an herb's relative safety.[7]

GENERAL SOURCES:

Mayell, M. *Off-the-Shelf Natural Health: How to Use Herbs and Nutrients to Stay Well.* New York: Bantam Books, 1995.

Tierra, M. *The Way of Herbs.* New York: Pocket Books, 1990.

Tyler, V.E. *The Honest Herbal.* Binghamton, NY: Haworth Press/Pharmaceutical Products Press, 1993.

Weiner, M.A., and J.A. Weiner. *Herbs That Heal: Prescription for Herbal Healing.* Mill Valley, CA: Quantum Books, 1994.

TEXT CITATIONS:

1. M. Tierra, *The Way of Herbs* (New York: Pocket Books, 1990).
2. F. de Oliveria et al., *Revista Farm Bioquim Univ Sao Paulo,* 20(1–2) (1980): 261–77.
3. V.E. Tyler, *The Honest Herbal* (Binghamton, NY: Haworth Press/Pharmaceutical Products Press, 1993).
4. S. Nakai et al., *Phytochemistry,* 23(8) (1984): 1703–5. T. Takemoto et al., *Tetrahedron Letters,* 24(10) (1983): 1057–60.
5. T. Takemoto and T. Odajima, Japanese Patent 59/184,198 (October 19, 1984).
6. Tyler, op. cit.
7. Ibid.

PRIMARY NAME:

SUPEROXIDE DISMUTASE

SCIENTIFIC NAME:
N/A

COMMON NAMES:
Orgotein, SOD

RATING:

Oral forms only: 4 = Research indicates that this substance will not fulfill the claims made for it, but that it is also unlikely to cause any harm.

What Is Superoxide Dismutase?

Nearly all living cells contain superoxide dismutase, an enzyme. Thanks to genetic engineering, it can also be taken as a dietary supplement. Orgotein represents the injectable form of superoxide dismutase and is commonly used in clinical trials.

What It Is Used For:

Superoxide dismutase (SOD) helps prevent cell damage by rendering inert certain toxic substances in the body called superoxide radicals that are produced as a result of inflammation. Because of this known property, manufacturers and others recommend taking supplements to improve overall health, slow the aging process (SOD levels are said to decline with age), melt away wrinkles, control arthritis, protect against radiation, and "revitalize" cells. Veterinarians have long used SOD in injectable form (intramuscularly or subcutaneously) for treating inflammatory disorders in horses and other animals.

Forms Available Include:

Injectable formulations (orgotein; not commonly available), tablet (plain or enteric-coated).

Dosage Commonly Reported:

To use commercial superoxide dismutase preparations, follow the package instructions.

Will It Work for You? What the Studies Say:

SOD has proved to be a valuable medicine when given in injectable form, but oral forms such as tablets have never been shown to affect human health in any way. This can probably be explained by the fact that SOD is a sensitive enzyme that stomach acids rapidly degrade. Some sources suggest selecting enteric-coated tablets for this reason, so that the active substances can survive the journey to the intestines intact, but no data indicate that this strategy works.[1] It certainly received no support from a 1983 study showing that animals placed on a diet containing high concentrations of SOD do not subsequently develop higher levels of SOD in their blood or body tissue than animals given a placebo.[2] The same fate awaits SOD ingested through foods, such as red meat and many vegetables. Most SOD tablets bought at health food stores contain much less SOD than indicated on the bottle, according to a 1981 analysis of twelve brands.[3]

Injectable forms of SOD (orgotein), on the other hand, have proved effective in treating a number of ailments, most notably local inflammation related to arthritic disorders. German physicians have used orgotein for years to reduce inflammation caused by osteoarthritis (particularly knee joint osteoarthritis),[4] rheumatoid arthritis,[5] and sports injuries.[6] Studies also indicate promise in treating infant respiratory distress syndrome, reducing rejection rates following kidney transplantation, treating complications of cancer radiation therapy such as chronic bladder inflammation and injury,[7] relieving symptoms of Peyronie's disease (abnormal tissue formation in the penis),[8] and controlling the progression of hepatic cirrhosis.[9]

Will It Harm You? What the Studies Say:

For obvious reasons, the safety of SOD in injectable form has been much more carefully examined than the safety of oral forms. Extensive animal testing of injectable forms indicates that they are very safe to use in recommended amounts,[10] although rare cases of severe allergic reactions have been reported.[11] The drug does not appear to interact with any other medicines in animals or humans, including steroids and nonsteroidal anti-inflammatory drugs (NSAIDs).[12] One can only presume that SOD in oral forms is relatively safe to take in moderation because the drug is never absorbed into the body.

GENERAL SOURCES:

Balch, J.F., and P.A. Balch. *Prescription for Nutritional Healing: A Practical A to Z Reference to Drug-Free Remedies Using Vitamins, Minerals, Herbs & Food Supplements.* 2nd ed. Garden City Park, NY: Avery Publishing Group, 1997.

Der Marderosian, A., and L. Liberti. *Natural Product Medicine: A Scientific Guide to Foods, Drugs, Cosmetics.* Philadelphia: George F. Stickley, 1988.

Lawrence Review of Natural Products. St. Louis: Facts and Comparisons, July 1995.

Tyler, V.E., L.R. Brady, and J.E. Robbers, eds. *Pharmacognosy.* Philadelphia: Lea & Febiger, 1988.

TEXT CITATIONS:

1. *Lawrence Review of Natural Products.* St. Louis: Facts and Comparisons, July 1995.
2. S. Zidenberg-Cherr et al., *American Journal of Clinical Nutrition*, 37 (1983): 5.
3. *Annual Stockholder Report*, DDI (Diagnostic Data, Inc.) (October 1991). V.E. Tyler, L.R. Brady, and J.E. Robbers, eds., *Pharmacognosy* (Philadelphia: Lea & Febiger, 1988).
4. B. Mazieres et al., *Journal of Rheumatology—Supplement*, 27 (1991): 134–37. H. McIlwain et al., *American Journal of Medicine*, 87(3) (1989): 295–300.
5. M.J. Borigini and H.E. Paulus, *Baillieres Clinical Rheumatology*, 9(4) (1995): 689–710.
6. *Lawrence Review of Natural Products*, op. cit. W. Huber, *Clinics in Rheumatic Diseases*, 6(3) (1980): 1.
7. F. Sanchiz et al., *Anticancer Research*, 16(4A) (1996): 2025–28. U. Maier and O. Zechner, *Zeitschrift für Urologie und Nephrologie*, 81(5) (1988): 305–8.
8. G. Primus, *International Urology & Nephrology*, 25(2) (1993): 169–72.
9. K.O. Lewis and A. Paton, *The Lancet*, 2(8291) (1982): 188.
10. *Lawrence Review of Natural Products*, op. cit.
11. A. Joral et al., *Journal of Investigational Allergology & Clinical Immunology*, 3(2) (1993): 103–4.
12. A.M. Michelson et al., *Superoxide Dismutases* (London: Academic Press, 1977).

SCIENTIFIC NAME:
Tamarindus indica L. Family:
Leguminosae (Fabaceae)

COMMON NAME:
Tamarindo

RATING:
3 = Studies on the effectiveness
of this substance are
conflicting, or there are not
enough studies to draw a
conclusion. It appears to be
safe to use.

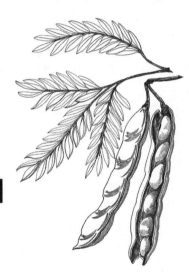

Tamarind
Tamarindus indica

What Is Tamarind?

The tamarind tree is native to tropical Asia and Africa and is cultivated world-wide, including in Florida. The partially dried, ripe fruit (the pod) of this large-trunked evergreen tree is used medicinally once its thin and easily breakable outer shell has been removed. The fruit, which typically contains up to twelve seeds, has a sweet-and-sour, stringy pulp. It is partially dried and preserved with sugar.

What It Is Used For:

Tamarind makes a refreshing drink that various cultures in the tropics have long considered good for cooling the body, especially during a fever, and as an effective laxative to treat constipation. Many cases of infectious diarrhea have reportedly been treated with it through the years. Traditional Chinese healers prescribe it for eradicating worms in children and reducing nausea during pregnancy.[1] Many Asian curries and pickling juices contain tamarind. It is also an ingredient in steak sauces, including Worcestershire sauce.

Forms Available Include:

Fruit (preserved in syrup or molded into cakes or balls), extracts.

Dosage Commonly Reported:

Tamarind is typically taken in doses of 4 to 8 grams a day.

Will It Work for You? What the Studies Say:

Tamarind contains large amounts of sugars (20 to 40 percent) and plant acids such as citric and tartaric acids. No evidence can be found to support the fruit's reputation as a fever-reducer, although the refreshing taste produced by these ingredients may offer a much appreciated cooling sensation.

Once listed in the *National Formulary*, tamarind has mild laxative properties that reportedly degrade upon cooking.[2] Its traditional use for infectious diarrhea, food poisoning, and other diarrhea-related illnesses is somewhat justified by laboratory findings indicating that it fights bacteria commonly responsible for these conditions, including *Escherichia coli*, *Bacillus subtilis*, and *Staphylococcus aureus*.[3] Tamarind reportedly also kills common disease-causing fungi such as *Candida albicans* and *Aspergillus niger*.

The Chinese tradition of fighting intestinal worms with tamarind gets some support from laboratory findings that liquid extracts (such as teas) are deadly to the parasitic organism *Schistosoma mansoni*.[4]

Will It Harm You? What the Studies Say:

The recent medical literature contains no reports of adverse reactions to tamarind. The FDA places it on its list of foods "Generally Recognized As Safe" (GRAS) for consumption.

GENERAL SOURCES:

Leung, A.Y., and S. Foster. *Encyclopedia of Common Natural Ingredients Used in Food, Drugs, and Cosmetics.* 2nd ed. New York: John Wiley & Sons, 1996.

Tyler, V.E., L.R. Brady, and J.E. Robbers, eds. *Pharmacognosy.* Philadelphia: Lea & Febiger, 1988.

Weiner, M.A., and J.A. Weiner. *Herbs That Heal: Prescription for Herbal Healing.* Mill Valley, CA: Quantum Books, 1994.

TEXT CITATIONS:

1. A.Y. Leung and S. Foster, *Encyclopedia of Common Natural Ingredients Used in Food, Drugs, and Cosmetics,* 2nd ed. (New York: John Wiley & Sons, 1996).
2. Ibid.
3. P.L. Lee et al., *Journal of Agricultural and Food Chemistry,* 23 (1975): 1195.
4. E.S. Imbabi et al., *Fitoterapia,* 63(6) (1992): 537.

PRIMARY NAME:

TANSY

SCIENTIFIC NAME:

Tanacetum vulgare L. Also known as *Chrysanthemum vulgare* L. Family: Asteraceae (Compositae)

COMMON NAMES:

Bitter buttons, parsley fern, scented fern, stinking willie

RATING:

5 = Studies indicate that there is a definite health hazard to using this substance, even in recommended amounts.

What Is Tansy?

This tall and hardy aromatic perennial is native to Europe and grows throughout North America. It belongs to the daisy family and features dense clusters of bright yellow flowers and feathery dark green leaves. The entire aboveground herb has been used medicinally.

What It Is Used For:

The word "tansy" stems from the Greek word for immortality; at one time people rubbed the strong-smelling herb onto corpses and burial shrouds to repel worms and other insects. The herb has been used extensively through the centuries to kill intestinal worms, including scabies, roundworm, and threadworm infections. A tansy ointment was applied to anal itching caused by worms.[1] The herb was also recommended to allay migraine headaches and nerve pains, stimulate menstruation, relieve gas, reverse appetite loss, and serve as a tonic, stimulant, and antispasmodic. Many—but not all—contemporary herbalists no longer recommend taking tansy in internal form, although some promote it as an external insect repellent. In the United States, tansy is approved as a food flavoring once certain toxic compounds have been removed.

Forms Available Include:

Infusion (for external use), oil, tea (in herbal blends). Prepared forms may not be readily available in the United States; sale of the dried herb (by botanical dealers or by mail order) is illegal.[2]

Dosage Commonly Reported:

Tansy should not be used medicinally, either internally or externally.

Will It Work for You? What the Studies Say:

While research in test tubes and with laboratory animals indicates that tansy may fight intestinal worms[3] and reduce intestinal tract spasms,[4] it is far too

T

Tansy

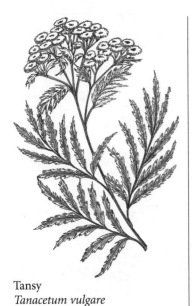

Tansy
Tanacetum vulgare

toxic to be considered a healing herb. Its essential oil (0.2 to 0.6 percent) contains varying amounts, depending on the species or subtype, of a very toxic substance called thujone. Some batches may contain no thujone at all,[5] but given the risk, neither internal nor external formulations of the herb should be used. German health authorities, citing concerns over safety as well as a lack of substantiating evidence, declined to approve of tansy (the flower or herb) for worms, migraine headaches, nerve pain, rheumatism, or appetite loss, and various other ailments.[6]

The risk of poisoning makes other research findings on tansy interesting but somewhat irrelevant, at least for the moment. For example, studies on humans have shown that tansy infusions and alcoholic extracts can stimulate bile activity—and thus reduce pain, improve digestion, and increase appetite—in people suffering from liver and gallbladder ailments.[7] Rabbit studies indicate that tansy extracts injected into the stomach may reduce blood lipid (fat) levels and influence blood-sugar concentrations.[8] Tansy has also demonstrated antibacterial[9] and antifungal properties in the test tube, shown antitumor activity in the test tube and in laboratory animals,[10] and displayed an ability to induce resistance to the encephalitis virus in infected mice.[11]

Will It Harm You? What the Studies Say:

Whether ingested or placed on the skin, tansy can cause severe toxic reactions, even with apparently common doses.[12] In one case, ten drops of the oil proved fatal, and in another, a person died after drinking tansy tea.[13] Pregnant or nursing women should avoid this herb assiduously; in addition to the risks applicable to everyone, animal studies indicate that it may affect the menstrual cycle and uterus.[14] Severe dermatitis may develop after handling the plant or its extracts.[15] Experts attribute tansy's toxicity to thujone; see **Wormwood** for more information about the potentially harmful and even lethal effects of this substance. Allergic reactions are also a risk, particularly for people sensitive to other members of the daisy family.

GENERAL SOURCES:

Blumenthal, M., J. Gruenwald, T. Hall, and R.S. Rister, eds. *The Complete German Commission E Monographs: Therapeutic Guide to Herbal Medicine.* Boston: Integrative Medicine Communications, 1998.

Dobelis, I.N., ed. *The Magic and Medicine of Plants: A Practical Guide to the Science, History, Folklore, and Everyday Uses of Medicinal Plants.* Pleasantville, NY: Reader's Digest Association, 1986.

Lawrence Review of Natural Products. St. Louis: Facts and Comparisons, September 1992.

Newall, C.A., et al. *Herbal Medicines: A Guide for Health-Care Professionals.* London: The Pharmaceutical Press, 1996.

Tyler, V.E. *The Honest Herbal.* Binghamton, NY: Haworth Press/Pharmaceutical Products Press, 1993.

Weiner, M.A., and J.A. Weiner. *Herbs That Heal: Prescription for Herbal Healing.* Mill Valley, CA: Quantum Books, 1994.

Weiss, R.F. *Herbal Medicine*, trans. A.R. Meuss, from the 6th German edition. Beaconsfield, England: Beaconsfield Publishers, Ltd., 1988.

TEXT CITATIONS:

1. R.F. Weiss, *Herbal Medicine*, trans. A.R. Meuss, from the 6th German edition. (Beaconsfield, England: Beaconsfield Publishers, Ltd., 1988).
2. C.A. Newall et al., *Herbal Medicines: A Guide for Health-Care Professionals* (London: The Pharmaceutical Press, 1996).
3. D.L.J. Opdyke, *Food & Cosmetics Toxicology*, 14 (1976): 869-71.
4. *Lawrence Review of Natural Products* (St. Louis: Facts and Comparisons, September 1992).
5. Ibid.
6. M. Blumenthal, J. Gruenwald, T. Hall, and R.S. Rister, eds., *The Complete German Commission E Monographs: Therapeutic Guide to Herbal Medicine* (Boston: Integrative Medicine Communications, 1998).
7. Newall, op. cit.
8. Opdyke, op. cit.
9. M. Holopainen and V. Kaupinnen, *Planta Medica*, 55 (1989): 102.
10. Newall, op. cit.
11. G.I. Fokina et al., *Voprosy Virusologii*, 36(1) (1991): 18.
12. Blumenthal et al., op. cit.
13. *Lawrence Review of Natural Products*, op. cit.
14. Newall, op. cit.
15. *Lawrence Review of Natural Products*, op. cit.

PRIMARY NAME:

TARRAGON

SCIENTIFIC NAME:

Artemisia dracunculus L.
Family: Asteraceae
(Compositae)

COMMON NAMES:

Dragon herb, estragon, French tarragon, herbe au dragon

RATING:

4 = Research indicates that this substance will not fulfill the claims made for it, but that it is also unlikely to cause any harm when used as recommended.

What Is Tarragon?

This thickly branched, aromatic perennial is cultivated worldwide for the distinctive, sweet-peppery flavor of its leaves. The narrow, lance-shaped leaves are also used medicinally once dried, as is the whole aboveground herb and the essential oil extracted from it. Some sources indicate that the root is used as well. Tarragon bears long clusters of greenish flower heads. Settlers planted tarragon shortly after they arrived in North America in the 1600s.

What It Is Used For:

Tarragon is a common ingredient in American kitchens, but probably no culture has incorporated it into the national diet as the French have; think, for example, of béarnaise sauce. Many commercially prepared foods and drinks have the herb added as a flavoring, and cosmetics contain the oil as a fragrance. Do not confuse the relatively flat-tasting Russian tarragon (*Artemisia redowskii*) with the refined, almost licorice-like flavor of French tarragon (*Artemisia dracunculus*).

As the herb dries, the critical aromatic oil dissipates. Perhaps for this very reason, tarragon's reputation as a healing herb apparently started to flag in the 1600s.[1] But it has recently undergone a revival by contemporary herbalists, who recommend it for ailments ranging from rheumatism and arthritis to poor appetite, aching teeth, sleeping trouble, delayed menstruation, and fluid retention (as a diuretic, or "water pill").

Forms Available Include:

Leaves (dried, fresh), tea, tincture.

T

Tarragon

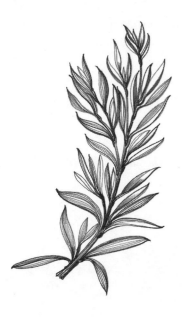

Tarragon
Artemisia dracunculus

Dosage Commonly Reported:

A tea made using 1 to 2 teaspoons of fresh or frozen tarragon leaves per cup of water is drunk up to three times a day. The tincture is taken in dosages of ½ to 1 teaspoon up to three times per day. The fresh leaves are chewed to relieve tooth pain.

Will It Work for You? What the Studies Say:

The purported healing element in tarragon is its volatile oil, contained in concentrations of about 0.25 to 1 percent in the aboveground herb and featuring such constituents as thujone and estragole (in concentrations up to 70 percent). The oil in the leaves dissipates with drying, so use only fresh ones. Research has shown that this oil fights many types of bacteria. But how this and other purported properties of the volatile oil aid healing is still unclear and poorly documented.

Russian tarragon contains the anesthetic chemical eugenol, which may explain why the ancients recommended rubbing that plant against aching teeth for temporary pain relief.

Will It Harm You? What the Studies Say:

Tarragon is safe to use in moderation as a medicinal herb. It does contain a substance, however, that has reportedly produced tumors in mice.[2] So far there have been no documented cases linking the herb to cancer in humans, but as a precaution, do not take more than typically recommended medicinal concentrations and avoid long-term, continued use. The oil does not irritate or sensitize human skin.[3] Although miscarriage has never been documented, pregnant women may want to avoid medicinal doses of the herb.

GENERAL SOURCES:

Bremness, L. *Herbs*. 1st American ed. Eyewitness Handbooks. New York: Dorling Kindersley Publications, 1994.

Castleman, M. *The Healing Herbs: The Ultimate Guide to the Curative Power of Nature's Medicines*. New York: Bantam Books, 1995.

Chevallier, A. *The Encyclopedia of Medicinal Plants: A Practical Reference Guide to More Than 550 Key Medicinal Plants & Their Uses*. 1st American ed. New York: Dorling Kindersley Publications, 1996.

Dobelis, I.N., ed. *The Magic and Medicine of Plants: A Practical Guide to the Science, History, Folklore, and Everyday Uses of Medicinal Plants*. Pleasantville, NY: Reader's Digest Association, 1986.

Leung, A.Y., and S. Foster. *Encyclopedia of Common Natural Ingredients Used in Food, Drugs, and Cosmetics*. 2nd ed. New York: John Wiley & Sons, 1996.

Tyler, V.E., L.R. Brady, and J.E. Robbers, eds. *Pharmacognosy*. Philadelphia: Lea & Febiger, 1988.

Weiss, R.F. *Herbal Medicine*, trans. A.R. Meuss, from the 6th German edition. Beaconsfield, England: Beaconsfield Publishers, Ltd., 1988.

TEXT CITATIONS:

1. M. Castleman, *The Healing Herbs: The Ultimate Guide to the Curative Power of Nature's Medicines* (New York: Bantam Books, 1995).

2. A.Y. Leung and S. Foster, *Encyclopedia of Common Natural Ingredients Used in Food, Drugs, and Cosmetics*, 2nd ed. (New York: John Wiley & Sons, 1996).

3. Ibid.

TEA, BLACK

SCIENTIFIC NAME:
Camellia sinensis (L.) Kuntze.
Family: Theaceae

COMMON NAME:
Tea

RATING:
3 = Studies on the effectiveness and safety of this substance are conflicting, or there are not enough studies to draw a conclusion.

What Is Black Tea?

Black tea is a beverage made from the dried bright green, toothed, oval leaves of the *Camellia sinensis* shrub. Although green and oolong teas are also made from these leaves and they share many of the same ingredients as black tea, the traditional methods used for preparing them account for complex chemical differences that give rise to the common as well as the unique medicinal properties of each. The fermentation to which black tea—but not green tea—is subjected accounts for its characteristic strong flavor and aroma. The bulk of the tea market is black tea, which is made of leaves that are dried and fermented. About 20 percent of the market is green tea, which is milder in flavor and consists of leaves that are steamed and dried. A small percentage of the market consists of a greenish-brown, semifermented tea called oolong. *Camellia sinensis*, a large, semitropical shrub or tree, is native to eastern Asia. It is not a garden herb in North America but has been cultivated for generations in Asia.

For information on green tea, see **Tea, Green**.

What It Is Used For:

After water, tea ranks as the second most popular beverage in the world. Europeans and Americans have long favored black tea over green tea, although green tea remains extremely popular in Asia and other parts of the world. Most people drink black tea as a stimulant as one would coffee. It is also has diuretic ("water pill") properties.

Traditional Chinese healers have used black tea for millennia. Contemporary Western herbalists have adopted a number of the traditional Chinese uses, suggesting that black tea may help treat diarrhea, coughs and colds, asthma and other respiratory conditions demanding a bronchial decongestant, as well as alleviate headache and even cut the risk of stroke. In folk medicine, black tea bags are sometimes placed on baggy eyes or made into a compress for tired eyes or headache. The tea bag has also been used as a wash for sunburn and to stop a tooth from bleeding. Tea extracts also serve as food and beverage flavorings.

Forms Available Include:

Infusions (made from loose tea or tea bags). Compresses or washes can be made with infusions or decoctions and used externally.

Dosage Commonly Reported:

An infusion is made using commercial tea bags or 1 to 2 teaspoons of dried herb per cup of water and is drunk up to three times per day. When taken as a stimulant, the infusion should be allowed to steep for two minutes or so. When taken for diarrhea, it should be allowed to steep for ten minutes.

Will It Work for You? What the Studies Say:

Black tea contains caffeine, a central nervous system stimulant. The average cup of black tea contains between 10 and 50 milligrams of caffeine, depending on the type of tea and the preparation method, while a cup of brewed coffee has about 100 milligrams. (Black tea contains far more caffeine than green tea.) The amount of caffeine that passes into the body depends in part on the way the beverage is prepared. To make as strong a stimulant tea as possible, a German textbook recommends allowing it to steep for two to ten minutes, and then straining it.[1] A method for significantly lowering the caffeine content is to steep the tea bag in a small amount of hot water for ten seconds, pour out the water, and then add more water to steep regularly.

In addition to caffeine, black tea contains the stimulant alkaloids theobromine and theophylline. In adequate concentrations, these substances will ease breathing by opening up the bronchial tubes, and many asthmatics take theophylline alone (as a prescription medicine) to treat their condition. To consume enough tea for this purpose would be impractical, however, given caffeine's stimulant effects. Moreover, asthma attacks can be life-threatening, so counting on tea in such situations is risky at best.

Caffeinated drinks such as black tea are widely recognized as mild diuretics, but are rarely used for any serious disorder, given the likelihood of intolerable side effects from the caffeine. Some sources recommend tea as a slimming aid, claiming that it raises body heat and promotes the burning of fat when taken regularly. There is little good evidence for this, and responsible herbalists do not recommend caffeine-containing products for weight reduction because any lost weight simply represents transitory fluid loss.

Black tea also contains tannins, astringent substances that constrict (tighten) skin tissue when applied topically. This property may help explain the logic behind putting tea bags on baggy or tired eyes and washes on sunburns and bleeding tooth sockets. The fluoride and tannins in black tea may also help prevent tooth decay, according to some sources. Unfortunately, tea can also stain teeth.

There are reports that tea (usually in the form of a strong decoction) can effectively treat infectious diarrhea due to bacteria or amoebas, acute gastroenteritis, and acute infectious hepatitis.[2] Tannins are again the key component, believed to control or stop diarrhea by reducing inflammation in the intestines. Theophylline also plays a role in controlling diarrhea.[3] When treating diarrhea unrelated to an underlying disease or grave infection, a German textbook recommends allowing the tea to steep for ten minutes and drinking a cup two to three times a day.[4]

Recent research on rats indicates that black tea has antidiabetic activity, with an extract significantly reducing blood sugar levels in both preventive and curative ways in rats with experimentally induced diabetes.[5] What this means for humans with diabetes requires further examination.

Will It Harm You? What the Studies Say:

Billions of people around the world drink black tea every day to no apparent ill effect. As with any caffeine-containing product, it can cause unwanted stimulant effects such as anxiety, nervousness, tremors, irritability, trouble sleeping, fast or irregular heartbeat, and stomach upset if taken in excessive doses or by people who are sensitive to caffeine. Caffeine is considered an addictive drug. Children, heart disease sufferers, and pregnant women should take caffeine-containing products in moderation or avoid them altogether.

Keep in mind that no tannin-rich drug should be used over long periods of time, given the potential, still not fully understood, of an increased risk of malignant (cancerous) changes. In addition, tannins are nutritionally counterproductive because they interfere with protein use, particularly when consumed in excess.[6] Some data show an increased risk for developing esophageal cancer in groups of people who consume excessive amounts of certain kinds of tannin-containing teas, including black tea.[7] Drinking the tea with milk may significantly reduce this risk, however, as it appears to neutralize the tannins.

A 1991 study in ten women indicated that the consumption of black tea inhibits the body's use of the vitamin thiamin, but does not affect the availability of niacin.[8]

GENERAL SOURCES:

Bisset, N.G., ed. *Herbal Drugs and Phytopharmaceuticals*. Stuttgart: medpharm GmbH Scientific Publishers, 1994.

Castleman, M. *The Healing Herbs: The Ultimate Guide to the Curative Power of Nature's Medicines*. New York: Bantam Books, 1995.

Leung, A.Y., and S. Foster. *Encyclopedia of Common Natural Ingredients Used in Food, Drugs, and Cosmetics*. 2nd ed. New York: John Wiley & Sons, 1996.

Tyler, V.E. *Herbs of Choice: The Therapeutic Use of Phytomedicinals*. Binghamton, NY: Haworth Press/Pharmaceutical Products Press, 1994.

TEXT CITATIONS:

1. N.G. Bisset, ed., *Herbal Drugs and Phytopharmaceuticals* (Stuttgart: medpharm GmbH Scientific Publishers, 1994).
2. A.Y. Leung and S. Foster, *Encyclopedia of Common Natural Ingredients Used in Food, Drugs, and Cosmetics*, 2nd ed. (New York: John Wiley & Sons, 1996).
3. Bisset, op. cit.
4. Ibid.
5. A. Gomes et al., *Journal of Ethnopharmacology*, 45(3) (1995): 223–26.
6. J.F. Morton, *Basic Life Sciences*, 59 (1992): 739–65.
7. Bisset, op. cit.
8. R.S. Wang and C. Kies, *Plant Foods for Human Nutrition*, 41(4) (1991): 337–53.

PRIMARY NAME:
TEA, GREEN

SCIENTIFIC NAME:
Camellia sinensis (L.) Kuntze.
Family: Theaceae

COMMON NAME:
Tea

RATING:

3 = Studies on the effectiveness
and safety of this substance are
conflicting, or there are not
enough studies to draw a
conclusion.

What Is Green Tea?

Green tea is a beverage made by drying and steaming the bright green, toothed, oval leaves of the *Camellia sinensis* shrub. Black and oolong tea are also made from the leaves of this large, semitropical shrub or tree native to eastern Asia; different methods of curing are used for each type. About 20 percent of the world's tea market consists of green tea. *Camellia sinensis* is not a garden herb in North America, but has been cultivated for generations in Asia.

For information on black tea, see **Tea, Black**.

What It Is Used For:

After water, tea ranks as the second most popular beverage in the world. Europeans and Americans have long favored black tea over green tea, but green tea remains extremely popular in Asia and other parts of the world. Most people drink it as a mild stimulant, as one would black tea or coffee. It also has diuretic ("water pill") properties, as those drinks do. Traditional Chinese healers have prescribed green tea for millennia as a bronchial decongestant for colds, cough, asthma, and other respiratory disorders, as well as for headache and diarrhea, including infectious diarrhea. They also regard it as a cure for cancer.

Contemporary Western herbalists tout green tea's antioxidant and attendant anticancer properties, and its ability to promote weight loss, prevent tooth decay, and lower cholesterol levels and high blood pressure. Extracts are said to help promote healthy heart function and relieve peptic ulcer pain.

Forms Available Include:

Capsule, dried leaves, extract (sometimes standardized for epigallocatechin gallate content and/or total polyphenol content), infusion (made from loose tea or tea bag).

Dosage Commonly Reported:

A common daily dosage of green tea polyphenols is 50 to 100 milligrams, or 100 to 200 milligrams of capsules standardized for 50 percent polyphenols. The polyphenol content of capsules may range from 15 to 50 percent. Three 333-milligram capsules of green tea extract (containing 50 milligrams of polyphenols each) are taken two times a day. A cup of brewed tea contains approximately 20 to 30 milligrams of polyphenols.

Will It Work for You? What the Studies Say:

Accumulating evidence, although still preliminary and requiring verification by large-scale follow-up studies, indicates that green tea may indeed help to prevent certain types of cancer.[1] More than a few scientists have noted that in Japan, where green tea is a very popular drink, cancer rates are lower than in many other parts of the world.[2] A large-scale study found that Chinese women who regularly drank green tea had a 60 percent lower risk of developing esophageal cancer than those who did not.[3] The investigators came to this conclusion after taking into consideration alcohol intake, smoking, and dietary habits. In another study, high intake of green tea was linked to a decreased risk of developing polyp-like growths in the lower colon, some of which can be precancerous.[4]

Not all population studies such as these have indicated a positive anticancer action for green tea, however, and definitive clinical trials would be useful but are hard to design, partly because cancer can take a long time to develop. Studies of animals that have had cancerous changes chemically induced have proved promising, however. The human population studies overall indicate positive results for cancers affecting the skin, lungs, stomach, liver, and pancreas in particular.[5]

There are several theories about why green tea may have cancer-protective actions. Many researchers attribute these reported properties to the presence of substances called polyphenols and flavonoids (compounds that purportedly function like antioxidants); the polyphenols have been shown to inhibit cancer by blocking the formation of nitrosamines, well-recognized cancer-causing substances.[6] They may help in other ways as well. Studies also indicate that green tea is an antioxidant, meaning it helps to control the formation of dangerous substances in the body called free radicals, which damage cells through oxidation. Some free radicals are believed to contribute to cancer cell formation. Increased antioxidant activity has been noted in animal studies: animals treated with tannin components of green tea and then subjected to chromosome abnormalities showed a greater ability to suppress these abnormalities in their bone cells than animals not pretreated with the tannin.[7]

Decreased total cholesterol levels have been linked to the consumption of large amounts of green tea (nine or more cups a day).[8] It did not, however, lower triglyceride levels or raise levels of the "good" HDL (high-density lipoprotein) cholesterol.

A 1995 population study reported that among the 3,625 Japanese subjects surveyed, increased consumption of green tea corresponded to relatively lower levels of ferritin and lipid peroxides in the blood, chemical markers that in elevated levels may be associated with certain disease processes such as atherosclerosis and liver ailments.[9]

Much of the value in green tea can be explained by the way it is typically prepared, being steeped for only short periods of time. As a result, the tea retains many of the important chemical substances present in the fresh leaf.[10] Do not brew or drink green tea scalding hot, as this may well destroy important components in the brew and cancel out potential medicinal benefits.

Green tea also contains caffeine, a central nervous system stimulant; and tannin, an astringent substance that helps control some types of diarrhea when taken internally and constricts skin tissue when applied topically. The fluoride and tannins in green tea may also help prevent tooth decay, according to some sources. In fact, reduced cavity rates were noted in rats fed the tea.[11] Unfortunately, tea can also stain teeth.

Will It Harm You? What the Studies Say:

Billions of people around the world drink green tea every day to no apparent ill effect. But as with any caffeine-containing product, it can cause unwanted stimulant effects such as anxiety, tremors, irritability, and trouble sleeping if taken in excessive doses or by people who are very sensitive to caffeine. These side effects appear to be relatively uncommon with green tea, however, perhaps because of the lower caffeine content produced by steeping the leaves for relatively short periods of time.

GENERAL SOURCES:

Balch, J.F., and P.A. Balch. *Prescription for Nutritional Healing: A Practical A to Z Reference to Drug-Free Remedies Using Vitamins, Minerals, Herbs & Food Supplements.* 2nd ed. Garden City Park, NY: Avery Publishing Group, 1997.

Castleman, M. *The Healing Herbs: The Ultimate Guide to the Curative Power of Nature's Medicines.* New York: Bantam Books, 1995.

Lawrence Review of Natural Products. St. Louis: Facts and Comparisons, May 1993.

Leung, A.Y., and S. Foster. *Encyclopedia of Common Natural Ingredients Used in Food, Drugs, and Cosmetics.* 2nd ed. New York: John Wiley & Sons, 1996.

Mayell, M. *Off-the-Shelf Natural Health: How to Use Herbs and Nutrients to Stay Well.* New York: Bantam Books, 1995.

Murray, M.T. *The Healing Power of Herbs: The Enlightened Person's Guide to the Wonders of Medicinal Plants.* Revised and expanded 2nd ed. Rocklin, CA: Prima Publishing, 1995.

TEXT CITATIONS:

1 *Lawrence Review of Natural Products* (St. Louis: Facts and Comparisons, May 1993).

2. C.S. Yang and Z.Y. Wang, *Journal of the National Cancer Institute,* 85(13) (1993): 1038–49.

3. M.T. Murray, *The Healing Power of Herbs: The Enlightened Person's Guide to the Wonders of Medicinal Plants,* revised and expanded 2nd ed. (Rocklin, CA: Prima Publishing, 1995).

4. S. Kono et al., *Journal of Clinical Epidemiology,* 44(11) (1991): 1255.

5. Murray, op. cit.

6. A. Komori et al., *Japanese Journal of Clinical Oncology,* 23(3) (1993): 186–90.

7. H. Imanishi et al., *Mutation Research,* 259(1) (1991): 79.

8. S. Kono et al., *Preventive Medicine,* 21(4) (1992): 526.

9. K. Imai and K. Nakachi, *British Medical Journal,* 310 (1995): 693–96.

10. *Lawrence Review,* op. cit.

11. S. Rosen et al., *Journal of Dental Research,* 63(5) (1984): 658.

PRIMARY NAME:

TEA TREE OIL

SCIENTIFIC NAME:

Melaleuca alternifolia (Maiden & Betche) Cheel. Family: Myrtaceae

COMMON NAMES:

Australian tea tree oil, cajeput, cajeput oil

What Is Tea Tree Oil?

This pleasant-smelling, pale yellow volatile oil is distilled from the leaves of *Melaleuca alternifolia,* a shrub or small tree found growing naturally in swampy or wet ground in parts of New South Wales and southern Queensland in Australia. The oil is also produced from other *Melaleuca* species, but this information pertains only to that from *Melaleuca alternifolia.*

What It Is Used For:

Although people native to Australia had long recognized its antiseptic and healing properties, tea tree oil earned widespread fame only in the 1700s, when Captain John Cook's expedition spread the word of its value in healing skin cuts and burns.[1] Settlers in Australia reportedly used the oil similarly for insect bites and other external ailments, and brewed a tea from the leaves. In World War II,

RATING:

2 = According to a number of well-designed studies and common use, this substance appears to be relatively effective and safe when used in recommended amounts for the indication(s) noted in the "Will It Work for You?" section.

Australian soldiers were issued tea tree oil as a disinfectant, and the oil was integrated into machine-cutting oils in ammunition factories to lower the risk of accident-related infections.[2]

It was in the late 1970s and early 1980s that real interest in tea tree oil developed in the United States with the encouragement of herbalists, traditional healers, and the tea tree oil industry. Today, the oil is widely touted as a topical antiseptic and general treatment for a dizzying array of ailments from sunburns to sores, cuts, pus-filled wounds, boils, muscle aches, varicose veins, arthritis, bruises, insect bites, lice, warts, vaginitis, acne, fungal infections, mouth ulcers, and dandruff.

Forms Available Include:

- *For external use:* Oil (diluted and undiluted). Tea tree oil appears in numerous ointments, creams, soaps, toothpastes, shampoos, and other commercial products.
- *For internal use:* Lozenges (commercially prepared).

Dosage Commonly Reported:

Externally, tea tree oil is applied in concentrations of 0.4 to 100 percent, depending on what part of the body it is applied to and for what purpose.

Will It Work for You? What the Studies Say:

Tea tree oil has been studied intensively. It has proven antiseptic properties, and a body of research is building to support its use for certain ailments. Although many of the clinical trials reported for this herb were conducted more than fifty years ago when study standards were frequently looser than they are today, a few more recent ones indicate that the oil may benefit skin and vaginal infections.[3]

Of the oil's many compounds, substances called terpenes figure the most prominently, and researchers have identified the primary germ-fighting ingredient as terpinen-4-ol. This compound both weakens bacteria so that the body can fight them off more effectively and kills a variety of germs, including some that other standard antibiotics are ineffective against.[4] A 1995 test-tube study indicates that relatively low concentrations of tea tree oil (lower than typical commercial concentrations) can both inhibit and kill certain antibiotic-resistant bacteria common in hospitals, such as *Staphylococcus aureus*.[5] The terpenes also endow the oil with its pleasant smell. In Australia there are standards for the minimum and maximum amounts of terpenes in tea tree oil products. It is important that the oil used is from *Melaleuca alternifolia* and not another *Melaleuca* species, as some contain a substance—cineole—that can irritate the skin and reduce terpinen-4-ol's antiseptic powers.[6]

Research indicates that skin infections such as athlete's foot, and corns, calluses, and bunions, respond to tea tree oil (usually diluted in solution form).[7] The oil effectively fights acne, according to a 1990 study involving 124 individuals with mild to moderate acne.[8] Five percent tea tree oil in a water-based gel did not work as quickly as a 5 percent benzoyl peroxide lotion in reducing acne lesions, but both significantly reduced the mean number of lesions by the end of three months. More important, perhaps, only 44 percent of those treated with tea tree oil reported such side effects as dryness, irritation, stinging, burning, itching, and redness, compared with 79 percent of those treated with benzoyl peroxide.

Various vaginal conditions also appear to respond to tea tree oil formulations. In one study, the condition of seven of thirteen women with chronic cystitis (bladder infection) improved somewhat when they took a tea tree capsule once a day.[9] In another, vaginal suppositories containing the oil proved effective in eliminating vaginal yeast infections.[10] Researchers have found that the oil fights organisms commonly responsible for vaginal infections, including *Trichomonas vaginalis* and *Candida albicans*.[11] Only specially prepared tea tree formulations will treat vaginal problems effectively, however.

Will It Harm You? What the Studies Say:

The oil may irritate sensitive skin but is for the most part considered safe to use in external form. It has caused vaginal irritation in some cases. While folk use suggests that internal use is not harmful, many modern herbalists recommend against ingesting the oil, given concerns about toxic reactions.

GENERAL SOURCES:

American Pharmaceutical Association. *Handbook of Nonprescription Drugs*. 11th ed. Washington, D.C.: American Pharmaceutical Association, 1996.

Lawrence Review of Natural Products. St. Louis: Facts and Comparisons, January 1991.

Leung, A.Y., and S. Foster. *Encyclopedia of Common Natural Ingredients Used in Food, Drugs, and Cosmetics*. 2nd ed. New York: John Wiley & Sons, 1996.

Murray, M.T. *The Healing Power of Herbs: The Enlightened Person's Guide to the Wonders of Medicinal Plants*. Revised and expanded 2nd ed. Rocklin, CA: Prima Publishing, 1995.

Tierra, M. *The Way of Herbs*. New York: Pocket Books, 1990.

Tyler, V.E. *Herbs of Choice: The Therapeutic Use of Phytomedicinals*. Binghamton, NY: Haworth Press/Pharmaceutical Products Press, 1994.

———. *The Honest Herbal*. Binghamton, NY: Haworth Press/Pharmaceutical Products Press, 1993.

Weiner, M.A., and J.A. Weiner. *Herbs That Heal: Prescription for Herbal Healing*. Mill Valley, CA: Quantum Books, 1994.

TEXT CITATIONS:

1. *Lawrence Review of Natural Products* (St. Louis: Facts and Comparisons, January 1991).
2. American Pharmaceutical Association, *Handbook of Nonprescription Drugs*, 11th ed. (Washington, D.C.: American Pharmaceutical Association, 1996).
3. A.L. Blackwell, *The Lancet*, 337 (1991): 300. V.E. Tyler, *The Honest Herbal* (Binghamton, NY: Haworth Press, 1992).
4. C. Carson et al., *Journal of Antimicrobial Chemotherapy*, 35 (1995): 421–24.
5. C. Carson et al., op. cit.
6. Tyler, op. cit.
7. M. Walker, *Current Podiatry* (April 1972). *Lawrence Review of Natural Products*, op. cit. M.T. Murray, *The Healing Power of Herbs: The Enlightened Person's Guide to the Wonders of Medicinal Plants*, revised and expanded 2nd ed. (Rocklin, CA: Prima Publishing, 1995).
8. B. Bassett et al., *Medical Journal of Australia*, 153 (1990): 455–58.
9. *Lawrence Review of Natural Products*, op. cit.
10. P. Belaiche, *Phytotherapie*, (1985): 15.
11. E.F. Pena, *Obstetrics & Gynecology*, 19 (1962): 793–95.

SCIENTIFIC NAME:
Thymus vulgaris L., *Thymus zygis* L. Family: Labiatae (Lamiaceae)

COMMON NAMES:
Common thyme, French thyme, garden thyme, rubbed thyme, *Thymus zygis:* Spanish thyme

RATING:
2 = According to a number of well-designed studies and common use, this substance appears to be relatively effective and safe when used in recommended amounts for the indication(s) noted in the "Will It Work for You?" section. However, see the safety warning regarding the oil in the "Will It Harm You?" section.

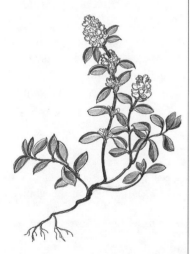

Thyme
Thymus vulgaris

What Is Thyme?

This aromatic perennial, a member of the mint family, has stiff, woody stems that give rise to small clusters of lilac or pink flowers. The whole aboveground herb, from these flowering tops to the narrow gray-green leaves, is used medicinally.

What It Is Used For:

This common American spice has a much broader range than the kitchen. Meats were preserved with it in ancient times, and medieval knights carried sprigs as a symbol of courage. Folk medicine traditions from Europe to China have prescribed the fresh and dried herb for centuries as an expectorant to control coughs and treat sore throat, acute bronchitis, and whooping cough. It has also been used to treat appetite loss, encourage smooth digestion, alleviate gas, and resolve chronic gastritis. Many have ascribed antiseptic, diaphoretic (sweat-inducing), diuretic ("water pill"), and worm-killing properties to it.

Some contemporary herbalists recommend thyme as their predecessors did for disinfecting wounds, eliminating skin parasites (crabs, lice), reducing aches and pains, and treating fungal infections such as athlete's foot. Some bath preparations contain thyme to treat skin ailments such as bruises and sprains, as well as to manage rheumatic symptoms. Aromatherapists consider the essential oil a powerful mood-enhancing herb for low spirits, fatigue, mental stress, and premenstrual tension.

An extract of the volatile oil in thyme—thymol—appears in numerous cough drops, gas remedies, counterirritant skin preparations, mouthwashes (it is the main ingredient in Listerine®, for example), antifungal medicines, dental formulations, and cosmetics.

Forms Available Include:

Elixir, herb (fresh and dried), infusion, liquid extract, oil, syrup, tea, tincture.

Dosage Commonly Reported:

An infusion made using 1 teaspoon herb per cup of water is drunk up to three times per day. Thyme syrup is taken by the teaspoonful several times per day. The liquid herb extract is taken in doses of 0.6 to 4 milliliters, and the elixir in doses of 4 to 8 milliliters. Externally, a few drops of the tincture are applied as an antiseptic. The essential oil is diluted in a carrier oil before being applied to the skin.

Will It Work for You? What the Studies Say:

The critical ingredient in this herb is an aromatic volatile oil (0.4 to 3.4 percent) that contains phenols called thymol and carvacrol. The actions of these two substances, as well as flavonoids, explain many of thyme's traditional uses.

Plant experts tend to agree that thyme will help reduce the symptoms of bronchitis, upper respiratory catarrh (congestion), and pertussis (whooping cough), all conditions for which the German health authorities have endorsed the herb.[1] Antispasmodic and expectorant properties in the herb explain why it is effective for these conditions, as they help to relax the respiratory tract and liquefy secretions so that they are easier to cough up.[2] A German textbook recommends inhaling the steam from thyme placed in hot water to obtain the same antispasmodic and bronchial-clearing effects.[3] The broad antibacterial and antifungal properties in the herb justify the use of thyme and its extract, thymol, in mouthwashes and gargles. The herb's antispasmodic actions may explain thyme's traditional use as a digestive aid. Many herbs containing volatile oils are used for this purpose.

Researchers have identified antiworm properties in thymol,[4] justifying this folk use. The toxicity of thymol has precluded the spread of this practice, however.

Thymol is most likely responsible for the herb's value in reducing aches and pain. When applied to the skin, it causes blood to rush to the area, spreading a sense of warmth and attendant relief from pain and inflammation.

Will It Harm You? What the Studies Say:

Although thyme is safe to use in culinary and medicinal concentrations, avoid ingesting the oil directly, as it is toxic. Even in modest amounts, such as a few teaspoonsful, the thymol may cause such adverse reactions as nausea, vomiting, weakness, stomach pain, dizziness, headache, convulsions, coma, and cardiac and respiratory arrest.[5]

Pregnant women may want to avoid ingesting large amounts of thyme, given its traditional use for altering the menstrual cycle.[6] People suffering from a thyroid condition should talk to their doctor before taking medicinal doses of thyme, because rat studies indicate that the herb may suppress the gland's normal activity.[7]

Applied externally, the herb can cause rashes in sensitive skin. Apply the oil only if it has been properly diluted in commercial formulations, or you may risk irritating the skin and mucous membranes.[8] Thyme oil in bath preparations has caused severe inflammation and hyperemia (blood collection in a particular part of the body). In toothpastes it can cause cracks in the corners of the mouth and a swollen tongue.

GENERAL SOURCES:

Blumenthal, M., J. Gruenwald, T. Hall, and R.S. Rister, eds. *The Complete German Commission E Monographs: Therapeutic Guide to Herbal Medicine.* Boston: Integrative Medicine Communications, 1998.

Castleman, M. *The Healing Herbs: The Ultimate Guide to the Curative Power of Nature's Medicines.* New York: Bantam Books, 1995.

Leung, A.Y., and S. Foster. *Encyclopedia of Common Natural Ingredients Used in Food, Drugs, and Cosmetics.* 2nd ed. New York: John Wiley & Sons, 1996.

Mayell, M. *Off-the-Shelf Natural Health: How to Use Herbs and Nutrients to Stay Well.* New York: Bantam Books, 1995.

Newall, C.A., et al. *Herbal Medicines: A Guide for Health-Care Professionals.* London: The Pharmaceutical Press, 1996.

Stary, F. *The Natural Guide to Medicinal Herbs and Plants.* Prague: Barnes & Noble, Inc., in arrangement with Aventinum Publishers, 1996.

Tierra, M. *The Way of Herbs*. New York: Pocket Books, 1990.

Tyler, V.E. *Herbs of Choice: The Therapeutic Use of Phytomedicinals*. Binghamton, NY: Haworth Press/Pharmaceutical Products Press, 1994.

Weiner, M.A., and J.A. Weiner. *Herbs That Heal: Prescription for Herbal Healing*. Mill Valley, CA: Quantum Books, 1994.

Weiss, R.F. *Herbal Medicine*, trans. A.R. Meuss, from the 6th German edition. Beaconsfield, England: Beaconsfield Publishers, Ltd., 1988.

TEXT CITATIONS:

1. M. Blumenthal, J. Gruenwald, T. Hall, and R.S. Rister, eds., *The Complete German Commission E Monographs: Therapeutic Guide to Herbal Medicine* (Boston: Integrative Medicine Communications, 1998).

2. C.O. Van den Broucke, *Fitoterapia*, 4 (1983): 171–74. N.G. Bisset, ed., *Herbal Drugs and Phytopharmaceuticals* (Stuttgart: medpharm GmbH Scientific Publishers, 1994).

3. R.F. Weiss, *Herbal Medicine*, trans. A.R. Meuss, from the 6th German edition (Beaconsfield, England: Beaconsfield Publishers, Ltd., 1988).

4. A.Y. Leung and S. Foster, *Encyclopedia of Common Natural Ingredients Used in Food, Drugs, and Cosmetics*, 2nd ed. (New York: John Wiley & Sons, 1996).

5. Ibid.

6. C.A. Newall et al., *Herbal Medicines: A Guide for Health-Care Professionals* (London: The Pharmaceutical Press, 1996).

7. Leung and Foster, op. cit.

8. Newall, op. cit.

PRIMARY NAME:

TIENCHI

SCIENTIFIC NAME:

Panax notoginseng (Burk.) F.H. Chen. Family: Araliaceae

COMMON NAMES:

Renshen sanqi, sanchi, sanchi ginseng, sanqi, shen sanqi, tianchi, tianqi, tian sanqi, tienchi-ginseng

RATING:

3 = Studies on the effectiveness and safety of this substance are conflicting, or there are not enough studies to draw a conclusion.

What Is Tienchi?

The tuberous root of this perennial Chinese shrub is used medicinally. Harvesters separate the roots from the young plants before flowers appear in spring, drying them in the sun, kneading them by hand, and further processing them to produce a dark and shiny root. Tienchi is widely cultivated in the Yunnan province of China. It is sometimes classified as a ginseng. For information on true Asian ginseng, see **Ginseng, Asian**.

What It Is Used For:

In traditional Chinese medicine, this sweet, slightly bitter-tasting root has been used for centuries as an antibleeding agent and heart tonic. Myriad types of bleeding have been treated with it, from wound-related bleeding to vomited blood and nosebleeds. Chinese and American airmen in World War II carried a tienchi-rich substance called yunnan bao yao to stop bleeding from wounds.[1] Coronary heart disease and stabbing chest or abdominal pain are thought to benefit from it as well. Tienchi has been ascribed painkilling and antiswelling properties. Contemporary Western herbalists recommend tienchi to prevent fatigue and bolster the system against stress, and suggest that it be taken in the form of a soothing tonic soup to normalize blood pressure, improve blood circulation, and steady the heart rate.

Some shampoos and skin-care products sold in Asia contain tienchi powder and extracts for their purported ability to erase dark skin spots and dilate vessels.[2]

Forms Available Include:

Capsule, root (whole, powdered; numerous grades of quality), tablet.

Dosage Commonly Reported:

Standard Chinese recommendations are for 1 to 3 grams of the powdered root daily.

Will It Work for You? What the Studies Say:

Chinese investigators have examined this traditional healing agent closely and discovered promising indications of its ability to control bleeding and beneficially affect the heart. The herb contains 7 to 10.8 percent crude saponins, some of which are identical to the ones found in Asian ginseng.[3]

Antibleeding properties have been noted in several animal studies; when taken internally, tienchi shortens the time it takes for blood to coagulate, which means that bleeding stops more quickly.[4] Interestingly, test-tube studies suggest that tienchi actually encourages the destruction of red blood cells in certain animals.[5] Whether the overall effect of these actions on the blood is positive or negative for humans requires further study.

Other research indicates that this "cardiac tonic" affects the cardiovascular system in a generally positive way, with the saponins lowering blood pressure in laboratory animals,[6] protecting against heart injury in rats, and demonstrating antiarrhythmic actions in rats, mice, and rabbits.[7] Other studies, virtually all of them done in China, indicate that tienchi also offers anti-inflammatory and immune-system-altering properties, among others. What any of these findings mean for human beings remains unclear, however.

Will It Harm You? What the Studies Say:

The data available indicate that tienchi is a safe herb to take internally. Countless Chinese have consumed it in the form of tonic soups. No reports of significant adverse reactions to the herb appear in the recent medical literature, and no adverse reactions or deaths were observed in mice fed tienchi powder in both short- and long-term trials.[8] On the other hand, no large-scale toxicity studies of humans appear to have been done so far.

GENERAL SOURCES:

Leung, A.Y., and S. Foster. *Encyclopedia of Common Natural Ingredients Used in Food, Drugs, and Cosmetics.* 2nd ed. New York: John Wiley & Sons, 1996.

Tierra, M. *The Way of Herbs.* New York: Pocket Books, 1990.

Tyler, V.E. *The Honest Herbal.* Binghamton, NY: Haworth Press/Pharmaceutical Products Press, 1993.

Tyler, V.E., L.R. Brady, and J.E. Robbers, eds. *Pharmacognosy.* Philadelphia: Lea & Febiger, 1988.

TEXT CITATIONS:

1. A.Y. Leung and S. Foster, *Encyclopedia of Common Natural Ingredients Used in Food, Drugs, and Cosmetics,* 2nd ed. (New York: John Wiley & Sons, 1996).
2. Ibid.

3. V.E. Tyler, *The Honest Herbal* (Binghamton, NY: Haworth Press/Pharmaceutical Products Press, 1993).
4. B.H. Zhang, *Zhongcaoyao*, 15(11) (1984): 34. Leung and Foster, op. cit.
5. J.D. Wang and J.X. Chen, *Acta Pharmacologica Sinica*, 5 (1984): 181.
6. Leung and Foster, op. cit.
7. S. Liu and J.X. Chen, *Acta Pharmacologica Sinica*, 5 (1984): 100. B.Y. Gao et al., *Yaoxue Xuebao*, 27 (1992): 641. Leung and Foster, op. cit.
8. B.H. Zhang, *Zhongcaoyao*, 15(11) (1984): 34. Tyler, op. cit.

PRIMARY NAME:
TONKA BEAN

SCIENTIFIC NAME:
Dipteryx odorata (Aubl.) Willd.
Family: Fabaceae
(Leguminosae)

COMMON NAMES:
Cumaru, tonco seed, tonga bean, tongo bean, tono bean, tonquin bean, torquin bean

RATING:
5 = Studies indicate that there is a definite health hazard to using this substance, even in recommended amounts.

What Is Tonka Bean?

This long, deeply wrinkled, single-seeded bean grows on tropical trees belonging to the genus *Dipteryx* in Venezuela, Brazil, and Guyana. The highly aromatic, nearly black-colored beans (technically, the fruit) are known as "black beans" (not to be confused with the common legumes sold as black beans) when dried. Upon processing, which sometimes involves softening them by letting them steep in rum, a frosting of white crystals containing a substance called coumarin develops. The bean, the processed bean, and the coumarin are all used medicinally.

What It Is Used For:

The coumarin on these beans imparts an odor reminiscent of vanillin, and it was long used in imitation vanilla flavorings in the United States.[1] The food industry used it widely until 1954, when the FDA, concerned about health risks, banned coumarin-containing tonka beans and their extracts in foods.[2] Synthetically produced coumarins have since taken over and are used as flavorings in foods and tobacco. Mexican vanilla may attribute its reputation for superior aromaticity to the continued use of "natural" coumarin from tonka beans.[3]

South American folk healers reportedly turned to tonka bean to treat cramps, nausea, spasms, whooping cough, and cachexia (wasting). Indigenous peoples concocted a nutty beverage from the seed paste and milk. North American outlets sometimes promote the bean's reputed "tonic" properties in teas.

Forms Available Include:

Liquid extract, seed (from the bean), seed oil.

Dosage Commonly Reported:

Tonka bean should not be used medicinally.

Will It Work for You? What the Studies Say:

Test-tube studies of the bean and its extracts have documented broad antimicrobial[4] and strong antioxidative[5] activity for the beans. (Antioxidants help control the formation of dangerous substances in the body called free radicals, which damage cells through oxidation. Some free radicals are believed to contribute to cancer-cell formation.) A 1937 study reports success in treating a case of tuberculous pulmonary lesions through internal administration and injections of tonka bean oil.[6] In the decades since then, few if any studies of humans appear to have been done. The potential healing properties of tonka bean are irrelevant in any case, given the clear health hazards associated with the contained coumarin.

Will It Harm You? What the Studies Say:

Although probably safe when taken in common flavoring concentrations,[7] tonka bean does pose distinct risks when ingested in higher amounts. The contained coumarin can cause severe liver damage, for example, which is why the FDA banned the use of the beans as a flavoring agent. It can also cause a tendency to bleed and abnormal blood clotting mechanisms. You may recognize the name coumarin in relation to the common anticoagulant warfarin, sold as Coumadin™, which is given in a controlled manner to alter the blood's clotting ability. The hazards of coumarin have been documented in laboratory animals, with rats and dogs fed the chemical developing liver damage, testicular atrophy, and retarded growth.[8] In large doses the fluid extract can reportedly paralyze the heart.[9]

GENERAL SOURCES:

Duke, J.A. *CRC Handbook of Medicinal Herbs.* Boca Raton, FL: CRC Press, 1985.

Lawrence Review of Natural Products. St. Louis: Facts and Comparisons, November 1995.

Pound, F.J. "History and Cultivation of the Tonka Bean (*Dipetryx odorata*) with Analyses of Trinidad, Venezuelan and Brazilian Samples." *Tropical Agriculture,* 15 (1938): 4–9, 28–32.

Tyler, V.E., L.R. Brady, and J.E. Robbers, eds. *Pharmacognosy.* Philadelphia: Lea & Febiger, 1988.

TEXT CITATIONS:

1. M.B. Jacobs, *American Perfumery,* 48(3) (1946): 56, 59.
2. *Lawrence Review of Natural Products* (St. Louis: Facts and Comparisons, November 1995).
3. G. Sullivan, *Texas Journal of Science,* 36(1) (1984): 17–23.
4. J.C. Maruzzella and M. Freundlich, *Journal of the American Pharmaceutical Association,* 48 (1959): 356–58.
5. T. Hirosue et al., *Nippon Shokuhin Kogya Gakkaishi,* 35(9) (1988): 630–33.
6. P. Sobrinho, *Revista da Flora Medicinal* (1937): 531–37.
7. *Lawrence Review of Natural Products,* op. cit.
8. J.A. Duke, *CRC Handbook of Medicinal Herbs* (Boca Raton, FL: CRC Press, 1985).
9. Ibid.

L-TRYPTOPHAN

SCIENTIFIC NAME:
N/A

COMMON NAME:
Tryptophan

RATING:
5 = Studies indicate that there is a definite health hazard to using this substance, even in recommended amounts.

What Is L-Tryptophan?

L-tryptophan is an essential amino acid. "Essential" means that your body cannot manufacture it on its own and must get it through the foods you eat.

What It Is Used For:

In addition to contributing to numerous other body functions, L-tryptophan serves as a precursor to the neurotransmitter serotonin, an important brain chemical involved in the regulation of sleep. Serotonin also affects mood. L-tryptophan appears in casein, a substance found in cow's milk, and was at one time thought to contribute to the sleepiness so many people experience with a bedtime glass of milk.[1] Numerous sources billed L-tryptophan as a sedative, and the amino acid enjoyed widespread popularity as a supplement until it was linked to the development of a serious blood disorder and banned by the FDA in 1989.

Although it is not available in supplement form in the United States anymore, many sources still cite L-tryptophan as a valuable amino acid for inducing sleep, combating anxiety and depression, treating migraine headache, reducing the risk of heart spasms, and alleviating stress, among other things.

Forms Available:

None available in the United States. However, this amino acid is easily obtained through foods such as bananas, turkey, milk, peanuts, and lentils.

Dosage Commonly Reported:

L-tryptophan should not be used medicinally.

Will It Work for You? What the Studies Say:

According to studies conducted in the 1960s and 1970s, 1-gram doses of L-tryptophan reduce the time it takes for both insomniacs and people without sleeping problems to fall asleep.[2] With aggressive marketing, and in much higher doses than this—500-milligram and even 667-milligram tablets and capsules were available at one point—L-tryptophan became a wildly popular sleep aid. Interestingly, the studies had shown that doses larger than 1 gram did not enhance the amino acid's sleep-inducing properties.

Relapses developed in individuals taking L-tryptophan supplements for chronic depression who could no longer get it after the British government banned it,[3] a testimony to the amino acid's ability to affect mood.

Will It Harm You? What the Studies Say:

The FDA banned L-tryptophan in 1989 because its use was linked to the development of a blood disorder, eosinophilia-myalgia syndrome, in people who had taken the amino acid in supplement form. This serious disorder is characterized by an elevated white blood cell count and symptoms such as muscular pain, fatigue, edema (swelling), rash, and respiratory problems. Several dozen deaths were attributed to the amino acid. A subsequent investigation revealed the true culprit: a contaminant introduced by improper processing and purification of the amino acid by a single manufacturer, the Japanese company Showa Denko K.K. The contaminant was most likely an unintended by-product of a new production process, a fusion of two L-tryptophan molecules that had been chemically linked.[4] Thus, many still consider uncontaminated L-tryptophan safe to use.

For more information on the wisdom and safety of taking single amino acid supplements, see **L-Tyrosine.**

GENERAL SOURCES:

Balch, J.F., and P.A. Balch. *Prescription for Nutritional Healing: A Practical A to Z Reference to Drug-Free Remedies Using Vitamins, Minerals, Herbs & Food Supplements.* 2nd ed. Garden City Park, NY: Avery Publishing Group, 1997.

Griffith, H.W. *Complete Guide to Vitamins, Minerals, Nutrients, & Supplements.* Tucson: Fisher Books, 1988.

Mayell, M. *Off-the-Shelf Natural Health: How to Use Herbs and Nutrients to Stay Well.* New York: Bantam Books, 1995.

Tyler, V.E. *The Honest Herbal.* Binghamton, NY: Haworth Press/Pharmaceutical Products Press, 1993.

Tyler, V.E., L.R. Brady, and J.E. Robbers, eds. *Pharmacognosy.* Philadelphia: Lea & Febiger, 1988.

TEXT CITATIONS:

1. V.E. Tyler, *The Honest Herbal* (Binghamton, NY: Haworth Press/Pharmaceutical Products Press, 1993).
2. E. Hartmann, *The Sleeping Pill* (New Haven: Yale University Press, 1978). Tyler, op. cit.
3. N. Ferrier et al., *The Lancet,* 336 (1990): 380–81.
4. A.N. Mayeno et al., *Science,* 250 (1990): 1707–8.

PRIMARY NAME:
TURMERIC

SCIENTIFIC NAME:
Curcuma longa L. Also referred to as *Curcuma domestica* Val. Family: Zingiberaceae

COMMON NAMES:
Curcuma, Indian saffron, yu jin

RATING:
3 = Studies on the effectiveness and safety of this substance are conflicting, or there are not enough studies to draw a conclusion.

What Is Turmeric?

Turmeric is the large, deep-yellow rhizome (underground stem) of *Curcuma longa,* a perennial shrub of the ginger family cultivated throughout Asia, China, India, and tropical regions of the world. The plant bears long green leaves and yellow flowers. The aromatic, pungent rhizomes are typically boiled or scalded, dried, and then pulverized before being used.

What It Is Used For:

Turmeric commands a venerable position in Indian and Asian medicine. Many ailments have been treated with it, from indigestion to jaundice, hepatitis, gallstones, and blood clots. In India it is considered a tonic for the whole body. It has been used as a diuretic ("water pill") and as an agent to promote the flow of bile into the intestines. Traditional Chinese healers prescribe it for liver problems and colic, among other ills. Topical formulations are applied to the skin to reduce pain and itching in small wounds and ringworm infections.

Contemporary American herbalists recommend turmeric for reducing the pain and inflammation of arthritis, enhancing liver function, preventing gallbladder disease, reestablishing menstrual regularity, reducing congestion, and controlling fever.

Turmeric is also used as a spice (it is a key ingredient in curry powder, and is also used in mustards), and as a yellow food coloring. Turmeric oil appears in perfumes. Before litmus paper was invented, lab scientists used turmeric to test for alkalinity.

Forms Available Include:

Capsule, liquid extract, powder, tincture.

Dosage Commonly Reported:

A standard dose of powdered turmeric is 0.5 to 1 gram taken several times a day between meals, or 1.5 to 3 grams per day taken dissolved in warm milk. The contained curcumin is taken in doses of 1,200 milligrams. The 300-milligram capsules are taken up to three times a day.

Will It Work for You? What the Studies Say:

Most Americans are probably unaware that in other parts of the world this distinctive yellow powder leads another life outside of the kitchen. Extensive analyses over the decades have uncovered a number of important facts about turmeric. It contains 4.2 to 14 percent of an orange-yellow volatile oil, bitter principles, and critical substances known as curcuminoids. The curcuminoids are held responsible for the herb's distinctive color and many of its medicinal effects.

Animal studies and laboratory findings indicate that there is some wisdom to taking turmeric to soothe stomach upset and reduce excess gas. In the test tube and in animals,[1] one of its three major curcuminoids—curcumin—fights a number of bacteria, including protozoans (microscopic creatures) responsible for illnesses such as infectious diarrhea.[2] Given such findings and centuries of use—there have apparently been no large clinical trials—German health authorities endorse the use of turmeric for indigestion.[3] Turmeric also has a long-standing reputation as a cholagogue, meaning that it stimulates the liver's output of bile into the intestines. Both curcumin and the volatile oil in turmeric are probably involved. Test-tube and animal studies also indicate that curcumin has a protective effect on the liver.[4] Whether these properties occur in humans to any beneficial measure has yet to be demonstrated, however.

Test-tube and animal studies suggest that there may be validity to the long-standing tradition in folk medicine, especially in India, of using turmeric to prevent and relieve inflammatory conditions such as arthritis. Anti-inflammatory and antiarthritic activity was observed in rats given curcuma oil from turmeric.[5] More research on the subject, with humans, is needed.

Recent findings have stimulated interest in treating certain kinds of cancers with turmeric. Test-tube experiments demonstrate the power of curcuminoids to kill particular kinds of cells, including certain tumor cells such as lymphoma, as well as their potential to fight external cancers.[6] Investigators believe that curcumin and other substances in turmeric also function as antioxidants, which means that they help remove toxic by-products that may contribute to the formation of cancer cells. A number of these properties have been verified in animal studies. Several studies indicate that turmeric may help prevent tumors.[7] In one, mice fed substances containing curcumin were less likely than those not given the substance to develop experimentally induced overgrowth in the colon.[8] Another investigator reported that in mice, curcumin inhibits unchecked cell growth involved in the early, progressive, and late stages of cancer.[9]

Hints of the same type of cancer-preventive effect in humans were demonstrated in a study involving smokers. Mutagens are substances that can increase the frequency or breadth of a mutation, a critical step in cancer development. In the study, significantly fewer mutagens were found in smokers given 1.5 grams of turmeric a day for thirty days than in the smokers not given turmeric.[10] Although these findings are intriguing, much more research is needed before conclusions can be made about turmeric's role as a cancer-fighter in humans.

Other research raises hopes that turmeric helps prevent blood clots, reduce cholesterol, and possibly protect against gallbladder disease. But as with so much of the research into this herb, these studies were done in test tubes or with animals, so their relevance for treating human disease remains hazy.

Will It Harm You? What the Studies Say:

Very little is known about the toxicity of turmeric. Certainly, millions have used it safely as a spice. It is not likely to cause side effects or interact negatively with other remedies.[11] Medicinal concentrations merit some caution, however. Turmeric in amounts higher than recommended can cause stomach upset. According to one investigator, the herb's curcuminoids may play a role in the formation of stomach ulcers, although not much more on the subject was heard after this was reported in 1980.[12]

German health authorities warn that an individual with a bile duct blockage should avoid medicinal concentrations, and that anyone with gallstones should talk to a doctor before using them.[13] An American herbalist likewise cautions individuals with blood clotting problems to steer clear of medicinal concentrations, given evidence of the herb's potential anticlotting actions.[14] Overall, however, turmeric as a folk remedy is considered safe.

Long-term consumption of turmeric extracts may be harmful. In test mice the extracts led to significant changes in the weight of the heart and lungs, and both red and white blood cell counts dropped significantly.[15] Although the results have not been reproduced, the findings also indicated that turmeric may affect fertility; sexual organs increased in weight, and the motility of sperm increased. What this means for humans remains unclear, although it must be kept in mind that these mice were fed large amounts of extracts every day for ninety days.

According to test-tube studies, curcuminoids in turmeric can potentially damage cells, producing chromosome changes in some cases. Scientists are still unclear about the relevance of this for humans without cancer.[16]

GENERAL SOURCES:

Bisset, N.G., ed. *Herbal Drugs and Phytopharmaceuticals.* Stuttgart: medpharm GmbH Scientific Publishers, 1994.

Blumenthal, M., J. Gruenwald, T. Hall, and R.S. Rister, eds. *The Complete German Commission E Monographs: Therapeutic Guide to Herbal Medicine.* Boston: Integrative Medicine Communications, 1998.

Castleman, M. *The Healing Herbs: The Ultimate Guide to the Curative Power of Nature's Medicines.* New York: Bantam Books, 1995.

Lawrence Review of Natural Products. St. Louis: Facts and Comparisons, February 1993.

Leung, A.Y. *Encyclopedia of Common Natural Ingredients Used in Food, Drugs, and Cosmetics.* New York: John Wiley & Sons, 1980.

Mindell, E. *Earl Mindell's Herb Bible.* New York: Simon & Schuster, 1992.

TEXT CITATIONS:

1. Y. Kiso et al., *Planta Medica,* 49 (1983): 185.
2. M. Tomoda et al., *Phytochemistry,* 29 (1990): 1083.
3. M. Blumenthal, J. Gruenwald, T. Hall, and R.S. Rister, eds., *The Complete German Commission E Monographs: Therapeutic Guide to Herbal Medicine* (Boston: Integrative Medicine Communications, 1998).
4. Kiso, op. cit.
5. D. Chandra and S.S. Gupta, *Indian Journal of Medical Research,* 60 (1972): 138.
6. R. Kuttan et al., *Tumori,* 73 (1987): 29. R. Kuttan et al., *Cancer Letters,* 29 (1985): 197.
7. M.A. Azuine and S.V. Bhide, *International Journal of Cancer,* 51 (1992): 412.
8. M.T. Huang et al., *Cancer Letters,* 64 (1992): 117.
9. M. Nagabhushan and S.V. Bhide, *Journal of the American College of Nutrition,* 11 (1992): 192.
10. K. Polasa, *Mutagenesis,* 7 (1992): 107.
11. N.G. Bisset, ed., *Herbal Drugs and Phytopharmaceuticals* (Stuttgart: medpharm GmbH Scientific Publishers, 1994).
12. B. Gupta et al., *Indian Journal of Medical Research,* 71 (1980): 806.
13. Blumenthal et al., op. cit.
14. M. Castleman, *The Healing Herbs: The Ultimate Guide to the Curative Power of Nature's Medicines* (New York: Bantam Books, 1995).
15. S. Quereshi et al, *Planta Medica,* 58 (1992): 124.
16. Bisset, op. cit.

PRIMARY NAME:
TURPENTINE OIL

SCIENTIFIC NAME:
Pinus palustris Mill., *Pinus pinaster* Aiton, *Pinus elliotti* Engelm, and various other *Pinus* species and varieties. Family: Pinaceae

COMMON NAMES:
Gum turpentine, purified turpentine, rectified turpentine, rosin, spirits of turpentine, turpentine

What Is Turpentine Oil?

Turpentine is the oleoresin (a natural product containing chiefly resin and essential oils) obtained from various pine tree (*Pinus*) species, particularly the longleaf pine (*Pinus palustris* Mill.). Only a high-quality form of turpentine is appropriate for medicinal use; never use commercial turpentine in paint solvents and other substances for medicinal purposes. Technically, spirits of turpentine and rectified turpentine oil represent the essential oil that has been steam-distilled from turpentine's oleoresin. A medicinal-quality resin called rosin (colophony) is also extracted from the oleoresin.

What It Is Used For:

Most people think of paint solvent when they hear "turpentine." But it also has a history as a starter for the synthesis of various chemicals including camphor and menthol, as a food flavor (in minute amounts), as an insect repellent, and as a resin for chewing gum and adhesives.[1] Few people know that the oil has also long been used in ointments and other topical forms as a counterirritant for alleviating various pains and aches such as pulled muscles, nerve pain, and stiff joints. In commercially prepared extracts in cough and cold remedies it serves as a stimulating expectorant to help expel phlegm (mucus). Other reported uses for spirits of turpentine include as a carminative (for excess gas), diuretic ("water pill"), colic remedy, and diarrhea treatment. Rheumatism sufferers were once reportedly encouraged to take turpentine baths. Today, it is a common home remedy in some parts of the country,[2] and various herbalists recommend its (cautious) use for certain ailments.

Forms Available Include:

Extracts, oil. Extracts appear in various commercial products. *Never use turpentine intended as a paint solvent to treat an illness.*

Dosage Commonly Reported:

For adults and children over the age of two, turpentine is applied externally in concentrations of 6 to 50 percent up to three or four times per day. For internal preparations, use commercial products only and follow dosage instructions carefully.

Will It Work for You? What the Studies Say:

Most of the folk claims for turpentine have not been closely examined, with the exception of two: as a topical treatment for pain, and as a cough and congestion remedy. Turpentine oil, when used carefully—given its risk for toxicity—appears to be an effective treatment for certain kinds of skin ailments. Classified as a counterirritant and rubefacient, it is intended to cause surface irritation and redness to increase circulation to the area and produce associated sensations of warmth and distraction from deeper pain.

In the United States, turpentine oil has long been used in over-the-counter preparations for minor pains, aches, and muscle sores. German health authorities approve of the use of purified topical turpentine oil preparations for pain caused by rheumatic and neuralgic (nerve pain) ailments.[4] Traditional Chinese healers have relied on gum turpentine and rosin in similar ways for centuries.[5] Along the same lines, turpentine baths have been given to Russians suffering from disseminated sclerosis, a painful collagen-vascular disease involving extensive inflammation and stiffening.[6] The safety of this treatment remains to be determined.[7]

German health authorities also approve of the use of purified topical turpentine oil preparations for chronic bronchial diseases involving heavy mucus secretions.[8] In the United States, certain commercially prepared products may contain turpentine oil or spirits to treat cough and cold symptoms.[9] Its effectiveness is somewhat questionable,[10] however, apparently never having been conclusively demonstrated in any study. In any case, do not risk using turpentine oil in these ways on your own; stick to commercial preparations.

Turpentine oil applied to severe wounds infested with fly larvae reportedly helps remove the dead skin tissue.[11] Given results of test-tube studies, it may also help fight certain bacteria.[12]

Will It Harm You? What the Studies Say:

Turpentine oil must be handled carefully to avoid toxic reactions and even fatal poisonings. Swallowed turpentine oil is a common source of childhood poisonings, accounting for one of the most frequent calls to poison control centers,[13] and proving fatal in some cases in doses as small as 15 milliliters.[14] Doses of 140 milliliters may be fatal to adults.[15] Poisoning may induce redness, rash, hives, headache, coughing, vomiting, bloody urine, insomnia, protein in the urine (albuminuria), and coma.[16]

If turpentine oil is applied to the affected skin area more than the recommended three or four times a day, local burning, irritation, gastrointestinal upset, and breathing problems may develop in certain individuals.[17] A 1995 article describes a fifty-six-year-old Mississippi man who developed hives, vomiting, and blistering eruptions after applying large amounts of turpentine oil to his skin to get rid of "seed ticks."[18] Pregnant women should not use turpentine oil in any form.

Turpentine applied to the skin of various animals over long periods of time has caused benign skin tumors to develop.[19]

Store turpentine products properly, because of their volatile nature; read package instructions carefully.

GENERAL SOURCES:

American Pharmaceutical Association. *Handbook of Nonprescription Drugs.* 11th ed. Washington, D.C.: American Pharmaceutical Association, 1996.

Blumenthal, M., J. Gruenwald, T. Hall, and R.S. Rister, eds. *The Complete German Commission E Monographs: Therapeutic Guide to Herbal Medicine.* Boston: Integrative Medicine Communications, 1998.

Lawrence Review of Natural Products. St. Louis: Facts and Comparisons, April 1993.

Leber, M.R., et al. *Handbook of Over-the-Counter Drugs and Pharmacy Products.* Berkeley, CA: Celestial Arts Publishing, 1994.

Leung, A.Y., and S. Foster. *Encyclopedia of Common Natural Ingredients Used in Food, Drugs, and Cosmetics.* 2nd ed. New York: John Wiley & Sons, 1996.

Tyler, V.E. *Herbs of Choice: The Therapeutic Use of Phytomedicinals.* Binghamton, NY: Haworth Press/Pharmaceutical Products Press, 1994.

Weiner, M.A., and J.A. Weiner. *Herbs That Heal: Prescription for Herbal Healing.* Mill Valley, CA: Quantum Books, 1994.

Weiss, R.F. *Herbal Medicine,* trans. A.R. Meuss, from the 6th German edition. Beaconsfield, England: Beaconsfield Publishers, Ltd., 1988.

TEXT CITATIONS:

1. A.Y. Leung and S. Foster, *Encyclopedia of Common Natural Ingredients Used in Food, Drugs, and Cosmetics,* 2nd ed. (New York: John Wiley & Sons, 1996).
2. *Lawrence Review of Natural Products* (St. Louis: Facts and Comparisons, April 1993).
3. American Pharmaceutical Association, *Handbook of Nonprescription Drugs,* 11th ed. (Washington, D.C.: American Pharmaceutical Association, 1996).
4. M. Blumenthal, J. Gruenwald, T. Hall, and R.S. Rister, eds., *The Complete German Commission E Monographs: Therapeutic Guide to Herbal Medicine* (Boston: Integrative Medicine Communications, 1998).
5. Leung and Foster, op. cit.

6. E.A. Ludianskii, *Voprosky Kurortologii Fiziolerapii i Lechebnoi Fizicheskoi Kul'tury*, 3 (1992): 34.
7. *Lawrence Review of Natural Products*, op. cit.
8. Blumenthal et al., op. cit.
9. I. Ziment, *Respiration*, 58 (1991): 37. *Lawrence Review of Natural Products*, op. cit.
10. Blumenthal et al., op. cit.
11. D.C. Agarwal and B. Singh, *Indian Journal of Ophthalmology*, 38 (1990): 187. *Lawrence Review of Natural Products*, op. cit.
12. Leung and Foster, op. cit.
13. K. Melis et al., *Nederlands Tijdschrift voor Geneeskunde*, 134 (1990): 811.
14. E.L. Boyd et al., *Home Remedies and the Black Elderly: A Reference Manual for Health Care Providers* (Levittown, PA: Pharmaceutical Information Associates, Ltd., 1991).
15. American Pharmaceutical Association, op. cit.
16. Leung and Foster, op. cit.
17. American Pharmaceutical Association, op. cit.
18. *Morbidity and Mortality Weekly Report*, Centers for Disease Control and Prevention, 44 (1995): 204–7.
19. *Lawrence Review of Natural Products*, op. cit. Leung and Foster, op. cit.

PRIMARY NAME:

L-TYROSINE

SCIENTIFIC NAME:

N/A

COMMON NAME:

Tyrosine

T

L-Tyrosine

RATING:

4 = Research indicates that this substance will not fulfill the claims made for it. Its safety remains undetermined. For important safety warnings, see the "Will It Harm You?" section.

What Is L-Tyrosine?

L-tyrosine is a nonessential amino acid. "Nonessential" means that the body produces it naturally.

What It Is Used For:

The body uses this amino acid to help produce dopamine, norepinephrine (noradrenaline), and epinephrine (adrenaline) in addition to performing other important functions. Advocates claim that taking tyrosine supplements will elevate mood and counter depression, reduce stress, fight chronic fatigue, stimulate the libido, boost brain function, suppress the appetite and help reduce body fat, possibly aid Parkinson's disease sufferers, and encourage the thyroid, pituitary, and adrenal glands to function normally.

Forms Available Include:

Capsule, powder.

Dosage Commonly Reported:

Some sources recommend 500 to 1,000 milligrams twice a day, taken with high-carbohydrate meals.

Will It Work for You? What the Studies Say:

Amino acids such as L-tyrosine contain nitrogen, carbon, oxygen, and hydrogen. They are the building blocks of proteins, the body's main structural component, crucial to proper growth and development. Despite the numerous claims made for the benefits of supplementing the diet with single amino acids such as L-tyrosine, however, there is little if any information in the recent medical literature to support them. In fact, there is scant evidence to substantiate the use of any single amino acid for generally healthy, well-nourished individuals; an amino acid supplement will not make such an individual healthier. Moreover, deficiencies do not occur in single amino acids; they develop in tandem with declines in other amino acids. A total protein deficiency will develop before the levels of a particular amino acid drop very low in most cases.

Vegetarians who avoid milk, fish, eggs, and meat are at increased risk of an amino acid deficiency but can easily correct this by varying their diet. Premature infants and people who have recently suffered from a severe burn or injury may represent another category of people who may benefit from properly supervised amino acid supplementation. Overall, however, such protein deficiency is rare in the United States and other industrialized nations today.

Will It Harm You? What the Studies Say:

The wisdom of taking any single amino acid in isolated doses is very controversial. Over time, an imbalance in other amino acids or their ability to function properly may occur. Interestingly, this is a particular risk for people whose diets are very poor. The deaths of dozens of people who took supplements containing a single amino acid—L-tryptophan (see **L-Tryptophan**)—in the late 1980s also haunt this practice. (The cases involved contamination of the supplements.) Much remains to be learned about the risks of taking any single amino acid in high doses over time.

Individuals who take monoamine oxidase (MAO) inhibitors, such as certain antidepressants, should limit their intake of tyrosine-containing foods and dietary supplements, given the risk of a potentially fatal increase in blood pressure. Foods rich in tyrosine include almonds, bananas, cheese, peanuts, and sesame seeds. Consult your doctor for dietary guidance.

GENERAL SOURCES:
Balch, J.F., and P.A. Balch. *Prescription for Nutritional Healing: A Practical A to Z Reference to Drug-Free Remedies Using Vitamins, Minerals, Herbs & Food Supplements.* 2nd ed. Garden City Park, NY: Avery Publishing Group, 1997.
Barrett, S., and V. Herbert. *The Vitamin Pushers: How the "Health Food" Industry Is Selling America a Bill of Goods.* Amherst, NY: Prometheus Books, 1994.
Griffith, H.W. *Complete Guide to Vitamins, Minerals, Nutrients & Supplements.* Tucson: Fisher Books, 1988.
Mayell, M. *Off-the-Shelf Natural Health: How to Use Herbs and Nutrients to Stay Well.* New York, NY: Bantam Books, 1995.

UVA URSI

SCIENTIFIC NAME:

Arctostaphylos uva ursi L. Spreng. Also referred to as *Arbutus uva ursi* L. The related plants *Arbutus adenotricha* and *Arbutus coactylis* Fern et Macbr. have also been referred to as uva ursi by some authors. Family: Ericaceae

COMMON NAMES:

Arbutus, bearberry, beargrape, hogberry, kinnikinnick, manzanita, mealberry, rockberry, upland cranberry

RATING:

3 = Studies on the effectivess and safety of this herb are conflicting, or there are not enough studies to draw a conclusion.

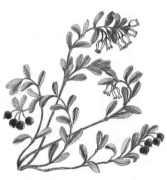

Uva Ursi
Arctostaphylos uva ursi

What Is Uva Ursi?

This low-growing evergreen shrub develops in colonies throughout the northern hemisphere from North America to Europe and Asia. Bright red or pink fruit the size of currants, as well as clusters of pink or white flowers, develop off the creeping stems. But it is the dark, fleshy, leathery dried leaves and extracts from them that are used medicinally. The plant is commonly known as bearberry in the United States.

What It Is Used For:

Uva ursi has long been used in folk medicine as a urinary antiseptic and astringent. Traditional healers through the decades and in far-flung parts of the globe have independently recommended it for toning the urinary tract in inflammatory conditions such as cystitis and urethritis, as well as for treating bronchitis, kidney infections, and kidney stones. The *U.S. Pharmacopoeia* listed the plant as a urinary antiseptic for more than a century from 1820 to 1936.

Contemporary herbalists carry on a tradition in recommending the herb as a diuretic ("water pill") for fluid retention, bloating, and swelling. In fact, few modern herbal diuretic herbal blends, many of them billed as weight-loss products, fail to contain this herb.[1] Homeopaths prescribe minute amounts for urinary tract inflammations, among other disorders. (See page 2 for a discussion of homeopathy.) Native Americans reportedly created a smoking mixture called kinnikinnick with tobacco and uva ursi leaves.

Forms Available Include:

Capsule, infusion, leaves, liquid extract, powdered solid extract, tea, tincture.

Dosage Commonly Reported:

The dried leaf is taken in single doses of 1.5 to 2.5 grams each, up to 10 grams a day, corresponding to 400 to 700 milligrams of an important ingredient called arbutin. Many sources recommend allowing the herb to soften in a cup of cold water overnight (which will reduce the level of bitter-tasting and potentially stomach-irritating tannins) and taking it over a period of a few days to one week. Consume a lot of vegetables and fruit during this period. One to three 505-milligram leaf capsules are taken three times a day. The liquid leaf extract is taken in doses of 2 to 4 milliliters.

Will It Work for You? What the Studies Say:

Test-tube research indicates that uva ursi fights organisms responsible for urinary tract infections, such as *Escherichia coli* and *Staphylococcus aureus*,[2] but whether this action is vigorous enough to eliminate a urinary tract infection remains unproven in human trials. The plant also has a mild diuretic action, meaning that it slightly increases urine output. This is considered beneficial in helping to flush out infectious organisms.

Both the antiseptic and the diuretic properties of uva ursi can largely be explained by the presence of glycosides in the leaves, particularly arbutin, which researchers identified in the mid-1800s in concentrations of 5 to 12 percent.

Once inside the urinary tract, arbutin is chemically transformed to release the critical chemical hydroquinone. This substance has proved itself as both a urinary astringent and an antiseptic,[3] but only if it is taken in hefty doses and in the presence of alkaline urine. To ensure alkaline urine, eat alkaline-rich foods such as milk, vegetables, noncitrus fruits, and even sodium bicarbonate, and avoid such acid-rich foods as citrus fruits and vitamin C supplements.[4] Apparently, preparations containing the crude drug are more effective as antiseptics and astringents than those containing only the extracted arbutin.[5] The astringent properties of the leaves can be attributed to the relatively high levels of tannin (15 to 20 percent).

The introduction of more powerful drugs for urinary tract infections ended the widespread use of uva ursi for this ailment. German health authorities, however, still approve of the plant for treating inflammatory conditions of the urinary tract.[6]

Some researchers have brought into question the diuretic powers of uva ursi, with one study indicating that it inhibits increased urine output.[7] But other scientists report the presence of additional diuretic components, such as ursolic acid.[8] Most responsible herbalists do not recommend diuretics for weight reduction, as any lost weight is transitory. In any case, most conditions requiring a diuretic are serious enough to merit consultation with a medical professional.

Will It Harm You? What the Studies Say:

Uva ursi appears to be relatively safe to take in recommended amounts for brief periods of time. It may turn the urine greenish-brown, but this is considered harmless. A small number of people may develop nausea and vomiting,[9] especially children and people with sensitive stomachs.[10] Avoid taking uva ursi for longer than a week, however, or in high doses, given the potentially stomach-irritating elements in the herb (the tannins) as well as the potential toxicity of hydroquinone. In very large doses—many times the 1 gram of crude uva ursi found in most commercial products—hydroquinone can cause adverse reactions including nausea, vomiting, tinnitus (ringing in the ears), cyanosis, convulsions, collapse, and death in some cases.[11]

Take all kidney and bladder infections seriously; they can cause complications if not promptly and properly treated. Call a doctor if symptoms of a urinary tract infection persist for more than forty-eight hours.[12] Pregnant and nursing women may want to avoid the herb altogether, given the lack of data on safety. In 1986, a branch of the Canadian government issued a report advising that food preparations containing uva ursi be labeled to alert pregnant women to avoid them.[13] The FDA had placed uva ursi on its formerly maintained list of "Herbs of Undefined Safety."

GENERAL SOURCES:

American Pharmaceutical Association. *Handbook of Nonprescription Drugs.* 11th ed. Washington, D.C.: American Pharmaceutical Association, 1996.

Blumenthal, M., J. Gruenwald, T. Hall, and R.S. Rister, eds. *The Complete German Commission E Monographs: Therapeutic Guide to Herbal Medicine.* Boston: Integrative Medicine Communications, 1998.

Bradley, P.C., ed. *British Herbal Compendium: A Handbook of Scientific Information on Widely Used Plant Drugs*, vol. 1. Bournemouth (Dorset), England: British Herbal Medicine Association, 1992.

Castleman, M. *The Healing Herbs: The Ultimate Guide to the Curative Power of Nature's Medicines*. New York: Bantam Books, 1995.

Dobelis, I.N., ed. *The Magic and Medicine of Plants: A Practical Guide to the Science, History, Folklore, and Everyday Uses of Medicinal Plants*. Pleasantville, NY: Reader's Digest Association, 1986.

Griffith, H.W. *Complete Guide to Vitamins, Minerals, Nutrients & Supplements*. Tucson: Fisher Books, 1988.

Lawrence Review of Natural Products. St. Louis: Facts and Comparisons, September 1987.

Leung, A.Y., and S. Foster. *Encyclopedia of Common Natural Ingredients Used in Food, Drugs, and Cosmetics*. 2nd ed. New York: John Wiley & Sons, 1996.

Murray, M.T. *The Healing Power of Herbs: The Enlightened Person's Guide to the Wonders of Medicinal Plants*. Revised and expanded 2nd ed. Rocklin, CA: Prima Publishing, 1995.

Newall, C.A., et al. *Herbal Medicines: A Guide for Health-Care Professionals*. London: The Pharmaceutical Press, 1996.

Tyler, V.E. *Herbs of Choice: The Therapeutic Use of Phytomedicinals*. Binghamton, NY: Haworth Press/Pharmaceutical Products Press, 1994.

———. *The Honest Herbal*. Binghamton, NY: Haworth Press/Pharmaceutical Products Press, 1993.

Weiner, M.A., and J.A. Weiner. *Herbs That Heal: Prescription for Herbal Healing*. Mill Valley, CA: Quantum Books, 1994.

Weiss, R.F. *Herbal Medicine*, trans. A.R. Meuss, from the 6th German edition. Beaconsfield, England: Beaconsfield Publishers, Ltd., 1988.

TEXT CITATIONS:

1. *Lawrence Review of Natural Products* (St. Louis: Facts and Comparisons, September 1987).
2. S.A. Moskalenko, *Journal of Ethnopharmacology*, 15 (1986): 31–59.
3. D. Forhne, *Planta Medica*, 178 (1970): 23–25. C.A. Newall et al., *Herbal Medicines: A Guide for Health-Care Professionals* (London: The Pharmaceutical Press, 1996).
4. V.E. Tyler, *The Honest Herbal* (Binghamton, NY: Haworth Press/Pharmaceutical Products Press, 1993).
5. Newall, op. cit.
6. M. Blumenthal, J. Gruenwald, T. Hall, and R.S. Rister, eds., *The Complete German Commission E Monographs: Therapeutic Guide to Herbal Medicine* (Boston: Integrative Medicine Communications, 1998).
7. B. Borkowski, *Planta Medica*, 8 (1960): 95–104.
8. Tyler, op. cit.
9. American Pharmaceutical Association, *Handbook of Nonprescription Drugs*, 11th ed. (Washington, D.C.: American Pharmaceutical Association, 1996).
10. Blumenthal et al., op. cit.
11. *Lawrence Review of Natural Products*, op. cit.
12. Newall, op. cit.
13. *Lawrence Review of Natural Products*, op. cit.

SCIENTIFIC NAME:
Valeriana officinalis L. and related *Valeriana* species, including *Valeriana wallichii.* Family: Valerianaceae

COMMON NAMES:
All-heal, Belgian valerian, common valerian, fragrant valerian, garden heliotrope, garden valerian, Indian valerian. *Valeriana wallichii:* radix valerianae

RATING:
1 = Years of use and extensive, high-quality studies indicate that this substance is very effective and safe when used in recommended amounts for the indication(s) noted in the "Will It Work for You?" section.

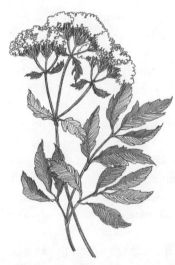

Valerian
Valeriana officinalis

What Is Valerian?

Valerian consists of the dried rhizomes (underground stems) and roots of *Valeriana officinalis,* a tall perennial that grows in temperate regions of North America, Europe, and Asia. Clusters of tiny white or reddish flowers bloom in summer. The herb emits an unpleasant odor as it dries. There are about 250 *Valeriana* species, but *V. officinalis* is the species most frequently cultivated for medicinal use.

Do not confuse valerian, which is essentially a mild sedative derived from plants, with Valium™, the trade name of a powerful synthetic drug.

What It Is Used For:

Valerian has been used for more than one thousand years as a sedative and calmative. In medieval Europe it was popular for treating epilepsy and plague. It is known as the "Valium of the nineteenth century." The *U.S. Pharmacopoeia* listed it as a tranquilizer from 1820 until 1942, when more powerful sedatives known as benzodiazepines took over. Valerian has a distinct advantage over benzodiazepines, however: it is not addictive.

Today, valerian continues to be recommended for treating anxiety, relaxing the body, promoting sleep, damping nervous tension, and helping to control panic attacks, headaches, and intestinal and menstrual cramps. More than one hundred drugs and teas sold in Europe contain valerian and its extracts. It is also a popular over-the-counter sedative in Japan. Topical formulations have been used to treat pimples and skin sores.

Forms Available Include:

- *For internal use:* Capsule, decoction, dried root, infusion, juice (from the pressed plant), liquid extract, tincture.
- *For external use:* Bath additive.

To ensure effectiveness, use only the highest-quality valerian product, one made from the fresh root that has been recently and carefully dried at a low temperature, for example.[1]

Dosage Commonly Reported:

Valerian is commonly taken in dosages of 2 to 3 grams one to three times per day. Three 475-milligram root capsules are taken three times a day or before going to bed. A tea is made using 1 teaspoon (2 to 3 grams) of the root per cup of water. The tincture or extract is taken in doses of ½ to 1 teaspoon, or 3 to 5 milliliters.

Will It Work for You? What the Studies Say:

Valerian is best characterized as a mild sedative. Numerous studies have borne this out.[2] Clinical trials have shown that the herb both improves the quality of sleep and shortens the time it takes to fall asleep.[3] The study assessing the quality of sleep involved 128 individuals who were given 400 milligrams of valerian extract—a commercial valerian product—or a placebo. Neither the subjects nor the investigators knew which subjects were taking the drug or the placebo, thus ruling out bias and strengthening the study findings. Interestingly, while the subjects taking valerian experienced improved quality of sleep, they woke up as often during the night and felt just as sleepy the next morning as the subjects who took a placebo. The study that showed shortened time to fall asleep unfortunately involved only eight subjects. In Germany, valerian is officially approved for treating sleep disturbances due to excitability and generalized restlessness.[4]

Despite intense research over the past decades, investigators have been unable to determine exactly which ingredients in valerian are responsible for its tranquilizing, sedative, and calmative effects. A mixture of compounds is probably responsible, rather than one ingredient in particular.[5] Animal studies indicate that the herb reduces blood pressure and may have anticonvulsant properties, but large-scale studies in human beings do not appear to have been done. Recent experiments show that valerian depresses (slows down) the central nervous system in laboratory animals,[6] probably owing to the effect of a group of compounds called valeportriates. These also have antispasmodic actions in laboratory animals.[7] The active constituents of valerian appear to bind weakly to benzodiazepine receptors in the body, which may be why it does not lead to the dependence or addiction seen with benzodiazepine sedatives such as diazepam and alprazolam.[8] It does not cause withdrawal symptoms.

Researchers conducting test-tube and animal studies have also found that valerian can fight certain bacteria and protect against experimentally induced liver necrosis (tissue death).[9] Whether these actions occur in humans taking valerian demands further investigation.

Will It Harm You? What the Studies Say:

So far, studies indicate that valerian, when used in recommended amounts, causes no significant side effects, although specific toxicity studies do not appear to have been done. It apparently does not cause loss of coordination,[10] and it is not addictive. In Europe, where valerian is widely used, authorities cite no contraindications to its use.[11] The FDA includes valerian on its list of foods "Generally Recognized As Safe" (GRAS).

Symptoms of overdose may include paralysis, weakening of the heartbeat, giddiness, light-headedness, blurred vision, restlessness, nausea, and possibly liver toxicity. A woman who attempted suicide with valerian—she swallowed forty to fifty capsules of powdered valerian containing 470 milligrams each (about twenty times the recommended amount)—experienced chest tightness, fatigue, stomach cramping, and tremors, but all passed within twenty-four hours.[12]

Even though alcohol and barbituates do not appear to significantly exaggerate the effects of valerian—a rodent study indicated that adding alcohol to valerian did not increase the sedative effect[13]—one should avoid taking them with valerian.[14] Exercise extra care when driving or operating machinery. Substances in valerian called valepotriates have shown cell-toxic and mutation-causing properties in test-tube studies,[15] but whether this puts the average user at risk is far from clear, particularly considering that valepotriates may well degrade in your body when you take them orally.[16]

Although no adverse reactions or birth defects have been linked to the use of valerian during pregnancy or nursing, the subject has not been properly studied[17]; err on the side of caution.

GENERAL SOURCES:

American Pharmaceutical Association. *Handbook of Nonprescription Drugs*. 11th ed. Washington, D.C.: American Pharmaceutical Association, 1996.

Blumenthal, M., J. Gruenwald, T. Hall, and R.S. Rister, eds. *The Complete German Commission E Monographs: Therapeutic Guide to Herbal Medicine*. Boston: Integrative Medicine Communications, 1998.

Bradley, P.C., ed. *British Herbal Compendium: A Handbook of Scientific Information on Widely Used Plant Drugs*, vol. 1. Bournemouth (Dorset), England: British Herbal Medicine Association, 1992.

Foster, S. *Valerian: Valeriana officinalis*. American Botanical Council's Botanical Series No. 312. 1990.

Leung, A.Y., and S. Foster. *Encyclopedia of Common Natural Ingredients Used in Food, Drugs, and Cosmetics*. 2nd ed. New York: John Wiley & Sons, 1996.

Mayell, M. *Off-the-Shelf Natural Health: How to Use Herbs and Nutrients to Stay Well*. New York: Bantam Books, 1995.

Murray, M.T. *The Healing Power of Herbs: The Enlightened Person's Guide to the Wonders of Medicinal Plants*. Revised and expanded 2nd ed. Rocklin, CA: Prima Publishing, 1995.

Newall, C.A., et al. *Herbal Medicines: A Guide for Health-Care Professionals*. London: The Pharmaceutical Press, 1996.

Stary, F. *The Natural Guide to Medicinal Herbs and Plants*. Prague: Barnes & Noble, Inc., in arrangement with Aventinum Publishers, 1996.

Tierra, M. *The Way of Herbs*. New York: Pocket Books, 1990.

Tyler, V.E. *Herbs of Choice: The Therapeutic Use of Phytomedicinals*. Binghamton, NY: Haworth Press/Pharmaceutical Products Press, 1994.

———. *The Honest Herbal*. Binghamton, NY: Haworth Press/Pharmaceutical Products Press, 1993.

Tyler, V.E., L.R. Brady, and J.E. Robbers, eds. *Pharmacognosy*. Philadelphia: Lea & Febiger, 1988.

Weiss, R.F. *Herbal Medicine*, trans. A.R. Meuss, from the 6th German edition. Beaconsfield, England: Beaconsfield Publishers, Ltd., 1988.

TEXT CITATIONS:

1. V.E. Tyler, *The Honest Herbal* (Binghamton, NY: Haworth Press/Pharmaceutical Products Press, 1993).

2. P.C. Bradley, ed., *British Herbal Compendium: A Handbook of Scientific Information on Widely Used Plant Drugs*, vol. 1 (Bournemouth [Dorset], England: British Herbal Medicine Association, 1992).

3. P.D. Leathwood et al., *Pharmacology, Biochemestry & Behavior*, 17 (1982): 65–71. P.D. Leathwood, *Planta Medica*, (1985): 144–48.

4. M. Blumenthal, J. Gruenwald, T. Hall, and R.S. Rister, eds., *The Complete German Commission E Monographs: Therapeutic Guide to Herbal Medicine* (Boston: Integrative Medicine Communications, 1998).

5. Tyler, op. cit. J. Krieglstein and D. Grusia, *Deutsche Apotheker Zeitung*, 128 (1988): 2041–46.

6. A.Y. Leung and S. Foster, *Encyclopedia of Common Natural Ingredients Used in Food, Drugs, and Cosmetics*, 2nd ed. (New York: John Wiley & Sons, 1996).

7. Ibid.

8. D.J. Brown, *Quarterly Review of Natural Medicine* (Fall 1994).

9. Leung and Foster, op. cit.

10. T. Sakamoto et al., *Chemical & Pharmaceutical Bulletin*, 40(3) (1992): 758–61.
11. Blumenthal et al., op. cit. Bradley, op. cit.
12. L.B. Willey, *Veterinary and Human Toxicology*, 37(4) (1995): 364–65.
13. K.W. Von Eickstedt, *Arzneimittel-Forschung*, 19 (1969): 995.
14. Bradley, op. cit.
15. C. Bounthanh et al., *Planta Medica*. 41 (1981): 21.
16. Leung and Foster, op. cit. Bradley, op. cit.
17. P.J. Houghton, *Pharmaceutical Journal*, 253 (1994): 95–96.

VERVAIN

SCIENTIFIC NAME:

Verbena officinalis L. (European) and *Verbena hastata* (North American). Family: Verbenaceae

COMMON NAMES:

Bastard balm, blue vervain, devil's medicine, enchanter's herb, herb-of-the-cross, holy wort, Indian hyssop, ma bian cao, pigeon's-grass, Simpler's joy, verbena

RATING:

3 = Studies on the effectiveness and safety of this substance are conflicting, or there are not enough studies to draw a conclusion.

V

Vervain

What Is Vervain?

Verbena officinalis and *Verbena hastata* represent only two of hundreds of species in the family Verbenaceae. These common perennials grow wild in temperate regions around the world. Slender flowering spikes emerge off thin, stiff stems; the lilac or blue color of the small flowers accounts for the common American name, "blue vervain." The flowers, the roots, and the oblong leaves are used medicinally.

What It Is Used For:

This ancient herb has a long and complicated history as a folk medicine and ceremonial herb. Many cultures attributed magical properties to it. Europeans, Chinese, and Native Americans reportedly used it widely, often as a cure-all. The multiplicity of uses for which contemporary herbalists recommend the herb is nearly as remarkable and often reflects popular past uses as a digestive aid, relaxing tonic, antidepressant, menstruation promoter, expectorant for cold symptoms (to clear congestion), diuretic ("water pill") for swelling, and breast-milk stimulator. Convalescents—especially those suffering from depression—were once fed vervain brews. Many of today's herbalists consider it a good choice for nervous exhaustion, jaundice, menstrual cramps, headaches (including migraines), depression, fever, and minor pains and inflammations. External formulations are recommended as astringents for wounds, acne, and skin ulcers. Vervain has even been used as a toothpaste.

Forms Available Include:

- *For internal use:* Herb, fresh and dried; infusion (of dried herb); liquid extract; tea bag; tincture.
- *For external use:* Compress, poultice, powder for toothpaste.

Dosage Commonly Reported:

An infusion made using 1 teaspoon dried herb in a cup of water is drunk up to four times per day. The liquid herb extract is taken in doses of 2 to 4 milliliters.

Will It Work for You? What the Studies Say:

Researchers have not focused on vervain since the 1930s and 1940s. Enthusiasts often cite findings from that time, when scientific research standards were somewhat different. The validity of some of the findings—as well as implications for human health—remains unclear. No study involved human subjects. Researchers in those years demonstrated that bitter iridoid glycosides in the herb, including verbenalin, have anti-inflammatory and painkilling actions in laboratory animals.[1] Investigators reported in 1938 that verbenaloside acts as a weak parasympathomimetic in laboratory dogs,[2] but whether this means that it will calm nervousness or reduce nervous exhaustion in humans, as some contemporary herbalists assert,[3] is far from clear.

In 1943, researchers reported that vervain has a diuretic action in rats,[4] and that the constituent verbenalin lowers blood pressure slightly and contracts the isolated uterus of the guinea pig.[5] The same year, investigators comparing vervain extracts in small animals found that certain formulations of the herb demonstrated superior anti-inflammatory or painkilling actions.[6] Many modern plant experts consider these findings inconclusive or poorly substantiated. German health authorities decline to approve of vervain for any ailment, although they note its potential value as a secretolytic for upper respiratory tract congestion (meaning that it will help break up secretions).[7] A relatively recent study indicates that verbenalin has anticough properties.[8]

Several studies indicate that the herb may affect the uterus, although much about this remains unclear. In 1974, Chinese researchers reported that rat uteruses placed in chemical baths started to develop contractions when exposed to the herb.[9] Years before, researchers had reported similar findings with rabbit intestines and guinea pig uteruses exposed to verbenaloside.[10] A substance in the herb called aucubin has been found to have galactagogue (breast-milk-stimulating) properties.[11] Interestingly, in tropical West Africa, extracts of the vervain fruit are used to stimulate breast milk and treat menstrual pain.[12]

Will It Harm You? What the Studies Say:

Vervain poses no known health risks when used in typically recommended doses,[13] but relatively little is known about its potential toxicity. Therefore, it should be used carefully. To be on the safe side, avoid using it in large or excessive amounts. This may be particularly important for those taking blood pressure medicine or on hormone therapy, as the herb may interfere with these.[14] Pregnant women should avoid the herb, given its still poorly defined effects on the uterus. The FDA places *Verbena officinalis* on its list of food ingredients "Generally Recognized As Safe" (GRAS), but it put *Verbena hastata* on its formerly maintained list of "Herbs of Undefined Safety."

GENERAL SOURCES:

Bisset, N.G., ed. *Herbal Drugs and Phytopharmaceuticals*. Stuttgart: medpharm GmbH Scientific Publishers, 1994.

Blumenthal, M., J. Gruenwald, T. Hall, and R.S. Rister, eds. *The Complete German Commission E Monographs: Therapeutic Guide to Herbal Medicine*. Boston: Integrative Medicine Communications, 1998.

Bremness, L. *Herbs*. 1st American ed. Eyewitness Handbooks. New York: Dorling Kindersley Publications, 1994.

Castleman, M. *The Healing Herbs: The Ultimate Guide to the Curative Power of Nature's Medicines*. New York: Bantam Books, 1995.

V

Vervain

Chevallier, A. *The Encyclopedia of Medicinal Plants: A Practical Reference Guide to More Than 550 Key Medicinal Plants & Their Uses.* 1st American ed. New York: Dorling Kindersley Publications, 1996.

Hallowell, M. *Herbal Healing: A Practical Introduction to Medicinal Herbs.* Garden City Park, NY, 1994.

Mowrey, D.B. *Proven Herbal Blends: A Rational Approach to Prevention and Remedy.* (Condensed from *The Scientific Validation of Herbal Medicine.*) New Canaan, CT: Keats Publishing, Inc., 1986.

Newall, C.A., et al. *Herbal Medicines: A Guide for Health-Care Professionals.* London: The Pharmaceutical Press, 1996.

Stary, F. *The Natural Guide to Medicinal Herbs and Plants.* Prague: Barnes & Noble, Inc., in arrangement with Aventinum Publishers, 1996.

Tierra, M. *The Way of Herbs.* New York: Pocket Books, 1990.

Weiss, R.F. *Herbal Medicine*, trans. A.R. Meuss, from the 6th German edition. Beaconsfield, England: Beaconsfield Publishers, Ltd., 1988.

TEXT CITATIONS:

1. N.G. Bisset, ed., *Herbal Drugs and Phytopharmaceuticals* (Stuttgart: medpharm GmbH Scientific Publishers, 1994).
2. J. Cheymol, *J Pharm Chim*, 27 (1938): 374–86.
3. D.B. Mowrey, *Proven Herbal Blends: A Rational Approach to Prevention and Remedy*, (Condensed from *The Scientific Validation of Herbal Medicine;* New Canaan, CT: Keats Publishing, Inc., 1986). A. Chevallier, *The Encylopedia of Medicinal Plants: A Practical Reference Guide to More Than 550 Key Medicinal Plants & Their Uses*, 1st American ed. (New York: Dorling Kindersley Publications, 1996).
4. K. Breitwieser, *Pharms Ind*, 10 (1943): 76–78.
5. C.J. Zufall and W.O. Richtmann, *Archives of Pharmacology Research*, 14 (1943): 65–80, 81–96.
6. S. Sakai, *Gifu Ika Daigaku Kiyo*, 11(1) (1963): 6–17.
7. M. Blumenthal, J. Gruenwald, T. Hall, and R.S. Rister, eds., *The Complete German Commission E Monographs: Therapeutic Guide to Herbal Medicine* (Boston: Integrative Medicine Communications, 1998).
8. C. Kui and R. Tang, *Zhongyao Tongbao*, 10 (1985): 467.
9. *Tung Wu Hsueh Pao*, Research Group on Reproductive Physiology, 20(4) (1974): 340–45.
10. Cheymol, op. cit.
11. M.F. Lahloub et al., *Planta Medica*, 52 (1986): 47.
12. C.A. Newall et al., *Herbal Medicines: A Guide for Health-Care Professionals* (London: The Pharmaceutical Press, 1996).
13. Blumenthal et al., op. cit.
14. Newall, op. cit.

WATERCRESS

SCIENTIFIC NAME:
Nasturtium officinale R. BR,
sometimes referred to as
Rorippa nasturtium-aquaticum.
Family: Cruciferae

COMMON NAME:
Water pepper

RATING:
3 = Studies on the effectiveness
and safety of this substance are
conflicting, or there are not
enough studies to draw a
conclusion.

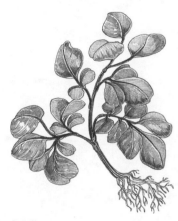

Watercress
Nasturtium officinale

What Is Watercress?

This hardy, well-known perennial has small, pungent leaflets and white flowers with yellow anthers and brown seeds. It belongs to the mustard family and grows in and around water throughout temperate regions of the world. The aboveground parts are used medicinally. Watercress bears no relation to the ornamental plant commonly referred to as nasturtium (*Tropaeolum majus*).

What It Is Used For:

Since ancient times, people have not only enjoyed the faintly spicy and slightly bitter taste of watercress in their salads and other foods, but have hailed it as a natural tonic and digestive aid. Watercress juice and other preparations have been touted as "spring cures" to stimulate the metabolism and nervous system, boost the appetite, relieve indigestion, increase urination (as a diuretic, or "water pill"), strengthen the body overall, cleanse the blood and skin, stave off scurvy (it contains high stores of vitamin C), combat nervousness, and relieve coughs and respiratory congestion. Extracts appear in European cholagogues (to increase bile flow).

Forms Available Include:

Fresh herb (whole or chopped), infusion, juice (freshly pressed). Also available as an ingredient in herbal blends sold in capsule form.

Dosage Commonly Reported:

Watercress is consumed as part of the diet, often in salads. From 20 to 30 grams of fresh herb is consumed daily. The freshly pressed juice is taken in daily doses of 60 to 150 grams. An infusion is made by pouring boiling water over 2 grams of the fresh herb and straining after ten minutes.

Will It Work for You? What the Studies Say:

Many of the traditional uses for watercress have not been examined. German health authorities endorse its use for respiratory tract congestion and inflammation.[1] This endorsement is presumably based on the presence of small amounts of mustard-oil glycosides, but the scientific justification for the decision is not clear.

Research indicates that watercress contains rich stores of a substance—gluconasturtiin, a precursor of phenethyl isothiocyanate (PEITC)—that may help prevent the development of lung cancer in smokers. PEITC is released upon chewing of watercress. It has been shown to be protective against lung cancer induced by a tobacco-specific carcinogen known as NNK. This was first observed in mice and then demonstrated in humans.[2] Research on this promising subject continues.

Watercress contains the vitamins A, B_1, B_2, C, and E, various minerals, mustard-oil glycosides, and other glucosinolates. A number of these vitamins and other important ingredients disintegrate with storage, which explains why many herbalists recommend the fresh juice.[3] Vitamin content appears to fluctuate throughout the year.

Will It Harm You? What the Studies Say:

Although widely considered a safe medicinal herb, stomach and intestinal upset can develop when watercress is eaten in large amounts or for extended periods of time. The mustard-oil glycosides are responsible for this irritation.[4] German health authorities advise that children under four and people with gastric and duodenal ulcers or inflammatory kidney disorders should avoid watercress in medicinal concentrations.[5]

There have also been several reports of a parasitic infection involving the liver— *Fasciola hepatica* infection—developing in people who consumed wild watercress.[6] Symptoms in many cases included fever, abdominal pain, weight loss, and generalized muscle and joint pain.[7] A number of these reports were from Mexico and South America.

GENERAL SOURCES:

Bisset, N.G., ed. *Herbal Drugs and Phytopharmaceuticals*. Stuttgart: medpharm GmbH Scientific Publishers, 1994.

Blumenthal, M., J. Gruenwald, T. Hall, and R.S. Rister, eds. *The Complete German Commission E Monographs: Therapeutic Guide to Herbal Medicine*. Boston: Integrative Medicine Communications, 1998.

Bremness, L. *Herbs*. 1st American ed. Eyewitness Handbooks. New York: Dorling Kindersley Publications, 1994.

Chevallier, A. *The Encyclopedia of Medicinal Plants: A Practical Reference Guide to More Than 550 Key Medicinal Plants & Their Uses*. 1st American ed. New York: Dorling Kindersley Publications, 1996.

Dobelis, I.N., ed. *The Magic and Medicine of Plants: A Practical Guide to the Science, History, Folklore, and Everyday Uses of Medicinal Plants*. Pleasantville, NY: Reader's Digest Association, 1986.

Hylton, W.H., ed. *The Rodale Herb Book: How to Use, Grow, and Buy Nature's Miracle Plants*. Emmaus, PA: Rodale Press, Inc., 1974.

Weiss, R.F. *Herbal Medicine*, trans. A. R. Meuss, from the 6th German edition. Beaconsfield, England: Beaconsfield Publishers, Ltd., 1988.

TEXT CITATIONS:

1. M. Blumenthal, J. Gruenwald, T. Hall, and R.S. Rister, eds., *The Complete German Commission E Monographs: Therapeutic Guide to Herbal Medicine* (Boston: Integrative Medicine Communications, 1998).

2. S.S. Hecht, *Advances in Experimental Medicine & Biology*, 401 (1996): 1–11. F.L. Chung et al., *Cancer Epidemiology, Biomarkers & Prevention*, 1(5) (1992): 383–85.

3. R.F. Weiss, *Herbal Medicine*, trans. A. R. Meuss, from the 6th German edition (Beaconsfield, England: Beaconsfield Publishers, Ltd., 1988). M.G. Serranillos and F. Zaragoza, *An Bromatol,* 23(4) (1971): 402–16.

4. N.G. Bisset, ed. *Herbal Drugs and Phytopharmaceuticals* (Stuttgart: medpharm GmbH Scientific Publishers, 1994).

5. Blumenthal et al., op. cit.

6. J. Sapunar et al., *Boletín Chileno de Parasitiología,* l47(3–4) (1992): 70–76. R. Alvarez-Chacón et al. *Boletín Médico del Hospital Infantil de México,* 49(6) (1992): 365–71. U. Bechtel et al., *Deutsche Medizinische Wochenschrift,* 117(25) (1992): 978–82.

7. M. De Gorgolas et al., *Enfermedades Infecciosas y Microbiología Clínica,* 10(9) (1992): 514–19.

WHITE COHOSH

SCIENTIFIC NAME:
Actaea alba (L.) Mill, sometimes referred to as *Alba pachypoda* or *Alba rubra* (Alt.) Willd. Family: Ranunculaceae

COMMON NAMES:
Coralberry, doll's eyes, red baneberry

RATING:
5 = Studies indicate that there is a definite health hazard to using this substance, even in recommended amounts.

What Is White Cohosh?

This tall perennial bears sharply toothed leaflets, red- or black-dotted white berries, and round clusters of small white flowers which bloom in late spring. *Alba rubra* grows throughout North America, while *Alba pachypoda* is found primarily on the East Coast. It is not clear which part of the plant was traditionally used medicinally.

What It Is Used For:

In times past, white cohosh had a reputation similar to those of black and blue cohosh[1] for treating menstrual irregularities such as delayed or painful periods, and for triggering and hastening labor. (See **Black Cohosh** and **Blue Cohosh** for information on those herbs.)

Forms Available Include:

Decoction.

Dosage Commonly Reported:

No part of this plant should be used medicinally.

Will It Work for You? What the Studies Say:

Other than identifying an essential oil, research has revealed little about the chemical makeup of this plant and even less about the effect it might have on the human body. The recent medical literature contains no references to studies in test tubes, animals, or humans.

Will It Harm You? What the Studies Say:

Only the roots and berries of white cohosh contain toxic substances (protoanemonin), but experts consider all parts of the plant poisonous and capable of causing headache, stomach cramps, vomiting, fast pulse, and shock (circulatory failure), among other adverse reactions.[2]

GENERAL SOURCES:
Der Marderosian, A., and L. Liberti. *Natural Product Medicine. A Scientific Guide to Foods, Drugs, Cosmetics.* Philadelphia: George F. Stickley, 1988.
Dobelis, I.N., ed. *The Magic and Medicine of Plants: A Practical Guide to the Science, History, Folklore, and Everyday Uses of Medicinal Plants.* Pleasantville, NY: Reader's Digest Association, 1986.
Lawrence Review of Natural Products. St. Louis: Facts and Comparisons, February 1986.

TEXT CITATIONS:
1. A. Der Marderosian and L. Liberti, *Natural Product Medicine. A Scientific Guide to Foods, Drugs, Cosmetics* (Philadelphia: George F. Stickley, 1988).
2. *Lawrence Review of Natural Products.* St. Louis: Facts and Comparisons, February 1986.

WILD CHERRY BARK

SCIENTIFIC NAME:

Prunus serotina Ehrh. Also referred to as *Prunus virginiana* Mill. Family: Rosaceae

COMMON NAMES:

Black cherry, choke cherry, rum cherry bark, Virginia prune bark, wild black cherry

RATING:

2 = According to a number of well-designed studies and common use, this substance appears to be relatively effective and safe when used in recommended amounts for the indication(s) noted in the "Will It Work for You?" section.

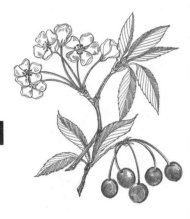

Wild Cherry
Prunus serotina

What Is Wild Cherry Bark?

The wild cherry is a native North American tree which can grow to eighty feet or more. The outer bark is rough and dark. The reddish-brown inner bark of the stems, once dried, is used medicinally. Shiny green oval leaves turn yellow or red in autumn, and long spokes of small white flowers give way to fleshy, blue-black fruits.

What It Is Used For:

Certain Native American tribes reportedly drank wild cherry bark tea to treat colds, coughs, and diarrhea, and valued it for its perceived tranquilizing and sedative effects. Cherokee women drank the tea to battle labor pains. Over time it became known as a general pain reliever. Early settlers picked up on its use for lung ailments in particular, treating whooping cough, bronchitis, pneumonia, and other similar disorders with it. Some were said to use it for cancers. By the 1800s, many Americans were familiar with wild cherry bark preparations. The *U.S. Pharmacopoeia* started listing it as a mild sedative and expectorant to clear congestion.

Herbalists today recommend wild cherry bark for respiratory ailments such as cough, cold, and bronchitis, and some consider it effective as a sedating infusion for anxiety, stress, or sleeplessness. Bark extracts appear in many commercial cough and cold syrups and other preparations, and in a wide array of foods.

The wood is highly valued for making fine furniture and musical instruments, and is used in building for ornamental detailing of such components as mantels, doors, and paneling. The fruit is used in preparing jellies and wines.

Forms Available Include:

Dried inner bark, infusion, syrup, tincture. The cough-relieving elements dissipate with high heat, so never boil it.

Dosage Commonly Reported:

An infusion made using 1 teaspoon powdered bark per cup of water is drunk up to three times per day. The tincture is taken in doses of ¼ to ½ teaspoon up to three times per day. The syrup is taken in doses of 2.5 to 10 milliliters.

Will It Work for You? What the Studies Say:

Wild cherry bark has long been popular in both herbal and conventional medicine to treat chronic dry and irritable coughs, and apparently with good reason. It contains a substance called prunasin which is believed to reduce the cough reflex. As an expectorant, it loosens sticky secretions so that they are easier to cough up. These properties also help explain why it was once commonly prescribed for bronchitis and other lung disorders.

The mild sedative and tranquilizing activity identified in a chemical in the plant—hydrocyanic acid—appears to be irrelevant given that the acid is a poison, at least at doses which would be considered effective in calming you or making you sleepy.[1]

Astringent tannins in the herb[2] may explain its traditional use for treating diarrhea; tannins are believed to control or stop diarrhea by reducing inflammation in the intestines.

Will It Harm You? What the Studies Say:

Taking typically recommended amounts of wild cherry bark has not been linked to serious adverse reactions in humans. However, the bark, leaves, and fruit do contain a chemical similar to cyanide (hydrocyanic acid) that in large doses can cause serious poisoning and even death. The amount of hydrocyanic acid present depends on numerous factors, such as the season in which the plant part was harvested; it has been found in wild cherry extracts.[3] *Never chew the raw bark* . Animals grazing on the leaves, which are more toxic than the bark, have suffered severe adverse reactions.

Pregnant women may want to avoid wild cherry bark preparations given reports of birth defects among offspring of female laboratory animals exposed to the herb, according to one source.[4]

GENERAL SOURCES:

Castleman, M. *The Healing Herbs: The Ultimate Guide to the Curative Power of Nature's Medicines.* New York: Bantam Books, 1995.

Chevallier, A. *The Encyclopedia of Medicinal Plants: A Practical Reference Guide to More Than 550 Key Medicinal Plants & Their Uses.* 1st American ed. New York: Dorling Kindersley Publications, 1996.

Hylton, W.H., ed. *The Rodale Herb Book: How to Use, Grow, and Buy Nature's Miracle Plants.* Emmaus, PA: Rodale Press, Inc., 1974.

Leung, A.Y., and S. Foster. *Encyclopedia of Common Natural Ingredients Used in Food, Drugs, and Cosmetics.* 2nd ed. New York: John Wiley & Sons, 1996.

Tierra, M. *The Way of Herbs.* New York: Pocket Books, 1990.

Weiner, M.A., and J.A. Weiner. *Herbs That Heal: Prescription for Herbal Healing.* Mill Valley, CA: Quantum Books, 1994.

TEXT CITATIONS:

1. A.Y. Leung and S. Foster, *Encyclopedia of Common Natural Ingredients Used in Food, Drugs, and Cosmetics*, 2nd ed. (New York: John Wiley & Sons, 1996).
2. L. Buchalter, *Journal of Pharmaceutical Sciences*, 58(10) (1969): 1272–73. Leung and Foster, op. cit.
3. Leung and Foster, op. cit.
4. M. Castleman, *The Healing Herbs: The Ultimate Guide to the Curative Power of Nature's Medicines* (New York: Bantam Books, 1995).

WILD OREGON GRAPE

SCIENTIFIC NAME:

Berberis aquifolium Pursh., sometimes referred to as

What Is Wild Oregon Grape?

This evergreen shrub is native to the Rocky Mountain regions. It has branched, holly-like leaves and can grow to ten feet or more. The dried rhizomes (underground stems) and roots are used medicinally. The plant is a relative of the European barberry (*Berberis vulgaris* L.); see **Barberry** for more information on that herb.

Mahonia aquifolium Nutt.
Family: Berberidaceae

COMMON NAMES:
California barberry, holly-leaf
barberry, Rocky Mountain
grape, trailing mahonia

RATING:
3 = Studies on the effectiveness
and safety of this substance are
conflicting, or there are not
enough studies to draw a
conclusion. However, see the
"Will It Harm You?" section for
dosage warnings.

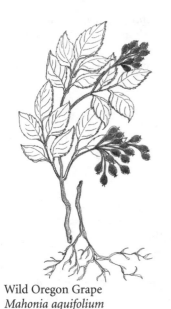

Wild Oregon Grape
Mahonia aquifolium

What It Is Used For:

Many Native American tribes made a decoction of parts of this plant to stimulate the appetite and treat cough, kidney disorders, ulcers, liver ailments, constipation, and fluid retention (as a diuretic, or "water pill"). They regarded it as a tonic for overall weakness. Settlers used it similarly and as a wash for bruises and cuts, and to treat acne, eczema, psoriasis, and other chronic skin conditions. The European **Barberry** (*Berberis vulgaris*), which the settlers introduced, was counted on for the same types of disorders, as was the closely related, indigenous goldenseal plant (*Hydrastis canadensis*; see **Goldenseal**).

Official U.S. pharmacopoeias listed the plant as a bitter tonic up until the middle of the twentieth century. Contemporary herbalists emphasize the plant's purported value in treating hepatitis, jaundice, and other liver conditions, as well as in "purifying" the blood (often a euphemism for venereal disease cures). They also still consider external formulations good for treating skin conditions, particularly psoriasis. Homeopaths prescribe it in minute doses for various ailments. (See page 2 for a discussion of homeopathy.)

Forms Available Include:

Compress, decoction, extract, powdered root bark, tincture, wash.

Dosage Commonly Reported:

A decoction made using ½ teaspoon powdered root bark per cup of water is drunk once per day or used in a compress. The liquid root extract is taken in 1- to 2-milliliter doses.

Will It Work for You? What the Studies Say:

Given the likeness in chemical makeup among wild Oregon grape, barberry, goldenseal, and other *Berberis* species, very similar pharmacological activity can be expected from them all. Most important, all contain high concentrations of berberine, a widely studied substance, and other isoquinoline alkaloids. See **Barberry** for more information on what to expect from wild Oregon grape.

Researchers have identified an apparently unique property in wild Oregon grape: an antioxidant action in the bark extract that appears to make the herb beneficial in treating psoriasis.[1] Investigators have also identified antifungal properties in the plant that may further explain its traditional use for skin disorders.[2] Astringent tannins are likely contribute as well by constricting (tightening) skin and mucous membrane tissue and reducing oozing, helping the skin to heal.

Will It Harm You? What the Studies Say:

Wild Oregon grape has not been carefully studied in humans, so no one knows whether or not it is truly safe. On the other hand, people have used it for generations. Berberine and berberine-containing plants overall are considered nontoxic at recommended doses. But higher berberine doses—greater than 0.5 grams—have been associated with skin and eye irritation, nosebleeds, shortness of breath, lethargy, nausea, vomiting, and diarrhea.[3] Kidney irritation and inflammation has also been reported, and there have been cases of fatal poisonings in humans.[4] Normal metabolism of vitamin B may be altered with high doses. Pregnant women should probably avoid the herb given still unconfirmed reports that it can stimulate the uterine muscles.

GENERAL SOURCES:

Balch, J.F., and P.A. Balch. *Prescription for Nutritional Healing: A Practical A to Z Reference to Drug-Free Remedies Using Vitamins, Minerals, Herbs & Food Supplements.* 2nd ed. Garden City Park, NY: Avery Publishing Group, 1997.

Castleman, M. *The Healing Herbs: The Ultimate Guide to the Curative Power of Nature's Medicines.* New York: Bantam Books, 1995.

Duke, J.A. *CRC Handbook of Medicinal Herbs.* Boca Raton, FL: CRC Press, 1985.

Blumenthal, M., J. Gruenwald, T. Hall, and R.S. Rister, eds. *The Complete German Commission E Monographs: Therapeutic Guide to Herbal Medicine.* Boston: Integrative Medicine Communications, 1998.

Hylton, W.H., ed. *The Rodale Herb Book: How to Use, Grow, and Buy Nature's Miracle Plants.* Emmaus, PA: Rodale Press, Inc., 1974.

Mindell, E. *Earl Mindell's Herb Bible.* New York: Simon & Schuster/Fireside, 1992.

Murray, M.T. *The Healing Power of Herbs: The Enlightened Person's Guide to the Wonders of Medicinal Plants.* Revised and expanded 2nd ed. Rocklin, CA: Prima Publishing, 1995.

Weiner, M.A., and J.A. Weiner. *Herbs That Heal: Prescription for Herbal Healing.* Mill Valley, CA: Quantum Books, 1994.

TEXT CITATIONS:

1. L. Bezakova et al., *Pharmazie*, 51(10) (1996): 758–61. U. Misik et al., *Planta Medica*, 61(4) (1995): 372–73. K. Muller et al., *Planta Medica*, 61(1) (1995): 74–75.
2. A.R. McCutcheon et al., *Journal of Ethnopharmacology*, 44(3) (1994): 157–69.
3. M. Blumenthal, J. Gruenwald, T. Hall, and R.S. Rister, eds., *The Complete German Commission E Monographs: Therapeutic Guide to Herbal Medicine* (Boston: Integrative Medicine Communications, 1998).
4. Ibid.

PRIMARY·NAME:

WILD STRAWBERRY

SCIENTIFIC NAME:

Fragaria vesca L. Family: Rosaceae

COMMON NAMES:

Woodland strawberry, wood strawberry

RATING:

4 = Research indicates that this substance will not fulfill the claims made for it, but that it is also unlikely to cause any harm.

What Is Wild Strawberry?

This low-growing perennial spreads by means of underground runners. Stems emerging above ground sport clusters of bright green three-part leaves. White-petaled flowers appear in May and fall off in late summer, at which point the flower receptacle becomes a bright red berry. The leaves, fruit, and root are used medicinally. The plant is native to temperate regions of Europe and Asia and can be found across North America. In Indiana it is classified as a rare and endangered plant.

What It Is Used For:

Wild strawberry leaves are a common substitute for ordinary tea. For generations the plant has also been put to work as a remedy for many ills. It has been widely used in infusion form as a mild astringent for diarrhea and stomach upset and to stimulate the appetite. Many European folk healers attribute cooling and "cleansing" diuretic properties to the leaves as well as the fruits, recommending them for such ailments as arthritis and gout. Contemporary herbalists continue to highly

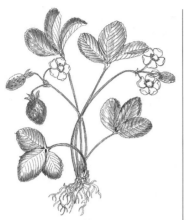

Wild Strawberry
Fragaria vesca

recommend the leaves as "cleansing" diuretics. Externally, leaf preparations have traditionally been used for rashes and wounds, and lotions have been made to apply to minor burns and scrapes. Gargles were concocted to treat sore throats.

The fruits once ranked as a popular cosmetic to whiten the complexion (even helping to lighten freckles), as well as to remove tartar and tooth stains. The fresh fruits are considered laxative. A poultice of crushed berries is applied to skin inflammations and sunburns.

Forms Available Include:

- *For internal use:* Fresh or dried leaves, infusion (of fresh or dried leaves), fruit (fresh), prepared tea. Also appears in numerous herbal blends.
- *For external use:* Fruits, gargle (made with leaves), leaves, poultice (made with fruits).

Dosage Commonly Reported:

An infusion is made using 1 teaspoon chopped leaves per cup of water. To control diarrhea it is drunk several times per day.

Will It Work for You? What the Studies Say:

There is very little scientific data to justify the use of wild strawberry for any of its proposed uses. Herbalists cite the presence of astringent tannins in the leaves to explain its traditional use as a sore throat gargle and diarrhea remedy; tannins constrict tissue and control bleeding and are believed to control or stop diarrhea by reducing inflammation in the intestines. Many other herbs contain higher concentrations of tannins than wild strawberry does, however, and research shows them to be more effective for these purposes. The only study cited in the recent medical literature was done in 1989, and described anti-ulcer properties of extracts (tannins, specifically) from wild strawberry.[1] This property has apparently never been studied in humans, however, and its implications are unclear.

Citing a lack of substantiating evidence, German health authorities declined to approve of wild strawberry leaf preparations for any of the proposed traditional uses, including externally for rashes and internally for diarrhea, stomach upset, congestion, night sweats, or to stimulate digestion or function as a diuretic.[2]

Will It Harm You? What the Studies Say:

No reports of significant adverse reactions have been linked to the use of wild strawberry as an herbal remedy, although no formal studies have apparently been done. Many national health authorities allow the plant as a food additive. If you are sensitive to regular strawberries, be aware that the wild strawberry leaves and fruits used in many teas and other preparations may cause an allergic reaction.

GENERAL SOURCES:

Bisset, N.G., ed. *Herbal Drugs and Phytopharmaceuticals.* Stuttgart: medpharm GmbH Scientific Publishers, 1994.

Bremness, L. *Herbs.* 1st American ed. Eyewitness Handbooks. New York: Dorling Kindersley Publications, 1994.

Chevallier, A. *The Encyclopedia of Medicinal Plants: A Practical Reference Guide to More Than 550 Key Medicinal Plants & Their Uses.* 1st American ed. New York: Dorling Kindersley Publications, 1996.

Dobelis, I.N., ed. *The Magic and Medicine of Plants: A Practical Guide to the Science, History, Folklore, and Everyday Uses of Medicinal Plants.* Pleasantville, NY: Reader's Digest Association, 1986.

Blumenthal, M., J. Gruenwald, T. Hall, and R.S. Rister, eds. *The Complete German Commission E Monographs: Therapeutic Guide to Herbal Medicine.* Boston: Integrative Medicine Communications, 1998.

Hylton, W.H., ed. *The Rodale Herb Book: How to Use, Grow, and Buy Nature's Miracle Plants.* Emmaus, PA: Rodale Press, Inc., 1974.

Ody, P. *The Herb Society's Complete Medicinal Herbal.* London: Dorling Kindersley Limited, 1993.

TEXT CITATIONS:
1. B. Vennat et al., *Pharmaceutica Acta Helvetiae*, 64(11) (1989): 316-20.
2. M. Blumenthal, J. Gruenwald, T. Hall, and R.S. Rister, eds., *The Complete German Commission E Monographs: Therapeutic Guide to Herbal Medicine* (Boston: Integrative Medicine Communications, 1998).

WILD YAM

SCIENTIFIC NAME:
Dioscorea villosa L. and other *Dioscorea* varieties such as *Dioscorea paniculata* L. Family: Dioscoreacea

COMMON NAMES:
Barbasco, colic root, rheumatism root, wild Mexican yam, wild yam root

RATING:
3 = Studies on the effectiveness and safety of this substance are conflicting, or there are not enough studies to draw a conclusion.

What Is Wild Yam?

This climbing perennial vine, a native of North and Central America now found in many regions of the world, has heart-shaped leaves and small green flowers. It produces large tubers that look like potatoes, although it bears no relation to the sweet potatoes or yams found in American supermarkets. The rhizomes (underground stems) and long, twisting roots are used medicinally.

What It Is Used For:

Wild yam was traditionally used by Native Americans, slaves, and early American physicians for clearing congestion (as an expectorant), promoting sweating, alleviating rheumatic pain, relaxing smooth muscles and thus reducing muscle spasms and colicky pain from gallstones and other ailments (hence the name, colic root), and, in large doses, inducing vomiting. Female complaints such as painful menstrual periods, ovarian cramping, menstrual and childbirth problems, and even pregnancy-related nausea and vomiting were reportedly once treated with the herb.

Some contemporary herbalists recommend wild yam for these kinds of disorders, often highlighting its purported antispasmodic, anti-inflammatory, and hormonal effects. The plant contains hormone precursors which many sources contend can help relieve inflammation and pain from inflammatory ailments such as arthritis. Topical "hormone" creams made from wild yam can be found on the market.

Forms Available Include:

Capsule, cream, decoction, drops, liquid extract, powder, tincture.

Dosage Commonly Reported:

The tincture is taken in doses of ½ teaspoon twice a day, and the liquid extract is taken in doses of 2 to 4 milliliters. Two 505-milligram root capsules are taken daily.

Will It Work for You? What the Studies Say:

The marketing of wild yam as a "natural progesterone" has stirred up considerable controversy among plant experts and herbalists, with a number voicing doubt about its practical value and concern over its potential toxicity.[1] At one time, wild yam proved to be a critical source of material (steroidal saponins) for synthesizing progesterone for steroid drugs such as cortisone, estrogens, oral contraceptives, and various steroid products. The key steroidal saponin is diosgenin. Technically, however, diosgenin is a hormonal precursor, which means it has to be chemically processed in a laboratory to render it valuable as a synthetic sex hormone such as testosterone or progesterone. Given the complex steps involved, it is far from clear that wild yam in the form of a simple decoction, tincture, or capsule can live up to the claim of functioning as a hormone in the body. The medical literature contains no references to clinical trials using wild yam to treat hormone-related (or any other) disorders, including menopausal symptoms or inflammatory diseases such as arthritis.

According to a 1996 study, supplementing the diet with dioscorea, a steroid extract of wild yams, did not increase levels of the steroid DHEA (dehydroepiandrosterone) in older adult volunteers.[2] (See **DHEA.**) But it did significantly lower triglyceride levels and increase levels of the "good" high-density lipoprotein (HDL) cholesterol, apparently through its ability to prevent the lipids from damaging the arterial lining (antioxidation). This study and its implications require further examination; it involved selected older adults, for example, and was not double-blind or placebo-controlled to rule out bias.

Will It Harm You? What the Studies Say:

Although generally regarded as nontoxic, the safety of wild yam remains a mystery. A number of critics are starting to express concern about the potential for adverse reactions with hormone precursors,[3] especially in the presence of hormone-sensitive conditions such as certain types of breast cancer. Even enthusiasts warn that pregnant women should take the herb only under a doctor's guidance.[4]

GENERAL SOURCES:

Balch, J.F., and P.A. Balch. *Prescription for Nutritional Healing: A Practical A to Z Reference to Drug-Free Remedies Using Vitamins, Minerals, Herbs & Food Supplements.* 2nd ed. Garden City Park, NY: Avery Publishing Group, 1997.

Chevallier, A. *The Encyclopedia of Medicinal Plants: A Practical Reference Guide to More Than 550 Key Medicinal Plants & Their Uses.* 1st American ed. New York: Dorling Kindersley Publications, 1996.

Dobelis, I.N., ed. *The Magic and Medicine of Plants: A Practical Guide to the Science, History, Folklore, and Everyday Uses of Medicinal Plants.* Pleasantville, NY: Reader's Digest Association, 1986.

Hylton, W.H., ed. *The Rodale Herb Book: How to Use, Grow, and Buy Nature's Miracle Plants.* Emmaus, PA: Rodale Press, Inc., 1974.

Mayell, M. *Off-the-Shelf Natural Health: How to Use Herbs and Nutrients to Stay Well.* New York: Bantam Books, 1995.

Mowrey, D.B. *Proven Herbal Blends: A Rational Approach to Prevention and Remedy.* Condensed from *The Scientific Validation of Herbal Medicine.* New Canaan, CT: Keats Publishing, Inc: 1986.

Ody, P. *The Herb Society's Complete Medicinal Herbal.* London: Dorling Kindersley Limited, 1993.

Tierra, M. *The Way of Herbs.* New York: Pocket Books, 1990.

Weiner, M.A., and J.A. Weiner. *Herbs That Heal: Prescription for Herbal Healing.* Mill Valley, CA: Quantum Books, 1994.

Weiss, R.F. *Herbal Medicine,* trans. A. R. Meuss, from the 6th German edition. Beaconsfield, England: Beaconsfield Publishers, Ltd., 1988.

TEXT CITATIONS:

1. *HerbalGram* # 37, The American Botanical Council, Summer 1996.
2. M. Araghiniknam et al., *Life Sciences,* 59(11) (1996): PL147–57.
3. P.L. Whitten et al., *Journal of Nutrition,* Mar 125(3 Suppl) (1995): 771S–76S.
4. P. Ody, *The Herb Society's Complete Medicinal Herbal* (London: Dorling Kindersley Limited, 1993).

PRIMARY NAME:
WILLOW BARK

SCIENTIFIC NAME:
Salix alba L. (white willow) and occasionally other species including *Salix purpurea* L., *Salix daphnoides* Villars, and *Salix fragilis* L. Family: Salicaceae

COMMON NAMES:
Common willow, European willow, white willow

RATING:
3 = Studies on the effectiveness and safety of this substance are conflicting, or there are not enough studies to draw a conclusion.

What Is Willow Bark?

There are several hundred species of willow tree. Many have been used in traditional healing, but in the United States the dried bark of the white willow (*Salix alba*) has been used most commonly. This tall, gray-barked tree has short silky leaves and bears long clusters of spring flowers.

What It Is Used For:

As early as 500 B.C., Chinese healers recommended willow bark to control pain. Centuries passed before Westerners started using the bark to reduce fevers and as a pain reliever for rheumatism and headaches. Independently of the rest of the world, Native American tribes turned to indigenous willows for similar purposes. The colonists introduced white willow to North America.

In the mid-1800s European chemists identified the active chemical in white willow—salicin—and subsequently purified a more potent substance from it called salicylic acid. They also found salicin (and salicylic acid) in other plants. Both substances proved capable of lowering fever and reducing pain and inflammation. A derivative of salicylic acid—acetylsalicylic acid—was subsequently taken from another plant altogether (see **Meadowsweet**) to make the first aspirin tablets. (Aspirin is now entirely synthetic.)

Some contemporary sources recommend willow bark as an aspirin substitute to break a fever, treat headache pain and gout, and control pain or inflammation caused by arthritis, rheumatism, and sprains. Many consider it a good choice for mild feverish colds and infections. Some manufacturers include it in weight-loss products.

Forms Available Include:

Bark (chopped, powdered), capsule, decoction (made with chopped or pow-dered bark), tincture.

Dosage Commonly Reported:

Willow bark is taken up to three times a day as a decoction made with 1 to 2 teaspoons powdered bark, as a tincture (1 to 2 milliliters containing 25 percent ethanol), or in a standardized form corresponding to 60 to 120 milligrams of salicin. Two or three 379-milligram capsules are taken every three hours, up to a total of eighteen a day.

Will It Work for You? What the Studies Say:

As a healing agent, willow bark has its promoters and its detractors. The bark reportedly shares many of the painkilling properties of aspirin (acetylsalicylic acid), but not many of its side effects.[1] But while no scientist questions the pres-ence of salicin, some challenge the notion that the active ingredient is present in adequate concentrations to soothe a headache, relieve muscle pain, reduce inflammation, or break a fever, for example.

Moreover, the concentration of salicin naturally varies from one batch to another (as well as among willow species), making its potency unreliable at best. To get an average painkilling dose, for example, a person would probably have to drink between three and twenty-one cups (0.75 to 5 liters) of willow bark tea, not a good idea considering the presence of tannin, an astringent sub-stance used for diarrhea that has potential cancer-causing properties in high doses.[2] An arthritis sufferer would have to imbibe 5½ gallons or so of the tea (20 liters) to get the amount of aspirin typically recommended for pain (an average dose of 4.5 grams).

Nonetheless, German health authorities endorse the use of willow bark for feverish illnesses, headaches, and rheumatic complaints.[3] It is notable, however, that in Germany, the concentration of active ingredients (total salicin) is stan-dardized and marked on the package, and aspirin is commonly taken along with it.[4] Such standardized products are not readily available in the United States. Advocates dismiss these criticisms, noting that not as much can be expected of willow bark as aspirin, but that one cannot deny that it still contains the critical painkilling, anti-inflammatory, and fever-reducing ingredients.

Some herbal manufacturers tout willow bark as a weight-loss agent. No sub-stantiating studies appear in the recent medical literature, however.

Will It Harm You? What the Studies Say:

As long as willow bark tea and other preparations are used in typically recom-mended amounts, they appear to pose no risk of harm. Some people may develop stomach upset because of the contained tannins, but this appears to be uncommon. It may not be a wise choice if you suffer from chronic stomach problems. The risk of interactions with other medicines, as can occur with aspirin, also appears to be negligible.[5] But overall, in addition to being far less potent than aspirin, willow bark poses much less risk of the side effects—

particularly stomach upset—that annoy many aspirin users. It appears to have no impact on blood platelet function, as aspirin does.[6]

Precisely because of the chemical similarity to aspirin, however, avoid willow bark if you have had any type of allergic reaction to aspirin. Although no direct link has ever been demonstrated, pregnant women may want to avoid the bark given evidence linking certain levels of aspirin use to birth defects and other complications. Do not give willow bark to children under sixteen with flu or chicken pox symptoms; this may pose a risk for the development of a rare but serious ailment called Reye's syndrome that has been associated with the use of aspirin under these conditions. The syndrome has never been directly linked to white willow use, however.

GENERAL SOURCES:

American Pharmaceutical Association. *Handbook of Nonprescription Drugs.* 11th ed. Washington, D.C.: American Pharmaceutical Association, 1996.

American Family Physician. 38 (1988): 197.

Bisset, N.G., ed. *Herbal Drugs and Phytopharmaceuticals.* Stuttgart: medpharm GmbH Scientific Publishers, 1994.

Blumenthal, M., J. Gruenwald, T. Hall, and R.S. Rister, eds. *The Complete German Commission E Monographs: Therapeutic Guide to Herbal Medicine.* Boston: Integrative Medicine Communications, 1998.

Bradley, P.C., ed. *British Herbal Compendium: A Handbook of Scientific Information on Widely Used Plant Drugs.* Vol. 1. Bournemouth (Dorset), England: British Herbal Medicine Association, 1992.

Castleman, M. *The Healing Herbs: The Ultimate Guide to the Curative Power of Nature's Medicines.* New York: Bantam Books, 1995.

Mayell, M. *Off-the-Shelf Natural Health: How to Use Herbs and Nutrients to Stay Well.* New York: Bantam Books, 1995.

Mindell, E. *Earl Mindell's Herb Bible.* New York: Simon & Schuster/Fireside, 1992.

Mueller, R.L., and S. Scheidt. *Circulation.* 89(1) (1994): 432–49.

Newall, C.A., et al. *Herbal Medicines: A Guide for Health-Care Professionals.* London: The Pharmaceutical Press, 1996.

Sallis, R.E. *American Family Physician.* 39 (1989): 209.

Tyler, V.E. *Herbs of Choice: The Therapeutic Use of Phytomedicinals.* Binghamton, NY: Haworth Press/Pharmaceutical Products Press, 1994.

Weiss, R.F. *Herbal Medicine,* trans. A. R. Meuss, from the 6th German edition. Beaconsfield, England: Beaconsfield Publishers, Ltd., 1988.

TEXT CITATIONS:

1. G. Weissman, *Scientific American,* January (1991): 58–64. C.A. Newall et al., *Herbal Medicines: A Guide for Health-Care Professionals* (London: The Pharmaceutical Press, 1996).
2. V.E. Tyler, *Herbs of Choice: The Therapeutic Use of Phytomedicinals* (Binghamton, NY: Hawthorn Press/Pharmaceutical Products Press, 1994).
3. M. Blumenthal, J. Gruenwald, T. Hall, and R.S. Rister, eds., *The Complete German Commission E Monographs: Therapeutic Guide to Herbal Medicine* (Boston: Integrative Medicine Communications, 1998).
4. Tyler, op. cit.
5. N.G. Bisset, ed., *Herbal Drugs and Phytopharmaceuticals* (Stuttgart: medpharm GmbH Scientific Publishers, 1994).
6. Weissman, op. cit.

PRIMARY NAME:

WINTERGREEN

SCIENTIFIC NAME:
Gaultheria procumbens L.
Family: Ericaceae

COMMON NAMES:
Boxberry, checkerberry,
mountain tea, partridgeberry,
spiceberry, teaberry

RATING:
1 = Years of use and extensive,
high-quality studies indicate
that this substance is very
effective when used in
recommended amounts for the
indication(s) noted in the "Will
It Work for You?" section.
Safety depends on judicious
use, however; see the "Will It
Harm You?" section.

What Is Wintergreen?

This shrublike, low-lying perennial is common to woody areas and bears small white or pale pink bell-shaped flowers that bloom in July and August and are followed by brilliant scarlet fruits, or "berries." The berries are used medicinally, along with the herb's glossy green and leathery leaves and an essential oil distilled from them.

What It Is Used For:

Native Americans reportedly brewed a tea from the leaves of this indigenous evergreen to alleviate rheumatic discomforts, headache, fever, sore throat, and various aches and pains. Settlers adopted a number of these uses and came up with some of their own, including taking wintergreen as a diuretic, or "water pill," for fluid retention. Herbalists today promote wintergreen tea taken internally as a balm for pain, colic, and excess gas.

External uses are more popular by far, however, with the oil's reputation as a pain reliever, astringent, diuretic, and stimulant enduring into modern herbal and conventional medicine guides. The oil is regularly applied to painfully swollen, inflamed, or sore muscles and joints, especially when caused by injuries or rheumatic ailments. The tea also finds use as a gargle.

The oil was once popular as a flavoring in candies, toothpastes, and food, as well as an aromatic agent in perfumes, but today manufacturers generally rely on synthetic formulations.

Forms Available Include:

- *For internal use:* Infusion.
- *For external use:* Gargle, liniment, oil, ointment. Wintergreen oil, often sold as methyl salicylate, appears in gels, liniments, lotions, ointments, and solutions.

Dosage Commonly Reported:

Formulations containing concentrations of methyl salicylate of 10 to 60 percent are applied externally up to four times per day. They should not be used after strenuous exercise or in conjunction with a heating pad. An infusion for internal use is made with one teaspoon of the leaves and flowering tops, steeped 5 to 20 minutes in boiling water. It is drunk cold, one mouthful at a time, not exceeding one cup per day.

Will It Work for You? What the Studies Say:

Wintergreen contains a high concentration of methyl salicylate, a compound medically accepted as a mild topical counterirritant for inflamed or irritated joints. Counterirritants cause superficial irritation and redness, thereby deflecting deeper pain and discomfort such as that caused by muscle injuries and arthritic joint pains. Methyl salicylate, which is also an ingredient in sweet birch oil (see **Birch** for more information on that substance), bears a chemical relationship to aspirin and should also help reduce inflammation. This substance can now be made synthetically.[1]

Wintergreen also contains astringent compounds called tannins, and a soothing and softening substance called mucilage. Such substances may help indirectly alleviate the soreness in muscles and joints, and may explain why a gargle is used for throat irritation and why some people take wintergreen tea to relieve stomach upset. No studies to examine wintergreen's direct impact on these types of conditions appear in the medical literature, however.

Wintergreen's reputation for reducing fever and treating inflammation and pain internally may also be explained by methyl salicylate's similarity to aspirin. No studies have apparently ever been done to explore the herb's practical use for these conditions, however, and adequate concentrations of the active ingredient—the methyl salicylate in the oil—quickly become toxic at certain dosages.

Will It Harm You? What the Studies Say:

Never take wintergreen oil internally (except as it appears in approved commercial formulations) because it is poisonous except in very small amounts, such as those used commercially for flavoring. Fatalities have been reported in children who drank the oil.[2] Do not even apply the oil to the skin of children under twelve unless directed to do so by a medical professional.

Likewise, never swallow methyl salicylate; it is much more toxic than most salicylates, such as the acetylsalicylic acid found in aspirin, and fatal poisonings in children have been reported.[3] A twenty-one-month-old boy who ate a lot of wintergreen-flavored candy suffered from toxic reactions (vomiting, lethargy, rapid breathing) to the contained methyl salicylate.[4] This substance has also been blamed for accidental poisonings[5] and suicides in adults.[6] Individuals taking warfarin, a blood thinner, may develop bleeding problems and other adverse reactions and may want to avoid methyl-salicylate-containing products altogether.[7]

Whether from wintergreen or synthesized in the laboratory, the oil sold as methyl salicylate should be used very cautiously as a counterirritant. Follow package instructions and avoid applying it after vigorous exercise or in hot and humid weather because dangerous amounts could get absorbed into your system.[8] It can also cause allergic contact dermatitis and anaphylactic (severe allergic) reactions.[9]

Wintergreen infusions are probably safe to take in moderation.

GENERAL SOURCES:

American Pharmaceutical Association. *Handbook of Nonprescription Drugs*. 11th ed. Washington, D.C.: American Pharmaceutical Association, 1996.

Balch, J.F., and P.A. Balch. *Prescription for Nutritional Healing: A Practical A to Z Reference to Drug-Free Remedies Using Vitamins, Minerals, Herbs & Food Supplements*. 2nd ed. Garden City Park, NY: Avery Publishing Group, 1997.

Chevallier, A. *The Encyclopedia of Medicinal Plants: A Practical Reference Guide to More Than 550 Key Medicinal Plants & Their Uses*. 1st American ed. New York: Dorling Kindersley Publications, 1996.

Dobelis, I.N., ed. *The Magic and Medicine of Plants: A Practical Guide to the Science, History, Folklore, and Everyday Uses of Medicinal Plants*. Pleasantville, NY: Reader's Digest Association, 1986.

Hylton, W.H., ed. *The Rodale Herb Book: How to Use, Grow, and Buy Nature's Miracle Plants*. Emmaus, PA: Rodale Press, Inc., 1974.

Leung, A.Y., and S. Foster. *Encyclopedia of Common Natural Ingredients Used in Food, Drugs, and Cosmetics.* 2nd ed. New York: John Wiley & Sons, 1996.

Tyler, V.E. *Herbs of Choice: The Therapeutic Use of Phytomedicinals.* Binghamton, NY: Haworth Press/Pharmaceutical Products Press, 1994.

Weiner, M.A., and J.A. Weiner. *Herbs That Heal: Prescription for Herbal Healing.* Mill Valley, CA: Quantum Books, 1994.

TEXT CITATIONS:

1. V.E. Tyler, *Herbs of Choice: The Therapeutic Use of Phytomedicinals* (Binghamton, NY: Haworth Press/Pharmaceutical Products Press, 1994).
2. I.N. Dobelis, ed., *The Magic and Medicine of Plants: A Practical Guide to the Science, History, Folklore, and Everyday Uses of Medicinal Plants.* Pleasantville, NY: Reader's Digest Association, 1986.
3. A.Y. Leung and S. Foster, *Encyclopedia of Common Natural Ingredients Used in Food, Drugs, and Cosmetics,* 2nd ed. (New York: John Wiley & Sons, 1996).
4. D.L. Howrie, et al., *Pediatrics,* 75(5) (1985): 869–71.
5. W.L. Cauthen and W.H. Hester, *Journal of Family Practice,* 29(6) (1989): 680–81.
6. T.Y. Chan, *Postgraduate Medical Journal,* 72(844) (1996): 109–12.
7. T.Y. Chan, *Human & Experimental Toxicology,* 15(9) (1996): 747–50.
8. Tyler, op. cit.
9. Chan, op. cit.

PRIMARY NAME:

WITCH HAZEL

SCIENTIFIC NAME:

Hamamelis virginiana L.
Family: Hamamelidaceae

COMMON NAMES:

Hamamelis, snapping hazel, spotted alder, tobacco wood, winter bloom

RATING:

2 = According to a number of well-designed studies and common use, this substance appears to be relatively effective and safe when used in recommended amounts for the indication(s) noted in the "Will It Work for You?" section. However, see the warning about witch hazel water in the "Will It Harm You?" section.

What Is Witch Hazel?

This unusual perennial shrub (or small tree) grows in eastern North American forests. Spidery golden yellow flowers bloom along its flexible branches following the loss of its oval leaves in autumn, often long after other trees have lost their color. Black seeds are ejected from capsules along the stem at the same time that the flowers bloom. The dried leaves, bark, and dormant twigs (partially dried) are used medicinally. Whereas hydroalcoholic extracts are commonly found in Europe, the most commonly available witch hazel product in the United States is distilled witch hazel extract, also called witch hazel water or hamamelis water, which is made by steam-distilling dormant twigs soaked and softened in water.[1]

What It Is Used For:

Native Americans introduced witch hazel to early settlers, who quickly picked up on the practice of applying a strained decoction of the leaves and twigs to small wounds, insect bites, sore muscles and joints, and bruised or irritated eyes. They also took up sipping witch hazel tea to control internal bleeding, soothe sore throats, and stem excessive menstrual flow. Over time, witch hazel became a valued cooling, topical astringent for these and other ailments, including varicose veins, hemorrhoids, abrasions, bruises, and other skin inflammations. Internal formulations were used for diarrhea.

By the late 1900s, however, American manufacturers were marketing a watered-down version of the highly astringent decoction the Native Americans had known. The new version, which was easier to prepare, consisted of steam-

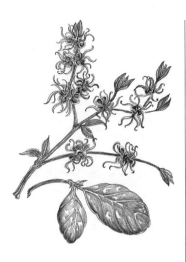

Witch Hazel
Hamamelis virginiana

distilled plant parts. Only minimal amounts of its astringent tannin—and, hence, of its healing powers—remained. Today's herbalists recommend witch hazel especially as a gargle for mouth inflammations and sore throat. But they suggest it only in the form of a bark decoction, not the form one finds on most drugstore shelves.

Forms Available Include:

Bark (chopped, powdered), bottled witch hazel water, decoction (for both internal and external use), extract, eyewash, leaf, ointment, poultice, suppository, tea, tincture. Plant extracts also appear in various over-the-counter products including face creams, shaving lotions, and eyewashes.

Dosage Commonly Reported:

A decoction made using 1 teaspoon (2 to 3 grams) chopped or powdered bark is drunk up to three times a day, applied externally, or gargled. Alternatively, a tea is made using 2 to 4 teaspoons (1 to 2 grams) chopped leaves. The tincture (made with the bark) is taken in doses of 2 to 4 milliliters.

Will It Work for You? What the Studies Say:

Witch hazel contains considerable amounts of an astringent substance called tannin (up to 10 percent in the leaf and 3 percent in the bark), which explains why it is effective in helping to soothe and heal minor skin injuries, skin and mucous membrane irritations such as gum inflammation (in the form of a mouthwash of the infusion), varicose veins, and hemorrhoids. Tannins constrict tissue and reduce oozing and bleeding. German health authorities approve of both leaf and branch preparations for these kinds of ailments.[2] A German textbook cites witch hazel as an excellent hemorrhoid remedy.[3]

Animal research shows that witch hazel extracts have anti-inflammatory, local styptic (stopping bleeding), and vasoconstrictive (blood-vessel-constricting) actions which are valuable for the above conditions as well.[4] Rabbit experiments show that injection of alcoholic fluid extracts can cause vein constriction,[5] which helps explain why Europeans sometimes treat varicose veins with witch hazel extracts,[6] although they take them orally. Alcoholic fluid extracts have proved far more potent than water extracts such as teas for this purpose.[7] Although the astringent tannins also explain the use of witch hazel bark for acute diarrhea, few sources recommend this practice. Tannins are believed to control or stop diarrhea by reducing inflammation in the intestines. German health authorities recommend leaf preparations for acute diarrhea not due to an underlying disease.[8]

The astringent property that can be attributed to witch hazel water—the steam distillate that contains essentially no tannins—is presumed to be due only to the added alcohol (about 14 percent).[9] The alcohol is likely responsible for the cooling and refreshing sensations witch hazel water produces when rubbed into the skin.

Will It Harm You? What the Studies Say:

Based on the ingredients identified and years of use by many people to no apparent ill effect, witch hazel preparations appear to be safe to use externally in recommended amounts. The health risks involved in taking witch hazel preparations internally are far less clear, however. Some susceptible individuals may develop stomach upset with possible nausea, vomiting, or constipation, and in rare cases the tannins in the bark may cause liver damage if enough are absorbed.[10] The volatile oil contains a known carcinogen (safrole), but in such small amounts that it is unlikely to pose any risk of harm.[11] Also keep in mind that no tannin-rich drug should be used over long periods of time given the potential, still not fully understood, of an increased risk of malignant (cancerous) changes. *Do not use witch hazel water internally.*

GENERAL SOURCES:

American Pharmaceutical Association. *Handbook of Nonprescription Drugs.* 11th ed. Washington, D.C.: American Pharmaceutical Association, 1996.

Bisset, N.G., ed. *Herbal Drugs and Phytopharmaceuticals.* Stuttgart: medpharm GmbH Scientific Publishers, 1994.

Blumenthal, M., J. Gruenwald, T. Hall, and R.S. Rister, eds. *The Complete German Commission E Monographs: Therapeutic Guide to Herbal Medicine.* Boston: Integrative Medicine Communications, 1998.

Castleman, M. *The Healing Herbs: The Ultimate Guide to the Curative Power of Nature's Medicines.* New York: Bantam Books, 1995.

Lawrence Review of Natural Products. St. Louis: Facts and Comparisons, September 1990.

Leung, A.Y., and S. Foster. *Encyclopedia of Common Natural Ingredients Used in Food, Drugs, and Cosmetics.* 2nd ed. New York: John Wiley & Sons, 1996.

Newall, C.A., et al. *Herbal Medicines: A Guide for Health-Care Professionals.* London: The Pharmaceutical Press, 1996.

Tierra, M. *The Way of Herbs.* New York: Pocket Books, 1990.

Tyler, V.E. *Herbs of Choice: The Therapeutic Use of Phytomedicinals.* Binghamton, NY: Haworth Press/Pharmaceutical Products Press, 1994.

———. *The Honest Herbal.* Binghamton, NY: Haworth Press/Pharmaceutical Products Press, 1993.

Weiner, M.A., and J.A. Weiner. *Herbs That Heal: Prescription for Herbal Healing.* Mill Valley, CA: Quantum Books, 1994.

Weiss, R.F. *Herbal Medicine,* trans. A. R. Meuss, from the 6th German edition. Beaconsfield, England: Beaconsfield Publishers, Ltd., 1988.

TEXT CITATIONS:

1. American Pharmaceutical Association, *Handbook of Nonprescription Drugs,* 11th ed. (Washington, D.C.: American Pharmaceutical Association, 1996).

2. M. Blumenthal, J. Gruenwald, T. Hall, and R.S. Rister, eds., *The Complete German Commission E Monographs: Therapeutic Guide to Herbal Medicine* (Boston: Integrative Medicine Communications, 1998).

3. R.F. Weiss, *Herbal Medicine,* trans. A. R. Meuss, from the 6th German edition (Beaconsfield, England: Beaconsfield Publishers, Ltd., 1988).

4. N.G. Bisset, ed., *Herbal Drugs and Phytopharmaceuticals* (Stuttgart: medpharm GmbH Scientific Publishers, 1994).

5. *J Pharm Beig,* 27 (1972): 505.

6. *Lawrence Review of Natural Products* (St. Louis: Facts and Comparisons, September 1990).

7. V.E. Tyler, *The Honest Herbal* (Binghamton, NY: Haworth Press/Pharmaceutical Products Press, 1993).
8. Bisset, op. cit.
9. American Pharmaceutical Association, op. cit. A.Y. Leung and S. Foster, *Encyclopedia of Common Natural Ingredients Used in Food, Drugs, and Cosmetics*, 2nd ed. (New York: John Wiley & Sons, 1996).
10. Bisset, op. cit. *Lawrence Review of Natural Products*, op. cit.
11. C.A. Newall et al., *Herbal Medicines: A Guide for Health-Care Professionals* (London: The Pharmaceutical Press, 1996).

PRIMARY NAME:
WOOD BETONY

SCIENTIFIC NAME:
Stachys officinalis (L.) Trev., sometimes referred to as *Stachys betonica* or *Betonica officinalis*. Family: Labiatae (Lamiaceae)

COMMON NAMES:
Betony, bishop's wort

RATING:
3 = Studies on the effectiveness and safety of this substance are conflicting, or there are not enough studies to draw a conclusion.

What Is Wood Betony?

This European and Asian perennial bears loose spikes of pink or white summer flowers and faintly pungent, hairy oval leaves. It favors open woodlands and meadows, and is popular for herb gardens. The dried aboveground parts of the plant and occasionally the roots are used medicinally.

What It Is Used For:

Many contemporary herbalists do not even bother mentioning this herb, once considered something of a cure-all. Magical powers for warding off evil spirits were attributed to wood betony in medieval Europe. Herbalists once regarded it highly for eliminating headaches, and its astringent actions were long put to use in treating diarrhea and mucous membrane irritations such as sore throats and inflamed gums. Herbalists today recommend it as a mild sedative and treatment for anxiety, nervous tension, nervous system disorders, indigestion, and premenstrual syndrome. Many contend it stimulates the liver and digestive system and functions as an overall tonic. Betony is often added to herbal tea blends as a flavoring.

Forms Available Include:

Infusion (for drinking, gargle, mouthwash), liquid extract, poultice, tincture. Also appears in numerous herbal blends.

Dosage Commonly Reported:

The liquid herb extract is taken in doses of 2 to 4 milliliters.

Will It Work for You? What the Studies Say:

The plant's high tannin content—about 15 percent—explains its traditional use as an astringent for skin and mucous membrane irritations such as sore throat, gum inflammation, and diarrhea.[1] Tannins constrict (draw together) skin tissue and reduce oozing and bleeding. They are believed to control or stop diarrhea by reducing inflammation in the intestines. Wood betony's mildly bitter taste is cited as evidence for its ability to stimulate the digestive system, but this property has not been well documented.

Over the years, Russian investigators have reported finding substances in

W

Wood Betony

wood betony with anti-inflammatory, cholagogic (increasing bile flow), and significant blood-pressure-lowering actions.[2] Whether these properties affect humans is far from clear. If they do, this may partially explain certain traditional uses for the herb, such as treating headaches and anxiety,[3] skin inflammations, and biliary problems. Clearly, much more research is needed.

Will It Harm You? What the Studies Say:

Serious adverse reactions have not been associated with typically recommended amounts of wood betony, although excessive doses may cause stomach irritation.[4] Keep in mind that any tannin-rich drug used over long periods may increase the risk of malignant (cancerous) changes.[5] A number of herbalists advise pregnant women to avoid the herb, although the reasons for this are unclear; some say the herb stimulates the uterus.

GENERAL SOURCES:

Bremness, L. *Herbs*. 1st American ed. Eyewitness Handbooks. New York: Dorling Kindersley Publications, 1994.

Chevallier, A. *The Encyclopedia of Medicinal Plants: A Practical Reference Guide to More Than 550 Key Medicinal Plants & Their Uses*. 1st American ed. New York: Dorling Kindersley Publications, 1996.

Lawrence Review of Natural Products. St. Louis: Facts and Comparisons, August 1991.

Mayell, M. *Off-the-Shelf Natural Health: How to Use Herbs and Nutrients to Stay Well*. New York: Bantam Books, 1995.

Ody, P. *The Herb Society's Complete Medicinal Herbal*. London: Dorling Kindersley Limited, 1993.

Tierra, M. *The Way of Herbs*. New York: Pocket Books, 1990.

Tyler, V.E. *The Honest Herbal*. Binghamton, NY: Haworth Press/Pharmaceutical Products Press, 1993.

Weiner, M.A., and J.A. Weiner. *Herbs That Heal: Prescription for Herbal Healing*. Mill Valley, CA: Quantum Books, 1994.

TEXT CITATIONS:

1. V.E. Tyler, *The Honest Herbal* (Binghamton, NY: Haworth Press/Pharmaceutical Products Press, 1993).
2. A.Y. Kobzar, *Khim Prir. Soedin*, 2 (1986): 239. T.V. Zinchenko, and I.M. Fefer, *Farmatscvtichnii Zhumal*, 17(3) (1962): 35–38.
3. Tyler, op. cit.
4. Ibid.
5. Ibid.

WOODRUFF, SWEET

SCIENTIFIC NAME:

Galium odoratum (L.) Scop., sometimes referred to as *Asperula odorata* L. Family: Rubiaceae

COMMON NAMES:

Master of the wood, woodruff, woodward

RATING:

3 = Studies on the effectiveness of this substance are conflicting, or there are not enough studies to draw a conclusion about it. Safety is a concern, however; see the "Will It Harm You?" section.

What Is Sweet Woodruff?

This small, spreading perennial, a common groundcover, grows to only about a foot high. It has lance-shaped leaves and bears loose clusters of small white flowers. Although native to Eurasia and North Africa, it can be found growing throughout North America. The whole, dried plant is used medicinally. It emits a scent of fresh-cut hay when it dries or is cut; this scent intensifies with time.

What It Is Used For:

This sweet-smelling herb has been used over the years as a diuretic ("water pill"), expectorant, sedative, sweat-inducer, digestive aid, liver tonic, and antispasmodic. Fresh leaves were once placed on small wounds. Contemporary herbalists recommend it for arthritis and constipation. Some German textbooks recommend it for varicose veins and thrombophlebitis (clots and swelling in the leg veins). Homeopaths prescribe minute amounts of the plant extract as an antispasmodic and for various other ailments. (See page 2 for more information on homeopathy.)

In another era, sweet woodruff's appealing scent was commonly encountered in homes and churches. The herb is a key ingredient in May wine and also appears in vermouth, bitters, candies, and certain foods as a flavoring.

Forms Available Include:

Decoction, extract, leaf (fresh), tea bag.

Dosage Commonly Reported:

No dosage information available.

Will It Work for You? What the Studies Say:

Sweet woodruff reportedly contains a blood-thinning substance called coumarin, although not all sources agree on this.[1] Whether the herb is therefore effective in preventing or treating such conditions as thrombophlebitis or blood clots remains unclear. In any case, these are serious conditions that should be under the care of a qualified medical professional.

An extract of the herb fared well in a classic animal test for inflammation, the chemically induced rat paw edema test.[2] The extract inhibited swelling by 25 percent when fed to the rats, comparing favorably with the 45 percent reduction in swelling seen with a standard anti-inflammatory medicine, indomethacin. Whether this means the herb will help reduce inflammation associated with such disorders as arthritis remains to be properly tested.

Also unclear is whether sweet woodruff's anti-inflammatory actions are of aid in treating skin wounds and inflammation. The presence of astringent tannins theoretically would contribute to healing as well; astringents typically tighten skin tissue and help reduce oozing and bleeding. Antibacterial properties have also been identified in the herb, possibly helping to prevent infection, although this, too, has yet to be properly tested in animals or humans.[3]

The herb reportedly contains a bitter principle; bitters typically stimulate salivation and gastric juices, aiding digestion.

Will It Harm You? What the Studies Say:

Although safe for use in foods, sweet woodruff may pose some risk of harm when taken in larger doses for medicinal purposes, largely because of its contained coumarin. Animals fed high doses of coumarin have developed blood-clotting problems, liver damage, growth inhibition, and wasting of the testicles.[4] A German textbook notes that these studies involved the extract only—not the whole plant, as herbalists are recommending—and at doses much higher than the average human would get.[5] A placebo-controlled study of pregnant rabbits administered medicinal doses of the herb intravenously did not indicate an increased risk of birth defects.[6] No reports of serious adverse reactions among humans appear in the recent medical literature, but moderation is probably a wise approach, as large doses of the tea reportedly can cause dizziness and vomiting, among other unpleasant responses.[7]

GENERAL SOURCES:

Dobelis, I.N., ed. *The Magic and Medicine of Plants: A Practical Guide to the Science, History, Folklore, and Everyday Uses of Medicinal Plants.* Pleasantville, NY: Reader's Digest Association, 1986.

Duke, J.A. *CRC Handbook of Medicinal Herbs.* Boca Raton, FL: CRC Press, 1985.

Lawrence Review of Natural Products. St. Louis: Facts and Comparisons, August 1991.

Leung, A.Y., and S. Foster. *Encyclopedia of Common Natural Ingredients Used in Food, Drugs, and Cosmetics.* 2nd ed. New York: John Wiley & Sons, 1996.

Weiss, R.F. *Herbal Medicine,* trans. A. R. Meuss, from the 6th German edition. Beaconsfield, England: Beaconsfield Publishers, Ltd., 1988.

TEXT CITATIONS:

1. A.Y. Leung and S. Foster, *Encyclopedia of Common Natural Ingredients Used in Food, Drugs, and Cosmetics,* 2nd ed. (New York: John Wiley & Sons, 1996).
2. N. Mascolo et al., *Phytotherapy Research,* 1 (1987): 28.
3. J.A. Duke, *CRC Handbook of Medicinal Herbs* (Boca Raton, FL: CRC Press, 1985).
4. Ibid. *Lawrence Review of Natural Products* (St. Louis: Facts and Comparisons, August 1991). R.F. Weiss, *Herbal Medicine,* trans. A. R. Meuss, from the 6th German edition (Beaconsfield, England: Beaconsfield Publishers, Ltd., 1988).
5. W. Grotz and J. Weinmann, *Arzneimittel-Forschung,* 23(9) (1973): 1319.
6. Weiss, op. cit.
7. I.N. Dobelis, ed., *The Magic and Medicine of Plants: A Practical Guide to the Science, History, Folklore, and Everyday Uses of Medicinal Plants* (Pleasantville, NY: Reader's Digest Association, 1986).

PRIMARY NAME:

WORMWOOD

SCIENTIFIC NAME:
Artemesia absinthium L. Family: Asteraceae (Compositae)

COMMON NAMES:
Absinthe, absinthites, absinthium, armoise, artemesia, wermut

What Is Wormwood?

The silky silvery leaves and greenish-yellow flowering tops of this strongly aromatic perennial are used medicinally once dried. It is native to Europe and grows plentifully in certain parts of North America.

What It Is Used For:

People have taken wormwood preparations to kill intestinal parasites since the earliest of times. Wormwood has also been regarded as a stomach tonic, digestive aid, appetite stimulant, sedative, sweat-inducer, liver remedy, menstrual stimulant, and topical antiseptic.[1]

RATING:

3 = Studies on the effectiveness of this substance are conflicting, or there are not enough studies to draw a conclusion about it. Safety is a major concern, however; see the "Will It Harm You?" section.

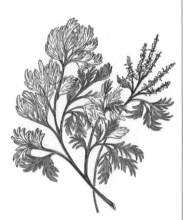

Wormwood
Artemesia absinthium

Most countries allow extracts of the herb's essential oil, which has a spicy and somewhat bitter taste, to be added to vermouth and other beverages once a toxic element, thujone, has been chemically removed. This precaution was initiated in the early part of the twentieth century when bizarre symptoms were noted in people (including the painter Vincent van Gogh) who had drunk an emerald-green, wormwood-flavored concoction called absinthe. The oil also finds use as an insecticide and fragrance.

Forms Available Include:

Decoction, dried flowers and leaves, infusion, liquid extract, powder, retention enema, rub, tea, tincture. Many of these are not available in the United States.

Dosage Commonly Reported:

An infusion made using 1 teaspoon of dried flowering tops of wormwood per cup of water is drunk before meals as an appetite stimulant or after meals as a digestive aid. The tincture is taken in doses of 4 to 16 milliliters, and the liquid herb extract in doses of 1 to 2 milliliters.

Will It Work for You? What the Studies Say:

The most important component in wormwood, the volatile oil, consists primarily of absinthol, the famous thujone (3 to 12 percent), and bitters. Thujone can paralyze roundworms, threadworms, and possibly other parasites, giving the body a chance to expel them.[2] Other wormwood components fight parasites as well, but because of the thujone, which can slow down the central nervous system, most experts consider the herb too dangerous for this purpose.

The presence of bitters in wormwood explains why the herb has been treasured for so many years as an appetite stimulant and gas remedy. German health authorities approve of thujone-free wormwood for these and other purposes, including to control spasms in the biliary tract,[3] which may reduce biliary colic.

Mouse studies indicate that wormwood has potential for preventing and curing liver damage due to overdoses of acetaminophen (e.g., Tylenol™),[4] and that it may fight the malaria bacteria.[5]

Will It Harm You? What the Studies Say:

Few scientists dispute the fact that the thujone in wormwood's volatile oil is very dangerous, capable of producing such uncomfortable and even terrifying symptoms as vomiting, severe diarrhea, stomach cramps, urinary retention, thirst, kidney damage, tremors, vertigo, seizures, intellectual deterioration, psychosis, hallucinations, stupor, and convulsions. In 1939, researchers showed that relatively low levels of thujone injected into rats could cause convulsions and that higher doses could kill them.[6] In humans, as little as 15 grams of the oil is considered toxic enough to cause loss of consciousness.[7]

Given these kinds of risks, one would imagine few people would dare touch the "remedy." But experts disagree on whether all wormwood preparations act similarly. Some contend that preparations such as teas put the average user at little risk because minimal amounts of the volatile oil (and hence thujone) make their way into the liquid. In Vincent van Gogh's time, on the other hand, the oil featured highly in the "sinister" intoxicating absinthe drink, which is why it proved so lethal. Many countries, while banning use of the herb's oil and alcoholic extracts, permit thujone-free preparations as well as liquid extracts such as teas. The FDA considers wormwood an unsafe herb and approves of thujone-free preparations only for use in foods. Even thujone-free wormwood preparations should be used in moderation, however. Side effects are unlikely when the herb is used as prescribed, although allergic reactions do occur, and anyone with stomach or intestinal disorders should probably avoid it altogether.[8]

Topical preparations may cause skin eruptions in sensitized individuals[9]; most members of the daisy plant family are allergenic.

GENERAL SOURCES:

Arnold, W.N. *Journal of the American Medical Association.* 260(20) (1988): 3042–44.

Bisset, N.G., ed. *Herbal Drugs and Phytopharmaceuticals.* Stuttgart: medpharm GmbH Scientific Publishers, 1994.

Blumenthal, M., J. Gruenwald, T. Hall, and R.S. Rister, eds. *The Complete German Commission E Monographs: Therapeutic Guide to Herbal Medicine.* Boston: Integrative Medicine Communications, 1998.

del Castillo, J., et al. *Nature.* 253 (1975): 365.

Dobelis, I.N., ed. *The Magic and Medicine of Plants: A Practical Guide to the Science, History, Folklore, and Everyday Uses of Medicinal Plants.* Pleasantville, NY: Reader's Digest Association, 1986.

Duke, J.A. *CRC Handbook of Medicinal Herbs.* Boca Raton, FL: CRC Press, 1985.

Heinerman, J. *Heinerman's Encyclopedia of Healing Herbs and Spices.* West Nyack, NY: Parker Publishing Co., 1996.

Lawrence Review of Natural Products. St. Louis: Facts and Comparisons, April 1991.

Sampson, F. *Journal of Pharmacology and Experimental Therapeutics.* 65 (1939): 275–80.

Tyler, V.E. *Herbs of Choice: The Therapeutic Use of Phytomedicinals.* Binghamton, NY: Haworth Press/Pharmaceutical Products Press, 1994.

———. *The Honest Herbal.* Binghamton, NY: Haworth Press/Pharmaceutical Products Press, 1993.

Vogt, D.D. *Journal of Ethnopharmacology.* 4(3) (1981): 337–42.

TEXT CITATIONS:

1. G.A. Conway and J.C. Solcumb, *Journal of Ethnopharmacology,* 1(3) (1979): 241–61. I.N. Dobelis, ed., *The Magic and Medicine of Plants: A Practical Guide to the Science, History, Folklore, and Everyday Uses of Medicinal Plants* (Pleasantville, NY: Reader's Digest Association, 1986).

2. W.N. Arnold, *Scientific American,* 260 (1989): 112.

3. M. Blumenthal, J. Gruenwald, T. Hall, and R.S. Rister, eds., *The Complete German Commission E Monographs: Therapeutic Guide to Herbal Medicine* (Boston: Integrative Medicine Communications, 1998).

4. A.H. Gilani and K.H. Janbaz, *General Pharmacology,* 26(2) (1995): 309–15.

5. M.M. Zafar and A. Hameed, *Journal of Ethnopharmacology,* 30(2) (1990): 223–26. *Lancet,* 339(8794) (1992): 649–51.

6. F. Sampson, *Journal of Pharmacology and Experimental Therapeutics,* 65 (1939): 275–80.

7. J.A. Duke, *CRC Handbook of Medicinal Herbs* (Boca Raton, FL: CRC Press, 1985).

8. N.G. Bisset, ed., *Herbal Drugs and Phytopharmaceuticals* (Stuttgart: medpharm GmbH Scientific Publishers, 1994).

9. *Lawrence Review of Natural Products* (St. Louis: Facts and Comparisons, April 1991).

YARROW

SCIENTIFIC NAME:
Achillea millefolium L. Family:
Asteraceae (Compositae)

COMMON NAMES:
Achillea, bad man's plaything,
bloodwort, herbe militaire,
milfoil, nosebleed, soldier's
herb, soldier's woundwort,
thousand weed

RATING:
2 = According to a number of
well-designed studies and
common use, this substance
appears to be relatively
effective and safe when used in
recommended amounts for the
indication(s) noted in the "Will
It Work for You?" section.

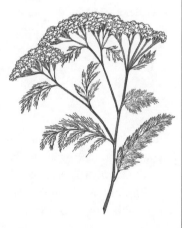

Yarrow
Achillea millefolium

What Is Yarrow?

The name yarrow has been applied to many barely distinguishable species and subspecies of plants. It can be broadly defined as a delicate perennial that grows wild in pastures, meadows, roadsides, and waste places across the United States, northern Asia, and Europe. It is also cultivated to meet demand. The profusion of narrow, divided leaves that emerge off the stem lends it a feathery or even lacy appearance. In summer, dense clusters of small white, pink, or yellow flowers appear on umbrella-like stalks (umbellate clusters). The entire aboveground plant—from the stems to the leaves and flower tops—are used medicinally. They have a mild aromatic odor and slightly bitter taste.

What It Is Used For:

Yarrow is perhaps most famed as a wound healer. The herb was reportedly enlisted as a wound treatment during the Trojan wars; "Achillea" is the Latin name for the Greek hero Achilles. Later, Romans wounded in battle reportedly rubbed the herb into injured tissue. Folk healers in medieval Europe stopped bleeding—including nosebleeds—with it. Native Americans collected yarrow to treat burns and wounds. Many of the folk uses for yarrow are the same as those for **Chamomile**.

Contemporary herbalists recommend yarrow externally for controlling inflammation and preventing infection in wounds, ulcers, inflamed joints (using the essential oil), rashes, and mucous membrane inflammations. Herbal moisturizers sometimes contain yarrow to take advantage of its reported soothing and healing actions.

The herb has a similarly long history for internal use, having been taken for centuries to treat digestive system upset (including diarrhea, cramps, and gall-bladder ailments), and to stimulate sagging appetites, lower fever by inducing perspiration, control urinary tract infections, manage high blood pressure, stop diarrhea, and reduce menstrual pains. Traditional Chinese and Indian (Ayurvedic) healers relied on it in many ways as well. Yarrow appears in numerous herbal blends—especially in Europe—for gastrointestinal upset, biliary problems, and cough and congestion, to name a few. It is believed to stimulate the flow of bile, fight inflammation, improve blood clotting, counter infection, and resolve spasms.

Forms Available Include:

- *For external use:* Baths, fresh leaves and flowering tops, infusion, liquid extracts. Extracts appear in various lotions, ointments, poultices, herbal blends, and other formulas.
- *For internal use:* Capsule, infusion (of dried leaves and flowering tops), juice from fresh plant, liquid extracts, tea, tincture. Add honey, lemon, or sugar to the liquid formulations to mask the bitter taste.

Dosage Commonly Reported:

An infusion made using 1 to 2 teaspoons of dried yarrow is drunk three or four times a day, or applied externally. A common daily dose of the juice is 3 teaspoons, and for the tincture, ½ to 1 teaspoon. A bath is made by adding 100 grams of yarrow to 20 liters of water. The fresh leaves and flowering tops are used in a poultice. Two 340-milligram flower capsules are taken two to three times a day. The liquid herb extract is taken in doses of 2 to 4 milliliters.

Will It Work for You? What the Studies Say:

Although no human studies appear to have been done, chemical analyses and animal studies indicate that yarrow may effectively treat a number of conditions. Trojan warriors who bound wounds with the fresh leaves may have been on to something, for example. Scientists have identified various useful wound-healing substances in yarrow, including antiseptics (tannins, terpeniol, cineol) active against a wide range of common disease-causing bacteria, pain relievers such as camphor and eugenol, and substances that help stop bleeding (achilletin, achilleine). Yarrow also contains a blue-colored, aromatic volatile oil called azulene that boasts anti-inflammatory properties; chamomile contains this oil as well, which explains why the two herbs are often used in the same way. A number of yarrow's healing properties, such as the anti-inflammatory properties of topical liquid extracts[1] and the ability to reduce inflammation in classic rat-paw tests[2] have been demonstrated in animal experiments.

Yarrow also contains substances that explain its enduring popularity for certain internal ills. These include bitter-tasting substances that encourage the appetite and ease digestion by increasing salivation and stimulating gastric juices, and antispasmodic properties (in the azulene) that help relax the smooth muscle of the digestive tract. Animal experiments have confirmed bile-stimulating properties, which may also encourage good digestion.[3] German health authorities approve of using yarrow internally for appetite loss and digestive system upset such as mild cramplike pains in the abdominal area.[4]

Yarrow's antispasmodic and anti-inflammatory properties may help resolve painful cramplike conditions in the pelvic area, such as back pain and painful menstruation, according to a German physician who recommends sipping the herb tea slowly for these discomforts.[5] Benefits may be felt only if the remedy is taken over extended periods of time.[6] German health authorities approve of yarrow bath (sitz) formulas for treating painful, cramplike conditions of psychosomatic origin in the lower parts of the female pelvis; however, no human studies on this subject can be found in the medical literature.

Yarrow will help induce sweating, a property once highly valued for reducing fever. Scientists also report that the herb can lower blood pressure, but this action has not been studied in humans and may be too weak or unreliable.[7] The hypnotic chemical thujone appears in yarrow in small amounts and according to some herbalists may account for its use as a sedative. The capacity of the volatile oil to depress (slow down) central nervous system activity has been demonstrated in mouse studies,[8] but no human studies appear to have been done. The same is true for a slight diuretic action (increased urination) observed in mice fed high doses of a liquid extract.[9]

Will It Harm You? What the Studies Say:

The risk for side effects with typically recommended doses of yarrow is low. Excessive doses, however, may cause skin irritation, faintness, sedation, diarrhea, increased urination, or other unwanted reactions. Yarrow may also interfere with anticoagulant and blood-pressure treatments. Stop using the herb if any adverse reactions occur.

Pregnant women should avoid the herb given the presence of trace amounts of thujone, a chemical that can cause miscarriage at certain doses.[10] People with epilepsy should also use the herb with caution.[11] German health authorities advise that anyone who is allergic to yarrow or other plants of the same botanical family, such as chamomile and ragweed, should avoid using yarrow, including yarrow tea, because it could cause a rash, blistering, anaphylaxis, or other serious allergic reaction.[12] Handling the flowers could cause a rash with small blisters, and more serious reactions if the allergy is severe.

The FDA considers yarrow safe to use in commercial beverages as long as all of the potentially toxic substance thujone has been removed.

GENERAL SOURCES:

Albert-Puelo, M. *Economic Botany.* 32 (1978): 71.

Bisset, N.G., ed. *Herbal Drugs and Phytopharmaceuticals.* Stuttgart: medpharm GmbH Scientific Publishers, 1994.

Blumenthal, M., J. Gruenwald, T. Hall, and R.S. Rister, eds. *The Complete German Commission E Monographs: Therapeutic Guide to Herbal Medicine.* Boston: Integrative Medicine Communications, 1998.

Bradley, P.C., ed. *British Herbal Compendium: A Handbook of Scientific Information on Widely Used Plant Drugs.* Vol. 1. Bournemouth (Dorset), England: British Herbal Medicine Association, 1992.

Busse, W.W., et al. *Journal of Allergy and Clinical Immunology.* 73 (1984): 801.

Castleman, M. *The Healing Herbs: The Ultimate Guide to the Curative Power of Nature's Medicines.* New York: Bantam Books, 1995.

Duke, J.A. *CRC Handbook of Medicinal Herbs.* Boca Raton, FL: CRC Press, 1985.

———. *HerbalGram.* 12 (1987): 7.

Heinerman, J. *Heinerman's Encyclopedia of Healing Herbs and Spices.* West Nyack, NY: Parker Publishing Co., 1996.

Leung, A.Y., and S. Foster. *Encyclopedia of Common Natural Ingredients Used in Food, Drugs, and Cosmetics.* 2nd ed. New York: John Wiley & Sons, 1996.

Mayell, M. *Off-the-Shelf Natural Health: How to Use Herbs and Nutrients to Stay Well.* New York: Bantam Books, 1995.

Middleton, E., and G. Drzewiecki. *Biochemical Pharmacology.* 33 (1984): 3333.

Newall, C.A., et al. *Herbal Medicines: A Guide for Health-Care Professionals.* London: The Pharmaceutical Press, 1996.

Ody, P. *The Herb Society's Complete Medicinal Herbal.* London: Dorling Kindersley Limited, 1993.

Sama, S.K., et al. *Indian Journal of Medical Research.* 64 (1976): 738.

Stary, F. *The Natural Guide to Medicinal Herbs and Plants.* Prague: Barnes & Noble, Inc., in arrangement with Aventinum Publishers, 1996.

Tyler, V.E. *The Honest Herbal.* Binghamton, NY: Haworth Press/Pharmaceutical Products Press, 1993.

Tyler, V.E., L.R. Brady, and J.E. Robbers, eds. *Pharmacognosy.* Philadelphia: Lea & Febiger, 1988.

Weiss, R.F. *Herbal Medicine,* trans. A. R. Meuss, from the 6th German edition. Beaconsfield, England: Beaconsfield Publishers, Ltd., 1988.

TEXT CITATIONS:

1. A.S. Goldberg et al., *Journal of Pharmaceutical Sciences*, 58 (1972): 938–41.
2. T. Shipochliev and G. Fournadjiev, *Probl Vutr Med*, 12 (1984): 99–107.
3. N.G. Bisset, ed., *Herbal Drugs and Phytopharmaceuticals* (Stuttgart: medpharm GmbH Scientific Publishers, 1994).
4. M. Blumenthal, J. Gruenwald, T. Hall, and R.S. Rister, eds., *The Complete German Commission E Monographs: Therapeutic Guide to Herbal Medicine* (Boston: Integrative Medicine Communications, 1998).
5. Weiss, R.F. *Herbal Medicine*, trans. A. R. Meuss, from the 6th German edition (Beaconsfield, England: Beaconsfield Publishers, Ltd., 1988).
6. Ibid.
7. A.Y. Leung and S. Foster, *Encyclopedia of Common Natural Ingredients Used in Food, Drugs, and Cosmetics*, 2nd ed. (New York: John Wiley & Sons, 1996).
8. F.W. Kudrzycka-Bieloszabska, and K. Glowniak, *Diss Pharm Pharmacol*, (1966): 449–54.
9. A.S. Goldberg et al., *Journal of Pharmaceutical Sciences*, 58 (1969): 938–41.
10. C.A. Newall et al., *Herbal Medicines: A Guide for Health-Care Professionals* (London: The Pharmaceutical Press, 1996).
11. Ibid.
12. M. Abramowicz, ed., *Medical Letter on Drugs and Therapeutics*, 21(7) (1979): 30.

PRIMARY NAME:
YELLOW DOCK

SCIENTIFIC NAME:
Rumex crispus L. Family: Polygonaceae

COMMON NAMES:
Curled dock, curly dock, narrow dock, rumex, sad dock, sour dock

RATING:
3 = Studies on the effectiveness of this substance are conflicting, or there are not enough studies to draw a conclusion. However, see the safety warnings in the "Will It Harm You?" section.

Y

Yellow Dock

What Is Yellow Dock?

This perennial flowering herb, a native of Europe now found growing throughout the United States, has distinctive slender, light green leaves with curly margins. It grows about three- to four-feet high. The dried yellow rhizomes (underground stems) and roots are used medicinally.

What It Is Used For:

Over the centuries, folk healers have relied on this herb as an astringent and laxative, using it to remedy a myriad of ailments including anemia (the roots are said to absorb iron from the soil), cancer, and tuberculosis. Once introduced to yellow dock, Native American tribes reportedly applied it to burns, bruises, skin lesions, and oral sores. They also treated venereal diseases with it.[1] Asian Indians applied the powdered root to diseased gums. Many people today choose it as a dentifrice.

Some contemporary herbalists recommend yellow dock as a tonic and a blood "purifier" and "cleanser"—typical euphemisms for syphilis or venereal disease remedies.[2] Many extol its value in treating inflammatory and gallbladder disorders, contending that it purifies the blood by increasing the capacity of the liver and other organs. Some also recommend it for chronic skin diseases such as psoriasis, eczema, hives, and acne.

The herb's tart spring greens are boiled and eaten as a potherb in salads.

Forms Available Include:

Capsule, decoction, liquid extract, powder (for external use), root (dried), tea, tincture.

Dosage Commonly Reported:

Two to three 505-milligram root capsules are taken three times a day.

Will It Work for You? What the Studies Say:

Experts have deemed yellow dock an effective laxative based on the presence of well-known chemicals in the plant called anthraquinones (emodin, chrysophanic acid, physcion; approximately 2 percent of each). Anthraquinones stimulate a bowel movement by increasing the volume of the bowel contents and initiating peristalsis, the wavelike contractions of the large intestine that we experience as "the urge." Anthraquinones are also responsible for the effectiveness of laxatives such as **Senna** and **Cascara Sagrada**, which contain higher concentrations than yellow dock does. Interestingly, in the case of yellow dock, tannins (5 percent) also confer astringent properties that may actually promote constipation. (Tannins are believed to control or stop diarrhea by reducing inflammation in the intestines.)

When applied to minor skin wounds and mucous membranes such as the gums, the astringent tannins in yellow dock likely encourage healing by drawing tissue together and controlling oozing. Extracts of the herb have shown slight antibacterial activity toward common disease-causing bacteria such as *Staphylococcus aureus* and *Escherichia coli*.[3] A substance in yellow dock called chrysophanic acid has long been used topically to treat fungal infections, psoriasis, and other skin disorders.[4] A chemical called rumicin, a rubefacient, stimulates nourishing blood flow to the skin, warming and reddening the area. Despite these astringent, antiseptic, and blood-stimulating properties, however, the value of yellow dock for treating skin conditions remains unclear and largely unverified.

No evidence can be found to justify the use of yellow dock as a "blood purifier" or venereal disease cure.[5]

Will It Harm You? What the Studies Say:

Research and collective experience indicate that yellow dock root and rhizome preparations are safe to use in recommended amounts, but that excessive doses can be dangerous. Laxative formulations in which the anthraquinones have not been standardized may be risky to take because their potency is unreliable. Overdoses may cause abdominal cramps, diarrhea, nausea, and excessive urination.

Given the way that yellow dock encourages bowel movements, avoid the herb if you have an intestinal obstruction. Abuse of a laxative such as this may eventually lead to poor intestinal function, potassium loss, and other complications. It is not a good choice for constipation in pregnant women. Long-term use of any tannin-rich plant may carry some cancer risk, although much remains to be learned about this. Sensitive individuals may develop allergic contact dermatitis after handling the plant.

The leaves contain substances called oxalate crystals that can irritate and even damage mucosal tissue, cause stomach and intestinal upset, and result in kidney damage and other adverse reactions. For these reasons, avoid ingesting mature and uncooked leaves (boiled young leaves are probably safe) or using the leaves in such a way that these toxins could get absorbed into the body, such as applying them to open skin wounds.[6] Livestock that have consumed large amounts of yellow dock have died.[7] Tannic acid such as that found in yellow dock was promoted as an effective burn treatment in the mid-1920s in America, but the practice was stopped about two decades later when experts realized that large amounts of the acid were being absorbed into the body through the injured skin, posing the risk of liver damage.[8]

GENERAL SOURCES:

Der Marderosian, A., and L. Liberti. *Natural Product Medicine. A Scientific Guide to Foods, Drugs, Cosmetics.* Philadelphia: George F. Stickley, 1988.

Duke, J.A. *CRC Handbook of Medicinal Herbs.* Boca Raton, FL: CRC Press, 1985.

Hallowell, M. *Herbal Healing: A Practical Introduction to Medicinal Herbs.* Garden City Park, NY: 1994.

Lawrence Review of Natural Products. St. Louis: Facts and Comparisons, September 1992.

Mayell, M. *Off-the-Shelf Natural Health: How to Use Herbs and Nutrients to Stay Well.* New York: Bantam Books, 1995.

Mowrey, D.B. *Proven Herbal Blends: A Rational Approach to Prevention and Remedy.* Condensed from *The Scientific Validation of Herbal Medicine.* New Canaan, CT: Keats Publishing, Inc: 1986.

Newall, C.A., et al. *Herbal Medicines: A Guide for Health-Care Professionals.* London: The Pharmaceutical Press, 1996.

Tierra, M. *The Way of Herbs.* New York: Pocket Books, 1990.

Tyler, V.E. *Herbs of Choice: The Therapeutic Use of Phytomedicinals.* Binghamton, NY: Haworth Press/Pharmaceutical Products Press, 1994.

———. *The Honest Herbal.* Binghamton, NY: Haworth Press/Pharmaceutical Products Press, 1993.

Weiner, M.A., and J.A. Weiner. *Herbs That Heal: Prescription for Herbal Healing.* Mill Valley, CA: Quantum Books, 1994.

TEXT CITATIONS:

1. J.A. Duke, *CRC Handbook of Medicinal Herbs* (Boca Raton, FL: CRC Press, 1985).
2. V.E. Tyler, *The Honest Herbal* (Binghamton, NY: Haworth Press/Pharmaceutical Products Press, 1993).
3. M. Miyazawa and H. Kameoka, *Yakagaku,* 32 (1983): 45–47.
4. Duke, op. cit.
5. Tyler, op. cit.
6. *Lawrence Review of Natural Products* (St. Louis: Facts and Comparisons, September 1992).
7. Ibid.
8. Duke, op. cit.

YERBA SANTA

Eriodictyon californicum (Hook. et Arn.) Torr. Family: Hydrophyllaceae

COMMON NAMES:
Bear's weed, consumptive's weed, eriodictyon, gum plant, holy herb, mountain balm, tarweed

RATING:
3 = Studies on the effectiveness and safety of this substance are conflicting, or there are not enough studies to draw a conclusion.

What Is Yerba Santa?

This aromatic, flowering evergreen shrub is native to mountainous regions of the American southwest. It bears clusters of bluish to lavender flowers, and has thick, lance-shaped leaves. The dried leaves are used medicinally.

What It Is Used For:

Various Native American tribes smoked or chewed the leaves of this indigenous plant to treat asthma and made a tea to counter congestion from coughs and colds. Spanish missionaries quickly adopted the herb, as did settlers. The priests held it in such high esteem that they started referring to it as yerba santa, or holy weed. Some treated tuberculosis, asthma, and genitourinary infections with it. Poultices and other external formulations were used to relieve rheumatic pains and treat wounds and inflammatory skin conditions such as poison ivy, dermatitis, and bruises, and skin rubs were used to lower fevers.[1]

Yerba santa was officially listed in and then removed several times from the *U.S. Pharmacopoeia* as an expectorant, although it remains in the *National Formulary*. Many contemporary herbalists recommend the herb for clearing upper respiratory congestion caused by coughs and colds, asthma, chronic bronchitis, and hay fever. External uses remain essentially the same.

The herb serves as a flavoring in many bitter-tasting drugs such as quinine, as well as in foods and beverages.

Forms Available Include:

- *For internal use:* Extract, herb (dried), infusion, syrup, tincture.
- *For external use:* Poultice, rub.

Dosage Commonly Reported:

An infusion is made with 1 tablespoon of dried herb per glass of hot water and drunk once a day. The extract is taken in dosages of 10 to 20 drops per day.

Will It Work for You? What the Studies Say:

Science has revealed little about the potential healing properties of this herb. A substance called eriodictyol, present in concentrations up to 0.6 percent, is said to have expectorant properties valuable in treating respiratory ailments and may explain the herb's enduring popularity as a decongestant. Scientists have identified other such constituents as well, including eriodictyonine (3 to 6 percent), other flavonoids, a volatile oil (trace amounts), tannin (an astringent), and resin.[2] But whether these substances are present in adequate concentrations or in a form that the human body can use is far from clear.

In 1992, investigators reported isolating twelve potential chemopreventive substances in the herb, specifically flavones that inhibit the metabolism of the cancer-causing chemical benzopyrene.[3] They recommend that these flavones be further investigated as potential cancer-preventing agents.

Will It Harm You? What the Studies Say:

Very little is known about the potential for adverse reactions to yerba santa, although no reports of toxicity can be found in the recent medical literature. The FDA approves of the herb as a food ingredient.

GENERAL SOURCES:

Hylton, W.H., ed. *The Rodale Herb Book: How to Use, Grow, and Buy Nature's Miracle Plants.* Emmaus, PA: Rodale Press, Inc., 1974.
Lawrence Review of Natural Products. St. Louis: Facts and Comparisons, March 1991.
Leung, A.Y., and S. Foster. *Encyclopedia of Common Natural Ingredients Used in Food, Drugs, and Cosmetics.* 2nd ed. New York: John Wiley & Sons, 1996.
Mindell, E. *Earl Mindell's Herb Bible.* New York: Simon & Schuster/Fireside, 1992.
Tierra, M. *The Way of Herbs.* New York: Pocket Books, 1990.

TEXT CITATIONS:

1. *Lawrence Review of Natural Products* (St. Louis: Facts and Comparisons, March 1991).
2. A.Y. Leung and S. Foster, *Encyclopedia of Common Natural Ingredients Used in Food, Drugs, and Cosmetics,* 2nd ed. (New York: John Wiley & Sons, 1996).
3. Y.L. Liu et al., *Journal of Natural Products,* 55(3) (1992): 357–63.

SCIENTIFIC NAME:

Taxus brevifolia Nutt. Related species in the United States include *Taxus canadensis* Marsh. and *Taxus floridana* Nutt., and in Europe, *Taxus bacatta* L. and *Taxus cuspidata* Sieb. and Zucc. Family: Taxaceae

COMMON NAMES:

California yew, ground hemlock, Pacific yew

RATING:

2 = According to a number of well-designed studies and common use, this substance appears to be relatively effective when used in recommended amounts for the indication(s) noted in the "Will It Work for You?" section. Its safety depends on proper and judicious use, however; see the "Will It Harm You?" section.

What Is Pacific Yew?

This slow-growing, flowering evergreen tree can be found throughout woods and forests from the shores of Alaska down along the coast to Washington, Oregon, and northern California, and into Idaho and Montana. It and related species, some of them bushes rather than trees, have reddish bark and flat, dark green, needlelike leaves with pale undersides. The bark is used medicinally. The trees have no cones. Female trees produce green to black seeds partially covered with a berrylike, fleshy red fruit called an aril.

What It Is Used For:

Legend has it that Druids planted the revered native yew species in holy sites and that Celts dipped their arrows in yew sap to poison their targets. Traditional healers reportedly administered very small amounts of leaf tinctures made with various yew species to remedy urinary, liver, and rheumatic complaints, but the plant's toxicity was readily recognized and the practice did not endure.

In recent times, the Pacific yew has captured the attention of the medical profession because the bark was found to contain small amounts (about 0.01 percent) of an anticancer compound designated paclitaxel, an alkaloid. (Taxol is the brand name for paclitaxel.) When given intravenously, paclitaxel has shown great promise in treating certain types of cancer. Other yew species have also been used. But given the scarcity of this material—concerns have been voiced over stripping the bark of many majestic yews to extract small amounts of the medicine—researchers have been investigating ways to cultivate precursors of the active ingredients from other parts of the tree, as well as from other yew species. Some have tried to synthesize the active ingredient.

Forms Available Include:

Injection solutions.

Dosage Commonly Reported:

The bark is not appropriate for home use.

Will It Work for You? What the Studies Say:

Paclitaxel has shown promise in treating various types of cancer, including those affecting the ovaries,[1] breasts,[2] cervix (squamous cervix cancers),[3] and skin (malignant melanomas).[4] In some cases, studies have used derivatives from other yew trees, such as taxotere from the English yew. Paclitaxel has a unique mechanism of action, preventing cells from dividing by interfering with a critical step in their reproductive process. As a result, cancer cells have less chance to continue their rapid division, growth, and spread through the body.

Clinical studies have been conducted both in the United States and abroad. The first few involved women with advanced ovarian cancer.[5] Recently, promising results have been reported in adding taxol to another chemotherapy drug, cisplatin, in women with advanced ovarian cancer.[6] Paclitaxel has become the preferred treatment (over estrogens) for treating metastatic breast cancer in postmenopausal women, with significant increases in disease-free survival in these women, particularly if they have hormone-receptor-positive tumors.[7]

Will It Harm You? What the Studies Say:

With the exception of the red aril, all parts of the yew are poisonous. Symptoms of poisoning that develop within an hour of ingesting the plant may include dizziness, dry mouth, pupil dilation, abdominal cramping, salivation, vomiting, rash, paleness in the face, and blueness of the lips.[8] Shortness of breath, slow heartbeat, and low blood pressure may develop, with possible coma and death due to cardiac or respiratory failure. A number of fatalities have been reported in people who drank yew tea or swallowed the leaves.[9]

On the other hand, most people appear to tolerate intravenous treatment with paclitaxel for cancer relatively well. Bone marrow suppression and hypersensitivity reactions presented problems particularly in earlier trials before investigators learned how to handle them better. Other adverse reactions have included muscle and joint pains, hair loss, diarrhea, nausea, vomiting, and peripheral neuropathy (abnormal sensations in the distal nerves of the body).[10] Sometimes administering the drug over a longer period of time reduces these types of reactions.

GENERAL SOURCES:

Bremness, L. *Herbs.* 1st American ed. Eyewitness Handbooks. New York: Dorling Kindersley Publications, 1994.

Chevallier, A. *The Encyclopedia of Medicinal Plants: A Practical Reference Guide to More Than 550 Key Medicinal Plants & Their Uses.* 1st American ed. New York: Dorling Kindersley Publications, 1996.

Dobelis, I.N., ed. *The Magic and Medicine of Plants: A Practical Guide to the Science, History, Folklore, and Everyday Uses of Medicinal Plants.* Pleasantville, NY: Reader's Digest Association, 1986.

Lampe, K.E., and M.A. McCann. *AMA Handbook of Poisonous and Injurious Plants.* Chicago: American Medical Association, 1985.

Lawrence Review of Natural Products. St. Louis: Facts and Comparisons, May 1993.

Mayell, M. *Off-the-Shelf Natural Health: How to Use Herbs and Nutrients to Stay Well.* New York: Bantam Books, 1995.

Tyler, V.E. *Herbs of Choice: The Therapeutic Use of Phytomedicinals.* Binghamton, NY: Haworth Press/Pharmaceutical Products Press, 1994.

TEXT CITATIONS:

1. T. Thigpen et al., *Seminars in Oncology*, 22(6 Suppl 14) (1995): 23–31. N.O. McGuire et al., *Annals of Internal Medicine*, 111(4) (1989): 273–79.
2. S.S. Legha, *Annals of Internal Medicine*, 109(3) (1988): 219–28.
3. W.P. McGuire et al., *Journal of Clinical Oncology*, 14(3) (1996): 792–95.
4. A.Y. Bedikian et al., *Journal of Clinical Oncology*, 13(12) (1995): 2895–99. S.S. Legha et al., *Cancer*, 65(11) (1990): 2478–81.
5. N.O. McGuire, et al., *Annals of Internal Medicine*, 111(4) (1989): 273–79.
6. W.P. McGuire et al., *New England Journal of Medicine*, 334(1) (1996): 1–6.
7. S.S. Legha, *Annals of Internal Medicine*, 109(3) (1988): 219–28.
8. K.E. Lampe and M.A. McCann, *AMA Handbook of Poisonous and Injurious Plants* (Chicago: American Medical Association, 1985).
9. *Lawrence Review of Natural Products* (St. Louis: Facts and Comparisons, May 1993).
10. N.O. McGuire et al., *Annals of Internal Medicine*, 111(4) (1989): 273–79.

PRIMARY NAME:

YOGURT

SCIENTIFIC NAME:
N/A

COMMON NAME:
N/A

Y

Yogurt

RATING:

2 = According to a number of well-designed studies and common use, this substance appears to be relatively effective and safe when used in recommended amounts for the indication(s) noted in the "Will It Work for You?" section.

What Is Yogurt?

The fermented milk product known as yogurt is made by adding "friendly" bacteria to heated whole or skimmed cow's milk. These bacteria act on the sugars in the milk to create a semisolid curdled or coagulated material. Typically, the live cultures of *Lactobacillus buglaricus* and *Streptococcus thermophilus* are used, although *Lactobacillus acidophilus* has become increasingly popular. Yogurt can be made at home with a special yogurt maker.

What It Is Used For:

People have been enjoying the taste and texture of yogurt for centuries. It is an excellent source of calcium and vitamins. It has been proposed as a remedy for various ailments, including vaginal yeast infections (*Candida*), and as a protective agent against high cholesterol and tumors. Some individuals intolerant to the lactose in (most) milk products—a condition called lactase deficiency syndrome—consume yogurt because they seem to be able to digest it more easily than other dairy products. Its "friendly" bacteria have been touted as valuable for restoring normal gastrointestinal flora after antibiotic therapy; see **Acidophilus** for more information about this, as well as for information on yogurt as a vaginal douche.

Forms Available Include:

Whole, low-fat, or nonfat; also available as a liquid and in capsule form.

Dosage Commonly Reported:

To combat vaginal yeast infections, 8 ounces of yogurt containing live acidophilus cultures are eaten daily.

Will It Work for You? What the Studies Say:

Researchers are still searching for the component in yogurt and other dairy products that explains an apparent lipid-lowering action. In one sixteen-week study, both calcium supplements and yogurt added to the high-cholesterol diets of rabbits eventually reduced cholesterol levels significantly more than in rabbits that were only given milk as a supplement.[1] In 1977, investigators reported that individuals whose normal diets were supplemented daily with yogurt (whole or skimmed) experienced significant drops in cholesterol levels within twenty days.[2] In comparison, the cholesterol levels in those given milk (whole or skimmed) generally did not fall. The amount of daily yogurt needed to protect against high cholesterol levels has yet to be established, however.[3]

Many sources have recommended eating yogurt to restore normal concentrations of healthy stomach flora after antibiotic therapy; antibiotics can adversely alter the gut's bacterial composition by promoting the activity of various fungi. Research has shown that yogurt also fights *Salmonella typhimurium*, *Staphylococcus aureus*, and other disease-causing organisms. In one study, yogurt reduced rates of infectious illnesses and death when given to rats intentionally infected with *Salmonella*.[4] But well-designed studies have yet to confirm the value of consuming yogurt to restore normal concentrations of healthy stomach and intestinal flora after antibiotic therapy. More than a decade ago, experts concluded that bacterial replacement therapy with live cultures was of no value in combating yeast infections.[5] Live bacteria in yogurt may not survive the trip to the gut, especially in older individuals.[6] Studies also indicate that the beneficial bacteria do not survive the journey to the colon in healthy individuals,[7] and therefore may be of no use in alleviating anal itching, for example.

Similarly, directly inserting yogurt into the vagina for yeast infections, as is recommended in several home remedy books, is generally ineffective.[8] However, a 1993 study in pregnant women with bacterial vaginosis—in which case the culprit is a bacterium rather than a yeast—found that commercial yogurt inserted into the vagina benefited the acidity of the vagina and *Lactobacillus flora*.[9] Although the women tolerated the treatment well, more well-controlled trials are needed before this strategy can be recommended.[10] For more information on yogurt and vaginal yeast infections, see **Acidophilus**.

Although requiring more controlled trials, preliminary research indicates that consuming yogurt may slightly lower the risk of colon, breast, and possibly other cancers. In a 1994 study, investigators found that increased consumption of fermented dairy products such as yogurt slightly decreased the risk of colorectal cancer in 120,852 Dutch men who were followed for three years.[11] In 1986 an analysis of alcohol and dairy produce consumption in nearly 3,000 individuals found that eating yogurt regularly was associated with a lower rate of new cases of breast cancer.[12] Investigators have also identified compounds in *Lactobacillus bulgaris*, a common yogurt ingredient, that inhibit the growth and development of tumors in laboratory animals.

As of yet, no firm conclusions can be drawn about whether individuals with lactase-deficiency syndrome can tolerate yogurt much better than milk,[13] although the studies done so far indicate that most can. The type and amount of yogurt consumed probably makes a big difference.[14] Yogurt contains about 3 percent lactose, milk contains 4.6 percent, and Bulgarian yogurt contains about 4.5 percent. In one study, neither unflavored nor flavored yogurt caused symptoms of lactose intolerance in lactase-deficient subjects.[15] Breath tests (of hydrogen) indicated that the subjects tolerated unflavored yogurt much better than milk and flavored yogurt moderately better than milk.

Will It Harm You? What the Studies Say:

People have been eating yogurt for centuries to no apparent ill effect. The greatest risk may be posed by contamination of yogurt batches with toxic bacteria, a very uncommon situation but one that can occur, especially with homemade yogurt.

GENERAL SOURCES:

American Pharmaceutical Association. *Handbook of Nonprescription Drugs*. 11th ed. Washington, D.C.: American Pharmaceutical Association, 1996.

Balch, J.F., and P.A. Balch. *Prescription for Nutritional Healing: A Practical A to Z Reference to Drug-Free Remedies Using Vitamins, Minerals, Herbs & Food Supplements*. 2nd ed. Garden City Park, NY: Avery Publishing Group, 1997.

Der Marderosian, A., and L. Liberti. *Natural Product Medicine. A Scientific Guide to Foods, Drugs, Cosmetics*. Philadelphia: George F. Stickley, 1988.

Lawrence Review of Natural Products. St. Louis: Facts and Comparisons, May 1995.

Tyler, V.E. *Herbs of Choice: The Therapeutic Use of Phytomedicinals*. Binghamton, NY: Haworth Press/Pharmaceutical Products Press, 1994.

TEXT CITATIONS:

1. M. Eichholzer and H. Stahelin, *International Journal of Vitamin and Nutrition Research*, 63(3) (1993): 159.
2. G.V. Mann, *Atherosclerosis*, 26(3) (1977): 335.
3. *Lawrence Review of Natural Products* (St. Louis: Facts and Comparisons, May 1995).
4. A.D. Hitchins et al., *Nutrition Reports Intern*, 31 (1985): 601.
5. *Medical Letter Drugs Ther*, 14(16) (192): 59. *Lawrence Review of Natural Products*, op. cit.
6. Ibid.
7. H.P. Bartram et al., *American Journal of Clinical Nutrition*. 59(2) (1994): 428.
8. American Pharmaceutical Association, *Handbook of Nonprescription Drugs*, 11th ed. (Washington, D.C.: American Pharmaceutical Association, 1996).
9. A. Neri et al., *Acta Obstet Gynecol Scand*, 72(l) (1993): 17.
10. *Lawrence Review of Natural Products*, op. cit.
11. E. Kampman et al., *Cancer Research*, 54(12) (1994): 3186.
12. M.G. Le et al., *Journal of the National Cancer Institute*, 77(3) (1986): 633.
13. *Lawrence Review of Natural Products*, op. cit.
14. A. Der Marderosian and L. Liberti, *Natural Product Medicine. A Scientific Guide to Foods, Drugs, Cosmetics* (Philadelphia: George F. Stickley, 1988).
15. M.C. Martini et al., *American Journal of Clinical Nutrition*, 46(4) (1987): 636.

YOHIMBE

SCIENTIFIC NAME:
Pausinystalia yohimbe (K. Schum.) Pierre, also referred to as *Corynanthe johimbi* Schum. Family: Rubiaceae

COMMON NAME:
Yohimbehe

RATING:
2 = According to a number of well-designed studies and common use, this substance appears to be relatively effective and safe when used in recommended amounts for the indication(s) noted in the "Will It Work for You?" section. See the "Will It Harm You?" section for precautions, however.

What Is Yohimbe?

The bark of this tall West African evergreen tree is used medicinally. It contains a mixture of chemicals called alkaloids, including the all-important yohimbine believed to be responsible for many of the bark's claimed effects. The tree has large, leathery leaves and white flowers arranged in clusters.

What It Is Used For:

West Africans have reportedly long enjoyed yohimbe bark tea as an aphrodisiac to stimulate sexual desire and performance. They also consider it a cure for impotence. Both the bark and a purified compound of yohimbine, for which there are now prescription formulations in some countries, have been used for these purposes. Impotence caused by psychogenic factors such as anxiety, fear, and feelings of inadequacy have been treated with it, although most of the focus is now on impotence due to organic problems such as diabetes.[1] The bark has been smoked as an hallucinogen. Folk healers have also prescribed it for angina (chest pain), high blood pressure, and to boost athletic performance. Yohimbe is available in minute doses in homeopathic form. (See page 2 for more information on homeopathy.)

Forms Available Include:

- *Yohimbe bark:* Capsule, concentrated drops, decoction, tablet, tea, tincture.
- *Yohimbine:* Tablet (available by prescription only).

Dosage Commonly Reported:

The alkaloid yohimbine should be taken only under a doctor's supervision.

Will It Work for You? What the Studies Say:

Both the bark and its contained alkaloid, yohimbine, an alpha-2-adrenergic blocking agent (it blocks certain nerve receptors), are active drugs, but more research has been conducted on yohimbine. Neither measure up as aphrodisiacs. The herb and its alkaloid dilate (open up) the blood vessels of the skin and mucous membranes, leading to an increased blood flow to the sexual organs and presumably resulting in an erection in males and arousal in females. There is also increased reflex excitability in the related region of the spinal cord, and increased nerve stimulation in the genital area.[2] But these substances also cause an often notable drop in blood pressure, depleting energy reserves for a sexual encounter. Citing both a lack of proven and consistent effectiveness and a high risk of adverse reactions, German health authorities have declined to approve of either yohimbe or yohimbine as a stimulant or male aphrodisiac.[3]

Interestingly, yohimbine also stimulates the central nervous system at low doses, causing sensations of anxiety in many users. This stimulation also explains the interest in the alkaloid as a treatment for male impotence. Recent reports indicate yohimbine may have some value in improving erectile function in men suffering from impotence (related to both psychogenic and organic causes) to the point at which they can carry through the act of sexual intercourse. Earlier studies typically relied on a prescription product (Afrodex) that produced unimpressive results; current thinking is that the dose must be higher (6 milligrams three times a day) than what was included in that formulation.[4] Several investigators have recommended yohimbine for impotence, contending that it is as effective and safe as other treatment strategies for the problem.[5] Yohimbine may be particularly beneficial for impotent men with diabetes; in one study involving eleven diabetics, ten of the twenty-three men benefited from the drug.[6] German health authorities, however, are still unimpressed with the numbers and have declined to approve of yohimbe or yohimbine as treatments for male impotence.[7]

Will It Harm You? What the Studies Say:

Yohimbe and its contained alkaloid, yohimbine, are powerful medicines that must be taken with care and respect. Responsible sources recommend taking them only under the guidance of a doctor. Caution is needed because the effective dose is very close to the toxic dose. Side effects may include agitation, nervousness, anxiety, panic attacks, tremors, sleeplessness, elevated blood pressure and heart rate, salivation, nausea, and vomiting. Some people may even develop hallucinations. Larger doses may cause severe low blood pressure, weakness, and ultimately central nervous stimulation and paralysis.

Even with proper professional supervision, neither yohimbe nor yohimbine should be taken if you have low blood pressure, chronic inflammation of the prostate gland or related organs, or heart, kidney, or liver disease. Because yohimbe is classified as a monoamine-oxidase (MAO) inhibitor, do not take it at the same time as consuming tyramine-containing foods such as cheese, red wine, and liver, or with nasal decongestants or phenylpropanolamine-containing diet aids. It should probably not be mixed with antidepressants or mood-altering drugs[8]; there is a risk of triggering psychoses in predisposed people, such as those with schizophrenia.[9]

The FDA has ruled yohimbine unsafe and ineffective for over-the-counter use, but both yohimbe and yohimbine can be found in health-food outlets. Some states such as Georgia have banned their sale in nonprescription form, however. A laboratory sampling of yohimbe capsules sold in the Netherlands revealed that the amount of the herb was misrepresented and that the capsules also contained several other active substances (alkaloids).

GENERAL SOURCES:

Balch, J.F., and P.A. Balch. *Prescription for Nutritional Healing: A Practical A to Z Reference to Drug-Free Remedies Using Vitamins, Minerals, Herbs & Food Supplements.* 2nd ed. Garden City Park, NY: Avery Publishing Group, 1997.

Bisset, N.G., ed. *Herbal Drugs and Phytopharmaceuticals.* Stuttgart: medpharm GmbH Scientific Publishers, 1994.

Blumenthal, M., J. Gruenwald, T. Hall, and R.S. Rister, eds. *The Complete German Commission E Monographs: Therapeutic Guide to Herbal Medicine.* Boston: Integrative Medicine Communications, 1998.

Lawrence Review of Natural Products. St. Louis: Facts and Comparisons, May 1993.

Leung, A.Y., and S. Foster. *Encyclopedia of Common Natural Ingredients Used in Food, Drugs, and Cosmetics.* 2nd ed. New York: John Wiley & Sons, 1996.

Mayell, M. *Off-the-Shelf Natural Health: How to Use Herbs and Nutrients to Stay Well.* New York: Bantam Books, 1995.

Tyler, V.E. *Herbs of Choice: The Therapeutic Use of Phytomedicinals*. Binghamton, NY: Haworth Press/Pharmaceutical Products Press, 1994.

———. *The Honest Herbal*. Binghamton, NY: Haworth Press/Pharmaceutical Products Press, 1993.

Tyler, V.E., L.R. Brady, and J.E. Robbers, eds. *Pharmacognosy*. Philadelphia: Lea & Febiger, 1988.

Weiner, M.A., and J.A. Weiner. *Herbs That Heal: Prescription for Herbal Healing*. Mill Valley, CA: Quantum Books, 1994.

TEXT CITATIONS:
1. *Lawrence Review of Natural Products* (St. Louis: Facts and Comparisons, May 1993).
2. A.Y. Leung and S. Foster, *Encyclopedia of Common Natural Ingredients Used in Food, Drugs, and Cosmetics*, 2nd ed. (New York: John Wiley & Sons, 1996).
3. M. Blumenthal, J. Gruenwald, T. Hall, and R.S. Rister, eds., *The Complete German Commission E Monographs: Therapeutic Guide to Herbal Medicine* (Boston: Integrative Medicine Communications, 1998).
4. *Lawrence Review of Natural Products*, op. cit. *Medical World News*, 23 (1982): 115.
5. K. Reid et al., *Lancet*, II (1987): 421–23.
6. A. Morales et al., *Journal of Urology*, 128 (1982): 45.
7. Blumenthal et al., op. cit.
8. Leung and Foster, op. cit.
9. V.E. Tyler, *The Honest Herbal* (Binghamton, NY: Haworth Press/Pharmaceutical Products Press, 1993). Ingram, C.G., *Clinical Pharmacology and Therapeutics*, 3 (1962): 345–52.

PRIMARY NAME:

YUCCA

SCIENTIFIC NAME:
Various *Yucca* species, including *Yucca glauca*, *Yucca schidigera* Roezl et Ortgies, and *Yucca brevifolia* Engelm. Family: Agavaceae

COMMON NAMES:
Adam's needle, dagger plant, Joshua tree, Our Lord's candle, soapweed, Spanish bayonet. (These common names refer to various *Yucca* species.)

RATING:
4 = Research indicates that this substance will not fulfill the claims made for it, but that it is also unlikely to cause any harm.

What Is Yucca?

As many as forty or more species of *Yucca* grow across North America, primarily in arid, warmer sections. Many of these hardy trees or shrubs have stiff, evergreen lance-shaped leaves that emerge off erect central stems, and candlelike white or greenish flowerheads. All rely on nocturnal yucca moths for pollination. The dried leaves and occasionally the dried root are used medicinally.

What It Is Used For:

For centuries, various Native American tribes relied on the yucca plant as a source for food, cloth, rope, and cleaning substances, and as a healing remedy for skin diseases and sores, inflammation, and bleeding. The many uses for which contemporary herbalists have recommended it include migraine headache and high blood pressure, although its purported value in relieving arthritic and rheumatic pains has been headlined the most vigorously. Yucca extracts can be found in shampoos, cleansers, flavorings, frothy drinks such as root beer (as a foaming agent), and other commercial products.

Forms Available:

Capsule, decoction, liquid extract, tablet, tincture.

Dosage Commonly Reported:

Three 490-milligram capsules are taken three times a day.

Y

Yucca

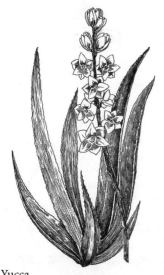

Yucca
Yucca glauca

Will It Work for You? What the Studies Say:

The value of treating arthritis and rheumatism with yucca preparations remains unclear. The plant's popular reputation was born with a 1975 study reporting success and safety in treating arthritis in test subjects who took a yucca extract (a saponin) four times a day.[1] The 75 to 150 arthritis sufferers reportedly experienced some relief from pain, swelling, and stiffness. The study suffered from several weaknesses, however, including that patients continued to take other medications.[2] Also, the investigators did not describe which part of the plant or which *Yucca* species they were using. Dosages and treatment periods also differed widely, from one week to fifteen months in some cases. The Arthritis Foundation released a statement declaring the study poorly designed and controlled and the conclusions based on inconsistent results. "There is no proper scientific evidence that yucca tablets are useful for treating rheumatoid arthritis or osteoarthritis," the statement read.[3] Apparently no well-designed studies in humans have been done since then to support or refute the results.

Interestingly, in the same arthritis study noted above, reductions in blood pressure and cholesterol levels were noted for the subjects who took the yucca extract for six months or more. The yucca extracts also improved circulation and offered some relief from headaches.[4] The importance of these findings has yet to be fully explored.

The primary active ingredients in yucca are steroidal saponins, which appear in varying amounts based on factors such as when the plant was harvested. Mouse studies found that liquid alcoholic extracts of the *Yucca glauca* plant are active against B^{16} melanoma[5]; melanoma is a serious type of skin cancer. Test-tube investigations indicate that a protein in the yucca leaf can inhibit the virus that causes oral and genital herpes eruptions (herpes simplex virus types 1 and 2) and also the human cytomegalovirus.[6] The implications of these and other research findings for treating tumors, herpes outbreaks, or other ailments in humans are still very hazy.

Will It Harm You? What the Studies Say:

Although yucca appears to be relatively safe to take as an herbal remedy, no human trials have been done specifically to determine its toxicity. Importantly, no signs of toxicity were noted in more than seven hundred subjects who took a saponin-containing extract in an arthritis study.[7] Rats fed yucca for twelve weeks displayed no signs of a toxic reaction.[8] Its traditional use as a food also bodes well for its safety.[9]

Scientists know that saponins often present in the plant in high concentrations can cause hemolysis (destruction of red blood cells) in the test tube and when injected into the body.[10] Some experts seem to consider the risk of this kind of a reaction quite remote when the herb is taken orally, largely because the yucca saponins are not thought to be absorbed into the body through the gastrointestinal tract.[11] Others seem to consider the reaction possible but probably weak.[12] So far there have been no reports of this hemolysis occurring in humans taking yucca.

GENERAL SOURCES:

Balch, J.F., and P.A. Balch. *Prescription for Nutritional Healing: A Practical A to Z Reference to Drug-Free Remedies Using Vitamins, Minerals, Herbs & Food Supplements.* 2nd ed. Garden City Park, NY: Avery Publishing Group, 1997.

Lawrence Review of Natural Products. St. Louis: Facts and Comparisons, March 1994.

Leung, A.Y., and S. Foster. *Encyclopedia of Common Natural Ingredients Used in Food, Drugs, and Cosmetics.* 2nd ed. New York: John Wiley & Sons, 1996.

Mindell, E. *Earl Mindell's Herb Bible.* New York: Simon & Schuster/Fireside, 1992.

Newall, C.A., et al. *Herbal Medicines: A Guide for Health-Care Professionals.* London: The Pharmaceutical Press, 1996.

Tierra, M. *The Way of Herbs.* New York: Pocket Books, 1990.

Tyler, V.E. *The Honest Herbal.* Binghamton, NY: Haworth Press/Pharmaceutical Products Press, 1993.

Tyler, V.E., L.R. Brady, and J.E. Robbers, eds. *Pharmacognosy.* Philadelphia: Lea & Febiger, 1988.

Weiner, M.A., and J.A. Weiner. *Herbs That Heal: Prescription for Herbal Healing.* Mill Valley, CA: Quantum Books, 1994.

TEXT CITATIONS:

1. R. Bingham et al., *Journal of Applied Nutrition,* 27(2–3) (1975): 45–51.
2. V.E. Tyler, *The Honest Herbal* (Binghamton, NY: Haworth Press/Pharmaceutical Products Press, 1993).
3. C.C. Benett, *Public Information Memo* (New York: The Arthritis Foundation. February 22, 1977).
4. *Lawrence Review of Natural Products* (St. Louis: Facts and Comparisons, March 1994).
5. M.S. Ali et al., *Growth,* 42 (1978): 213.
6. K. Hayashi et al., *Antiviral Research,* 17 (1992): 323.
7. C.A. Newall et al., *Herbal Medicines: A Guide for Health-Care Professionals* (London: The Pharmaceutical Press, 1996).
8. B.L. Oser, *Food & Cosmetics Toxicology,* 4 (1966): 57.
9. Newall, op. cit.
10. *Lawrence Review of Natural Products,* op. cit.
11. R. Bingham et al., *Journal of Applied Nutrition,* 27 (1975): 45–51. Newall, op. cit.
12. *Lawrence Review of Natural Products,* op. cit.

RATING:

2 = According to a number of well-designed studies and common use, this substance appears to be relatively safe when used in recommended amounts for the indication(s) noted in the "Will It Work for You?" section. However, see the warnings in the "Will It Harm You?" section.

What Is Zinc?

Zinc is a trace mineral obtained through the diet that the body uses in a number of fundamental ways.

What It Is Used For:

Zinc is essential to normal cellular immune function and stabilization of membrane structure and contributes to the synthesis of DNA and RNA. The body regulates this trace mineral very efficiently. Most Americans get their zinc (about 70 percent) from meats and other animal products.[1] High-protein foods such as peanuts, whole-grain cereals, and oysters are also good sources.

Recently, dietary supplement manufacturers and other sources have started to recommend taking zinc supplements prevent and treat a variety of disorders, including colds, skin diseases, infertility, alcoholism, and ulcers. Some suggest taking it to help wounds heal, increase "brain power," encourage weight loss, prevent or treat certain serious eye disorders, promote beautiful skin and heightened senses, reduce cancer risk, boost the immune system, detoxify the liver, and increase male sexual potency. Others hail it as an antioxidant.

Forms Available Include:

Capsule, lozenge, tablet. Also appears in many multivitamin and multimineral supplements.

Dosage Commonly Reported:

The Recommended Daily Allowance for zinc is 15 milligrams for adult men, 12 milligrams for adult women, 10 milligrams for children, and 5 milligrams for infants. Because zinc is only partially absorbed from the gastrointestinal tract, taking 220 milligrams of zinc sulfate (50 milligrams of elemental zinc) supplies 5 to 20 milligrams of zinc.

Will It Work for You? What the Studies Say:

Low zinc levels have been linked to slow wound healing, growth retardation in children, appetite loss, skin problems, night blindness, delayed sexual development, sensory impairments, and complications in child birth. Zinc deficiencies in the United States today are uncommon, however. Most Americans probably get 20 to 50 milligrams of zinc in their diet every day, as much as or more than the Recommended Daily Allowance (RDA)[2]

Vegetarians do not generally suffer from low zinc levels. Serious zinc deficiencies generally occur only in individuals with gastrointestinal tract problems such as fistulas or severe diarrhea, or in individuals on IV feeding tubes.[3] A number of conditions may cause zinc levels to be lower than ideal, including major surgery, heart attack, infection, alcoholism, cirrhosis of the liver, and malabsorption syndrome. Pregnant and lactating women need to ensure that they get adequate amounts of this and other important vitamins and minerals. Except for a few notable exceptions, no evidence in the scientific literature can be found to substantiate claims that zinc above RDA levels will prevent or treat any ailment or condition in an otherwise healthy individual. The exceptions to this are in the treatment of the common cold and in wound healing. If taken within hours of cold symptoms developing, zinc lozenges may reduce the severity of symptoms, according to a handful of studies.[4] More research is needed to substantiate these promising findings. There is also evidence that supplementing the diet with zinc may help individuals who have wounds that are not healing properly.[5]

Will It Harm You? What the Studies Say:

Zinc can cause gastrointestinal upset and vomiting at high doses (2 grams, or 2,000 milligrams). Talk to a medical professional before taking more than 15 milligrams a day over long stretches of time.[6] Signs of zinc toxicity include vomiting and potential abdominal pain, dizziness, dehydration, and muscle incoordination.

Zinc may decrease the absorption of tetracycline or lower levels of copper (with high zinc doses), so avoid taking zinc at the same time as taking these substances. Conversely, foods high in calcium, phosphate, or phytate may decrease the absorption of zinc, as may bran and dairy products.

GENERAL SOURCES:

American Pharmaceutical Association. *Handbook of Nonprescription Drugs.* 11th ed. Washington, D.C.: American Pharmaceutical Association, 1996.

Balch, J.F., and P.A. Balch. *Prescription for Nutritional Healing: A Practical A to Z Reference to Drug-Free Remedies Using Vitamins, Minerals, Herbs & Food Supplements.* 2nd ed. Garden City Park, NY: Avery Publishing Group, 1997.

Mayell, M. *Off-the-Shelf Natural Health: How to Use Herbs and Nutrients to Stay Well.* New York: Bantam Books, 1995.

TEXT CITATIONS:

1. American Pharmaceutical Association, *Handbook of Nonprescription Drugs*, 11th ed. (Washington, D.C.: American Pharmaceutical Association, 1996).
2. Ibid.
3. Ibid.
4. G.A. Eby et al., *Antimicrobial Agents & Chemotherapy*, 25 (1984): 20–24. J.C. Godfrey et al., *Journal of International Medical Research*, 20 (1992): 234–46. American Pharmaceutical Association, op. cit.
5. American Pharmaceutical Association, op. cit.
6. Ibid.

Index of Symptoms

Note: Substances recommended to treat the following indications are listed under each symptom or condition. Always check the actual entry before using a natural medicine for any reason.

ABDOMINAL PAIN
acidophilus
allspice
peppermint

ACNE
basil
fruit acids
pansy

AIDS/HIV
aloe vera
cucumber, Chinese
marijuana
scullcap

ALCOHOLISM
kudzu

ALLERGIES
dong quai
gingko
nettle
reishi mushroom

ALZHEIMER'S DISEASE
gingko
lecithin

ANEMIA
anise (and star anise)
chive

ANESTHETICS
allspice
arnica

ANTISEPTICS
agrimony
allspice
arnica
honey
oak bark
red clover
tea tree oil
uva ursi
yarrow

APHRODISIACS
damiana
deer antler

APPETITE DEPRESSANTS
glucomannan
maté

APPETITE STIMULANTS
angelica
bay, sweet
bee pollen
bitter orange
blessed thistle
bogbean
caraway
cinnamon (and cassia)
coriander

APPETITE STIMULANTS (continued)

dandelion
devil's claw
fenugreek
gentian
hops
horehound
Iceland moss
mugwort
quassia
rosemary
wormwood
yarrow

APPETITE SUPPRESSANTS

gymnema

ARTHRITIS

borage
chamomile, German
echinacea
evening primrose oil
ginger
glucosamine
nettle
New Zealand green-lipped
    mussel
peppermint
rehmannia
superoxide dismutase
willow bark
yucca

ASTHMA

aloe vera
coltsfoot
devil's dung
forskolin (and coleonol)
gingko
kola (cola)
picrorhiza
poppy

ATHEROSCLEROSIS

alfalfa
coenzyme Q10

garlic
ginseng, Siberian
onion
pycnogenol
reishi mushroom
saffron

BACK PAIN

cod-liver oil
yarrow

BACTERIAL INFECTIONS

agrimony
allspice
anise (and star anise)
barberry
basil
bay, sweet
boneset
burdock root
camphor
chamomile, German
cranberry
eucalyptus
garlic
goldenseal
honey
honeysuckle
hops
horseradish
ivy
jujube, common
kombucha (Manchurian
    mushroom)
linden flower
marshmallow
meadowsweet
mugwort
neem
nutmeg (and mace)
onion
passionflower
peony, white
peppermint
prickly ash
propolis

rosemary
sage
tamarind
tea tree oil
thyme
yarrow
yellow dock

BILIARY DISORDERS

artichoke
bayberry
dandelion
fumitory
milk thistle
wormwood

BLEEDING

tienchi
yarrow

BLOATING

caraway
evening primrose oil
fennel
gentian
lovage
peppermint
rosemary

BLOOD PRESSURE, HIGH

barberry
forskolin (and coleonol)
garlic
ginseng, Siberian
hawthorn
kudzu
motherwort
olive leaf
onion
yucca

BLOOD PRESSURE, LOW

broom

BODY COMPOSITION

chromium picolinate

BOILS

slippery elm

BOWEL IRREGULARITY

black walnut
glucomannan
Irish moss
peppermint
psyllium

BREAST TENDERNESS

evening primrose oil

BRONCHITIS

apricot pit
horseradish
ivy
licorice
mullein
thyme

BURNS

aloe vera
gotu kola
honey
pineapple
St. John's wort
slippery elm
L-tyrosine

CANCER

almond, sweet
aloe vera
apricot pit
asparagus
astragalus
barley (and barley grass)
basil
beta-carotene
bugleweed
carrot

foxglove
garlic
green tea
nutmeg (and mace)
onion
pycnogenol
quassia
red bush
red clover
rehmannia
reishi mushroom
rosemary
saffron
scullcap
selenium
watercress
yew, Pacific
yogurt

CARDIOVASCULAR DISORDERS, *SEE*
HEART AND CARDIOVASCULAR
DISORDERS

CAVITIES

tea, black
tea, green

CHEST CONGESTION

anise (and star anise)
camphor
cowslip, European
elecampane
eucalyptus
fennel
horseradish
hyssop
ivy
licorice
mullein
mustard
red clover
savory
senega root
spearmint
thyme
turpentine oil

vervain
watercress
yerba santa

CHOLESTEROL, HIGH

acidophilus
activated charcoal
alfalfa
almond, sweet
artichoke
barley (and barley grass)
L-carnitine
evening primrose oil
flax
garlic
glucomannan
guggul
lecithin
oats
onion
psyllium
reishi mushroom
saffron
tea, green
wild yam
yogurt
yucca

CIRCULATION DISORDERS

bilberry
broom
butcher's broom
camphor
gingko
gotu kola
grape seed extract
hawthorn
kudzu
pycnogenol
rosemary
salvia
yucca

COLDS

black currant
cowslip, European

COLDS (*continued*)

echinacea
elder
elecampane
garlic
hyssop
Iceland moss
ipecac
Labrador tea
linden flower
maté
meadowsweet
mullein
peppermint
soapwort
turpentine oil
zinc

COLD SORES

balm
echinacea
goldenseal
marjoram, sweet
peppermint

COLIC

anise (and star anise)
caraway
fennel
fumitory

CONSTIPATION

almond, sweet
aloe vera
apple
blueberry
boldo
cascara sagrada
castor oil
cleavers
dandelion
dong quai
elder
flax

fo-ti
glucomannan
hibiscus
Irish moss
rhubarb, Chinese
senna
sheep's sorrel
tamarind
yellow dock

CONTRACEPTIVES

neem

COUGH

anise (and star anise)
camphor
coltsfoot
couch grass
cowslip, European
elecampane
eucalyptus
fennel
Iceland moss
ipecac
licorice
linden flower
marshmallow
mullein
oregano
peppermint
poppy
red clover
savory
senega root
slippery elm
squill
thyme
turpentine oil
vervain

COUGH, DRY

coltsfoot
horehound
Iceland moss
wild cherry bark

COUNTERIRRITANTS

arnica
birch
camphor
mustard
peppermint
red pepper
rosemary
turpentine oil
wintergreen

DANDRUFF

jojoba oil
pansy

DEPRESSION

DHEA
evening primrose oil
gingko
St. John's wort

DIABETES

agrimony
artichoke
barley (and barley grass)
DHEA
ginseng, Siberian
glucomannan
gymnema

DIARRHEA

acidophilus
agrimony
apple
barberry
bilberry
blackberry
black currant
black haw
blueberry
borage
fennel
guarana
lady's mantle
meadowsweet
Mormon tea
mullein

DIARRHEA (continued)

nutmeg (and mace)
oak bark
poppy
psyllium
raspberry
rhatany
rhubarb, Chinese
savory
slippery elm
squaw vine
tamarind
tea, black
tea, green
wild cherry bark
wild strawberry
wood betony
yellow dock

DIGESTIVE AIDS

acidophilus
allspice
angelica
anise (and star anise)
artichoke
bitter orange
blessed thistle
bogbean
bromelain
caraway
cinnamon (and cassia)
gentian
ginger
goldenseal
hops
olive oil
oregano
papaya
passionflower
peppermint
pineapple
quassia
red bush
red pepper
rhubarb, Chinese
rosemary

spearmint
thyme
turmeric
yarrow

DIGESTIVE SYSTEM UPSET

activated charcoal
angelica
artichoke
balm
basil
bay, sweet
betel nut
bilberry
bitter orange
boldo
cardamom
chamomile, German
coriander
dandelion
devil's claw
dill
fennel
fenugreek
flax
fumitory
garlic
gentian
ginger
Iceland moss
Irish moss
juniper berry
lavender
lovage
marijuana
marjoram, sweet
meadowsweet
milk thistle
mugwort
parsley
peppermint
rosemary
sage
St. John's wort
savory
slippery elm

turmeric
yarrow

DIURETICS

alfalfa
artichoke
asparagus
birch
boldo
buchu
celery seed
cleavers
corn silk
couch grass
dandelion
dong quai
goldenrod
hibiscus
horsetail
hydrangea
lovage
maté
meadowsweet
nettle
parsley
sarsaparilla
squill
tea, black
uva ursi

EAR DISORDERS

gingko

ECZEMA

arnica
birch
chamomile, German
oak bark

EYE COMPLAINTS

bilberry
carrot
oak bark

FATIGUE

ginseng, Siberian

FEVER

elder
neem
sage
willow bark
yarrow

FLATULENCE

activated charcoal
anise (and star anise)
gentian

FLU

black currant
elder
garlic
linden flower
maté
propolis

FUNGAL INFECTIONS

agrimony
allspice
barberry
bay, sweet
bitter orange
black walnut
burdock root
chamomile, German
cinnamon (and cassia)
English walnut leaf
garlic
hops
ivy
jewelweed
mugwort
nutmeg (and mace)
onion
oregano
passionflower
peony, white
prickly ash
propolis
rosemary

scullcap
tamarind
thyme

GAS

allspice
angelica
anise (and star anise)
balm
basil
bay, sweet
caraway
cinnamon (and cassia)
dandelion
devil's dung
fennel
fenugreek
glucomannan
lavender
lovage
parsley
peppermint
rosemary
savory
spearmint
turmeric
wormwood

GLAUCOMA

marijuana

GUMS

allspice
bloodroot
chamomile, German
clove
neem
oak bark
witch hazel
wood betony
yellow dock

HAIR DYE

henna

HEADACHES

gingko
willow bark
yucca

HEART AND CARDIOVASCULAR DISORDERS

astragalus
beta-carotene
broom
L-carnitine
coenzyme Q10
DHEA
foxglove
garlic
ginseng, Siberian
guggul
hawthorn
motherwort
onion
prickly ash
pycnogenol
saffron
salvia
squill
tienchi

HEMORRHOIDS

agrimony
aloe vera
arnica
bayberry
blackberry
black walnut
butcher's broom
cascara sagrada
cod-liver oil
collisonia
horse chestnut
mullein
oak bark
psyllium
rhatany
rhubarb, Chinese
witch hazel

HERPES

balm
echinacea
marjoram, sweet
peppermint
propolis

HORMONAL IMBALANCES

black cohosh
bugleweed
chaste tree berry
false unicorn root
fennel
flax
melatonin

HYPERTHYROIDISM

bugleweed

HYPOGLYCEMIA

artichoke
barley (and barley grass)
fenugreek
garlic
ginseng, Asian
glucomannan
gymnema
kudzu
olive leaf
reishi mushroom

IMMUNE SYSTEM DISORDERS

astragalus
boneset
cat's claw
chamomile, German
DHEA
echinacea
ginseng, Asian
marshmallow
pangamic acid
rehmannia
reishi mushroom
shiitake mushroom

IMPOTENCE

gingko
yohimbe

INFECTIONS

clove

INFLAMMATIONS

arnica
ashwagandha
beta-carotene
boswellin
calendula
cat's claw
chamomile, German
comfrey
devil's claw
garlic
ginger
gingko
glucosamine
goldenrod
gotu kola
guggul
honeysuckle
horse chestnut
licorice
marijuana
marshmallow
meadowsweet
neem
nutmeg (and mace)
peony, white
picrorhiza
pineapple
prickly ash
propolis
red clover
reishi mushroom
rhubarb, Chinese
saw palmetto
scullcap
soapwort
superoxide dismutase
thyme
willow bark

wintergreen
witch hazel
yarrow

INHALANTS

camphor
cedar, eastern red
eucalyptus

ITCHING

apricot pit
camphor

JET LAG

melatonin

JOINT PAIN

birch
borage
cod-liver oil
devil's claw
evening primrose oil
glucosamine
mustard
rosemary
wintergreen

KIDNEY AILMENTS

artichoke
asparagus
birch
cranberry
goldenrod
horsetail
nettle

LACTATION

chaste tree berry
jasmine
zinc

LACTOSE INTOLERANCE

acidophilus
yogurt

LEPROSY

gotu kola

LICE

anise (and star anise)

LIVER DISORDERS

aloe vera
bayberry
boldo
lecithin
milk thistle
picrorhiza
reishi mushroom
schisandra
superoxide dismutase

LUNG AILMENTS

coltsfoot
cowslip, European
devil's dung
echinacea
Iceland moss
ipecac
ivy
Labrador tea

MEMORY

L-carnitine
gingko
ginseng, Asian
lecithin

MENOPAUSE

black cohosh
kava

MENSTRUAL DISCOMFORT

black cohosh
black haw
ginger
passionflower
pulsatilla
yarrow

MENSTRUAL IRREGULARITIES

chaste tree berry
lady's mantle

MENTAL DISTURBANCES

L-carnitine
lecithin

MENTAL PERFORMANCE

ginseng, Asian

MIGRAINE HEADACHES

feverfew
kola (cola)

MORNING SICKNESS

ginger

MOTION SICKNESS

ginger

MOUTH INFECTIONS

blackberry
English walnut leaf
goldenseal

MOUTH INFLAMMATIONS

blueberry
calendula
chamomile, German
clove
coltsfoot

MUSCLE ACHES AND PAINS

allspice
camphor
horseradish
mustard
St. John's wort
wintergreen

MUSCLE TENSION

bitter orange
catnip
chamomile, German
cramp bark

dill
dong quai
fennel
fumitory
ginger
goldenrod
ivy
kava
peony, white
peppermint
poppy
reishi mushroom

NASAL CONGESTION

agrimony
peppermint
red pepper
soapwort
spearmint
vervain

NAUSEA

artichoke
ginger
marijuana

NEUROLOGIC DISORDERS

lecithin
marijuana

PAIN

arnica
camphor
cinnamon (and cassia)
clove
cod-liver oil
devil's claw
ivy
kava
marijuana
mustard
neem
peony, white
peppermint
poppy
prickly ash

PAIN (*continued*)

red pepper

reishi mushroom

rhubarb, Chinese

rosemary

soapwort

thyme

turpentine oil

willow bark

wintergreen

yarrow

PARASITES

allspice

basil

elecampane

ivy

POISONING

activated charcoal

**PREGNANCY, UNPLEASANT
EFFECTS OF**

glucomannan

PREMENSTRUAL SYNDROME

black cohosh

chaste tree berry

evening primrose oil

PROSTATE DISORDERS

cucurbita

nettle

saw palmetto

RASHES

agrimony

oak bark

RINGWORM

black walnut

SCABIES

anise (and star anise)

neem

SCURVY

chickweed

**SKIN, DRY, ROUGH,
OR INFLAMED**

agrimony

almond, sweet

aloe vera

calendula

castor oil

couch grass

English walnut leaf

fenugreek

flax

fruit acids

jojoba oil

jujube, common

Labrador tea

marshmallow

mullein

myrrh

oats

olive oil

St. John's wort

slippery elm

SKIN INFECTIONS

allspice

SKIN PROBLEMS

aloe vera

cedar, eastern red

chamomile, German

cleavers

gotu kola

ivy

neem

oats

pansy

papaya

peony

tea tree oil

turpentine oil

wild Oregon grape

SLEEPLESSNESS

ashwagandha

balm

barberry

hops

ivy

lavender

lettuce opium

marijuana

melatonin

passionflower

peony, white

reishi mushroom

valerian

SORES

black walnut

slippery elm

SORE THROAT, *SEE* **THROAT, SORE**

STIMULANTS

betel nut

cardamom

cocoa

guarana

kola (cola)

maté

tea, black

tea, green

STRESS

ashwagandha

ginseng, Asian

ginseng, Siberian

kava

schisandra

SUNBURNS

aloe vera

jojoba oil

tea, black

SWEATING, PROMOTION OF

elder

linden flower

SWEATING, PROMOTION OF (continued)

sarsaparilla

yarrow

SWEATING, REDUCTION OF

English walnut leaf

sage

SWELLING

horse chestnut

horsetail

lovage

pineapple

saw palmetto

THROAT, SORE

agrimony

bayberry

bilberry

blackberry

blueberry

calendula

clove

coltsfoot

echinacea

eucalyptus

fenugreek

goldenrod

hyssop

Iceland moss

licorice

marshmallow

mullein

myrrh

oak bark

peppermint

raspberry

rhatany

rose hip

rose oil (and rose water)

sage

savory

slippery elm

wild strawberry

wood betony

THYROID PROBLEMS

kelp

motherwort

rehmannia

TONICS

codonopsis

ginseng, Asian

nux vomica

TOOTHACHE

allspice

ULCERS

bayberry

chamomile, German

honey

Irish moss

licorice

neem

slippery elm

URINARY TRACT INFECTIONS

acidophilus

barberry

birch

cranberry

echinacea

goldenrod

horseradish

horsetail

superoxide dismutase

tea tree oil

uva ursi

URINARY TRACT INFLAMMATIONS

asparagus

birch

couch grass

goldenrod

horsetail

nettle

uva ursi

VARICOSE VEINS

butcher's broom

gingko

horse chestnut

rosemary

witch hazel

VIRAL INFECTIONS

agrimony

allspice

aloe vera

bay, sweet

echinacea

eucalyptus

peony, white

peppermint

propolis

scullcap

VITAMIN SOURCES

carrot

chickweed

chlorella

dandelion

honey

maté

pangamic acid

parsley

raspberry

red bush

red pepper

rose hip

shiitake mushroom

spirulina

watercress

VOMITING, INDUCTION OF

ipecac

squill

WARTS

mayapple, American

WORMS

betel nut

cucurbita

garlic

WORMS (*continued*)

ivy

oregano

prickly ash

WOUNDS

agrimony

aloe vera

balm

barberry

basil

black walnut

calendula

chamomile, German

comfrey

echinacea

English walnut leaf

gentian

goldenrod

gotu kola

honey

horsetail

Labrador tea

lady's mantle

lavender

mullein

neem

oak bark

peppermint

pineapple

propolis

rhatany

rhubarb, Chinese

St. John's wort

slippery elm

yarrow

yellow dock

zinc

YEAST INFECTIONS

acidophilus

agrimony

allspice

barberry

chamomile, German

cleavers

echinacea

passionflower

tea tree oil

yogurt

Index of Remedies

Note: Substances are followed by the indications for which they have been widely recommended. Always check the actual entry before using a natural medicine for any reason.

ACIDOPHILUS
abdominal pain
diarrhea
digestive aids
lactose intolerance
urinary tract infections
yeast infections

ACTIVATED CHARCOAL
cholesterol, high
digestive system upset
flatulence
poisoning

AGRIMONY
antiseptics
astringents
bacterial infections
diabetes
diarrhea
fungal infections
hemorrhoids
nasal congestion
rashes
skin inflammations
throat, sore
viral infections
wounds
yeast infections

ALFALFA
atherosclerosis
cholesterol, high
diuretics

ALLSPICE
abdominal pain
anesthetics
antiseptics
bacterial infections
digestive aids
fungal infections
gas
gums
muscle aches and pains
parasites
skin infections
toothache
viral infections
yeast infections

ALMOND, SWEET
cancer
cholesterol, high
laxatives
skin, dry, rough, or inflamed

ALOE VERA
AIDS/HIV
asthma
burns
cancer
constipation
hemorrhoids
liver disorders
skin, dry, rough, or inflamed
skin problems
sunburns

ALOE VERA (*continued*)

viral infections

wounds

ANGELICA

appetite stimulants

digestive aids

digestive system upset

gas

ANISE (AND STAR ANISE)

anemia

bacterial infections

chest congestion

colic

cough

digestive aids

flatulence

gas

lice

scabies

APPLE

constipation

diarrhea

APRICOT PIT

bronchitis

cancer

itching

ARNICA

anesthetics

antiseptics

counterirritants

eczema

hemorrhoids

inflammations

pain

ARTICHOKE

biliary disorders

cholesterol, high

diabetes

digestive aids

digestive system upsets

diuretics

hypoglycemia

kidney ailments

nausea

ASHWAGANDHA

inflammations

sleeplessness

stress

ASPARAGUS

cancer

diuretics

kidney ailments

urinary tract inflammations

ASTRAGALUS

cancer

heart and cardiovascular
disorders

immune system disorders

BALM

cold sores

digestive system upsets

gas

herpes

sleeplessness

wounds

BARBERRY

bacterial infections

blood pressure, high

diarrhea

fungal infections

sleeplessness

urinary tract infections

wounds

yeast infections

BARLEY (AND BARLEY GRASS)

cancer

cholesterol, high

diabetes

hypoglycemia

BASIL

acne

bacterial infections

cancer

digestive system upsets

gas

parasites

wounds

BAY, SWEET

appetite stimulants

bacterial infections

digestive system upsets

fungal infections

gas

viral infections

BAYBERRY

biliary disorders

hemorrhoids

liver disorders

throat, sore

ulcers

BEE POLLEN

appetite stimulants

BETA-CAROTENE

cancer

heart and cardiovascular
disorders

inflammations

BETEL NUT

digestive system upsets

stimulants

worms

BIFIDOBACTERIUM, *SEE* **ACIDOPHILUS**

BILBERRY

circulation disorders

diarrhea

digestive system upsets

eye complaints

throat, sore

BIRCH

counterirritants
diuretics
eczema
joint pain
kidney ailments
urinary tract infections
urinary tract inflammations

BITTER ORANGE

appetite stimulants
digestive aids
digestive system upsets
fungal infections
muscle tension

BLACKBERRY

diarrhea
hemorrhoids
mouth infections
throat, sore

BLACK COHOSH

hormonal imbalances
menopause
menstrual discomfort
premenstrual syndrome

BLACK CURRANT

colds
diarrhea
flu

BLACK HAW

diarrhea
menstrual discomfort

BLACK WALNUT

bowel irregularity
fungal infections
hemorrhoids
ringworm
sores
wounds

BLESSED THISTLE

appetite stimulants
digestive aids

BLOODROOT

gums

BLUEBERRY

constipation
diarrhea
mouth inflammations
throat, sore

BLUE COHOSH: *DEFINITE HEALTH HAZARD*

BOGBEAN

appetite stimulants
digestive aids

BOLDO

constipation
diuretics
liver disorders
stomach upsets

BONESET

bacterial infections
immune system disorders

BORAGE

arthritis
diarrhea
joint pain
skin, dry, rough, or inflamed

BOSWELLIN

inflammations

BROMELAIN

digestive aids

BROOM

blood pressure, low
circulation disorders

heart and cardiovascular
disorders

BUCHU

diuretics

BUGLEWEED

cancer
hormonal imbalances
hyperthyroidism

BURDOCK ROOT

bacterial infections
fungal infections

BUTCHER'S BROOM

circulation disorders
hemorrhoids
varicose veins

CALAMUS: *DEFINITE HEALTH HAZARD*

CALENDULA

inflammations
mouth inflammations
skin inflammations
throat, sore
wounds

CAMPHOR

bacterial infections
chest congestion
circulation disorders
cough
counterirritants
inhalants
itching
muscle aches and pains
pain

CARAWAY

appetite stimulants
bloating
colic

CARAWAY (*continued*)
digestive aids
digestive system upsets
gas

CARDAMOM
digestive system upsets
stimulants

L-CARNITINE
cholesterol, high
heart and cardiovascular
    disorders
memory
mental disturbances

CARROT
cancer
eye complaints
vitamin sources

CASCARA SAGRADA
constipation
hemorrhoids

CASSIA, *SEE* CINNAMON

CASTOR OIL
constipation
skin, dry, rough, or inflamed

CATNIP
muscle tension

CAT'S CLAW
immune system disorders
inflammations

CEDAR, EASTERN RED
inhalants
skin problems

CELERY SEED
diuretics

CHAMOMILE, GERMAN
arthritis
bacterial infections
digestive system upsets
eczema
fungal infections
gums
immune system disorders
inflammations
mouth inflammations
muscle tension
skin problems
ulcers
wounds
yeast infections

CHAPARRAL: *DEFINITE HEALTH HAZARD*

CHASTE TREE BERRY
hormonal imbalances
lactation
menstrual irregularities
premenstrual syndrome

CHICKWEED
scurvy
vitamin sources

CHICORY
appetite stimulants
digestive system upsets

CHIVE
anemia

CHLORELLA
vitamin sources

CHLOROPHYLL, *SEE* CHLORELLA

CHROMIUM PICOLINATE
body composition

CINNAMON (AND CASSIA)
appetite stimulants
digestive aids
fungal infections
gas
pain

CLEAVERS
constipation
diuretics
skin problems
yeast infections

CLEMATIS: *DEFINITE HEALTH HAZARD*

CLOVE
gums
infections
mouth inflammations
pain
throat, sore

CLUB MOSS: *DEFINITE HEALTH HAZARD*

COCOA
stimulants

COD-LIVER OIL
back pain
hemorrhoids
joint pain
pain

CODONOPSIS
tonics

COENZYME Q10
atherosclerosis
heart and cardiovascular
    disorders

COLEONOL, *SEE* FORSKOLIN

COLLISONIA
hemorrhoids

COLTSFOOT
asthma
cough
cough, dry
lung ailments
mouth inflammations
throat, sore

COMFREY
inflammations
skin, dry, rough, or inflamed
wounds

CORIANDER
appetite stimulants
digestive system upsets

CORN SILK
diuretics

COUCH GRASS
cough
diuretics
skin, dry, rough, or inflamed
urinary tract inflammations

COWSLIP, EUROPEAN
chest congestion
colds
cough
lung ailments

CRAMP BARK
muscle tension

CRANBERRY
bacterial infections
kidney ailments
urinary tract infections

CUCUMBER, CHINESE
AIDS/HIV

CUCURBITA
prostate disorders
worms

DAMIANA
aphrodisiacs

DANDELION
appetite stimulants
biliary disorders
constipation
digestive system upsets
diuretics
gas
vitamin sources

DEADLY NIGHTSHADE: *DEFINITE HEALTH HAZARD*

DEER ANTLER
aphrodisiacs

DEVIL'S CLAW
appetite stimulants
digestive system upsets
inflammations
joint pain
pain

DEVIL'S DUNG
asthma
gas
lung ailments

DHEA
depression
diabetes
heart and cardiovascular
    disorders
immune system disorders

DILL
digestive system upsets
muscle tension

DONG QUAI
allergies
constipation
diuretics
muscle tension

ECHINACEA
arthritis
colds
cold sores
herpes
immune system disorders
lung ailments
throat, sore
urinary tract infections
viral infections
wounds
yeast infections

ELDER
colds
constipation
fever
flu
sweating, promotion of

ELECAMPANE
chest congestion
colds
cough
parasites

ENGLISH WALNUT LEAF
fungal infections
mouth infections
skin, dry, rough, or inflamed
sweating, reduction of
wounds

EPHEDRA: *DEFINITE HEALTH HAZARD*

EUCALYPTUS
bacterial infections
chest congestion
cough
inhalants
throat, sore
viral infections

EVENING PRIMROSE OIL
arthritis
bloating

EVENING PRIMROSE OIL (*continued*)
breast tenderness
cholesterol, high
depression
joint pain
premenstrual syndrome

EYEBRIGHT: *DEFINITE HEALTH HAZARD*

FALSE UNICORN ROOT
hormonal imbalances

FENNEL
bloating
chest congestion
colic
cough
diarrhea
digestive system upsets
gas
hormonal imbalances
muscle tension

FENUGREEK
appetite stimulants
digestive system upsets
gas
hypoglycemia
skin, dry, rough, or inflamed
throat, sore

FEVERFEW
migraine headaches

FLAX
cholesterol, high
constipation
digestive system upsets
hormonal imbalances
skin, dry, rough, or inflamed

FORSKOLIN (AND COLEONOL)
asthma
blood pressure, high

FO-TI
constipation

FO-TI-TIENG, *SEE* GOTU KOLA; KOLA

FOXGLOVE
cancer
heart and cardiovascular
   disorders

FRUIT ACIDS
acne
skin, dry, rough, or inflamed

FUMITORY
biliary disorders
colic
digestive system upsets
muscle tension

GARLIC
atherosclerosis
bacterial infections
blood pressure, high
cancer
cholesterol, high
colds
digestive system upsets
flu
fungal infections
heart and cardiovascular
   disorders
hypoglycemia
inflammations
worms

GENTIAN
appetite stimulants
bloating
digestive aids
digestive system upsets
flatulence
wounds

GINGER
arthritis
digestive aids
digestive system upsets
inflammations
menstrual discomfort
morning sickness
motion sickness
muscle tension
nausea

GINGKO
allergies
Alzheimer's disease
asthma
circulation disorders
depression
ear disorders
headaches
impotence
inflammations
memory
varicose veins

GINSENG, AMERICAN, *SEE* GINSENG, ASIAN

GINGSENG, ASIAN
hypoglycemia
immune system disorders
memory
mental performance
stress
tonics

GINSENG, SIBERIAN
atherosclerosis
blood pressure, high
diabetes
fatigue
heart and cardiovascular
   disorders
stress

GLUCOMANNAN

appetite depressants
bowel irregularity
cholesterol, high
constipation
diabetes
gas
hypoglycemia
pregnancy, unpleasant effects of

GLUCOSAMINE

arthritis
inflammations
joint pain

L-GLUTAMINE, SEE L-TYROSINE

GOLDENROD

diuretics
inflammations
kidney ailments
muscle tension
throat, sore
urinary tract infections
urinary tract inflammations
wounds

GOLDENSEAL

bacterial infections
cold sores
digestive aids
mouth infections

GOTU KOLA

burns
circulation disorders
inflammations
leprosy
skin problems
wounds

GRAPE SEED EXTRACT

circulation disorders
see also pycnogenol

GUARANA

diarrhea
stimulants

GUGGUL

cholesterol, high
heart and cardiovascular
disorders
inflammations

GYMNEMA

appetite suppressants
diabetes
hypoglycemia

HAWTHORN

blood pressure, high
circulation disorders
heart and cardiovascular
disorders

HENNA

hair dye

HIBISCUS

constipation
diuretics

HONEY

antiseptics
bacterial infections
burns
ulcers
vitamin sources
wounds

HONEYSUCKLE

bacterial infections
inflammations

HOPS

appetite stimulants

bacterial infections
digestive aids
fungal infections
sleeplessness

HOREHOUND

appetite stimulants
cough, dry

HORSE CHESTNUT

hemorrhoids
inflammations
swelling
varicose veins

HORSERADISH

bacterial infections
bronchitis
chest congestion
muscle aches and pain
urinary tract infections

HORSETAIL

diuretics
kidney ailments
swelling
urinary tract infections
urinary tract inflammations
wounds

HYDRANGEA

diuretics

HYSSOP

chest congestion
colds
throat, sore

ICELAND MOSS

appetite stimulants
colds
cough
cough, dry

ICELAND MOSS (*continued*)

digestive system upset

lung ailments

throat, sore

IPECAC

colds

cough

lung ailments

vomiting, induction of

IRISH MOSS

bowel irregularity

constipation

digestive system upset

ulcers

IVY

bacterial infections

bronchitis

chest congestion

fungal infections

lung ailments

muscle tension

pain

parasites

skin problems

sleeplessness

worms

JASMINE

lactation

JEWELWEED

fungal infections

JOJOBA OIL

dandruff

skin, dry, rough, or inflamed

sunburns

JUJUBE, COMMON

bacterial infections

skin, dry, rough, or inflamed

JUNIPER BERRY

digestive system upset

KAVA

menopause

muscle tension

pain

stress

KELP

thyroid problems

KOLA (COLA)

asthma

migraine headaches

stimulants

KOMBUCHA (MANCHURIAN MUSHROOM)

bacterial infections

KUDZU

alcoholism

blood pressure, high

circulation disorders

hypoglycemia

LABRADOR TEA

colds

lung ailments

skin, dry, rough, or inflamed

wounds

LADY'S MANTLE

diarrhea

menstrual irregularities

wounds

LADY'S SLIPPER: *THE ETHICS OF USING THIS NOW RARE PLANT ARE QUESTIONABLE*

LAVENDER

digestive system upset

gas

sleeplessness

wounds

LECITHIN

Alzheimer's disease

cholesterol, high

liver disorders

memory

mental disturbances

neurologic disorders

LETTUCE OPIUM

sleeplessness

LICORICE

bronchitis

chest congestion

cough

inflammations

throat, sore

ulcers

LIFE ROOT: *DEFINITE HEALTH HAZARD*

LINDEN FLOWER

bacterial infections

colds

cough

flu

sweating, promotion of

LOBELIA: *DEFINITE HEALTH HAZARD*

LOVAGE

bloating

digestive system upset

diuretics

gas

swelling

L-LYSINE, *SEE* **L-TYROSINE**

MARIJUANA

AIDS/HIV

MARIJUANA (*continued*)

digestive system upset
glaucoma
inflammations
nausea
neurologic disorders
pain
sleeplessness

MARJORAM, SWEET

cold sores
digestive system upset
herpes

MARSHMALLOW

bacterial infections
cough
immune system disorders
inflammations
skin, dry, rough, or inflamed
throat, sore

MATÉ

appetite depressants
colds
diuretics
flu
stimulants
vitamin sources

MAYAPPLE, AMERICAN

warts

MEADOWSWEET

bacterial infections
colds
diarrhea
digestive system upset
diuretics
inflammations

MELATONIN

hormonal imbalances
jet lag
sleeplessness

MENTHOL, *SEE* PEPPERMINT

MILK THISTLE

biliary disorders
digestive system upsets
liver disorders

MISTLETOE: *DEFINITE HEALTH HAZARD*

MORMON TEA

diarrhea

MOTHERWORT

blood pressure, high
heart and cardiovascular
    disorders
thyroid problems

MUGWORT

appetite stimulants
bacterial infections
digestive system upset
fungal infections

MULLEIN

bronchitis
chest congestion
colds
cough
diarrhea
hemorrhoids
skin, dry, rough, or inflamed
throat, sore
wounds

MUSTARD

chest congestion
counterirritants
joint pain
muscle aches and pains
pain

MYRRH

skin, dry, rough, or inflamed
throat, sore

NEEM

bacterial infections
contraceptives
fever
gums
inflammations
pain
scabies
skin problems
ulcers
wounds

NETTLE

allergies
arthritis
diuretics
kidney ailments
prostate disorders
urinary tract inflammations

NEW ZEALAND GREEN-LIPPED MUSSEL

arthritis

NUTMEG (AND MACE)

bacterial infections
cancer
diarrhea
fungal infections
inflammations

NUX VOMICA

tonics

OAK BARK

antiseptics
diarrhea
eczema
eye complaints
gums

OAK BARK (*continued*)

hemorrhoids
rashes
throat, sore
wounds

OATS

cholesterol, high
skin, dry, rough, or inflamed
skin problems

OLIVE LEAF

blood pressure, high
hypoglycemia

OLIVE OIL

digestive aids
skin, dry, rough, or inflamed

ONION

atherosclerosis
bacterial infections
blood pressure, high
cancer
cholesterol, high
fungal infections
heart and cardiovascular
    disorders

OREGANO

cough
digestive aids
fungal infections
worms

PANGAMIC ACID

immune system disorders
vitamin sources

PANSY

acne
dandruff
skin problems

PAPAYA

digestive aids
skin problems

PARSLEY

digestive system upset
diuretics
gas
vitamin sources

PASSIONFLOWER

bacterial infections
digestive aids
fungal infections
menstrual discomfort
sleeplessness
yeast infections

PAU D'ARCO: *DEFINITE HEALTH HAZARD*

PEONY

skin problems

PENNY ROYAL: *DEFINITE HEALTH HAZARD*

PEONY, WHITE

bacterial infections
fungal infections
inflammations
muscle tension
pain
sleeplessness
viral infections

PEPPERMINT

abdominal pain
arthritis
bacterial infections
bloating
bowel irregularity
colds
cold sores
cough

counterirritants
digestive aids
digestive system upset
gas
herpes
muscle tension
nasal congestion
pain
throat, sore
viral infections
wounds

PERIWINKLE, LESSER: *DEFINITE HEALTH HAZARD*

L-PHENYLALANINE, *SEE* L-TYROSINE

PICRORHIZA

asthma
inflammations
liver disorders

PINEAPPLE

burns
digestive aids
inflammations
swelling
wounds

PLEURISY ROOT: *DEFINITE HEALTH HAZARD*

POKEWEED: *DEFINITE HEALTH HAZARD*

POPPY

asthma
cough
diarrhea
muscle tension
pain

PRICKLY ASH (NORTHERN AND SOUTHERN)

bacterial infections
fungal infections

PRICKLY ASH (NORTHERN AND SOUTHERN) (*continued*)

heart and cardiovascular disorders
inflammations
pain
worms

PROPOLIS

bacterial infections
flu
fungal infections
herpes
inflammations
viral infections
wounds

PSYLLIUM

bowel irregularity
cholesterol, high
diarrhea
hemorrhoids

PULSATILLA

menstrual discomfort

PYCNOGENOL

atherosclerosis
cancer
circulation disorders
heart and cardiovascular disorders

QUASSIA

appetite stimulants
cancer
digestive aids

RASPBERRY

diarrhea
throat, sore
vitamin sources

RED BUSH

cancer

digestive aids
vitamin sources

RED CLOVER

antiseptics
cancer
chest congestion
cough
inflammations

RED PEPPER

counterirritants
digestive aids
nasal congestion
pain
vitamin sources

REHMANNIA

arthritis
cancer
immune system disorders
thyroid problems

REISHI MUSHROOM

allergies
atherosclerosis
cancer
cholesterol, high
hypoglycemia
immune system disorders
inflammations
liver disorders
muscle tension
pain
sleeplessness

RHATANY

diarrhea
hemorrhoids
throat, sore
wounds

RHUBARB, CHINESE

constipation

diarrhea
digestive aids
hemorrhoids
inflammations
pain
wounds

ROSE HIP

throat, sore
vitamin sources

ROSEMARY

appetite stimulants
bacterial infections
bloating
cancer
circulation disorders
counterirritants
digestive aids
digestive system upsets
fungal infections
gas
joint pain
pain
varicose veins

ROSE OIL (AND ROSE WATER)

throat, sore

RUE: *DEFINITE HEALTH HAZARD*

SAFFRON

atherosclerosis
cancer
cholesterol, high
heart and cardiovascular disorders

SAGE

bacterial infections
digestive system upsets
fever
sweating, reduction of
throat, sore

ST. JOHN'S WORT
burns
depression
digestive system upset
muscle aches and pains
skin, dry, rough, or inflamed
wounds

SALVIA
circulation disorders
heart and cardiovascular
disorders

SARSAPARILLA
diuretics
sweating, promotion of

SASSAFRAS: *DEFINITE HEALTH HAZARD*

SAVORY
chest congestion
cough
diarrhea
digestive system upsets
gas
throat, sore

SAW PALMETTO
inflammations
prostate disorders
swelling

SCHISANDRA
liver disorders
stress

SCULLCAP
AIDS/HIV
cancer
fungal infections
inflammations
viral infections

SELENIUM
cancer

SENEGA ROOT
chest congestion
cough

SENNA
constipation

SHEEP'S SORREL
constipation

SHIITAKE MUSHROOM
immune system disorders
vitamin sources

SLIPPERY ELM
boils
burns
cough
diarrhea
digestive system upset
skin, dry, rough, or inflamed
sores
throat, sore
ulcers
wounds

SOAPWORT
colds
inflammations
nasal congestion
pain

SPEARMINT
chest congestion
digestive aids
gas
nasal congestion

SPIRULINA
vitamin sources

SQUAW VINE
diarrhea

SQUILL
cough
diuretics
heart and cardiovascular
disorders
vomiting, induction of

SUPEROXIDE DISMUTASE
arthritis
inflammations
liver disorders
urinary tract infections

TAMARIND
bacterial infections
constipation
diarrhea
fungal infections

TANSY: *DEFINITE HEALTH HAZARD*

TEA, BLACK
cavities
diarrhea
diuretics
stimulants
sunburns

TEA, GREEN
cancer
cavities
cholesterol, high
diarrhea
stimulants

TEA TREE OIL
antiseptics
bacterial infections
skin problems
urinary tract infections
yeast infections

THYME
bacterial infections
bronchitis

THYME (*continued*)

chest congestion
cough
digestive aids
fungal infections
inflammations
pain

TIENCHI

bleeding
heart and cardiovascular
    disorders

TONKA BEAN: *DEFINITE HEALTH
HAZARD*

L-TRYPTOPHAN: *DEFINITE HEALTH
HAZARD*

TURMERIC

digestive aids
digestive system upset
gas

TURPENTINE OIL

chest congestion
colds
cough
counterirritants
pain
skin problems

L-TYROSINE

burns

UVA URSI

antiseptics
diuretics
urinary tract infections
urinary tract inflammations

VALERIAN

sleeplessness

VERVAIN

chest congestion
cough
nasal congestion

WATERCRESS

cancer
chest congestion
vitamin sources

WHITE COHOSH: *DEFINITE HEALTH
HAZARD*

WILD CHERRY BARK

cough, dry
diarrhea

WILD OREGON GRAPE

skin problems
see also barberry

WILD STRAWBERRY

diarrhea
throat, sore

WILD YAM

cholesterol, high

WILLOW BARK

arthritis
fever
headaches
inflammations
pain

WINTERGREEN

counterirritants
inflammations
joint pain
muscle aches and pains
pain

WITCH HAZEL

gums
hemorrhoids
inflammations
varicose veins

WOOD BETONY

diarrhea
gums
throat, sore

WORMWOOD

appetite stimulants
biliary disorders
gas

YARROW

antiseptics
appetite stimulants
back pain
bacterial infections
bleeding
digestive aids
digestive system upsets
fever
inflammations
menstrual discomfort
pain
sweating, promotion of
wounds

YELLOW DOCK

bacterial infections
constipation
diarrhea
gums
wounds

YERBA SANTA

chest congestion

YEW, PACIFIC

cancer

YOGURT
cancer
cholesterol, high
lactose intolerance
yeast infections

YOHIMBE
impotence

YUCCA
arthritis

blood pressure, high
cholesterol, high
circulation disorders
headaches

ZINC
colds
lactation
wounds

Appendix A: Sources Used for Compiling the Dosage Information

American Pharmaceutical Association. *Handbook of Nonprescription Drugs. 11th ed.* Washington, DC: American Pharmaceutical Association, 1996.

Bensky, D., and A. Gamble. *Chinese Herbal Medicine—Materia Medica.* Rev. edit. Seattle: Eastland Press, 1993.

Bisset, N. G., ed. *Herbal Drugs and Phytopharmaceuticals.* Stuttgart: medpharm GmbH Scientific Publishers, 1994.

Blumenthal, M., J. Gruenwald, T. Hall, and R. S. Rister, eds. *The Complete German Commission E Monographs: Therapeutic Guide to Herbal Medicine.* Boston: Integrative Medicine Communications, 1998.

Bradley, P. C., ed. *British Herbal Compendium. A Handbook of Scientific Information on Widely Used Plant Drugs.* Vol. 1. Bournemouth (Dorset), England: British Herbal Medicine Association, 1992.

Carper, J. *The Food Pharmacy.* New York: Bantam/Doubleday, 1989.

Castleman, M. *The Healing Herbs. The Ultimate Guide to the Curative Power of Nature's Medicines.* New York: Bantam Books, 1995.

Chevallier, A. *The Encyclopedia of Medicinal Plants: A Practical Reference Guide to More Than 550 Key Medicinal Plants & Their Uses.* 1st American ed., New York: Dorling Kindersley Publications, 1996.

Der Marderosian, A., and L. Liberti. *Natural Product Medicine: A Scientific Guide to Foods, Drugs, Cosmetics.* Philadelphia: George F. Stickley, 1988.

Mayell, M. *Off-the-Shelf Natural Health. How to Use Herbs and Nutrients to Stay Well.* New York: Bantam Books, 1995.

Mindell, E. *Earl Mindell's Herb Bible.* New York: Simon and Schuster/Fireside, 1992.

Murray, M. T. *The Healing Power of Herbs: The Enlightened Person's Guide to the Wonders of Medicinal Plants.* Revised and expanded 2nd ed. Rocklin, CA: Prima Publishing, 1995.

Newall, C. A., et al. *Herbal Medicines: A Guide for Health-Care Professionals.* London: The Pharmaceutical Press, 1996.

Ody, P. *The Herb Society's Complete Medicinal Herbal.* London: Dorling Kindersley Limited, 1993.

The Review of Natural Products. (Before October 1996, known as *The Lawrence Review of Natural Products.*) St. Louis, MO: Facts and Comparisons.

Tyler, V. E. *Herbs of Choice. The Therapeutic Use of Phytomedicinals.* Binghamton, NY: Haworth Press/Pharmaceutical Products Press, 1994.

Tyler, V. E. *The Honest Herbal.* Binghamton, NY: Haworth Press/Pharmaceutical Products Press, 1993.

The University of California at Berkeley Wellness Letter, eds. *The New Wellness Encyclopedia: The Best-Selling Guide to Preventing Disease and Maintaining Your Health and Well-Being.* New York: Houghton Mifflin Co., 1995.

Vidya B. Bhavan's Swami Prakashanandra Ayurveda Research Centre Combay for CHEMEXCIL. *Selected Medicinal Plants of India: A Monograph of Identity, Safety, and Clinical Usage.* Bombay: CHEMEXCIL, 1992.

Weiss, R. F. *Herbal Medicine*, trans. A. R. Meuss, from the 6th German edition. Beaconsfield, England: Beaconsfield Publishers, Ltd., 1988.

Williamson, E. M., and F. J. Evans. *Potter's New Cyclopedia of Botanical Drugs and Preparations.* Rev. ed. Essex, England: Saffron Walden, The C. W. Daniel Co., Ltd., 1989.

Dosage information was compiled separately using the above sources.

Appendix A

Appendix B: Sources Frequently Consulted

Several books and periodicals were particularly valuable in researching natural medicines, either because of their scientifically sound and objective perspective or the insight they offered into what is being recommended to consumers. We would like to acknowledge our debt to these sources.

American Pharmaceutical Association. *Handbook of Nonprescription Drugs.* 11th ed. Washington, DC: American Pharmaceutical Association, 1996.

Balch, J. F., and P. A. Balch. *Prescription for Nutritional Healing: A Practical A to Z Reference to Drug-Free Remedies Using Vitamins, Minerals, Herbs & Food Supplements.* 2nd ed. Garden City Park, NY: Avery Publishing Group, 1997.

Barret, S., and V. Herbert. *The Vitamin Pushers: How the "Health Food" Industry Is Selling America a Bill of Goods.* Amherst, NY: Prometheus Books, 1994.

Bensky, D., and A. Gamble. *Chinese Herbal Medicine—Materia Medica.* Rev. ed. Seattle: Eastland Press, 1993.

Bisset, N. G., ed. *Herbal Drugs and Phytopharmaceuticals.* Stuttgart: medpharm GmbH Scientific Publishers, 1994.

Blumenthal, M., J. Gruenwald, T. Hall, and R. S. Rister, eds. *The Complete German Commission E Monographs: Therapeutic Guide to Herbal Medicine.* Boston: Integrative Medicine Communications, 1998.

Bradley, P. C., ed. *British Herbal Compendium. A Handbook of Scientific Information on Widely Used Plant Drugs.* Vol. 1. Bournemouth (Dorset), England: British Herbal Medicine Association, 1992.

Bremness, L. *Herbs.* 1st American ed. Eyewitness Handbooks. New York: Dorling Kindersley Publications, 1994.

Castleman, M. *The Healing Herbs. The Ultimate Guide to the Curative Power of Nature's Medicines.* New York: Bantam Books, 1995.

Chevallier, A. *The Encyclopedia of Medicinal Plants: A Practical Reference Guide to More Than 550 Key Medicinal Plants and Their Uses.* 1st American ed. New York: Dorling Kindersley Publications, 1996.

Der Marderosian, A., and L. Liberti. *Natural Product Medicine. A Scientific Guide to Foods, Drugs, Cosmetics.* Philadelphia: George F. Stickley, 1988.

Dobelis, I. N., ed. *The Magic and Medicine of Plants. A Practical Guide to the Service, History, Folklore & Everyday Use of Medical Plants.* Pleasantville, NY: Reader's Digest Association, 1986.

Duke, J. A. *CRC Handbook of Medicinal Herbs.* Boca Raton, FL: CRC Press, 1985.

Foster, S., and J. A. Duke. *The Peterson Field Guide Series: A Field Guide to Medicinal Plants. Eastern and Central North America.* Boston: Houghton Mifflin Company, 1990.

Hoffman, D. *The Information Sourcebook of Herbal Medicine.* Freedom, CA: The Crossing Press, 1994.

Lampe, K. E., and M. A. McLean. *AMA Handbook of Poisonous and Injurious Plants.* Chicago: American Medical Association 1985.

Leung, A. Y. *Encyclopedia of Common Natural Ingredients Used in Food, Drugs, and Cosmetics.* New York: John Wiley & Sons, 1980.

Leung, A. Y., and S. Foster. *Encyclopedia of Common Natural Ingredients Used in Food, Drugs, and Cosmetics.* 2nd ed. New York: John Wiley & Sons, 1996.

Mayell, M. *Off-the-Shelf Natural Health. How to Use Herbs and Nutrients to Stay Well.* New York: Bantam Books, 1995.

Mindell, E. *Earl Mindell's Herb Bible.* New York: Simon and Schuster/Fireside, 1992.

Murray, M. T. *The Healing Power of Herbs: The Enlightened Person's Guide to the Wonders of Medicinal Plants.* Revised and expanded 2nd ed. Rocklin, CA: Prima Publishing, 1995.

Newall, C. A., et al. *Herbal Medicines: A Guide for Health-Care Professionals.* London: The Pharmaceutical Press, 1996.

Ody, P. *The Herb Society's Complete Medicinal Herbal.* London: Dorling Kindersley Limited, 1993.

The Review of Natural Products. St. Louis: Facts and Comparisons. (Before October 1996, known as *The Lawrence Review of Natural Products.*)

Stary, F. *The Natural Guide to Medicinal Herbs and Plants.* Prague: Barnes & Noble, Inc., in arrangement with Aventinum Publishers, 1996.

Tierra, M. *The Way of Herbs.* New York: Pocket Books, 1990.

Trease, G. E., and W. C. Evans. *Trease and Evan's Pharmacognosy.* 13th ed. Philadelphia: Balliere Tindall, 1989.

Tyler, V. E. *Herbs of Choice. The Therapeutic Use of Phytomedicinals.* Binghamton, NY: Haworth Press/Pharmaceutical Products Press, 1994.

Tyler, V. E. *The Honest Herbal.* Binghamton, NY: Haworth Press/Pharmaceutical Products Press, 1993.

Tyler, V. G., L. R. Brady, and J. E. Robberts, eds. *Pharmacognosy.* Philadelphia: Lea & Febijer, 1988.

Weiner, M. A., and J. A. Weiner. *Herbs That Heal: Prescriptions for Herbal Healing.* Mill Valley, CA: Quantum Books, 1994.

Weiss, R. F. *Herbal Medicine,* trans. A. R. Meuss, from the 6th German edition. Beaconsfield, England: Beaconsfield Publishers, Ltd., 1988.